PRINCIPLES AND PRACTICE OF STRESS MANAGEMENT

Principles and Practice of
Stress
Management

Edited by
Paul M. Lehrer
Robert L. Woolfolk
Wesley E. Sime

Foreword by David H. Barlow

THE GUILFORD PRESS
New York   London

Printed in the United States of America

This book is printed on acid-free paper.

Last digit is print number: 9 8 7 6 5 4 3 2 1

The authors have checked with sources believed to be reliable in their efforts to provide
information that is complete and generally in accord with the standards of practice that are
accepted at the time of publication. However, in view of the possibility of human error or
changes in medical sciences, neither the authors, nor the editor and publisher, nor any other
party who has been involved in the preparation or publication of this work warrants that the
information contained herein is in every respect accurate or complete, and they are not
responsible for any errors or omissions or the results obtained from the use of such
information. Readers are encouraged to confirm the information contained in this book with
other sources.

Library of Congress Cataloging-in-Publication Data

Principles and practice of stress management / edited by Paul M. Lehrer, Robert L. Woolfolk,
Wesley E. Sime ; foreword by David H. Barlow.—3rd ed.
   p. ; cm.
   Includes bibliographical references and index.
   ISBN-10: 1-59385-000-X ISBN-13: 978-1-59385-000-5 (cloth: alk. paper)
   1. Stress management. I. Lehrer, Paul M. II. Woolfolk, Robert L. III. Sime, Wesley E.
   [DNLM: 1. Stress, Psychological—prevention & control. 2. Stress, Psychological—
therapy. 3. Relaxation Techniques. WM 172 P957 2007]
   RA785.P75 2007
   155.9′042—dc22
                                                            2007024866

We dedicate this volume to Dr. Edmund Jacobson.
He was one of the great founders of psychosomatic medicine
and one of the first researchers to examine both the effectiveness
and the mechanism for salutary effects of a standardized,
scientifically derived stress management method.
He also was coinventor of the first device to measure relaxation
by surface electromyography, and thus became a grandfather
of a major branch of stress psychophysiology and biofeedback.
He was our teacher and our inspiration.

To David, Sylvie, and Ariana.
There is no greater source of joy and well-being
than playing with beautiful grandchildren.

—P. M. L.

To Col. R. L. Woolfolk, USA

—R. L. W.

To Maxine, Natalie, Danika, Brandon, Andrea, and Craig
for making my life special and all the work worthwhile

—W. E. S.

About the Editors

Paul M. Lehrer, PhD, is a clinical psychologist and Professor of Psychiatry at the University of Medicine and Dentistry of New Jersey–Robert Wood Johnson Medical School. He has published more than 100 articles and chapters, mostly on biofeedback, psychophysiology, and cognitive-behavioral therapy. Dr. Lehrer is past president of the Association for Applied Psychophysiology and Biofeedback and has received their Distinguished Scientist Award. He has also recently served as president of the International Society for the Advancement of Respiratory Psychophysiology and of the International Stress Management Association—USA Branch.

Robert L. Woolfolk, PhD, is Professor of Psychology and Philosophy at Rutgers, The State University of New Jersey, and Visiting Professor of Psychology at Princeton University. He has published numerous papers and several books on psychotherapy, psychopathology, and the philosophical foundations of psychology. A practicing clinician for more than 30 years, Dr. Woolfolk has sought in both his work with patients and his scholarly endeavors to integrate the scientific and humanistic traditions of psychotherapy. He is the coauthor of *Stress, Sanity, and Survival* and *Treating Somatization: A Cognitive-Behavioral Approach*, and the author of *The Cure of Souls: Science, Values, and Psychotherapy*.

Wesley E. Sime, PhD, is a health psychologist and stress physiologist and Professor in the Department of Nutrition and Health Science at the University of Nebraska–Lincoln. He is past chair of both the Biofeedback Certification Institute of America (BCIA) and the International Stress Management Association—USA Branch (ISMA-USA). He was one of the founders of the Stress Management Certification program through BCIA and continues to work with ISMA-USA. Dr. Sime was an early contemporary of Hans Selye and Edmund Jacobson and continues to facilitate stress management developments with Paul Rosch, Charles Spielberger, and James Quick. He is also a consultant in medical and sports performance settings.

Contributors

Lesley A. Allen, PhD, Department of Psychiatry, University of Medicine and Dentistry of New Jersey–Robert Wood Johnson Medical School, Piscataway, New Jersey

Frank Andrasik, PhD, Institute for Human and Machine Cognition, University of West Florida, Pensacola, Florida

Aaron T. Beck, MD, Department of Psychiatry, University of Pennsylvania, Philadelphia, Pennsylvania

Douglas A. Bernstein, PhD, Department of Psychology, University of South Florida, Tampa, Florida

Joke Bradt, PhD, The Arts and Quality of Life Research Center, Temple University, Philadelphia, Pennsylvania

Charles R. Carlson, PhD, Department of Psychology, University of Kentucky, Lexington, Kentucky

Patricia Carrington, PhD, Department of Psychiatry, University of Medicine and Dentistry of New Jersey–Robert Wood Johnson Medical School, Piscataway, New Jersey

Kevin Chen, PhD, Center for Integrative Medicine, University of Maryland School of Medicine, Baltimore, Maryland

Paul Davis, MEd, Department of Agricultural Leadership, Education, and Communication, University of Nebraska–Lincoln, Lincoln, Nebraska

Cheryl Dileo, PhD, Department of Music Education and Therapy, and The Arts and Quality of Life Research Center, Temple University, Philadelphia, Pennsylvania

Erika J. Eisenberg, MA, Ferkauf Graduate School of Psychology, Yeshiva University, New York, New York

Steven L. Fahrion, PhD, Life Sciences Institute of Mind–Body Health, Topeka, Kansas (retired)

Jonathan M. Feldman, PhD, Ferkauf Graduate School of Psychology, Yeshiva University, New York, New York

Eduardo Gambini-Suárez, BA, Ferkauf Graduate School of Psychology, Yeshiva University, New York, New York

Richard N. Gevirtz, PhD, California School of Professional Psychology, Alliant International University, San Diego, California

Nicholas D. Giardino, PhD, Department of Psychiatry, University of Michigan Medical School, Ann Arbor, Michigan

Lee Hyer, EdD, Department of Psychiatry, Mercer University School of Medicine and Georgia Neurosurgical Institute, Macon, Georgia

Robert A. Karlin, PhD, Department of Psychology, Rutgers, The State University of New Jersey, New Brunswick, New Jersey

Sat Bir S. Khalsa, PhD, Division of Sleep Medicine, Department of Medicine, Brigham and Women's Hospital, Harvard Medical School, Boston, Massachusetts

Jean L. Kristeller, PhD, Department of Psychology, Indiana State University, Terre Haute, Indiana

Bonnie Kushner, PhD, private practice, Toronto, Ontario, Canada

Paul M. Lehrer, PhD, Department of Psychiatry, University of Medicine and Dentistry of New Jersey–Robert Wood Johnson Medical School, Piscataway, New Jersey

Wolfgang Linden, PhD, Department of Psychology, University of British Columbia, Vancouver, British Columbia, Canada

Angele McGrady, PhD, Department of Psychiatry, University of Toledo, Toledo, Ohio

F. J. McGuigan, PhD (deceased), Institute for Stress Management, U.S. International University, San Diego, California

Donald Meichenbaum, PhD, Department of Psychology, University of Waterloo, Waterloo, Ontario, Canada (emeritus); Melissa Institute for Violence Prevention and Treatment of Victims of Violence, Miami, Florida

Jack H. Nassau, PhD, Bradley/Hasbro Children's Research Center, Department of Psychiatry and Human Behavior, The Warren Alpert Medical School of Brown University, Providence, Rhode Island

Patricia A. Norris, PhD, Life Sciences Institute of Mind–Body Health, Topeka, Kansas (retired)

Leo O. Oikawa, PhD, Department of Psychiatry, University of Medicine and Dentistry of New Jersey–Robert Wood Johnson Medical School, Piscataway, New Jersey

Laszlo A. Papp, MD, Department of Clinical Psychobiology, New York State Psychiatric Institute, College of Physicians and Surgeons, Columbia University, New York, New York

James L. Pretzer, PhD, Cleveland Center for Cognitive Therapy, Behavioral Health Associates, Inc., Beachwood, Ohio

James Robertson, MS, Department of Sports Studies, St. Andrews Presbyterian College, Laurinburg, North Carolina

John E. Schmidt, PhD, Department of Psychology, University of Kentucky, Lexington, Kentucky

Wesley E. Sime, PhD, Department of Health and Human Performance, University of Nebraska–Lincoln, Lincoln, Nebraska

Jonathan C. Smith, PhD, The Stress Institute, Department of Psychology, Roosevelt University, Chicago, Illinois

Lynda Thompson, PhD, Biofeedback Institute of Toronto, Toronto, Ontario, Canada

Michael Thompson, MD, Biofeedback Institute of Toronto, Toronto, Ontario, Canada

Jan van Dixhoorn, MD, PhD, The Center for Breathing Therapy, Amersfoort, The Netherlands; Kennemer Hospital, Haarlem, The Netherlands

Robert L. Woolfolk, PhD, Department of Psychology, Princeton University, Princeton, New Jersey

Foreword

From the fight–flight response identified by the great physiologist Walter Cannon and the classic stages of the stress response described by Hans Selye, to the intriguing and uniquely feminine "tend-and-befriend" response to stress described by Shelly Taylor (Taylor et al., 2000), the concept of stress is universal. While the prevalence of physical disease and psychopathology is relatively small for each disorder, the deleterious effects of stress are something that almost everyone experiences from time to time. The consequences of excessive stress, ranging from increased vulnerability to the common cold to clearly established excessive mortality from various disease processes (Cohen, Doyle, & Skoner, 1999; Vaillant, 1979), are issues that concern societies around the world.

The universality of stress is never more evident than in Robert Sapolsky's eloquent description of stress in the animal kingdom, specifically his extensively studied free-ranging baboons in East Africa (Sapolsky, 1990, 2000). In a series of elegant observational studies, he chronicles the life-shortening and brain-altering effects of finding oneself at the bottom of the social hierarchy and/or fighting continually to keep a more elevated spot in the hierarchy. It has been widely acknowledged that levels and intensity of stress in our daily lives increase over time, particularly levels of stress occasioned by fragmenting systems of social support. But how should we as a society ensure that we do not find ourselves systematically replicating the experience of Sapolsky's baboons by suffering the ravages of hypercortisolemia, never knowing when the next attack or challenge will occur, and with little or no confidence that we can cope when they do?

The long-range answer to this most basic of all human dilemmas is to reorganize the priorities in society to maximize social and community support and minimize the extent of those challenges and burdens from our day-to-day life that are beyond our reasonable capabilities. These fundamental societal changes will be a long time coming. In the meantime, societies around the world, reflecting the universality of stress, have originated their own procedures to reduce stress or increase one's capacity to cope with the sometimes unbearable burdens of life. Perhaps the best known of these strategies are the mindfulness and meditation practices of the great Eastern religions. In their totality, these tactics have come to be known as stress management procedures and comprise an important part of our lives, sometimes permeating our cultures. In this excellent compendium, strategies from around the world that have received empirical support for successfully managing and reducing stress are described in such a way as to enable practicing clinicians to incorporate them into their practice.

Procedures described in this book range from some of the old standbys in Western cultures, such as Jacobson's progressive muscle relaxation, to the aforementioned mindfulness and meditation procedures, to yoga and Qigong as therapeutic interventions. Add to this modern applications of music for the purpose of reducing stress, a strategy that is widely used by different cultures around the world, as well as more biologically based procedures such as neurofeedback and medication, and the clinician has as comprehensive a set of procedures as could be found anywhere. Yet the editors of this volume have organized these contributions in such a way as to guide the clinician in selecting appropriate techniques and implementing them in the context of a therapeutic relationship. Each chapter also details potential limitations and impediments to therapeutic success, as well as problem-solving strategies for when the inevitable resistance arises. Whether one approaches the system of stress by changing appraisals of threats or challenges in the environment (which then might affect biological responsiveness to stress) or by directly altering brain function (which then should affect attributions and appraisals), the importance of matching the chosen strategy in a way that best meets the individual's need is highlighted.

Much has been made lately of the burdens of evidence-based practice (EBP) in the clinical arena; indeed, this concept has sometimes been misused by policy makers and insurance providers to unnecessarily restrict clinical practice. And yet EBP, correctly applied, always centers directly on individuals who require the intervention; it is better considered as a strategic way of intervening for the benefit of the individual rather than a simple list of techniques. A recent policy statement on this topic by the American Psychological Association (APA; APA Presidential Task Force on Evidence-Based Practice, 2006) describes the development of two different concepts, to which I add a third. First, as noted by the APA, *empirically supported treatment* is a strategy that focuses on a specific intervention and communicates the extent of existing evidence for that intervention in the context of a given disorder. To this I would add that *clinical practice guidelines* should go beyond empirically supported treatments to focus on a specific problem or disorder (rather than a treatment procedure) by outlining an optimal strategy for going forward with a set of "best practices" for the assessment and treatment of that disorder. But EBP, unlike the preceding two concepts, focuses only on the individual (or groups of individuals) and brings to bear all of the evidence on how best to proceed with that individual to alleviate suffering or to enhance functioning. This may or may not include utilizing empirically supported treatments and/or following closely a nomothetic clinical practice guideline. In practice, this means that the clinician faced with the individual seeking help should, after a careful assessment, consider which empirically supported treatments might be appropriate and then implement the treatment if it best matches the needs of the individual seeking help. To make this judgment, the clinician must consider not only the set of symptoms or disorder with which the patient presents but also the patient's individual characteristics, including his or her preferences, that would maximize the possibility of success. It would always be up to the clinician, working closely with the patient, to make these decisions. If the clinician then started with an empirically supported treatment and found, through careful monitoring of outcomes, that it was not succeeding in the expected time frame, it would be incumbent on the clinician to consider carefully the next step, which might include an alternative approach. Thus EBP requires that clinicians be accountable to themselves, to their clients, to insurance providers, and to society at large by making their clinical judgment explicit and providing data and outcomes supporting the decisions they make. This is a far cry from the rigid predetermined approach to intervention that has become the caricature of EBP.

From this book, clinicians from around the world now have available a description of the leading empirically supported stress management procedures accompanied by descriptions by the world's experts on how to best implement the procedures in their practices. As our understanding of the nature of stress and its manifestations unfolds in the future, these procedures will surely evolve into what may be a more select but more flexibly applied set of strategies. In the meantime, clinicians of all stripes can lead the way by creatively extracting from this book the most powerful set of techniques for use in their own practice.

DAVID H. BARLOW, PhD
Center for Anxiety and Related Disorders
Boston University

REFERENCES

APA Presidential Task Force on Evidence-Based Practice. (2006). Evidence-based practice in psychology. *American Psychologist, 61*(4), 271–285.

Cohen, S., Doyle, W. J., & Skoner, D. P. (1999). Psychological stress, cytokine production, and severity of upper respiratory illness. *Psychosomatic Medicine, 61,* 175–180.

Sapolsky, R. M. (1990). Stress in the wild. *Scientific American, 262*(1), 116–123.

Sapolsky, R. M. (2000). Glucocorticoids and hippocampal atrophy in neuropsychiatric disorders. *Archives of General Psychiatry, 57,* 925–935.

Taylor, S. E., Klein, L. C., Lewis, B. P., Gruenewald, T. L., Gurung, R. A. R., & Updegraff, J. A. (2000). Biobehavioral responses to stress in females: Tend-and-befriend, not fight-or-flight. *Psychological Review, 107,* 411–429.

Vaillant, G. E. (1979). Natural history of male psychological health. *New England Journal of Medicine, 301,* 1249–1254.

Preface

It is both with a sense of satisfaction and with some trepidation that we have undertaken a third edition of this volume. In many circles, the previous editions have become standard texts for teaching stress management methods. We believe and hope that this occurred because of our attempts to provide both clinical richness and empirical grounding for each of the methods we present and from the accomplishments and reputations of the contributing authors, many of whom were originators of methods they wrote about and whose names are inextricably associated with their methods. We are aware that some of the chapters represent classic descriptions of well-known methods and that "updating" them may reflect bowing to changing academic and clinical fads as much as to genuine progress in the field. In other cases, particularly our own review chapters, the field has indeed marched on. In some cases, we have attempted to grow and change with it; in others, we hope we have recognized that new perspectives are required from people with newer and deeper expertise. In all chapters, we now review new results that have appeared since the last edition.

In the years since the second edition, a number of changes have taken place. The sheer number of empirical studies of stress management methods has skyrocketed. Procedures and criteria for evaluating empirical validation of clinical methods have been developed and become widely accepted. New stress management methods have appeared that meet our criteria for clinical acceptance and empirical validation. New applications have been explored for stress management methods. More has been discovered about the basic processes of stress itself. Finally, with some poignancy, we realize that leadership in the field is beginning to pass to a new generation of researchers and clinicians. Where new advances in the field require it or where original contributors no longer are available, we have invited new contributors.

In assembling this edition, we have tried to balance multiple demands: faithfulness to classic clinical techniques, respect for their originators, combining the clinical "how-to" with empirical validation, and including a comprehensive compendium of the well-accepted and well-validated stress management methods in use today. In this edition we also evaluate the empirical validation of various methods according to recently promulgated criteria by the Association for Applied Psychophysiology and Biofeedback and/or the American Psychological Association. In approaching our revision, we hope that the current edition will continue to serve the needs both of graduate students and of clinicians who are mindful of empirical validation.

In addition to updates and changes in authorship of particular chapters, we have added a coeditor, Wesley E. Sime, who has special expertise in applying stress management methods to athletics and improvement of human performance. We have added a chapter on the psychology and psychophysiology of stress as a backdrop to understanding various stress management techniques. In place of our own reviews of stress management literature, which focused heavily on specific effects of various methods, these chapters now focus more on effectiveness of stress management methods for resolving particular kinds of problems. Additionally, some chapters are entirely new, describing methods that have been devised, validated, and/or widely used more recently. This includes Jan van Dixhoorn's chapter on breathing retraining (Chapter 12), which describes a method that is a standard stress management and cardiac rehabilitation strategy in parts of Europe. We hope this first English-language exposition of the method will make it more widely available. Similarly, Paul Davis, Wesley Sime, and James Robertson have contributed a new chapter on performance enhancement (Chapter 23), Lee Hyer and Bonnie Kushner a chapter on eye movement desensitization and reprocessing (Chapter 21), Kevin Chen a chapter on Qigong (Chapter 16), Jean Kristeller a chapter on mindfulness meditation (Chapter 15), and Michael and Lynda Thompson a chapter on neurofeedback (Chapter 11).

We hope that the current volume will be considered as useful and definitive as the previous editions. To the extent that our aim has been achieved, we as editors thank the contributors, whose number include some of the most prominent contributors to our field. We humbly thank them for their willingness to contribute to this venture. Where our aims have not been met, we, as editors, bear responsibility both for our own contributions and for oversight of the enterprise.

Contents

PART III. INTEGRATION

PART I

INTRODUCTION

CHAPTER 1

Conceptual Issues Underlying Stress Management

ROBERT L. WOOLFOLK
PAUL M. LEHRER
LESLEY A. ALLEN

RESEARCH VERSUS CLINICAL PRACTICE IN STRESS MANAGEMENT

In the midst of the hoopla and ballyhoo that have surrounded the burgeoning public concern with stress and its deleterious consequences, meticulous scientists have systematically investigated the effects of numerous stress reduction techniques. Their efforts are the basis on which we warrant and legitimize the methods employed to solve varied and complex human problems. Applications of general knowledge to unique, concrete human situations, however, are always problematic. In the treatment of stress-related disorders, bridging the gap between laboratory and clinic presents numerous challenges to which the research literature is an insufficient guide.

The clinician who attempts to learn therapeutic strategies by reading the empirical literature on stress management techniques inevitably experiences disappointment. The descriptions of treatment methods are cursory and terse; only those already intimately familiar with the interventions studied can understand clearly what procedures were involved. Treatments typically are not adapted to individual cases but are uniform for all participants. Frequently the "clinical version" of the treatment undergoes some modification so that a standardized form, suitable for testing, can be achieved. Moreover, stress reduction techniques often are abbreviated to make them easier to teach, easier to learn, and consistent with control or comparison conditions on such dimensions as length of training or amount of therapist contact.

Due to the presence of experimental controls necessary for the preservation of internal validity, treatment outcome studies do not provide a veridical picture of the clinical practice of stress management. Furthermore, because of the methodological requirements of research designs seeking to isolate causal influences, a given group of participants often is administered a single stress management technique. Overly recalcitrant or disturbed participants may be excluded at the outset, or they may become casualties of experimental attrition, resulting in their data being removed or statistically imputed in the final data analysis. The exigencies of research often dictate the random assignment of participants to treatment conditions, making it impossible to observe the interactions among individual differences and factors related to treatments. Stress problems are intertwined in complicated ways with other pathological life circumstances and personal characteristics; the standard factorial design is not well suited to an examination of these complexities.

In behavioral science experiments, the emphasis on statistical significance, or even an effect size, as an index of treatment success creates a different emphasis from that in the world of clinical application. It is, of course, necessary to demonstrate that differences between treatment and control conditions are unlikely to have occurred as a result of chance factors. Efficacy when compared with a control condition in a laboratory setting is a necessary but insufficient basis for a technique to be considered clinically effective in "real-world" settings. Efficacy when compared with a control condition in a well-controlled study indicates that a technique was found superior to a control in a study with high internal validity. The real word utility of a therapeutic method—its effectiveness—requires, on the other hand, that the impact of therapeutic techniques be demonstrated in a study with high external validity. Effectiveness research, exemplified by the recent generation of "services research" studies, attempts to examine the impact of clinical interventions in everyday real-world contexts. In such research the external validity of the research may be accorded more importance than considerations of internal validity, resulting in the use of systematic naturalistic methods or quasi-experimental designs. Out in the real world of clinical services, a therapy technique not only must be better than nothing, but it must also be clinically powerful enough to justify its use. It must provide sufficient relief of suffering and enhanced ability to function to make it worth the time and effort to invoke it. It must be sufficiently acceptable to the client population to generate a high rate of treatment adherence. It must also be cost-effective.

In the years since the previous edition of this volume, the distinction between the efficacy of an intervention and its effectiveness has come to be sharply drawn. Many of the issues germane to clinical practice in the real world have proved to be amenable to systematic study via empirical methods. Improvement rates are calculated, degree of improvement assessed, and cost–benefit analyses conducted. It is doubtful, however, that any number of such studies can provide answers to all the questions that arise in the course of clinical practice. Applications of scientific knowledge to the clinical arena will inevitably contain elements of art and of pedagogy. A mistake made often by newcomers to this field is to assume that the extensive scientific foundation of self-regulation technology obviates the necessity for clinical sensitivity, perspicacity, and wisdom. Although stress reduction techniques are more standardized and explicit than some other therapeutic methods, their success is no less dependent on the tacit skills and know-how that experienced and effective clinicians develop as they face the intricate and thorny problems clients present to them.

THE IDIOGRAPHIC NATURE OF STRESS MANAGEMENT

An important distinction that must be drawn at the outset is that between the nomothetic and the idiographic. Nomothetic knowledge is general; idiographic knowledge is specific to a particular case. Much knowledge in psychiatry and psychology is generic. Most knowledge that the therapist possesses is of generalities and is derived from theory, research, and personal experience. Psychotherapy is an application of this general knowledge to a specific case that is always, in some respects, unique. Therapeutic interventions, interpretations, and prescriptions are always directed toward an idiograph: an individual person, couple, family, or group. The therapist is always in the position of asking him- or herself, "What is going on here with this particular case I am treating?"

In both assessment and treatment, the therapist must make many decisions, such as whether to use Treatment A or Treatment B with a client or whether the discontent within a marriage is due to the couple's poor conflict resolution skills or to some more basic incompatibilities. For a client to accept a therapeutic interpretation, he or she must decide that it is true not of most people but of him- or herself. The challenge of any given case in psychotherapy is determining which generalities apply to that particular case, and to what degree. Such determinations always involve some uncertainty, and may require some trial and error.

Even in applied fields derived from such systematic and unimpeachable disciplines as physics and chemistry, application to specific cases is not entirely straightforward. Mishaps occur frequently, and some practical knowledge about the particular arena of application often is required to effect a successful translation from theory to practice. Newly created airplanes may not perform as aerodynamically as expected, climate-control systems may not produce the temperatures intended, tunnels may collapse, winds may cause buildings to sway unacceptably, and torpedoes may bounce off the hulls of enemy ships without detonating.

Biological and psychological phenomena are more complex and variable than those of the physical sciences. They are more difficult to classify and measure. The truth about them is harder to discover and more difficult to confirm. Most research results are subject to conflicting interpretations, and debate about the clinical significance of almost any research finding often seems endless. When we do find an unchallenged truth, it commonly comes in the form of a stochastic or probabilistic generalization, for example, that smokers are twice as likely to develop heart disease or that treatment A is effective 60% of the time whereas treatment B works 45% of the time. The external and ecological validities of clinical research are rarely established for the clinician. Can the treatments be implemented? Was the sample representative? Will the results generalize? These elementary questions often have no clear answers.

Now this is not to say that nomothetic research findings are without import. Often they are the very best we can do in the absence of knowledge about the particular case with which we are concerned. Most often we simply will want to play the odds, rather than function without any rational basis for choice. For example, we would be rational to use exposure methods instead of three-times-a-week psychoanalysis for the treatment of simple phobias and to stop smoking rather than risk that we will be among the lucky ones who escape disease. Such decisions are sensible and prudent in the absence of more certain knowledge about the case in question; for example, based on numerous unsuccessful attempts to employ tricyclic antidepressants with a particular patient, a treating psychiatrist concludes that this patient cannot tolerate the side effects of this class of drug. But whatever the particulars may be, the logic of applying nomothetic research findings to an essentially idiographic situation, such as psychotherapy, requires that we recognize the uncertain and probabilistic nature of the application.

When we are confronted with an individual patient, even one with a clear *Diagnostic and Statistical Manual of Mental Disorders* (DSM) diagnosis, we are still very much in the dark and may become enlightened only after the fact, after we have tried and either succeeded or failed. Yet, even after the fact, clarity may not emerge. The analysis of individual cases with the aim of developing valid idiographic knowledge also is fraught with logical pitfalls, as any text on single-subject research methodology will attest. For example, a client can never know, for sure, whether it was a particular cognitive intervention that lifted his or her spirits or the cumulative impact of the caring and empathy provided by his or her therapist. Such inferences, always, are subject to the fallacy of *post hoc ergo propter hoc*.[1]

Given the plethora of methods and the claims on their behalf circulating through the mental health culture and society at large, clinicians and students interested in the treatment of stress problems need not only to learn techniques but also to evaluate the clinical worth of those techniques. This volume includes not only descriptions of clinical methods but also material on the empirical research that validates the technique. The book is designed primarily to serve the clinician rather than the researcher. Although each of our contributors has research credentials, we have asked them to refrain from providing comprehensive and exhaustive surveys of the empirical literature; such reviews are readily available in scientific journals.

Our contributors are consummate artists of their crafts, each a master of his or her respective area. We have commissioned them to make personal statements based on their clinical experience and to hold in abeyance some of the circumspection and reserve that might characterize their activities as scientists. Our charge to them has been to wear their clinical hats—to communicate to their fellow clinicians those aspects of clinical acumen, artistry, and sagacity that so often are missing from descriptions of stress management methods. We have asked our contributors to become teachers—not only to convey the readily specifiable technical aspects of their crafts but also to explicate those seemingly ineffable therapeutic nuances and intuitive rules of thumb that are the hallmarks of clinical virtuosos. We have asked them also to describe pertinent research findings regarding therapeutic and adverse consequences of their techniques and to show how they utilize research findings to guide their practice.

All of the contributions to this volume address the basic clinical questions that cut across techniques: assessment; selection of appropriate techniques; the client–therapist relationship; the limitations of stress management technology; potential impediments to therapeutic success; and client cooperation, resistance, and adherence to therapeutic regimens. The clinical experience of our contributors represents a unique and invaluable repository of knowledge—the kind of practical knowledge and clinical rules of thumb that can only be acquired through experience.

THE CONCEPT OF STRESS

History

The word *stress* dates back to the 14th century, and its origins to that time when the English language developed from an intermingling of Norman French and Anglo-Saxon (Simpson & Weiner, 1989, 1993; Proffitt, 1997). *Stress* derives from the Middle French word *destresse* ("distress"), which in turn derives from the Latin *strictus* ("compressed"). Various forms of word originally denoted hardship or adversity. By the 16th century the word was employed to indicate subjecting an entity "(a material thing, a bodily organ, a mental faculty) to stress or strain; to overwork, fatigue" (Simpson & Weiner, 1989). In the 19th century, *stress* became a precise scientific term employed within physics, used to refer to force applied to objects that could potentially result in deformation or strain.

The great physiologist Walter Cannon (1939), although he used the term *stress* infrequently, originated our modern biomedical concept of stress as involving a perturbation of somatic homeostasis by external threats that induce a mobilization of bodily resources to contend with the circumstances. Cannon coined the term *fight or flight response* to describe a mobilization of the organism that prepares it more effectively to aggress or to flee. Cannon located the genesis of the response in the limbic system and presented to us the ironic conception of the modern human being, located in a complex contemporary world in which physical danger is minimal yet equipped with antiquated reptilian response system disposed to mobilize the organism for fight or flight even though, for most contemporary threats, neither fleeing nor combat is a viable option.

The next great figure in the history of stress was Hans Selye (1956), the man who promulgated the concept of stress within medicine and biology and made it a household word among the general public. Selye expanded on Cannon's work and described three stages of the stress response: the alarm stage, the adaptive–resistance stage, and the exhaustion stage. The alarm stage is equivalent to Cannon's fight-or-flight response, the adrenomedullary response that prepares the individual to respond to an emergency or threat. During the second, adaptive–resistance, stage, homeostatic processes cause the body to return to its state prior to arousal, when the stressor is no longer present. The exhaustion stage is sometimes called "burnout" and results from extended excessive metabolic demands of a protracted alarm stage. The resulting depletion of bodily resources makes the organism prone to infirmity, or even death.

Whereas Cannon tended to view stress primarily in terms of a disruption of homeostasis during the elicitation of the fight-or-flight response, recent, more complex formulations of the response to stress have suggested that stress may activate bodily mechanisms whose function it is to maintain stability in the face of a changing internal or external environment. The term *allostasis*, which literally means the maintenance of stability through change, was conceived by Sterling and Eyer (1988) in characterizing the functioning of the cardiovascular system in its adjustment to various levels of bodily activity.

The concept of allostasis has been incorporated into a model of stress by McEwen and colleagues (Goldstein & McEwen, 2002; McEwen, 1998) that emphasizes the complex and multifarious functions of the glucocorticoids and the catecholamines. A related concept, allostatic load, refers to the "wear and tear" on the organism that results from multiple cycles of allostasis, as well as from less than optimal initiation and cessation of allostatic cycles. A classic example of animals manifesting allostatic load is male cynomologus monkeys striving for status in an unstable dominance hierarchy who encounter repeated and continuous confrontations and conflicts with other animals. These monkeys exhibit accelerations in atherosclerotic plaque formation that are associated with rises in blood pressure and raised catecholamine levels (Manuck, Kaplan, Adams & Clarkson, 1995). Another example would be the class study that showed that serum cholesterol levels rose and blood-clotting time was reduced in accountants during the peak workload of tax season (Friedman, Rosenman, & Carroll, 1958).

One Stress Response or Many?

Although the response to stress is most often formulated in terms of the individual organism defending itself against threat by fighting or fleeing, a number of kinds of response to stress have been observed. The antithesis of behavioral activation, a "freeze–hide" response, also has been widely observed. Evolutionary biologists sometimes refer to the tendency to produce an active versus a passive response to stress as a distinction between "hawks" and "doves" and between "hawk" and "dove" strategies for acquiring resources and enhancing inclusive fitness (Korte, Koolhaas, Wingfield, & McEwen, 2005). Hawks are proactive and bold, whereas doves favor a response style that emphasizes passivity, reactivity, nonaggression, and caution. Each style has its evolutionary advantages.

Korte et al. (2005) have suggested that hawks exhibit Cannon's fight-or-flight response, the sympathetic adrenomedullary response that produces elevated epinephrine in the bloodstream, increased levels of synaptic norepinephrine, and, during fight, the activation of a hypothalamic–pituitary–gonadal response that produces an increase in plasma testosterone. In response to stress, doves manifest the activation of the hypothalamic–pituitary–adrenal axis and the concomitant production of corticotropin-releasing factor that stimulates the pituitary gland to secrete adrenocorticotropic hormone into the blood. As a result the adrenal cortex releases cortisol. Although much of the research underlying the hawk–dove formulation is based on studies of infrahumans, the possibility that the stress response may be more differented than originally assumed is an intriguing possibility for future research and theory.

Tend-and-Befriend

In a series of recent articles, Taylor and her colleagues (Taylor et al., 2000; Taylor et al., 2002) have argued that males and females may respond to stress differently. In particular, they described a response to stress that is posited to be an alternative to fight or flight. This response is labeled "tend and befriend" and is thought to be characteristic of the female of various species. According to the model, the tend-and-befriend response is selected for by evolution and reflects the proclivity of females toward affiliation, cooperation, and caretaking:

> Tending involves nurturant activities designed to protect the self and offspring that promote safety and reduce distress; befriending is the creation and maintenance of social networks that may aid in this process. (Taylor et al., 2000, p. 411)

The tend-and-befriend response putatively derives from females' attachment and caregiving propensities. The biological underpinnings of the response, adduced from human and animal studies, appear to involve oxytocin operating in concert with female reproductive hormones and endogenous opioid peptide mechanisms. Aggression in males seems to be mediated by arousal of the sympathetic nervous system, whereas in females, aggression has not been linked reliably linked to sympathetic arousal, suggesting that, in females aggression may not be a component of the adrenomedullary "initial alarm" stage of the response to stress. The possibility that the stress response may be "gendered" further complicates our picture of the stress response.

Active and Passive Coping; Social Coping versus Fight–Flight

Gender differences in the stress response are reflected in underlying psychophysiological patternings of the stress response, which affect both genders equally. Although the autonomic substrate of the stress response is often characterized as the fight-or-flight reflex, it is rare indeed that everyday stress requires either fighting or fleeing. We rarely experience situations that require either physical combat or escape. Most everyday stress involves managing social judgment and exercising skill in maneuvering through social hierarchies. More subtle physical activity may play a part in such functioning, particularly relating to body posture and facial expression. Nuances in facial coloration and expression are powerful agents of social communication and play a more important role in managing the social environment than sympathetic mobilization. Such physiological events are mediated by parasympathetic, rather than sympathetic, function through a network of vagal–trigeminal interactions, as described by Gevirtz (Chapter 9, this volume).

Even more gross vegetative responses may be parasympathetic in nature. Although active stress coping may be accompanied by sympathetic activation and parasympathetic inhibition, passive coping with stress tends to be associated with the opposite. Thus Aboussafy, Campbell, Lavoie, Aboud, and Ditto (2005) demonstrated a parasympathetic reaction and consequent deterioration in asthma (in which parasympathetic arousal causes bronchoconstriction) among asthmatic patients exposed to situations involving passive response to stress. Similar response occurs in experimentally induced sadness among asthmatic children (Miller & Wood, 1997). Other studies showing asthma exacerbation as a stress response have tended to use social stressors that could not be managed (e.g., psychological abuse by an authoritarian figure; Isenberg, Lehrer, & Hochron, 1992). Exposure to blood and gore also seems to evoke a parasympathetic response (Bosch, de Geus, Veerman, Hoogstraten, & Nieuw Amerongen, 2003), perhaps a reflex reflecting preparation for shock to preserve blood supply. The "play dead" response also may be reflected in a parasympathetic discharge, a paradigmatic stress response. It is found massively in passive stress responses in rodents (Belser, 1983; Richter, Schumann, & Zwiener, 1990; Zwiener, Richter, Schumann, Glaser, & Witte, 1990), but is also found in humans (Heslegrave & Furedy, 1978). Such "vasovagal" stress reactions can even be life threatening at times (Chamarthi, Dubrey, Cha, Skinner, & Falk, 1997; Samniah, Iskos, Sakaguchi, Lurie, & Benditt, 2001).

Stress management approaches to this complex of stress responses involving social responsivity, particularly when characterized by passivity and/or sadness or a blood phobic–anticipatory shock response, might well include components designed to modulate this pattern. These could include social skills training, aspects of cognitive therapy, exercise, and control of respiration and heart rate variability.

Contemporary Revisions of the Stress Concept

In recent years, the concept of psychosocial stress has proliferated and become widespread in both scientific and popular usage, not only in the United States but also around the world. Public awareness of the adverse effects of stress has never been higher. In fact, one could argue that the awareness has become a preoccupation. Many magazine covers, including that of *Time*, have featured stress, and countless self-help books on the topic have been printed. So great is the importance attributed to stress in the etiology of disease that laypersons occasionally regard it as more central to health than it may actually be. For example, in surveys, stress reliably emerges as the risk factor the public considers most important in the etiology of coronary heart disease, more important than smoking or hypertension (French, Senior, Weinman, & Marteau, 2001). And, indeed, stress is listed more frequently than tobacco consumption as a cause of cancer (Maskarinec, Gotay, Tatsumura, Shumay, & Kakai, 2001).

The concept of stress has been criticized for its lack of precision and questioned as to what exactly it refers to. Indeed, stress is sometimes used to refer to what was, at one time in psychology, called *external stimuli*. Under this usage, stress is in the environment, part of the external world. Another usage defines stress not as the stimulus but as the perceived or processed stimulus. This is the stance of those such as Richard Lazarus (1994) and other subscribers to a cognitive-appraisal model of stress. Still others conceive of stress as the response, rather than the stimulus. Stress can be chronic or episodic, positive or negative, a problem or a challenge.

What is one to do with such a plurality of meanings? *Stress*, in fact, is probably best thought of as a generic, nontechnical term, analogous to *disease* or to *addiction*. At times the term *stress* may function as little more than a rather crude metaphor. But stress is a useful umbrella concept in that it helps identify and categorize a multiplicity of diverse phenomena, although without supplying much in the way of theoretical guides to a deeper understanding of the phenomena. It is part of an idiom that allows laypersons to describe life's perturbations without using such potentially undesirable terms as *anxiety* or *depression*. It is also an umbrella term that fosters communication and heuristically beneficial grounds for scientific collaboration (Woolfolk, 2001). The intellectual functions of the concept of stress often seem to be analogous to those of other biopsychosocial concepts that occur at similar levels of abstraction, for example, disorder, trauma, and addiction, that organize objects of scientific research conveniently but without clear theoretical utility. For example, the stress label seems to work as a symbol for communication among scientists and clinicians, although the notion of stress management, which is the common denominator of this volume, does not denote a narrow set of techniques with straightforward and consistent defining characteristics. Yet those of us who operate within the subculture of stress management recognize the affinities or "family resemblances" among the different endeavors that we pursue. The concept of stress may eventually be replaced by a set of more precise terms, such as *allostasis*. Until that time, however, *stress* is a term just nebulous enough to facilitate communication among diverse practitioners and to provide a rubric that has allowed a valuable set of scientific and clinical efforts to develop and to flourish.

Cultural Influences on Stress and Stress Management

Although people from all places and cultures experience stress and its sequelae, the sources of stress, the quality of the experience, and the acceptability of various treatment methods may vary considerably. For example, it has been widely reported that, compared with Anglos, people from Hispanic backgrounds tend to respond to trauma and stress with more somatic symptoms (Hulme, 1996), although a specific stress syndrome *without* somatic component has been described as a folk illness in Peru (Dobkin de Rios, 1981). A somatic stress "syndrome" has been noted in Korean culture (Pang, 1990). Askew and Keyes (2005) have theorized that direct expression of emotional distress would be considered more deviant in more collectivist cultures, such as Korea, than in more individualist cultures, such as the United States, and hence that symptoms of stress tend to be experienced somatically more frequently in Asian cultures.

Cultural biases in symptom expression are mirrored in approaches to treatment. Patients with emotional illness *without* somatic components tend to receive more treatment opportunities in the United States than in South Korea, whereas this disparity disappears for patients with a major somatic component in their symptomatology, suggesting a cultural bias in treatment methods (Keyes & Ryff, 2003). Thus treatment methods described in this book that originate in Asia tend to have more of a somatic focus. This is particularly true for yoga and Qigong, but it also applies to mindfulness meditation, in which the mental focus often is on body sensations. Although it is less true for mantra meditation, all of these methods have been influenced by Eastern religious values, emphasizing feelings of inner peace and "oneness" with the environment. Although Western in origin, autogenic training shares some of this philosophy. Indeed, Johanees Schultz spent considerable time in Japan while formulating the method (see Chapter 7, this volume) and explicitly acknowledges his debt to yoga and Zen.

In contrast, although somatic in focus, the philosophies behind progressive relaxation, pharmacotherapy, and biofeedback are more Western: technological, physiological, and mechanistic. Less focused on a state of inner being, they are more oriented toward fixing particular problems, and their origins are more directly tied to Western parametric research. Edmund Jacobson (1938) specifically eschewed any connection between his progressive relaxation method and the methods of yoga. Cognitive therapy and stress inoculation methods are similarly quintessentially "Western," focused on rational discourse and on purging oneself of irrational and maladaptive tendencies of thought.

PHILOSOPHICAL AND SOCIOCULTURAL ASPECTS OF STRESS MANAGEMENT

Despite the impressive array of clinical wisdom and empirical data accumulated to date about modifying stress responses in individuals, it is likely that some issues related to stress management can be comprehended only at the levels of history, society, and culture. The stressors, diets, toxins, and activity patterns of industrialized urban life take their toll on our minds and on our bodies. Diseases such as coronary heart disease, hypertension, and cancer, which are rare among primitive peoples, are our chief causes of death and disability. A major reason for the rise of the degenerative physical diseases, as well as the high levels of psychological distress in contemporary Western societies, may well be the stress of modern life. This stress seems inescapable; no matter what we do, we cannot avoid it entirely.

Why should stress be such a problem in the contemporary world? Were there not terrible happenings and awful circumstances that troubled our ancestors, just as our current frustrations and tribulations beset us? Clearly, premodern life was (and still is, in contemporary developing nations) very difficult. Wars, pestilence, and dangers from the elements have undoubtedly produced emotional arousal throughout human history. And indeed, life often has been viewed as too much for us; too difficult to bear. The first noble truth of Buddhism avers that life is *dukkha* (usually translated as "suffering," but occasionally translated as "stress"). Many centuries ago the Stoics developed a philosophy based on the view that extraordinary training was necessary for one not to be undone by the ubiquitous perturbations of this existence.

Yet there are key differences in the sociocultural environment of the modern world that can foster a kind of unremitting tension in modern individuals—at levels that are chronic and multilayered, as opposed to the less complex stressors that were (and are) more characteristic of less complicated societies. The modern world is fundamentally and qualitatively different from that of the past. These differences provide some important clues to the capacity of contemporary Western society to create great distress and tension in its citizens.

Among the distinctive features of modernization are the ordering of life by the clock and a large increase in time-pressured work. Caplan, Cobb, French, Harrison, and Pinneau (1975) found that machine-paced assembly workers reported more somatic complaints and anxiety than did assemblers who were not machine-paced. Levi and his colleagues (Levi, 1972) reported that piecework pressure produced increases in noradrenalin levels and in blood pressure. Tax accountants were found to show substantial increases in serum cholesterol and reductions in blood-clotting latency when working under the pressure of deadlines (Friedman, Rosenman, & Carroll, 1958).

As Alvin Toffler (1970) and various other observers have pointed out, not only is modern society an ever-changing panorama, but also the rate of that change is ever-increasing. Many of the implications of this condition are rather straightforward. An individual is constantly required to make adjustments to a varying sociocultural matrix. We have earlier reported how such social disruptions can elevate levels of stress. In the areas of job skills, interpersonal relationships, management of personal finances, and sex roles, to name just a few, such rapid and fundamental changes have occurred that old assumptions are in continual need of revision.

Three hundred years ago it was possible for one individual, the German philosopher Gottfried Wilhelm von Leibniz, to assimilate the entire scope of human knowledge. Seventy-five years ago, an individual could know the entire fledgling field of psychology. Today, however, the knowledge explosion makes it impossible for one person to possess a significant fraction of the pertinent information in even a small domain of that field or any other, and the pool of knowledge is growing every day. Professionals who are not inclined toward voracious reading within their specialties are soon out of date, their knowledge obsolete. Life is a little like this for all of us: We must keep changing, ceaselessly adapting to a world that transforms itself more rapidly each day. We must move faster and faster just to maintain our places.

One effect of industrialization and modernization is almost universally regarded as beneficial—that of enhancing the freedom and material well-being of individuals. The removal of many of the economic and social barriers to personal growth and self-expression presents the modern individual with a dazzling array of choices, as well as an awesome set of responsibilities. Today we choose our own careers, our circles of friends, our places of residence, and, perhaps most important, our own values. We must make decisions on a number of issues that would have been given or fixed in prior eras. We decide everything, from whether to alter our appearances through dieting, exercise, or cosmetic surgery to what religion (if any) to follow. We are able to create for ourselves the rules that will govern relations with both intimates and acquaintances. The plasticity of the human being is such that even alteration of gender is now possible. Very little is set, fixed, or taken for granted. In the absence of some generally agreed-on set of values or beliefs that provides practical wisdom to guide the making of choices, too many options can be difficult to bear. The great French sociologist Emile Durkheim (1897/1958), writing at the turn of the century, called this lack of values and norms "anomie"; he demonstrated that under anomic conditions, suicide rates rise dramatically.

The sociologist Ferdinand Tonnies (1963), in describing the changes in society that took place at the time of the Industrial Revolution, outlined two basic kinds of social organization. Modern American sociologists often continue to call them by the German words *gemeinschaft* and *gesellschaft*, or, literally, "community" and "society." The *gemeinschaft* form of social organization is the preindustrial form. It is characterized by group cohesiveness and coherent social order, but little freedom. In communal cultures, status is ascribed, and jobs, wealth, and marriage are determined on the basis of who a person is, rather than what he or she can do. *Gemeinschaft* contains small social units (e.g., the family, the small village), as well as diffuse relationships in which various social roles (e.g., family member, boss, friend, teacher, healer, and church member) are extensively intermixed within the same small group of individuals.

In contrast, the *gesellschaft* form encourages individual freedom and ambition, but at the price of social isolation and anomie. It is characterized by achieved rather than ascribed statuses. Units of social organization are large, so that even many of the people in a particular congregation or factory workforce, let alone in a neighborhood or town, may not be known to each other. This form is also distinguished by role specificity; thus we pray with one group of people, work with another, and socialize with a third. Few, if any, formalized activities take place within the extended family. The extended family all but disappears, and even the nuclear family is weakened. Social isolation and anomie are significant sources of stress in this more modern form of society (Nisbet, 1973).

In the contemporary West, individuals continually are thrown back on themselves and their own psychic resources. The German sociologist and philosopher Arnold Gehlen (1980) has written that one of the functions of society is to protect the individual from the burden of excessive choice. If this is so, then contemporary industrialized societies are less than completely successful in this function. Never before has such a large percentage of the population been without durable and dependable social support.

The loss of community is related to the lack of meaning that is so often described by sociologists and existential philosophers as a concomitant of contemporary life. The premodern worldview was communal and spiritual, as contrasted with the individualistic and materialistic consciousness of contemporary times. Premoderns felt themselves to be useful and necessary elements of a cosmological order that had inherent purpose and meaning (Taylor, 1975). But the replacement of religion by science as the ultimate source of epistemic authority, the desacralization of nature, the ascendancy of technology and its associated rationality and means–ends perspective, and the relativization of values have disrupted the human security that emanated from a sense of belonging and the confidence that each individual life had some larger purpose and meaning (Richardson, Fowers, & Guignon, 1999). Existential writers such as Albert Camus have described this shift in human self-perception in compelling terms: "In a universe suddenly divested of illusions and lights, man feels an alien, a stranger. His exile is without remedy since he is deprived of the memory of a lost home or the hope of a promised land" (Camus, 1960, p. 5).

There is much evidence that people who find some purpose in existence, who believe that their activities are meaningful, and who view life as possessing coherence and lawfulness are less likely to manifest stress-related reactions (Antonovsky, 1987; Kobasa, 1979; Shepperd & Kashani, 1991). This evidence brings to mind the writings of the great sociologist Max Weber and his concept of "theodicy." Theodicies are elements of a cultural worldview that explain and confer meaning on experiences of suffering and wrongfulness. Berger, Berger, and Kellner (1973) have pointed out that despite the great changes that have accompanied modernization, the "finitude, fragility, and mortality" of the human condition is essentially unchanged; at the same time, those previous definitions of reality that made life easier to bear have been seriously weakened by modernization.

Psychotherapy and stress management (especially the cognitive aspects) may very well be in the business of supplying secular theodicies to people who look to science and scientifically grounded professionals to alleviate the discomforts of life (Woolfolk, 1998). The worldviews we proffer typically are justified on the basis of some instrumental criterion: They reduce stress, promote health, enhance happiness, or the like. Determining the beliefs that reduce the stress of life is, however, not equivalent to establishing the truth or legitimacy of those beliefs. Any worldview that is advanced solely on the basis of its instrumental benefits to health and happiness will be subject to various forms of criticism. One such criticism is the ethical rejoinder suggesting that many beliefs may be worth being stressed for—indeed, worth dying for. A worldview whose ultimate claim to authority is pragmatic may be inherently self-limiting and self-defeating if an "inherent" sense of purpose is what provides people with the capacity to withstand the corrosive aspects and vicissitudes of living.

The activities of stress management professionals are orchestrated within the sociocultural matrix and also—along with the ubiquitous mental health and self-improvement industry of which they are part—serve to constitute this matrix. It would seem important for practitioners to have a grasp of the moral and sociohistorical aspects of their role. With respect to existential issues, they may not possess any ultimate answers, but they should at least know what the questions are.

NOTE

1. The Latin expression is translated "After that, therefore because of that" and refers to the logical error of inferring that event A causes event B simply because A occurs before B. *Post hoc ergo propter hoc* is a special case of the fallacy of the "false cause" (Copi, 1961). A related instance of the false-cause fallacy familiar to behavioral scientists is that of inferring causation from mere correlation.

REFERENCES

Aboussafy, D., Campbell, T. S., Lavoie, K., Aboud, F. E., & Ditto, B. (2005). Airflow and autonomic responses to stress and relaxation in asthma: The impact of stressor type. *International Journal of Psychophysiology, 57*, 195–201.

Antonovsky, A. (1987). The salutogenic perspective: Toward a new view of health and sickness. *Advances, 4*, 47–55.

Askew, R. A., & Keyes, C. L. M. (2005). Stress and somatization: A sociocultural perspective. In K. V. Oxington (Ed.), *Psychology of stress* (pp. 129–144). Hauppage, NY: Nova Biomedical Publishers.

Belser, R. C. (1983). Psychophysiological coping-response specificity (Unpublished doctoral dissertation, Rutgers University). *Dissertation Abstracts International, 44*(5-B), 1631–1632.

Berger, P. L., Berger, B., & Kellner, H. (1973). *The homeless mind.* New York: Random House.

Bosch, J. A., de Geus, E. J., Veerman, E. C., Hoogstraten, J., & Nieuw Amerongen, A. V. (2003). Innate secretory immunity in response to laboratory stressors that evoke distinct patterns of cardiac autonomic activity. *Psychosomatic Medicine, 65*, 245–258.

Cannon, W. B. (1939). *The wisdom of the body.* New York: Norton.

Caplan, R. D., Cobb, S., French, J. R. P., Jr., Harrison, R. V., & Pinneau, S. R., Jr. (1975). *Job demands and worker health* (DHEW Publication No. NIOSH 75–160). Washington, DC: U.S. Government Printing Office.

Chamarthi, B., Dubrey, S. W., Cha, K., Skinner, M., & Falk, R. H. (1997). Features and prognosis of exertional syncope in light-chain associated AL cardiac amyloidosis. *American Journal of Cardiology, 80*, 1242–1245.

Copi, I. M. (1961). *Introduction to logic.* New York: Macmillan.

Dobkin de Rios, M. (1981). Saladerra: A culture-bound misfortune syndrome in the Peruvian Amazon. *Culture, Medicine and Psychiatry, 5*, 193–213.

Durkheim, E. (1958). *Suicide.* Glencoe, IL: Free Press. (Original work published 1897)

French, D., Senior, V., Weinman, J., & Marteau, T. (2001). Causal attributions for heart disease: A systematic review. *Psychology and Health, 16*, 77–98.

Friedman, M., Rosenman, R. H., & Carroll, V. (1958). Changes in serum cholesterol and blood clotting time in men subjected to cyclic variation of occupational stress. *Circulation, 17*, 852–861.

Gehlen, A. (1980). *Man in the age of technology.* New York: Columbia University Press.

Goldstein, D. S., & McEwen, B. (2002). Allostasis, homeostasis, and the nature of stress. *Stress, 5*, 55–58.

Heslegrave, R. J., & Furedy, J. J. (1978). Anticipatory HR deceleration as a function of perceived control and probability of aversive loud noise: A deployment of attention account. *Biological Psychology, 7*, 147–166.

Hulme, P. A. (1996). Somatization in Hispanics. *Journal of Psychosocial Nursing and Mental Health Services, 34*(3), 33–37.

Isenberg, S. A., Lehrer, P. M., & Hochron, S. (1992). The effects of suggestion and emotional arousal on pulmonary function in asthma: A review. *Psychosomatic Medicine, 54*, 192–216.

Jacobson, E. (1938). *Progressive relaxation.* Chicago: University of Chicago Press.

Keyes, C. L., & Ryff, C. D. (2003). Somatization and mental health: A comparative study of the idiom of distress hypothesis. *Social Science and Medicine, 57*, 1833–1845.

Kobasa, S. (1979). Stressful life events, personality, and health: An inquiry into hardiness. *Journal of Personality and Social Psychology, 37*, 1–11.

Korte, S. M., Koolhaas, J. M., Wingfield, J. C., & McEwen, B. S. (2005). The Darwinian concept of stress: Benefits of allostasis and costs of allostatic load and the trade-offs in health and disease. *Neuroscience and Biobehavioral Reviews, 29,* 3–38.

Lazarus, R. S. (1994). *Emotion and adaptation.* New York: Oxford University Press.

Levi, L. (1972). *Stress and distress in response to psychosocial stimuli.* Elmsford, NY: Pergamon Press.

Manuck, S. B., Kaplan, J. R., Adams, M. R., & Clarkson, T. B. (1995). Studies of psychosocial influences on coronary artery atherosclerosis in cynomolgus monkeys. *Health Psychology, 7,* 113–124.

Maskarinec, G., Gotay, C. C., Tatsumura Y., Shumay, D. M., & Kakai, H. (2001). Perceived cancer causes: Use of complementary and alternative therapy. *Cancer Practice, 9,* 183–190.

McEwen, B. S. (1998) Stress, adaptation, and disease: Allostasis and allostatic load. *Annals of the New York Academy of Sciences, 840,* 33–44.

Miller, B. D., & Wood, B. L. (1997). Influence of specific emotional states on autonomic reactivity and pulmonary function in asthmatic children. *Journal of the American Academy of Child and Adolescent Psychiatry, 36,* 669–677.

Nisbet, R. (1973). *The social philosophers: Community and conflict in Western thought.* New York: Crowell.

Pang, K. Y. (1990). *Hwabyung:* The construction of a Korean popular illness among Korean elderly immigrant women in the United States. *Culture, Medicine and Psychiatry, 14,* 495–512.

Proffitt, M. (Ed.). (1997). *Oxford English dictionary additions series* (Vol. 3). Oxford, UK: Oxford University Press.

Richardson, F. C., Fowers B. J., & Guignon, C. B. (1999). *Re-envisioning psychology: Moral dimensions of theory and practice.* San Francisco: Jossey-Bass.

Richter, A., Schumann, N. P., & Zwiener, U. (1990). Characteristics of heart rate fluctuations and respiratory movements during orienting, passive avoidance and flight–fight behaviour in rabbits. *International Journal of Psychophysiology, 10,* 75–83.

Samniah, N., Iskos, D., Sakaguchi, S., Lurie, K. G., & Benditt, D. G. (2001). Syncope in pharmacologically unmasked Brugada syndrome: Indication for an implantable defibrillator or an unresolved dilemma? *Europace, 3,* 159–163.

Selye, H. (1956). *The stress of life.* Toronto: McGraw-Hill.

Shepperd, J. A., & Kashani, J. V. (1991). The relationship of hardiness, gender, and stress to health outcomes in adolescents. *Journal of Personality, 59,* 747–768.

Sterling, P., & Eyer, J. (1988). Allostasis: A new paradigm to explain arousal pathology. In J. Fisher & J. Reason (Eds.), *Handbook of life stress, cognition and health* (pp. 629–649). New York: Wiley.

Taylor, C. (1975). *Hegel.* Cambridge, UK: Cambridge University Press.

Taylor, S. E., Klein, L. C., Lewis, B. P., Gruenewald, T. L., Gurung, R. A. R., & Updegraff, J. A. (2000). Biobehavioral responses to stress in females: Tend-and-befriend, not fight-or-flight. *Psychological Review, 107,* 411–429.

Taylor, S. E., Lewis, B. P., Gruenewald, T. L., Gurung, R. A. R., Updegraff, J. A., & Klein, L., C. (2002). Sex differences in biobehavioral responses to threat: Reply to Geary and Flinn. *Psychological Review, 109,* 751–753.

Toffler, A. (1970). *Future shock.* New York: Random House.

Tonnies, F. (1963). *Community and society.* New York: Harper & Row.

Woolfolk, R. L. (1998). *The cure of souls: Science, values, and psychotherapy.* San Francisco: Jossey-Bass.

Woolfolk, R. L. (2001). The concept of mental illness: An analysis of four pivotal issues. *Journal of Mind and Behavior, 22,* 161–178.

Zwiener, U., Richter, A., Schumann, N. P., Glaser, S., & Witte, H. (1990). Heart rate fluctuations in rabbits during different behavioural states. *Biomedica Biochimica Acta, 49,* 59–68.

CHAPTER 2

Psychophysiological Mechanisms of Stress
A Foundation for the Stress Management Therapies

ANGELE McGRADY

Stress pervades human existence, from the prenatal period to birth until the end of life. The brain is hardwired to perceive experiences, to identify them as negative, neutral, or positive, and to react to them. Volumes have been written on the physiology and biochemistry of the stress response, which are not covered in such detail in this chapter. However, understanding the stress response is critical to effective implementation of the stress management therapies that are discussed in this book. This chapter presents summaries of the theories of stress, a description of the stress responses organized in the central and autonomic nervous systems and the endocrine and immune systems, and the linkages among these major systems. Responses to stress are discussed from a developmental perspective, beginning with the interaction of heredity and environment, and examples of stressors most likely to be encountered in each age range are provided. Factors contributing to the valence of perceptions are discussed, including individual differences in the stress response. Finally, examples of maladaptive responses to stress in control systems are addressed, along with the long-term consequences that lead to the development of medical and psychiatric illness.

DEVELOPMENTAL PERSPECTIVE

Genetics and environment interact to determine responses to stress. It has been consistently observed that individuals exposed to similar stressful situations react differently; some adapt successfully, whereas others experience long-term emotional problems. Two different examples of variable reactions to life stress highlight the effect of genetics on physiological and emotional responses to environmental demands. Individuals with different genetic makeup in the serotonin gene are at higher or lower risk for depressive disorders. Specifically, with a short allele in the promoter region of the serotonin transporter gene, persons tend to be depressed and to have suicidal thoughts after stress compared with those who are homozygous for the long allele (Caspi et al., 2003). Those born with the short allele who are abused as children are also at significantly higher risk for adult clinical depression when exposed to stress. Rosmond, Bouchard, and Björntorp (2002) studied the impact of a polymorphism in the alpha-adrenergic receptor gene promoter on blood glucose levels. This variation was associated with lower than expected cortisol response to stimulation with dexamethasone and higher blood glucose, implying that suppressed reactivity is also related to risk of illness.

Certain stressful situations are more likely to occur during particular developmental periods. Environmental attacks of a psychological nature on the neonate increase the vulnerability for later dysfunction in both the emotional and physical domains. Maladaptive reactions to stress can already be identified in the infant, depending on whether its mother's pregnancy went to term. Neonates who were born prematurely have lower heart rate variability (an index of neural feedback mechanisms) than full-term infants. Low heart rate variability and vagal tone in these infants imposes vulnerabilities to later stress (Porges, 1992). When infants did not decrease vagal tone (the vagal brake) during a social attention task at 9 months of age, they manifested more behavioral problems at 3 years of age (Porges, Doussard-Roosevelt, Portales, & Greenspan, 1996). In fact, mastery of each subsequent developmental stage is influenced by parental guidance and support of children's attempts at the required tasks. Early life experiences that lack the nurturing quality of healthy parent–child relationships may produce structural deviations from normal development in the brain. Thus early experience has a strong influence on subsequent behavior and health via the effects on the developing brain.

One of the first interactions between primary caregiver and infant is facial expression. The amygdala in the brain interprets the smiles and frowns, allowing the infant to learn to associate certain expressions and sounds with emotion. Autonomic reactivity mediates appropriate behavioral and emotional responses to positive or negative stimuli (Porges, Doussard-Roosevelt, & Maiti, 1996). Soothing actions by mother toward child decrease the stress response and associated activation of the brain and endocrine system. The child's cries are answered, and the uncomfortable experiences of hunger, thirst, overstimulation, or loneliness are decreased by mom's attention and touch (McEwen, 2003a). During maturation, the goal is for the infant to learn mom's comforting techniques in such a way that the infant can in time self-soothe with thumb, pacifier, or blanket. This process sets the stage for later responses to stress. In contrast, some families behave aggressively toward the baby or fail to interact, thereby detaching from or neglecting the newborn. The neglected infant becomes desperate in the short term, later fails to attach to significant persons, and has difficulty responding appropriately to most social interactions (Schore, 2002). The infant withdraws from the mother and others and becomes passive. Adults may conclude that the baby is finally quiet and not so difficult. However, the baby's emotion has burrowed under the skin, producing internal biological responses that reflect the desperation. Negative fearful experiences are overconsolidated, turning states into traits. Physical and psychological effects emerge, such as failure to thrive, sleep problems, and childhood depression. In summary, during the first years of life, both positive and negative experiences have the power to change the brain.

Besides the direct effects of caregivers on children, parents' psychological states influence symptoms in their children. Morris, Blount, Brown, and Campbell (2001) found that when parents were anxious or depressed, their children had more frequent episodes of syncope. The worry and concern over having a child with asthma can increase parents' negative affect and overall stress level, escalating the tendency for respiratory symptoms in the child. Infants whose parents demonstrate high distress have more episodes of wheezing (Wright, Cohen, Carey, Weiss, & Gold, 2002). Thus children sense their parents' tension in nonverbal ways, as well as by the timbre and pitch in their voices or by their actions. Finally, adults who had poor attachment as children are likely to have more physical problems, more unexplained symptoms, and associated greater utilization of medical services (Ciechanowski, Walter, Katon, & Russo, 2002).

Patterns of behavior and emotional reactivity settle in during late adolescence and fully mature during early adulthood. Between the ages of 13 and 19, teens are faced with dramatic changes in their bodies and the challenges of making difficult decisions while dealing with the influence of their peers. Humiliation or embarrassment can be devastating, even to a generally secure girl or boy (Kendler, Hettema, Butera, Gardner, & Prescott, 2003). For example, a classroom joke or an embarrassing moment of illness makes such an impression that a neural network is permanently altered in the brain without conscious awareness. Memory of that event is overconsolidated; that is, emotional reactions to that stressor are conditioned by replaying of the images and their accompanying physiological responses. Emotional development seems to be arrested, with concomitant difficulties in identifying internal states and regulating arousal. Later, the adult overreacts to a slight criticism, with little understanding of the behavior, not realizing that at the unconscious level, the clock has been turned back years.

During the natural aging of a healthy person, some systems become more vulnerable to stress as physical strength and resiliency decline. Genetics plays a larger role again, as it did in infancy and childhood. Behavior patterns have had their effect; positive or negative, healthy or unhealthy eating and sleeping patterns are set. If physical activity was a significant part of stress control, the elderly may be more stress-response prone if movement is compromised due to injury or other disease (Cacioppo et al., 2000). During the last years of life, health status is moderated in a negative direction by depressive symptoms and in a positive manner by use of health control strategies, some of which were learned earlier (Wrosch, Schulz, & Heckhausen, 2002).

Once neuronal plasticity was demonstrated in the laboratory, then modulation of neural transmission and synaptic events by environmental factors was conceptually possible. Subsequent research showed that throughout the lifespan, changes in thinking, emotion, and psychophysiological responses to stress are occurring constantly and have the capacity to modify the brain (Sapolsky, 2003). Reflex control systems, like the baroreceptor-based blood pressure control system, can also undergo modifications in strength and timing of responses. Positive, healthy modifications promote more efficient regulation through the expansion of neural networks. Chronic negative stress and the associated release of stress hormones limit the growth of new neurons, interfering with regulation of or balance among physiological systems (i.e., dysregulation; McEwen, 2003c).

The age at which events happen in an individual's life has a strong influence on brain development. The younger the person, the more likely it is that negative events exert permanent damage to the brain (Perry & Pollard, 1998). Adult women who were abused as children have more physical symptoms, are more likely to overuse alcohol than women never abused, and, in fact, had the same risk for substance abuse as women currently being abused as adults (McCauley et al., 1997). There is a group of neurons in the hypothalamus that secrete corticotropin-releasing factor (CRF), a neurohormone that stimulates release of cortisol from the adrenal cortex. These neurons are more sensitive in people with history of trauma. In response to current stress, higher levels of CRF are released that, combined with genetic predisposition, dramatically increase the risk of emotional illnesses such as anxiety or depression (Heim et al., 2000).

THE STRESS RESPONSE TRIAD: NERVOUS, ENDOCRINE, AND IMMUNE SYSTEMS

Responses to stress are observed in multiple psychophysiological systems, with linkages between the brain, endocrine, and immune systems forming the collective heart of the stress response (Cacioppo, 1994). Response patterns are superbly designed to respond to acute stimuli across the whole range of severity and to recover after the stimulus, so that the organism is ready to respond the next time. The sympathetic nervous system and adrenal hormones are activated during acute stress responses; within seconds, norepinephrine is released from nerve endings and binds to postsynaptic receptors, and epinephrine leaves the adrenal medulla to circulate in the blood. Adrenergically mediated cardiovascular reactions—blood pressure and heart rate—in addition to faster respiration, tense muscles, decreased gastrointestinal activity, and alertness, are rapid adaptive responses to short-term challenges (Cacioppo, 1994). In addition, the adrenal cortex releases glucocorticoids, such as cortisol, relatively quickly to increase metabolic rate and inhibit the inflammatory response, as indicated by release of proinflammatory cytokines (Miller, Cohen, & Ritchey, 2002).

Plasticity, the ability to modify responses to repeated stimuli, and efficiency are the hallmarks of the feedback system (Björntorp, Holm, & Rosmond, 2000). Cells of the three systems have receptors on their cell membranes that react to information transmitted in one or more ways from the other two (Dantzer, 2001). Feedback loops constantly monitor information and organize physiological responses and actions, proceeding from brain to endocrine to immune cells and back. More neuronal space in the brain is devoted to inhibition, because the tendency of the brain is to be active, firing off multiple nerve impulses. Many interneurons are inhibitory, forming a neurotransmitter brake to the tendency of the excitatory neurons to continue firing action potentials.

In addition, the systems can also be modified by quite diverse factors, some positive (physical exercise, social support) and some negative (substance abuse and isolation). Normal feedback loops become deranged under conditions of repeated bombardment or slowed recovery time. The hypothalamic–pituitary–adrenal (HPA) axis, a three-component biological system comprising the hypothalamus and pituitary regions of the brain and the adrenal glands, evolves into a hypersensitive system. Whereas activation of the sympathetic nervous system and release of catecholamines from the adrenal medulla may solve a short-lasting problem, chronic mobilization of stress neurotransmittors and hormones creates a higher risk for physical problems, such as insulin resistance and inflammatory disease (Björntop, Holm, & Rosmond, 1999). Abnormal cortisol responses programmed early in life may speed up the process of development of the metabolic syndrome (discussed later), leading to the development of obesity and hyperglycemic symptoms at a younger age.

Most people experience stressful situations as time-consuming and mentally exhausting. Cognitive energy is devoted to thinking about the stressor and how it will affect oneself and loved ones. Perception of challenges from the environment within the context of awareness of personal ability occurs constantly, focusing attention and directing behavior, motivating the organism. Approach or avoidance behaviors actually reflect the person's assessment of the valence of the situation and the amount of energy directed to arousal and the subsequent behavior. The person's ability to judge the demands of the environment, to select the stimulus that requires attention and apply skills based on his or her own capabilities, determines the appropriateness of the behavioral and emotional response.

Self-care behaviors are often compromised so that adherence to a prescribed medical regimen decreases. One of the best examples of stress negatively affecting self-care is in diabetes, the most behaviorally demanding of the chronic illnesses. As persons with diabetes redirect their time and attention toward coping with the stressor, they may forget to take their insulin, skip meals or settle for fast food, discontinue their exercise routines, and fail to monitor blood glucose. Within a week, glycemic control is affected, resulting in increasingly negative mood, associated physiological stress responses, and further compromise in self-care (Rubin & Peyrot, 2001). Furthermore, self-destructive behaviors increase in frequency during long-term stress, as people turn to alcohol, cigarettes, and excess consumption of carbohydrates in attempts to improve mood.

Of the health behaviors, the modifying influence of the sleep cycle is often ignored despite the fact that normal sleep is related to efficiency and responsiveness of the HPA axis. Acute sleep loss alters the cortisol secretion profile. Higher cortisol levels compared with normal ones were measured in the evening after sleep deprivation, implying a disruption in the normal feedback regulation system for cortisol (Leproult, Copinschi, Buxton, & Van Cauter, 1997). Those who live in lower socioeconomic neighborhoods are frequently subjected to nighttime traffic noise, which shortens and disrupts sleep. In turn, the sleep–wake cycle strongly influences eating schedules; sleep-deprived children are more prone to overeat, particularly carbohydrates. Serotonin levels in the brain mediate sleep, appetite, and mood, with high-calorie foods increasing serotonin levels more than low-calorie healthy choices (Bear, Connors, & Paradiso, 2001). Obviously, the association among sleep, eating patterns, and stress-related illness is potentially an active area for investigation.

Stress modifies both short- and long-term memory through multiple brain areas, including the hippocampus, amygdala, cingulate cortex, medial prefrontal cortex, and the dorsolateral prefrontal cortex (Bremner & Narayan, 1998). The perception of situations as neutral, positive, or threatening affects short- and long-term memory. Incidents of forgetting increase even during mild short-term stress. Following an argument with a spouse, small bits of information, such as the location of the car keys, are difficult to retrieve. The hippocampus is particularly well supplied with glucocorticoid receptors, which, when constantly stimulated, result in impaired branching of nerve cell dendrites and deficits in memory for facts and events (Sapolsky, 2003). Excessive activation of protein kinase C has been proposed as one of the mediators of stress interference on working memory in the prefrontal cortex (Birnbaum et al., 2004). Some stressful memories are seemingly engraved on a person's brain and are replayed repeatedly over subsequent months and years, with some modifications. Those suffering from posttraumatic stress disorder (PTSD) unconsciously modify the memories of the events up to years afterward. These traumatic memories, although they change over time, remain connected with their emotional valence and sensory accompaniments, to the great distress of those who experienced the traumatic event (Arnsten, 1998). It is increasingly clear, based on animal studies and brain scans of survivors of trauma, that stress-related neuronal damage is real. Changes in neurotransmitter concentration, such as decreased serotonin and decreased volume of the hippocampus, are two examples of the effects of stress on the brain (Bremner, 1999).

The interrelationship between the immune and nervous systems is complex yet critical to understanding maladaptive responses to acute and chronic stress and the benefits of the stress management therapies. The suppression of immune responses is adaptive; however, after the stressor is resolved, prolonged activation of the sympathetic nervous system and the stress hormones and immune suppression become counterproductive (Thayer & Lane, 2000). Negative emotions, such as depressed mood, heightened anxiety, and pervasive worry, have the capacity to up- or down-regulate the release of pro-inflammatory cytokines, markers of chronic inflammation (Kiecolt-Glaser, McGuire, Robles, & Glaser, 2002).

Stress affects the response to immunization more convincingly in the secondary immune response (strong, rapid reaction facilitated by memory cells that recognize the antigen), in contrast to the weak effects on the primary response (weak, short, slower response activated at the first encounter with the antigen; Cohen, Miller, & Rabin, 2001). Specifically, high stress was suggested to reduce the secondary response. The stressors found to be most relevant in this context were high degree of negative affect and chronic personal problems (Cole, Kemeny, Weitzman, Schoen, & Anton, 1999).

Individuals who are socially inhibited demonstrate a predisposition to hyper-responsiveness (greater induration response in delayed-type hypersensitivity to tetanus), which was observed only during specific conditions of social engagement. Stress hormones affect the synthesis and release of the cytokines by leukocytes; acute stress can suppress the responses (virus-specific and T-cell) to hepatitis B vaccine. The poorer responses to vaccines are particularly relevant to older adults (Glaser, Rabin, Chesney, Cohen, & Natelson, 1999). Chronic illness takes a long time to develop, so the question of stability of changes in immune function linked to disease is challenging to study. Cell division takes place at varying rates in different tissues, in addition to differing recovery rates of organ systems after stress. The chronic stress of caring for an ill spouse has provided a useful model for study of long-term stress responses (Kiecolt-Glaser, McGuire, Robles, & Glaser, 2002). Burleson et al. (2003) found consistency for 1 year in immune variables such as leukocyte subsets, total T lymphocytes, and the CD4/CD8 (types of lymphocytes) ratio in middle-aged and older women. In summary, psychological processes influence the immune/brain system in a bidirectional manner in a variable time frame (Kiecolt-Glaser et al., 2002; Maier, Watkins & Fleshner, 1994; Raison & Miller, 2003).

The respiratory system is another target for the deleterious effects of stress. Both sympathetic and parasympathetic fibers innervate the lungs, with bronchodilation resulting from sympathetic stimulation and bronchoconstriction mediated by parasympathetic nerves. During stress, the person may hyperventilate (rapid, shallow breathing), and sympathetic stimulation may be followed by a rebound activation of the parasympathetic system (Lehrer, Song, Feldman, Giardino, & Schamling, 2002). Hyperventilation exposes the system to more total air flow than is necessitated by metabolism, reduces the levels of carbon dioxide (hypocapnia), and increases oxygen concentration. Vasoconstriction of the cerebral blood vessels ensues, setting the stage for numerous physical and affective symptoms, including dizziness, tingling in the limbs, noncardiac chest pain, and affective symptoms such as anxiety, fear, and panic (Gevirtz & Schwartz, 2003). Breathing rate correlates with oscillations in heart rate, called heart rate variability (HRV); slower breathing at about six breaths per minute induces greater variability (Lehrer, 2003). The importance of HRV lies in the influence of variability on other physiological reflexes such as the baroreceptors and the relationship between low variability and illness. In addition, HRV is subject to conditioning and can be increased with training (Lehrer et al., 2003). People with panic disorder have higher heart rates and lower HRV than nonanxious controls (Friedman & Thayer, 1998). In some patients with asthma, specific stress responses, such as embarrassment, can trigger bronchoconstriction. Asthma is a complicated illness characterized by airway obstruction, inflammation, and increased airway responsiveness. Asthma symptoms may be intensified by panic in people with few self-management skills and through stress-induced neuroimmunological pathways. Repeated practice of slow, deep breathing increases HRV and has been suggested to benefit the cardiovascular and respiratory systems, in particular, in patients with asthma and hypertension. In addition, the baroreflex mechanism that underlies normal regulation of blood pressure can be modified with training and practice such that sensitivity and efficiency are improved (Lehrer et al., 2003). Clearly, understanding the psychophysiology of respiration is essential for the practitioner who wishes to apply the stress management therapies appropriately.

The connection between stress and psychophysiology is rarely more evident than in the response of the muscular system to both challenge (positive) and negative events. Athletes train their minds to focus, concentrate, and override painful sensations from their active muscles in order to achieve optimal performance. In contrast, the skeletal muscles are also targets for dysfunction when chronic or severe stress impedes recovery from sustained contraction. Sympathetic activity affects the muscular system by way of neural input to the muscle spindle and hypersensitization of muscle tissue trigger points, resulting in pain (Gevirtz, Hubbard, & Harpin, 1996). Yet central sensitization also contributes to the development of chronic pain. Psychological factors, such as a tendency to view situations as negative and mood and anxiety disorders, affect the perception of pain. Patients with chronic pain reported more pain during voluntary muscle tension, focused more acutely on physical signals, and performed poorly on discrimination tasks (Flor, 2001). Catastrophizing about pain was correlated with missing more days from work and with higher medication use in people with current musculoskeletal pain (Severeijns, Vlaeyen, van den Hout, & Picavet, 2004).

THEORIES OF STRESS

Fundamental to applying the psychophysiological mechanisms of stress is an understanding of the major theories of stress. Although the reader is referred to more comprehensive texts for details, three major theories are summarized here: Selye's general adaptation syndrome (GAS), Lazarus's model based on differential perception of stress, and McEwen's allostasis theory. Underlying the GAS is the concept of stereotyped, physical (largely endocrine) responses to stress that comprise three phases: alarm, adaptation, and exhaustion. A stress-related disease would occur if the system does not adjust or compensate for the stressor. Thus Selye enunciated the link between stress and disease (in fact, death), although his understanding and examples were limited to physical illness. In terms of behavior, Cannon proposed fight, flight, and freeze as stereotyped responses to stress, again emphasizing physiological activity, particularly the mobilization of the muscular system and release of stress hormones from the adrenal medulla (Everly & Lating, 2002). These stress responses are understood to evolve from our animal ancestors and were adaptive within the context of short-term, physical stressors common in lower primates. The animal that can use camouflage and remain motionless increases its chances for survival, as long as the predator does not continue its vigilance for a long time. Instinct drives rabbits to run to successfully escape from a recognized danger, but this response is limited by the amount of energy available. So these early stress theories fostered decades of research and hundreds of scientific papers, yet they were limited to descriptions of nonspecific, physical responses. The individual's capacity to cognitively process an event and withstand long-term, serious stress to emerge relatively unscathed was unexplained.

Lazarus (1984) proposed that perception of stress (which he called *appraisal*) determines whether there is any response or not and then whether there is a positive or negative response. Stress occurs when there is a discrepancy between the expected events and reality. This concept brought psychological factors into the stress model and opened the possibilities for variable responses to the same stressful event. *Reappraisal* refers to the individual's assessment of his or her ability to manage or cope with the stressor. Those who cannot cope maintain arousal longer than those who adapt to new experiences more quickly (Eriksen, Olff, Murison, & Ursin, 1999).

More than three decades ago, Holmes and Rahe (1967) postulated that events in a person's life could be prognostic factors for illness in the future and incorporated major events into the Social Readjustment Scale (SRS). The events were listed with a multiplying factor that indicates the magnitude of adaptation that each event requires. The SRS has been revised and updated (Hobson & Delunas, 2001; Miller & Rahe, 1997), and thus it retains relevance to understanding the effects of accumulated stress on prognosis for disease. Assessment of recent life events was incorporated into the model of threat perception as it correlates with somatization symptoms (Wickramasekera, 1995). Attempts to quantify the impact of these stressors or to develop a linear relationship based on the amount of adaptation necessary to cope with varying degrees of stress have been more challenging.

Allostasis, the optimal operation of regulatory systems, links the central nervous system with the endocrine and immune systems (McEwen & Wingfield, 2003). Brain regions such as the amygdala and hippocampus interpret the surroundings in light of past experience and current psychological state and signal the cortex to organize an appropriate response. Allostatic load develops as a result of wear and tear on the body due to chronic stress or poor recovery, moderated by a mismatch between demand and coping. The distinction between short-term adaptation and long-term distress is clear when conditions of frequent or enduring stress are considered or when the system loses its capacity to return to baseline after the stress is terminated.

McEwen and Lasley (2003) summarize several scenarios regarding responses to stress that are modified by lifestyle factors of varying valence, for example, sleep quality and quantity, diet, smoking, and alcohol. Perceived lack of control over stressful situations increases arousal; the person must always be on guard against potential harm, sometimes resulting in insomnia as the person continues to worry about unresolved problems. Responses to stress protect and, in fact, are critical to survival but can also harm the person, eventually causing death. Frequently, habituation occurs with repeated exposure, but some people continue to react as if they were seeing this particular stressor for the first time (McEwen, 1998). Mental escape techniques, such as imagery or relaxation therapy, can help decrease arousal, but learning is essential to adaptation.

Genetics may have the strongest influence on which specific bodily or psychological systems react (anxiety or depression; hypertension or irritable bowel syndrome). For example, family history of hypertension is an important factor in the recovery of elevated blood pressure after the end of a stress (McEwen & Wingfield, 2003). In some types of situations, such as social conflict, escape is not appropriate or not possible, but the person prepares for escape nonetheless. Instinctive reactions are driven by self-preservation and personal defense, but they can later be at least modified by cognitive processing and learning. Even the knee jerk, a spinal reflex, can be controlled to some extent by higher brain centers.

In summary, chronic stress affects psychological, physiological, cognitive, and behavioral systems. The central nervous system coordinates behavioral and immune responses to stress via CRF either with healthy adaptation or pathological adaptation (maladaptation). An appropriately directed acute response may develop over time into chronic illness, as physical energy supplies are depleted and psychological coping resources become exhausted. Cognitive adaptation fails if the person cannot efficiently process new information or recall information learned in the past.

INDIVIDUAL DIFFERENCES IN RESPONSES TO STRESS

The types of stress that affect humans vary with their age and stage of development (Seymour & Black, 2002). Having considered the biochemical and physiological activities that underlie the acute and chronic stress responses in general terms, it is worthwhile to emphasize some of the differences. In contrast to the stereotyped responses to stress described in the preceding section, person-specific and stress-specific responses to stressful triggers were also proposed. Individual-response stereotypy refers to the consistent physiological responses to most situations that a person encounters, although strength or duration of the response may differ (Andreassi, 1995).

Dickerson and Kemeny (2004) reviewed more than 200 studies of acute stress, including public speaking, noise, and cognitive tasks, with the primary outcome measure being plasma cortisol. It was clear that there are stress-specific responses of varying magnitude and duration. Stress perceived as uncontrollable and performance tasks evaluated by others were associated with the largest response in cortisol, adrenocorticotropic hormone (ACTH, released from the pituitary gland) and the longest time to recovery. This research facilitates our understanding of the effects of acute embarrassment on adolescents, which can continue to influence the adult's thinking for years afterward.

Individuals with similar chronic health problems report widely variable levels of disability, service utilization, and emotional distress resulting from the physical problem. Low socioeconomic status, poor sleep, questionable food choices, lack of exercise, and nonrestorative sleep are examples of behavioral factors that modulate the individual's perception of stimuli and his or her ability to cope. Negative affect is related to physical symptoms, tendency toward somatization, and service utilization (McGrady, Lynch, Nagel, & Wahl, 2003). Patients who were high utilizers of services at a gastroenterology clinic (in the absence of organic disease) were those who had more frequent somatic symptoms, greater psychological distress, and a history of sexual abuse (Bass, Alison, Gill, & Sharpe, 1999). Gender differences in how depression manifests itself are related to types of life stress. Women report more stress-producing events and have different vulnerabilities than men (Sherrill et al., 1997). Women have a higher prevalence of major depressive disorder and phobias and restrict their activities due to illness more than men do.

The experience of anxiety, excessive worry, grief, and depression crosses gender, socioeconomic status, and culture. However, rules that govern display of emotions, recognition of mental illness, and types of suitable providers (physicians, folk healers, counselors, or ministers) exist in all cultures and will affect presentation of symptoms. Depending on the person's culture and ethnicity, depression and anxiety may be conceptualized as biological illness, somatized conflict, or the result of lifestyle or may be labeled as moral problems (Kirmayer, 2001). Immigration to a new country has been studied as a model of adaptation (maladaptation). Whether the person is in fact an immigrant who decided to move or a refugee who was forced to flee determines in large part the difficulty involved in integration into the community. Other important factors are the magnitude of the difference between old culture and new culture, financial resources, and marketable skills, in addition to physical and emotional health. Some immigrants attempt to remain connected with the old world and search for communities where they can do so, such as "Little Italy" or "Chinatown." History of a traumatic event in immigrants' lives increases the risk for psychiatric illness and subsequent utilization of medical resources (Holman, Silver, & Waitzkin, 2000).

How individuals perceive stress and how stress fits into their worldviews influences their physiological and biochemical responses to stress. When a pessimistic view of the world predominates, the person constantly finds evidence that the current situation will have a poor outcome, seeing potential harm everywhere and in everyone. The high-risk model of threat perception (HRMTP) proposed that those with negative affect—a tendency to magnify the negative aspects of a situation—with few compensating buffers (social support and positive coping) were at higher risk for tendency to somatize distress into physical symptoms (Wickramasekera, 1995). The model was initially studied in a psychiatric population; later the predisposing factors of the model were tested in a family practice population (McGrady, Lynch, Nagel, & Zsembik, 1999). Patients with somatoform pain disorder had more chronic physical problems and higher negative affect. In a study of personality factors in patients with chronic pain, extraversion was linked to less disability. Patients with high neuroticism scores and depression had the most blatantly negative health outcomes. Health status comprised disability, utilization, and pain. For somatization and anxiety disorders, severity of depression and higher neuroticism were predictors (Russo et al., 1997).

Individual differences in the effects of stress on the immune system are often observed, as shown in the following example. Grief and depression, two negative emotions, are characterized by differences in natural killer cells and the proliferation response to antigens (Kemeny & Laudenslager, 1999). Some types of stress produce the largest responses, specifically uncontrollable stress and the social evaluative stressors in cases in which one's performance is judged by others (Dickerson & Kemeny, 2004; Kemeny & Laudenslager, 1999). Seventy-two male firefighters were studied using repeated measurements of cortisol and testosterone under varying stress levels in their jobs during 1 year. As daily stress decreased, salivary cortisol increased and testosterone levels decreased. Workers with the highest strain had the lowest levels of cortisol whereas workers with greater ability to make decisions had the highest levels. A pattern of down-regulation of cortisol after increased stress is suggested (Roy, Kirschbaum, & Steptoe, 2003).

Some of the deleterious effects of stress are avoided for short periods of time by defense mechanisms, such as repression. For example, repressors are described as those who have a decreased capacity to attend to and recall negative emotions, instead having preferential memory for positive emotional states. Individuals may avoid dealing with psychological issues or emotional challenges and may demonstrate lack of awareness of feelings and inability to express them. Nonetheless, the autonomic nervous and immune systems respond appropriately, leading to uncoupling of physiology and feelings (Lane, Sechrest, Riedel, Shapiro, & Kaszniak, 2000). In summary, multiple individual and stimulus-specific factors affect the extent and duration of the stress response.

MALADAPTIVE RESPONSES TO STRESS

Posttraumatic Stress Disorder

Two broad categories of responses to trauma comprise hyperarousal and dissociation. Posttraumatic stress disorder (PTSD) exemplifies both of these reactions at different times. Recreating and reexperiencing the original traumatic event challenges the system, increasing over time the sensitivity of the individual to situations reminiscent of the initial event (Sadock & Sadock, 2003). Normal psychophysiological reactions to acute and chronic stress are modified after trauma. Repeated activation of the HPA pathways can cause sensitization and exaggerated responses to even mild stressors (Perry & Pollard, 1998; Perry, Pollard, Blakley, Baker, & Vigilante 1995). Noradrenergically mediated hyperarousal responses are more commonly observed in adolescents and men, in contrast to the opioid, vagally mediated dissociation responses seen in younger children and women (Perry, 2002). Memory for traumatic events is very vivid, and the most difficult life experiences are recalled in great detail. Stimulation of the noradrenergic system enhances memory for emotional material, whereas less recall is associated with blockade of the noradrenergic system (O'Carroll, Drysdale, Cahill, Shajahan, & Ebmeier, 1999). The dissociative response numbs the pain experience temporarily, but symptoms frequently evolve into chronic headaches, back pain, or gastrointestinal distress. PTSD has effects similar to rapid aging, affecting physiology, mood, and behavior and decreasing the capacity for learning (Bremner & Narayan, 1998).

Chronic stress in infants alters the normal stress response in such a way that, as adults, these people appear unconcerned about daily hassles or major life events. In fact, their physiological response, as well as their emotional response, to stress has been numbed (Peeters, Nicholson, & Berkhof, 2003). The derealization, reminiscent of the "freeze" pattern of responses in lower animals, creates an internal world in which the abused feels safer. The person wishes that time could be turned back to before the trauma occurred. "I stood there frozen. Some part of me believed that if I didn't move, I could just hold my place, like a bookmark, so that someone could open time and move back to the pages he had missed, perhaps to put the book down again and forget to go on to the part where the world shattered" (Prince-Hughes, 2004, p. 14).

Some poorly forgotten memories are of situations that were so stressful that they are overconsolidated; therefore, they continue to perturb the internal environment. The effects of such memories, unconscious or conscious, constantly affect the way in which the person reacts to particular stimuli. Reactions take place without insight or understanding and affect the person's responses to other illnesses. For example, history of trauma (broadly defined) during childhood and adulthood compromised the ability of male patients to manage their pain (Spertus, Burns, Beth, Lofland, & Lance, 1999). Similarly, clinicians frequently observe the delayed and more complicated recovery from even a minor automobile accident in patients with a history of past trauma.

Cardiovascular Disease

The etiology of cardiovascular disease is complex, comprising genetic, physical, and psychosocial factors that includes excessive stress reactivity, reduced heart rate variability, unhealthy behaviors (e.g., smoking), depression, and anxiety. The type A behavior pattern, particularly hostility, in addition to high life stress and poor social networks, increases the risk for acute cardiovascular events and long-term coronary artery disease (Manuck, Kaplan, & Matthews, 1986; Tennant, 1999). Reduced heart rate variability and higher heart rates over a range of severity in depressed persons are mediated by altered autonomic function, a relative paucity of parasympathetic activity, and more adrenergic activity. The glucocorticoid arm of the stress response is also relevant to the function of the cardiovascular system, affecting the arterial baroreceptor reflex control system in a way that is partially independent of changes in arterial blood pressure (Scheuer & Mifflin, 2001).

Increased risk for mortality in depressed patients can be partially explained by autonomic dysregulation, although health maintenance behaviors are also compromised in severe depression (Stein et al., 2000). Patients who have difficulty motivating themselves to take care of their basic responsibilities have little energy for exercise and for planning low-fat meals. The lack of motivation inherent in depression prevents exercise and social interaction, which might in other circumstances buffer the effects of disease (Wulsin & Singal, 2003).The link between symptoms of depression and reduced heart rate variability was also seen in physically healthy individuals exposed to acute stress in the laboratory. It is suggested that altered responses in depressed persons are not the result of already present cardiac disease but are, in fact, an independent biochemical effect of depression (Hughes & Stoney, 2000).

A review of 10 studies highlights the link between coronary disease and depression. Although there are more than 200 risk factors for heart disease, depression acts as an independent risk factor, conferring greater risk than passive smoking but less than active smoking. The increased cardiac morbidity and mortality in depressed patients must account for the observation that, in depression, increased serotonin mediated platelet activation, hyperactive platelet 5-HT_{2A} receptor signaling, magnifies the risk for thromboembolic events (Schins, Honig, Crijns, Baur, & Hamulyak, 2003).

As was discussed previously, acute stress may produce withdrawal behaviors in an attempt to decrease the impact of stress instead of the classic activation of the system. A diphasic response may occur, beginning with sympathetic arousal and followed by parasympathetic dominance, leading to decreases in blood pressure and heart rate. Syncope may result if adequate levels of blood pressure are not maintained. Medically unexplained syncope is strongly linked to psychiatric illness (Linzer et al., 1992). Psychiatric causes of syncope include anxiety, somatoform disorders, and PTSD (McGrady & McGinnis, 2005). Depression has been related to lower systolic blood pressure, particularly in women with a positive tilt table test for neurocardiogenic syncope (McGrady, Kern-Buell, Bush, Khuder, & Grubb, 2001). An extreme form of stress response (withdrawal) is sudden death due to cardiac arrest (Samuels, 1997). This reaction is called "voodoo death" because it occurs during extreme fright with underlying mechanisms of ventricular arrhythmia and sympathetic overactivity with catecholamine toxicity.

The Metabolic Syndrome: Essential Hypertension, Type 2 Diabetes, Hyperlipidemia, and Obesity

Development of the metabolic syndrome has been correlated with repeated activation of the HPA axis and the sympathetic nervous system (hypothalamic arousal syndrome) in genetically at-risk persons. Repeated stress increases the tendency to develop insulin resistance, central obesity, essential hypertension, and dyslipidemia. The environmental factors most likely to perturb the normal feedback system during stress are depressive and anxious traits, alcohol consumption, and smoking (Björntorp et al., 1999, 2000).

The relationship between activation of the stress response and the risk for the metabolic syndrome is mediated by CRF, by locus ceruleus–norepinephrine autonomic systems, by the HPA axis, and by peripheral effectors (Chrousos, 2000.) When the stressor is presented, the stimulus is put into the context of past experience, the availability of social support is considered, and arousal occurs. For example, a married couple experiences situations that lead to disagreement and hostility; over time the negative feeling between the husband and wife has detrimental effects on health, including elevated blood pressure, in addition to the previously discussed immune dysfunction (Kiecolt-Glaser et al., 1993). The CARDIA study explored psychosocial risk factors in the incidence of hypertension in young, healthy adults (Yan et al., 2003). In a substudy of CARDIA, two measurements of job strain and blood pressure were taken 8 years apart. Those workers who had little control over everyday job demands and a high level of responsibility were more likely to develop high blood pressure (Markovitz, Matthews, Whooley, Lewis, & Greenlund, 2004). Borderline hypertension and sustained elevated blood pressure both exemplify autonomic imbalance as the central etiological component. Additional maladaptive pathways of excess sympathetic activity and decreased parasympathetic tone develop into type 2 diabetes mellitus, arrhythmia, thrombosis, and arterial vessel hypertrophy (Brook & Julius, 2000).

Cortisol concentration and variability in daily secretion patterns were tested in an attempt to ascertain the pathways responsible for the development of the metabolic syndrome. Stress-related cortisol secretion was strongly related to obesity factors, such as cholesterol and low-density lipoprotein, as well as blood pressure and deposition of fat in the abdominal region. In seriously overweight people, morning cortisol levels are low, and the diurnal variation is blunted. Therefore, relationships can be demonstrated among the endocrine and hemodynamic systems when cortisol regulation is disrupted such that variability is low and normal suppression of cortisol by the experimental agent dexamethasone is lowered (Rosmond, Dallman, & Björntorp, 1998). Increased cortisol stimulates appetite and decreases serotonin, reminiscent of the need for extra energy in response to physical stress. Stress also contributes to obesity in behavioral ways, in that eating is not motivated by physiological need for calories but driven by need for comfort, warmth, and consolation.

Depression

An abnormally functioning HPA axis, high cortisol, and disruption of normal endocrine rhythms are characteristic of depressive illness (Raison & Miller, 2003). About half of patients with depression do not show the expected suppression of cortisol secretion response to dexamethasone, which may be relevant to the choice of antidepressants in treatment (Pariante & Miller, 2001). The physical symptoms of poor sleep and loss of appetite are controlled by the hypothalamus–pituitary axis and neuronal serotonin (Morin, Rodrigue, & Ivers, 2003). Sleep problems predict later depression, but the lack of deep sleep also seems to magnify sensory experience, particularly pain. Poor sleepers overreact to minor stressors and perceive their lives as more stressful than those who have restorative sleep, even though both groups report equal numbers of stressful circumstances. Noise and light awakens poor sleepers more easily, and they report more sensitivity to pain. A vicious cycle ensues, in which poor sleep increases sensitivity and hyperarousal makes it harder for the person to fall asleep.

There is clear evidence that depression has many physiological manifestations besides those that are part of the diagnostic interview. Cardiac autonomic imbalance is manifested by decreased HRV in depressed patients (Nahshoni et al., 2004). Early trauma in women with and without current diagnosed depression affected their responses to a mild stressor such as public speaking (Heim et al., 2000). In major depressive disorder, cortisol does not always increase in response to negative events; actually, some individuals demonstrate a blunted response, more evident in people with a family history of mood disorders (Peeters et al., 2003). In that case, recovery from stress may be indicated by increased cortisol responses, as was shown in a group of people who meditated regularly (MacLean et al., 1997).

If a person lacks words to describe feelings (alexithymia), his or her vocabulary for communicating distress consists of physical symptoms. Somatization of feelings into stomachache or migraine is likely to occur. In addition, severity of depression was associated with alexithymia (Bankier, Aigner, & Bach, 2001). Although alexithymia is thought to be a stable trait, Honkalampi, Hintikka, Laukkanen, Lehtonen, and Viinamäki (2001) found that it is inconsistent when the state is part of major depressive disorder and thus may be the target of psychotherapy.

Activity in the hippocampus, which contains corticosteroid receptors, has the capacity to inhibit many aspects of HPA activity, including the onset and termination of stress responses (Jacobson & Sapolsky, 1991). Altered declarative memory in major depressive disorder has been suggested to be due to alternations in glucocorticoid receptor signaling in the hippocampus (Bremner et al., 2004). The relationship between depression and arthritis exemplifies the links between psychological responses to stress and immune dysregulation. Common pathways involving signaling by peripheral cytokines and activation of stress-related hormones and neurohormones may mediate disorders that are manifested by both emotional and inflammatory dysregulation (Sternberg, Chrousos, Wilder, & Gold, 1992).

Anxiety Disorders

Anxiety is experienced as simultaneous physiological responses of tachycardia, hyperventilation, and sweating and the emotional experience of intense arousal, derealization, and difficulty concentrating (Sadock & Sadock, 2003). In children, anxious emotion is observed as crying, tantrums, or freezing or clinging responses to feared though sometimes neutral stimuli without the realization that the fears are unreasonable. Although the adult is aware that the same fear is not realistic, the reactions continue to be disturbing. Anxiety may overlap with mood disorders, manifested in agitation, sleep disturbances, fatigue, restlessness, and irritability (Roy-Byrne, 1997). When coping capacity is exhausted, the person may feel hopeless and depressed emotionally; at the same time, the ability of the HPA axis to respond through normal feedback mechanisms is also altered (Olff, 1999).

Thayer and Lane (2000) proposed that anxiety reactions result from faulty disinhibition associated with dysregulated attention, defensive responses, and sustained alertness. Neutral stimuli are perceived as stressful, and the defenses fail to identify safety zones and nonthreatening situations and people. Clinical anxiety, anxious alarm, and sustained apprehension are the emotional manifestations of neuronal hypersensitivity (Barlow, 1988). However, the increase in arousal and chronic worry coexists with lower heart rate variability, indicating decreased inhibition by the parasympathetic system. Reduced autonomic flexibility is implicated as a major factor in chronic anxiety, whereas the normally functioning person exhibits reactivity, flexibility, and resiliency in response to arousal-producing situations (Friedman & Thayer, 1998). The association between anxiety and disease is more convincing for the less serious illnesses, such as colds and flu. The interrelationship among psychological factors and serious diseases is more variable, perhaps due to the complexities involved in the etiology and progression of cancer and AIDS (Cohen & Herbert, 1996).

PROTECTION AGAINST THE EFFECTS OF STRESS

Emotional dysregulation may lead to psychopathology and stress-related physical disorders as seemingly diverse as generalized anxiety disorder, essential hypertension, major depressive disorder, and coronary heart disease. In contrast, personal direction, goal setting, being passionate about an activity, and having a sense of purpose allow the person to ignore the rapid heart rate, labored breathing, and the tightened gut, sometimes transforming stress responses into fulfillment of one's life's passion.

Many stress buffers decrease the effects of stress on physiological and psychological states. Some examples are social support, positive coping, optimism, prayer, exercise, and the acquired techniques discussed later in this book. Some of the stress-buffering methods must be learned, whereas hardiness or resiliency seems to be mainly inborn. Exercise has the potential to buffer the potential negative consequences of low social support and depression (psychosocial risk) in patients who recently suffered heart attacks. In a large trial of ethnically diverse men and women (the ENRICH trial), those with varying degrees of depression showed similar exercise-related survival benefits. It was suggested that regular physical aerobic exercise functions as an antidepressant, as evidenced by decreased scores on the Beck Depression Inventory after 6 months of exercise (Blumenthal et al., 2004).

Coping is defined as a cognitive process that results in a reduced secretion of adrenal glucocorticoid during what is expected to be a stressful situation. Persons gain control of their environment as healthy defenses are mobilized, followed by stress-specific behaviors. Because the brain retains some capacity to replace neurons or to expand the dendritic tree, learning new behaviors and adaptation occur despite old age (McEwen, 2003b). According to Ray (2004), four categories of coping skills—knowledge, inner resources, social support and spirituality—mediate the direction of mental effects on the body, that is, toward health or illness. Higher levels of active coping were correlated with a greater proliferation response to stimulation with experimental mitogens, a healthy immune response (Stowell, Kiecolt-Glaser, & Glaser, 2001). The presence of familiar partners and significant social relationships assists coping, in contrast to the influence of critical evaluators of one's performance (Levine, 1993). Stress in a group has less potent effects than in situations that must be confronted alone, as indicated by the severe psychological effects of solitary confinement. Greater frequency of experience of positive emotion is linked to a decreased number of incidents of the common cold (Cohen, Doyle, Turner, Alper, & Skoner, 2003). Even as severe a stressor as abuse in childhood is not necessarily irreversible in adulthood because loving relationships in later life may decrease the burden of traumatic memories and lessen allostatic load and the risk of illness (McEwen, 2003c).

Social support is a multidimensional construct; support may be familial or emotional in nature (Uchino, Cacioppo, & Kiecolt-Glaser, 1996). Higher quantities and better quality of social support was correlated with higher natural killer cell activity and stronger proliferation responses to stimulation by mitogens (Kiecolt-Glaser, McGuire, Robles, & Glaser, 2002). Persons who are hardy or resilient despite socioeconomic disadvantage may still have relatively low allostatic load because positive social relationships may serve as buffers to the negative effects of low income and poor education (Singer & Ryff,

1999). The power of protection by social relationships was tested by Bloor, Uchino, Hicks, and Smith (2004), who had participants recall and speak about relationships. Women demonstrated more cardiovascular reactivity to recalling and speaking about negative relationships than men did. It should be noted that cognitive representations of relationships are available in memory and can constitute a pathway through which social relationships affect health. Remembering and writing about feelings (journaling) related to stressful experiences decreases the consequences of the stress response, particularly with regard to physical illness (Pennebaker, Kiecolt-Glaser, & Glaser, 1988).

In the normative aging study of male veterans, optimism was associated with better mental health and lower levels of pain; in contrast, depression was correlated with lower levels of functioning over all SF-36 (quality of life) domains (Achat, Kawachi, Spiro, DeMolles, & Sparrow, 2000). Optimism can also buffer the effects of acute stress on the immune system (Cohen et al., 1999). The combination of social support and positive coping decreased the tendency toward frequent physical symptoms, as measured by the PRIME-MD, a short screening questionnaire designed for use in primary care. Individuals who had high scores on total social support and who rarely used avoidance coping had fewer office visits in a primary care setting (McGrady et al., 2003).

The effects of stress are also buffered by attendance at church, such that regular church attendees recover more quickly from physical illness (Koenig, 1997). However, religion also has the potential of interfering with positive coping. Religious struggle increased the risk of death in elderly ill men when they acknowledged thoughts of abandonment by God or attribution of the illness to the devil (Pargament, Koenig, Tarakeshwar, & Hahn, 2001). Nonetheless, although the mechanisms underlying the effects of religious practice on health are unknown, social support, positive imagery, relaxation, and optimism may all contribute to the beneficial effects.

SUMMARY

This chapter describes aspects of the stress response that are fundamental to applying stress management interventions to physical and emotional illness. A developmental framework was utilized, because many stressors that occur in childhood and adolescence have long-term repercussions in adulthood and old age. Knowledge of the mechanisms by which the brain is transformed as a result of stress can be applied to the choice of treatment. The clinician must understand the stress response and its physiological and psychological ramifications in order to match the most effective therapy to the patient and his or her illness. Similarly to the individual differences in the stress response, diversity in reactions to stress management is more the norm than the exception. Thus the practitioner requires an exhaustive knowledge of the different types of relaxation techniques and the applicability to specific illnesses. Patients' reactions to stress may seem stereotyped and unchanging, giving credence in this century to Selye's theories of the past century, yet many people are desirous and capable of reversing their course in life. Despite genetic influences that increase risk, people can learn to appraise stressful situations in a different way and can increase their utilization of stress buffers. Within the context of a psychotherapeutic relationship, a disastrous past can evolve into a stable present and a successful future. New ideas and experience, using techniques discussed in this book, have the potential to change the brain, using neurophysiological pathways similar to those that react to stress. The different psychopharmacological and psychotherapeutic modalities alter functioning of specific brain sites. Each therapy discussed in this book is based on some aspect of the stress responses described in this chapter, further matched to its major target organ. For some, mechanisms and supporting empirical evidence are strong, whereas others have less evidence. However, similarly to the explosion of knowledge about neurotransmitters in the brain, drug effects at the molecular level, and genetic underpinnings of disease, the research on the mechanisms of the therapies discussed in this book will grow at an exponential pace.

REFERENCES

Achat, H., Kawachi, I., Spiro, A., DeMolles, D. A., & Sparrow, D. (2000). Optimism and depression as predictors of physical and mental health functioning: The normative aging study. *Annals of Behavioral Medicine, 22,* 127–130.

Arnsten, A. (1998). The biology of being frazzled. *Science, 280*(5370), 1711–1712.

Andreassi, J. L. (1995). Concepts in psychophysiology. In J. L. Andreassi (Ed.), *Psychophysiology: Human behavior and physiological response* (3rd ed., pp. 336–349). Hillsdale, NJ: Erlbaum.

Bankier, B., Aigner, M., & Bach, M. (2001). Alexithymia in DSM-IV disorder. *Psychosomatics, 42,* 235–240.

Barlow, D. H. (1988). *Anxiety and its disorders.* New York: Guilford Press.

Bass, C., Alison, B., Gill, D., & Sharpe, M. (1999). Frequent attenders without organic disease in a gastroenterology clinic: Patient characteristics and health care use. *General Hospital Psychiatry, 21,* 30–38.

Bear, M. F., Connors, B. W., & Paradiso, M. A. (Eds.). (2001). *Neuroscience: Exploring the brain* (2nd ed.). Baltimore: Lippincott Williams & Wilkins.

Birnbaum, S. G., Yaun, P. X., Wang, M., Vijayraghavan, S., Bloom, A. K., Davis, D. J., et al. (2004). Proteinkinase cover activity impairs prefrontal cortical regulation of working memory. *Science, 306,* 882–884.

Björntop, P., Holm, G., & Rosmond, R. (1999). Hypothalamic arousal, insulin resistance and type 2 diabetes mellitus. *Diabetic Medicine, 16,* 373–383.

Björntop, P., Holm, G., & Rosmond, R. (2000). Metabolic diseases: The hypothalamic arousal syndrome. In D. I. Mostofsky & D. H. Barlow (Eds.), *The management of stress and anxiety in medical disorders* (pp. 282–289). Boston: Allyn & Bacon.

Bloor, L. E., Uchino, B. N., Hicks, A., & Smith, T. W. (2004). Social relationships and physiological function: The effects of recalling social relationships on cardiovascular reactivity. *Annals of Behavioral Medicine, 28,* 29–38.

Blumenthal, J. A., Babyak, M. A., Carney, R. M., Huber, M., Saab, P. G., Burg, M. M., et al. (2004). Exercise, depression, and mortality after myocardial infarction in the ENRICHD trial. *Medicine and Science in Sports & Exercise, 36,* 746–755.

Bremner, J. D. (1999). Does stress damage the brain? *Biological Psychiatry, 45,* 797–805.

Bremner, J. D., & Narayan, M. (1998). The effects of stress on memory and the hippocampus throughout the life cycle: Implications for childhood development and aging. *Development and Psychopathology, 4,* 871–885.

Bremner, J. D., Vythilingam, M., Vermetten, E., Anderson, G., Newcomer, J. W., & Charney, D. S. (2004). Effects of glucocorticoids on declarative memory function in major depression. *Biological Psychiatry, 55,* 811–815.

Brook, R. D., & Julius, S. (2000). Autonomic imbalance, hypertension, and cardiovascular risk. *American Journal of Hypertension, 13,* 112–122.

Burleson, M. H., Poehlmann, K. M., Hawkley, L. C., Ernst, J. M., Berntson, G. G., Malarkey, W. B., et al. (2003). Neuroendocrine and cardiovascular reactivity to stress in mid-aged and older women: Long-term temporal consistency of individual differences. *Psychophysiology, 40,* 358–369.

Cacioppo, J. T. (1994). Social neuroscience: Autonomic, neuroendocrine, and immune responses to stress. *Psychophysiology, 31,* 113–128.

Cacioppo, J. T., Burleson, M. H., Poehlmann, K. M., Malarkey, W. B., Kiecolt-Glaser, J. K., Berntson, G. G., et al. (2000). Autonomic and neuroendocrine responses to mild psychological stressors: Effects of chronic stress on older women. *Annals of Behavioral Medicine, 22,* 140–148.

Caspi, A., Sugden, K., Mofitt, T., Taylor, A., Craig, I. W., Harrington, H., et al. (2003). Influence of life stress on depression: Moderation by a polymorphism in the 5-HTT gene. *Science, 301,* 386–389.

Chrousos, G. P. (2000). The role of stress and the hypothalamic–pituitary–adrenal axis in the pathogenesis of the metabolic syndrome: Neuro-endocrine and target tissue-related causes. *International Journal of Obesity and Related Metabolic Disorders, 24,* S50–S55.

Ciechanowski, P. S., Walker, E. A., Katon, W. J., & Russo, J. E. (2002). Attachment theory: A model for health care utilization and somatization. *Psychosomatic Medicine, 64,* 660–667.

Cohen, F., Kearney, K. A., Zegans, L. S., Kemeny, M. E., Neuhaus, J. M., & Stites, D. P. (1999). Differential immune system changes with acute and persistent stress for optimists vs. pessimists. *Brain Behavior and Immunity, 13,* 155–174.

Cohen, S., Doyle, W. J., Turner, R. B., Alper, C. M., & Skoner, D. P. (2003). Emotional style and susceptibility to the common cold. *Psychosomatic Medicine, 65,* 652–657.

Cohen, S., & Herbert, T. B. (1996). Health psychology: Psychological factors and physical disease from the perspective of human psychoneuroimmunology. *Annual Review of Psychology, 47,* 113–142.

Cohen, S., Miller, G. E., & Rabin, B. S. (2001). Psychological stress and antibody response to immunization. *Psychosomatic Medicine, 63,* 7–18.

Cole, S. W., Kemeny, M. E., Weitzman, O. B., Schoen, M., & Anton, P. A. (1999). Socially inhibited individuals show heightened DTH response during intense social engagement. *Brain Behavior and Immunity, 13,* 187–200.

Dantzer, R. (2001). Can we understand the brain and coping without considering the immune system? In D. M. Broom (Ed.), *Coping with challenge: Welfare in animals including humans* (Vol. 7, pp. 102–110). Berlin, Germany: Dahlem University Press.

Dickerson, S. S., & Kemeny, M. E. (2004). Acute stressors and cortisol responses: A theoretical integration and synthesis of laboratory research. *Psychological Bulletin, 130,* 355–391.

Eriksen, H. R. A., Olff, M., Murison, R., & Ursin, H. (1999). The time dimension in stress responses: Relevance for survival and health. *Psychiatry Research, 85,* 39–50.

Everly, G., Jr., & Lating, J. (2002). The link from stress arousal to disease. In *A clinical guide to the treatment of the human stress response* (2nd ed., pp. 49–61). New York: Kluwer Academic/Plenum Press.

Flor, H. (2001). Psychophysiological assessment of the patient with chronic pain. In D. C. Turk & R. Melzack (Eds.), *Handbook of pain assessment* (2nd ed., pp. 76–96). New York. Guilford Press.

Friedman, B. H., & Thayer, J. F. (1998). Anxiety and autonomic flexibility: A cardiovascular approach. *Biological Psychology, 47,* 243–263.

Gevirtz, R. N., Hubbard, D., & Harpin, E. (1996). Psychophysiologic treatment of chronic low back pain. *Professional Psychology: Research and Practice, 27*(6), 561–566.

Gevirtz, R. N., & Schwartz, M. S. (2003). The respiratory system in applied psychophysiology. In M. S. Schwartz & F. Andrasik (Eds.), *Biofeedback: A practitioner's guide* (3rd ed., pp. 212–244). New York: Guilford Press.

Glaser, R., Rabin, B., Chesney, M., Cohen, S., & Natelson, B. (1999). Stress-induced immunomodulation implications for infectious diseases? *Journal of the American Medical Association, 281,* 2268–2270.

Heim, C., Newport, D. J., Heit, S., Graham, Y., Wilcox, M., Bonsall, R., et al. (2000). Pituitary–adrenal and autonomic responses to stress in women after sexual and physical abuse in childhood. *Journal of the American Medical Association, 284,* 592–597.

Hobson, C. J., & Delunas, L. (2001). National norms and life-event frequencies for the revised Social Readjustment Rating Scale. *International Journal of Stress Management, 8,* 299–314.

Holman, E. A., Silver, R. C., & Waitzkin, H. (2000). Traumatic life events in primary care patients. *Archives of Family Medicine, 9,* 802–810.

Holmes, T. H., & Rahe, R. H. (1967). The social readjustment rating scale. *Journal of Psychosomatic Research, 11,* 213–218.

Honkalampi, K., Hintikka, J., Laukkanen, E., Lehtonen, J., & Viinamäki, H. (2001). Alexithymia and depression: A prospective study of patients with major depressive disorder. *Psychosomatics, 42,* 229–234.

Hughes, J. W., & Stoney, C. M. (2000). Depressed mood is related to high-frequency heart rate variability during stressors. *Psychosomatic Medicine, 62,* 796–803.

Jacobson, L., & Sapolsky, R. (1991). The role of the hippocampus in feedback regulation of the hypothalamic–pituitary–adrenocortical axis. *Endocrine Reviews, 12,* 118–134.

Kemeny, M. E., & Laudenslager, M. L. (1999). Beyond stress: The role of individual difference factors in psychoneuroimmunology. *Brain, Behavior, and Immunity, 13,* 73–75.

Kendler, K. S., Hettema, J. M., Butera, F., Gardner, C. O., & Prescott, C. A. (2003). Life event dimensions of loss, humiliation, entrapment, and danger in the prediction of onsets of major depression and generalized anxiety. *Archives of General Psychiatry, 60,* 789–796.

Kiecolt-Glaser, J. K., Malarkey, W. B., Chee, M., Newton, T., Cacioppo, J. T., Mao, H. et al. (1993). Negative behavior during marital conflict is associated with immunological down-regulation. *Psychosomatic Medicine, 55,* 395–409.

Kiecolt-Glaser, J. K., McGuire, L., Robles, T. F., & Glaser, R. (2002). Psychoneuroimmunology: Psychological influences on immune function and health. *Journal of Consulting and Clinical Psychology, 70,* 537–547.

Kirmayer, L. J. (2001). Cultural variations in the clinical presentation of depression and anxiety: Implications for diagnosis and treatment. *Journal of Clinical Psychiatry, 62*(Suppl. 13), 22–28.

Koeing, H. G. (1997). *Is religion good for your health? The effects of religion on physical and mental health.* New York: Hayworth Pastoral Press.

Lane, R., Sechrest, L., Riedel, R., Shapiro, D., & Kaszniak, A. (2000). Pervasive emotion recognition deficit common to alexithymia and the repressive coping style. *Psychosomatic Medicine, 62,* 492–501.

Lazarus, R. S. (1984). On the primacy of cognition. *American Psychologist, 39,* 124–129.

Lehrer, P. (2003). Applied psychophysiology: Beyond the boundaries of biofeedback (Mending a wall, a brief history of our field, and applications to control of the muscles and cardiorespiratory systems). In F. Andrasik (Ed.), *Applied Psychophysiology and biofeedback* (Vol. 28, pp. 291–304). New York: Kluwer Academic/Plenum Press.

Lehrer, P., Song, H.-S., Feldman, J., Giardino, N., & Schmaling, K. (2002). Psychological aspects of asthma. *Journal of Consulting and Clinical Psychology, 70,* 691–711.

Lehrer, P. M., Vaschillo, E., Vaschillo, B., Lu, S.-E., Eckberg, D. L., Edelberg, R., et al. (2003). Heart rate variability biofeedback increases baroreflex gain and peak expiratory flow. *Psychosomatic Medicine, 65,* 796–805.

Leproult, R., Copinschi, G., Buxton, O., & Van Cauter, E. (1997). Sleep loss results in an elevation of cortisol levels the next evening. *Sleep, 20,* 865–870.

Levine, S. (1993). The influence of social factors on the response to stress. *Psychotherapy and Psychosomatics, 60,* 33–38.

Linzer, M., Varia, I., Pontinen, M., Divine, G. W., Grubb, B. P., & Estes, N. A. M., III. (1992). Medically unexplained syncope: Relationship to psychiatric illness. *American Journal of Medicine, 92*(Suppl. 1A), 18S–25S.

MacLean, C. R. K., Walton, K. G., Wenneberg, S. R., Livitsky, D. K., Mandarino, J. P., Waziri, R., et al. (1997). Effects of the transcendental meditation program on adaptive mechanisms: Changes in hormone levels and responses to stress after 4 months of practice. *Psychoneuroendocrinology, 22,* 277–295.

Maier, S. F., Watkins, L. R., & Fleshner, M. (1994). Psychoneuroimmunology: The interface between behavior, brain, and immunity. *American Psychologist, 49,* 1004–1017.

Manuck, S. B., Kaplan, J. R., & Matthews, K. A. (1986). Behavioral antecedents of coronary heart disease and atherosclerosis. *Arteriosclerosis, 6,* 2–14.

Markovitz, J. H., Matthews, K. A., Whooley, M., Lewis, C. E., & Greenlund, K. J. (2004). Increases in job strain are associated with incident hypertension in the CARDIA study. *Annals of Behavioral Medicine, 28,* 4–9.

McCauley, J., Kern, D. E., Kolodner, K., Dill, L., Schroeder, A. F., DeChant, H. K., et al. (1997). Clinical characteristics of women with a history of childhood abuse: Unhealed wounds. *Journal of the American Medical Association, 277,* 1362–1368.

McEwen, B., & Lasley, E. N. (2003). Allostatic load: When protection gives way to damage. *Advances, 19,* 28–33.

McEwen, B. S. (1998). Protective and damaging effects of stress mediators. *New England Journal of Medicine, 338,* 171–179.

McEwen, B. S. (2003a). Early life influences on life-long patterns of behavior and health. *Mental Retardation and Developmental Disabilities Research Reviews, 9,* 149–154.

McEwen, B. S. (2003b). Interacting mediators of allostasis and allostatic load: Towards an understanding of resilience in aging. *Metabolism, 52,* 10–16.

McEwen, B. S. (2003c). Mood disorders and medical illness: Mood disorders and allostatic load. *Biological Psychiatry*, *54*, 200–207.

McEwen, B. S., & Wingfield, J. C. (2003). The concept of allostasis in biology and biomedicine. *Hormones and Behavior*, *43*, 2–15.

McGrady, A., Kern-Buell, C., Bush, E., Khuder, S., & Grubb, B. P. (2001). Psychological and physiological factors associated with tilt table testing for neurally mediated syncopal syndromes. *Pacing and Clinical Electrophysiology*, *24*(3), 296–301.

McGrady, A., Lynch, D., Nagel, R., & Wahl, E. (2003). Application of the high-risk model of threat perception to medical illness and service utilization in a family practice. *Journal of Nervous and Mental Disease*, *191*, 255–259.

McGrady, A., Lynch, D., Nagel, R., & Zsembik, C. (1999). Application of the high-risk model of threat perception for a primary care patient population. *Journal of Nervous and Mental Disease*, *187*, 369–375.

McGrady, A., & McGinnis, R. (2005). Psychiatric disorders in patients with syncope. In B. Grubb & B. Olshansky (Eds.), *Syncope: Mechanisms and management* (2nd ed., pp. 214–224). Malden, MA: Blackwell Futura.

Miller, G. E., Cohen, S., & Ritchey, A. K. (2002). Chronic psychological stress and the regulation of pro-inflammatory cytokines: A glucocorticoid-resistance model. *Health Psychology*, *21*, 531–541.

Miller, M. A., & Rahe, R. H. (1997). Life changes scaling for the 1990s. *Journal of Psychosomatic Research*, *43*, 279–292.

Morin, C., Rodrigue, S., & Ivers, H. (2003). Role of stress, arousal, and coping skills in primary insomnia. *Psychosomatic Medicine*, *65*, 259–267.

Morris, J. A. B., Blount, R. L., Brown, R. T., & Campbell, R. M. (2001). Association of parental psychological and behavioral factors and children's syncope. *Journal of Consulting and Clinical Psychology*, *5*, 851–857.

Nahshoni, E., Aravot, D., Aizenberg, D., Sigler, M., Zalsman, G., Strasberg, B., et al. (2004). Heart rate variability in patients with major depression. *Psychosomatics*, *45*, 129–134.

O'Carroll, R. E., Drysdale, E., Cahill, L., Shajahan, P., & Ebmeier, K. P. (1999). Stimulation of the noradrenergic system enhances and blockade reduces memory for emotional material in man. *Psychological Medicine*, *29*, 1083–1088.

Olff, M. (1999). Stress, depression and immunity: The role of defense and coping styles. *Psychiatry Research*, *85*, 2.

Pargament, K. I., Koenig, H. G., Tarakeshwar, M. A., & Hahn, J. (2001). Religious struggle as a predictor of mortality among medically ill elderly patients. *Archives of Internal Medicine*, *161*, 1881–1885.

Pariante, C., & Miller, A. (2001). Glucocorticoid receptors in major depression: Relevance to pathophysiology and treatment. *Biological Psychiatry*, *49*, 391–404.

Peeters, F., Nicholson, N., & Berkhof, J. (2003). Cortisol response to daily events in major depressive disorder. *Psychosomatic Medicine*, *65*, 836–841.

Pennebaker, J. W., Kiecolt-Glaser, J. K., & Glaser, R. (1988). Disclosure of traumas and immune function: Health implication for psychotherapy. *Journal of Consulting and Clinical Psychology*, *56*(2), 239–245.

Perry, B. (2002). Childhood experience and the expression of genetic potential: What childhood neglect tells us about nature and nurture. *Brain and Mind 3*, 79–100.

Perry, B., & Pollard, R. (1998). Homeostasis, stress, trauma, and adaptation: A neurodevelopmental view of childhood trauma. *Child and Adolescent Psychiatric Clinics of North America*, *7*(1), 33–51.

Perry, B., Pollard, R., Blakley, T., Baker, W., & Vigilante, D. (1995). Childhood trauma, the neurobiology of adaptation, and "use-dependent" development of the brain: How "states" become "traits." *Infant Mental Health Journal*, *16*(4), 271–291.

Porges, S. W. (1992). Vagal tone: A physiologic marker of stress vulnerability. *Pediatrics*, *9*(3) 498–504.

Porges, S. W., Doussard-Roosevelt, J. A., Portales, A. L., & Greenspan, S. I. (1996). Infant regulation of the vagal "brake" predicts child behavior problems: A psychobiological model of social behavior. *Developmental Psychobiology*, *29*, 697–712.

Porges, S. W., Doussard-Roosevelt, J. A., & Maiti, A. K. (1996). Vagal tone and the physiological regulation of emotion. *Monographs of the Society for Research in Child Development*, *39*, 167–186.

Prince-Hughes, D. (2004). *Songs of the gorilla nation: My journey through autism.* New York: Harmony Books.

Raison, C., & Miller, A. (2003). When not enough is too much: The role of insufficient glucocorticoid signaling in the path physiology of stress-related disorders. *Psychiatry, 160,* 1554–1565.

Ray, O. (2004). How the mind hurts and heals the body. *American Psychologist, 59*(1), 29–40.

Rosmond, R., Bouchard, C., & Björntorp, P. (2002). A C-1291G polymorphism in the a_{2A}-adrenergic receptor gene (ADRA2A) promoter is associated with cortisol escape from dexamethasone and elevated glucose levels. *Journal of Internal Medicine, 251,* 252–257.

Rosmond, R., Dallman, M. F., & Björntorp, P. (1998). Stress-related cortisol secretion in men: Relationships with abdominal obesity and endocrine, metabolic and hemodynamic abnormalities. *Journal of Clinical Endocrinology and Metabolism, 83*(6), 1853–1859.

Roy, M., Kirschbaum, C., & Steptoe, A. (2003). Intraindividual variation in recent stress exposure as a moderator of cortisol and testosterone levels. *Annals of Behavioral Medicine, 26*(3), 194–200.

Roy-Byrne, J. (1997). Generalized anxiety disorder in primary care: The precursor/modifier pathway. *Journal of Clinical Psychiatry, 58*(3), 34–38.

Rubin, R. R., & Peyrot, M. (2001). Psychological issues and treatments for people with diabetes. *Journal of Clinical Psychology, 57,* 457–478.

Russo, J., Katon, W., Lin, E., Korff, V., Bush, T., Simon, G., et al. (1997). Neuroticism and extraversion as predictors of health outcomes in depressed primary care patients. *Psychosomatics, 38,* 339–348.

Sadock, B. J., & Sadock, V. A. (2003). Anxiety Disorders. In *Synopsis of psychiatry* (9th ed.). Philadelphia: Lippincott Williams & Wilkins.

Samuels, M. A. (1997). "Voodoo" death revisited: The modern lesions of neurocardiology. *Neurologist, 3,* 293–304.

Sapolsky, R. M. (2003). Stress and plasticity in the limbic system. *Neurochemical Research, 28,* 1735–1742.

Schins, A., Honig, A., Crijns, H., Baur, L., & Hamulyak, K. (2003). Increased coronary events in depressed cardiovascular patients: 5-HT$_{2A}$ receptor as missing link? *Psychosomatic Medicine, 65,* 729–737.

Scheuer, D. A., & Mifflin, S. W. (2001). Glucocorticoids modulate baroreflex control of renal sympathetic nerve activity. *American Journal of Physiology: Regulatory, Integrative and Comparative Physiology, 280,* R1440–1449.

Schore, A. N. (2002). Dysregulation of the right brain: A fundamental mechanism of traumatic attachment and the psychopathogenesis of posttraumatic stress disorder. *Australian and New Zealand Journal of Psychiatry, 36,* 9–30.

Severeijns, R., Vlaeyen, J. W. S., van den Hout, M. A., & Picavet, J. S. J. (2004). Pain catastrophizing is associated with health indices in musculoskeletal pain: A cross-sectional study in the Dutch community. *Health Psychology, 23,* 49–57.

Seymour, D. J., & Black, K. (2002). Stress in primary care patients. In F. V. DeGruy III, W. P. Dickinson, & E. W. Staton (Eds.), *Twenty common problems in behavioral health* (pp. 65–88). New York: McGraw-Hill.

Sherrill, J. T., Anderson, B., Frank, E., Reynolds, C. F., Tu, X. M., Patterson, D., et al. (1997). Is life stress more likely to provoke depressive episodes in women than in men? *Depression and Anxiety, 6,* 95–105.

Singer, B., & Ryff, C. D. (1999). Hierarchies of life histories and associated health risks. *Annals of the New York Academy of Sciences, 896,* 96–115.

Spertus, I. L., Burns, J., Beth, G., Lofland, K., & Lance, M. (1999). Gender differences in associations between trauma history and adjustment among chronic pain patients. *Pain, 82,* 97–102.

Stein, P. K., Carney, R. M., Freeland, K. E., Skala, J. A., Jaffe, A. S., Kleiger, R. E., et al. (2000). Severe depression is associated with markedly reduced heart rate variability in patients with stable coronary heart disease. *Journal of Psychosomatic Research, 48,* 493–500.

Sternberg, E. M., Chrousos, G. P., Wilder, R. L., & Gold, P. W. (1992). The stress response and the regulation of inflammatory disease. *Annals of Internal Medicine, 117,* 854–866.

Stowell, J. R., Kiecolt-Glaser, J. K., & Glaser, R. (2001). Perceived stress and cellular immunity: When coping counts. *Journal of Behavioral Medicine, 24,* 323–339.

Tennant, C. (1999). Life stress, social support and coronary heart disease. *Australian and New Zealand Journal of Psychiatry, 33,* 636–641.

Thayer, J., & Lane, R. (2000). A model of neurovisceral integration in emotion regulation and dysregulation. *Affective Disorders Journal, 61,* 201–216.

Uchino, B. N., Cacioppo, J. T., & Kiecolt-Glaser, J. K. (1996). The relationship between social support and physiological processes: A review with emphasis on underlying mechanisms and implications for health. *Psychological Bulletin, 119,* 488–531.

Wickramasekera, I. (1995). Somatization: Concepts, data, and predictions from the high-risk model of threat perception. *Journal of Nervous and Mental Disease, 183,* 15–23.

Wright, R. J., Cohen, S., Carey, V., Weiss, S. T., & Gold, D. R. (2002). Parental stress as a predictor of wheezing in infancy: A prospective birth-cohort study. *American Journal of Respiratory and Critical Care Medicine, 165,* 358–365.

Wrosch, C., Schulz, R., & Heckhausen, J. (2002). Health stresses and depressive symptomatology in the elderly: The importance of health engagement control strategies. *Health Psychology, 21*(4), 340–348.

Wulsin, L. R., & Singal, B. M. (2003). Do depressive symptoms increase the risk for the onset of coronary disease? A systematic quantitative review. *Psychosomatic Medicine, 65,* 201–210.

Yan, L. L., Liu, K., Matthews, K. A., Daviglus, M. L., Ferguson, T. F., & Kiefe, C. I. (2003). Psychosocial factors and risk of hypertension: The Coronary Artery Risk Development in Young Adults (CARDIA) study. *Journal of the American Medical Association, 290,* 2138–2148.

CHAPTER 3

The Psychology of Relaxation

JONATHAN C. SMITH

People relax in many ways and for many reasons. One might take a walk to enjoy nature, listen to music for pleasure, or contemplate sacred scriptures for spiritual comfort. Our concern is with formal and passive relaxation exercises that involve a degree of withdrawal—for example, yoga, progressive muscle relaxation, and meditation. Such techniques have been the subject of thousands of empirical studies and are perhaps the most popular tools in stress management. But what is relaxation and how does it work?

For over a century, neurophysiological perspectives have dominated the field. As early as 1853 James Braid defined hypnosis, a forerunner to some contemporary approaches to relaxation, as "neuro-hypnotism" (sleep of the nerves). In the 20th century, Jacobson (1938) and Schultz (1932) introduced progressive muscle relaxation and autogenic training as methods for moderating neuromuscular and autonomic processes. In the 1970s Benson (1975) popularized the "relaxation response" as the global physiological process underlying all approaches to professional relaxation. Today, concepts of nonspecific or specific arousal reduction continue to dominate the profession.

Neurophysiological models of relaxation have served us well and continue to form the primary justification for relaxation training in most stress management programs. These models are persuasive and easy to explain to practitioners. Research consistently finds reduced arousal to be associated with a wide range of health and performance outcomes. Arousal models have lifted techniques from the darkness of religion, pseudoscience, and the occult to genuine professional credibility.

However, an exclusive emphasis on neurophysiology risks missing something important. Most practitioners of relaxation appear to master arousal-reducing skills in a month or so; yet many go on to practice for years and decades (Smith, 1990). Often masters of meditation and yoga claim to progress deeper in their practice even after a lifetime of practice. Clearly, such individuals are discovering something more than reduced heart rate.

As is apparent in this volume, psychological theory forms the basis of other forms of stress management. Learning theory underlies desensitization. Cognitive psychology provides the foundation for cognitive therapy, stress inoculation training, and exposure treatments. Constructs from social psychology are central to anger management and conflict resolution. The list goes on. In contrast, relaxation has been viewed more similarly to exercise, diet, or psychopharmacology, defined by what happens in the body. But are the experiences of a lifelong meditator in any way analogous to the experiences of a lifelong consumer of vegetables? How much do we really learn by comparing prayer to Prozac or Mozart to a marathon run? For practitioners of relaxation, more is going on than can be measured in the body or brain.

Two decades ago (Smith, 1985, 1986), I proposed the beginnings of what I now call psychological relaxation theory (Smith, 2005). In this chapter, I introduce the latest version of this theory, review a sampling of empirical studies, and offer a psychologically based approach to teaching relaxation.

R-STATES AND RELAXATION

Psychological relaxation theory begins with a simple question remarkably few trainers or researchers ask: What do you experience when you relax? If you ask students of progressive muscle relaxation, yoga stretching, breathing exercises, autogenic training imagery, meditation, or mindfulness, you will quickly encounter a rich and diverse rainbow of positive psychological states. Some feel "peaceful" or "rested." Others feel "sleepy" and "far away," or even "energized" and "joyful." And practitioners of strictly secular approaches may have deeply spiritual feelings. Such reports are not of passing consequence, akin to an occasional itch or giggle. They point to the very heart and soul of relaxation.

My first step in developing psychological relaxation theory was to systematically identify and map the positive psychological states associated with relaxation, or, as I prefer, "R-States" (relaxation states). I started with an exhaustive catalog of 400 words used in more than 200 core textbooks on progressive muscle relaxation, autogenic training, yoga, breathing exercises, imagery, creative visualization, tai chi, self-hypnosis, meditation, contemplation, and prayer. Nine published factor analytic studies, involving 6,077 participants and more than 40 relaxation techniques and activities, currently point to at least 12 basic R-States (Smith, 1999, 2001a, 2005):

1. Accepting
2. At Ease/Peaceful (Mentally Relaxed)
3. Aware/Focused/Clear
4. Disengaged (feeling distant, indifferent, far away)
5. Joyful
6. Mystery (experiencing the "deep mystery" of things)
7. Optimistic
8. Physically Relaxed
9. Quiet (mind still, without thought)
10. Reverent/Prayerful
11. Sleepy
12. Timeless/Boundless/Infinite/At One

These words can be seen as the beginnings of a basic lexicon or universal "natural language" of psychological relaxation. But how should they be organized? What underlying processes do they reflect? My current thinking is that they reflect four categories of relaxation experience: *basic relaxation*, *core mindfulness*, *positive energy*, and *transcendence*.

Basic Relaxation

Popular models of relaxation focus on reduced neurophysiological arousal. Four R-States make up an analogous category of reduced psychological arousal or Basic Relaxation: Sleepy, Disengaged, Physically Relaxed, and At Ease/Peaceful. Note that each depicts one aspect of reduced psychological tension, which may or may not have neurophysiological correlates. For example, one might experience intense peacefulness after resolving a fight. Such peace may well manifest as considerable brain activity while being experienced as reduced psychological tension.

Core Mindfulness

Mindfulness meditation is currently the most widely researched approach to relaxation. My own PsycINFO search for 2001–2007 found 388 studies citing mindfulness topping all forms of relaxation, including: meditation other than mindfulness or transcendental meditation (292 citations), massage (201), hypnosis for relaxation/stress management (110), biofeedback for relaxation/stress management (109), visualization/imagery for relaxation/stress management (104), progressive muscle relaxation/progressive relaxation (83), autogenic training (78), tai chi/qigong/tao yin (77), music and relaxation (73) breathing exercises/diaphragmatic breathing (43) transcendental meditation (39), saunas/hot tubs/baths (28), acupuncture for relaxation (20), yoga stretching/Hatha, (10), prayer for stress management/relaxation (7), laughter/humor therapy (7), art therapy for relaxation (6), herbal supplements/vitamins and relaxation (2) relaxation flotation (sensory deprivation) tanks (1), aromatherapy (1), Benson's meditation (1), and clinically standardized meditation (0).

Typically, *mindfulness* is defined as sustained focus, an absence of elaborative thought, and nonjudgmental acceptance (Bishop et al., 2004). These dimensions appear similar to the R-States of Aware/Focused/Clear, Quiet, and Accepting.

Positive Energy

Substantial research links positive affect with health and longevity (Pressman & Cohen, 2005). Most studies have focused on "happiness" and "optimism," corresponding to the R-States of Joyful and Optimistic. Together they suggest a core relaxation dimension of positive energy. Broadly defined, positive energy may include a rainbow of highly correlated states, including beauty, harmony, happiness, and mirth, among others

Transcendence

R-State Reverent/Prayerful, Mystery, as well as Timeless/Boundless/Infinite/At One, clearly are spiritual states in which one experiences something that cannot be put into words and is larger or greater than oneself. The experience of transcendence does not require belief in a theistic God and can emerge in those moments of relaxation when one quietly confronts the beauty and grandeur of the universe.

I have organized these R-States into a "window of renewal" (See Figure 3.1). This schema includes additional hypothesized R-States of Rested/Refreshed (basic relaxation), Energized (positive energy), Thankful/Loving (positive energy), Innocent (core mindfulness), Centering (core mindfulness), Awakening (core mindfulness), and Awe and Wonder (transcendence). Although these R-States have yet to emerge as separate factors in published research, I have found them to have considerable clinical utility.

TRANSCENDENCE	
Timeless / Boundless / Infinite / At One Mystery Reverent / Prayerful Awe and Wonder*	

CORE MINDFULNESS	POSITIVE ENERGY
Quiet Aware / Focused / Clear Accepting Innocent* Centering* Awakening*	Joyful Optimistic Energized* Thankful/Loving*

BASIC RELAXATION	
At Ease / Peaceful(Mentally Relaxed) Physically Relaxed Disengaged ("Far Away, Indifferent") Sleepy Rested / Refreshed*	

*, hypothesized R-States.

Note. Over the years, my listing of R-States has varied slightly depending on which inclusion criteria I deployed. The present listing is based on published factor analytic research. All R-States are assessed by the Smith Relaxation States Inventory–3 (SRSI-3) available at *www.lulu.com/stress.*

FIGURE 3.1. The window of renewal: categories of relaxation states (R-States). Copyright 2007 by Jonathan C. Smith. Reprinted by permission.

The Value of R-States

What good are R-States? First, I propose that R-States are powerful reinforcers for starting and maintaining relaxation practice. By explaining, measuring, and discussing R-States, one sensitizes clients to potential rewards of continued practice. Second, R-States may be central to positive relaxation outcomes as society often discounts R-States as distractions from true productivity, as laziness, as a needless indulgence to be enjoyed only after work, or at best as good feelings that are as inconsequential as a passing memory of a good meal. Positive psychology has shown clearly that positive states have a direct impact on health, immune system functioning, and even longevity. Perhaps the most important task of a relaxation trainer is to persuade a client that R-States are not trivial and passing moods but a fundamental and powerful part of all relaxation.

R-States help clients articulate their relaxation goals and integrate relaxation with the rest of life. If relaxation is simply viewed as physical stress relief, then it is little more than a nap. One practices a technique and returns to work. By considering the full rainbow of R-States, clients can consider the value of relaxation for goals beyond stress relief and ways of integrating relaxation with activities and concerns beyond the practice session. Let me elaborate.

Psychological relaxation theory proposes four groups of potential relaxation goals: negative goals (enhancing sleep, managing stress, enhancing the healing process), positive–practical goals (enhancing health and energy; calm, directed action; productivity, and effectiveness), positive–expressive goals (spontaneous enjoyment, creativity, and insight), and transcendent goals (god-based spirituality, meditation, and mindfulness). This formulation was derived through numerous factor analytic studies (Smith, 2001c, 2005).

Our R-State window of renewal (Figure 3.1) sheds light on how various relaxation goals can be approached. When clients and trainees are given a full range of techniques, the paths they discover are typically highly individualized and show remarkable creativity. One program of mindfulness may combine meditation, yoga, and imagery, and focus on R-States Disengaged, Aware/Focused/Clear, Quiet, and Accepting. A hypertension client may desire R-States Physically Relaxed, At Ease/Peaceful, and Accepting, and fashion a program of progressive muscle relaxation, breathing exercises, and imagery. A harried student may create a rest break exercise of yoga and autogenic training that targets R-States Joyful, Optimistic, and Quiet. A religious group may consider prayerful imagery and breathing exercises as a path to R-States Reverent/Prayerful, Optimistic, and Mystery. An insomniac may blend progressive muscle relaxation and autogenic training for R-States Disengaged and Sleepy. When one considers the psychology of relaxation, the possibilities are endless.

THE SIX FAMILIES OF RELAXATION

Many health professionals sort the myriad of existing relaxation techniques into more or less six groups: yoga stretching, progressive muscle relaxation, breathing exercises, autogenic training, imagery/positive self-statements, and meditation/mindfulness. I propose that this differentiation is no accident but an inevitable consequence of the very nature of psychological and physiological processes that underlie stress arousal (Smith, 2005). According to psychological relaxation theory, we can trigger and sustain psychological and physiological stress arousal through six forms of *self-stressing*, elaborated below. Each form of self-stressing suggests a corresponding family of relaxation techniques:

- *Stressed posture and position.* When confronted with stress, people often assume a variety of defensive or aggressive postures or positions (standing, crouching, bending over a desk) for an extended time. This, combined with sustained immobility, can evoke skeletal muscle tension, joint stress, and reduced blood flow and contribute to tension, fatigue, and decreased energy.
- *Stressed skeletal muscles.* When threatened, one clenches, grips, and tightens skeletal muscles to prepare for attack or escape. When chronic, such tension can contribute to pain and fatigue.
- *Stressed breathing.* Under stress one is more likely to breathe in a way that is shallow, uneven, and rapid, deploying greater use of the intercostal (ribcage) and trapezius (shoulder) muscles and less use of the diaphragm. Hyperventilation is a second form of stressed breathing in which inhalation and exhalation is excessively rapid and deep.
- *Stressed body focus.* Simply attending to and evoking thoughts and images about a specific body part or process can evoke related neurophysiological changes. An individual facing a threat may notice her rapidly beating heart or churning stomach. Attending to and thinking about these somatic reactions can aggravate them.
- *Stressed emotion.* We often motivate and energize ourselves for a stressful encounter with affect-arousing cognitions. We entertain fantasies and repeat words and self-statements that can evoke anxiety, anger, or depression.
- *Stressed attention.* When dealing with a threat, we actively and effortfully concentrate on attacking, defending, or running. In addition, we often direct our attention to multiple targets, including competing tasks (as in multitasking), a targeted task versus worried preoccupation, or self-stressing efforts (thinking about how one is breathing,

TABLE 3.1. Relaxation Access Skills and Relaxation Families

Initial Self-Stressing Target	Family of Relaxation Technique
Stressed posture and position	Stretching (Hatha yoga)
Stressed muscles	Progressive muscle relaxation
Stressed breathing	Breathing exercises
Stressed body focus	Autogenic training
Stressed emotion	Imagery/positive self-talk
Stressed attention	Meditation/mindfulness

maintaining a stressed posture or position, thinking about related fantasies or negative emotions, etc.) rather than the task at hand.

Self-stressing specificity theory suggests that the hundreds of passive relaxation techniques now available can be organized into six general family groups, each targeting as its initial and defining effect a parallel category of self-stressing. For example, yoga stretching initially targets stressed joints, progressive muscle relaxation works for striated muscle tension, breathing exercises reduce stress-related breathing symptoms, and so on. It should be emphasized that the parallel targeted effect may be temporary and initial; in time, exercises have an impact on other forms of self-stressing. Whereas progressive muscle relaxation may initially result in reduced muscle tension, it may later affect breathing and emotional stress. Also, numerous combination approaches blend family groups. For example, tai chi may combine slow stretching, breathing, meditation, and imagery. What is often presented as mindfulness meditation is actually a mix of mindfulness, breathing, and yoga stretching. Yoga programs frequently combine just about every approach (see Table 3.1).

OTHER FEATURES OF PSYCHOLOGICAL RELAXATION THEORY

One chapter cannot describe all the features of psychological relaxation theory. I list here six additional elements and invite the reader to explore elsewhere (Smith, 2005):

1. R-Beliefs (relaxation beliefs) are personal philosophies and spiritual perspectives hypothesized to enhance the practice of relaxation. They include Deeper Perspective, Belief in God, and Belief in Inner Wisdom. These were derived through numerous factor analytic studies (Mui, 2001).
2. R-Attitudes are negative attitudes toward relaxation that can interfere with practice. Examples include fears about disengagement, relaxation-induced anxiety, the possibility of losing control, having an unqualified trainer, and religious or hypnotic control. These were derived through factor analytic research (Smith, 2001b).
3. R-Dispositions reflect the enduring propensity to report R-States.
4. R-Motivations reflect the desire to experience more (or less) of an R-State.
5. IRCs (idiosyncratic reality claims) are irrational/paranormal/supernatural beliefs that may enhance certain R-States. The list includes literal Christianity; magic (astrology, crystals, new age beliefs, etc.); communication with the dead; miraculous powers of meditation, prayer, and belief; and space aliens. These were derived through factor analysis (Smith, 2001a; Smith & Karmin, 2002).
6. N-states (negative states) are aversive distracting thoughts, feelings, or sensations that can emerge in relaxation and that are paradoxically associated with the practice of relaxation.

RESEARCH

When relaxation techniques are viewed in terms of physiological variables, relatively few differences emerge. However, in dramatic contrast, every single study that has compared R-States has found significant, consistent, and dramatic differences among techniques (Table 3.2). In this section I present a sample of studies that have deployed the Smith Relaxation States Inventory–3 (SRSI-3; Smith, 2007), which includes basic R-States, as well as various exploratory R-States, including Rested/Refreshed, Awe and Wonder, Thankful/Loving, and Energized.

Gender, Ethnic, and Racial Differences

Males, females, and individuals from various cultural groups report different patterns of R-States, especially during what they describe as their "preferred and most effective" form of casual self-relaxation. Males report basic relaxation, whereas females are more likely to report positive energy, especially the hypothesized R-State Thankful/Loving. Dramatically, African American females report the largest number and widest range of R-States, including Disengaged, Physically Relaxed, Energized and Aware (combined), At Ease/Peaceful, Quiet, Joyful, Thankful/Loving, Reverent, and Timeless, Boundless/Infinite/At One (Bowers, Darner, Goldner, & Sohnle, 2001; McDuffie, 2001; Smith, McDuffie, Ritchie, & Holmes, 2001).

Personality Correlates of R-States

The personality correlates of R-States are complex. We focus on three fundamental R-States that appear to be particularly intriguing: Disengaged, At Ease/Peaceful, and Energized (in early research, combined with Aware/Focused/Clear).

Disengaged

Perhaps one of the most important fruits of R-State research has been the discovery of the R-State Disengaged. In factor analysis, the core of Disengaged is defined by three dimensions: spatial, attitudinal, and somatic. Each reflects withdrawal from and reduced

---

TABLE 3.2. Published Research on psychological relaxation theory (1996–2004)

Anderson (2001)	Rice, Cucci, & Williams (2001)
Bang (1999)	Ritchie, Holmes, & Allen (2001)
Bowers, Darner, Goldner, & Sohnle (2001)	Smith (1986)
Gaff (2001)	Smith (2001c)
Gonzales (2001)	Smith (2001d)
Ghonchec, Byers, Sparks, & Wasik (2001)	Smith, Amutio, Anderson, & Aria (1996)
Ghonchec & Smith (2004)	Smith, Goc, & Kinzer, (2001)
Gillani & Smith (2001)	Smith & Karmin (2002)
Hughes (2001)	Smith & Jackson (2001)
Khasky & Smith (1999)	Smith & Joyce (2004)
Leslie & Clavin (2001)	Smith, McDuffie, Ritchie, & Holmes (2001)
Lewis(2001a)	Smith & Sohnle (2001)
Lewis (2001b)	Smith et al. (2000)
Matsumoto & Smith (2001)	Sohnle (2001)
McDuffie (2001)	Sonobe (2001)

awareness of the world. Terms such as feeling "distant," "far away," and "in my own world" are primarily spatial. In contrast, statements such as feeling "detached," "indifferent," "not caring about anything," "unmoved," or "unbothered" represent an attitude of withdrawal. As relaxation progresses, one may display a type of disengagement in which one becomes less aware of one's limbs and parts of one's body. A client may realize that he or she has lost awareness of hands, arms, legs, or feet. More dramatically, one may have an "out of body experience" in which one feels as though, or actually hallucinates, floating above and observing one's physical body. Clinically, one might view R-State Disengaged at least in part as low-level, potentially adaptive dissociation.

I summarize some of the many correlates of the disengaged state, and then offer some interpretation. Disengaged correlates negatively with the Sixteen Personality Factor (16PF) factors of emotional stability and positively with vigilance, abstractedness, apprehension, and anxiety (Leslie & Clavin, 2001). On the Millon Index of Personality Styles, it correlates positively with persevering, accommodating, introversing, hesitating, dissenting, and complaining (Sohnle, 2001). On the Symptom Checklist–90—Revised, Disengaged correlates positively and highly with all scales of psychopathology except paranoid ideation (Anderson, 2001).

This and other research suggests that Disengagement (like Sleepiness) is a fundamental R-State. Possibly those under distress are most likely to conceptualize effective relaxation as simply "getting away from it all," "tuning out," or becoming "indifferent," all of which are defining descriptors of Disengaged. In addition, Disengaged appears to be one of the first R-States that emerge in relaxation training, especially progressive muscle relaxation, and it may be a prerequisite to becoming successfully Physically Relaxed. To relax the body, one must first learn to disengage from the stressors of the world. Progressive muscle relaxation (and, I hypothesize, rudimentary autogenic standard exercises) may well be among the most effective tools for becoming Disengaged. Yoga stretching and Breathing exercises appear less likely to evoke R-State Disengaged (Ghonchec & Smith, 2004; Matsumoto & Smith, 2001) and perhaps less effective at evoking deep muscle relaxation.

At Ease/Peaceful and Energized and Aware

At Ease/Peaceful is perhaps the one R-State most people think of when they define what relaxation means to them (the exception is individuals under extreme duress or suffering from psychopathology, who tend to think of relaxation in terms of R-State Disengaged. The items that load on factor At Ease/Peaceful help us understand the nature of this construct: "at ease, calm, carefree, contented, laid back, peaceful, relaxed, soothed." Dictionary definitions connote an absence or resolution of tension ("calm, relaxed"), conflict ("peaceful"), worry ("carefree"), desire and frustration ("contented"), pain ("soothed"), or effort ("at ease, laid back"). In sum, such terms reflect a basic psychological experience of release of and recovery from sources of tension manifested as an alleviation of conflict, worry, desire, pain, and effort. R-State Energized and Aware (combined) is additionally defined by terms such as "strengthened," "confident," "aware," "focused," "clear," and "awake." Generally, I see Energized and Aware as related to self-efficacy.

Both At Ease/Peaceful and Energized and Aware appear to be associated with health status, including fewer reported illnesses and less somatic stress (Gaff, 2001), a greater propensity to report active coping and planning (Sonobe, 2001), and claimed enhancements in general health (Smith, 2001c).

Relaxation Treatments and Activities

One of the most consistent findings of R-State research has been that relaxation techniques differ. Progressive muscle relaxation is initially associated with R-States Disengaged and Physically Relaxed, whereas both yoga stretching and breathing exercises are more associated with Energized and Aware (Ritchie, Holmes, & Allen, 2001; Rice, Cucci, & Williams, 2001; Smith & Jackson, 2001; Ghonchec & Smith, 2004; Matsumoto & Smith, 2001; Boukydis, 2004).

Ghonchec and Smith (2004), Matusmoto and Smith (2001), and Boukydis (2004) have used a promising new design for evaluating techniques. These researchers assigned participants to one of two approaches. Ghonchec and Smith (2004) compared progressive muscle relaxation and yoga stretching whereas Boukydis (2004) and Smith and Matsumoto (2001) looked at progressive muscle relaxation and breathing exercises. Participants practiced their assigned technique once a week for 5 weeks in a supervised group setting, using standardized matched 28-minute recordings (Smith, 2005, Smith, 1999). Samples were diverse. Matsumoto and Smith (2001) examined college undergraduates; Ghonchec and Smith (2004) used banking employees; and Boukydis (2004) used a clinical sample of outpatients who had been in therapy for an average of 6 years for anxiety and depression.

R-States were assessed before and after each session. At weeks 1 and 5, R-State "aftereffects" were assessed. An aftereffect (Smith, 1999) is a relaxation state that emerges after a 3-minute pause at the end of training and after an initial posttest. During the intervening 3 minutes, participants are instructed to casually think about the forthcoming day and week's activities. All studies found that PMR consistently evokes R-States Physically Relaxed and (except for Boukydis, 2004) Disengaged. Interestingly, for all studies, some effects took 4 or 5 weeks to emerge and did not show up on an immediate posttest but as an aftereffect 3 minutes after posttesting. For example, both Ghonchec and Smith (2004) and Matsumoto and Smith (2001) found that R-States Quiet and Joyful emerge as an aftereffect.

Little research has examined the impact of combining relaxation techniques. Two cross-cultural studies on senior citizens provide some intriguing leads. Bang (1999) examined relaxation scripting on 22 non-English-speaking Korean American nursing home residents. Half were assigned to a no-treatment control group and half received the "relaxation scripting" strategy described later in this chapter. Specifically, scripting participants were taught a different technique each day for 6 days (progressive muscle relaxation, autogenic training, breathing, yoga, imagery, and meditation). On the seventh day a group combination script was constructed incorporating exercise components that participants voted to include. The group script was then practiced for the remaining 14 days. Gonzales (2001) repeated this design on 24 senior citizens in Rio Piedras, Puerto Rico. Both studies found significantly reduced Beck Depression Inventory scores and increased scores on R-States Sleepy, Disengaged, and Physically Relaxed. In addition, Bang (1999) found increased scores on R-States Joyful and Thankful/Loving whereas Gonzales (2001) found higher levels of Quiet, Rested/Refreshed, and At Ease/Peaceful. Both studies report a larger number of R-State effects than any other R-State study yet conducted. Of course, this may be the result of variables other than the combination treatment (such as daily practice over a 2-week period; a sample consisting of seniors; use of a non-Western culture). More research is needed.

Additional technique studies are worthy of brief note. Gillani and Smith (2001) found that advanced Zen meditators report higher levels of Quiet, Thankful/Loving, and Reverent/Prayerful. Smith and Joyce (2004) compared the relaxing impact of Mozart's music, new age music, and reading popular magazines. Individuals who selected and listened to Mozart's "Eine Kleine Nachtmusik" reported higher levels of Quiet, Awe and Wonder, and Mystery. Both Mozart listeners and listeners to new age music (Halpern's "Serenity Suite") reported higher levels of At Ease/Peaceful and Rested/Refreshed, and Thankful/Loving, suggesting that these R-States may come from a general relaxing effect of music.

TRAINING IMPLICATIONS

What are the implications of psychological relaxation theory for training and practice? The finding that different approaches to relaxation have different effects should prompt trainers of all approaches to take a new look at what they are doing and pay attention to what their trainees say about their experience of relaxation.

Training options should be considered with care and targeted to client strengths, needs, and interests. However, training specificity is meaningful only the extent to which the procedural components of various approaches can be differentiated. For example, it makes little sense to contrast the effects of hatha yoga, progressive muscle relaxation, mindfulness, and breathing exercises when all of these approaches incorporate breathing exercises. Of all approaches, hatha yoga is perhaps the most difficult to research, given that it often incorporates not only breathing exercises but also meditation, letting go (a variant of progressive muscle relaxation), imagery, and an occasional autogenic suggestion. Thus I find it virtually impossible to interpret nearly all studies on yoga.

Of course, no global family is a pure representation of any one access skill. This leads to the central practical hypothesis of psychological relaxation theory:

> *Different approaches to relaxation evoke different patterns of R-States. Relaxation training that deploys multiple techniques will cultivate a greater range of R-States and contribute to greater treatment compliance, effectiveness, and generalization beyond the practice session.*

Combination Formats

Careful examination of what master trainers of relaxation actually do (as opposed to what they say they do) reveals a preference for combining approaches. Many forms of progressive muscle relaxation blend letting go with an occasional quick stretch, often paced with inhaling and releasing breath, incorporated with some imagery ("imagine a tight wad of string slowly unwinding") and physically targeted suggestions ("Let the tension melt away . . . "). Traditional hatha yoga is a rich mixture of stretching, breathing, physically targeted suggestion, and, often, letting go. Autogenic standard exercises deploy physically targeted suggestion and passive breathing exercises. More advanced autogenic exercises introduce imagery. And all approaches to relaxation incorporate a bit of targeted and sustained "meditative" focus (Smith, 2005).

Although expert trainers may combine approaches, often they do so without a clear rationale. A good example of this is the preference among many well-known meditation and mindfulness instructors for preparatory stretching or breathing exercises. Why not use progressive muscle relaxation as a preparation? Indeed, our research (Ghonchec & Smith, 2004; Matsumoto & Smith, 2001) has found that progressive muscle relaxation (and not stretching or breathing) can evoke R-State Quiet, which is strongly associated with the practice of meditation (Gillani & Smith, 2001). Indeed, Jacobson (1938) himself described his approach as a neuromuscular method for reducing worry or, as meditators prefer, "distracting thought." Devotees of various schools of meditation or mindfulness may bristle at any deviation from millennia of "time-tested" tradition. However, we need to be mindful that such tradition often reflects the popularity of charismatic "masters" (and their favorite techniques), the endurance of pseudoscientific beliefs (and associated relaxation exercises), religious dogma, and unsystematic and careless trial and error. There are no substitutes for rigorous research.

How I Teach Relaxation

Although I have devised a number of relaxation training protocols (Smith, 1985, 1990, 1999, 2005, 2006), all have three important elements in common.

1. I prefer to teach techniques from several families of relaxation.
2. I initially emphasize relatively "pure" versions of techniques so that clients can differentiate and identify the unique effects of a technique family. For example, when teaching progressive muscle relaxation, I do not draw attention to breathing ("Let go as you breathe out") or imagination ("Image tension unwinding like a tight ball of string"). Thus clients can identify the unique R-States associated with tensing up and letting go.
3. Only after teaching several families of relaxation do I combine families of relaxation into an individualized program. For example, it is at this stage that imagery and breathing might be incorporated with progressive muscle relaxation.

Some additional differences between my approach to specific families of relaxation and traditional training methods can be noted:

• *Yoga form stretching.* As mentioned earlier, I emphasize simple stretching that can be accomplished safely with little supervision. Most traditional hatha yoga exercises require professional supervision, and some are associated with risk of injury.

• *Progressive muscle relaxation.* I teach both a more active version similar to what is popular today and a version similar to Jacobson's relatively passive strategy.

• *Breathing exercises.* I teach three approaches: bowing and breathing, active diaphragmatic exercises ("place your hands on your abdomen and press in as you breathe out"), and passive breath-flow exercises ("breathe out through your lips").

• *Autogenic training.* I focus on only four standard suggestions: heaviness, warmth, calmly beating heart, and abdominal warmth. The remaining breathing and forehead-cooling exercises are redundant with exercises presented elsewhere (breathing, meditation). Also, I present two versions of beginning autogenic exercises: verbal and visual. Verbal exercises rely on the passive repetition of suggestive words (*warm* and *heavy*). Visual exercises rely on simple images suggestive of somatic change ("warm sun on hands, heavy sand pulling hands down").

• *Imagery.* In initial training, I devote considerable time to helping clients construct an individualized imagery sequence. We first sample a range of images from four themes (travel, nature/outdoor, water, indoor). Once an image is selected, it is checked for possible negative associations and revised. Then possible sense details are considered (what you see, hear, feel, smell). The client is then instructed to engage in self-directed imagery based on the theme and details selected. Note that during the first half of imagery training, the training is directive, with the trainer providing all the details for sample themes. During the last half of training, the trainer remains silent, and the client engages in imagery in silence. This division appears to accommodate those clients who prefer high levels of instructor direction and patter, and those who wish to engage in imagery in silence.

• *Meditation/mindfulness*. I strongly disagree with the prevailing practice of teaching one modality of meditation (e.g., mantra meditation, breathing, mindfulness). My approach is to teach no fewer than eight types of meditation, giving each equal time and emphasis. The eight meditations are:

1. Body sense meditation ("attend to the pleasant physical sensations associated with relaxation, such as warmth in your abdomen")
2. Rocking meditation
3. Breathing meditation
4. Mantra meditation
5. Meditation on an internally generated image
6. Meditation on a simple external sound
7. Meditation on a simple external visual stimulus
8. Mindfulness

Having taught this sequence to several thousand individuals, I can report that no one approach has emerged as "most preferred" or "most effective." There is a slight trend for beginners to prefer rocking meditation. Once clients have the opportunity to learn all eight approaches (over two or three sessions), they pick one or two types of meditation to continue practicing. Virtually all trainees have clear preferences.

Psychological relaxation theory suggests nine formats for incorporating multiple techniques and access skills (for details, see Smith, 2005). They are as follows.

• *Revised traditional format*. Exercises that incorporate supplementary skills are woven into a traditional sequence. For example, one might augment progressive muscle relaxation with substantial breathing and imagery elements, closing with meditation.

• *Mini-scripts*. A client creates a 5-minute abbreviated version of a complete relaxation script (described below).

• *Package programs*. Based on initial assessment, clients are assigned three to five approaches to relaxation. After 2 more weeks of rotated practice, clients determine which approaches work best.

• *World tour*. Clients receive training in six families of relaxation, one per week, and then determine which approaches work best.

• *Access zone scanning*. In a 30-minute exercise, clients are exposed to six families of relaxation demonstrating six different relaxation skills. Five-minute samples of each family are presented in a logical and coherent sequence.

• *Spot relaxation*. After exploring several families of relaxation, clients target brief (1–2 minutes) relaxation exercises for specific situations (breathing deeply before an exam, engaging in imagery before a dental visit, tensing and letting go after an argument, etc.).

• *Workshops*. The six families of relaxation are explained and demonstrated in a group workshop format.

• *Group relaxation*. Individual families of techniques, or an entire scripting sequence, is taught to groups of individuals.

• *Relaxation scripting*. This is our most comprehensive approach to relaxation. First, clients are taught all six families of relaxation. Then an individualized recording is made that includes elements of preferred exercises, R-States, and R-Beliefs tailored to the client. The goal is to create a coherent relaxation sequence that is both interesting and meaningful, rather than a mechanical health chore or fitness routine.

CONCLUSION

Relaxation is often treated like a generic anxiety pill. Any brand will do because all have the same overall effect. In contrast, I suggest we think of relaxation as a balanced diet, one that carefully selects from various basic families of approaches. Each relaxation family is a "basic food group" of exercises that targets a different set of relaxation skills and psychological states. Yoga may evoke feelings energy, progressive muscle relaxation may foster physical relaxation, meditation may be good for quieting the mind, and so on. Complete relaxation is an individualized and balanced blend of exercises selected to match practitioner needs and goals.

However, psychological relaxation theory presents a more encompassing challenge to relaxation trainers, researchers, and practitioners. Most programs of relaxation, meditation, and mindfulness taught outside of the health professions go beyond neurophysiological arousal. Each promotes its own favorite goals and R-States. A mindfulness system might emphasize R-States Thankful/Loving, Quiet, and Accepting. A group practicing centering prayer may focus on Reverent/Prayerful, At Ease/Peaceful, Optimistic, and Accepting. A yoga monastery might teach Energy, Physically Relaxed, and Timeless/Boundless/Infinite/At One. It is useful to ask how programs pick their guiding R-States and ignore others. Surprisingly, it is almost always the opinion of an early program leader. And typically such opinions are informed not by fact but by the shifting sands of history, dogma, bias, and tradition. Our window of renewal presents an empirically derived set of R-States not based on any particular tradition. Such a universal lexicon challenges and invites us to look beyond our favored techniques and consider the larger universe of relaxation and renewal.

AUTHOR NOTE

Jonathan C. Smith is a licensed clinical psychologist, professor of psychology at Roosevelt University, Chicago, and founding director of the Roosevelt University Stress Institute. He has authored more than 20 books and three dozen articles on relaxation, mediation, mindfulness, and stress management. Dr. Smith's stress, relaxation, and mindfulness inventories, as well as his self-training manuals and work on the Flying Spaghetti Monster, are available on his web site, *www.lulu.com/stress*. Professional recordings of yoga stretching, progressive muscle relaxation, breathing exercises, autogenic training, imagery, meditation, and mindfulness are available at *drsmith.deltalprinting.com*.

REFERENCES

Anderson, K. P. (2001) The Symptom Checklist–90—Revised and relaxation states during one's preferred relaxation activity. In J. C. Smith (Ed.), *Advances in ABC relaxation: Applications and inventories* (pp. 138–140). New York: Springer.

Bang, S. C. (1999). *ABC relaxation training as a treatment for depression for the Korean elderly*. Unpublished master's thesis, Roosevelt University, Chicago.

Benson, H. (1975). *The relaxation response*. New York: Morrow.

Bishop, S. R., Lau, M., Shapiro, S., Carlson, L., Anderson, N. D., Carmody, J., et al. (2004). Mindfulness: A proposed operational definition. *Clinical Psychology: Science and Practice, 11*, 230–241.

Boukydis, N. N. (2004). *Progressive muscle relaxation, breathing exercises, and ABC relaxation training in an outpatient clinical population.* Unpublished master's thesis, Roosevelt University, Chicago.

Bowers, R., Darner, R. M., Goldner, C. L., & Sohnle, S. (2001). Gender differences for recalled relaxation states, dispositions, beliefs, and benefits. In J. C. Smith (Ed.), *Advances in ABC relaxation: Applications and inventories* (pp. 111–113). New York: Springer.

Braid, J. (1853). *Neurypnology or the rationale of nervous sleep considered in relation with animal magnetism.* London: Churchill

Gaff, J. L. (2001). Health status, stress and relaxation dispositions, motivations, and beliefs. In J. C. Smith (Ed.), *Advances in ABC relaxation: Applications and inventories* (pp. 145–148). New York: Springer.

Ghonchec, S., Byers, K., Sparks, S. E., & Wasik, M. A. (2001). The relationship between relaxation beliefs and relaxation dispositions, motivations, and recalled states for one's preferred relaxation activity. In J. C. Smith (Ed.), *Advances in ABC relaxation: Applications and inventories* (pp. 176–179). New York: Springer.

Ghonchec, S., & Smith, J. C. (2004). Progressive muscle relaxation, yoga stretching, and ABC relaxation theory. *Journal of Clinical Psychology, 60*, 131–136.

Gillani, N. B., & Smith, J. C. (2001). Zen meditation and ABC relaxation theory: An exploration of relaxation states, beliefs, dispositions, and motivations. *Journal of Clinical Psychology, 57*, 839–846.

Gonzales, R. (2001). ABC relaxation training as a treatment for depression for Puerto Rican elderly. In J. C. Smith (Ed.), *Advances in ABC relaxation: Applications and inventories* (pp. 209–211). New York: Springer.

Hughes, R. F. (2001). The NEO Personality Inventory—Revised and relaxation dispositions, motivations, and beliefs. In J. C. Smith (Ed.), *Advances in ABC relaxation: Applications and inventories* (pp. 126–131). New York: Springer.

Jacobson, E. (1938). *Progressive relaxation* (2nd ed.). Chicago: University of Chicago Press.

Khasky, A. D., & Smith, J. C. (1999). Stress, relaxation states, and creativity. *Perceptual and Motor Skills, 88*, 409–416.

Leslie, K. A., & Clavin, S. L. (2001). The Sixteen Personality Factor Questionnaire and recalled relaxation states in one's preferred relaxation activity. In J. C. Smith (Ed.), *Advances in ABC relaxation: Applications and inventories* (pp. 122–125). New York: Springer.

Lewis, J. E. (2001a). R-States, beliefs, attitudes, and concerns. In J. C. Smith (Ed.), *Advances in ABC relaxation: Applications and inventories* (pp. 180–182). New York: Springer.

Lewis, J. E. (2001b). Recalled relaxation states and preferred relaxation activities: II. In J. C. Smith (Ed.), *Advances in ABC relaxation: Applications and inventories* (pp. 190–192). New York: Springer.

Matsumoto, M., & Smith, J. C. (2001). Progressive muscle relaxation exercises, breathing exercises, and ABC relaxation theory. *Journal of Clinical Psychology, 57*, 1551–1557.

McDuffie, S. R. (2001). Race, gender, and ABC relaxation theory. In J. C. Smith (Ed.), *Advances in ABC relaxation: Applications and inventories* (pp. 117–121). New York: Springer.

Mui, P. (2001). The factor structure of relaxation beliefs. In J. C. Smith (Ed.), *Advances in ABC relaxation: Applications and inventories* (pp. 165–166). New York: Springer.

Pressman, S. D., & Cohen, S. (2005). Does positive affect influence health? *Psychological Bulletin, 131*, 925–971.

Rice, S., Cucci, L., III, & Williams, J. (2001). Practice variables as predictors of stress and relaxation dispositions for yoga and meditation. In J. C. Smith (Ed.), *Advances in ABC relaxation: Applications and inventories* (pp. 193–196). New York: Springer.

Ritchie, T. D., Holmes, R. C., III, & Allen, D. (2001). Preferred relaxation activities and recalled relaxation states. In J. C. Smith (Ed.), *Advances in ABC relaxation: Applications and inventories* (pp. 187–189). New York: Springer.

Schultz, J. H. (1932). *Das autogene training—Konzentrative Selbstentspannung.* Leipzig, Germany: Thieme.

Smith, J. C. (1985). *Relaxation dynamics: Nine word approaches to self-relaxation.* New York: Springer

Smith, J. C. (1986). Meditation, biofeedback, and the relaxation controversy: A cognitive-behavioral perspective. *American Psychologist, 41*, 1007–1009.

Smith, J. C. (1990). *Cognitive-behavioral relaxation training: A new system of strategies for treatment and assessment*. New York: Springer.

Smith, J. C. (1999). *ABC relaxation theory*. New York: Springer.

Smith, J. C. (2001a). *Advances in ABC relaxation: Applications and inventories*. New York: Springer.

Smith, J. C. (2001b). The factor structure and correlates of negative relaxation attitudes. In J. C. Smith (Ed.), *Advances in ABC relaxation: Applications and inventories* (pp. 167–171). New York: Springer.

Smith, J. C. (2001c). The factor structure and correlates of claimed relaxation benefits. In J. C. Smith (Ed.), *Advances in ABC relaxation: Applications and inventories* (pp. 172–175). New York: Springer.

Smith, J. C. (2001d). ABC relaxation theory and yoga, meditation and prayer: Relaxation dispositions, motivations, beliefs, and practice patterns. In J. C. Smith (Ed.), *Advances in ABC relaxation: Applications and inventories* (pp. 197–201). New York: Springer.

Smith, J. C. (2005). *Relaxation, meditation, and mindfulness: A mental health professional's guide to new and traditional approaches*. New York: Springer.

Smith, J. C. (2006). *Relaxation, meditation and mindfulness: Free Internet exercises*. Morrisville, NC: Lulupress.

Smith, J. C. (2007). *The Smith Relaxation States Inventory–3 (SRSI-3)*. Morrisville, NC: Lulupress.

Smith, J. C., Amutio, A., Anderson, J. P., & Aria, L. A. (1996). Relaxation: Mapping an uncharted world. *Biofeedback and Self-Regulation, 21*, 63–90.

Smith, J. C., Goc, N. L., & Kinzer, D. J. (2001). Initial trial of the Smith Intercentering Inventory: Progressive muscle relaxation versus yoga stretching versus breathing relaxation. In J. C. Smith (Ed.), *Advances in ABC relaxation: Applications and inventories* (pp. 212–214). New York: Springer.

Smith, J. C., & Jackson, L. (2001). Breathing exercises and relaxation states. In J. C. Smith (Ed.), *Advances in ABC relaxation: Applications and inventories* (pp. 202–204). New York: Springer.

Smith, J. C., & Joyce, C. A. (2004). Mozart vs. new age music: Relaxation states, stress, and ABC relaxation theory. *Journal of Music Therapy, 41*, 215–224.

Smith, J. C., & Karmin, A. D. (2002). Idiosyncratic reality claims, relaxation dispositions, and ABC relaxation theory: Happiness, literal Christianity, miraculous powers, metaphysics, and the paranormal. *Perceptual and Motor Skills, 95*, 1119–1128.

Smith, J. C., McDuffie, S. R., Ritchie, T., & Holmes, R. H., III. (2001). Ethnic and racial differences in relaxation states for recalled relaxation activities. In J. C. Smith (Ed.), *Advances in ABC relaxation: Applications and inventories* (pp. 115–116). New York: Springer.

Smith, J. C., & Sohnle, S. (2001). Stress, relaxation dispositions, and recalled relaxation states for one's preferred relaxation activity. In J. C. Smith (Ed.), *Advances in ABC relaxation: Applications and inventories* (pp. 143–144). New York: Springer.

Smith, J. C., Wedell, A. B., Kolotylo, C. J., Lewis, J. E., Byers, K. Y., & Segin, C. M. (2000). ABC relaxation theory and the factor structure of relaxation states, recalled relaxation activities, dispositions, and motivations. *Psychological Reports, 86*, 1201–1208.

Sohnle, S. (2001). The Millon Index of Personality Styles and recalled relaxation states for one's preferred relaxation activity. In J. C. Smith (Ed.), *Advances in ABC relaxation: Applications and inventories* (pp. 132–137). New York: Springer.

Sonobe, Y. (2001). Coping styles and relaxation dispositions, motivations, and beliefs. In J. C. Smith (Ed.), *Advances in ABC relaxation: Applications and inventories* (pp. 149–154). New York: Springer.

PART II

STRESS MANAGEMENT METHODS

Muscle Relaxation

CHAPTER 4

Progressive Relaxation
Origins, Principles, and Clinical Applications

F. J. McGUIGAN
PAUL M. LEHRER

HISTORY

Influences on Jacobson

In 1905 Edmund Jacobson, the originator of progressive relaxation (PR), was sent to graduate school at Harvard University by Walter Dill Scott, psychologist and president of Northwestern University, to study with three of the great minds of the day: William James, Josiah Royce, and Hugo Münsterberg. All three had a considerable influence on him: James by exhorting him to study "the whole man"; Royce by nurturing his philosophical paper on truth; and Münsterberg in a negative way that, however, was beneficial for PR. Münsterberg discharged Jacobson as his assistant because, as Jacobson later related, the data he collected were at odds with Münsterberg's theory. Thus freed to work on his own, Jacobson studied the startle reaction to an unexpected loud noise. He found that there was no obvious startle to sudden noise in more relaxed participants. This was the first systematic study of relaxation, and it marked the birth of PR.

After graduating from Harvard, Jacobson worked with Edward Bradford Titchener at Cornell University. He probably was influenced by Titchener in two very important ways: through Titchener's expertise in introspection and through his context theory of meaning. Titchener's context theory held that the meanings of words originate, in part, in bodily attitudes (postures) involving the skeletal muscle system. Related to these two avenues of influence, two contemporary applications of PR for clinical purposes are (1) de-

---

This is an update of F. J. McGuigan's chapter for earlier editions of this book. Dr. McGuigan, a major contributor to psychology and, particularly, to the understanding of stress and its treatment, passed away before work on this revision had been begun. Dr. McGuigan was Edmund Jacobson's most articulate and longest term student. He devoted much of his professional life to teaching Jacobson's method and performing research studies on various correlates of Jacobson's theory. As someone who also had the privilege of working under Dr. Jacobson's tutelage, I (PML) have undertaken a revision of this chapter. This is done with great humility, because the original work was quite definitive. Updates include a review of more recent research literature, as well as some minor editorial changes.

tailed observation of ("introspection" on) minute kinesthetic sensations and accompanying mental processes; and (2) clinical interpretation of localized bodily tensions as meanings of acts that occur in one's imagination.

Objective Measurement of Tension

After leaving Cornell, Jacobson received his MD and worked in the Department of Physiology at the University of Chicago from 1926 until 1936; he also conducted a private clinical practice. At Chicago, Jacobson, collaborating with A. J. Carlson, discovered an objective measure of tension: They found that the amplitude of knee-jerk reflexes varied directly with the degree of patients' tension. Consequently, as overly tense patients learned to relax, the amplitude of their knee-jerk reflexes decreased. Jacobson's (1938) further research on several reflexes established that chronic tonus (sustained tension) of the skeletal muscles increased the amplitude of reflexes and decreased their latency; conversely, reflexes diminished in amplitude and increased in latency as patients relaxed. As general skeletal muscle tone decreased, the involuntary startle reflex also was eliminated. Charles Sherrington (1909) also made this point when his research established that it was not possible to evoke the patellar tendon reflex in an absolutely toneless muscle. More generally, Sherrington concluded that the appearance of reflexes depended on the presence of tone in the muscles constituting part of the reflex arc. (After about 2 months in our own PR classes, we sometimes drop a large book onto the floor when the students are well into their relaxation period. Seldom is there even a blink of the eye in these well-relaxed students.)

As successful as it was, measuring the knee-jerk reflex was cumbersome. Through arduous efforts with the aid of scientists at Bell Telephone Laboratories, Jacobson eventually was able to measure tension directly. He recorded electrical muscle action potentials as low as one microvolt, a unit previously unmeasurable by the physiologists of the day. Thus quantitative electromyography (EMG) was launched. The resultant use of objective measures of degree of relaxation and tension guided Jacobson to develop and validate PR.

Measuring Mental Events

With this new instrumentation, Jacobson made important discoveries about how the mind and body function. He found that, in a relaxed person, just the *thought* of moving a limb was accompanied by unique covert EMG responses in that limb. For example, if the individual imagined hitting a nail with a hammer three times, there were three unique EMG bursts in the preferred arm. Through extensive research he concluded that all thought is accompanied by skeletal muscle activity, though response amplitude may be extremely low. The eye and speech muscles, he found, were especially important during visual and speech imagery. Conversely, his data indicated that mental processes diminished and even disappeared as the skeletal musculature relaxed toward zero. As Jacobson concluded, "It might be naive to say that we think with our muscles, but it would be inaccurate to say that we think without them" (cited in McGuigan, 1978, p. iii).

Therapeutic Consequences

Jacobson's research showed that to relax the mind and the body, one must relax all of the skeletal musculature. Jacobson applied this basic principle of PR for more than 70 years, with immense therapeutic consequences. His numerous scientific and clinical studies gave the world effective methods for directly controlling the various systems of the body, including those that generate mental processes. We now turn to an exposition of these methods.

THEORETICAL UNDERPINNINGS

PR begins with the ancient and venerable concept of rest. Physicians have long known the value of rest, frequently prescribing it in the form of "bed rest." However, many people who are instructed to rest in bed simply toss and turn. Mere prescription is not sufficient; patients may be told to rest but do not know how. These patients must diligently learn habits of effective rest. Such habits may enable them to prevent the development of a serious tension malady and to use bodily energy with greater efficiency. When relaxation is applied therapeutically, it has often helped restore the body to a normally functioning condition, providing, of course, that the tension malady is reversible. How tension develops in the body is a straightforward physiological event.

How Stressors Evoke Tension

Each stressful situation ("stressor") that people meet in everyday life reflexively evokes the primitive startle pattern of rising (covertly or overtly) on the balls of the feet and hunching forward. The entire skeletal musculature reacts immediately. Within a matter of 100 or so milliseconds, people thereby ready themselves for fight or flight, as Walter Cannon (1929) theorized. This startle reaction, followed by complex autonomic and endocrine changes, has had great survival value. However, it is often prolonged beyond the immediate emergency, resulting in a condition of chronic overtension and continued hyperactivity of the systems of the body. In particular, consistent, excessive covert tightening of the skeletal musculature overdrives the central nervous system and increases activity of the autonomic, cardiovascular, endocrine, and other systems. Prolonged, heightened skeletal muscle tension may then result in any of a variety of pathological conditions, as we soon explain. To reverse the process of overtension, a person needs to learn to relax the skeletal musculature, whereupon activity in the other systems of the body is reduced.

Principles and Physiology of Progressive Relaxation

In learning PR, one cultivates the ability to make extremely sensitive observations of the world beneath the skin. To acquire such heightened internal sensory observation, which is a kind of physiological introspection, one first learns to recognize subtle states of tension. When a muscle contracts (tenses), volleys of neural impulses are generated and carried to the brain along afferent neural pathways. This muscle–neural phenomenon, the generation of afferent neural impulses, constitutes the local sign of tension that one learns to observe. This tension sensation is the "muscle sense of Bell," which was reported in the early 19th century by the eminent physiologist Sir Charles Bell.

Tension is the contraction of skeletal muscle fibers that generates the tension sensation. *Relaxation* is the elongation (lengthening) of those fibers, which then eliminates the tension sensation. After learning to identify the tension sensation, one learns to relax it away. For this, one learns to allow the muscle fibers that generated the tension to elongate. In the learning process, one contrasts the previous tension sensation with the later elimination of tension. This general procedure of identifying a local state of tension, relaxing it away, and marking the contrast between the tension and ensuing relaxation is then applied to all of the major muscle groups. In PR one thus learns to control all of the skeletal musculature so that any portion thereof may be systematically relaxed or tensed as one chooses. Those familiar with EMG biofeedback may wish to think of PR as a method of "internal biofeedback" in which the learner internally monitors feedback signals from the muscle instead of perceiving their representations on external readout systems.

The Skeletal Muscles Control Other Bodily Systems through Neuromuscular Circuits

In the 19th century, the famous psychologist Alexander Bain (e.g., Bain, 1855) claimed that the skeletal musculature is the only physiological system over which a person has direct control. Hence, as Bain, Jacobson, and others held, skeletal muscles are "the instrument of the will." They contain the only receptor cells in the body that can be directly shut off, which is accomplished merely by lengthening muscle fibers. A synonym for *skeletal muscles* is *voluntary muscles*, precisely because when one wishes to perform an act, one systematically contracts and relaxes the voluntary muscles. For instance, a person who decides to walk contracts muscles to put one foot in front of the other. This point is so obvious that it does not need elaboration. What is not so obvious is that the internal (covert) functions of the body are similarly controlled by means of the skeletal muscles. PR is predicated on the principle that covert functions of the body can also be controlled through slight muscle tensions.

Thus the tension sensation (the muscle sense of Bell) is called the *control signal* because it literally controls the body's activities. Muscles exercise such control as they interact with the brain through "neuromuscular circuits" (Jacobson, 1964). When volleys of neural impulses generated by contracting muscles feed back to the brain, extremely complex events result, following which neural impulses return to the muscles along efferent neural pathways. The muscles then further contract, directing additional neural impulses to and from the brain, and so on. Numerous neuromuscular circuits throughout the body simultaneously reverberate in this way to carry out the body's functions. By learning internal sensory observation, one can become quite proficient in recognizing control signals wherever they may occur throughout the skeletal musculature. Through practice, those controls may be activated or relaxed. Relaxation of the skeletal muscle controls produces a state of rest throughout the neuromuscular circuits, including reduced activity of the brain itself. The long-range goal of PR is for the body to instantaneously monitor all of its numerous control signals and to automatically relieve tensions that are not desired. The trained body has an amazing capacity to monitor the many neuromuscular circuits that reverberate in parallel fashion throughout the body. The ultimate goal is to develop "automaticity," wherein one automatically, unconsciously, and effortlessly identifies and relaxes unwanted tensions.

Jacobson (1964) emphasized the control functions of PR when he used *self-operations control* as a synonym for PR. *Self-operations control* was a precedent for contemporary use of such terms as *self-regulation* and *stress management*. Its aims are to increase behavioral efficiency by programming oneself to eliminate tensions that interfere with one's primary purposes. A person can thereby control blood pressure, emotional life, digestive processes, mental processes, and the like, as we later illustrate.

The Concept of Neuromuscular Circuits Has a Venerable History

The concept of reverberating neuromuscular circuits driven by muscle controls is ancient. Dating from the period of the early Greeks, its evolution can be impressively traced through the writings of philosophers, through the scientific Renaissance, through the research of later physiologists and psychologists, and into the very forefront of contemporary scientific and clinical thinking (see McGuigan, 1978). Some of our the most prominent thinkers have recognized that the human body functions in terms of information generated and transmitted between the muscle systems and the brain. One of the most influential presentations of this concept was provided by Norbert Wiener (1948) in his classic book *Cybernetics*. In greater depth than all others before him, Wiener developed the model that the body functions according to principles of feedback circuits. As he put it:

> The central nervous system no longer appears as a self-contained organ, receiving inputs from the senses and discharging into the muscles. On the contrary, some of its most characteristic activities are explicable only as circular processes, emerging from the nervous system into the muscles, and re-entering the nervous system through the sense organs, whether they be proprioceptors or organs of the special senses. (Wiener, 1948, p. 15)

A similar neuromuscular concept was put forth by Alexander Bain in 1855:

> The organ of mind is not the brain by itself; it is the brain, nerves, muscles, and organs of sense. . . . We must . . . discard forever the notion of the sensorium commune, the cerebral closed, as a central seat of mind, or receptacle of sensation and imagery. (cited in Holt, 1937, pp. 38–39)

More recently, a considerable number of research findings have shown a close connection between skeletal muscle innervation and the sympathetic nervous system (e.g., Delius, Hagbarth, Hongell, & Wallin, 1972) such that increased muscle tension triggers a burst of sympathetic activity, causing constriction of blood vessels within the muscle tissue. These vascular effects are regulated by the baroreflexes (Kienbaum, Karlssonn, Sverrisdottir, Elam, & Wallin, 2001), which also are important modulators of autonomic stress responses (cf. Chapter 10, this volume).

Neurophysiology of Relaxation

In various publications, Gellhorn (e.g., Gellhorn, 1958; Gellhorn & Kiely, 1972) sought to specify the neural mechanisms by which the skeletal musculature leads to relaxation of the body. Gellhorn was especially impressed with Jacobson's method, and Jacobson approved of Gellhorn's theorizing as to those neural mechanisms (Jacobson, 1967). Gellhorn started with the basic fact that PR decreases afferent neural impulses from the skeletal musculature. He then noted that the reticular formation receives considerable innervation from those skeletal muscles, so that relaxation reduces activity there. The reticular formation, in turn, functions in circuits with the posterior hypothalamus and thence with the cortex. Consequently, muscular relaxation reduces proprioceptive input to the hypothalamus, with a resulting lessening of hypothalamic–cortical and autonomic discharges. Gellhorn concluded that lessened emotional reactivity during muscular relaxation is the result of reduced proprioceptive impulses to the hypothalamus, which then decreases excitability of the sympathetic nervous system. Jacobson summarized research by Bernhaut, Gellhorn, and Rasmussen (1953) as follows:

> These findings suggest that a relaxation of the skeletal musculature is accompanied by a diminution in the state of excitability of the sympathetic division of the hypothalamus and, through a reduction in the hypothalamic–cortical discharges, by a similar reduction in the state of excitability of the cerebral cortex. (Jacobson, 1967, p. 155)

In these ways, then, the skeletal muscles can control other systems of the body, including the reduction and elimination of mental (including emotional) events.

More recent research on muscle relaxation therapy has documented decreases in sympathetic arousal, including a decrease in circulating norepinephrine levels and myocardial contractility (Davidson, Winchester, Taylor, Alderman, & Ingels, 1979), as well as decreased electrodermal activity and heart rate levels and reactivity (Lehrer, 1978; Lehrer, Schoicket, Carrington, & Woolfolk, 1980; McGlynn, Moore, Lawyer, & Karg, 1999; Shapiro & Lehrer, 1980). The close connection between the skeletal muscles and the sympathetic nervous system has received much empirical attention. The muscles are an important element in a complex feedback system that controls physiological arousal. Perception of muscle sensations and afferent feedback from the muscles are provided by active sensory cells called *muscle spindles*. The muscle spindles are active in that they may expand or contract independently of actual muscle tension. Efferents to the muscle spindles may therefore control the amount of afferent feedback provided by muscle tension. Activity in the muscle spindles is strongly influenced by the sympathetic system (Grassi & Passastore, 1988; Roatta, Windhorst, Ljubisavljevic, Johansson, & Passatore, 2002). Jacobson's emphasis on training people to perceive very low levels of muscle tone through his *method of diminishing tensions* may provide specific training in perception of low-level afferent feedback from the muscle spindles. By controlling this activity, one may directly alter the feedback loop between the muscles and the sympathetic system during PR training. Perception and control of muscle spindle activity may be an important mechanism behind the effects of PR in diminishing sympathetic arousal.

Differential Relaxation

Differential relaxation (DR) is the optimal contraction of only those muscles required to accomplish a given purpose. Those and only those muscles should contract, and they should contract only to the extent required to accomplish the purpose at hand. All other (irrelevant) muscles of the body should be relaxed. In the moment-to-moment monitoring of tensions throughout the day, people can often catch themselves wasting energy. Some needlessly clasp their hands together; others tap their fingers and feet, wrap their legs around the legs of a chair, or needlessly rock back and forth. In learning DR, while studying a particular tension signal that is to be controlled, the learner recognizes other tensions elsewhere in the body. These are unwanted tensions that can be relaxed away when the learner later practices on that part of the body. By learning to differentially relax 24 hours a day, a person can save considerable energy, so that relevant tensions can be more efficiently directed toward the accomplishment of specific goals. Later we consider some specific applications of the principle of DR.

The Method of Diminishing Tensions

In developing control over one's muscles, it is necessary (eventually) to detect the most subtle control signals. For this purpose, PR starts with relatively obvious control signals generated in the dorsal surface of the forearm by raising the hand at the wrist to nearly a 90° angle. Thus the learner initially perceives a localized sensation of tension in the forearm. With the "method of diminishing tensions," one then studies tensions of ever-decreasing intensity. Thus, after the control signal generated by raising the hand vertically at the wrist is studied, for the next practice the hand is raised only half as much—at a 45° angle from the horizontal. Then the third practice position is to raise the hand only half as high as before (at about a 20° angle); on successive practice positions the hand is raised less and less until movement is imperceptible, but perception of tension persists. The eventual goal is to identify tension signals of perhaps 1/1000th the intensity of those with which the learner began. Such signals are common in the minute muscles of the tongue and eyes, but occur in nearly all muscles.

Some practitioners give instructions to generate high-intensity tensions (e.g., to clench the fist tightly). We believe that this practice is counterproductive for learning to perceive and control *low-intensity* tensions. Many covert responses are below 1 μV. To control small tensions, one should study *them* rather than large tensions.

Avoiding Suggestion

In learning PR, trainees are never told that they are doing well, that they are getting better, that they are relaxing, that their hands feel heavy, that they are getting sleepy, or the like. No attempt is made to convince the individual that he or she will be "cured" in any sense of the word. Instead, the trainees are aided by instructions, just as in any other learning procedure. Thus a teacher may interrupt a trainee's practice with criticism whenever the individual is failing to relax.

Jacobson (1938) listed a number of reasons for avoiding suggestion. As with the placebo effect, any method will accomplish something (although usually only temporarily) if it instills into the person the belief that he or she will benefit from its application. Jacobson pointed out that relaxation is a fundamental physiological occurrence that consists of learning to elongate muscle fibers systematically. He specified definitive physiological changes in the body that differ from those occurring during suggestion. The trainee may be skeptical in regard to the procedure, but he or she still can learn very well when presented with objective evidence of progress. Moreover, the person learns to be independent of the therapist; in "suggestion" therapies, by contrast, dependence on therapists is engendered. As Lehrer, Woolfolk, and Goldman (1986) added,

> [Jacobson held that] the danger of suggestion . . . is that it may make the individual feel that relaxation is taking place even when it is not. The *perception* of relaxation is not so important as actual physical relaxation, according to Jacobson. Therefore, suggestion may be deleterious because a person may stop devoting the time and concentration necessary to learn relaxation if he or she [incorrectly] feels relaxed already. (Lehrer et al., 1986, p. 202; italics in original)

Tape-Recorded Relaxation Instructions and Biofeedback

Just as Jacobson eschewed the use of suggestion in relaxation instructions, he also avoided the use of tape-recorded instructions. He did this primarily because he thought that tape-recorded instructions might offer more suggestion than training. In support of this position, a literature review by Lehrer (1982) found that taped training did not produce physiological effects that were measurable outside of training sessions.

Jacobson also recommended against using surface EMG biofeedback, even though he was the first to use this technique (see Jacobson, 1978, fig. 25, p. 146). He thought that people should not depend on external sources of biological information but should develop their own powers to sense very low levels of muscle tension and to relax in all situations, even when a biofeedback machine is not available.

However, modern technology has made surface EMG biofeedback a much easier and cheaper methodology. People now can afford to have home monitors, which may be used as teaching aids for attaining more sensitive perception and greater control of the muscles. Jacobson's objections to biofeedback may no longer apply.

Relaxation Practice Is Not an Exercise

Many suggestions for how to relax use a lay meaning of the term, which is inappropriate in a scientific/clinical context. For instance, advice to exercise is not advice to relax, because exercise is work. Exercise is very advisable on other grounds. For the same reason, terms such as *relaxation exercises* or *relaxation response* are self-contradictory, because *exercise* and *response* are "work words." The essence of relaxing is to allow the muscle fibers to elongate, which is physiologically impossible when one *tries* (through exercising or responding) to accomplish it. One simply cannot make an *effort* to relax, because an effort to relax is a failure to relax.

Is There a Shortcut?

From a naive learner's point of view, the amount of time required to learn PR may seem excessive. Indeed, one needs to learn to control a large mass of muscle that makes up almost half the body weight. Recognizing the desire on the part of the learner for brevity, Jacobson spent many years attempting to shorten the method. However, he abandoned his attempt because patients did not sufficiently generalize from what they learned in the clinic to everyday life. His conclusion was that there simply is no satisfactory brief method for learning to relax a body that has been practicing overtension for decades. Nevertheless, Jacobson (1964) did offer a "briefer course," reducing the time devoted to each muscle group. For instance, instead of practicing for 3 hours on a single position, one practices three positions in 1 hour, starting with the first three in Table 4.2 (later in the chapter). Similar abridgements have been made for other muscle groups. The complete course can thus be shortened to one-third of the time it ordinarily takes. However, in this world "you get what you pay for," so that you learn considerably less control from a briefer than from a longer course. An appropriate analogy is learning to play the piano: Certainly you can practice for shorter periods, but your competence is thereby reduced. Nevertheless, in clinical practice, the method has been routinely shortened to six or fewer sessions by combining training in several muscle groups in a single session (e.g., muscles of the arms in one session, then the legs in another, the trunk in a third, the face and neck in the fourth, and differential relaxation training in the fifth and sixth).

Jacobson's research in school systems and in clinical work led him to conclude that children learn PR quite rapidly. His reasoning was that they have not spent so many years acquiring maladaptive tension habits that must be reversed. Teaching PR in elementary school has been done on a large scale in Sweden (Setterlind, 1983).

With this explanation of the principles of PR, we now turn to the psychologically important topic of clinical control of mental (cognitive) processes. To establish a basis, we first consider the scientific nature of mind and its component mental events.

A Psychophysiological Model of Mind

Mental (cognitive) events are generated by the selective interaction of reverberating neuromuscular circuits. Various functions of the everyday notion of "mind" are indicated by such terms as *ideas, images, thoughts, dreams, hallucinations, fears, depression,* and *anxieties.* According to the present model, all such mental (cognitive) events are generated when selective systems of the body interact through highly integrated neuromuscular circuits. Most mental processes are generated when muscles of the eyes and speech regions tense, whereupon specialized circuits to and from the brain are activated. Other pathways are activated also, including those involving the somatic musculature and the autonomic system. A detailed presentation of and perhaps the most extensive documentation for this neuromuscular model of the generation of mental events are provided in McGuigan (1978).

1. *Muscular events are present during cognition.* McGuigan's (1978) summary of relevant research over an 80-year period provides a firm basis for the conclusion that muscular contraction in selected regions of the body corresponds to the nature of the mental activity present. During visual imagery, the eyes are uniquely active (e.g., when one is imagining the Eiffel Tower, the eyes move upward in imaginal scanning as detected through electro-oculography). During imagining, somatic activity EMG readings detect localized covert responses (e.g., imagining lighting a cigarette produces a distinct covert response in the active arm). Covert muscular responses have been recorded in the speech musculature during a great variety of thinking tasks; for example, there was heightened tongue EMG while participants were performing a verbal mediation task using Tracy Kendler's paradigm (McGuigan, Culver, & Kendler, 1971). In addition, there is heightened speech muscle activity in both children and adults during silent reading; increased speech muscle activity covertly occurs while individuals are engaged in cursive handwriting; in deaf children, covert responses occur in the fingers, which are the locus of their "speech" region, while they think; rapid, phasic speech muscle activity occurs during night dreams involving auditory content; heightened speech muscle activity occurs in patients with paranoid schizophrenia during auditory hallucinations; and so on for other mentalistic activities (see especially McGuigan, 1978, Ch. 10). Conversely, there is no conscious awareness at all when people are well relaxed, as objectively determined by a lack of tension measured through EMG readings (Jacobson, 1938).

The reasoning here is that because specific muscle activity occurs during cognitive activity, and because cognitive activity disappears when this muscle activity is reduced to zero, it may be concluded that muscle activity is a critical component of those cognitive events.

2. *Numerous covert reactions during cognition are related by neuromuscular circuits.* Although there are foci of muscular activity in selective regions of the body depending on the nature of the cognitive activity, other covert responses are simultaneously occurring throughout the skeletal musculature. For example, while participants in one study processed a silent answer to a question, events were simultaneously recorded in the arms, lips, neck, and eyes, as well as in the left temporal lobe and left motor area of the brain (McGuigan & Pavek, 1972). The conclusion is that these unique, simultaneously occurring events throughout the body are not independent. Rather, they are related by means of rapidly reverberating neuromuscular circuits between the brain and the extensive skeletal musculature. Because those widespread events occur simultaneously with the silent thought, it is assumed that the neuromuscular circuits generate that thought. We turn now to how such a verbal thought is generated.

3. *There are general linguistic, visual, and somatic components of cognition.* Focusing on linguistic cognition, research has indicated that speech muscles generate a phonetic code, which is presumably transmitted to and from the linguistic regions of the brain (see especially McGuigan & Winstead, 1974; McGuigan & Dollins, 1989). When those speech muscles and linguistic brain regions function in unison, perceptual understanding of linguistic cognitions occurs. No doubt similar processing occurs to generate nonlinguistic cognitive activity. Thus circuits between the eyes and the brain generate visual imagery, and circuits between the nonspeech skeletal musculature and the brain generate somatic components of thoughts (see McGuigan, 1989, 1991b).

Control of Cognitions

From a practical point of view, this model of the mind makes it abundantly clear how people can volitionally control their emotions and other cognitive activities, as well as other bodily functions. That is, if cognitive activities are identical with the energy expended when neuromuscular circuits reverberate, those cognitive events can be eliminated when the neuromuscular circuits cease to be active. They stop reverberating when a person relaxes the skeletal muscle components.

The Meaning and Purpose of Tensions

Recalling Titchener's context theory of meaning, a compatible basic principle of PR is that every tension has a purpose—that every tension means something. This point is obvious in many instances. For example, the purpose of the tension in the upper surface of the forearm while bending back the hand at the wrist is simply to raise the hand. Similarly, the purpose of tensions in the muscles of the legs while walking is simply to move the body. What is not so obvious is the interpretation of subtle muscular tensions in the application of clinical PR.

Distinguishing between "Meaning" and "Process"

To interpret control signals, one learns that *process* is the way in which meaning is generated—process is the actual tension sensation that one observes within one's body. *Meaning* designates the purpose of the tension, the reason why one tenses. In generating mental events, "process" consists of the muscular contractions within neuromuscular circuits that generate the relevant images, sensations, and so on. "Meaning" is thus the content of those mental processes.

In therapy, a patient is first carefully trained in detecting (proprioceptively introspecting on) subtle tensions throughout the body that constitute process. Then she or he is carefully trained in developing the ability to introspect on and report the content of mental activity in considerable detail. Process usually occurs in unexpected places in the body. The patient first identifies the nature and locality of process. When these are identified, the question to be answered by clinician and patient working together is this: Why do those tensions occur in particular regions and during a given kind of mental activity? Establishing the meaning of the tensions can give the patient better understanding of and control over his or her difficulties. For example, while learning to relax, a man observed subtle tensions throughout his entire right leg. That was process. After some study, the tensions were interpreted as follows: The man was tensing *as if* he were about to fall out of a tree house and crash into a board with the leg. The mental content generated by the covert tensions in the leg was his remembrance of actually having fallen out of a tree house when he was a boy. As the muscles in the leg covertly contracted in the present, he relived that experience in his memory as if it were overtly occurring. Rolfers report similar experiences when muscles are stimulated.

Consider a case of a woman whose complaints included anemia, chronic constipation, nervous tension with inability to sit quietly, slight dizzy spells during excitement, and a slight discharge from the nose (Jacobson, 1938). After training, she reported the process of sitting stiffly and formally. The meaning of this apparently was that she sought to maintain proper posture in her back because of a fear of developing a habit of faulty posture. That is, the purpose served by maintaining a stiff and formal posture was the prevention of an incorrect everyday posture. To control the tension on the meaning level, she came to understand the reasons why she held herself stiffly and was persuaded to change; on the process level, she learned how to relax the relevant controlling muscles.

In clinical work, it may take a long time to identify tensions characteristic of the "nervous" condition of the patient, to interpret those tensions, and to deal with them effectively. But the history of clinical PR is one of considerable success in following this paradigm. For example, anxiety is regarded as a fearful condition represented in the skeletal musculature. Once the clinician can ascertain the meaning of the skeletal muscle representations, it is then possible to relax those critical tensions, whereupon the state of anxiety can be diminished or eliminated. We return to anxiety later in this chapter.

ASSESSMENT

Applications of the Method

There are two general purposes of tension control—prophylactic and therapeutic. By learning to relax differentially 24 hours a day, a person can increase the likelihood of preventing a stress or tension disorder. For a person already thus victimized, clinical PR can often ease or eliminate the condition.

Stress and tension disorders fall into two classic categories: cognitive ("psychiatric") and somatoform ("psychosomatic") disorders. Elsewhere (McGuigan, 1991a), applications within the first category are discussed. This includes such neurotic disorders as anxiety state, panic disorder, phobic disorders, neurotic depression, and neurasthenia, as well as lesser fears and worries. The second category includes such disorders as irritable bowel syndrome with accompanying diarrhea and constipation, teeth grinding (bruxism), essential hypertension, coronary heart disease, rheumatological pathologies, chronic fatigue, and such pains as those of headaches and backaches.

For over seven decades, Jacobson (e.g., 1938, 1970) collected an abundance of scientific and clinical data that validated the therapeutic application of PR for "psychiatric tension pathologies" (his term). These included nervous hypertension, acute insomnia with nervousness, "anxiety neurosis" (what we now would consider to be panic disorder, generalized anxiety disorder, or one of the other anxiety disorders), cardiac neurosis, chronic insomnia, cyclothymic disorder, obsessive–compulsive disorder, hypochondria, fatigue states, and dysthymia. Somatoform disorders to which he successfully applied PR included convulsive tic; esophageal spasm; various bowel disorders including colitis, irritable bowel, and chronic constipation; arterial hypertension; and tension headaches. More recent controlled studies have found improvement in a variety of disorders after at least eight sessions of training in Jacobson's technique, including chronic pain (Gay, Philippot, & Luminet, 2002), headache (Murphy, Lehrer, & Jurish, 1990), anxiety

(Lehrer, 1978; McCann, Woolfolk, & Lehrer, 1987), and generalized stress (Carrington et al., 1980; Lehrer, Atthowe, & Weber, 1980; Woolfolk, Lehrer, McCann, & Rooney, 1982). Effects on asthma, although *statistically* significant, tend not to be of *clinically* significant magnitude (Lehrer et al., 2004).

Therapy

Cognitive (psychiatric) and somatoform (psychosomatic) disorders, as well as lesser conditions, are characterized by excessive, chronic tension and may be reversed by relaxing the skeletal muscles. To summarize, practice in the gradual lengthening of skeletal muscle fibers can result in a generalized state of relaxation, which in turn can produce a state of relative quietude throughout the central nervous system. Consequently, the viscera can also relax, as evidenced by a lowering of blood pressure, a reduction of pulse rate, and a loosening of the gastrointestinal tract. In this way, numerous somatoform disorders can be alleviated or eliminated.

The rationale for treating cognitive aspects of neurotic and related disorders is to interrupt the reverberation of neuromuscular circuits, preventing undesired thoughts from occurring. Some drugs can interrupt neuromuscular circuits by acting on the brain. However, the most natural way to cause these circuits to be tranquil is to relax the tense muscles that are their peripheral components (a "natural tranquilizer"). Verbal components of undesired thoughts, such as those of phobias and worries, can be eliminated by relaxing the speech muscles (tongue, lips, jaws, throat, and cheeks). The eye muscles are the focus for eliminating the visual imagery of thoughts. When the eye muscles are totally relaxed, one does not visually perceive anything; the eyeballs must move in order for visual perception or visual imagery to occur. Thoroughly relaxing all of the muscles of the body can bring all undesired mental processes to zero.

Developing Emotional Control

Jacobson (1938) demonstrated that relaxation and the experience of emotions are incompatible—that it is impossible to experience emotions while simultaneously relaxing. The paradigm for controlling emotions, as for controlling other mental events, is to control the skeletal musculature that generates them when neuromuscular circuits are selectively activated.

The goal is to determine rationally when to experience and when not to experience particular emotions. One can thus be wisely emotional by wisely tensing to allow favorable emotions to flow freely and inhibiting negative emotions such as temper tantrums or anxiety states. As has been observed clinically in numerous cases, patients who learn to control the skeletal musculature in both its tonic and phasic activity diminish undesired emotions, such as proneness to anger, resentment, disgust, anxiety, or embarrassment. Conversely, as general tension increases, the proprioceptive impulses thereby generated increase emotionality by exciting the central nervous system, the autonomic system, the endocrine system, and so on, presumably through the pathways specified by Gellhorn (Gellhorn, 1958; Gellhorn & Kiely, 1972).

Both increased and decreased emotionality are objectively evidenced by the amplitude and latency of patients' reflexes, as discussed earlier. Everyday examples of this point are obvious, such as when a saucer is accidentally dropped at a tea party. The excessively tense guest will emit an exaggerated startle reflex with heightened emotionality, whereas the well-relaxed person may not even blink or interrupt ongoing conversation.

Individuals who are excessively anxious often continually rehearse their griefs, worries, and difficulties with life. If they can acquire control of the skeletal muscle tensions that key this internal speech, they can consequently control their emotions and other negative mental processes. These controls occur principally in the eye muscles, for visualizing their difficulties, and in the speech muscles, for verbalizing their problems, though the remaining mass of skeletal musculature also helps to control mental processes. Thorough training in PR makes it possible to change gradually away from a condition of continually attending to difficulties and to develop a habit of turning attention from those issues. Anxious individuals thus become better able to verbalize relevant contingencies and to react to problems more rationally. That is to say, instead of reacting reflexively to a difficulty, they can stop and reason about the problem (unless, of course, it is something like an onrushing truck). As they become relaxed, then, they attend less frequently to disturbing issues and can instead focus on other matters and become less emotionally disturbed about problems. A trained person can stop, momentarily relax, and assess a situation—verbalizing, for instance, that "this other person seems to be yelling and screaming at me, and it is to his advantage as well as to mine if I do not yell and scream back."

Specific Applications of DR

The term *tension control* does not mean the same thing as *tension reduction*, because people could not function in life without tensions. The purpose is not to eliminate all tensions but to control them so that they can be wisely used. In other words, the purpose is to relax differentially, which can be prophylactic as well as therapeutic.

For instance, relaxed eating behavior is as appropriate for healthy people as it is for patients with ulcers. Many people exhibit bizarre, often frantic, eating patterns. Such an individual may be hunched over a plate with elbows on the table, eating tools grasped in the hands, tensed legs, and bent shoulders—all as if the eater is ready to leap in animalistic protection of the food should an adversary momentarily appear. The eating process is often a continuous shoveling of food from plate to mouth, with no interruption of the chewing process. Conversation, if any, is through half-ground food, with particles exuded in the direction of the listener. Such overtense eating habits most assuredly do not contribute to smooth digestion. People should be differentially relaxed when eating in order to help prevent a variety of gastrointestinal difficulties, as well as to enjoy dining as a pleasant process.

Similarly, a major industry that dispenses a wide variety of products dedicates itself to helping people alleviate their sleep problems. The complaints of such people include not getting to sleep when they first get in bed, as well as waking up during the night and not getting back to sleep. One patient reported that he had only about 2 hours of actual sleep over a period of 4 nights in bed. The consequences of night after night of inadequate sleep can be catastrophic, producing chronic fatigue and inefficient work performance. Nonprescription medicines, opaque blinds for the windows, earplugs, and covers over the eyes are meant to satisfy complaints that the room is "too hot," "too noisy," "too bright," "too cold," and so forth. The effective solution for the insomniac's problems is to learn to practice DR 24 hours a day, which includes sleeping at night. By applying the principles of DR, one can carry the habit of automatic relaxation into the sleeping state.

Several other common applications of DR discussed by McGuigan (1991a) include relaxing while hurrying; conquering the fear of flying by differentially relaxing on an airplane; controlling one's own temper; and learning how to deal with unreasonable people by controlling the tempers of others, too.

Support for Various Applications: Problems in the Literature

Jacobson's clinical applications of PR are impressive indeed. However, there apparently are no experimental (vs. clinical) data that validate the method, probably because of the extensive methodological difficulties in conducting an experiment. That is, a true experimental test would require randomly assigning a sufficient number of patients to two or more groups and giving the experimental group(s) extensive training over an extended period of time with an hour of practice each day. A procedure approximating that of the clinical case study presented at the end of this chapter would have to be employed with a number of experimental participants—a demanding requirement indeed. The problem of comparable activity in a control group (or groups) to contrast with such an extensive treatment presents another difficult issue.

Although the literature on various forms of relaxation therapy is impressive, descriptions of the length and nature of training indicate either that the research has not used Jacobson's PR procedure or that this procedure has been confounded with other methods. Several examples should illustrate. Nicassio and Bootzin (1974) gave their participants four 1-hour individual sessions using something of an approximation to PR; however, in a short training period, "the entire sequence of muscles was covered at each session" (p. 255). Such a compressed learning session must have been overwhelming to the participants and is contrary to Jacobson's directions. Murphy, Lehrer, and Jurish (1990) taught participants a combination of PR training and autogenic training and used a headache diary, a cognitive questionnaire, and an expectancy measure for their dependent variables. Because their participants learned both methods, however, specific conclusions about PR are precluded. Schaer and Isom (1988) confused PR with hypnosis, stating that "progressive relaxation has some similarities to hypnosis" (p. 513), and used a scale of hypnotic susceptibility to specify participants who were "susceptible to progressive relaxation."

Despite the lack of experimental data on this original version of PR, extensive clinical and related data nevertheless lend credence to the effectiveness of the method. There also is a large body of experimental literature on other methods that involve briefer muscle training (consult Chapters 5, 24, 25, this volume). Because of the relative intensiveness of Jacobson's original method, there is reason to believe that its effects may be considerably more robust than those of the briefer methods.

Limitations and Contraindications

We have seen that PR can be appropriately applied to the reduction of everyday tensions, as in DR, and clinically to the elimination of syndromes related to stress and tension. We have discussed a number of cognitive and somatoform disorders, along with other tension-related maladies, that have been shown empirically to benefit from PR. This specification of potentially beneficial applications means that other applications are probabilistically excluded; these would constitute the limitations of the method. One thus could not expect to use relaxation directly to remove a cancer or to cure a viral infection. At the same time, PR can be an adjunctive therapy that can ease discomfort resulting from any malady. There do not appear to be any contraindications to its use.

PR does not induce anxiety. Some investigators have reported an adverse effect of relaxation therapy, referring to it as "relaxation-induced anxiety" (e.g., Heide & Borkovec, 1984; Lazarus & Mayne, 1990). It is reported that learners become frightened of sensations, fear losing control, fear the experience of anxiety, engage in worrisome cognitive activity, and the like. "Relaxation-induced anxiety" apparently results from the use of methods of relaxation that differ from PR. Lehrer, Batey, Woolfolk, Remde, and Garlick

(1988) specified several differences between what they called "post-Jacobsonian progressive relaxation techniques" and Jacobson's PR. "Briefer methods," in which learners engage in large tensions, do not use the method of diminishing tensions, and rely heavily on suggestion, clearly depart from PR. "Relaxation-induced anxiety" apparently results from such other methods of relaxation, but it rarely if ever occurs using this approach to PR and is not a contraindication for PR. What sometimes does happen in PR during the early stages of learning to observe and control internal tension signals is that patients say such things as "I think my body is floating." In the initial stages of learning to control anxiety, a learner experiences the world beneath the skin for the first time and lacks words to describe novel sensations adequately. However, these experiences are minor, causing no undue discomfort. In any event, they are forgotten after the first month or two of training, when such ambiguous statements are replaced with more precise reports of process, such as "Tension in my lower left calf."

Another event that sometimes occurs early in the learning process is the "predormescent start," in which the trunk and limbs may give a convulsive jerk. Apparently it takes place in individuals who have been hypertense during the day's activities or are experiencing a traumatic event. The physiological mechanism may be similar to that of a nervous start, so that it disappears as relaxation progresses but may appear again after exciting experiences. In any event, some months later the learner usually does not recall having made the predormescent start.[1]

THE METHOD

Introducing the Method to the Client

The basic physiology of neuromuscular circuits and the nature of tension and relaxation are explained to the learner. Muscles, the learner is told, contain muscle fibers that are about the diameter of the human hair and are aligned in parallel. Their action is very simple, in that they can do only two things: by sliding alongside each other, they can either contract (tense) or lengthen (relax). When muscles contract, they generate the control signal that is used within neuromuscular circuits to control the functions of the body. Relaxation of the body is achieved when a person learns how to allow the muscle fibers to elongate.

The learner is provided with a realistic estimate of how far an overly tense individual has to go. It is explained that there are some 1,030 striated muscles in the human body, which make up almost half of the body weight. A lifetime of injudicious use of such a mass of muscle simply cannot respond to "quick and easy cures" for tension maladies. Just as the learner has spent a lifetime learning how to misuse the muscles, it is reasonable to expect that prolonged practice is required to reeducate them. It simply takes time and practice to learn to reverse long-standing maladaptive muscular habits. Fortunately, this cultivation of a state of bodily rest can be achieved in much less time than it took to learn deleterious muscle habits in the first place.

A frequently asked question is "How long will it take me to learn to relax?" A reasonable answer is to counter with the question "How long would it take you to learn to play the piano [or become a good golf, chess, or tennis player]?" The answer, of course, depends on where one starts and on how proficient one wishes to become. An answer more acceptable to the prospective learner is that the basic course specified in Jacobson (1964) and in McGuigan (1991a) is about 13 weeks in length. In our experience, students who take a university course covering those practice positions become quite proficient by the end of a semester. For those who have a neurotic disorder such as a phobic reaction, 6 months or a year of therapy may be required.

A disadvantage of PR is that some people complain that "it takes too much time." Such individuals simply do not understand the physiology of excessive tension and the disastrous consequences thereof. To do a proper job, as we have discussed earlier, there is no shortcut. People who complain that they "don't have enough time to practice an hour a day" can only suffer the consequences. If they let their bodies get into the painful condition of being phobic, having intense headaches, having bleeding ulcers, or the like, then they might wish that they had learned preventive PR. Jacobson's clinical experience led him to conclude that learning PR sufficiently early can add 20 years to a person's life. If one totals up all of the hours of practice and compares that with an additional 20 years of life, the practice time would seem well worthwhile. Other suggestions include the one that Jacobson gave a coauthor of this chapter, Paul Lehrer—to awaken an hour earlier each day for practice; the relaxation would give him or her the extra rest he or she needed. Certainly if one is practicing DR 24 hours a day, a considerable amount of energy *is* saved.

These are some of the essential points to get across to the beginning learner. To a large extent, the success or failure of the application depends on the learner's self-discipline—on his or her willingness to practice the method for the prescribed hour each day.

The Physical Environment and Equipment

The physical environment for teaching PR can be varied. Groups have been taught in such places as gyms, dance studios, and classrooms. The learners should have something reasonably soft to lie on, such as a thick carpet, gym mats, blankets, or sleeping bags. In clinical treatment, individual rooms in relative quietude with cots, pillows, and blankets are provided. An adept clinician can treat several patients simultaneously, one in each individual room. But whatever the learning situation, no effort is made to eliminate external distractions completely. The goal is to learn to relax in a "normal" environment, which is usually somewhat noisy. The learner should anticipate and eliminate any possible distraction during the hour of practice and should cover the body with a blanket at the start to prevent chilling (with successful relaxation, the body temperature may fall noticeably through decreased metabolic rate).

EMG Confirmation of Progress

Ideally, the clinician obtains objective EMG tension profiles as treatment progresses over the weeks. This is done to confirm any therapeutic observations of potential progress, especially reports of diminishing complaints from the patient. For illustration, abbreviated tension profiles for a nervous individual and for a relatively relaxed participant are presented in Table 4.1. This table indicates that the goal for a nervous individual is to achieve a tension profile typical of normotensives. One simplistic way of characterizing this application of PR is that it may turn a "type A" individual into a "type B"; the person's excessively tense body regions then become relatively relaxed. Observation of the nervous participant with the naked eye would typically yield such traits as the following: wrinkled forehead, frown, darting eyes, exaggerated breathing, rapid pulse and respiration, and habits of fidgeting. But even the experienced clinical eye may not properly diagnose an excessively tense individual when such obvious symptoms are absent. EMG readings are required for proper diagnosis.

**TABLE 4.1. Tension Profiles of a "Nervous"
versus a Normotensive ("Normal") Participant**

Measures	Nervous subject	Normotensive subject
Brow EMG (µV)	8.68	2.95
Left-arm EMG (µV)	2.10	0.58
Tongue EMG (µV)	5.57	2.75
Right-arm EMG (µV)	3.10	0.59
Right-leg EMG (µV)	1.36	0.53
Pulse/minute	70	69
Respirations/minute	17	15
Blood pressure (mm Hg)	117/71	96/70

Note. Adapted from Jacobson (personal communication, 1978). EMG values are based on peak-to-peak measurement.

The Therapist–Client Relationship

I have emphasized that the clinical application of PR minimizes suggestive effects so as to produce definitive and permanent, rather than fleeting, physiological changes—changes that differ from those that result from suggestion and the placebo effect. Thus the hypochondriac who continually seeks reassurance is not suggestively reassured. Instead, if the patient starts to discuss maladies during the instruction period, he or she is merely told to relax the relevant tensions away. The patient should become as independent of the clinician as possible. The teacher emphasizes that it is the learner who successfully eliminates the control signal, thus putting emphasis on the learner rather than the instructor. The clinician as teacher merely guides the learner. PR is a trial-and-error process that has to be learned step by step, with moments of success and failure. Through this process, relaxation, like any other habit, can become permanent.

Description of the Method

Preparation

The psychological set with which the learner starts each practice period is critical. This is the period in which the patient is to do absolutely nothing at all but learn to relax. The session is planned in a quiet room, free from intrusion, so that practice may be continuous for an hour without interruption from telephones, doorbells, or people entering. Any unnecessary movement, such as getting up or fidgeting, is discouraged, because these added tensions retard progress. An hour-long practice period seems optimal because the individual progressively relaxes, achieving lower and lower intensity tensions throughout the body as the hour progresses.

Program Overview

The 1,030 or so skeletal muscles in the body are studied in groups. Another meaning of "progressive relaxation" is that an individual progressively relaxes regions of the body, progressing from one muscle group to the next in a specific order. The muscle groups progressively studied are first those in the arms, then those in the legs, followed by those in the trunk, neck, and eye region, and finally by those in the speech musculature. There are, for instance, six localized muscle groups in the left arm to be studied. Table 4.2 describes the practice program for the left and right arms.

Often, the amount of instruction covered can be concentrated, if necessary, with several parts of the body covered in a single session. Lehrer and Carr (1996) have written a manual for relaxation training across only seven sessions of training.

The First Practice Session

The learner starts by lying on a couch, bed, floor, or mat with arms alongside the body. Only one position is practiced each hour, the control signal being observed three times in each period (as specified in Table 4.2). The eyes are open for several minutes and then gradually allowed to close. (The specific amount of time that elapses is not important, as the learner should not concentrate on timing or anything else. Nor should the individual actively close the eyes, as that would be work; he or she simply allows the muscle fibers around the eyes to lengthen.) When the eyes have remained closed for another several minutes, the learner raises the hand at the wrist steadily, without fluctuation; there should be no seesawing or wiggling. While the hand is being bent back, the vague sensation in the upper surface of the left forearm, a "tightness," is the signal of tension—the control signal—that the individual is to learn to recognize. The learner holds the position for a minute or two, studying the tension sensation. Then "power goes off" for a few minutes.

Thus the learner studies each major muscle group as follows: (1) identifying the control signal, and thereupon (2) relaxing the control signal away. The learner is not told where the control signal is but should find it for herself or himself. For example, when the instruction is to raise the hand vertically at the wrist, the learner comes to identify the control signal at the dorsal surface of the forearm. As the learner searches for the control signal, there may be some uncertainty about what is being sought. Some people identify the control signal immediately, whereas others have great difficulty. It is very subtle, and only a vague guess as to its location may be sufficient, but with repeated practice the control signal can become as obvious as a loud noise. Even the subtle tension sensations in the small muscles of the tongue and eyes can eventually be identified easily.

During this initial learning phase, a number of irrelevant tensions may be identified, whereupon the instructor merely informs the learner that he or she is incorrect, and searching must continue. Often the learner will erroneously report that the control signal is at the base of the wrist; this sensation, which is more prominent than the subtle control signal, is "strain." Strain is the *result* of tension and is generated by receptor cells in the

TABLE 4.2. Practice Program for the Arms

Day	Left arm	Day	Right arm
1	Bend the hand back.	8	Bend the hand back.
2	Bend the hand forward.	9	Bend the hand forward.
3	Relax only.	10	Relax only.
4	Bend the arm at the elbow.	11	Bend the arm at the elbow.
5	Press the wrist down on books.	12	Press the wrist down on books.
6	Relax only.	13	Relax only.
7	Progressive tension and relaxation of the whole arm (general, residual tension).	14	Progressive tension and relaxation of the whole arm (general, residual tension).

Note. Practice is for one period each day, performing the indicated tension three times at intervals of several minutes. Then go negative for the remainder of each period. Thus, on day 1, bend the left hand back. On day 2, bend the left hand forward, and on day 3 do nothing at all. After 14 days, you are ready to go on to the leg. From McGuigan (1991a, p. 155), as adapted from Jacobson (1964). Copyright 1991 by F. J. McGuigan. Reprinted by permission of the author's estate.

tendons and joints. That is, tension in the muscles pulls on the tendons and joints, so that tension causes strain, which is sometimes easier to perceive than muscle sensations. One cannot learn to run oneself by means of effects (strain), but only by causes (which are tension signals). Consequently, one must learn to control the body through the tension signals.

An effort to relax is a failure to relax. The process of relaxing is one in which an individual gives up the tension—just lets it go and allows the muscle fibers to elongate. Instructions that are synonymous to "relax the tension away" are to "let the power go off" and "go in the negative direction." It is to be emphasized that no work is required to allow "power off." All the learner needs to do is to discontinue working; no effort is required to follow the instruction "Just don't bother to do anything at all." Untrained people often fail to relax because they work to relax. Typically, at first the learner works the hand down, which is merely adding tension. The key is that one cannot *try* to relax; all one does is to discontinue tensing. Instruction largely consists of preventing the beginner from doing the wrong thing—that is, making an effort to relax. For instance, when the muscle fibers in the dorsal surface of the forearm elongate, the hand simply collapses like a limp dishrag that is released. When successful, all sensations in the relaxed area cease because receptor cells in the muscles "shut off." Although the learner cannot cease activity of the eyes or the ears, the muscle fibers can be instructed to stop generating signals.

In Jacobson's more intensive method, only this single instruction is given in the first instructional session. This sequence is repeated two more times. At the end of the session the therapist reviews progress and other matters of interest to the patient, answering any questions raised. A program of practice can then be scheduled for the patient; for example, following Table 4.2, the individual can be instructed to practice for 14 days on the positions specified. At the end of 2 weeks, the patient may then be asked to return to go on to the next practice area. The precise schedule and length of time between visits to the therapist can vary, depending on the requirements of patient and therapist.

After the First Practice Period

On day 2, the learner bends the left hand forward instead of backward (see Table 4.2), and so on for 14 days. As in Jacobson (1964) and McGuigan (1991a), the entire practice sequence while lying down is as follows: left arm, 7 days; right arm, 7 days; left leg, 10 days; right leg, 10 days; trunk, 10 days; neck, 6 days; eye region, 12 days; visualization, 9 days; speech region and speech imagery, 19 days.

The last region to be studied, the speech musculature, is critically important. As shown in Table 4.3, specific practice positions for the various parts of the speech musculature are presented in the first 8 days. Then the concluding days are spent in practicing developing speech imagery, so that the individual can learn to control the linguistic components of mental activities. In an analogous way, the individual learns to control the visual components of thoughts through eye control with imaginal practice of visual scenes (the "visualization" practice noted in the preceding paragraph).

After these positions are practiced lying down, they are practiced again in the same order, but in a sitting position. Repetition is the keynote of PR.

Generalized and Localized Tension

In Table 4.2, days 7 and 14 call for practice with generalized, residual tensions. In addition to localized tension (that confined to specific muscle groups), the body also gen-

TABLE 4.3. Speech Region Practice

Day	Instruction
1	Close your jaws somewhat firmly.
2	Open the jaws.
3	Relax only.
4	Show your teeth (as if smiling).
5	Pout.
6	Relax only.
7	Push your tongue forward against your teeth.
8	Pull your tongue backward.
9	Relax only.
10	Count out loud.
11	Count half as loudly.
12	Relax only.
13	Count very faintly.
14	Count imperceptibly.
15	Relax only.
16	Imagine that you are counting.
17	Imagine that you are saying the alphabet.
18	Relax only.
19	Imagine saying your name three times.
	Imagine saying your address three times.
	Imagine saying the name of the president three times.

Note. In Jacobson's preferred method, one position is to be practiced on each day, performing the indicated tension three times at intervals of several minutes. Then go negative for the remainder of each period. Thus, on day 1, close jaws somewhat firmly. On day 2, open jaws, and on day 3 do nothing at all. In practice, however, these instructions are often combined in a single session, including practice with the method of diminishing tensions and instructions to become aware of residual tension sensations. From McGuigan (1991a, p. 194), as adapted from Jacobson (1964). Copyright 1991 by F. J. McGuigan. Reprinted by permission of the author's estate.

erates a more widespread kind of tension that is carried chronically throughout the skeletal musculature. This general tension is a residual tension in which there is fine, continuous contraction of the muscle fibers. Localized relaxation allows the individual to relax a particular group of muscles, but a different technique is required for general tension. An effective procedure for controlling this widespread phenomenon is very slightly, gradually, and uniformly to stiffen (tense) an entire limb for perhaps 30 seconds or a minute. The learner then studies this sensation, which is uncomfortable and insidious. General tension differs from local tension in another respect—namely, that it appears to have no useful purpose. After the learner studies the general tension for a brief period, the muscle is then gradually relaxed over an extended period of time. If the general tension is built up within the first 15 minutes or so of the period, the remainder of the hour may be spent reducing the general tension in the limb so that the learner gradually relaxes over an extended period of time. The learner also will usually experience some residual tension sensations after thinking that the muscles are completely relaxed. Becoming aware of this residual tension and allowing it to dissipate while doing *nothing* (because *doing* is a form of tension) is one of the critical components of Jacobson's technique and differentiates it from briefer methods of training. This procedure, with sufficient practice, can allow the individual to relax residual tension down to zero, which can be verified by objective EMG measurements. Needless to say, the untrained person is not directly aware of either localized or generalized tension.

A Learner Can Relax!

Sometimes a learner asserts that he or she *cannot* relax; the point is that the learner *did not* relax. To make the point vividly, the instructor can ask the learner to push down the wall of a room. The learner fails to do so, it can be further explained, because such an act violates the laws of physics. On the other hand, elongating the muscle fibers does not violate the laws of physics. The fact that the person *did not* relax does not mean that the person *cannot* relax.

A learner who complains that he or she finds it hard to lie quietly at practice is confused about what is wanted, for there has never been an instruction to hold still *(holding* still is not relaxing). It is never "hard" to relax, for "hard" implies effort. If a learner stiffens when requested to relax, she or he is making a task of it, which is not relaxation but only an unsuccessful attempt. When the learner replaces a statement that "Relaxing makes me nervous" with the statement that "I am beginning to enjoy it," this indicates progress.

If Thoughts Occur

Some learners ask, "What shall I think about when I lie down?" They are instructed not to think, not to bother to *make* the mind blank, not to focus on anything. If they find themselves thinking about something, they should merely "let the power go off" in all the muscle regions on which they have practiced. If the thinking recurs, they should go negative again, no matter how often. But since they do not yet have control of all of their muscles, they should not expect perfection; complete elimination of thoughts can come later if they are diligent.

Also, patients should not think frequently about their symptoms as they continue relaxation training. Signs of progress may appear soon after they start, or there may be a delay, depending on such matters as how tense they are and what everyday pressures they experience. The essential point is to practice daily; if they do that, they can expect improvement. Furthermore, they should be aware that learning relaxation skills is like learning any other performance skill: two steps forward and one step back, two steps forward and one step back.

Resistance, Compliance, and Maintenance of Behavior Change

Perhaps half of those individuals who take the first step in learning PR go on to succeed in developing reasonably adequate control over their bodies, including their mental processes. This estimate covers a wide variety of potential learners, including patients who come to clinics; heterogeneous members of the community in evening classes; college, medical, and graduate students; and even professionals who participate in specialized workshops. To explain this difference in behavior would require a complex research project. Short of that, it can be said that some people have the discipline to see themselves through the program, whereas others simply do not. Clearly, the difference cannot be explained according to the need to relax, for many with the greatest need have shunned the opportunity immediately after requesting it. I (FJM) recall the president of a successful company who came for treatment of a peptic ulcer. In our second session, he confessed that he had not practiced a single day since our first instruction period. His explanation was that he had spent his life giving other people ulcers and now he resented having to deal with one for himself. It was agreed that further "treatment" would be a waste of time for all concerned.

Healthy individuals seem to learn more quickly than do patients in distress. Those with neurotic disorders, for instance, are distracted, and their learning is thus prolonged. People who are engaged in cultist activities and fads are especially suggestible and dependent, which makes it more difficult for the teacher to get them to rely on themselves. They have many bizarre ideas that interfere with their learning to relax, and much time can be lost if the teacher chooses to argue with them. Similarly, people who have excessive faith in the clinician also generally fail to observe tensions for themselves and take longer to relax than do average individuals.

Such illustrations of resistance and failure to comply could be enumerated indefinitely, but the problem is not unique to PR. In many spheres of life people behave in a self-destructive fashion, even when they can verbalize the contingencies between their behavioral inadequacies and the consequences thereof. Failure to take prescribed medication for high blood pressure, drug (including alcohol) abuse, and smoking are examples of such self-destructive behaviors. There is often little anyone can do for individuals who engage in denial processes, such as the hospital nurse who asserted that her cigarette smoking was healthy for her. For those individuals who can verbalize the contingencies, perhaps there is some limited hope if they will at least try to discipline themselves in efforts to develop self-operations control—in other words, to enhance their "willpower" (McGuigan, 1991a).

On the other hand, many of those individuals who have dedicated themselves to daily practice and to regular instruction have made amazing progress. A wide variety of symptoms have been alleviated or eliminated, with lasting effects, as shown by follow-up testing (Jacobson, 1938, 1970). The following is adapted from a classic illustrative case reported by Jacobson (1970).

CASE EXAMPLE:
A CASE OF ANXIETY, EXHAUSTION, AND ACROPHOBIA

Summary

A middle-level manager for a large bank, 32 years old, believed that he had overworked to the point of permanent exhaustion; in his words, he felt "burned out" for life. He was uneasy, irritable, and often dizzy and could not speak in front of colleagues or drive a car for fear of fainting or other discomfort. His fears kept him from high places. "Reasoning" and "fighting" these "ridiculous" symptoms only made them worse. The symptoms had first appeared about 4 or 5 years previously. Instruction in progressive relaxation was begun, omitting all reassurance and other "suggestive therapy." Soon he discontinued treatment and went elsewhere; but after several weeks he returned. Gradually with persistence he developed excellence in observating and reporting on his tension patterns. Voluntarily he acted as a participant in electrophysiological studies on mental activities. Action-potential measurements indicated increasing skill in maintaining relaxed states, when lying, when sitting quietly, or when reading. He "made it a rule to relax any phobia or disturbing thought-act." Two years later, his symptoms and complaints had diminished; he was able to resume public speaking appearances and to drive without nervous difficulties. He was then discharged anxiety-free. Evidently acrophobia was no longer present, for without telling the doctor he took another position, located in the tower of a high building. Twenty-nine years thereafter he reports that he still practices progressive relaxation, although not so regularly as he should. Throughout this period there has been no recurrence of the anxiety, phobias, or other disabilities about which he had complained initially.

Complaints

An exceedingly busy middle-level bank manager, 32 years of age, was referred by a relative, a physician, for an anxiety state that included fears of heights and of dizziness, general uneasiness and irritability, and headache at the vertex and the occiput. He stated that he had been living at high tension all day long and in his opinion was "burned out" for life. Walking down the street or speaking at corporate meetings, he was suddenly beset by fears of dizziness, making him feel very uncomfortable. At times he felt as if he were about to faint, and because he had never fainted, he felt that this was "all ridiculous." "Fighting" the aforementioned symptoms had only made them worse; he had tried to reason matters out and had tried to relax, he had tried to get his mind off of himself, but all had been in vain. He was particularly concerned because when speaking at meetings about his areas of responsibility, he suddenly began to fear becoming dizzy. In consequence, he had been caused to avoid these meetings, delegating speaking responsibilities to a subordinate, feeling, however, that sometime he would return.

Onset

The onset had been 4 or 5 years previously, in the middle of a presentation, when confronted by a challenging and somewhat abusive superior. At the time he suffered from pain in the left lower portion of his thorax, both subcardially and laterally. He successfully completed his presentation, however, and his recommendations were accepted by the group. The symptoms disappeared after the use of belladonna plasters and the administration of a tonic. But he had begun to feel anxious about one set of matters, and the anxiety turned gradually to others. His relative, the doctor, had suggested that if he would pay no attention to his symptoms, they would disappear. Accordingly, he had said to himself, "Get your mind off it. Forget it." This seemed to bring him relief for about 6 months. Then, however, the symptoms insidiously recurred.

Personal History

Among previous diseases had been a severe case of influenza 9 years previously. Two months prior to symptom recurrence, he suffered from cystitis following cystoscopy, and since then occasional blood cells had appeared in his urine. As a rule he slept well, but there were exceptions of late when he continued to worry. He had been married for 9 years and had two children, a boy and a girl, both well. His parents were well, except that his mother was rheumatic and worrisome.

General Examination and Clinical Laboratory Tests

General examination disclosed a fairly well-nourished man looking the age stated. His pulse was regular at the rate of 96 in the sitting posture, and his blood pressure was 130/96. His temperature was 98.6°F. He was 5 feet 7 inches tall and weighed about 157 pounds. General examination revealed a somewhat pendulous abdominal wall but otherwise no significant findings, aside from an extremely lively foot-flexion reflex. Laboratory tests supplied by his relative indicated Wasserman and Kahn reactions negative; basal metabolism, −12; blood nonprotein nitrogen, 27 mg%; urea nitrogen, 15 mg%; blood sugar, 84 mg%; red blood count, 4,310,000; white count, 6,500; hemoglobin, 75% with a color index of 0.8. The differential count fell within normal limits. Fluoroscopy of the chest proved negative. Urine analysis was completely negative, aside from a few mucous threads.

Instruction Begun

Instruction in progressive relaxation was begun. At this time, over a 10-year period, I [Edmund Jacobson] was attempting to rule out from our procedures all use of any form of suggestive therapy, so far as this might be possible. To this end, I tried to avoid not only reassurance to the patient in any possible form but also unnecessary conversation. I attempted to confine our relationship to instruction in the forms of progressive relaxation appropriate to the patient's needs in my judgment. Accordingly, when the patient asked questions bearing upon the outcome of the instruction, hoping that it might prove favorable, or when he was in doubt that the instruction really applied to his case, I avoided answers that might possibly be interpreted by him suggestively. In reaction to this, the patient lost confidence after a month or two of instruction, suddenly leaving to go elsewhere for "psychiatric treatment." After 3 weeks of absence with little ado or comment on either side, he returned to complete his course.

Second month of treatment. He has been learning. He states that when emotionally disturbed he localizes the tension patterns and lets them go.

Eighth month of treatment. Instruction devoted to review of tension patterns in the eyelids and eyeballs. Practice is given in observing tension patterns and going negative upon looking in various directions with eyelids closed and looking from finger to finger with eyelids open.

Visualization Found Impossible during Complete Eye Muscle Relaxation

Visualization training. He is requested to imagine that he is seeing the fingers held about 10 feet away from his eyes, but at the same time to remain perfectly relaxed. He reports that he finds this instruction impossible to carry out. He finds it necessary to exert effort tensions of the eyes, that is, to look in specific directions, if he is to imagine objects seen. This request and report are typical of our endeavors to secure objective reports from highly trained patients, without leading them to anticipate the answers. Indeed, these autosensory observations with patients have been carried out under strictly controlled methods characteristic of laboratories of experimental psychology.

Autosensory Observation during Emotion

One week later. He mentions fear of being in a high building, but fails to give a clear-cut sensory and imaginal report, evidently not yet prepared to describe his experiences, but losing himself in the emotion. He is given further instruction in observing and in reporting matters of visual imagination of indifferent affect.

The following weeks. He continues to be emotionally disturbed from time to time. Training is devoted to the musculature of speech, with particular reference to steady or static tensions.

Two months later. He states that today he has suffered from phobia of high places. Instruction is given in verbal imagination. As yet he fails to recognize tension patterns in the various muscles of speech and to state their locations.

Autosensory Observation during Unemotional Experiences

One week later. He enters the clinic exultant over his personal discovery that attention to the object of fear diminishes the fear. Instruction today begins in the lying posture with the request, "Think of infinity." He fails to report the imaginal, the tension, and other signal patterns, stating only the meaning of his reflection. However, when requested to engage in simple multiplication, as of 14 by 42, he gives a complete report, not only of the meaning but also of the tension pattern. He is given repeated practice in observation of sensory experiences, distinguishing the report thereof from the interpretation or meaning.

Anger Tension Relaxed

He announces that he now relaxes spells of anger and has been gaining in weight; and, as noted by his family physician, he no longer fidgets as he did formerly upon receiving a hypodermic injection. Upon being requested to describe an experience of phobia, he still engages in the "stimulus error" but to a lesser extent than formerly.

One month later. Differential relaxation is begun, with training devoted to the right arm. He has been at home with a fever of 101°F at times, due to an infection of the right kidney and of the bladder.

Instruction during the 4 following weeks. Instruction on the limbs is continued in the sitting posture. At times during the period while sitting, he is on the verge of sleep.

Efficiency

At the end of this time, he asserts that now he does his work effectively and without nervous excitement in a manner which had never previously been possible.

One week later. He complains of tension in the right side of the scalp, mistaking pull or strain on the scalp for muscular tension. After drill in wrinkling of the forehead, he reports relief.

One week later. Instruction is devoted to the abdomen and back in the sitting posture.

One month later. He affirms that his nerves are greatly improved. At times a little phobia persists, but he is becoming accustomed to observe tension patterns at such moments and to relax them. His relative, the doctor, recently was amazed at his calmness in public speaking, in contrast with his extreme excitability in former years. Friends who do not know of the instruction which he has been receiving spontaneously say to him that he is a changed man.

Phobic Tension Patterns Now Recognized and Relaxed

The following 2 weeks. He states that he has been in very good nervous condition and has been efficient. He makes it a rule to relax any phobia or disturbing thought-act. Instruction concerns brow tensions. He often sleeps during the period.

The following 4 weeks, sequentially. Repeated practice is given on imagining falling objects of indifferent affect. The purpose here is to teach him to observe the pattern of mental processes when any object falls. Thus a first step is taken in his learning to observe what he does in high places when he imagines himself jumping and falling. Thus, without telling him, we proceed in the treatment of acrophobia.

Return of Ability to Present at Meetings

Six weekly sessions, beginning 2 months later. For the first time in years, he speaks in public without nervous difficulties. His phobia at meetings has disappeared. Instruction is devoted to musculature of speech.

Return of Ability to Drive and to Go on Trips; No Acrophobia

One week later. He reports that for the first time in about 7 years he has taken a long drive. Previously fearful, but not knowing why, he now finds that he enjoys driving. Previous to present instruction, he dreaded and avoided speaking outside of his city. Recently, in contrast, he has gone on three long trips with no difficulty. Nowadays, he travels enjoyably, whereas previously he did it with dread. The phobia of jumping from high places has been completely absent. Last month was a very difficult time in his business, because large loans for which he was responsible came due at the height of the panic and bank failures of the Great Depression. Nevertheless, he was relaxed and not nervous. He adds that he relaxes concerns about business meetings. He no longer mentally argues business strategies, but he instead "relaxes the whole thought." Instruction is devoted to tension signals from the tongue and relaxation of tongue muscles.

The following 3 weeks. Instruction concerns imagining making various statements. He is still slow to relax to the point at which he is ready to observe and report. However, his reports are clear.

One month later. Instruction is begun relaxing the left arm as much as possible while reading.

Nine successive sessions. Instruction on reading is continued, while observing tension patterns and learning to relax muscles not required for the reading. He fails to report verbal tensions during reading, claiming that there are none, but only visual images and ocular tension patterns. Obviously his training is not yet sufficient, but he is not so informed.

One month later. His brother-in-law died suddenly. Instruction is devoted to exposing a single printed stimulus word within the instruction to read and get the meaning. At first his reports are confused: He gives interpretations in place of observations. Finally he begins to report more accurately, as follows: "Ocular tension in seeing the word. Ocular tension in imagining what the word indicates. Tensions in the tongue as in saying the word."

Slight Relapse, yet Patient Not Told What to Look For

One week later. Yesterday he experienced some nervous distress at a business meeting. Upon relaxing, the unnecessary emotions disappeared. He has been through various trying ordeals. For 2 months he has failed to report tensions in the organs of speech while reading. Accordingly he is requested to count while reading, employing the method of diminishing tensions. Finally he succeeds in observing the speech tensions. This occurs with no hint from the instructor that he has been omitting anything.

Relaxes Differentially

One week later. There have been four deaths in the family, which ordinarily would have disturbed him much more, he believes. However, in place of engaging in fears and worries each morning, now he goes to work relaxing and preparing himself to relax during the day. He has found that he does not have to postpone relaxation to the weekend but can relax during the work of each day. Accordingly he is greatly relieved.

Discharged

The following 2 weeks. Instruction is given in reading aloud, relaxing as much as possible during this occupation. He is discharged, apparently free from emotional disturbance. Electrical recording has shown excellent technique.

Freedom from Acrophobia

Following this patient's discharge, the phobia of high places had so evidently disappeared that, without suggestion from the doctor, he took a position with an office in the tower of a very high office building. In his new office, he felt no fear or phobia. Regarding his nervous condition, he considered himself well. He practices differential relaxation every day. On some days he fails to lie down, but as a rule, after dinner he practices in a lying posture for 45 to 90 minutes. On about half of these occasions he falls asleep. If he awakens at night and finds himself tense, he locates the tension patterns and relaxes accordingly. Uneasiness no longer is experienced, and he no longer shows marked irritability. When engaged in difficult matters, he relaxes so as to avoid becoming irritated. He has no dizziness, no fears, and no headaches. His technique shows excellent form.

Two years later. Electrical recording is performed with the eyes open. The right thigh averages little over 0.5 μV. The right biceps averages little over 0.075 μV with little variability (V). The right jaw muscles average in the neighborhood of 0.2 (V. The eye regions average about 3.5 μV. The values are fair for a trained individual except that variability is a little high.

Five years later. He reports that for the first time in his life, he has completely lost fear of being in high places. He flew in an airplane and at first was fearful when breathing through tubes of oxygen provided for this purpose, but he used his relaxation technique and enjoyed the flying trip from then on. He relaxes differentially to an extent that is readily appreciated by a professional observer.

Persistent Freedom from Anxiety Tension, Although Difficulties Remain

Five years afterward (10 years after discharge). He relates that he was "wonderfully well" for many years following the instruction. Ten years previously his daughter married, but the next year she became very unhappy, which was a "terrific jolt" to him. "During that whole year I suffered from worry, hoping that the situation would straighten out." His daughter was operated on for appendicitis and recovered. She joined him for a few weeks only, after which she returned home, because her husband needed her. "This," continued our patient, "took quite a bit out of me. Then my son was drafted for the war; usually parents worry about that. That year, loose [bowel] movements had occurred once or twice a year and I didn't know what started them. Certain medication overcame any spell promptly. Also I could avert the spells by avoiding raw fruits and vegetables. Five years later the spells became more intense and frequent. My brother-in-law got me into a business of his own, in which I sunk time and a small fortune. Two years later I foolishly let him leave the partnership. Thereafter he enticed the plant manager away, which proved irritating and took my time and interfered with my full-time position. Engineers called in to help the business gave bad counsel with resulting further loss. Later that year I sold the business for a pittance."

Irritable Colon

During the period of gastrointestinal distress, a severe spell of diarrhea was followed by X-ray examination and a diagnosis of duodenal ulcer. The symptoms disappeared after a short period of diet restriction and medication. Since then, there have been only two light spells and one severe spell with burning in the rectum.

Practice Neglected

"It was in the attempt to get rid of nervous disturbance that I sold the plant and returned to more or less regular periods of relaxation, which I had been neglecting, and to which I ascribed alone my lasting improvement. My downfall had been that practice was not regular."

Refresher, 10 years after discharge. A brief refresher course is begun.

First week. Roentgenological examination indicates negative findings as to duodenal ulcer. The colon, however, is found to be spastic. A similar examination made previously suggested that possibly there had been an early ulcer. At this time, however, he has been relaxing a little more frequently than before and has been able to partake once more of solids.

Fourteen weekly sessions. Review practice is given on limb tension patterns and relaxation.

Ten years after the refresher. His wife writes from her observations in retrospect that through relaxation training he had learned "a new way of life."

The following year. He reports that he has been free from anxiety tension, phobias, fears, and other emotional disturbances these many years. He is able to speak at meetings and public forums where and when he desires and has continued to be generally more relaxed than he had ever been in the decade before he reached the age of 32, when instruction had begun.

COMMENTS

The contemporary scene has been flooded with stress management procedures, varying from thinking certain colors while breathing through one nostril to repetitiously talking to oneself. There are a variety of muscular relaxation procedures, too, that are generally acknowledged as having flowed from PR. In the last analysis, which methods are most effective must be empirically determined. The primary criterion for assessing the effectiveness of a stress management procedure that purports to teach a person to relax is the extent to which the individual is able to selectively allow his or her muscle fibers to elongate on command—that is, to relax differentially in the face of stress. Once the person can thereby exercise self-operations control, he or she can more rationally deal with the stressful situation instead of just reflexively responding to it.

Edmund Jacobson spent over seven decades collecting data documenting the effectiveness of PR clinically and scientifically, including the use of EMG. We should all be indebted to him for giving the world PR, the grandfather of all relaxation methods. We can think of no better way to close this chapter than to quote Jacobson as follows:

> Until I see proof I incline in the direction of skepticism. Progressive relaxation, as developed in our laboratory and clinic, was to me a matter of skepticism at every step. Thirty years ago as I went from room to room trying to get individuals with different maladies to relax, I recall saying to myself, "What kind of nonsense is this that you are practicing?" The careful accumulation of data has vindicated the procedure. (1977, p. 123)

NOTE

1. In my own (FJM) experience, one day after some years of training, Jacobson instructed me to recall the most terrible even in my life. My reaction, similar to the predormescent start, was that my legs involuntarily flew directly into the air. My recollection was of a horrible event involving the use of my legs on the brakes of an automobile. (Later I asked Jacobson whether that was a normal reaction, but apparently I was being used as a guinea pig, because he said he had never given that instruction before.)

ACKNOWLEDGMENTS

We are deeply indebted to Edmund Jacobson for so many things that it would be impossible to list them all here. First and foremost, though, we would specify the innumerable hours and limitless energy that he spent in personally training both of us in PR. More specifically for this chapter, we are indebted to him for the ideas, principles, and applications and, in fact, often even for the use of his words, which have become part of our own repertoire.

REFERENCES

Bain, A. (1855). *The senses and the intellect.* London: Parker.

Bernhaut, M., Gellhorn, E., & Rasmussen, A. T. (1953). Experimental contributions to the problem of consciousness. *Journal of Neurophysiology, 16,* 21–35.

Cannon, W. B. (1929). *Bodily changes in pain, hunger, fear, and rage.* New York: Appleton-Century.

Carrington, P., Collings, G. H., Jr., Benson, H., Robinson, H., Wood, L. W., Lehrer, P. M., et al. (1980) The use of meditation-relaxation techniques for the management of stress in a working population. *Journal of Occupational Medicine, 22,* 211–231.

Davidson, D. M., Winchester, M. A., Taylor, C. B., Alderman, E. A., & Ingels, N. B., Jr. (1979). Effects of relaxation therapy on cardiac performance and sympathetic activity in patients with organic heart disease. *Psychosomatic Medicine, 41,* 303–309.

Delius, W., Hagbarth, K. E., Hongell, A., & Wallin, B. G. (1972). General characteristics of sympathetic activity in human muscle nerves. *Acta Physiologica Scandinavica, 84,* 65B81.

Gay, M.-C., Philippot, P., & Luminet, O. (2002). Differential effectiveness of psychological interventions for reducing osteoarthritis pain: A comparison of Erickson hypnosis and Jacobson relaxation. *European Journal of Pain, 6,* 1–16.

Gellhorn, E. (1958). The physiological basis of neuromuscular relaxation. *Archives of Internal Medicine, 102,* 392–399.

Gellhorn, E., & Kiely, W. F. (1972). Mystical states of consciousness: Neurophysiological and clinical aspects. *Journal of Nervous and Mental Disease, 154,* 399–405.

Grassi, C., & Passatore, M. (1988). Action of the sympathetic system on skeletal muscle Italian. *Journal of Neurological Sciences, 9,* 23–28.

Heide, F. J., & Borkovec, T. D. (1984). Relaxation-induced anxiety: Mechanisms and theoretical implications. *Behaviour Research and Therapy*, 22, 1–12.

Holt, E. B. (1937). Materialism and the criterion of the psychic. *Psychological Review*, 44, 33–53.

Jacobson, E. (1938). *Progressive relaxation* (2nd ed.). Chicago: University of Chicago Press.

Jacobson, E. (1964). *Self-operations control: A manual of tension control*. Chicago: National Foundation
for Progressive Relaxation.

Jacobson, E. (1967). *Biology of emotions*. Springfield, IL: Thomas.

Jacobson, E. (1970). *Modern treatment of tense patients*. Springfield, IL: Thomas.

Jacobson, E. (1977). The origins and development of progressive relaxation. *Journal of Behavior Therapy and Experimental Psychiatry*, 8, 119–123.

Jacobson, E. (1978). *You must relax* (4th ed.). New York: McGraw-Hill.

Kienbaum, P., Karlssonn, T., Sverrisdottir, Y. B., Elam, M., & Wallin, B. G. (2001). Two sites for modulation of human sympathetic activity by arterial baroreceptors? *Journal of Physiology*, 531, 861–869.

Lazarus, A. A., & Mayne, T. J. (1990). Relaxation: Some limitations, side effects, and proposed solutions. *Psychotherapy*, 27, 261–266.

Lehrer, P. M. (1978). Psychophysiological effects of progressive relaxation in anxiety neurotic patients
and of progressive relaxation and alpha feedback in non-patients. *Journal of Consulting and Clinical Psychology*, 46, 389–404.

Lehrer, P. M. (1982). How to relax and how not to relax: A reevaluation of the work of Edmund Jacobson. *Behaviour Research and Therapy*, 20, 417–428.

Lehrer, P. M., Atthowe, J. M., & Weber, E. S. (1980). Effects of progressive relaxation and autogenic
training on anxiety and physiological measures, with some data on hypnotizability. In F. J.
McGuigan, W. Sime, & J. M. Wallace (Eds.), *Stress and tension control* (pp. 171–184). New York:
Plenum Press.

Lehrer, P. M., Batey, D. M., Woolfolk, R. L., Remde, A., & Garlick, T. (1988). The effect of repeated
tense–release sequences on EMG and self-report of muscle tension: An evaluation of Jacobsonian
and post-Jacobsonian assumptions about progressive relaxation. *Psychophysiology*, 25, 562–569.

Lehrer, P. M., & Carr, R. (1996). Progressive relaxation. In W. T. Roth (Ed.), *Treating anxiety disorders*
(pp. 83–116). San Francisco: Jossey-Bass.

Lehrer, P. M., Schoicket, S., Carrington, P., & Woolfolk, R. L. (1980). Psychophysiological and cognitive
responses to stressful stimuli in subjects practicing progressive relaxation and clinically standardized meditation. *Behavior Research and Therapy*, 18, 293–303.

Lehrer, P. M., Vaschillo, E., Vaschillo, B., Lu, S.-E., Scardella, A., Siddique, M., et al. (2004). Biofeedback
treatment for asthma. *Chest*, 126, 352–361.

Lehrer, P. M., Woolfolk, R. L., & Goldman, N. (1986). Progressive relaxation then and now: Does
change always mean progress? In R. J. Davidson, G. E. Schwartz, & D. Shapiro (Eds.), *Consciousness and self-regulation* (Vol. 4, pp. 183–216). New York: Plenum Press.

McCann, B. S., Woolfolk, R. L., & Lehrer, P. M. (1987). Specificity in response to treatment: A study of
interpersonal anxiety. *Behaviour Research and Therapy*, 25, 129–136.

McGlynn, F. D., Moore, P. M., Lawyer, S., & Karg, R. (1999). Relaxation training inhibits fear and
arousal during in vivo exposure to phobia-cue stimuli. *Journal of Behavior Therapy and Experimental Psychiatry*, 30, 155–168.

McGuigan, F. J. (1978). *Cognitive psychophysiology: Principles of covert behavior*. Englewood Cliffs.
NJ: Prentice-Hall.

McGuigan, F. J. (1989). Managing internal cognitive and external environmental stresses through progressive relaxation. In F. J. McGuigan, W. Sime, & J. M. Wallace (Eds.), *Stress and tension control:
3. Stress management* (pp. 3–11). New York: Plenum Press.

McGuigan, F. J. (1991a). *Calm down: A guide for stress and tension control* (Rev. ed.). Dubuque, IA:
Kendall/ Hunt.

McGuigan, F. J. (1991b). Control of normal and pathological cognitive functions through neuromuscular
circuits: Applications of principles of progressive relaxation. In J. G. Carlson & A. R. Seifert (Eds.),
International perspectives on self-regulation and health (pp. 121–131). New York: Plenum Press.

McGuigan, F. J., Culver, V. L., & Kendler, T. S. (1971). Covert behavior as a direct electromyographic
measure of mediating responses. *Conditional Reflex*, 6, 145–152.

McGuigan, F. J., & Dollins, A. B. (1989). Patterns of covert speech behavior and phonetic coding. *Pav-
lovian Journal of Biological Science*, 24, 19–26.

McGuigan, F. J., & Pavek, G. V. (1972). On the psychophysiological identification of covert nonoral language processes. *Journal of Experimental Psychology, 92,* 237–245.

McGuigan, F. J., & Winstead, C. L., Jr. (1974). Discriminative relationship between covert oral behavior and the phonemic system in internal information processing. *Journal of Experimental Psychology, 103,* 885–890.

Murphy, A. I., Lehrer, P. M., & Jurish, S. (1990). Cognitive coping skills training and relaxation training as treatments for tension headaches. *Behavior Therapy, 21,* 89–98.

Nicassio, P., & Bootzin, R. (1974). A comparison of progressive relaxation and autogenic training as treatments for insomnia. *Journal of Abnormal Psychology, 83,* 253–260.

Roatta, S., Windhorst, U., Ljubisavljevic, M., Johansson, H., & Passatore, M. (2002). Sympathetic modulation of muscle spindle afferent sensitivity to stretch in rabbit jaw closing muscles. *Journal of Physiology, 540,* 237–248.

Schaer, B., & Isom, S. (1988). Effectiveness of progressive relaxation on test anxiety and visual perception. *Psychological Reports, 63,* 511–518.

Setterlind, S. (1983). Teaching relaxation in physical education lessons. I. Psychological results from empirical studies on school. *Scandinavian Journal of Sports Sciences, 5,* 56–59.

Shapiro, S., & Lehrer, P. M. (1980). Psychophysiological effects of autogenic training and progressive relaxation. *Biofeedback and Self-Regulation, 5,* 249–255.

Wiener, N. (1948). *Cybernetics.* New York: Wiley.

Woolfolk, R. L., Lehrer, P. M., McCann, B. S., & Rooney, A. J. (1982). Effects of progressive relaxation and meditation on cognitive and somatic manifestations of daily stress. *Behaviour Research and Therapy, 20,* 461–468.

CHAPTER 5

Progressive Relaxation
Abbreviated Methods

DOUGLAS A. BERNSTEIN
CHARLES R. CARLSON
JOHN E. SCHMIDT

In each of the previous editions of this volume, we began this chapter by noting that we live in a world full of tension and anxiety in which relaxation is a much-sought-after goal. The chapter for the second edition (Bernstein & Carlson, 1993) was written during the time of the Persian Gulf War, and the chapter for this edition was written after the invasion of Iraq and the third anniversary of the 9/11 terrorist incidents. Although much has changed during the decade between versions of this chapter, the search for relaxation remains important, especially for those in whom emotional arousal produces severe subjective distress, overt behavioral problems, and damage to various organ systems. Clinicians and researchers seeking nonpharmacological methods of promoting relaxation and combating anxiety have developed a number of useful procedures, the most popular of which is referred to as *progressive relaxation training*. As noted in the introductory chapters of this volume, progressive relaxation training is not a single method but a group of techniques that vary considerably in procedural detail, complexity, and length. Our goal in this chapter is to focus attention on the form known as abbreviated progressive relaxation training (APRT) and to update the scientific literature that has been developed over the past 10 years concerning the use of APRT.

HISTORY

The history of APRT as we now know it originates in the work of Edmund Jacobson during the early part of this century. The course of its development and use in Jacobson's laboratory and clinic has been reviewed by McGuigan and Lehrer in Chapter 4 of this volume. Jacobson's technique can be lengthy and painstaking. The entire training in all muscle groups may sometimes require 100 or more sessions over a period of several months or even years.

A considerably condensed version of progressive relaxation training was presented by Joseph Wolpe (1958) in the context of the classic work on counterconditioning methods for fear reduction, which ultimately led to the development of systematic desensitization. Wolpe saw relaxation not as an end in itself but as one of several responses (including assertiveness and sexual arousal) that are incompatible with, and thus capable of inhibiting, anxiety. Accordingly, he shortened Jacobson's original procedures to make them fit within the framework of systematic desensitization. "The reason why I have not resorted to Jacobson's intensive program is that by the desensitization method . . . I have been able to overcome anxieties . . . on the basis of such relaxation as is attained by my brief method of training" (Wolpe, 1958, p. 136).

In contrast to Jacobson's program, which focused on a single muscle group for several sessions before moving on to the next muscle group, Wolpe's brief method taught the client to relax several of 16 major muscle groups in each of about seven sessions. By shortening the procedure in this way, Wolpe was able to get on more quickly to the main component of treatment—namely, desensitization proper. Wolpe's methods also contrasted with Jacobson's in offering instructions and suggestions (such as "smooth it out" or "let it go further") about what the client should do following tension release.

The APRT methods described in this chapter represent a further modification of Jacobson's procedures as described by Paul (1966) and first formalized by Bernstein and Borkovec (1973). Among these modifications are tension-release cycle times that are considerably shorter than Wolpe's; inclusion of practice with all 16 muscle groups in every training session; introduction of the "pendulum" analogy to explain the need for tension cycles; and much more elaborate and active verbal input from the therapist (in the form of indirect relaxation suggestions) during training. These changes came about in the late 1960s and early 1970s and represented not only an effort to streamline progressive relaxation further for use in systematic desensitization but also to supplement and facilitate other methods (such as participant modeling) in the then-burgeoning list of behavioral approaches to anxiety-related problems.

THEORETICAL FOUNDATION

The theoretical basis of APRT is consistent with the rationale presented in Chapter 4 for Jacobson's progressive relaxation training. Briefly, it is assumed that anxiety and other emotional states involve subjective, behavioral, and physiological components that interact to create the ongoing emotional experience (Lang, 1977, 1979). For example, when physiological activation is perceived and labeled as "fear" or "anxiety," the client reports being afraid or anxious or nervous. Such reports and/or the cognitions preceding or accompanying them may act as additional fear-provoking stimuli that further amplify the autonomic arousal. This can lead to increased subjective discomfort and even more physiological activation in a continuing spiral that may culminate in panic, cognitive flooding, or a variety of other behavioral and physiological consequences.

APRT is believed to intervene in this process by providing a way of reducing autonomic activation. The early laboratory research of Jacobson (1938) and Gellhorn (1958; Gellhorn & Kiely, 1972) suggested that overactivation of the sympathetic branch of the autonomic nervous system is primarily responsible for excessive skeletal muscle activity. When skeletal muscle activity is reduced with progressive relaxation, Gellhorn (1958) proposed that there is a corresponding reduction in sympathetic nervous system activity as a result of negative feedback from the skeletal muscle proprioceptors to the ascending reticular activation system and hypothalamus. Resting muscles send little or no feedback information from the skeletal muscle proprioceptors to central brain structures; the lack of feedback information is believed to result in decreased autonomic activation. Direct supportive evidence from human studies of this model has been sparse. However, indirect evidence (e.g., decreased heart rate and blood pressure) from human research supports the efficacy of APRT in reducing autonomic activation (see reviews by Borkovec & Sides, 1979; Carlson & Hoyle, 1993; King, 1980; Lehrer, 1982; Luebbert, Dahme, & Hasenbring, 2001). Once autonomic activity is reduced, the client should be more capable of (1) providing meaningful assessment information to the clinician, (2) tolerating fear-provoking stimuli, (3) learning more adaptive responses to such stimuli, and (4) learning or using rational cognitions that help to forestall or eliminate subsequent problematic activation.

APRT seeks to reduce the autonomic activation component of anxiety by altering one of its manifestations—namely, skeletal muscle tension. As muscle tension drops, other, less directly accessible aspects of autonomic activation, such as heart rate and blood pressure, are also lowered. It is unclear whether alteration of peripheral muscle tension alone is sufficient to explain the effects of progressive relaxation training. For example, it has been argued that central nervous system events—primarily focused attention and pleasant cognitions—may be vital to clinically significant reductions in autonomic activation (Benson, 1975; Davison, 1966; King, 1980). When a client learns how to tense and release muscle groups and to use other relaxation techniques (to be described later), he or she is, at the very least, developing a set of voluntary skills that can then be used to reduce maladaptive autonomic activation and to prevent such activation from reaching a troublesome level in the first place.

It is worth noting that the skills the client learns through APRT represent but one way of achieving a state of deep relaxation. There are many other routes to that state (e.g., biofeedback, controlled breathing, autogenic training, stretch-based relaxation, and quiet meditation), all of which appear to capitalize on similar or related psychophysiological mechanisms (see Smith, 1985). Thus the choice of APRT for use in a given clinical situation must be made not because it leads to a relaxed state that is unique but because it meets the needs of the client and clinician.

ASSESSMENT

Clinical Indications

APRT has been successfully used, alone or in combination with other methods, to deal with a wide range of behavior problems in adults and children. Reviews of the progressive relaxation literature (see Borkovec & Sides, 1979; Carlson & Hoyle, 1993; Hyman, Feldman, Harris, Levin, & Malloy, 1989; King, 1980; Lehrer, 1982; Lehrer & Woolfolk, 1984) consistently affirm the clinical efficacy of progressive relaxation training for insomnia, generalized anxiety and stress, specific anxieties and phobias, hypertension, and tension headache. The list sometimes includes asthma in children (Borkovec & Sides, 1979; King, 1980, Lehrer & Woolfolk, 1984), aversion to chemotherapy and spasmodic dysmenorrhea (Lehrer & Woolfolk, 1984), and chronic pain (Hyman et al., 1989). Unfortunately, however, not all of these reviews have distinguished between APRT and other forms of progressive relaxation.

In order to update the current status of research on the effectiveness of APRT, we conducted a computer search of papers published since 1991 that concern progressive relaxation. The "Methods" sections of 24 of the resulting studies indicated that APRT was employed as the primary independent variable. Of these studies, 12 specified the treatment population and used multiple controls (a placebo or attention-treatment comparison group, a waiting-list control group, and/or a no-treatment control group). These 12 studies are summarized in Table 5.1 and generally suggest that APRT can lead to improvement in quality of life for cancer patients; reduction of symptoms of posttraumatic stress disorder; increased sleep quality; reduced stress and anxiety in persons with generalized anxiety disorder, women with urinary dysfunction, and people without dysfunctions; reduced blood pressure in persons with hypertension; and reduction in headache symptoms. In the other 12 studies that did not include multiple controls, improved behavioral performances in patients with Alzheimer's could be added to the list of positive responses to APRT (see Table 5.2). Given the converging evidence of these outcome studies and the conclusions of earlier reviews, we can place increased confidence in the clinical utility of APRT for selected disorders in which reduced physiological activation and improved psychological functioning are desired.

The use of APRT is governed by the judgment that maladaptive levels of autonomic arousal are at least partly responsible for the development and maintenance of the problems that bring the client to treatment. However, recognition of the fact that APRT can play a beneficial role in dealing with many diverse human problems must not lead to the conclusion that it will always be useful or that it is the treatment of choice for all clients whose complaints match those reported in the clinical literature. It is imperative that clinicians be sensitive to the needs of their clients in determining whether or not APRT may be of benefit.

It is generally safe to say that in the vast majority of cases involving clinical problems similar to those listed previously, the use of APRT is probably going to be of some help and is not likely to do harm even if a client is unprepared for the very small possibility of undesirable side effects (discussed later in this chapter). Furthermore, the time spent in teaching relaxation skills may provide a positive experience for both therapist and client; such an experience helps establish a good, task-oriented working relationship. Still, it must be recognized that time spent on APRT for, say, general tension cannot be spent in working directly with other problems, which in a given case may require immediate attention.

Thus, as is true for any clinical method, the decision to employ APRT must be based on careful evaluation of the full range of causal, contributing, maintenance, and complicating factors that may be related to a client's complaints. The information gathered in assessment should determine whether APRT is the intervention of choice, alone or in combination with other treatment modalities (e.g., assertiveness training), or whether the client's problems reflect factors (e.g., basic skill deficits) that call for more appropriate initial interventions. Relaxation training is most effectively used when it addresses client needs that are recognized and understood by both the therapist and the client.

The questions outlined next do not constitute an exhaustive list of items to consider in assessment, but they do provide a basic framework for inquiry that can easily be elaborated according to the dictates of each unique situation.

1. *Is there evidence that the client's complaints are related to anxiety, tension, or other aspects of maladaptive emotional arousal?* In some cases, this is a relatively easy question to answer: The client reports being tense and anxious, and there are obvious physiological and behavioral signs that coincide with the subjective experience. In other

TABLE 5.1. Clinical Efficacy of APRT: Designs Including Multiple Controls

Study	Treatment target	% female	Design	Dependent variables	Posttreatment effect size	Major findings
Phillips, Fenster, & Samson (1992)	Urinary dysfunction	100	$N = 30$ Mean age: 32 Conditions: APRT EMG biofeedback Wait-list control # of sessions: Varied Mode of training: Individual Practice: 2 times/day Practice tapes: Yes Compliance: Not reported APRT dropout: Not reported	Depression, anxiety, pain, weak urine flow	Depression $r = .41$ $d = 0.91$ Anxiety (state) $r = .40$ $d = 0.86$ Anxiety (trait) $r = .29$ $d = 0.61$ Pain $r = .34$ $d = 0.79$ Weak urine flow $r = .54$ $d = 1.28$	2-month posttreatment follow-up: Depression $r = .61$ $d = 1.55$ Anxiety (state) $r = .59$ $d = 1.45$ Anxiety (trait) $r = .56$ $d = 1.35$ Pain $r = .44$ $d = 0.99$ Weak urine flow $r = .59$ $d = 1.46$
Borkovec & Costello (1993)	Generalized anxiety disorder	57	$N = 63$ Mean age: 37.5 Conditions: APRT Nondirective therapy Cognitive-behavioral therapy # of sessions: 12 Mode of training: Individual Practice: 2 times/day Practice tapes: No Compliance: Not reported APRT dropout: 10%	Anxiety, worry, depression	Anxiety $r = .87$ $d = 3.50$ Worry $r = .66$ $d = 1.74$ Depression $r = .60$ $d = 1.49$	6-month posttreatment follow-up: Anxiety $r = .89$ $d = 3.95$ Worry $r = .64$ $d = 1.67$ Depression $r = .62$ $d = 1.59$
Vaughan et al. (1994)	Posttraumatic stress disorder (PTSD)	64	$N = 36$ Mean age: 40 Conditions: APRT Frontal EMG	PTSD symptoms, depression	PTSD symptoms $r = .29$ $d = 0.61$ Depression $r = .28$	3-month posttreatment follow-up: PTSD symptoms $r = .45$ $d = 1.00$ Depression

			Trapezius EMG # of sessions: 7Mode of training: Individual Practice: 2 times/day Practice tapes: Yes Compliance: Not reported APRT dropout: Not reported		$d = 0.58$	$r = .65$ $d = 1.73$

Arena, Bruno, Hannah, & Meador (1995)	Tension-type headache	80	$N = 24$
			Mean age: 32
			Conditions:
			  APRT
			  Image habituation training
			  Eye movement desensitization
			# of sessions: 4
			Mode of training: Individual
			Practice: 2 times/day
			Practice tapes: No
			Compliance: Not reported
			APRT dropout: Not reported
				Headache index	Headache index
					$r = .21$
					$d = 0.43$
					(3 months posttreatment)
						No other follow-up reported

Eller (1995)	HIV	12	$N = 69$
			Mean age: 37
			Conditions:
			  APRT
			  Guided Imagery
			  No treatment control
			# of sessions: 1
			Mode of training: Individual
			Practice: Once daily
			Practice tapes: Yes
			Compliance: Not reported
			APRT dropout: Not reported
				Fatigue, depression, cellular immunity (CD4, CD8, CD16 lymphocyte count)	Fatigue
					$r = .01$
					$d = 0.02$
					Depression
					$r = .05$
					$d = 0.11$
					CD4
					$r = .13$
					$d = 0.26$
					CD8
					$r = .01$
					$d = 0.03$
					CD16
					$r = .18$
					$d = 0.37$
						No follow-up reported

(continued)

TABLE 5.1. (continued)

Study	Treatment target	% female	Design	Dependent variables	Posttreatment effect size	Major findings
Yung & Keltner (1996)	Hypertension	50	N = 30 Mean age: 49 Conditions: APRT Stretch release Cognitive relaxation No treatment control # of sessions: 8 Mode of training: Individual Practice: Once daily Practice tapes: Yes Compliance: Not reported APRT dropout: Not reported	Systolic blood pressure (SBP), diastolic blood pressure (DBP), heart rate (HR)	SBP r = .94 d = 5.70 DBP r = .53 d = 1.26 HR r = .25 d = 0.52	1-month posttreatment follow-up: SBP r = .91 d = 1.39 DBP r = .68 d = 1.84 HR r = .16 d = 0.33
Amigo, Gonzalez, & Herrera (1997)	Hypertension	47	N = 45 Mean age: 43 Conditions: APRT Isotonic physical exercise No treatment control # of sessions: 8 Mode of training: Individual Practice: Once daily Practice tapes: No Compliance: Not reported APRT dropout: 2%	SBP, DPB, HR	SBP r = .54 d = 1.27 DBP r = .42 d = 0.93 HR r = .29 d = 0.60	6-month posttreatment follow-up: SBP r = .34 d = 0.77 DBP r = .45 d = 1.00 HR r = .20 d = 0.40
Kroner-Herwig, Hohm, & Pothmann (1998)	Pediatric headache	60	N = 50 Mean age: 11 Conditions: APRT EMG biofeedback Self-monitoring control	Headache frequency, intensity, and duration	Frequency r = .18 d = 0.37 Intensity r = .13 d = 0.13	6-month posttreatment follow-up: Frequency r = .29 d = 0.61 Intensity r = .29

				Results	Follow-up
		# of sessions: 6 Mode of training: Individual Practice: Once daily Practice tapes: Yes Compliance: Daily diaries APRT dropout: None		Duration $r = .02$ $d = 0.03$	$d = 0.60$ Duration $r = .16$ $d = 0.33$

Eller (1999)	13
	
	HIV
		$N = 69$
		Mean age: 36
		Conditions:
		  APRT
		  Guided imagery
		  No treatment control
		# of sessions: 1
		Mode of training: Individual
		Practice: Once daily
		Practice tapes: Yes
		Compliance: Daily log
		APRT dropout: None
			Quality of life (QoL), perceived health status (PHS)	QoL
				$r = .06$
				$d = 0.13$
				PHS
				$r = .08$
				$d = 0.16$
					No follow-up reported

Edinger,
Wohlgemuth,
Radke, March,
& Quillian
(2001)
	86
	
	Chronic
	insomnia
		$N = 75$
		Mean age: 55
		Conditions:
		  APRT
		  Cognitve-behavioral therapy
		  No treatment control
		# of sessions: 6
		Mode of training: Individual
		Practice: Once daily
		Practice tapes: Yes
		Compliance: Not reported
		APRT dropout: 2%
			Dysfunctional Beliefs and Attitudes about Sleep Scale (DBAS-SF) Total Score and Factors: Effects, Needs, Preoccupation, and Medication use	Total
				$r = .13$
				$d = 0.27$
				Effects
				$r = .16$
				$d = 0.33$
				Needs
				$r = .01$
				$d = 0.01$
				Preoccupation
				$r = .13$
				$d = 0.27$
				Meds
				$r = .07$
				$d = 0.15$
					No follow-up reported

(continued)

TABLE 5.1. (continued)

Study	Treatment target	% female	Design	Dependent variables	Posttreatment effect size	Major findings
Lohaus, Klein-Hesling, Vogele, & Kuhn-Hennighausen (2001)	Children	50	N = 64 Age range: 9–13 Conditions: APRT Imagery Neutral Story Control # of sessions: 5 Mode of training: Individual Practice: Not reported Practice tapes: No Compliance: Not reported APRT dropout: Not reported	Mood, physical well-being	Mood $r = .79$ $d = 2.60$ Physical well-being $r = .25$ $d = 0.52$	No follow-up reported
Loewe et al. (2002)	Myocardial infarction	25	N = 60 Mean age: 63 Conditions: APRT Feldenkrais therapy Treatment as usual control # of sessions: 2 Mode of training: Individual Practice: No Practice tapes: No Compliance: Not reported APRT dropout: None	Anxiety, depression, physical well-being, emotional well-being, self-efficacy	Anxiety $r = .04$ $d = 0.09$ Depression $r = .07$ $d = 0.14$ Physical well-being $r = .18$ $d = 0.36$ Emotional well-being $r = .07$ $d = 0.14$ Self-efficacy $r = .13$ $d = 0.26$	No follow-up reported

instances, the emotional arousal may not be the focus of the client's report, nor are there obvious signs that maladaptive arousal is at issue. For example, an adult client may report reduced energy level, lack of motivation, significant absenteeism from work, and mild depression. Though tension or anxiety is not mentioned spontaneously, it may not take much exploration to determine that new job pressures or other events may have threatened, frightened, or stressed the client.

Perhaps the client's initial response to the stress involved some obvious tension or anxiety, but by the time help is sought, an avoidance strategy may have been developed to mask the more fundamental problem. As is well known, anxiety may also play a role in the appearance of other escape or avoidance behaviors, such as alcohol or drug abuse, somatoform disorders, and a wide variety of interpersonal conflicts. Other subtle behavioral signs of anxiety can include insomnia, sexual dysfunction, restlessness, irritability, compulsive or stereotyped response patterns, and changes in appetite.

Physiological indicators of maladaptive arousal may include nausea, back pain or headache, unusual or irregular bowel activity (or other gastrointestinal problems), genitourinary system problems, hypertension, and a variety of other psychophysiological disorders. Subjectively, anxiety and its consequences may appear in the form of inability to concentrate, loss of memory, confusion, "flooding," or obsessional thoughts.

2. *Is anxiety or tension the primary focus of treatment?* Anxiety may play a significant role in a client's problems, but before choosing APRT as a component of treatment, the clinician should be satisfied that it is an appropriate initial treatment target. It is in regard to this issue that a distinction between "conditioned" and "reactive" anxiety must be made (Paul & Bernstein, 1973). If the client's overarousal has developed primarily through a series of unfortunate learning experiences (e.g., fear of driving stemming from having been in several serious auto accidents), new learning experiences (including the use of APRT) may help alleviate the problem, assuming that the client possesses adequate driving skills. However, if the client's fundamental problem primarily involves a reaction to punishment brought about by a lack of driving skills and/or the presence of maladaptive cognitive habits (e.g., "I'll never learn to drive safely"), APRT may be of little more than temporary help. In fact, if treatment does not focus on the development of new cognitive and overt behavioral skills, the disappointing effects of supplemented relaxation procedures could have a negative influence on the client's motivation to continue working with the therapist.

Recognition of the "conditioned versus reactive" dimension requires the clinician to go beyond the client's self-reports of discomfort to look for indications of skill deficits or for other problems that may be responsible for overarousal. This can be done in a variety of ways, including interviews with family members, *in vivo* behavioral observations, role playing, and informal observation during routine interviews. In most cases, the clinician is likely to find that anxiety-related problems have both conditioned and reactive components. The point to keep in mind is that unless relaxation training is needed as an immediate rapport-building procedure, it may be postponed or eliminated altogether when assessment reveals anxiety that is primarily reactive. If a significant conditioned residue remains after this aspect of the problem is dealt with, relaxation training may then be brought to bear.

3. *Are there organic components in tension-related problems?* It should go without saying that before progressive relaxation (or any psychologically oriented intervention) is chosen to help deal with physical problems apparently brought on by tension, the client should be examined by appropriate medical personnel in order to rule out organic causal factors. This is especially important when the client complains of such

TABLE 5.2. Clinical Efficacy of APRT: Designs Not Including Multiple Controls

Study	Treatment target	% female	Design	Dependent variables	Posttreatment effect size	Major findings

Blanchard, Green, Scharff, & Schwarz-McMorris (1993)	Irritable bowel syndrome	75	N = 16
			Mean age: 40
			Conditions:
			  APRT
			  Treatment as usual
			# of sessions: 8
			Mode of training: Individual
			Practice: Once daily
			Practice tapes: Yes
			Compliance: Not reported
			APRT dropout: 7, continued recruiting until 8 finished in each group
				Symptoms of irritable bowel syndrome: abdominal pain, diarrhea, nausea	Abdominal pain
					  r = .29
					  d = 0.55
					Diarrhea
					  r = .16
					  d = 0.32
					Nausea
					  r = .30
					  d = 0.62
						No follow-up reported

Haaga et al. (1994)	Hypertension	0	N = 43
			Mean age: 45.3
			Conditions:
			  APRT
			  Education only
			# of sessions: 7
			Mode of training: Group
			Practice: Once daily
			Practice tapes: Yes
			Compliance: Not reported
			APRT dropout: Not reported
				Percent change in blood pressure (SBP, DBP) and heart rate (HR), hostility, anger	SBP
					  r = .40
					  d = 0.88
					DBP
					  r = .36
					  d = 0.77
					Hostility
					  r = .11
					  d = 0.22
					Anger
					  r = .23
					  d = 0.47
						No follow-up reported

Echeburua, de Corral, Sarasua, & Zubizarreta (1996)	Sexual assault	100	N = 20
			Mean age: 22
			Conditions:
			  APRT
			  Cognitive restructuring/coping skills training
			# of sessions: 5
			Mode of training: Individual
			Practice: Not reported
			Practice tapes: Not reported
				PTSD symptoms (Global PTSD Scale)	PTSD symptoms
					  r = .68
					  d = 01.85
						1-month posttreatment follow-up:
						PTSD symptoms
						  r = .79
						  d = 2.55

Study					
Myers, Wittrock, & Foreman (1998)	Headache	100	Compliance: Not reported APRT dropout: None reported N = 30 Mean age: 20 Conditions: APRT Headache-free controls # of sessions: 1 Mode of training; Individual Practice: Not reported Practice tapes: Not reported Compliance: Not reported APRT dropout: None reported	Headache pain (VAS), subjective headache rating scale (SRS)	VAS $r = .58$ $d = 1.41$ SRS $r = .51$ $d = 1.19$	No follow-up reported
Greeff & Conradie (1998)	Alcoholics with insomnia	0	N = 16 Mean age: 46 Conditions: APRT Wait-list control # of sessions: 10 Mode of training; Group Practice: Once daily Practice tapes: Not reported Compliance: Not reported APRT dropout: None reported	Sleep quality	Sleep quality $r = .74$ $d = 2.19$	No follow-up reported
Suhr, Anderson, & Tranel (1995)	Alzheimer's disease	Not reported	N = 34 Mean age: 76 Conditions: APRT Guided imagery # of sessions: As necessary; mean of 5 Mode of training; Individual with caregiver Practice: Twice daily for 2 months Practice tapes: Not reported Compliance: Mean # sessions: 38 APRT dropout: 8%	Psychiatric and behavioral difficulties, cognitive performance	Psychiatric $r = .20$ $d = 0.40$ Behavioral $r = .62$ $d = 1.57$ Cognitive $r = .26$ $d = 0.54$	No follow-up reported

(continued)

99

TABLE 5.2. (continued)

Study	Treatment target	% female	Design	Dependent variables	Posttreatment effect size	Major findings

Matsumoto & Smith (2001)	Undergraduates	67	Mean age: 20
			Conditions:
			  APRT
			  Deep breathing
			# of sessions: 5
			Mode of training: Group
			Practice: Not reported
			Practice tapes: Not reported
			Compliance: Not reported
			APRT dropout: Not reported
				Physical relaxation	Physical relaxation
					$r = .80$
					$d = 2.70$
						No follow-up reported

Pawlow & Jones (2002)	Impact on stress indices	50	Mean age: 23
			Conditions:
			  APRT
			  Quiet sitting
			# of sessions: As necessary; mean of 2
			Mode of training: Individual
			Practice: Daily
			Practice tapes: Yes
			Compliance: Not reported
			APRT dropout: Not reported
				Salivary cortisol, anxiety	Cortisol
					$r = .24$
					$d = 0.49$
					Anxiety
					$r = .58$
					$d = 1.41$
						No follow-up reported

Cheung, Molassiotis, & Chang (2003)	Colorectal cancer, poststoma surgery	32	Mean age: 58
			Conditions:
			  APRT
			  Treatment as usual
			# of sessions: 2
			Mode of training: Not reported
				Quality of life (QoL), anxiety	QoL
					$r = .65$
					$d = 1.73$
					Anxiety
					$r = .97$
					$d = 8.20$
						No follow-up reported

100

Study	Population	N	Treatment	Outcome measures	Effect sizes	Follow-up
			Practice: 2–3 times/week for 10 weeks Practice tapes: Yes Compliance: Phone contact every 2 weeks APRT dropout: 10%			No follow-up reported
Veins, De Koninck, Mercier, St. Onge, & Lorrain (2003)	Insomnia	70	Mean age: 20 Conditions: APRT Anxiety management training # of sessions: 1 Mode of training: Individual Practice: 2 times/day Practice tapes: Yes Compliance: Visit by therapist once every 2 weeks APRT dropout: Not reported	Sleep-onset latency, anxiety, depression	Sleep-onset latency $r = .31$ $d = 0.65$ Anxiety $r = .52$ $d = 1.22$ Depression $r = .27$ $d = 0.55$	
Ghoncheh & Smith (2004)	Normals	63	Mean age: 34 Conditions: APRT Yoga training # of sessions: 5 Mode of training: Group Practice: Not reported Practice tapes: Not reported Compliance: Not reported APRT dropout: Not reported	Physical relaxation	Physical relaxation $r = .50$ $d = 1.17$	No follow-up reported

"traditional" psychophysiological disorders as pain in the head, neck, or lower back; cardiac symptoms (such as chest pain, tachycardia, or arrhythmia); asthma; and gastrointestinal difficulties. However, this consideration should also be kept in mind in cases in which a complaint could have a less obvious organic base. Examples include disorders of memory, concentration, logic, or other cognitive functions; depression; irritability; and aggressiveness. Furthermore, if the client has an illness or disease for which he or she is taking regular medication (e.g., insulin), a physician who is knowledgeable about relaxation effects should provide medical approval before relaxation treatment is begun.

Adverse Effects

In the general clinical population, significant adverse effects of relaxation training are uncommon. Edinger and Jacobsen (1982) surveyed 116 clinicians—who had conducted relaxation training with an estimated 17,542 clients—and noted that intrusive thoughts were the most frequently encountered problem (15%), followed by fear of losing control (9%), disturbing sensory experiences (4%), muscle cramps or spasms (4%), sexual arousal (2%), and emergence of psychotic symptoms (0.4%). Among clients with generalized anxiety disorder, Heide and Borkovec (1983) found that 30% reported increased tension during APRT. Bernstein and Borkovec (1973) noted from their clinical experience that problems with APRT included client coughing and/or sneezing, excessive movement, muscle cramps and spasms, sleep, anxious thoughts, laughter, and sexual arousal. In general, then, relaxation training does not appear to have significant and frequent adverse effects, but clinicians should be wary of any potential side effects and ready to address them. More is said in later sections about coping with common problems in relaxation training.

Adverse effects of relaxation training have been described as representing either "relaxation-induced anxiety" (RIA) or "relaxation-induced panic" (RIP; Adier, Craske, & Barlow, 1987). RIA refers to the gradual increase in behavioral, physiological, and psychological components of anxiety during relaxation training. RIP describes the rapid development of severe anxiety during relaxation training. Both of these phenomena might better be understood as procedurally induced than as relaxation-induced, given the general meaning of "relaxation." Nonetheless, the "relaxation-induced" nomenclature is more commonly used in the empirical literature.

Several mechanisms have been proposed to account for the development of RIA and RIP. These include fear of losing control (Bernstein & Borkovec, 1973; Carrington, 1977), fear of relaxation sensations (Borkovec, 1987; Borkovec, 1987), and interoceptive conditioning (Adier et al., 1987). Ley (1988) hypothesized that RIA and RIP phenomena are actually minute episodes of hyperventilation in persons who are susceptible to these because of unusually low concentrations of carbon dioxide (CO_2) in the blood. When the concentration of CO_2 is unusually low, very small changes in CO_2 production from metabolism or variations in respiration rate or volume can precipitate the sensations of hyperventilation. Symptoms of hyperventilation include breathlessness, rapid heart rate, muscle contractility, and palpitations. Ley (1988) believes that these symptoms of hyperventilation may be triggered during relaxation by slight increases in the volume of inspired air or by reduction in CO_2 production as a result of the lower metabolic activity produced by the abrupt change in physical activity level when a person rests quietly. As of yet, however, there is not a consistent body of evidence to support either the hyperventilation theory or the various other theories developed to account for the adverse effects of relaxation training.

Management of Adverse Effects

Effective management of adverse effects associated with relaxation training begins with a careful evaluation of the client and recognition of the potential for side effects. Clients with a history of generalized anxiety disorder or panic disorder are likely to experience adverse side effects; so, too, are persons with a history of hyperventilation. Extra effort should be made to inform such clients of the potential complications, and steps can be taken to reduce the likelihood of difficulties. For example, teaching clients diaphragmatic breathing skills prior to APRT may preempt difficulties, as well as provide skills to control any panic or anxiety that may result from breathing changes occurring during therapy. Providing clients with a thorough description of APRT may also aid in reducing adverse responses; if clients feel as though they have been prepared for the experiences they encounter during relaxation, they will be more likely to manage them effectively. Moreover, a therapist can remind a client that in the unlikely event that difficulties occur, they may actually serve as an important assessment tool; that is, they may clarify more fully the client's presenting complaint.

If adverse effects should occur despite the therapist's best efforts, several courses of action can be pursued, depending on the needs of the client. One strategy is to pause and reassure the client that the symptoms are transitory and will gradually subside with continued relaxation practice (Cohen, Barlow, & Blanchard, 1985; DeGood & Williams, 1982). Another strategy is to switch to an alternative relaxation technique. Several authors (Adier et al., 1987; Heide & Borkovec, 1983) suggest decreasing the focus on somatic experiences if adverse effects should emerge. Lastly, APRT can be discontinued if adverse effects persist or if the client is unwilling to carry on. The clinician's calm management of adverse reactions is important to enabling the client to continue working toward alleviation of his or her presenting complaints.

Contraindications

In spite of the generally benign and pleasant nature of APRT, the clinician considering its use should take care to ensure that no past or current physical conditions exist that would contraindicate some of the required tension–release cycles. Consultation with the client and his or her physician about this matter is especially important in cases in which certain muscles or connective tissues have been damaged or are chronically weak. In some cases, medical advice may suggest that it would be better to focus on strengthening certain muscle groups (e.g., in the lower back) than on learning to relax them. In such instances, APRT may still be feasible, but it would have to be modified to delete or alter procedures for problematic muscle groups (see Bernstein & Borkovec, 1973). The same is true in the case of an individual who, as the result of a neuromuscular disability, is incapable of exercising voluntary control over all muscles in the body (see Cautela & Groden, 1978). Finally, if the client is taking medication regularly (e.g., insulin for diabetes or propanolol for hypertension), medical consultation is necessary prior to beginning APRT, because relaxation training could change the amount of medication needed for management of the symptoms.

Beyond these considerations, the clinician should also ensure that the client is both able and willing to (1) maintain focused attention during relaxation training, (2) follow

instructions regarding tension–release cycles, and (3) engage in regular home practice between treatment sessions. If serious obstacles to any of these three basic requirements exist, it may be wise to work on eliminating those obstacles before beginning a relaxation
program.

Compliance, Resistance, and Maintenance

Like most other clinical procedures, APRT requires willingness on the part of the client to
comply with the training regimen. In the second edition of this chapter (Bernstein &
Carlson, 1993), we noted that of the 29 APRT studies described, the average number of
training sessions was 9, with training conducted at least twice weekly in 12 studies and
once per week in the remaining 17 studies. Home practice was assigned in virtually every
study, with the majority of studies encouraging at least one practice session per day. Seventeen of the 29 studies provided participants with audiotapes for home practice. Compliance rates for daily home practice could be determined from data for five studies and
ranged from 32 to 82%.

In three studies, home practice tapes were played on tape machines fitted with devices to count the number of "plays" (Hoelscher, Lichstein, & Rosenthal, 1986;
Hoelscher, Lichstein, Fischer, & Hegarty, 1987; Wisniewski, Genshaft, Mulick, Coury,
& Hammer, 1988). Hoelscher et al. (1986) noted that participants reported an average
of 120 minutes of practice per week, whereas the timing device indicated an average of
only 100 minutes of practice per week; they also reported that only 32% of participants actually practiced relaxation daily as prescribed. In a second study, Hoelscher et
al. (1987) again found that their participants overreported practice times (150 minutes
vs. 126 minutes). Wisniewski et al. (1988) found that their adolescent participants
overreported practice sessions by almost 70%. In a study not reviewed in this chapter
because of methodological limitations, Taylor, Agras, Schneider, and Allen (1983) reported that adherence to practice instructions was 39% according to the electronic record and 71% according to self-report. Taken together, these results suggest that compliance does vary and that clients are likely to overestimate the frequency of their
practice. Still, significant improvements in symptom status have been achieved in these
studies, despite discrepancies between self-report and actual practice.

One research program (Borkovec, 1987) has evaluated the relationship between frequency of self-reported practice and treatment outcome. The results are mixed, with one
study (Borkovec et al., 1987) finding no effect of reported practice frequency on outcome
and the other study (Borkovec & Mathews, 1988) finding that more frequent practice
was associated with greater decreases in symptom severity. In another report concerning
the use of APRT for reduction of muscle contraction headache (Blanchard, Steffek,
Jaccard, & Nicholson, 1991), there was an indication that home practice may lead to
greater reductions in headache activity than clinic practice of APRT only. However, these
results were marginally significant and based on a small sample size. At this point, it is
not clear to what extent practice frequency is linked to symptom improvement, but, obviously, less than full compliance with a prescribed practice regimen need not be lethal to
treatment effects. It seems important, therefore, to develop individualized criteria for relaxation and to determine the extent to which frequency of practice influences clinical
progress in given cases.

Another way to conceptualize compliance is to examine data regarding dropouts
from treatment. In the sample of studies summarized in Bernstein and Carlson (1993),

dropout rates from the APRT conditions ranged from 0 to 30%, with an average of 9% during the training periods. These results suggested that the role of the therapist may be important in influencing compliance with APRT. However, compliance may also be related to the presenting problems or the client's motivation. Therapist behaviors related to creating and maintaining a positive therapeutic environment, engaging the client's personal expectations, goals, and plans, and employing principles of learning (i.e., reinforcement) are likely to be important factors influencing compliance. Further research is needed, however, to identify more clearly the role that these behaviors may play in promoting compliance with APRT.

As mentioned earlier, the average number of APRT sessions across the 30 studies we reviewed in 1993 was 9, with the frequency ranging from 2 to 33. As that collection of studies illustrated, some clinical problems may require fewer training sessions, and some may require more training sessions than the average number calculated across representative studies. Long-term follow-up data available for 8 of those studies (average length of follow-up: 11.8 months) were encouraging, with the majority of studies indicating maintenance of treatment gains. Still, additional research is needed on the long-term utility of APRT.

METHOD

Introducing Relaxation to the Client

Once appropriate assessment has been completed and APRT has been decided on as a treatment of choice, the method and its specific procedures must be explained to the client in enough detail to promote cooperation and understanding. This presentation should include an explanation of (1) the role that anxiety seems to play in the client's problem and (2) the ways in which APRT may help. The level of discourse and amount of detail involved in this introductory session should vary from client to client in accordance with individuals' capacities to absorb and integrate the content and concepts involved. At the very least, the clinician should attempt to establish in the client a basic appreciation of how tension is manifested, how it can be reduced, and how that reduction can help alleviate some of the presenting problems. Without such basic understanding, the client's interest in learning and practicing relaxation is not likely to be strong enough for him or her to develop useful skills. Most clients find the idea of APRT intrinsically appealing; however, there will be those who continue to express doubts. If a client remains skeptical but is willing to try APRT seriously, the training itself may relieve the skepticism.

Once the client understands and at least provisionally accepts the conceptualization of his or her problems as partly involving maladaptive levels of tension, the clinician can present a more detailed rationale for the choice of APRT as a part of treatment. This rationale should provide (1) a brief overview of the history of progressive relaxation; (2) a description of APRT as a method whereby one learns a skill, in much the same manner as one learns other skills (such as swimming) that involve muscle control; (3) the stipulation that APRT will require regular practice, so that the client can learn to recognize and control the distinctly different sensations of tension and relaxation; and (4) the clear message that the therapist will not be doing anything to the client—rather, that the client will be developing a capability within himself or herself that can then be used independently.

A sample rationale is provided here. It is given merely as an illustration, not as a script. Each therapist should present this material in his or her own natural style.

The procedures I have been discussing in terms of reducing your tension are collectively called "progressive relaxation training." They were first developed in the 1930s by a physiologist named Jacobson, and in recent years we have modified his original technique in order to make it simpler and easier to learn. Basically, progressive relaxation training consists of learning to tense and then to relax various groups of muscles all through the body, while at the same time paying very close and careful attention to the feelings associated with both tension and relaxation. That is, in addition to teaching you how to relax, I will also be encouraging you to learn to recognize and pinpoint tension and relaxation as they appear in everyday situations, as well as in our sessions here.

You should understand quite clearly that learning relaxation skills is very much like learning any other kind of skill, such as swimming or golfing or riding a bicycle; thus, in order for you to get better at relaxing, you will have to practice doing it just as you would have to practice other skills. It is very important that you realize that progressive relaxation training involves learning on your part; there is nothing magical about the procedures. I will not be doing anything to you; I will merely be introducing you to the technique and directing your attention to various aspects of it, such as the presence of certain feelings in the muscles. Thus, without your active cooperation and regular practicing of the things you will learn today, the procedures are of little use.

Now I mentioned earlier that I will be asking you to tense and then to relax various groups of muscles in your body. You may be wondering why, if we want to produce relaxation, we start off by producing tension. The reason is that, first of all, everyone is always at some level of tension during his or her waking hours; if people were not tense to some extent, they would simply fall down. The amount of tension actually present in everyday life differs, of course, from individual to individual, and we say that each person has reached some "adaptation level"—the amount of tension under which he or she operates day to day.

The goal of progressive relaxation training is to help you learn to reduce muscle tension in your body far below your adaptation level at any time you wish to do so. In order to accomplish this, I could ask you to focus your attention, for example, on the muscles in your right hand and lower arm and then just to let them relax. Now you might think you can let these muscles drop down below their adaptation level just by "letting them go" or whatever, and to a certain extent, you probably can. However, in progressive relaxation, we want you to learn to produce larger and very much more noticeable reductions in tension, and a way to do this is first to produce a good deal of tension in the muscle group (i.e., to raise the tension well above adaptation level) and then, all at once, to release that tension. We believe the release helps to create a "momentum" which allows the muscles to drop well below adaptation level. The effect is like that which we could produce with a pendulum which is hanging motionless in a vertical position. If we want it to swing far to the right, we could push it quite hard in that direction. It would be much easier, however, to start by pulling the pendulum in the opposite direction and then letting it go. It will swing well past the vertical point and continue in the direction we want it to go.

Thus tensing muscle groups prior to letting them relax is like giving ourselves a "running start" toward deep relaxation through the momentum created by the tension release. Another important advantage to creating and releasing tension is that it will give you a good chance to focus your attention upon and become clearly aware of what tension really feels like in each of the various groups of muscles we will be dealing with today. In addition, the tensing procedure will make a vivid contrast between tension and relaxation and will give you an excellent opportunity to compare the two directly and to appreciate the difference in feeling associated with each of these states.

Do you have any questions about what I've said so far?

Instead of memorizing this kind of presentation, the therapist may want to use an outline of the main topics to be covered. This is likely to make the material sound less "canned" (see Bernstein & Borkovec, 1973, pp. 61–62, for a sample outline).

After any questions about the rationale have been answered, the therapist should begin working with the client to develop optimal tension–release procedures for each of the 16 muscle groups that will be the initial focus of training. These groups and a typical tensing strategy for each are given in the following list.

Muscle group	Method of tensing
1. Dominant hand and forearm	Make a tight fist while allowing upper arm to remain relaxed.
2. Dominant upper arm	Press elbow down against chair.
3. Nondominant hand and forearm	Same as dominant.
4. Nondominant upper arm	Same as dominant.
5. Forehead	Raise eyebrows as high as possible.
6. Upper cheeks and nose	Squint eyes and wrinkle nose.
7. Lower face	Clench teeth and pull back corners of mouth.
8. Neck	Counterpose muscles by trying to raise and lower chin simultaneously.
9. Chest, shoulders, upper back	Take a deep breath; hold it and pull shoulder blades together.
10. Abdomen	Counterpose muscles by trying to push stomach out and pull it simultaneously.
11. Dominant upper leg	Counterpose large muscles on top of leg against two smaller ones underneath (specific strategy will vary considerably).
12. Dominant calf	Point toes toward head.
13. Dominant foot	Point toes downward, turn foot in, and curl toes gently.
14. Nondominant upper leg	Same as dominant.
15. Nondominant calf	Same as dominant.
16. Nondominant foot	Same as dominant.

In order to facilitate transfer to the actual training situation, it is generally a good idea to have the client assume a reclining position while these tensing strategies are introduced and attempted. It is also advisable to work on the tension–release cycles for each muscle group in the same order as that to be used in subsequent training. When done in this way, the initial "run-through" can provide a reassuring preview of the procedures to come.

Inevitably, some clients will have difficulty achieving tension in the "standard" manner described here. In such a case, the therapist must work with the client to devise alternative methods to achieve significant tension. The client may also find it difficult to tense one muscle group without tensing other groups at the same time. This problem tends to disappear with practice, but the therapist should continue to observe the client and should be ready to provide helpful suggestions and instructions.

Finally, some clients feel self-conscious or silly while tensing certain muscle groups, particularly those involving the face. The therapist can usually put such a client at ease by demonstrating all tensing methods before asking the client to try them.

Description of the Method

Once the relaxation rationale has been presented and discussed, and once a set of muscle-tensing strategies has been agreed on, a few final instructions should be given. These are presented next in the form a "typical" therapist might employ. Naturally, the specific wording should be adjusted to suit one's own style.

1. I will be instructing you to focus your attention on one muscle group at a time. Please pay attention only to what I am saying and to the sensations you are experiencing in that muscle group, allowing the rest of your body to remain relaxed. I will ask you to tense and relax each of the muscle groups in the same order as we used when we practiced the tensing procedures.
2. When I ask you to tense a group, I will say, for example, "Tense the muscles in your forehead by raising your eyebrows, now." "Now" will be the cue word for you to tense the muscles. Do not tense the muscles until I say "now."
3. When I want you to relax a muscle group, I will say, "OK, relax the muscles in your forehead." When I say that, let all the tension go all at once, not gradually.
4. I will ask you to tense and relax each muscle group twice. After the second time, I will ask you to signal if the muscle group is completely relaxed. Please signal by raising the index finger on your right hand [whichever hand is visible to the therapist], but do not signal unless the muscles really feel completely relaxed.
5. During the session, try not to move any more than is necessary to remain comfortable. In order to gain the most benefit from relaxation, it is preferable not to move any muscles that have already been relaxed. This prevents tension from reappearing in those muscles.
6. In order to maintain as much relaxation as possible, I am going to ask you not to talk to me during our session unless it is absolutely necessary. We will mainly use your finger signal as a means of communication, and we will talk about how the session went after we finish today. Questions you may have can be discussed after completion of the relaxation.
7. Our session today will take about 45 minutes, so if you would like to use the restroom before we start, please do so.
8. Now I would like to have you remove or loosen any items (e.g., glasses or tight belts) that may cause discomfort during the session.
9. Do you have any further questions? Is there anything about which you are not clear?
10. OK, get in a comfortable position in your chair—fine. Now please close your eyes and keep them closed during the session. I will dim the lights now to minimize visual stimulation.

At this point, relaxation training can begin. Following the same sequence as the muscle groups presented previously, the therapist should treat each muscle group as follows:

1. Instruct the client to focus attention on the muscle group.

2. Using the predetermined "now" cue, instruct the client to produce tension in that group, repeating the instructions for tensing that group. For example, say, "By making a tight fist, tense the muscles in your right hand and lower your arm, now." Allow the client to maintain the tension for 5 to 7 seconds while describing the sensations of tension to the client. Use a shorter tension duration for the feet or other muscles in which the client may experience cramping.

3. Using the predetermined "relax" cue, instruct the client to relax the muscle group all at once (not gradually) and to attend to the sensations of relaxation. Allow the client to focus on the relaxation for 30 to 40 seconds while giving him or her some relaxation "patter" to highlight the sensations (see example following this list).

4. Repeat steps 2 and 3. After the second tension–release cycle, allow the client to maintain the relaxation and to focus on the sensations for 45 to 60 seconds.

5. Before moving on to the next muscle group, ask the client to signal if the current muscle group is completely relaxed. If not, repeat the tension and relaxation steps a third time. If the client still does not signal that the group is relaxed, the procedure may be repeated again. However, if relaxation is not achieved in four or five attempts, alternative means for achieving relaxation may be required. One alternative would be to instruct the client to allow those muscles to relax as much a possible while moving on to other groups and to return to them at a later point.

6. When the focus is on the chest, shoulders, and upper back, emphasis on breathing should be introduced as part of the procedure. Instruct the client to take deep breath and hold it while the muscles are tensed and to exhale when instructed to relax. From this point on, breathing cues should be included as a part of the tension–release procedure for all muscle groups. Furthermore, mention of slow, regular breathing can be incorporated into the relaxation "patter."

When these steps are combined, they go something like this:

> OK, Leslie, I would like you to focus all of your attention on the muscles of your chest, shoulders, and upper back. And by taking a deep breath and holding it and by pulling your shoulder blades back and together, I'd like you to tense the muscles of the chest, shoulders, and upper back, now. Good, notice the tension and the tightness, notice what the tension feels like, hold it . . . and relax.
>
> Fine, just let all that tension go. Notice the difference between the tension you felt before and the pleasant feelings of relaxation. Just focus all your attention on those feelings of relaxation as they flow into your chest, shoulders, and back. Just focus on your slow and regular breathing and go right on enjoying the relaxation.
>
> [Tension–release cycle is repeated after 30–45 seconds.]
>
> OK, Leslie, I would like you to signal if the muscles in the chest, shoulders, and upper back are as deeply relaxed as those of the neck (i.e., the previous group). OK, fine, just go on relaxing.

When all 16 muscle groups have been relaxed, the therapist should review each group, reminding the client that these muscles have been relaxed and asking him or her to continue to allow them to relax while attending to the accompanying sensations. The client should then be asked to signal if all the groups are indeed completely relaxed. If the client does not signal, the muscle groups should be named, one at a time, and the client should be instructed to signal when the group or groups that are not totally relaxed are mentioned. A tension–release cycle can then be repeated for these groups. Once again, the client should be instructed to signal if any tension remains. Once a signal of total relaxation is given, the client should be allowed simply to enjoy this totally relaxed state for a minute or two before the session is terminated.

To terminate the relaxation session easily and gradually, the therapist can count backward from 4 to 1. The client can be asked to move his or her feet and legs on the count of 4, to move hands and arms on the count of 3, to move head and neck on the count of 2, and to open the eyes and sit up on the count of 1. At this point, the therapist should ask open-ended questions such as "How do you feel?" or "How was that?" to encourage the client to discuss the feelings of relaxation and any problems that may have been encountered. If the client does not spontaneously report problems, the therapist should ask whether there were any muscle groups the client had difficulty in relaxing and whether the client has any questions about the procedure. The client should be asked whether any particular aspects of the "patter" helped or hindered relaxation.

If the client feels that some muscles were not well relaxed, it may be necessary for the therapist to suggest an alternative means of tensing those muscles and to incorporate the new method at the next session.

The therapist should arrange for the client to practice relaxation skills twice a day for 15 to 20 minutes each time. The therapist may help the client to decide on appropriate times and places for practice, attending to the same issues as those considered in selecting the location for APRT (see next section). If the client has difficulty determining a time and place for relaxation practice, it may be necessary to engage in problem solving about these matters with the client, in order to maximize the likelihood that he or she will practice regularly.

Environmental Factors

Environmental factors can have a marked influence on the effectiveness of relaxation training, especially in the early stages. Factors of particular importance include the location at which training and home practice are conducted, the chair or other furniture the client uses, the client's wearing apparel, and the tone of voice used by the therapist.

The therapist should provide a location for training where there will be minimum of extraneous stimuli. Particular care should be taken to prevent loud noises or the sound of conversation from reaching the treatment room. A sign should be placed on the door to prevent interruptions. Windows and drapes should be closed, and dim lighting should be used. If the client expresses reservations or feels discomfort in this type of environment, the therapist should discuss and resolve these concerns before proceeding.

If the environmental conditions just described cannot be created for some reason, effective APRT is still possible, though it may progress more slowly than usual. It is also true that relaxation skills may be more helpful to some clients if, once learned, they are practiced under somewhat less than optimal conditions. The assumption is that if a client can reach and maintain a state of deep relaxation in the face of some distractions, the relaxation skills will be more robust and useful in dealing with *in vivo* stress or imagined stimuli (as in systematic desensitization). An extreme example of this phenomenon was provided by one of our clients who was very successfully trained in progressive relaxation (and subsequently desensitized to performance anxiety) during sessions accompanied by the continuous and occasionally deafening sounds of construction coming from a building site next door.

As to the client's location during training and practice, a good reclining chair is ideal. It should provide full support for the entire body, so that as the skeletal muscles relax, various limbs do not slip off the chair into uncomfortable positions. For some clients, a small pillow may be needed to provide added lower back support or to prevent head turns. Sometimes a client may be more comfortable with a pillow under the knees. The therapist should encourage the client to experiment with a number of chair positions (and body orientations in each) until the best, most comfortably supportive combination is found.

Prior to the first relaxation session, the client should be advised to wear loose-fitting, comfortable clothing during relaxation training and at-home practice. He or she should remove contact lenses or glasses and should remove or loosen other articles (such as shoes, belts, or jewelry) that may cause discomfort. During APRT, the therapist's voice should initially have a normal, conversational tone, volume, and pace. As the session proceeds, it should become smoother, quieter, and more monotonous. During instructions to tense muscles, the voice should have more tension, volume, and speed than during instructions to relax. This discrepancy helps to contrast the sensations of tension and relaxation.

Therapist–Client Relationship

All successful therapeutic endeavors are based, to some degree, on a good working relationship between client and therapist in which each understands his or her roles and responsibilities. APRT is certainly no exception. Although APRT consists of a specific package of techniques, it should be conducted as part of a broader cooperative learning experience for the client, not as the mere dispensation of a "treatment." Indeed, if the therapist focuses entirely on the techniques of relaxation, at the expense of integrating the methods into an overall approach to helping the client to deal actively with problems, a "medication mentality" may develop. That is, the client may get the idea that the "relaxation exercises" guided by the therapist will, in some independent and mysterious way, solve the problems that are the focus of concern. This point of view not only may detract from the active practice and utilization of APRT but may also cast the therapist in the role of a remote technician who is simply applying a remedial procedure to a malfunctioning organism. As noted earlier, this problem can be prevented in large measure by placing APRT in its proper perspective during the presentation and discussion of the rationale. When this objective is achieved, and especially when generally good rapport exists between client and therapist, APRT is most likely to contribute to a beneficial outcome.

A word should also be said about the ways in which APRT can aid in the development of the therapeutic relationship. APRT is often useful early in treatment as a means of helping a very tense or confused client to calm down enough to organize his or her thoughts or discuss emotionally volatile material. One or two sessions of APRT can provide a pleasant experience as part of what has been anticipated to be a very trying therapy enterprise; in addition, it can be very impressive to the client. Helping a very tense, emotionally overaroused person to reach an unfamiliar state of deep relaxation rapidly may leave the client feeling more confident in the therapist's ability and more willing to "open up" regarding matters that might otherwise have remained private much longer.

This rapport-building aspect of APRT stems not only from the pleasant experiences that it engenders but also from the fact that it provides an opportunity for the therapist to communicate actively and clearly his or her interest in, caring for, and sensitivity to the client. These things can be conveyed in the care with which the therapist presents and explains APRT, answers questions about it, and expresses optimism about the client's ability to learn and use it. During training itself, a warm, caring attitude can be obviously reflected in the numerous requests for assurance that each muscle group is deeply relaxed and in instructions designed to reassure the client that he or she has no need to do anything but relax. Finally, postsession discussion of progress and problems usually centers on encouragement of the client's efforts, but, perhaps more important, it may center on minor points of difficulty that the therapist may have detected but that the client may have thought too trivial to warrant attention. Recognition that the therapist is truly "tuned in" to what is going on can be a very impressive and beneficial experience for the client.

Assessing Progress

In most cases, the client's self-report is the main source of information about the overall success of a program of APRT. Critical positive indicators in such reports include (1) appropriate frequency and regularity of home practice sessions; (2) decreasing time required to reach deep relaxation; (3) changes in general tension; (4) utilization of relaxation to deal with specific stressors; (5) corroborating self-monitoring records, if available; and (6) general references to satisfaction with the procedures. Such reports carry added weight when accompanied by changing in-session signs such as the following:

1. Decreased total time to achieve relaxation during training sessions.
2. No need to employ more than two tension–release cycles for any muscle group.
3. Increasing depth of relaxation (as indicated by such features as a slack jaw, splayed foot position, slowed relaxation signals, and less vigorous signals).
4. Sleep episodes.
5. Absence of gross motor movement.
6. Apparent total relaxation prior to coverage of all muscle groups.
7. Appearance of drowsiness on termination of session.

Combining Muscle Groups

If, after approximately three formal training sessions (with regular daily practice at home), assessment indicates that the client has become skillful at achieving deep relaxation using 16 muscle groups, a shorter procedure using only seven muscle groups can be introduced. The 16 muscle groups can be combined into seven groups as follows:

1. Dominant hand, forearm, and upper arm.
2. Nondominant hand, forearm, and upper arm.
3. All facial muscles.
4. Neck.
5. Chest, shoulders, upper back, and abdomen.
6. Dominant upper leg, calf, and foot.
7. Nondominant upper leg, calf, and foot.

These muscles can be tensed by using combinations of the tensing mechanisms prescribed for the 16 groups, or the therapist can work out some alternate means for achieving optimal tension.

The procedure for relaxation with seven muscle groups is the same as that for 16 muscle groups. If the client does not achieve satisfactory relaxation after a week or two with this shorter procedure (and regular at-home practice), the therapist should determine which combined groups are not becoming relaxed and should temporarily divide these into their original components before resuming use of the seven groups. The same type of questioning that follows relaxation with 16 groups should be used after relaxation with seven groups, in order to encourage the client to express any concerns or questions.

If all goes well, a high level of proficiency in relaxation with seven muscle groups should be attained after about 2 weeks of practice. However, the therapist should assess the client's skill before moving on to the next abbreviating step—namely, four muscle groups. The transition to four muscle groups should be treated in the same manner as the transition to seven muscle groups. The client should be capable of achieving deep relaxation with seven groups before attempting to use this even shorter procedure. The seven muscle groups are combined into four as follows:

1. Both arms and both hands.
2. Face and neck.
3. Chest, shoulders, back, and abdomen.
4. Both legs and both feet.

Using this four-group procedure, relaxation should take approximately 10 minutes. As with the seven-group method, questioning should follow each relaxation session. It is to be expected that the client will require continual, regular practice to achieve deep relaxation using only four muscle groups.

Releasing Tension by Recall

When the client is capable of achieving deep relaxation using the four-group procedure, relaxation through recall can be attempted. In this procedure, each of the four muscle groups is focused on individually, as before; however, the tension stage is eliminated. The client is asked to achieve relaxation by merely recalling the sensations associated with the release of tension. Mastery of this step is essential to the ultimate goal of relaxation training, which is to enable the client to control excess tension as it occurs in "real life" situations. Obviously, the client will not always be able to stop and run through even a short relaxation procedure every time tension occurs. The use of recall, along with other steps yet to be discussed, should ultimately enable the client to maintain minimum levels of tension in anxiety-provoking situations.

The therapist's procedure for teaching relaxation through recall is as follows:

1. Instruct the client to focus on a muscle group (each of the four muscle groups is to be dealt with individually) and to attend to any tension that may be present in that group.
2. Instruct the client to recall the sensations associated with the release of tension.
3. Using the cue word (*now*) as before, instruct the client to relax the muscle group.
4. Allow the client to focus on the relaxation process for 30 to 45 seconds while making statements to help the client attend to the feelings in the muscles.
5. Ask the client to signal if the muscle group is completely relaxed.
6. If the client signals that relaxation has been achieved, proceed to the next muscle group. If the client has not achieved relaxation, repeat the procedure, once again instructing the client to identify the remaining tension in the muscle group and to focus on releasing that tension.

Taken together, these procedures might sound like this:

OK, Jill, I would like you to focus all of your attention on the muscles of your arms and hands. And I want you to pay close attention to how those muscles feel and notice any feelings of tightness or tension that might be present in those muscles. OK, now just let those muscles relax, just recalling what it felt like when you let all that tension go. Just let that tension go now and allow the muscles of your arms and hands to become more and more relaxed. [Continue "patter" for 30–45 seconds.]

OK, if the muscles of your arms and hands feel completely relaxed. I'd like you to signal. . . . OK, fine, just go right on relaxing.

If the client experiences a great deal of difficulty achieving relaxation in any group with the recall procedure, it may be necessary to use a tension–release cycle for that group. However, a tensing strategy should be used only for that group and only in the training session. The other groups should be relaxed using recall alone, and the client should try to use recall for all groups when practicing at home. In most cases, relaxation through recall will improve with regular practice.

Termination of the session and questioning is the same for the recall procedures as they are for previous sessions.

Recall with Counting

A "counting" method can be introduced at the end of a recall session, once the recall procedure is a well-established method of achieving relaxation. It should be presented to the client as a simple procedure that will promote even deeper muscle relaxation.

To incorporate counting into the training session, the therapist should instruct the client to continue relaxing and to allow the relaxation to become deeper with each number as the therapist counts from 1 to 10. The counting should be timed to coincide with the client's exhalations. The therapist should provide some "patter" about the sensations of relaxation between counts. For example, after a signal of complete relaxation has been received, the therapist might say:

> OK, as you go right on relaxing, I am going to count slowly from 1 to 10, As I count, I would like you to allow all the muscles in your body to become even more deeply and completely relaxed. Just focus on your muscles as they relax more and more on each count.
>
> OK, 1 . . . 2. Let your arms and hands relax even more. 3 . . . 4. Focus on the muscles of the neck and face as they relax. 5 . . . 6. Allow the muscles of the chest, shoulders, back, and abdomen to become even more relaxed. 7 . . . 8. Let the muscles in your legs and feet relax more and more. 9 . . . 10. You are relaxing more and more all through your body.

If the client likes this procedure, he or she can be instructed to subvocalize a 1–10 count after relaxation by recall when practicing at home.

Counting Alone

When the client has developed a strong association between counting and relaxation, counting can be used alone to achieve relaxation, both in the consulting room and at home. The counting-alone procedure entails the same basic methods just described, except that the steps for relaxation by recall are eliminated. The therapist merely counts from 1 to 10, timing the counts with the client's exhalations, while presenting brief relaxation "patter" between counts. Once the counting is finished, the client should be asked to signal if any tension remains. If so, the remaining tension should be identified and released through recall (or, in rare cases, through a tension–release cycle).

At this point, the client possesses well-developed skills at relaxation. Practice may be decreased to once a day, but the client should be encouraged to continue practicing regularly to maintain proficiency.

Timetable

The following is an idealized timetable for progress in an abbreviated relaxation training program (Bernstein & Borkovec, 1973). Many clients will follow this ideal schedule, but it need not be strictly maintained. Indeed, the pace of progress must be adjusted (especially slowed) for clients who are having various kinds of problems in mastering the procedures. There is a corresponding tendency to want to speed things up for clients who are having no trouble, but in the interest of ensuring adequate learning (and with the exception of the recall-with-counting procedure), each step should be employed by the therapist in at least two formal training sessions. The therapist should never proceed to a more advanced step until he or she is satisfied that the one being used has been mastered by the client.

Procedure	Session
16 muscle groups, tension–release	1, 2, 3
7 muscle groups, tension–release	4, 5
4 muscle groups, tension–release	6, 7
4 muscle groups, recall	8
4 muscle groups, recall and counting	9
Counting	10

Potential Problems

Many problems may appear in the course of relaxation training. In some cases, the therapist may have to find his or her own unique solutions to them. However, some of the more common problems and some workable solutions are given here.

Muscle Cramps

As mentioned previously, cramping may occur in some muscle groups. If this happens, the client should move the affected muscles to alleviate the cramping, while allowing the rest of the body to remain as relaxed as possible. For areas of the body in which the client experiences frequent cramping, alternative tension means should be employed, along with shorter tension periods (e.g., 3–5 seconds). Once the cramp is relieved, the therapist should provide indirect suggestions to help the client regain the previous level of relaxation.

Movement

Frequent gross motor movement during a session may indicate that the client is not relaxing. The client should be reminded not to move any more than is necessary to remain comfortable and not to move any parts of the body that have already been relaxed. The therapist may wish to rephrase the relaxation instructions and present them again. Movement may also represent the presence of a serious problem relating to the client's acceptance of the method being used. If so, this issue should be discussed before proceeding.

Laughter

The client may laugh during relaxation, especially in the first session. This, however, should probably not be a cause for stopping the training session. A client's laughter may indicate something about motivation, feelings, or responses that may be helpful to the therapeutic process. Accordingly, it may be useful to explore the meaning of the laughter with the client after the relaxation training session is completed. There is also a possibility that the therapist is eliciting the laughter. Again, discussing the reasons underlying the laughter with the client may clarify the issues and enable further relaxation training sessions to proceed without interruption by laughter.

Talking

Talking by the client should be ignored unless the client is reporting a serious problem. It may be necessary to repeat the instructions not to talk.

Muscle Twitches

Clients sometimes experience involuntary muscle twitches during relaxation. If such a client seems to be concerned, the therapist should assure the client that such twitches are common, that they indicate deepening relaxation, and that the client should not try to control them.

Anxiety-Producing Thoughts

If the client reports anxiety-producing thoughts during training, the therapist should first try repeating the instructions to focus only on his or her voice and the sensations experienced in the muscles. The therapist can also increase the amount of "patter" during relaxation; this helps distract the client from unpleasant thoughts. Or the therapist and the client together may decide on some pleasant imagery on which the client can focus during the session. This imagery can be incorporated in the relaxation "patter," or the therapist can describe to the client the technique of "thought switching," in which the client deliberately changes the focus of his or her thoughts by concentrating on a pleasant image during the release phase of the relaxation training. Another approach may be to assist the client in altering the rate and/or depth of breathing patterns, as described by van Dixhoorn in Chapter 12 of this volume.

Sexual Arousal

The APRT setting and procedure (a dimly lit room, soft voice, pleasant feelings) can have sexual overtones for some clients. The presence of sexual thoughts and consequent arousal can, in most cases, be dealt with routinely as another form of intrusive thinking that may interfere with the relaxation process. The therapist should recognize and accept the problem, while assuring the client that it is unlikely to remain once the focus of attention is fully on relaxation in the muscles. Naturally, if the problem persists and more substantive interpersonal issues appear to be involved, a more extended discussion outside the context of APRT may be required.

Sleep

Some clients may fall asleep during relaxation. The therapist can determine whether the client is sleeping by first asking him or her to signal if relaxed, and then, if no signal is made, by asking the client to signal if not relaxed. Obviously, the client, if awake, should signal after one of these requests. To awaken the client, the therapist should gradually increase voice volume, repeating the request for a signal, until the client wakes. The therapist should be careful not to startle the client by making sudden, loud statements. It is also important to use an increasing voice volume as the strategy for awakening the client. It is not appropriate to touch the client, because such a move can have multiple interpretations for the client and because the therapist should make every effort to provide the client with a calm and relaxed environment.

Coughing and Sneezing

A client's coughing or sneezing may occasionally interrupt relaxation. Infrequent coughing or sneezing will usually not interfere with the procedure, but if the client has a cold or other ailment and coughing or sneezing is frequent, the relaxation should probably be postponed. A smoker's cough can be very disruptive to a relaxation session. Because deep breathing can trigger coughing for heavy smokers, the client can be asked to take only shallow breaths during tension or, alternatively, to maintain normal breathing during tension and relaxation. Sometimes a change in body position can help reduce the likelihood of coughing.

A CASE EXAMPLE

As noted throughout this chapter, APRT can be used alone or in combination with other treatment methods to deal with a broad range of human problems. For purposes of clarity, we have chosen a case example that illustrates the way in which APRT can work as the primary method of intervention when the presenting problems are rather severe but the time available for treatment is artificially short. Had circumstances allowed, a more elaborate, multidimensional treatment program would probably have been preferable, but these same circumstances created a formidable test of the value of APRT in isolation.

The client in this case was Mr. N, a professional man in his 50s. He had a wife, two children, and a "high-pressure" job, which he felt was in large measure responsible for his psychological and physical problems. At the first session, Mr. N described himself as suffering from "chronic tension." He was well aware of the fact that he was "high strung," irritable, aggressive, and generally difficult to get along with. He was also in considerable pain most of the time as the result of a severe stomach ulcer, which his physician had attributed to stress. For several years, Mr. N had been taking antacids and other prescribed ulcer medication. He also had a supply of prescription tranquilizers, which he took several times each day to combat his chronically high level of general tension.

Mr. N told the therapist that he was planning to move to the East Coast in less than 2 months in order to start a new and even more demanding job. He sought help at this time because he was afraid that the combined stress of the relocation and the new position might be "too much" for him. There was no question of his reassessing the decision to move, so the therapist was faced with the choice of either rejecting the case or seeking to help the client develop some tension-reduction skills—namely, through APRT.

The latter course was chosen, but only on the condition that the client would agree to a consultation between the therapist and Mr. N's physician about discontinuing the tranquilizer medication. This was more than acceptable to the client and, as it turned out, a long-term goal of the physician, as neither was happy with the idea of an open-ended pharmacological approach to the problem of tension. (We should add that the therapist was just as unhappy with a narrow and time-limited approach to psychological treatment, but by this time that issue had been resolved.) The primary purpose in getting the tranquilizing drugs out of the picture was to increase the probability (1) that any relaxation effects observed would be a function of APRT; (2) that the client could learn to experience sensations of relaxation fully without interfering drug effects; and (3) that the skills acquired during APRT would not have to be transferred to a nondrugged state, with possible loss of potency.

Only five training sessions could be scheduled in the time available before the client's departure, so the sequence of events was compressed somewhat. The therapist's goal was merely to teach the client basic relaxation skills and to bring him to a level of competence with them that might serve to combat general tension. Anything more, such as differential or cue-controlled relaxation (see Bernstein & Borkovec, 1973), was clearly unrealistic under the circumstances. Fortunately, the training sessions went very smoothly. The client was, as one might expect, highly motivated and cooperative. He practiced the procedures faithfully between sessions, and at the fifth session he was able to achieve deep relaxation through the recall method.

Somewhat to the therapist's surprise, but certainly to his delight, the client reported a number of immediate and significant benefits that he attributed to his newly acquired capability for relaxation. The client claimed to be far less generally tense and irritable than before, and he stated that he did not miss his tranquilizers (to our knowledge, he has never resumed their use). In addition, Mr. N said that he was finding it easier to deal with stressful events at work and at home by using relaxation "breaks" at the office and at the end of each day. The reduction in general and specific tension was also accompanied by reports of greatly reduced gastric discomfort. Some combination of increased physical comfort and decreased tension (and, perhaps, the prospect of a job change) created a noticeable improvement in Mr. N's behavior in relation to his family. Specifically, he began to appear less irritable, more understanding and tolerant, and easier to live with in general. It seems reasonable to suppose that the changes just described, although not brought about directly by APRT alone, were greatly facilitated by it.

COMMENTS AND REFLECTIONS

After four decades of development, clinical use, and experimental evaluation, APRT remains a major component of social learning approaches to behavior change. It is easy to see why this should be the case. The methods involved are relatively simple, straightforward, and easily adapted for use in isolation or along with more elaborate intervention packages of various kinds. Furthermore, clients usually enjoy learning and practicing the procedures and seem to make good use of the skills that evolve.

At the same time, the clinicians and researchers who use and investigate APRT have become more and more sophisticated about it. For one thing, there is far less defensiveness about the method. It is now seen not as a semimagical method that "makes desensitization work" but as one of several related methods through which autonomic overarousal and maladaptive subjective states can be effectively managed. Accordingly, there is now less emphasis on what is "special" about APRT and more emphasis on how it relates to other relaxation-inducing methods (such as yoga or biofeedback) and what common physiological and cognitive mechanisms might account for all of them (see Carlson & Hoyle, 1993; Smith, 1985; Tarler-Benlolo, 1978). There also appears to be a less rigid adherence to procedural orthodoxy in APRT. Whereas at one time only certain specific relaxation methods were seen as clinically useful, there is a broadening awareness that a single set of procedures, no matter how carefully developed and presented, may not meet the needs (or may "overtreat" the problems) of all clients. Thus, although "live," client-controlled relaxation methods may be desirable in general (e.g., Borkovec & Sides, 1979), there may be clients for whom and circumstances for which less elaborate procedures may be useful as well (see Carlson, Collins, Nitz, Sturgis, & Rogers, 1990; King, 1980). For example, having clients focus their attention during APRT on the physiological sensations of tension and relaxation may be important only for clients reporting certain kinds of problems and may actually decrease the benefits of training in some cases (e.g., Borkovec & Hennings, 1978).

The latter provides but one illustration of the way in which clinicians and researchers have turned their attention to individual differences in clients and their problems in the selection of APRT and variations thereof. As another example, it has been suggested that some anxiety or "tension" problems may involve a strong physiological component, that others may incorporate a significant cognitive component, and that still others may include both. Relaxation may be more useful in some cases than in others (e.g., Davidson & Schwartz, 1976; Lehrer, Woolfolk, & Goldman, 1986).

Finally, it should be pointed out that APRT, in whatever client-specific form it may be administered, has enjoyed an expansion of applications—not only in terms of the target problems for which it is used but also in the way it is used. Originally suggested as a relatively passive state that is incompatible with anxiety, relaxation through APRT has also been conceptualized as an active coping skill (e.g., Goldfried & Trier, 1974) that the client can bring to bear in handling stressful situations. As before, it is seen as potentially useful alone (e.g., as in cue-controlled relaxation) or as an adjunct to the development and use of more elaborate cognitive coping skills (King, 1980).

As illustrated by the examples given here, the flexibility and adaptability that are inherent in APRT represent two of its most attractive characteristics. These features, when combined with APRT's convenience, clinical utility, and apparent benefits, suggest that ever-expanding versions and applications of the original Jacobson and Wolpe methods will continue to be an important part of social learning approaches to human problems.

REFERENCES

Adier, C. M., Craske, M. G., & Barlow, D. H. (1987). Relaxation-induced panic (RIP): When resting isn't peaceful. *Integrative Psychiatry, 5*, 94–112.

Amigo, I., Gonzalez, A., & Herrera, J. (1997). Comparison of physical exercise and muscle relaxation training in the treatment of mild essential hypertension. *Stress Medicine, 13*, 59–65.

Arena, J. G., Bruno, G. M., Hannah, S. L., & Meador, K. J. (1995). A comparison of frontal electromyographic biofeedback training, trapezius electromyographic biofeedback training, and progressive muscle relaxation therapy in the treatment of tension headache. *Headache, 35*, 411–419.

Benson, H. (1975). *The relaxation response.* New York: Morrow.

Bernstein, D. A., & Borkovec, T. D. (1973). *Progressive relaxation training: A manual for the helping professions.* Champaign, IL: Research Press.

Bernstein, D. A., & Carlson, C. R. (1993). Progressive relaxation: Abbreviated methods. In P. M. Lehrer & R. L. Woolfolk, *Principles and practice of stress management* (2nd ed., pp. 53–87). New York: Guilford Press.

Blanchard, E. B., Greene, B., Scharff, L., & Schwarz-McMorris, S. (1993). Relaxation training as a treatment for irritable bowel syndrome. *Biofeedback and Self-Regulation, 18*(3), 125–132.

Blanchard, E. B., Steffek, B. D., Jaccard, J., & Nicholson, N. L. (1991). Psychological changes accompanying non-pharmacological treatment of chronic headache: The effects of outcome. *Headache: The Journal of Head and Face Pain, 31*, 249–253.

Borkovec, T. D. (1987). Commentary. *Integrative Psychiatry, 5*, 104–106.

Borkovec, T. D., & Costello, E. (1993). Efficacy of applied relaxation and cognitive-behavioral therapy in the treatment of generalized anxiety disorder. *Journal of Consulting and Clinical Psychology*, *61*(4), 611–619.

Borkovec, T. D., & Hennings, B. L. (1978). The role of physiological attention-focusing in the relaxation treatment of sleep disturbance, general tension, and specific stress reaction. *Behaviour Research and Therapy, 16*, 7–19.

Borkovec, T. D., & Sides, J. K. (1979). Critical procedural variables related to the physiological effects of progressive relaxation: A review. *Behaviour Research and Therapy, 17*, 119–125.

Carlson, C. R., Collins, F. L., Nitz, A. J., Sturgis, E. T., & Rogers, J. L. (1990). Muscle stretching as an alternative relaxation training procedure. *Journal of Behavior Therapy and Experimental Psychiatry, 21*, 29–38.

Carlson, C. R., & Hoyle, R. (1993). Efficacy of abbreviated progressive muscle relaxation training: A quantitative review. *Journal of Consulting and Clinical Psychology, 61*, 1059–1067.

Carrington, P. (1977). *Freedom in meditation*. Garden City, NY: Doubleday.

Cautela, J. R., & Groden, J. (1978). *Relaxation: A comprehensive manual for adults, children, and children with special needs*. Champaign, IL: Research Press.

Cheung, Y. L., Molassiotis, A., & Chang, A. M. (2003). The effect of progressive muscle relaxation training on anxiety and quality of life after stoma surgery in colorectal cancer patients. *Psychooncology, 12*(3), 254–266.

Cohen, A. S., Barlow, D. H., & Blanchard, E. B. (1985). Psychophysiology of relaxation-associated panic attacks. *Journal of Abnormal Psychology, 94*, 96–101.

Davidson, R. J., & Schwartz, G. E. (1976). The psychobiology of relaxation and related states: A multiprocess theory. In D. I. Mostofsky (Ed.), *Behavior control and modification of physiological activity* (pp. 395–442). Englewood Cliffs, NJ: Prentice Hall.

Davison, G. C. (1966). Anxiety under total curarization: Implications for the role of muscular relaxation in the desensitization of neurotic fears. *Journal of Nervous and Mental Disease, 143*, 443–448.

DeGood, D. E., & Williams, E. M. (1982). Parasympathetic rebound following EMG biofeedback training: A case study. *Biofeedback and Self-Regulation, 7*, 461–465.

Echeburua, E., de Corral, P., Sarasua, B., & Zubizarreta, I. (1996). Treatment of acute posttraumatic stress disorder in rape victims: An experimental study. *Journal of Anxiety Disorders, 10*(3), 185–199.

Edinger, J. D., & Jacobsen, R. (1982). Incidence and significance of relaxation treatment side effects. *Behavior Therapist, 5*, 137–138.

Edinger, J. D., Wohlgemuth, W. K., Radtke, R. A., Marsh, G. R., & Quillian, R. E. (2001). Does cognitive-behavioral insomnia therapy alter dysfunctional beliefs about sleep? *Sleep, 24*(5), 591–599.

Eller, L. S. (1995). Effects of two cognitive-behavioral interventions on immunity and symptoms in persons with HIV. *Annals of Behavioral Medicine, 17*(4), 339–348.

Eller, L. S. (1999). Effects of cognitive-behavioral interventions on quality of life in persons with HIV. *International Journal of Nursing Studies, 36*, 223–233.

Gellhorn, E. (1958). The influence of curare on hypothalamic excitability and the electroencephalogram. *Electroencephalography and Clinical Neurophysiology, 10*, 697–703.

Gellhorn, E., & Kiely, W. F. (1972). Mystical states of consciousness: Neurophysiological and clinical aspects. *Journal of Nervous and Mental Disease, 154*, 399–405.

Ghoncheh, S., & Smith, J. C. (2004). Progressive muscle relaxation, yoga stretching, and ABC relaxation theory. *Journal of Clinical Psychology, 60*(1), 131–136.

Goldfried, M. R., & Trier, C. S. (1974). Effectiveness of relaxation as an active coping skill. *Journal of Abnormal Psychology, 83*, 348–355.

Greeff, A. P., & Conradie, W. S. (1998). Use of progressive relaxation training for chronic alcoholics with insomnia. *Psychological Reports, 82*, 407–412.

Haaga, D. F., Davison, G. C., Williams, M. E., Dolezal, S. L., Haliblian, J., Rosenbaum, J., et al. (1994). Mode-specific impact of relaxation training for hypertensive men with type A behavior pattern. *Behavior Therapy, 25*, 209–223.

Heide, F. J., & Borkovec, T. D. (1983). Relaxation-induced anxiety: Paradoxical anxiety enhancement due to relaxation training. *Journal of Consulting and Clinical Psychology, 51*, 171–182.

Hoelscher, T. J., Lichstein, K. L., Fischer, S., & Hegarty, T. B. (1987). Relaxation treatment of hypertension: Do home relaxation tapes enhance treatment outcome? *Behavior Therapy, 18*, 33–37.

Hoelscher, T. J., Lichstein, K. L., & Rosenthal, T. L. (1986). Home relaxation practice in hypertension treatment: Objective assessment and compliance induction. *Journal of Consulting and Clinical Psychology, 54,* 217–221.

Hyman, R. B., Feldman, H. R., Harris, R. B., Levin, R. F., & Malloy, G. B. (1989). The effects of relaxation training on clinical symptoms: A meta-analysis. *Nursing Research, 38,* 216–220.

Jacobson, E. (1938). *Progressive relaxation* (2nd ed.). Chicago: University of Chicago Press.

King, N. J. (1980). Abbreviated progressive relaxation. In M. Hersen, R. M. Eisler, & P. M. Miller (Eds.), *Progress in behavior modification* (pp. 147–182). New York: Academic Press.

Kroner-Herwig, B., Mohn, U., & Pothmann, R. (1998). Comparison of biofeedback and relaxation in the treatment of pediatric headache and the influence of parent involvement on outcome. *Applied Psychophysiology and Biofeedback, 23*(3), 143–157.

Lang, P. J. (1977). Imagery in therapy: An information processing analysis of fear. *Behavior Therapy, 92,* 276–306.

Lang, P. J. (1979). A bio-informational theory of emotion imagery. *Psychophysiology, 16,* 495–512.

Lehrer, P. M. (1982). How to relax and how not to relax: A re-evaluation of the work of Edmund Jacobson: 1. *Behaviour Research and Therapy, 20,* 417–428.

Lehrer, P. M., & Woolfolk, R. L. (1984). Are stress reduction techniques interchangeable, or do they have specific effects? A review of the comparative empirical literature. In R. L. Woolfolk & P. M. Lehrer (Eds.), *Principles and practice of stress management* (1st ed., pp. 404–477). New York: Guilford Press.

Lehrer, P. M., Woolfolk, R. L., & Goidman, N. (1986). Progressive relaxation then and now: Does change always mean progress? In R. J. Davidson, G. E. Schwartz, & D. Shapiro (Eds.), *Consciousness and self-regulation* (Vol. 4, pp. 183–216). New York: Plenum Press.

Ley, R. (1988). Panic attacks during relaxation and relaxation-induced anxiety: A hyperventilation interpretation. *Journal of Behavior Therapy and Experimental Psychiatry, 19,* 253–259.

Lohaus, A., Klein-Hessling, J., Vogele, C., & Kuhn-Hennighausen, C. (2001). Psychophysiological effects of relaxation training in children. *British Journal of Health Psychology, 6,* 197–206.

Lowe, B., Breining, K., Wilke, S., Wellmann, R., Zipfel, S., & Eich, W. (2002). Quantitative and qualitative effects of Feldenkrais, progressive muscle relaxation, and standard medical treatment in patients after acute myocardial infarction. *Psychotherapy Research, 12*(2), 179–191.

Luebbert, K., Dahme, B., & Hasenbring, M. (2001). The effectiveness of relaxation training in reducing treatment-related symptoms and improving emotional adjustment in acute non-surgical cancer treatment: A meta-analytical review. *Psycho-oncology, 10,* 490–502.

Matsumoto, M., & Smith, J. C. (2001). Progressive muscle relaxation, breathing exercises, and ABC relaxation theory. *Journal of Clinical Psychology, 57*(12), 1551–1557.

Myers, T. C., Wittrock, D. A., & Foreman, G. W. (1998). Appraisal of subjective stress in individuals with tension-type headache: The influence of baseline measures. *Journal of Behavioral Medicine, 21*(5), 469–484.

Paul, G. L. (1966). *Insight versus desensitization in psychotherapy.* Stanford, CA: Stanford University Press.

Paul, G. L., & Bernstein, D. A. (1973). *Anxiety and clinical problems: Treatment by systematic desensitization and related techniques.* New York: General Learning Press.

Pawlow, L. A., & Jones, G. E. (2002). The impact of abbreviated progressive muscle relaxation on salivary cortisol. *Biological Psychology, 60*(1), 1–16.

Phillips, H. C., Fenster, H. N., & Samson, D. (1992). An effective treatment for functional urinary incoordination. *Journal of Behavioral Medicine, 15*(1), 45–63.

Smith, J. C. (1985). *Relaxation dynamics: Nine world approaches to self-relaxation.* Champaign, IL: Research Press.

Suhr, J., Anderson, S., & Tranel, D. (1999). Progressive muscle relaxation in the management of behavioral disturbance in Alzheimer's disease. *Neuropsychological Rehabilitation, 9*(1), 31–44.

Tarler-Benlolo, L. (1978). The role of relaxation in biofeedback training: A critical review of the literature. *Psychological Bulletin, 85,* 727–755.

Taylor, C. B., Agras, W. S., Schneider, J. A., & Allen, R. A. (1983). Adherence to instructions to practice relaxation exercises. *Journal of Consulting and Clinical Psychology, 51,* 952–953.

Vaughan, K., Armstrong, M. S., Gold, R., O'Connor, N., Jenneke, W., & Tarrier, N. (1994). A trial of eye movement desensitization compared to image habituation training and applied muscle relaxation in post-traumatic stress disorder. *Journal of Behavioral Therapy and Experimental Psychiatry, 25*(4), 283–291.

Viens, M., De Koninck, J., Mercier, P., St. Onge, M., & Lorrain, D. (2003). Trait anxiety and sleep-onset insomnia: Evaluation of treatment using anxiety management training. *Journal of Psychosomatic Research, 54*(1), 31–37.

Wisniewski, J. J., Genshaft, J. L., Mulick, J. A., Coury, D. L., et al. (1988). Relaxation therapy and compliance in the treatment of adolescent headache. *Headache: The Journal of Head and Face Pain, 28,* 612–617.

Wolpe, J. (1958). *Psychotherapy by reciprocal inhibition.* Stanford, CA: Stanford University Press.

Yung, P. M. B., & Keltner, A. A. (1996). A controlled comparison on the effect of muscle and cognitive relaxation procedures on blood pressure: Implications for the behavioral treatment of borderline hypertensives. *Behavioral Research and Therapy, 34*(10), 821–826.

Hypnotic Methods

CHAPTER 6

Hypnosis in the Management of Pain and Stress
Mechanisms, Findings, and Procedures

ROBERT A. KARLIN

HYPNOSIS: A (VERY) BRIEF HISTORY

Hypnosis may be seen as the oldest psychotherapeutic procedure still used in mainstream psychotherapy. Although claims for the use of hypnotic phenomena in more remote periods are common, we can certainly trace the roots of modern hypnotic procedures to the medical practice in Vienna and Paris of Franz Anton Mesmer (1734–1815) during the 1770s. Mesmer, a qualified physician, thought that there was an invisible force, the animal magnetic fluid, that he could accumulate in his own body, then transmit to ill people and thereby restore them to health.

Mesmer's methods were a combination of laying-on-of-hands and the application of magnets to the patient's body. In fact, they bore a close relationship to exorcism, a procedure that he, as a scientist–practitioner, derided. Mesmer's treatment often resulted in epileptiform seizures, followed by a sleep from which the patient awakened cured of symptoms. Interestingly, despite Mesmer's theory of an animal magnetic fluid—absurd in light of the science of our time and falsified by the scientists of the 1780s (Franklin et al., 1784/1970)—he cured illnesses and ameliorated symptoms that more orthodox practitioners found untreatable (Ellenberger, 1970).

Mesmer moved to Paris in 1777 and soon acquired proponents for his views, eventually including the Marquis de Puységur, the head of one of France's oldest and wealthiest families. Mesmer retreated to Switzerland after a scientific commission, chaired by Benjamin Franklin, showed Mesmer's theory about the fluid to be incorrect. However, Puységur and other members of the mesmeric Societies of Harmony carried on Mesmer's work. Within the next 30 years, Puységur and his colleagues had demonstrated all the major hypnotic phenomena, including amnesia, analgesia, motor catalepsies and automatisms, positive and negative hallucinations, and posthypnotic effects of suggestion (Ellenberger, 1970). Additionally, they demonstrated enduring individual differences is response to hypnotic suggestion (Shor, 1979).

Hypnosis went through a number of ups and downs during the first three-quarters of the 19th century (including having animal magnetism and mesmerism renamed *neuro-hypnosis* by James Braid in 1843). The modern study of hypnosis began with the work of two French neurology professors, Jean Charcot in Paris (Charcot & Richer, 1882/1978) and Hippolyte Bernheim in Nancy (Bernheim, 1884). Presaging the state–no-state controversy of the last half of the 20th century, Bernheim emphasized the lack of difference between waking suggestion and response to hypnosis, whereas Charcot (erroneously) delineated specific stages of hypnosis and their unique signs. Freud studied with both Charcot and Bernheim. He then returned to Vienna, used hypnosis in his neurology practice, and then abandoned it. In fact, hypnosis was the first victim of Freud's problematic symptom substitution hypothesis (Ellenberger, 1970).

Interest in hypnosis continued throughout the 20th century. In addition to Freud, Charcot, and Bernheim, a highly regarded group of psychologists and psychiatrists spent some part of their careers working on hypnosis during the years from 1878 through 1945. Among others, these included Vladimir Bechterev, Henri Bergson, Alfred Binet, Eugen Bleuler, Sandor Ferenczi, Clark Hull, William James, Pierre Janet, William McDougall, Henry Murray, Ivan Pavlov, Morton Prince, Charles Richet, and Wilhelm Wundt (Laurence & Perry, 1988). The second half of the 20th century was dominated by another group of superb researchers: Theodore Barber, Milton Erickson, Erika Fromm, Ernest and Josephine Hilgard, Martin and Emily Orne, and Phillip Sutcliffe. Their students (e.g., Kenneth and Patricia Bowers, Gail Gardner, Campbell Perry, Ronald Shor, and Nicolas Spanos) and their students' students (e.g., Jean-Roch Laurence and Kevin McConkey), as well as other talented and careful young scholars (e.g., Irving Kirsch, Steven Lynn, and Judith Rhue), have spent their careers studying hypnosis. As well as elucidating the domain of hypnosis, their careful investigations have increased understanding of the potential pitfalls that appear in many forms of experimentation with human research participants (cf. Orne, 1970).

Modern experimental studies of hypnotic phenomena have involved such issues as the existence of a "trance" state (cf. Barber, 1969; Kirsch & Lynn, 1995), the modifiability of hypnotizability (cf. Gfeller, Lynn, & Pribble, 1987; Gorassini, Sowerby, Creighton, & Fry, 1991; Perry, 1977) , the role of social and cognitive factors in hypnotic phenomena (cf. Lynn & Rhue, 1991) and neural correlates of hypnotic phenomena (cf. Horton & Crawford, 2004; Karlin & Orne, 2001; Raz, 2004; Vaitl et al., 2005). It is well beyond the scope of this chapter to deal with these issues, although a section on the mechanisms of hypnosis will allow a brief description of some of the relevant findings. Modern clinical work on hypnosis has involved an integration of science, art, and clinical lore (cf. Lynn, Kirsch, & Rhue, 1996) and to some degree has attempted to deal with the differentiation of specific versus common effects of clinical hypnosis (Rhue, Lynn, & Kirsch, 1993). I suggest later that the specific effects of hypnosis in clinical situations encompass both a cognitive ability called *hypnotizability* (which is related to the ability or inability to hallucinate in response to verbal suggestion) and effects specific to the social role of hypnotized patient, irrespective of measured response to hypnotic suggestibility scales (cf. Bowers & Kelly, 1979; Karlin, 2002). These latter specific effects derive from the history and widely accepted mythology about hypnosis. These beliefs, such as the notion that hypnosis is necessarily very relaxing, are factually incorrect, but widely believed. As a result they influence behavior and expectancies in ways that may be more difficult to achieve with other techniques. Both these beliefs and hallucinatory ability then combine with the interpersonal and situational effects common to all psychotherapies.

In contemporary practice, hypnotic suggestion is used to ameliorate a variety of physical and psychological disorders, as a stress management tool, and as a highly specific treatment for organically based acute and chronic pain (cf. Flammer & Bongartz, 2003). Unfortunately, since the 1970s, in clinical settings we have also seen hypnosis and hypnotic-like procedures influence the reconstruction of memories. Used naively, hypnosis has been used to evoke false memories of incestuous child abuse and to iatrogenically create a malignant form of multiple personality disorder (cf. McNally, 2003).

THEORETICAL FOUNDATIONS

Typical Response to Hypnotic Suggestions

A contemporary observer, watching a demonstration of hypnosis with highly hypnotizable research participants (highs), sees a series of simple verbal suggestions that result in relatively spectacular alterations of behavior, thought, emotion, and perception. For example, the hypnotized burn patient lies quietly and reports no pain, seemingly relaxing while his or her dressings are changed (a highly painful procedure). If he or she responds well to hypnosis, the laboratory research participant, asked to reexperience the distant past, seems to become childlike, entirely captured by the delusion that it is many years earlier. Asked to hallucinate the absence of an obstacle between where the participant sits and some other place, such a participant claims to see nothing in the intervening space. But when asked to walk to that place (and thus through the obstacle whose absence is being hallucinated), he or she walks around the obstacle without seeming to notice doing so. Asked to look back and see that there is nothing there, he or she agrees that there is nothing there and shows no seeming sense that walking around the obstacle has just contradicted this statement. Asked to forget all that has happened until a pencil is tapped twice, he or she will later "awaken" with reversible amnesia.

Thus, in response to brief verbal suggestions, the highly hypnotizable individual seems to see, hear, feel, smell, and taste in apparent contradiction to the stimuli actually present. His or her thinking seems to tolerate logical incongruities more easily than usual. Memory, the sense of volition, mood, and even awareness of self may be altered. With appropriate suggestions, such effects may be extended for some time into the posthypnotic period.

Hypnotic phenomena are easy to elicit and robust. A graduate student, given 2 or 3 hours of training and a standardized script (such as the one for the Stanford Hypnotic Susceptibility Scale, Form C; Weitzenhoffer & Hilgard, 1962), can elicit all the major hypnotic phenomena in a psychology laboratory. There, they can be studied under controlled conditions. Note that for all practical purposes, hypnotic suggestions are likely to be carried out only in settings seen as culturally appropriate. These include therapeutic, classroom, entertainment, research, and forensic settings.

What Clinically Relevant Basic Research on Hypnosis Has Shown Us about the Phenomena over the Past Half Century

A number of issues have been central to experimental research on and theorizing about hypnosis over the past 50 years. Those aspects of recent research and theory that seemingly have the most relevance for the clinical issues are discussed next.

There seem to be two factors that account for the efficacy of hypnosis. First, people manifest stable differences in response to hypnotic instructions (cf. Piccione, Hilgard, & Zimbardo, 1989). Some are highly hypnotizable (called "highs"), some are moderately hypnotizable (called "moderates"), and a few are not hypnotizable at all ("lows").[1] Highs can be expected to report hallucinations in response to simple verbal suggestion.

When brain activity is examined with a variety of imaging techniques, it is consistent with these reports (cf. Karlin, Morgan, & Goldstein, 1980; Karlin & E. Orne, 2001; Spiegel, 1989). Second, hypnotic trance shows no evidence of being a unique "state." Rather, it involves a definition of one's experience as hypnotic and purely subjective changes (cf. Kirsch & Lynn, 1995). However, trance is critically important in the clinical context. When patients define their experience as involving hypnosis, all the cultural beliefs and expectancies about hypnosis are brought into play, including the belief that patients are being influenced by a highly effective and powerful technique (cf. Goldstein, 1981; Rhue et al., 1993).

Factor 1: Stable Differences in Hypnotizability

Susceptibility to hypnosis is defined by participants' responses to standardized scripts for the induction of hypnosis followed by a standardized series of suggestions. There have been a number of attempts to create such scales, but most recent research has used the Stanford Scales (Weitzenhoffer & Hilgard, 1959, 1962, 1967) or one of its derivatives. Scales directly derived from or strongly correlated with the Stanford Scales have been used in a variety of situations and with a variety of different populations. For example, there are self-scored group scales, scales for children, scales to be administered without formal induction, and scales for clinical rather than experimental settings. In general, the scales have contained 5–12 suggestions that sample the realm of hypnotic phenomena. These suggestions range from easy suggestions (to which most willing participants respond with the suggested behavior and experience) to difficult suggestions that are "passed" by only a small minority. Easy suggestions include requests for motor movement without seeming volition (e.g., "As you feel the (hallucinated) force pulling your hands together, your hands will begin to actually move together"). Slightly harder items involve challenges to motor catalepsy (e.g., "Your arm is so heavy you cannot lift it. Try to lift it. Just try"). The most difficult suggestions require a direct change in cognition, perception, affect, or memory. Suggestions for positive and negative hallucinations, amnesia, and the like fall into this category. For example, one might present a display board showing three colored squares and suggest that participants open their eyes and see the two colored squares on the board. A highly hypnotizable participant will be aware of only two squares, not three squares, in response to that suggestion.

Responsiveness to hypnosis is usually scored by the observing the presence or absence of a key behavioral response to each suggestion (although experiential scoring can also be used). For example, the "hands together" suggestion starts with the hands about a foot apart. The suggestion takes less than a minute to make. If at the end of that period the hands are 6 or fewer inches apart, the item is scored as a pass. Similarly, if someone is asked to hallucinate a voice asking a question over a loudspeaker, passing or failing is determined by whether or not the participant verbally responds to the imaginary question. Score on the total scale is simply the number of items passed. Point–biserial correlations between passing or failing a single item and the number of other items passed on a scale range from about .4 to .7, and average about .6 (Hilgard, 1965). So there is good evidence for an underlying hypnotizability factor similar to "G."

Hypnotizability is a very stable difference among individuals. Hilgard and his colleagues have found that test–retest reliability of hypnotizability scales usually averages about +.90 over periods of 1 week and about +.70 over 25 years (Piccione et al., 1989). Among personality traits, the reliability of hypnotizability measurement is exceeded only by multitask measures of intelligence. As interpersonal dimensions are not this stable, the stability of hypnotizability is part of the argument that, basically, it is a cognitive, not an interpersonal, dimension. Another way to view this is that, whereas interpersonal issues may lower willingness to be hypnotized and therefore response to hypnosis, all the willingness in the world will not allow someone who is not very hypnotizable to hallucinate an elephant in the hypnotist's hand. Such a person can imagine the elephant quite clearly, but it will not be experienced as a percept, as highs seemingly experience it.[2]

Hypnotizability is not easily modifiable and governs the large majority of the variance in most experimental studies of hypnotic phenomena (cf. Perry, 1977).[3] It is important to note that what has come to be called "hypnotizability" is observable in response to suggested alterations in perception, memory, and/or cognition with or without formal hypnosis. That is, motivational instructions and/or creation of appropriate set and setting can abrogate the need for the formal induction of hypnosis when making suggestions usually seen as "hypnotic" (cf. Barber, 1969).

Are there truly differences between highs and their less hypnotizable counterparts other than self-reported hallucinations? Although peripheral physiological measures show no differences unique to hypnosis or specific hypnotic suggestions, several studies indicate that hypnotic suggestions to hallucinate alter central nervous system (CNS) activity among highs but not among moderates or lows. Using a number of measures of brain function, one finds that highs differ from their less hypnotizable counterparts in ways consistent with their reported hallucinatory experiences. For example, in evoked-response studies involving both visual and auditory stimuli and across experiments, highs showed evoked response whose components were consistent with suggested hallucinations. When positive hallucinations were suggested, highs showed augmented or faster positive components of evoked potentials and/or decreased or delayed negative components of the evoked potentials. Conversely, when negative hallucinations were suggested,[4] highs, compared with their less hypnotizable counterparts, show decreased or delayed positive components of evoked potentials and/or augmented or faster negative evoked potentials (cf. Karlin & E. Orne, 2001; Spiegel, 1989). In sum, highly hypnotizable participants show brain activity consistent with their reports of hypnotic hallucinations.

This chapter is interested in the effects of hypnotic analgesia instructions, the most clinically relevant negative hallucination. Instructions to not experience pain when exposed to a painful stimulus have been studied with a variety of measures of brain activity, including functional magnetic resonance imaging (fMRI), cerebral blood flow using ^{133}xenon, single photon emission computed tomography (SPECT), and integrated electro-encaphalography (EEG) measures (cf. Karlin et al., 1980; Rainville, Carrier, Hofbauer, Bushnell, & Duncan, 1999; Raz, 2004), as well as with the evoked potentials discussed previously (e.g., Spiegel, 1989). Such studies confirm the pattern seen in the evoked potential studies: Instructions to experience analgesia lead to measurable changes in brain function, indicating central amelioration of the painful stimuli among highly hypnotizable participants but not in lows or moderates (Horton & Crawford, 2004; Karlin & E. Orne, 2001).[5]

Factor 2: Trance versus No Trance, a Definition of the Situation

People commonly speak of being "hypnotized" or in a hypnotic "trance." The underlying assumption is that hypnosis is a distinct, altered state of consciousness. Most early theorizing (and much current clinical thought) about the hypnotic state employed circular reasoning that goes something like this: Q: Why do you say that person is hypnotized?

A: Because he is responding to hypnotic suggestions. Q: Why does he respond to hypnotic suggestions? A: Because he is hypnotized.

In fact, the hypnotized participant acts as shared cultural expectations suggest (Orne, 1970). The deeply relaxed hypnotic participant, sitting quietly while listening attentively to the hypnotist's voice, is demonstrating only one of many forms that hypnosis has assumed. Mesmer's Parisian patients often had epileptiform seizures during hypnosis. A century later, Charcot's Parisian patients demonstrated first catalepsy, then lethargy, and finally somnambulism (but generally did not have seizures) when deeply hypnotized. At the same time, in the south of France, Bernheim's hypnotized patients simply restfully reclined (Ellenberger, 1970). Most modern research participants and patients sit quietly and look very relaxed during hypnosis, although hypnosis is sometimes induced through aerobic exercise (Banyai & Hilgard, 1976).

Peripheral neural activity during these varying hypnotic activities differs widely, reflecting the activity, not hypnosis. Nor has there been any evidence of differential brain activity that accompanies either induction or the entire hypnotic experience. After 50 years of modern research, the lack of evidence for any unique psychophysiological marker of a hypnotic trance state is one of the factors that have led researchers to largely abandon the concept of a hypnotic trance as a causal explanation for response to hypnotic suggestions (cf. Kirsch & Lynn, 1995).

As noted earlier, the ability to respond to hallucinatory suggestions lies largely in the participant, not in the skill or will of the hypnotist, the particular wording of an induction, nor the evocation of a deep trance. Reports of being hypnotized or in a trance and reports about the depth of trance experienced are seen as reflecting a subjective experience that is one of the many effects of cognitive and emotional set, social and historical setting, and suggestion (Lynn & Rhue, 1991). However, these reports are important. When patients define their experience as a hypnotic trance and therefore see themselves as hypnotized, their expectancies are raised, and, as we see later, their outcomes are improved (cf. Goldstein, 1981).

Hypnotizability in the Clinical Context

Stable individual differences in hypnotizability allow interesting interpretations of clinical efficacy studies. Lows, who show a clear lack of responsiveness to hypnosis, are relatively rare in clinical practice. Their failure to respond may reflect intrapsychic or interpersonal factors, a lack of the cognitive ability to respond, or a combination of the two. Thus the responses of lows to both hypnotic induction and to treatment present interpretative problems. Alternatively, moderates, who constitute the large majority of patients seen in clinical practice, are motivated to experience hypnosis and garner its benefits but are unable to experience major hallucinations in response to verbal suggestions. With all the goodwill in the world, they do not see the suggested elephant in one's hand that is plainly visible to the highs. However, they do respond to easier suggestions with both objective movement and subjective experience. For example, it is the relatively rare patient who will not report a force pulling his or her hands together when one is suggested or feeling one arm getting lighter and the other heavier when that is suggested. This allows the moderates to experience themselves as hypnotized and to expect themselves to improve accordingly.

When one compares the treatment responses of highs and moderates, any differences that emerge seem related to the presence or absence of major hallucinatory ability. Alternatively, comparing the responses of patients exposed to hypnotic versus nonhypnotic treatment will tell us largely about the social role and expectancy effects generated by being hypnotized. Finally, when comparisons can be made both between highs and moderates and between hypnotic and nonhypnotic conditions in the same study, it is possible to view the additive effect of the two mechanisms underlying clinical response.

ASSESSMENT OF THE EFFICACY OF HYPNOSIS[6]

Hypnosis is used to ameliorate a very wide range of problems in behavioral medicine and psychotherapy (cf. Flammer & Bongartz, 2003). Direct hypnotic suggestions are employed to provide relief from or amelioration of symptoms of a variety of medical conditions, ranging from acute pain to asthma, from irritable bowel syndrome to warts. It is used for the hyperemesis of pregnancy and the anticipatory and consequent side effects of chemotherapy. Hypnosis is used in psychotherapy to aid psychoanalysis and cognitive-behavioral therapy (CBT). It is used alone or as an adjunct to other approaches for addictive disorders. Finally, and most unfortunately, during the past 30 years it has been used to "refresh recollection" in forensic settings, to create false memories of childhood sexual abuse, and both to set the stage for and treat a malignant, iatrogenic form of multiple personality disorder (cf. McNally, 2003).

Given that this volume is centrally concerned with stress management, discussion of the efficacy of hypnosis will be limited to an exploration of only two of these areas. First, I examine the effectiveness of hypnotic analgesia instructions, in which hypnosis is used to directly ameliorate the perception of the stressor. Second, I look at the adjunctive use of hypnosis with CBT, including relaxation training.[7] Here hypnosis can intensify the effects of beliefs and expectancies common to all psychotherapies (cf. Wampold, 2001).

Hypnotic Analgesia

Given that hypnotic analgesia is of interest both to experimental hypnosis researchers, who view it as a negative hallucination, and to clinicians interested in ameliorating pain and distress, it is unsurprising that the largest single body of research on the clinical efficacy of hypnosis has been in this area. As discussed before in regard to physiological correlates of specific hypnotic suggestions, researchers have given us an interesting view of the possible brain and attentional mechanisms that underlie the hallucinatory aspect of hypnotic analgesia among highly hypnotizable patients. But the ability to hallucinate and thereby banish or ameliorate painful sensation is far from the whole story in regard to clinical phenomena.

Highly hypnotizable individuals make up 0.3–30% of the population, depending on how strictly one sets the criteria for being a "high." Lows, about 15% of the population in experimental settings, are quite rare in clinical settings, making up no more than 2–5% of patients hypnotized in the course of treatment. The large majority of patients will be moderately hypnotizable; they will be cooperative and doing their best but unable to engage in hallucinatory control of pain. For this large majority, other mechanisms than hallucination, specifically beliefs, expectancies, and distraction, will have to ameliorate the pain.

Montgomery, DuHamel, & Redd (2000) did a meta-analysis of the effect of hypnotic analgesia instructions on reported pain using 27 effect sizes from 18 studies. After weighting effect sizes and variability for sample size, they found that hypnosis had a moderate effect on reported pain ($D = 0.67$, Var$D = .26$, $p < .01$) when hypnotic and nonhypnotic conditions were compared. Ten of the 27 effect sizes came from patient samples, whereas 17 effect sizes came from studies with student volunteers. There was no significant difference between the two (clinical, $D = 0.74$; experimental, $D = 0.64$).[8] Additionally, meta-analytic examination allowed comparison among high ($D = 1.16$), moderate ($D = 0.64$), and low ($D = -0.01$) hypnotizability groups.

Notice that the overall effect size of .67 is almost identical to that seen among the moderates ($D = 0.64$). As noted, moderates make up the large majority of patients, and they cannot meaningfully hallucinate the absence of painful stimulation. Thus this effect must be based on the beliefs, expectancies, and distraction inherent in hypnotic analgesia instructions. Among the highs ($D = 1.16$), we get another half a standard deviation of effect size. Allowing for sampling fluctuation, this suggests two additive effects in the range of 0.5–0.7, one related to defining the situation as hypnosis and the other related to the hallucinatory abilities of the highs when being treated for a condition to which hallucinatory ability is relevant. Thus hypnosis provides a setting for and a social role in which suggestions to control pain are seen as reasonable and appropriate. Moreover, hypnosis changes expectancies about controlling pain and provides the kind of relaxation and cognitive distraction that help patients do so. Finally, for those who can actually alter perception in response to verbal suggestion, an additional, hallucinatory effect emerges. This view is in line with the results of the most careful investigations of experimental pain (e.g., McGlashan, Evans, & Orne, 1969).

There have been two more recent reviews of the hypnotic analgesia literature. Montgomery, David, Winkel, Silverstein, & Bovbjerg (2002) examined the efficacy of hypnosis as an adjunct to standard nursing care and anesthesia for surgical patients. They found 20 relevant studies, one of which had three types of hypnosis groups. So there were 22 comparisons between hypnotic and control conditions involving a total of 1,624 patients. In 13 of the studies, assignment to group was random; in 9, it was not. A single mean effect size for all dependent variables was calculated for each hypnotic–control comparison. When the effect sizes were then weighted for sample size, a quite large effect emerged ($D = 1.20$, Var$D = 0.83$), indicating that the average patient in the hypnosis group did better than 89% of the patients in the control group. This large effect size may have been mediated by the weighted impact of the two largest samples, neither of which involved random assignment. (As is shown later, Flammer & Bongartz, 2003, have demonstrated that hypnotic outcome studies with nonrandom assignment can be expected to have significantly higher effect sizes than randomized controlled trials [RCTs].)[9,10] Finally, hypnosis had a positive effect on mood, pain, required analgesic medication, recovery time, and length of time taken by the surgical procedure.

Patterson and Jensen (2003) provided a comprehensive and thoughtful "box score" review of the literature on controlled trials of hypnosis and pain in clinical settings, ignoring the experimental studies with student volunteers that were included in the Montgomery et al. (2000) report. They began with studies of acute pain in which there was clear tissue damage or during a painful medical procedure. (Acute pain can be expected to be largely eliminated when the tissue damage is resolved or the procedure ends.) There were 17 studies identified, which comprised 12 comparisons of hypnosis and a control condition and eight comparisons of hypnosis with an alternative psychological treatment. Most of the 17 acute clinical pain studies were based on painful medical interventions (e.g., bone marrow aspirations, burn wound care, or surgery) or on childbirth. In the 12 comparisons in which a hypnotic intervention was compared with a control condition (waiting list, standard care, or attention placebo), hypnosis was more effective in 8 comparisons and equivalent in 3 studies. The twelfth study had mixed results, with hypnosis significantly improving observer ratings of distress, pain, and anxiety but not the verbal rating of their experience by the 3- to 6-year-old children undergoing bone marrow aspirations. In the 8 comparisons between hypnosis and alternative psychological treatments (CBT, relaxation training, distraction, and emotional support), hypnosis was superior in 4 and did not differ significantly in the other 4. There was no case in which hypnosis was inferior in regard to pain severity as assessed by patient report. In light of these findings, it seems appropriate to classify hypnotic analgesia instructions for acute pain as "efficacious and specific."[11]

Then Patterson and Jensen (2003) looked at chronic pain studies, in which no specific tissue damage was causally related to the pain. Most of these studies focused on headache pain. In this area, hypnosis was equivalent, but not superior, to other treatments, such as relaxation or autogenic training. The authors identified four RCTs involving nonheadache chronic pain (breast cancer, mixed etiologies, and refractory fibromyalgia). Two of these studies showed hypnosis to be superior to an alternative treatment (group supportive treatment for breast cancer pain and physical therapy for refractory fibromyalgia). Alternatively, two studies involving patients with mixed etiologies (most usually back pain) provided equivocal results.

Several explanations for the difference between the clear effectiveness of hypnosis for acute pain and its far less clear effects on chronic pain might be suggested. Distraction will have some effects on chronic pain but not enough to free one of the effects of pain. Moreover, most chronic pain patients will already have done what they can to distract themselves. The reduction of anxiety with hypnosis, also central to its success with moderates in the face of acute pain, is also less useful with chronic pain. In acute pain, anything that relieves anxiety helps with pain. In chronic pain, depression rather than anxiety is central, and one often strives to substitute achievement and consequent sense of mastery and self-efficacy for being pain-free as the goal of treatment. Finally, both the ability to hallucinate the absence of pain and positive expectancies may well fail over the long term when confronted with chronic pain.

In this vein, Patterson and Jensen (2003) suggest that chronic pain is a complex problem, with behavioral and physiological consequences as well as experiential ones. Jensen is presently pursuing a broad-spectrum approach to the use of hypnosis and other interventions with a population of patients with chronic pain, and the results of this program of research are eagerly awaited.

Hypnosis as an Adjunct to CBT

In a highly influential meta-analysis, Kirsch, Montgomery, and Sapirstein (1995) found 18 studies in which similar CBT treatments were administered in a social context that was either hypnotic or nonhypnotic.

The 18 studies that were analyzed in Kirsch et al. (1995) comprised 20 comparisons of hypnotic with nonhypnotic CBT groups, with a total of 90 effects and 577 participants. Larger positive effects tended to occur in larger samples. Two large-group studies of obesity with extremely high positive effect sizes (5.57, $n = 40$; 3.65, $n = 109$) were windsorized.[12] Even after they were windsorized, weighted effect was 0.66, so that the average person receiving CBT in a hypnotic context did as well as the person at the 75th percentile of those receiving CBT without hypnosis. Notice that this effect size is almost identical to that for the overall effect and the effect size for moderately hypnotizable participants in the Montgomery et al. (2000) review.

Analyses of subgroups of special interest can also be made. Kirsch et al. (1995) identified 14 studies in which suggestions were identical in both hypnotic and nonhypnotic conditions. In these studies, the only difference between hypnotic and nonhypnotic conditions was the use of the word *hypnosis* during relaxation instructions and training. Thus differential outcomes reflected changes in the expectancy and related effects of interventions caused by labeling each intervention *hypnotic*. The average weighted effect size for interventions labeled *hypnotic* compared with the same intervention without the label *hypnosis* for these 14 studies was $D = 0.63$. Thus labeling an intervention *hypnotic* increases its efficacy by more than half a standard deviation.

Seven studies analyzed by Kirsch et al. (1995) comprised 157 patients and compared the effectiveness of hypnotic versus nonhypnotic studies in the treatment of anxiety or anxiety-related disorders. There were two studies each of anxiety, insomnia, and hypertension and one of snake phobia. Using Table 1 in Kirsch et al. (1995), one can compute an average weighted effect size for these 7 studies as $D = 0.54$. So internal analyses provide a similar picture to the one provided by the analysis of all 18 studies; defining a situation as hypnotic results in an increase in efficacy of about 0.6.[13]

One other paper should be mentioned. Goldstein (1981) was one of the two windsorized studies reviewed by Kirsch et al. (1995). It compared behavior modification with two hypnosis conditions in the treatment of obesity. In one hypnosis condition, Goldstein used an arm-levitation suggestion to prove to patients that they had really been hypnotized. This group did far better than the other hypnotized group, whose experience afforded no subjectively convincing proof of being hypnotized. Thus the ability to convincingly define one's experience as hypnotic seemingly played a large role in the differential success of the two hypnotic groups in this study.

Recent Overall Snapshot of the Effects of Hypnosis

In the preceding discussion, the results seemingly support the notion that hypnosis has two specific effects, one related to hypnotizability and the other related to the particular history, myths, and role-related expectancies associated with hypnosis. One more meta-analysis is worth examining. Flammer and Bongartz (2003) provide the most comprehensive overall view of the literature on the effects of hypnosis in clinical situations. This review also looks more briefly at the relationship of hypnotizability with outcome. From a database of 444 reports, the authors found 57 RCTs involving between-groups comparisons. The results of this meta-analysis yielded an overall weighted effect size of $D = 0.56$.[14] Examining 6 studies that measured hypnotizability, they found a significant correlation of $r = .44$ between hypnotizability and symptom relief. The studies included one on symptom reduction in irritable bowel syndrome, three on pain control, one on warts, and the last on smoking cessation (which had an r of .16, n.s.). Thus, if we omit the study on smoking cessation, in which no relationship to hypnotizability should be expected, the other studies all focus on the use of hypnosis with uncomfortable physical symptoms and show a relatively large effect related to hypnotizability.

Flammer and Bongartz (2003) then examined another 76 studies of the original 444 that allowed computation of effect sizes. They found 18 studies with randomized designs in which effect sizes were computed from pre- to postdifference scores. These 18 studies had a mean weighted effect size of $D = 0.93$. Nonrandomized trials with between-groups comparisons (22 studies) had an average effect size of $D = 0.98$. The remaining 36 studies were nonrandomized trials using pre- and postdifference scores. These had a much larger effect size ($D = 2.29$). Experimenters who also have clinical practices often complain that the large effects they see in the clinic are seldom reflected in their own RCTs. In this light, it is intriguing to realize that clinical practice involves interaction similar to that found in trials with nonrandomized, pre–post designs.

Problems with the Evidence Base on CBT and Hypnosis

In RCTs, nonblind advocates for a technique compare its efficacy to "no treatment," "less credible placebo," and/or "less favored therapy" conditions. Such experiments are dissimilar to phase 3 multicenter, double-blind pharmaceutical trials. Thus, for the most part, we do not know whether our techniques work as well as or better than a pill placebo, especially a pill that causes minor side effects that add to the pill's credibility as an active medication. We also do not know, with rare exceptions, to what degree an arbitrarily chosen set of structured learning experiences would do as well as current "empirically supported" interventions if presented with a credible rationale by a nice, properly credentialed, intelligent believer (cf. Wampold, 2001). For example, if someone came up with a believable theory that the basis of psychopathology in the modern world was lack of courage, might teaching a (scientific sounding) version of white-water canoeing or rock climbing have equivalent effects to those obtained with CBT with or without hypnosis?

CONTRAINDICATIONS AND CAVEATS

Aside from the occasional short-term headache or sense of being lightheaded, there are essentially no negative effects of hypnosis in experimental settings, in which no long-term consequences of hypnotic suggestion are sought or expected. Unfortunately, hypnosis can be associated with serious negative effects in forensic and clinical settings. The use of hypnotic age regression to "refresh recollection" has caused a good deal of iatrogenic harm and must be approached with great caution. Recall that hypnotic age regression is often vivid and detailed. It is also more factually wrong than ordinary recall, and gaps in memory are often filled in with postevent information or with material generated by fears and beliefs. Moreover, using hypnosis to influence memory abrogates the usual relationship between certainty and accuracy, with people becoming quite sure of entirely inaccurate information. Thus hypnotic age regression procedures can create a vivid, detailed, fictive narrative that often cannot be distinguished from ordinary memory by the patient or the hypnotist (cf. Orne, Soskis, Dinges, & E. Orne, 1984).

In the forensic arena, hypnotic age regression has resulted in testimony that is far more prejudicial than probative (cf. McKonkey & Sheehan, 1995). Especially when used to "refresh recollection" for the facial features of the perpetrator of a criminal act, it can result in a major miscarriage of justice (Karlin, De Filippo, & E. Orne, 2003). In the clinical arena, it has resulted in "recovered memory therapy" in which people, usually women, "discovered" that they had been the victims of incest, usually by their biological fathers, at a very early age. For a variety of reasons, recovering "repressed memories" of early, entirely forgotten trauma is highly problematic (cf. McNally, 2003).[15] The effect on both patients and their families was often devastating.

In addition to finding repressed memories of early childhood incest, in the 1980s and 1990s hypnosis combined with recovered-memory therapy resulted in an epidemic of multiple personality disorder.[16] The "remembered" etiology of the disorder frequently turned out to be satanic ritual abuse during childhood. As there are no widespread satanic cults kidnapping children and equipping them with self-destructive "alters," a rash of lawsuits by patients who had spent years in treatment slowed this fad. While it flourished, however, it provided a new way for patients with borderline, narcissistic, or histrionic personality disorder to play a dramatic role that engaged heroic amounts of therapist attention (cf. Karlin & Orne, 1996). Unfortunately, this iatrogenic version of possession resulted in quite negative outcomes for vulnerable patients and therapists alike (cf. McNally, 2003; Yapko, 1994).

HYPNOSIS: A MINI-MANUAL

Many standardized hypnotic inductions and suggestions are available (cf. Hammond, 1990; Lynn et al., 1996). In the following version I have included an induction mostly based on the Stanford Hypnotic Clinical Scale (Hilgard & Hilgard, 1975) and then followed it with some specific suggestions.[17]

Discussing and Modeling Hypnosis as Anticipatory Socialization for Hypnotic Treatment

Clinicians often tend to be quite concerned about inducing hypnosis; experimentalists rarely have such concerns. In the experimental context, if a research participant fails to respond to hypnotic suggestions and does not experience anything that he or she will define as "being hypnotized" or being in a "trance," nothing is lost. The participant has contributed useful data. On the other hand, in a clinical setting, there is a good deal at stake when inducing hypnosis for the first time. Failure wastes two precious commodities—time and hope. One invests time in explaining how hypnosis works and how it may help the patient in a variety of ways. If nothing happens, one has to backtrack and convince the patient that other techniques will work. Second, patients often come to treatment because internal forces are getting them to react in embarrassing, uncomfortable, and/or ineffective ways in important situations and with important others in their lives. If, in the presence of the therapist, the patient is unable to respond to hypnosis, the credibility of treatment is threatened, and the patient again finds him- or herself blocked by inimical internal forces that, in this case, the therapist cannot help with. Thus one wants each patient to experience something that both the patient and the therapist can define as hypnosis.

To avoid "failure" at hypnosis, the clinician should inquire about previous hypnotic experiences and discuss any myths about hypnosis that may interfere with the patient's response or expectancies (e.g., that during hypnosis, people entirely lose touch with their surroundings and/or control of their behavior or that deep trance is required for a positive effect). In my own practice, if the patient seems skeptical or if I simply feel it will be helpful, I will ask the patient whether he or she has seen someone in a hypnotic state close up. Answered in the negative, I will give myself audible suggestions and put myself into a light self-hypnotic state, using a counting technique and having my hands move together in ways similar to those that I will use and then teach during the patient's hypnosis. This models hypnotic behavior for the patient and lowers patient embarrassment and other interfering thoughts and emotions. I will then introduce and induce hypnosis using a relatively standard hypnotic induction, a modified version of that created by Hilgard and Hilgard (1975).

Introductory Remarks

In just a moment, we will begin hypnosis. Remember that although you will be hypnotized, you will at all times be able to hear me. You may be less or more aware of your surroundings than you are now. It doesn't matter. What does matter is that you listen to my voice, pay attention to my voice. Then, just let happen whatever you find is happening, even if it isn't what you expect. Remember that at all times you will stay in complete control, no matter how deeply hypnotized you become. You will always be able to talk aloud, if quietly, without disturbing your concentration. If at any time you wish to ignore a suggestion, you can say "no" aloud, and the suggestion will have no effect. Similarly, if, for whatever reason is sufficient to you, you wish to come out of trance, you simply say "three, two, one, out," and you will come out relaxed and alert, feeling fine. You give yourself these instructions *aloud*, so that you can't get confused by merely thinking about coming out of the trance and wondering what effect that will have. In this state, we aren't much concerned with what you are thinking, but we are very concerned about what instructions you are getting. Giving instructions aloud allows you to clearly tell the difference between thoughts and instructions. Later, I will be giving you instructions that allow you to learn to put yourself into hypnosis. When you do that, you always give yourself instructions aloud. [*I turn on an audio tape recorder at this point, so that the patient also may listen to the instructions at home.*]

Now, please close your eyes [*at this point I close my eyes, modeling the behavior I want*] and listen carefully to what I say. Let yourself relax as best you can in your chair. Let the chair hold all of your weight, so all your muscles can relax. As you continue to listen to my voice, you may feel more or less wide awake than you do now. But no matter how deeply involved in hypnosis you become, you will at all times be able to hear me. You may be less or more aware of your surroundings than you are now. It doesn't matter. What does matter is that you listen to my voice, pay attention to my voice. You will always be able to hear me and to respond to suggestions that are good for you. Just let happen whatever you find is happening, even if it isn't what you expect.

Hypnotic Induction

[*Speaking more slowly.*] Now focus on your right arm and hand and let all the muscles relax. Let the muscles in the upper arm become limp. The muscles around the right elbow and forearm becoming loose and comfortable. And all the muscles in the hand letting go, letting go. Completely letting go. [*Pause.*] Now allow yourself to pay close attention to the left arm and hand. Let all the muscles in the upper arm become warm and heavy, soothed and comfortable. And let a feeling of deep relaxation flow down into the elbow, forearm, and wrist. Now the left hand and fingers are entirely relaxing as you move into a quiet, easy state of mind. [*Pause.*]

You may find that the mind relaxes along with the body. It becomes possible to put all worries aside. Do that now. Let go of all concerns for now and just let your body and mind relax. Allow yourself to become more and more comfortable as you continue to listen to my voice. Just keep your thoughts on what I am saying . . . [18] more and more relaxed, perhaps even drowsy, but at no time will you have any trouble hearing me.

Blue mountain lake.[19] Just some keywords for entering hypnosis, a pleasant image to delineate this state of mind from other states. I'm going to count from one to twenty, and as I count, you go ever deeper into this quiet relaxed state of mind. You will be able to do all sorts of things that I suggest, things that will be interesting and acceptable to you. You will be able to do them without breaking the pattern of complete relaxation that is gradually coming over you. And you can move around to make yourself comfortable at any time without it disturbing you or breaking the pattern of relaxation. One . . . Two . . . three. Let your legs relax now. Start with the right leg. Feel the muscles in the right thigh relaxing, easing and quieting, let the muscles around the knee and foreleg ease and relax as well. Now feel the muscles in the foot become warm and heavy, warm and heavy. [*Pause.*] Now feel that relaxation flowing through your left leg. The thigh . . . Knee . . . Foreleg . . . Foot . . . toes, all the muscles relaxing and easing as you calm and quiet, become eased and comfortable.

Four . . . five . . . six. Now the trunk of your body, your shoulders and chest, all the muscles in your abdomen loosening and letting go. Letting go, letting go, fully letting go.

Now the back. Imagine yourself breathing through every pore in your body, breathing in a million points of healing light with each breath. With each breath in, relaxation, ease, and health flow into your body. Focus for a moment on the muscles in your back. Imagine them opening to greet the air as it flows through your back directly into your lungs. And as you imagine this, the muscles in the back become easier and more relaxed and let you float more deeply into your chair. Now the muscles of your scalp and face and neck relax. The muscles around the jaw letting go. Letting go. [*Observe whether the mouth opens slightly. If so, the person is truly relaxing, as he or she is violating a norm about appropriate behavior in a public setting. Mouth opening isn't necessary, but it is nice when it happens.*] With each breath out, any remaining tension leaves you. This happens easily and naturally. There is nothing you have to do, no need to try, no need to hurry. As you allow yourself to become deeply, fully, and completely relaxed, nothing will disturb you. You can move about to respond to suggestions or simply to make yourself more comfortable without disturbing your concentration or relaxation in the slightest.

Seven . . . , eight . . . , nine . . . Ten. . . . Now bring both arms straight out in front of you, arms about shoulder height, hands about a foot apart, palms facing inward toward each other. That's good. Hands about a foot apart. Palms facing inward. Now, please imagine a force pulling your hands together. You can imagine that force any way you like. Perhaps you can imagine rubber bands pulling the hands together. Perhaps the force is like having magnets in each hand pulling your hands together. However you imagine it, imagine that force as fully as possible.[20] [*Pause.*]

Now something may begin to happen. You may be able to begin to really feel the force pulling your hands together. Slowly at first, your hands may begin to slowly move together. [*Pause, then as soon as there is any movement, say "Good."*] More and more together. Coming slowly together. And as they come together, you go deeper and deeper into this quiet state of mind, deeper and deeper into hypnosis. Don't try to help. Just let happen whatever you find is happening, as the hands move together, more and more together and you go deeper and quieter. And when your hands touch, that will be our signal that the deeper parts of your mind are open and responsive to suggestions that are good for you. When the hands touch, that will be our signal that you are deep enough to benefit from the suggestions that you will receive. [*Continue to give suggestions that the hands are moving together. When they get close say:*] Soon the hands will touch, soon they will touch. And when they do, that will be our signal of openness and readiness to receive and respond to suggestions that are good for you. Then the force will release and the hands can return to their resting position in your lap. The hands will return to their resting position. Soon they will touch. . . . Now, the hands return to their resting position in your lap.[21] Remember, you will always hear me distinctly no matter how hypnotized you are. [*At this point the formal induction of hypnosis has been completed.*][22]

Stress Reduction: Relaxation and General Healing Suggestions

Eleven . . . Twelve . . . thirteen . . . fourteen. *Magic garden, secret garden.* Please imagine a beautiful garden on a pleasant late spring or summer morning. The garden is a special place of enormous natural beauty. Look at the trees and flowers and grass. Imagine the slight pleasant breeze on your face. And somewhere in the garden you will see a couch or padded bench or specially soft patch of grass, someplace where you can lie down comfortably and absorb the calm and beauty and utter safety of this place. When you see the place to lie down, raise one finger of your right hand to let me know you are there. [*Wait for the signal.*] . . . Good . . . Now, please go to that place and lie down on it and during the next long minute, spend the rest of that morning resting and relaxing in the utter beauty and safety of that garden. Take a long minute and spend the rest of the morning there relaxing and absorbing the essence of beauty in the garden. [*Allow 60 seconds to pass.*]

Fifteen . . . sixteen . . . seventeen. Now you get up from the bench or couch and feel yourself drawn inexorably to the very center of the garden, where there is a body of water. Perhaps it is that mountain lake I spoke of, or perhaps it is a pond or a stream or a brook. Whatever it is, you are drawn toward it. And when you reach the water, just raise one finger of your right hand again to signal me that you are there. [*Wait for the signal*] . . . Good . . . Now please make contact with the water. You might bathe in it, or swim in it, or drink some of it, or simply wash with it. Whichever you do, you will find that the water is a healing balm, a healing fluid that penetrates every solid and permeates every subtle part of your body and mind. The healing balm flows everywhere in you, giving health and strength and ease to every aspect of your mind and body. [*Pause.*]

All right, now look around this place and find something to bring back with you, perhaps a twig or a leaf or a stone . . . something you can reach out and touch with your mind's eye that will connect you back to this place of peace and healing. And, please, safely tuck it away so that it comes back with you, so in the midst of other things you can always reach out and touch it and connect to this source of inner healing within yourself. And when you have done that, again raise one finger to let me know. [*Wait for the signal.*] . . . Good.

Eighteen . . . Nineteen. . . . Twenty, Twenty, Twenty, Twenty. Fully relaxed and fully hypnotized. You are able to incorporate into the deeper parts of yourself any suggestions that are good for you, and in this state you will only be open to suggestions that are good for you, and the deeper parts of yourself easily discriminate such suggestions.

General Self-Esteem Suggestions[23] and Specific Suggestions Designed for the Particular Patient

You are now very deeply relaxed . . . and everything that I tell you . . . will make a deep and lasting impression on your mind and affect your thoughts . . . your feelings . . . and your actions.

As a result of this deep relaxation . . . you are going to feel physically stronger and fitter in every way. You will find yourself to be more alert . . . more wide awake . . . more energetic. You will become and you will remain much less easily tired . . . much less easily fatigued . . . much less easily discouraged . . . much less easily depressed.

Every day . . . your nerves will become stronger and steadier . . . your mind calmer and clearer . . . more composed . . . more peaceful . . . more tranquil. You will become and you will remain much less easily worried . . . much less easily agitated . . . much less easily agitated . . . much less fearful and apprehensive . . . much less easily upset.

You will become and you will remain able to think more clearly . . . able to concentrate more easily and more fully. As a result . . . you will be able to see things in their true perspective . . . without magnifying them . . . without ever allowing them to get out of proportion.

[*Specific CBT instructions can be inserted here. This can be very useful if there are specific automatic thoughts that need to be corrected. For example, one might say:*] The ability to see things in their true perspective will make you more effective and happier in a variety of situations. So you will find that anytime you begin to feel disturbed by thoughts of making a mistake at work, you will remember all the good evaluations you have received and realize there is no evidence that you are in danger of getting fired. Rather, the reverse is true, and you will allow yourself to accept and appreciate the respect you have generated in others around you by your hard work. [*What follows is a return to Hartland, 1971.*]

As you become and as you remain able and willing to keep things in their true perspective, you will be emotionally much calmer . . . much more at peace with yourself and with the whole world. So you find yourself developing more and more confidence in yourself and your abilities . . . you find yourself able to do the things each day . . . the things you want to do and the things you ought to do. You do these things without fear of failure . . . without fear of consequences . . . without unnecessary anxiety . . . without uneasiness.

And everyday . . . you will feel a greater feeling of personal well-being . . . and a greater feeling of personal safety and security . . . than you have felt for a long, long time. Perhaps more than ever before. And all these things will begin to happen . . . exactly as I tell you they will happen . . . more and more rapidly, powerfully, and completely each day. And as you continue to listen to these suggestions and do the self-hypnosis I'm about to teach you, that feeling of being at peace with yourself and the universe will grow stronger and stronger until it becomes as much a part of you as the air that you breathe.

Instruction in Self-Hypnosis and Termination of Hypnosis

In a few minutes I am going to ask you to come back . . . come back awake, alert, with no headache or any other aftereffects . . . bringing back with you all the good things from this place. But before I do, please realize that you can enter this place on your own. You will have a tape of what we have done that you can play. But besides that you will to be able to enter hypnosis on your own and give yourself any appropriate instructions that are *good for you*. Remember, in this state, you will only respond to suggestions that are good for you, and the deeper parts of you can clearly distinguish them.

When you want to enter a trance, you will simply shut your eyes and say aloud "*blue mountain lake.*" Then say aloud, "*Hands together . . . one . . . two . . . three.*" Then, as you did before, raise your arms to about shoulder height so your hands are about a foot apart. Then, as you did, just imagine a force pulling your hands together and find that they come together until, when they touch, you are ready to receive suggestions that are good for you. When that happens and the hands touch, the force goes away, and your hands go back to a resting position. You then count *aloud* slowly from four to twenty and repeat "*blue mountain lake.*" Then you can then say "*magic garden*" and go to the garden to have several hours of rest during a long minute. Or you may wander to the pool or brook at the center of the garden and make contact with that healing fluid. Or you may give yourself any suggestion that is good for you. Remember, in self-hypnosis you give yourself all instructions aloud so as to distinguish between what you are suggesting to yourself and what you are merely thinking. You can say the suggestions softly, but you must say them aloud. Finally, you can come out of this state by doing just what we are about to do: count backward from ten to one and then say "out." At "three," not sooner, allow your eyes to open. When you reach "one," you follow it by saying "out," and you bring back all the good things that you have experienced during hypnosis.

Now I'm going to ask you to come back, out of hypnosis. I'm going to count from ten to one and then say "Out." You will gradually come back. At three, you allow your eyes to open. When I say "Out," you will be fully awake, bringing back with you the good things from the place you have been. All right now, ten . . . nine . . . eight . . . seven . . . six, half way . . . five . . . four . . . three allow your eyes to open . . . two . . . one . . . OUT. Coming back relaxed and alert, feeling good. [*End the audiotape recording here.*]

Practicing Self-Hypnosis and the Posthypnotic Discussion

[*If I am working on teaching self-hypnosis, I will immediately segue into it, repeating the instructions I gave before.*] Let's be sure the self-hypnosis part is set. Simply shut your eyes and say aloud "*blue mountain lake.*" Then, as you did today, you raise your arms to about shoulder height so your hands are about a foot apart. Next, say aloud, "*Hands together . . . one . . . two . . . three,*" and, as you did today, just imagine a force pulling your hands together and find that they come together until, when they touch, you are ready to receive suggestions that are good for you. Remember, in self-hypnosis you give yourself all instructions aloud so as to distinguish between what you are suggesting to yourself and what you are merely thinking. You can say the suggestions softly, but you must say them aloud. [*Closing my own eyes, I say:*] Do that now. Put yourself in a self-hypnotic state and bring yourself back just as I did with you, except this time the whole thing shouldn't take more than a couple of minutes altogether.

I will then prompt the patient to say "*Hands together,*" "*magic garden,*" and so on, and to repeat specific CBT suggestions, helping them with both the phrasing and the timing of their suggestions.

Whether or not we practice self-hypnosis in this session or another session depends on the patient and the situation. For example, severely depressed patients may not be able to do much more the first week or two than to listen to the positive suggestions on a tape recording of the hypnotic session.

After the end of the hypnosis session, have the patient describe what he or she experienced. People tend to elaborate hypnotic suggestions in idiosyncratic ways and often need reassurance that they are "doing it right." So, when asked to go to the Magic Garden, the patient may have gone to a specific garden that he or she has really been to and finds peaceful. That garden may have no water or water at a place other than the center of the garden. The patient needs to know that that is OK. It is important to emphasize that it is the essence of the experience that is important, not the wording of specific suggestions or how a suggestion is related to the person's own life. If the patient has been taught self-hypnosis, I usually communicate that self-hypnosis has been very useful in my life, citing an innocuous incident such as being stuck while writing a paper and using self-hypnosis to get past that point. Next, we schedule times for the patient to play the tape for him- or herself. I will ask him or her to keep the tape in a safe place, out of the hands of children, thus emphasizing the power of the instructions. If he or she is to listen to it while in bed, I explain that it will not harm him or her to fall asleep with the tape playing. He or she will simply come out of hypnosis during sleep. Finally, I will usually suggest that the person practice self-hypnosis once or twice a day but for no more than 2–3 minutes at a time.

HYPNOSIS AS PART OF STRESS MANAGEMENT AND CBT TREATMENT IN A CASE OF SEVERE DEPRESSION

As noted earlier, hypnosis is often used to facilitate CBT. The following case, involving long-term therapy, illustrates how the two can be used synergistically. Given the length of treatment, it is impossible to do this session by session. Rather, a broader overview should aid the reader in understanding how hypnosis is used in the framework of a fairly active and directive psychotherapy. Note that this patient, like the vast majority of clinical patients, was not highly hypnotizable. He was a moderate, compliant and willing to "go along," but not someone who was able to hallucinate with hypnosis. It was the context effects of hypnosis, not its ability to alter perception, memory, or cognition that was important here.

Mr. A suffered from a quite severe and chronic unipolar depression. In the 9 months before seeing me, Mr. A had had a relatively lengthy course of electroconvulsive therapy (ECT) during psychiatric hospitalization, with little, if any, lasting effect. He had been treated with a variety of antidepressants and, over the years, with a number of forms of psychotherapy. Like many others with severe, chronic depression, he arrived in my office strongly believing that any new treatment, like those in the past, would do him no good.

There were several major problem areas, but one key area was managing work stress. I briefly discussed cognitive therapy with him. He knew about it, had some minor experience with it, and dismissed it as "Pollyanna bullshit." Insisting on the utility of such techniques when a patient adopts this type of stance has been shown to be countertherapeutic (Castonguay, Goldfried, Wiser, Raue, & Hayes, 1996).

The one thing that created some hope was a discussion of hypnosis as a treatment modality. He felt unable to do anything for himself or to fight his depression any longer. Hypnosis, he believed, allowed him to be passive and listen to suggestions that might benefit him; he felt he could do that. Although it is clear that hypnosis does not require physical passivity (Banyai & Hilgard, 1976), the format of a standard relaxation induction supports such culture-wide beliefs.

In response to his view, I induced hypnosis using a format very close to that I detailed previously, including using the "hands-together" suggestion to ensure that he viewed the situation as hypnotic. I gave him tapes of our hypnotic sessions to listen to at home but, at the beginning, avoided self-hypnosis and specific CBT instructions. Passively listening to the tapes was in his repertoire. As his mood slightly improved, he was encouraged that "something was working." I was then able to address his belief that others at his job could sense how incompetent he was and therefore felt hostile toward him. In this regard, I used hypnosis to introduce (cognitively oriented) suggestions that he was becoming able to separate his interpretations of the events from the events themselves. He began to see that others were more indifferent to him than hostile. This led to an ability to employ rational disputation, using Beck's (1996) version of the dysfunctional thought record. Disputing the notion that "no one likes me," he recalled that some people at work had engaged in positive overtures that he had turned away.[24]

Now more able to perceive others' positive feelings, he began to socialize a little with his coworkers. These changes, and the sense that something was helping, made him willing to try other behavioral and cognitive procedures. We returned to behavioral activation and momentum-building strategies, along with cognitive techniques. His Beck Depression Inventory (BDI) scores soon moved from the 40s and 50s to under 20. Throughout this period he continued to use recorded hypnotic instructions, asking for suggestions that directly addressed problems he was having at work.

Soon thereafter, the company decided that they did not have enough work in his specialty to keep him busy. They therefore assigned him a job negotiating contracts. His history suggested that this was a job for which he was entirely ill suited. Nevertheless, with the help of hypnotically framed suggestions and the cognitive and momentum-building techniques he had learned, he was able to manage the resultant stress and keep basically positive during the next year, with his mood largely reflecting environmental events. When he felt overwhelmed, disheartened, and too paralyzed to use other procedures, he used hypnosis to allow a temporary passivity that soon led to more active, and actually quite heroic, coping. Note that we would discuss the specific suggestions that he thought might be helpful. Thus for months he was able to do a job for which he was unsuited by training and temperament. His courage, hypnosis, and cognitive therapy all helped him continue to manage the stress and strive hard to do a good job during this period.

Ultimately, the misfit between my patient and the work available in his company resulted in his being laid off. Understandably, he became quite depressed (BDI score over 40). Again, he used hypnosis to feel slightly better and then was able to use cognitive and behavioral techniques to move himself past feelings of worthlessness, hopelessness, and futility. Within a month of losing his job, his BDI scores had returned to well within the normal range. During this period, he was actively searching for a job and prepared for and took a difficult professional examination that significantly enhanced his resume. Eventually, he found a permanent job in a difficult work environment. Despite the difficulties, he is doing reasonably well, and a promotion to vice president is quite possible. He continues to use hypnosis along with the cognitive and behavioral techniques he has learned. Hypnosis is seen as a safety net, as well as a current aid, something that is always there should he need it.

In this case, I used a variety of techniques, including direct advice (cf. Karlin, 2002; Woolfolk, 1998), cognitive and behavioral procedures, and others. But hypnosis, seemingly, made them all possible. Hypnosis was useful because of culture-wide beliefs about it, not because of this patient's specific ability to respond to hypnotic suggestions. Deep hypnosis was not required, simply the sense that something different was going on. Instruction in the role of hypnotic subject was not required; it is well known enough in our culture to seem a natural response to hypnotic induction. Cognitive notions framed as hypnotic suggestions were never subjected to the skeptical appraisal of someone with whom many therapies had failed. Rather, he could listen to and absorb them with faith in the notion that "deeper parts of the mind" would be affected and that, at least at the beginning, only his passive attention was required for efficacy.

SUMMARY AND CONCLUSIONS

As we have seen, hypnosis has two sets of specific effects: those related to the ability to hallucinate in response to simple verbal suggestion and those related to the setting created by and beliefs about hypnosis. In clinical settings the large majority of patients are moderately hypnotizable; they are compliant and able to experience minor hypnotic phenomena but are incapable of real hallucinations. Therefore, unless one is dealing with acute pain and, perhaps, some other physical problems, the hallucinatory element plays little part in actual treatment. Instead, one depends on the ability to use beliefs about hypnosis, many of them both strongly rooted in the culture and factually incorrect, to create situations that are good for the patient. This is true whether stress management or the treatment of psychopathology is the therapist's concern. For example, an anxious patient, who has tried and failed to relax using breathing or progressive-relaxation-oriented procedures, will often relax during hypnosis because he or she doesn't have to try to relax. Instead, he or she naturally relaxes as he or she occupies the social role of hypnotized subject. Similarly, a severely depressed patient may listen passively to instructions and expect large benefits from his inactivity. Finally, wrapped in the mantle of hypnosis, positive self-statements and other CBT techniques may be perceived as stronger and have more credibility, a greater likelihood of being utilized, and greater effectiveness.

Hypnosis is a wonderfully flexible procedure, utilizable in directive behaviorally oriented therapy and in evocative treatment. However, especially in the latter arena, beliefs about the effects of hypnosis on memory have led to its use in creating inaccurate memories of childhood sexual abuse, memories that have driven families apart. The inappropriate use of hypnosis has also resulted in a small epidemic of a quite malignant, iatrogenic form of multiple personality disorder. In forensic settings, hypnotic age regression has led to detailed, convincing, inaccurate testimony resulting in major and minor miscarriages of justice. Thus the use of hypnosis to "refresh recollection" in both clinical and forensic settings should be approached very cautiously, if at all.

Lastly, a joint consideration of the hypnosis literature and the literature on the effectiveness of CBT yields some interesting directions for thought. Attempts to transport CBT into field settings have met with mixed success. Overall, obsessive–compulsive disorder and phobias have yielded the best effectiveness and transportability trials for CBT. These are disorders treated with exposure, and exposure works. Far less success has been seen with other disorders, with even the outcome of CBT for depression giving one reason to pause (cf. Elkin et al., 1989).

Similarly, with hypnosis, control of acute pain in response to hypnotic analgesia suggestions has two mechanisms to account for its success: the ability of highs to hallucinate (with its reflection in measurements of brain function) and the effect of the ritual of hypnosis as a distraction and as a historically and culturally credible means of reducing perceived pain. These add to the change in expectancies and attention concurrent with the use of any technique made credible by expert administration. Thus, for hypnotic analgesia and exposure-based CBT, we not only have RCTs but we also have believable mechanisms that underlie the success of the procedure across settings. I have noted earlier my concerns with the evidence base for "evidence-based" psychotherapy. Going forward, perhaps we should require elucidation of such mechanisms before claiming that a treatment is evidence-based.

Alternatively, we might focus on the contextual elements that make most psychotherapies generally beneficent and on avoiding tempting collusions, such as blaming easy targets outside the therapy dyad, that may do harm. Moreover, an understanding of the power of context and of people's beliefs about our techniques (as illustrated by hypnosis) and a recognition of the logic of emotions, the realities of interpersonal problems, and the utility of common sense might be seen as directions for future progress.

NOTES

1. The distinctions between highs, moderates, and lows can be made in a variety of ways. The simplest is to define hypnotizability levels in terms of response to a standardized hypnosis scale, such as the Stanford Hypnotic Susceptibility Scales—Forms A, B & C (SHSS-A, B & C; Weitzenhoffer & Hilgard, 1959, 1962) and related scales. These scales each comprise 12 standardized suggestions; each suggestion is scored as pass or fail. Most frequently, high, moderate, and low hypnotizability are defined in terms of number of suggestions passed. For example, with the SHSS-A, low hypnotizability is usually defined as passing 0–4 of the suggestions, moderate hypnotizability as passing 5–8 of the suggestions, and high hypnotizability as passing 9–12. A less frequently used method of distinguishing highs, moderates, and lows is to make diagnostic ratings of "plateau hypnotizability" over a number of sessions using clinical techniques for relaxing participants and maximizing their responses (cf. Orne & O'Connell, 1967). Such ratings indicate five levels of response: (1) no response, (2) response to suggestions for unobstructed movement, (3) objective and subjective inability to perform a movement when challenged, (4) responses to suggestions to hallucinate, and (5) reversible amnesia and true posthypnotic response. Each level assumes success at the previous level. The distinction of most importance in this chapter involves the ability to respond to cognitive and hallucinatory suggestions using both behavioral and subjective criteria. Highs routinely respond positively to such suggestions; moderates and lows do not.

2. It should probably be noted that there are no gender differences in response to hypnosis. With the exception of a relatively weak relationship to "absorption" (cf. Tellegen & Atkinson, 1974), hypnotizability seems unrelated to any measured personality dimension.

3. For an opposing view about the modifiability of hypnotizability, see the work of Lynn and his colleagues (e.g., Gfeller et al., 1987) and the work of Spanos and his colleagues (e.g., Gorassini et al., 1991). It is clearly possible to alter responses to hypnotic scales so that relatively unhypnotizable participants can soon learn to pass far more items on standardized scales than they did before. The question is whether such individuals also respond in other ways like highly hypnotizable participants. For example, do they show brain function changes during reported hypnotic hallucinations similar to those seen among untrained highly hypnotizable participants? Given the extraordinary stability of hypnotizability over time, I doubt it. I think the situation akin to a preparatory course for an IQ test. Certainly test performance can be improved with appropriate preparation, but it is not clear that one would still be measuring "G" when prepared participants are measured. In this line, Lynn and Raz are presently planning to conduct research that examines brain function among lows trained to respond as highs to stan-

dardized hypnotizability testing. Whether or not their brain function becomes similar to that of untrained highs may go some ways to settling this thorny issue.

4. In suggesting a positive hallucination, one suggests the presence of stimuli that are not, in fact, present. For example, during the age-regression suggestion on the Stanford C scale, one suggests that a voice will be heard coming from a school loudspeaker. Alternatively, for negative hallucinations, one can ask participants to hallucinate the absence of stimuli that are present (e.g., see two colored boxed on a poster that shows three boxes). Both analgesia and amnesia suggestions are viewed as suggestions for negative hallucinations in this context.

5. It may also be noteworthy that other studies indicate that hypnotic analgesia is not mediated by endogenous opiate systems.

6. The April 2000 issue (48[2]) of the International Journal of Clinical and Experimental Hypnosis, the primary specialty journal, was a special issue titled The Status of Hypnosis as an Empirically Validated Clinical Intervention. Almost all authors who had recently written major review articles or meta-analyses appeared in this volume. Taken together, the articles in this issue equitably represent the general conclusions of hypnosis researchers about what had been demonstrated to that point. Little of substance has changed since. The interested reader can obtain this issue of IJCEH from Sage Publications, 2455 Teller Rd., Thousand Oaks, CA 91320.

7. As is illustrated in the case study section of this chapter, among other things, the role of hypnotized participant can elicit relaxation and willingness to listen expectantly to positive suggestions and provide a context for improvement when a patient feels paralyzed by stress.

8. Where D is effect size (d) weighted by sample size.

9. Montgomery et al. (2002) report nonsignificant differences between randomized and nonrandomized studies. However, the results verge on significance ($p < .15$) and given that there were 13 randomized trials and 9 nonrandomized trials, the lack of statistical significance may well be explained as a type 2 error caused by low power. Another such type 2 error probably accounts for the lack of significant differences between the 14 studies in which a health professional was present to give the instructions ($D = 1.4$) and the 8 interventions that used audiotape ($D = 0.55$). Although audiotape may serve very well in experimental settings, a reassuring professional taking the time to be there in person probably enhances the effects of hypnosis for surgical patients.

10. RCTs are studies of the efficacy of an intervention. Patients who meet predetermined criteria for a specific disorder and who are not excluded due to the presence of undesirable comorbidity or other factors are randomly assigned to treatment or control groups. Therapist behavior during treatment and control conditions is usually governed by a treatment manual that specifies which interventions will occur in each treatment or control condition and which will not. Control conditions may include no-treatment, wait-list, supportive attention–placebo, and conventional treatment. RCTs are used to distinguish the specific effect of the techniques constituting the active treatment from more general effects found in most, if not all, therapeutic interactions, such as a positive change in patient expectancies, desire to please the therapist, and so on. The degree to which RCTs succeed at this goal and their generalizability to ordinary clinical settings are both problematic. Despite their problems, RCTs are often the best evidence available about the utility of a technique.

11. Even the general lack of manuals for treatments in these studies is little barrier to this designation. As Chambless and Hollon (1998) noted, relatively simple interventions may not require manuals. Hypnotic analgesia instructions for acute pain, involving distracting imagery or sensations and/or direct suggestions for analgesia, require only very brief training. They are about as simple an intervention as one can find.

12. Windsorizing data is a way to deal with outliers in a data set so that they do not distort the distribution of sample means and support unwarranted conclusions. In this case, windsorizing the two outlier studies was essentially equivalent to excluding them from further consideration in the analysis reported here.

13. Many of the studies reviewed by Kirsch et al. (1995) were done in the 1970s and early 1980s.

Thus methodological concerns are possible and have been expressed by one of Kirsch's colleagues (Schoenberger, 2000), who called for further RCTs to demonstrate the effectiveness of hypnosis as an adjunct to CBT. However, a recent study (Bryant et al., 2005) has supported the conclusions of Kirsch et al. (1995).

14. Flammer and Bongartz (2003) claim that their meta-analysis is very conservative and may well underestimate effect size because they included dependent variables that could not reasonably be expected to change with hypnosis. They are probably right, especially in regard to pain-related studies. Also, they excluded follow-up effect sizes (available from 22 of the 57 randomized studies). Interestingly, these effect sizes are often larger than those found immediately posttreatment.

15. Given that during age regression we are creating memories—memories that provide narrative, not historical truth—it should come as no surprise that one can age-regress people to the womb and beyond (cf. Spanos, 1996). One can also "age progress" a willing research participant well into the future or to a future life. However, I have yet to be able to age-progress someone to next month, have them pick up a newspaper, and accurately relate the prices of shares of IBM, Merck, or Ford. Unhappily in this case, fantasy has its limits.

16. DSM-IV was published in 1994, and multiple personality disorder (MPD) became known as dissociative identity disorder (DID). So it may seem anachronistic to use the older name for the disorder at this late date. The problem is that the older nomenclature is better. First, it is a description of the disorder as both the public and most clinicians understand it. Second, the term *dissociative identity disorder* indicates a mechanism that supposedly underlies the overt manifestation of the disorder, dissociation. However, I do not believe that dissociation, a much overused and highly problematic term, underlies most expressions of the syndrome (cf. Karlin & Orne, 1996). Rather than reflecting complex lesions in memory, MPD seems to involve (almost always) a dramatic social role adopted by patients with borderline, narcissistic, or histrionic personality disorder. Being a "multiple personality" allows such patients to focus away from unpleasant affects inherent in their disorders and to avoid responsibility for their behavior.

Let's briefly look at the evidence. For well over a century, cases of multiple personality were very rare and evidenced one or two alters. The usual alters were a somewhat withdrawn and morose personality and a somewhat flamboyant one. This older and milder version of MPD was still seen as recently as the 1950s. For example, Thigpen and Cleckley's (1957) *The Three Faces of Eve* portrayed a patient whose alters were rigid versus naughty. Moreover, Eve's disorder was traceable to her parents' well-meaning demand that she kiss her dead grandmother good-bye, hardly a case of incestuous abuse. Incidentally, Cleckley claims that of the thousands of putative multiples that have been referred to him since Eve, only one was a true multiple personality.

It was not until *Sybil* (Schrieber, 1973), the story of Cornelia Wilbur's patient, became a best-seller and then a movie, that we began to see the multilayered numerous alters that are common today. Sybil had numerous alters, some suicidal, and her disorder was caused by sadistic sexual abuse by her mother. Unfortunately, Sybil seems to have become the prototype for epidemic MPD (Ganaway, 1995). At present, MPD is a severe and malignant syndrome, with self-destructive alters being routine. It has also become increasingly rare to find patients with just two or three personalities. Having more than 10 alters has become commonplace, and more than 100 have been discovered in several patients.

The changing and malleable nature of this disorder suggests that we are seeing underlying pathology expressed in a manner shaped by the expectations and demand characteristics of the clinical setting. The geographic distribution of this disorder, which is observed largely among North American women and among women from a small set of Western European countries, also suggests that this symptom profile is shaped by cultural expectations and the availability of the role. Next, given that children are often observed by adults, the infrequency of childhood cases of MPD suggests that the disorder is an iatrogenic, adult expression of psychopathology, not a defense employed by overwhelmed children.

Finally, consider the rarity of simple psychogenic amnesia and that simple fugues are the equivalent of hen's teeth. For example, in more than 50 years of combined practice in hypnosis, Martin Orne and I reported having seen a total of three cases of simple psychogenic amnesia outside the forensic setting (Karlin & Orne, 1996). In that light, consider putative lesions in memory such that A knows about B and D, but not C, whereas C knows about all of them except G and H, and so on. Each of the personalities requires a fugue more complex than any seen before the publication of Sybil. Moreover, the notion that such complex fugue states are both relatively common and come and go on demand is absurd. It is similar to being told of a previously undiscovered talent that allows large groups of people to run 3-minute miles and jump 20 vertical feet. The organism simply isn't built that way. In light of these factors, the belief that MPD symptoms are purely the product of defensive dissociative states, rather than a dramatic social role legitimized by the media and therapists, seems naive. Hypnotic treatment based on that belief can be quite destructive.

17. The suggestions include a large section condensed from Hartland's (1971) ego strengthening technique, some paraphrased versions of suggestions or techniques taught by Martin Orne, Arnold Lazarus, or Herbert Spiegel, those I ran across elsewhere and liked, as well as occasional phrasing of my own. When I am aware of the source of the paraphrased suggestion, I have noted it. But I have been doing this so long that it is certain that some of what I consider original was, in fact, a gift from others. I ask their pardon for not citing them.

18. The symbol . . . Indicates a brief pause.

19. My arbitrarily chosen, signal phrase, "blue mountain lake," is used to delineate hypnotic and nonhypnotic periods. Although I use this phrase in heterohypnosis, I consider the phrase most useful in the context of self-hypnosis. Using it allows the patient to specify that the instructions that follow are hypnotic.

20. There is a trade-off here that is very important to understand. Although one never wants to give a suggestion to which the patient does not respond, at the same time suggestions should ask that something unusual occur so that the patient will attribute the unusual event to entering hypnotic trance. Thus I tend to avoid inductions involving naturally occurring phenomena, events that the patient can reasonably expect to occur, trance or no trance. For example, I would not induce trance by having someone gaze fixedly at a point above eye level. The eye fatigue and eye closure that routinely follow are too easily (and correctly) attributed to simple muscle fatigue. Thus I routinely use a hands-together suggestion to induce the experience of trance. There are a number of ways of minimizing the (quite minor) risks of having a patient not experience seemingly involuntary movement of the hands, but they are largely beyond the scope of the present discussion. However, let me mention one way to avoid the problem. One can give the hands-together suggestion without formally inducing hypnosis. Rather, the suggestion can be presented as a prehypnotic"test." One says, "Just let me see something. Allow your eyes to shut and hold both hands straight out in front of you," and so on. Because you can't fail at something you never tried, if the suggestion does not result in a positive response, the patient has not failed to respond to hypnosis. One then proceeds cautiously to determine the cause of the problem. However, such lack of response is rare. When a positive response occurs, as it does with the overwhelming majority of patients, one can easily segue from the nonhypnotic test into hypnosis with a patient who has already experienced an "involuntary" response. In my view, it is hard to overemphasize the importance of the patient perceiving her- or himself as hypnotized. The large differences in outcomes between the obesity patients who did hypnosis with or without a self-convincing arm levitation item in Goldstein's (1981) study seem to support this view.

21. When asking for a movement at any point in the procedure, repeat the last sentence, or last few words of the sentence, as needed, pausing between repetitions, until the movement occurs or it is clear it isn't going to occur. Incidentally, at this point, we are leaving the Stanford Hypnotic Clinical Scale (Hilgard & Hilgard, 1975). What follows for a while is my phrasing.

22. Similar techniques, such as a hand-levitation suggestion, are used to deepen hypnosis, if neces-

sary. For example, "Your arm feels lighter and lighter, as if it were being pulled upward by a buoyant balloon. Feel your arm become lighter and lighter. Pulled upward. And as your hand and arm rise upward, you go deeper and deeper, deeper and deeper, until, when you have reached the proper depth for you here and now, your arm will return to its resting position in your lap. Its resting position in your lap." Incidentally, this is the type of suggestion advocated by Orne and O'Connell (1967) to maximize hypnotic responsiveness.

23. These general suggestions are paraphrased and condensed from Hartland (1971).

24. From my point of view, there were two critical elements here. First, my patient had "tried" cognitive therapy and "it didn't work." So he was unwilling to try to actively dispute his strongly held, irrational cognitions. Moreover, he felt incapable of actively disputing them, even had he wanted to do so. Unlike most approaches, hypnosis allowed him to be passive and merely listen a number of times to the suggestion that he was becoming able to separate events and their interpretation. He could not repeatedly listen to that suggestion without understanding that his interpretations could be and should be separated from the events he was experiencing. Further, the suggestion said that he was more and more capable of making this differentiation. It then became reasonable to ask him about what had occurred during the week and to simply note that the behavior of his colleagues seemed more inattentive than hostile. Once hypnosis had planted the seed and discussion had paved the way, he came up with the (just noted) instances in which his colleagues had made positive overtures to him. At that point, he began to see his cognitions as irrational and became willing to dispute them in a standard CBT format enhanced by further hypnotic suggestions about emerging changes.

REFERENCES

Banyai, E., & Hilgard, E. (1976). A comparison of active-alert hypnotic induction with traditional relaxation induction. *Journal of Abnormal Psychology, 85*, 218–224.

Barber, T. (1969). *Hypnosis: A scientific approach.* New York: Van Nostrand Reinhold.

Beck, J. (1996). *Cognitive therapy worksheet packet.* Bala Cynwyd, PA: Beck Institute.

Bernheim, H. (1884). *De la suggestion dans l'etat hypnotique et dans l'etat de vielle.* Paris: Doin.

Bowers, K., & Kelly, P. (1979). Stress, disease, psychotherapy, and hypnosis. *Journal of Abnormal Psychology, 88*, 490–505.

Bryant, R., Moulds, M., Guthrie, R., & Nixon, R. (2005). The additive benefit of hypnosis and cognitive-behavioral therapy in treating acute stress disorder. *Journal of Consulting and Clinical Psychology, 73*, 334–340.

Castonguay, L., Goldfried, M., Wiser, S., Raue, P., & Hayes, A. (1996). Predicting the effect of cognitive therapy for depression: A study of unique and common factors. *Journal of Consulting and Clinical Psychology, 64*, 497–504.

Chambless, D., & Hollon, S. (1998). Defining empirically supported therapies. *Journal of Consulting and Clinical Psychologist, 66*, 7–18.

Charcot, J., & Richer, P. (1978). Contributions de l'hypnotisme chez les hysteriques. In *The origins of psychiatry and psychoanalysis: Pre-Freudian psychology series—France.* (Vol. 28). Nendeln/ Lichtenstein: Kraus-Thompson. (Original work published 1882)

Elkin, I., Shea, T., Watkins, J., Imber, S., Sotsky, S., Collins, J., et al. (1989). National Institute of Mental Health treatment of depression collaborative research program: General effectiveness of treatments. *Archives of General Psychiatry, 46*, 971–982.

Ellenberger, H. (1970). *The discovery of the unconscious: The history and evolution of dynamic psychiatry.* New York: Basic Books.

Flammer, E., & Bongartz, W. (2003). On the efficacy of hypnosis: A meta-analytic study. *Contemporary Hypnosis, , 20*, 179–197.

Franklin, B., de Bory, G., Lavoisier, A., Bailly, J., Majault, M., Sallin, J., et al. (1784). *Rapport des Commissionaires charges par le Roy de l'examen du magnetisme animal.* Paris: Bibliotheque Royale. (English reprint) *Foundations of hypnosis: From Mesmer to Freud*, pp. 82–128, by M. Tinterow, Ed., 1970. Springfield, IL: Thomas.

Ganaway, G. (1995). Hypnosis, childhood trauma, and dissociative identity disorder: Toward an integrative theory. *International Journal of Clinical and Experimental Hypnosis, 43,* 127–144.

Gfeller, J., Lynn, S., & Pribble, W. (1987). Enhancing hypnotic susceptibility: Interpersonal and rapport factors. *Journal of Personality and Social Psychology, 52,* 586–595.

Goldstein, Y. (1981). The effect of demonstrating to a subject that she is in a hypnotic trance as a variable in hypnotic interventions with obese women. *International Journal of Clinical and Experimental Hypnosis, 29,* 15–23.

Gorassini, D., Sowerby, D., Creighton, A., & Fry, G. (1991). Hypnotic suggestibility enhancement through brief cognitive skill training. *Journal of Personality and Social Psychology, 61,* 289–297.

Hammond, D. (Ed.). (1990). *Handbook of hypnotic suggestions and metaphors.* New York: Norton.

Hartland, J. (1971). Further observations on the use of "ego-strengthening" techniques. *American Journal of Clinical Hypnosis, 14,* 1–8.

Hilgard, E. (1965). *Hypnotic susceptibility.* New York: Harcourt Brace Jovanovich

Hilgard, E., & Hilgard, J. (1975). *Hypnosis in the relief of pain.* Los Altos, CA: Kaufmann.

Horton, J., & Crawford, H. (2004). Neurophysiological and genetic determinants of high hypnotizability. In M. Heap, R. Brown, & D. Oakley (Eds.), *The highly hypnotizable person: Theoretical, experimental and clinical issues*(pp. 133–51). London: Routledge.

Karlin, R. (2002). Advice and consent: Demand characteristics, ritual, and the transmission of practical wisdom in the clinical context. *Prevention and Treatment, 5,* Article 44.

Karlin, R., De Filippo, F., & Orne, E. (2003, November). *Eyewitness identification in murder cases where memory was "refreshed" by hypnosis: Armstrong and Kempinski.* Paper presented at the annual meeting of the Society for Clinical and Experimental Hypnosis, Chicago.

Karlin, R., Morgan, D., & Goldstein, L. (1980). Hypnotic analgesia: A preliminary investigation of quantitated hemispheric EEG and attentional correlates. *Journal of Abnormal Psychology, 31,* 227–234.

Karlin, R., & Orne E. (2001). Neural basis of hypnosis. In N. Smelser & P. Baltes (Eds.), *International encyclopedia of the social and behavioral sciences* (Vol. 10, pp. 7101–7105). New York: Elsevier Science.

Karlin, R., & Orne, M. (1996). Hypnosis, social influence, incestuous child abuse, and satanic ritual abuse: The iatrogenic creation of horrific memories for the remote past. *Cultic Studies Journal, 13,* 42–94.

Kirsch, E., & Lynn, S. (1995). The altered state of hypnosis: Changes in the theoretical landscape. *American Psychologist, 50,* 846–858.

Kirsch, I., Montgomery, G., & Sapirstein, G. (1995). Hypnosis as an adjunct to cognitive-behavioral psychotherapy: A meta-analysis. *Journal of Consulting and Clinical Psychology, 63,* 214–220.

Laurence, J., & Perry, C. (1988). *Hypnosis, will, and memory: A psycho-legal history.* New York: Guilford Press.

Lynn, S., Kirsch, I., & Rhue, J. (1996). *Casebook of clinical hypnosis.* Washington, DC: American Psychological Association.

Lynn, S., & Rhue, J. (1991). *Theories of hypnosis: Current models and perspectives.* New York: Guilford Press.

McGlashan, T., Evans, F., & Orne, M. (1969). The nature of hypnotic analgesia and placebo response to experimental pain. *Psychosomatic Medicine, 31,* 227–246.

McKonkey, K., & Sheehan, P. (1995). *Hypnosis, memory, and behavior in criminal investigation.* New York: Guilford Press.

McNally, R. (2003). *Remembering trauma.* Cambridge, MA: Harvard University Press.

Montgomery, G., David, D., Winkel, G., Silverstein, J., & Bovbjerg, D. (2002). The effectiveness of adjunctive hypnosis with surgical patients. *Anesthesia and Analgesia, 94,* 1639–1645.

Montgomery, G., DuHamel, K., & Redd, W. (2000). A meta-analysis of hypnotically induced analgesia: How effective is hypnosis? *International Journal of Clinical and Experimental Hypnosis, 48,* 138–153.

Orne, M. (1970). Hypnosis, motivation, and the ecological validity of the psychological experiment. In W. Arnold & M. Page (Eds.), *Nebraska Symposium on Motivation* (pp. 187–265). Lincoln: University of Nebraska Press.

Orne, M., & O'Connell, D. (1967). Diagnostic ratings of hypnotizability. *International Journal of Clinical and Experimental Hypnosis, 15,* 125–133.

Orne, M., Soskis, D., Dinges, D., & Orne, E. (1984). Hypnotically induced testimony. In G. Wells & E. Loftus (Eds.), *Eyewitness testimony: Psychological perspectives*(pp. 171–213). New York: Cambridge University Press.

Patterson, D., & Jensen, M. (2003). Hypnosis and clinical pain. *Psychological Bulletin, 129*, 495–521.

Perry, C. (1977). Is hypnotizability modifiable? *International Journal of Clinical and Experimental Hypnosis, 25*, 125–146.

Piccione, C., Hilgard, E., & Zimbardo, P. (1989). On the degree of stability of measured hypnotizability over a 25-year period. *Journal of Personality and Social Psychology, 56*, 289–295.

Rainville, P., Carrier, B., Hofbauer, R., Bushnell, M., & Duncan, G. (1999). Dissociation of sensory and affective dimensions of pain using hypnotic modulation. *Pain, 82*, 159–171.

Raz, A. (2004, November). *Multiple assays of highly- and less-hypnotizable individuals.* Paper presented at the annual meeting of the Society for Clinical and Experimental Hypnosis, Santa Fe, NM.

Rhue, J., Lynn, S., & Kirsch, I. (1993). *Handbook of clinical hypnosis.* Washington, DC: American Psychological Association.

Schoenberger, N. (2000). Research on hypnosis as an adjunct to cognitive-behavioral psychotherapy. *International Journal of Clinical and Experimental Hypnosis, 48*, 154–169.

Schreiber, F. (1973). *Sybil.* Chicago: Regnery.

Sheehan, P., & Perry, C. (1976). *Methodologies of hypnosis: A critical appraisal of contemporary paradigms of hypnosis.* Hillsdale, NJ: Erlbaum.

Shor, R. (1979). The fundamental problem in hypnosis research as viewed from historic perspectives. In E. Fromm & R. Shor (Eds.), *Hypnosis: Developments in research and new perspectives* (pp. 15–41). Hawthorne, NY: Aldine.

Spanos, N. (1996). *Multiple identities and false memories: A sociocognitive perspective.* Washington, DC: American Psychological Association.

Spiegel, D. (1989). Cortical event-related evoked potential correlates of hypnotic hallucinations. In V. Gheorghiu, P. Netter, H. Eysenck, & R. Rosenthal (Eds.), *Suggestion and suggestibility: Theory and research*(pp. 183–189). New York: Springer-Verlag.

Tellegen, A., & Atkinson, G. (1974). Openness to absorbing and self-altering experiences ("absorption"), a trait related to hypnotic susceptibility. *Journal of Abnormal Psychology, 83*, 268–277.

Thigpen, C., & Cleckley, H. (1957). *The three faces of Eve.* New York: McGraw-Hill.

Vaitl, D., Birbaumer, N., Gruzelier, J., Jamieson, G., Kotchoubey, B., Kubler, A., et al. (2005). Psychobiology of altered states of consciousness. *Psychological Bulletin, 131*, 98–127.

Wampold, B. (2001) *The great psychotherapy debate: Models, methods, and findings.* Mahwah, NJ: Erlbaum.

Weitzenhoffer, A., & Hilgard, E. (1959). *Stanford Hypnotic Susceptibility Scales: Forms A and B.* Palo Alto, CA: Consulting Psychologists Press.

Weitzenhoffer, A., & Hilgard, E. (1962). *Stanford Hypnotic Susceptibility Scales: Form C.* Palo Alto, CA: Consulting Psychologists Press.

Weitzenhoffer, A., & Hilgard, E. (1967). *Revised Stanford Profile Scales of Hypnotic Susceptibility: Forms I and II.* Palo Alto, CA: Consulting Psychologists Press.

Woolfolk, R. (1998). *The cure of souls: Science, values, and psychotherapy.* San Francisco: Jossey-Bass.

Yapko, M. (1994). Memories of the future: Regression and suggestions of abuse. In J. Zeig (Ed.), *Erickson's approach to multiple personality: A cross-cultural perspective* (pp. 482–494). New York: Brunner/Mazel.

CHAPTER 7

The Autogenic Training Method of J. H. Schultz

WOLFGANG LINDEN

THE HISTORY OF AUTOGENIC TRAINING

In a field as young as clinical psychology or the even younger one of stress management, autogenic training (AT) is almost a "grandmother"; it is one of the oldest biobehavioral techniques known and used. Although widely practiced all over Europe, in Russia, and in Japan, AT is much less popular in North America.

The German neurologist Johannes Heinrich Schultz (1884–1970) is credited with the development and promulgation of AT, which he himself described as a self-hypnotic procedure. During his medical training in dermatology and neurology, Schultz became fascinated with heterohypnosis, which, however, had a dubious image to many of his medical supervisors and peers at that time. Initially, Schultz worked with hypnosis only on his own time, outside of his regular clinic duties. The dominant therapeutic approach then for mental and psychosomatic problems was psychoanalysis, but Schultz rejected analysis as a promising treatment for psychosomatic disturbances. In a brief biography, Schaefgen (1984, p. 58) cites Schultz as having said that "it is complete nonsense to shoot with psychoanalytic guns after symptom-sparrows."

The breakthrough of AT came after Schultz opened his own medical practice in neurology and psychiatry in Berlin in 1924, where he promulgated AT without the constraints of medical superiors who did not share his vision. His first formal presentation of his experiences with AT was in 1926, in front of his colleagues in the Medical Society; his first book followed 6 years later (Schultz, 1932). In all, he is accredited with over 400 publications, numerous books, and translations of these into six languages. His groundbreaking book on AT had seen 18 editions by 1984.

The development of AT as a novel technique appears to be based on two sources: Schultz's own experiences with clinical hypnosis and Oskar Vogt's observations in brain research. Schultz himself noted that his hypnotized patients regularly reported two distinct sensations—an unfamiliar heaviness, especially in the limbs, and a similarly strange sensation of warmth. He was convinced that hypnosis was not something that the hypnotist actively did to the patient but something that the patient permitted to happen and, in that sense, actually did to himself or herself. In order for the patient to enter this state, there had to be a "switch," a point of change. Provoking this switch—placing the control in the hands of the patient—was what Schultz wanted to achieve. Oskar Vogt's experiences further strengthened Schultz's belief that it was possible to reliably trigger an autogenic state, because Vogt, a brain researcher, had reported to Schultz that his patients could volitionally produce the sensations of heaviness and warmth and could switch into self-hypnotic trance. Herein lay the seed for the autogenic formulas. Over several years, Schultz further developed the idea of formulas to reliably achieve deep relaxation and its accompanying sensations in various parts of the body. The publication of his 1932 book on AT was the culmination of his efforts to standardize the procedure.

AT remained essentially unknown on the other side of the Atlantic Ocean until one of Schultz's followers, Wolfgang Luthe, a physician, emigrated to Canada and began clinical work, teaching, and research on AT in English. A benchmark article appeared in the *American Journal of Psychotherapy* (Luthe, 1963), and this was later followed by a hefty six-volume book series that Luthe coauthored with Schultz (Luthe, 1970a, 1970b, 1970c; Luthe & Schultz, 1969a, 1969b; Schultz & Luthe, 1969). These volumes provide extensive descriptions of supporting experimental research, case studies, and clinical success reports of AT for a wide range of clinical problems. For the reader with a strong empiricist bent, however, reading the original works will likely be a frustrating task, because in the ultimate evaluation of AT's effectiveness no distinction is made by Schultz and Luthe among opinions, single-case reports, and controlled studies (of which there were precious few). For a more detailed description of the background research and applications, I refer the reader to my book *Autogenic Training: A Clinical Guide* (Linden, 1990), and for diligent reports on outcome the reader may want to peruse Stetter and Kupper's (2002) excellent meta-analysis or my detailed review that combines a narrative with a meta-analytic review approach (Linden, 1994).

THEORETICAL UNDERPINNINGS

Given the apparent similarities among meditation, hypnosis, biofeedback, muscular relaxation training, and AT (Benson, 1975), it requires a fine-grained analysis to reveal differences in underlying rationale, technique, and—possibly—outcome. Mensen (1975) aptly described AT as the "legitimate daughter" of hypnosis. AT, however, should not simply be equated with hypnosis; nor is it simply another form of relaxation therapy. Among the many descriptors used are "a psychophysiological self-control therapy" (Pikoff, 1984, p. 620) and "a psychophysiologic form of psychotherapy which the patient carries out himself by using passive concentration upon certain combinations of psychophysiologically adapted stimuli" (Luthe, 1963, p. 175). Although these latter two definitions may seem wordy, they emphasize AT's uniqueness as an autonomic self-regulation therapy. The emphasis is on "self-control" and "which the patient carries out." This also explains why AT manuals do not come with a cassette or CD that the patient can (or should) take home. In contrast, progressive muscular relaxation (PMR) as described by Bernstein and Borkovec (1973) combines the written manual with a record (later, tapes were offered) to facilitate relaxation practice. In this sense, AT is more similar to Jacobson's (1938) original PMR technique (see McGuigan & Lehrer, Chapter 4, this volume).

The term *autogenic* is derived from the Greek words *autos* and *genos* and can aptly be translated as "self-exercise" or "self-induction therapy." It is furthermore important to present in detail how in AT a conceptually sensible, physiological rationale and self-hypnotic suggestions are woven into a type of intervention linking "mind" and "body."

The creator of AT, Johannes Heinrich Schultz, was a firm believer in the self-regulatory capacities and ultimately the self-healing powers of the body if it were only left alone to do its "programmed" work. Homeostatic models (Cannon, 1933) and more recent formulations of biological self-regulation theory (Linden, 1988; Schwartz, 1977) were foreshadowed by Schultz when he conceptualized AT (Schultz, 1932). Although the most typical application of AT is to reduce excessive autonomic arousal (i.e., it serves as a relaxation technique), the AT rationale embraces a bidirectional homeostatic model, suggesting that AT should be equally useful in also raising dysfunctionally low levels of an autonomic function (e.g., low heart rate variability). The objective of AT is to permit self-regulation in either direction (i.e., deep relaxation or augmentation of a physiological activity) through "passive concentration," also described as "self-hypnosis."

In AT, the patient (or trainee) concentrates on his or her body sensations in a passive manner, without trying to directly or volitionally bring about change. *Passive concentration* may sound paradoxical, in that *concentration* usually suggests effort. What it means in AT is that the trainee is instructed to concentrate on inner sensations rather than environmental stimuli, and this is indeed somewhat effortful especially for the novice. If this concentration does not come easily, the trainee is told to let thoughts wander for a while, or to rearrange the body position for more comfort, rather than to force inner concentration. Not forcing, allowing sensations to happen, and being an observer rather than a manipulator are what *passive* refers to. The AT trainee is warned that trying too hard is counterproductive: It may lead to negative reactions such as muscle spasms, and it stands in the way of acquiring the necessary passive attitude.

The principle of passive concentration clearly differentiates AT from Jacobson's (1938) PMR and biofeedback (Schwartz & Andrasik, 2003), in which patients actively attempt to acquire control over physiological functions. A feature that AT shares with biofeedback, however, is the assumption that bidirectional change (increase or decrease of a physiological activity) is possible and, in some instances, desirable as well. Although AT is considered self-hypnotic, the differences between self-hypnosis and heterohypnosis need to be stressed. In heterohypnosis, the hypnotic trance is induced by another individual (i.e., the hypnotist), who will typically make relaxation and trance suggestions, followed by suggestions for behavioral changes, such as stopping smoking or feeling release from pain (see Karlin, Chapter 6, this volume). The key differences are self- versus other-control and dependence versus independence from a therapist. AT is designed to strengthen independence and to give control back to the patient, thus eliminating the need for either physiological feedback devices (as in biofeedback) or a hypnotherapist.

The claimed uniqueness of AT is supported by (1) experimental studies showing that biobehavioral methods have differential effects on a variety of clinical problems (a summary is provided later in this chapter) and (2) basic experimental findings that relaxation and hypnosis can be psychophysiologically distinguished from autogenic states. Diehl et al. (1989) investigated regional cerebral blood flow in 12 healthy male volunteers during autogenic training and during hypnosis. Hypnotic states were verified via successfully performed arm levitation and persistent catalepsy of the right arm. These researchers observed that global hemispheric blood perfusion increased significantly, relative to the participants' own baseline resting values. Perfusion during AT was significantly less than during hypnosis.

Shapiro and Lehrer (1980) contrasted psychophysiological effects in participants who had learned either PMR or AT in a 5-week training program. All active training reduced anxiety, depression, and reports of physical symptomatology, but only AT triggered self-perceived heaviness and warmth, as well as changes in depth of breathing. Similarly, in a contrast of the benefits of AT to those of PMR (Lehrer, Atthowe & Weber,

1980) for anxiety reduction, subjective reports revealed reduced anxiety for both active treatments, whereas AT showed additional advantages via heart rate reductions not seen in progressive relaxation. Unfortunately, few published studies indicate effect specificity for AT. The three studies described here support the potential of distinct physiological and subjective effects for various self-regulation methods without, however, offering conclusive evidence.

The core ingredients of AT that make it distinct as a method are six standard formulas that refer to specific body sensations. The formulas are subvocally repeated by the patient; in addition, the patient is encouraged to develop vivid, personally meaningful images to accompany and enhance these formulas. An important feature that also distinguishes AT from PMR (Jacobson, 1938) and meditation (Wallace, 1970) is the inherent claim of specific effects for each formula. Each formula targets a specific bodily function, and the sensations and images suggested by the formulas are derived from patient reports of deep relaxation and trance states rather than being theoretically derived. The formulas suggest sensations that a relaxed trainee is likely to experience anyway, and they create positive expectations of distinct somatic experiences; their occurrence then reinforces the effort and lends further credibility to the formulas. The "magic" of hypnosis is thereby tied to a focus on and increasing awareness of somatic sensations.

Experimental support is growing for the claim of AT propagators that AT may not only affect sympathetic tone but may also achieve some of its benefits through its impact on parasympathetic activation. To examine the hypothesis that the AT response is associated with an increase in cardiac parasympathetic tone, the frequency components of heart rate variability during relaxation training were investigated in 16 college students (Sakakibara, Takeuchi, & Hayano, 1994). Electrocardiograms and pneumograms were recorded during a 5-minute baseline period followed by three successive 5-minute sessions of AT (relaxation) or by the same periods of quiet rest (control), while participants in both groups breathed synchronously with a visual pacemaker (0.25 Hz). Although neither the magnitude nor the frequency of respiration showed a significant difference between relaxation and control, the amplitude of the high-frequency component of heart rate variability increased only during relaxation ($p = .008$). There was no significant difference in the ratio of the low-frequency (0.04–0.15 Hz) to the high-frequency amplitudes. The increased high-frequency amplitude without changes in the respiratory parameters indicates enhanced cardiac parasympathetic tone. Enhanced cardiac parasympathetic tone may explain an important mechanism underlying the beneficial effect of the relaxation response.

The assumption of AT that somatic imagery can trigger underlying physiological activity is also consistent with Lang's (1979) theory of emotional imagery coding and experience-based somatic–visceral responding. In a series of studies (Lang, Kozak, Miller, Levin, & McLean, 1980; Lang, Levin, Miller, & Kozak, 1983), Lang and his collaborators showed experimentally that focusing in imagination on a distinct physiological response (e.g., sweating or heart rate) did indeed provoke the imagined visceral response with reasonable specificity.

The heaviness formula in AT is directed at muscular relaxation and has been found to be associated with reduction in muscle tone, reductions in blood pressure, and increases in skin resistance (Fischel & Mueller, 1962; Ohno, 1965; Schultz, 1973; von Siebenthal, 1952; Wallnoefer, 1972). The warmth formula is directed at vascular dilation, and researchers have observed peripheral vasodilation in hands and face with an accompanying increase in skin temperature, as well as occasional light sweating (Dobeta, Sugano, & Ohno, 1966; Pelliccioni & Liebner, 1980; Polzien, 1953; Schwarz & Langen, 1966). Practice of the heart regulation formula has been associated with reduction in heart rate, reduced cardiac output with simultaneously improved CO_2 utilization, and stabilization of labile electrocardiogram signals (Luthe, 1970a; Polzien, 1953). Participants practicing the breathing regulation formula displayed reduced breathing rates and volume and showed shifts from predominantly thoracic to more abdominal breathing patterns (Ikemi et al., 1965; Linden, 1977; Luthe, 1970a; Polzien, 1953). Practice of the "sun rays" formula is supposed to regulate visceral organ activity, and researchers have indeed reported normalization of dysfunctional stomach and intestinal function; increased blood flow to the gastric mucous and vasodilation of peripheral blood vessels have also been noted (Ikemi et al., 1965; Sapir & Reverchon, 1965; Lantzsch & Drunkenmoelle, 1975). Finally, the "cool forehead" formula, which is meant to regulate brain activity and forehead blood flow, has been associated with reduced frequencies of beta waves and increased frequencies of alpha and theta waves in the electroencephalogram (Israel & Rohmer, 1958; Jus & Jus, 1968; Katzenstein, Kriegel, & Gaefke, 1974). Dierks, Maurer, and Zacher (1989) also reported increased theta and reduced beta wave activity; alpha wave activity, however, increased slightly with AT practice. Furthermore, Dierks et al. (1989) noted that the reduction in beta wave activity was specific to the right hemisphere, which is commonly presumed to be the site of emotional function.

A phenomenon not described in the literature for other self-regulation techniques is that of "autogenic discharges," which are seen as a sudden and unpredictable form of "unloading" of pent-up thoughts, sensory processes, and muscular activity (Luthe, 1970b). Although AT is presumed to have an overall gentle, slow effect on autonomic self-regulation, the concept of autogenic discharges incorporates the idea that some of the self-regulation may occur through short bursts of central nervous system activity. Luthe (1970b) differentiates (1) reactive discharges (i.e., responses to acute provocation); (2) normally occurring spontaneous discharges (e.g., motor discharges during presleep stages); (3) discharges that originate from the brain and characterize forms of pathology (e.g., epilepsy); and (4) discharges that may occur during sensory deprivation and during the practice of AT.

Luthe (1970b) also reported that some autogenic discharges are experienced as pain memories from previous injuries, illnesses, or operations. Similarly, there have been reports that the quality of the autogenic discharge may be related to the particular formula being practiced at the time. This can take on the form of a discharge sensation experienced in the body part that is currently being concentrated on and may be functionally related (although typically in the opposite direction) to the target sensation (e.g., heart palpitations during the heart regulation formula).

Unfortunately, the discharge phenomenon is experienced with considerable variation in intensity and can take on many different forms. In consequence, one can debate whether trainees who do not report sudden discharges nevertheless experience them with little direct awareness (Luthe's position; Luthe, 1970b) or whether the discharges do not occur at all. Also, given that the discharges may take on different forms, it cannot be ruled out that the label *autogenic discharge* may simply cover a variety of phenomena with heterogeneous underlying neuro- or psychophysiological origins. One thing, however, is clear: Autogenic discharges, when noticed by trainees, are usually interpreted as bothersome and unwanted side effects of the procedure. The traditional view in the AT literature, however, is that autogenic discharges are necessary in a "hydraulic" sense and are considered signs of progress, because they suggest a reduction in physiological and psychological inhibition and provide an opportunity for release of excessive pressure in the system. It is important for the AT instructor to interpret discharge experiences for confused trainees and to provide sensible, comforting explanations.

Data collected by Luthe (1970b) on two experimental groups may further serve to explain the phenomenon and illustrate the variety of possible autogenic discharge experiences. The two groups of participants were all AT trainees who could be classified either as openly sexually active or as sexually deprived because of their particular life situations (i.e., they were members of the clergy or were otherwise prohibited by their religions from being sexually active). The two groups were apparently similar in male–female proportion, age, clinical condition, and level of professional achievement. The experimental prediction was that the sexually deprived individuals would display more sexuality-related autogenic discharges. Luthe's (1970b) observations suggested that the sexually deprived group indeed had more sexuality-related and general discharge symptoms than did the controls. The sexually deprived group reported more itching, tingling, pain, and muscular twitches; they also reported more erections and vaginal spasms, as well as more sexual fantasies. The perceived sites of the most frequent sensory and motor discharges were the thighs, lower abdomen, and genital regions.

Autogenic discharges are similar in some ways to phenomena described in connection with other techniques (e.g., "relaxation-induced anxiety" as described in the PMR literature; see Bernstein, Carlson, & Schmidt, Chapter 5, this volume; the "side effects of tension release" described by Carrington, Chapter 14, this volume). The AT literature, however, presents a much more detailed picture of these phenomena than does the literature on other techniques and gives more specific suggestions for how to manage them when they occur.

ASSESSMENT

Studies of therapy effectiveness typically provide statistical demonstrations of between-group means (based on comparisons of treated patients with themselves before training or with waiting-list or other treatment controls) as demonstrations of a positive outcome (Linden & Wen, 1990). Hidden in such mean change comparisons, however, is considerable variability in treatment response: Some patients benefit, whereas others do not change or get even worse (Jacobson, Follette, & Revenstorf, 1984). A particularly striking demonstration of treatment effect variability is provided by Aivazyan, Zaitsev, and Yurenev (1988), who randomly assigned hypertensive patients to either AT or a no-treatment control condition. When mean changes were broken down into "percentage improved" ratings, the following figures emerged: In the AT-treated group, 32% improved, 59% remained unchanged, and 9% deteriorated; in the control group, 59% also remained unchanged, 11% improved, and 30% deteriorated. Clearly, therapy did little for the majority of patients, whereas the between-group difference is effectively attributable to treatment effects consisting of both direct improvement and the prevention of worsening. Thus valuable health care funds may be better invested if patients who are not going to benefit from treatment can be identified *a priori* and left out of the treatment comparison.

Especially in light of these observations on treatment outcome variability, a clinician treating individual patients cannot be satisfied with knowing that a statistically significant mean change of a treated group occurred; instead, the practitioner needs to attend to each individual's progress. Therefore, it is of great importance for practitioners using AT to be aware of what kind of patient can learn and benefit from AT and to know in advance whether AT is indeed the best method of treatment for a given patient. The question of AT's suitability, given certain patient characteristics, is addressed in this section.

The literature and my own experience indicate clearly that the mechanics of AT can be taught to a wide variety of individuals; nonetheless, some caveats are in order. Adults of all ages and many children have learned AT, but children below school age lack the discipline to master AT. Depending on a child's maturity, intelligence, and imaginative abilities, the youngest age at which AT can be taught effectively is between 6 and 10 years. Individuals with mental retardation, with acute central nervous system disorders, and with uncontrolled psychoses are also likely to be unable to process and follow the instructions. Thus, with these relatively few exceptions, AT can be taught effectively to a wide range of populations.

Although few individuals are unable to learn the mechanical aspects of autogenics, this does not mean that every learner will necessarily show clinical benefit, and the practitioner has to consider the possibility that AT is not the treatment of choice for a given person. Three lines of research contribute valuable information in this respect. The first is research on relaxation-induced anxiety (Heide & Borkovec, 1984). A second pertinent area of research has attempted to predict relaxation training success by considering differences in initial resting levels (Jacob, Chesney, Williams, Ding, & Shapiro, 1991) and interindividual differences in response to the first training sessions (Vinck, Arickx, & Hongenaert, 1987). And finally, personality factors as predictors of success have been specifically targeted (Badura, 1977).

Heide and Borkovec (1983) offer a number of potential explanations for the paradoxical effect of anxiety increase during relaxation. The first explanation is that during relaxation a shift toward greater parasympathetic dominance occurs, which results in peripheral vasodilation and feelings of warmth and heaviness (the first and second formulas in AT; Budzynski, Stoyva, & Pfeffer, 1980). The unfamiliarity with parasympathetic activity sensations may be particularly disturbing to chronically tense or anxious individuals. Also, relaxation frequently brings about unfamiliar spontaneous muscular–skeletal events such as myoclonic jerks, spasms, twitches, or restlessness ("autogenic discharges" in AT). Another explanation centers on the notion of fear of loss of control. Chronically anxious individuals may have learned to control their anxieties in the past by never letting go; they typically work in a compulsive, rigid manner and cannot permit themselves to relax (Martin, 1951). Finally, Ley (1985), on the basis of his work with panic disorder, has proposed that relaxation-induced anxiety may be linked to "relative hyperventilation" (*relative* in this context means that the perceived pace of one's own breathing is above what would be metabolically needed in a given situation). The discrepancy between perceived need and actual respiration pace serves as an alarm cue that triggers additional anxiety cognitions, which may then create an upward spiral toward even more arousal.

These findings suggest that such patient characteristics as having had an anxiety experience can predict differential relaxation treatment outcome and deserve consideration in individual treatment plans involving relaxation therapy. Unfortunately, the replicated findings in this research domain involve only meditation, exercise, and PMR, and it is not clear how AT outcome may be affected by individual predispositions such as pretreatment anxiety levels.

The second and third lines of research deal with pretreatment or early-treatment differences between individuals. Vinck et al. (1987) attempted to predict blood pressure treatment responses in normotensives who learned either PMR (Jacobson, 1938) or AT. Training was provided weekly for 6 weeks. Relaxation effects were measured as within-session changes during the first treatment session, as overall changes in resting values from the first to the last treatment session, and as within-session changes during the last treatment session. Although no differential effects for PMR relative to AT were reported, Vinck et al. (1987) did replicate Jacob, Kraemer, and Agras's (1977) findings that higher initial blood pressure levels also predicted the greatest reduction after relaxation training. A recent review and a controlled trial of therapy outcome for hypertension treated via relaxation strategies (Jacob et al., 1991; Linden, Lenz, & Con, 2001) clearly confirms the earlier (Jacob et al., 1977) contention that patients with initially high blood pressure show greater reductions.

Vinck et al. (1987) also found that trainees with the smallest changes within the first training session of either AT or PMR were the ones who showed the greatest reductions during the last training sessions. Attempts to predict blood pressure treatment response via personality indices was unsuccessful. Vinck el al. (1987) may have failed to identify personality factors as predictors of AT success because their participants were healthy individuals who probably reflected a relatively narrow range of associated personality features. No such range restriction was apparent in the work of Badura (1977), who related Minnesota Multiphasic Personality Inventory (MMPI) profiles to AT outcome in 200 patients who displayed neurotic, functional, and/or psychosomatic symptomatologies. Badura's patients were subdivided into "successes" and "failures" on the basis of their reported ability to achieve formula-specific autogenic sensations. Patients in the "failure" group were characterized by relative elevations on the Hypochondriasis, Depression, Hysteria, and Social Introversion subscales. Discriminant function analysis indicated that with these distinct MMPI profiles, 80% of the success–failure incidences in AT could be correctly classified.

A number of conclusions and suggestions appear justified. Patients with pronounced, stable sympathetically induced arousal (e.g., as seen with high blood pressure) profit more from AT (or other relaxation therapies) than those with lower resting states; similarly, those patients who show the least initial response to treatment improve relatively more over time. Also, clinical elevations on the MMPI scales noted in the previous paragraph predict lack of success with AT. Such individuals may be better served with another form of psychotherapy.

METHOD

The Training Format

AT can be taught individually or in groups. The advantages of each mode of training are fairly obvious and are the same as for other forms of psychological therapy. Individual training is much more expensive, but training can also be easily adjusted to likely differences in the pace of learning and other individual needs (this is especially true when AT is taught as part of a complex intervention package). The existence of a personal therapeutic relationship may also enhance compliance and credibility. Group training is more cost-effective but permits less individualized attention and may thus reduce compliance. On the other hand, groups also have the potential to develop cohesion and serve as mutual support systems, which in turn will have a positive impact on compliance. My personal preference is to teach AT in groups of 8–12 participants, as long as the group can be expected to have more or less homogeneous needs and learning paces. As far as between-session intervals are concerned, I recommend 1 week, but this is not based on any empirical evidence; it is mostly done to provide a reasonable length of time for practice and because a once-a-week pattern tends to match well with people's natural habit of looking for routines.

Another important point that cuts across the whole learning process is that of realistic expectations. At the outset of AT, trainees should be alerted to the probability that learning will be slow. The great majority of practitioners feel little, if anything, during their first practices, and it is perfectly normal for the desired sensations to remain weak for the first week or two of practice. This is true even for the avid practitioner who is fully compliant with the instruction to practice twice per day.

The Physical Setting

The ideal physical setting is one of comfort, with minimal likelihood of interruption, a room temperature of 20–24°C, a couch or exercise mattress (plus pillows) to stretch out on, and adjustable lighting conditions (a slightly darkened room is best). Training success is facilitated by an environment that permits trainees to concentrate on their inner sensations. Accordingly, any speech while training impedes the basic principle of "*auto*genics." If the trainer talks during the exercise or plays a record or cassette, the trainee cannot really learn to exercise autogenically (i.e., independently); instead, he or she will go through a light heterohypnosis. Therefore, autogenic training necessitates tranquility. In a tranquil setting, AT, with its focus on six functional systems (muscles, blood vessels, heart, breathing, inner organs, and the head), can be learned best.

In order to go through the training procedure, a very comfortable sitting—or, even better, lying—position is necessary. The entire body position must be comfortable, because body position itself may lead to muscle tension, which will interfere with progress in the exercises. It is most advantageous to exercise in a supine position, so that the neck especially is well supported. When lying down, the arms should be placed flat beside the body with slightly bent elbows, and the tips of the feet should fall slightly to the outside.

If lying down is not possible (e.g., if a trainee wants to practice in the clinician's office), a chair with a high back and armrests is best, so that the head and arms are supported. The elbows should be bent at nearly a right angle, because this will ensure that the stretching and bending muscles in each arm will be in a balanced state. The entire back and the back of the head should be fully supported. Small pillows may facilitate this support. The feet should rest flat on the floor and close to each other, and the knees should fall slightly to the outside, which will help to prevent mechanical tension in the thigh musculature. Most people will tend to close their knees even while sitting, although this position is often associated with unconscious muscular tension.

When it is not possible either to sit comfortably or to lie down, a third position may be used for the exercises: A trainee can sit on a bench or a chair without back support. In this position the head should be allowed to sink into the torso, so that the arms will hang at the sides and the head will be in a perfectly vertical position over the spine. It is important for the trainee not to bend forward; instead, the torso must be in a vertical position, although somewhat reduced in height. In this position, no muscular activity is necessary and no muscular tension is created, because the skeleton is held by the spine and its tendons. Now the arms can be moved loosely and can be supported on the widely spread thighs, so that the underarms (close to the elbow) will be supported by the thighs. The arms are again bent in the previously described manner. The body now hangs without any muscular work in its own bone structure.

These positions need to be assumed carefully before the exercises begin. In one of these positions (preferably lying down), the trainee can now begin with the first exercise. The eyes should be closed to facilitate passive concentration, and the trainee should now try to imagine the sensation in the formula as well as possible, without making any movement or trying to speak or do anything else. The ideas, images, and memories that will necessarily develop in each individual should not be fought off, because this attempt in itself would lead to tension. Ideas and images other than the formula-based sensations should be ignored.

Content and Sequence of Exercises

First Exercise: The Heaviness Experience (Muscular Relaxation)

The first AT exercise involves the musculature, because muscle activity is familiar to people and is most easily influenced by conscious efforts; in addition, experience with hypnosis and relaxation suggestions has shown that notable muscular relaxation can be achieved rapidly. Muscular relaxation is experienced as a heaviness of the extremities. Intentional concentration on outside stimulation is associated with muscular tension (e.g., looking, speaking, and reaching out are based on muscular movement). Attentional anticipation can also justifiably be called "tension," as muscles are already tensed in anticipation of movement. Even profound thinking may be associated with muscular activity, because many individuals crease the forehead while thinking. Each intention, or even vivid imagination, of a motion will result in increased tone of the musculature in the extremities.

It is not advisable to use the entire body as an object of training at once, because in this case the necessary focus would be difficult to achieve. The training should begin with the dominant arm. If this arm has been trained for a reasonable period of time, the experience of heaviness during muscle relaxation will generalize to the other arm, the legs, and other body systems, because all extremities and organs are accessed by the same nervous system. The exercise is executed on the arm until it has generalized to the other three extremities. It is important to achieve a maximal concentration in the one arm first and to permit a generalized overflow of relaxation into the other extremities before good results can be expected.

The steps in the heaviness formula are as follows: (1) "The right (left) arm is heavy" (this is repeated six times); (2) "I am very quiet" (this is said only once, and then alternates with the first step until six cycles have been completed). In normal individuals a noticeable experience of heaviness will develop soon, particularly in the area of the elbow and lower arm. After the heaviness formula is practiced, the instructions are "taken back." "Taking back" refers to a systematic set of activities designed to bring the trainee gradually from a state of relaxed, low muscle tone back to an alert state. This needs to be performed in a consistent manner to facilitate the reflex nature of the process. It is executed in the following steps: (1) Participants are asked to make fists repeatedly, holding the tension briefly and then letting go; (2) the arm is bent and stretched a few times with an energetic pull; (3) the individual takes a few deep breaths; and (4) the eyes are opened.

It is important that the trainee pay attention to the timing of the exercise. Training should be repeated in two practice sessions per day. In each training session, the person can practice the heaviness formula twice for about 1 minute each. If in the beginning the individual steps are extended—because many trainees want to do the exercise particularly well—semiconscious tensions may arise. Trainees will realize that the experience of heaviness, instead of increasing, decreases more and more with excessively long practices.

Within the first week of training, the feeling of heaviness in the trained arm will be more pronounced and will occur more rapidly; also, the same feeling will be experienced in the other extremities, usually at the same time as in the other arm. When the experience of heaviness in both arms is quite pronounced, the formula can now be changed into "Arms are heavy." The taking-back procedure for both arms involves a count from 1 to

4, in which each number is associated with a specific instruction: (1) "make a couple of fists"; (2) "bend the arms a few times"; (3) "breathe in deeply"; and (4) "open the eyes and sit up." Heaviness experience in the legs does not necessitate a particular taking-back procedure, because legs function more autonomically. Normally, within a week, the exercise has proceeded so far that with only a brief moment of inner concentration arms and legs can be perceived as quite heavy. It is then time to approach the second exercise.

Second Exercise: Experience of Warmth (Vascular Dilation)

Muscular exercises are something that the naive individual finds natural, because muscular activity is typically considered to be a voluntary act. It is a more novel idea that blood vessels may constrict or dilate through intentional effort. However, it should be noted that all emotional activity tends to be associated with a change in blood flow (i.e., flushing or paleness). Furthermore, there are systematic types of activities (e.g., a sauna) in which individuals systematically train blood vessels; these activities are reasonably familiar to many individuals. The second AT exercise, which aims at the warmth experience, affects the entire peripheral cardiovascular system: It affects blood flow through arteries, capillaries, and veins in the skin, organs, and musculature. The distribution of blood in the vessels is regulated through constriction and dilation, which take place as a response to nervous system innervation; their magnitude and direction are determined by physical activity, general state of arousal, and inhibition.

Once the first exercise with the heaviness experience has been well trained and can be induced rapidly and reliably, training sessions can then be extended by inclusion of the second formula, as follows:

1. "Arms (legs) are heavy" (this is repeated for a total of six times).
2. "I am very quiet" (this is said once).
3. "The right (left) arm is pleasantly warm" (this is repeated six times; the term *quiet* is then repeated once).

A normal individual will notice an inner streaming, flowing sensation of warmth very rapidly, typically in the area of the elbow and the lower arm. Quite frequently, trainees who master the heaviness sensation will also spontaneously report warmth sensations before they are instructed to imagine them. Specific instructions for "taking back" the experience of warmth are not necessary, because the blood vessels are elastic and governed by a compensatory self-regulation, which will trigger a return to their usual position in an autonomous manner.

The first and second training exercises are executed in the same manner for a period of at least 1 week, until warmth is experienced easily and rapidly in the trained arm first and then in all four extremities. The experience of heaviness and warmth will then also generalize to the entire body. The blood vessel dilation and associated relaxation have a particularly tranquilizing and sleep-inducing effect. Training exercises directed at blood vessel dilation are not necessarily innocuous, as the changed distribution of blood influences the entire organism. The exercise should be instituted only in healthy individuals for whom no vascular risks are known to exist.

When a new exercise step is added in AT (e.g., when the experience of warmth is added to the feeling of heaviness, as shown), the participant should always concentrate initially on the already learned exercises and should add a new exercise for only brief periods (typically 1 minute). New exercises are added for only brief periods in order to keep the overall exercise length brief and to prevent trainees from attempting to achieve "perfect success" (i.e., taking it too seriously). The choice of 1-minute segments is somewhat arbitrary; it is suggested because 1 minute is an even unit of time and because when all training steps are added together they amount to a reasonable practice length of 10–15 minutes. Once heaviness and warmth are achieved rapidly and reliably, the third exercise can be added.

Third Exercise: Regulation of the Heart

The awareness of heart activity varies considerably among people. How does one feel heart activity? Many individuals are aware of it in times of strain, excitement, and fever, but many others do not feel heart activity without prior training. These trainees need to be sensitized to their own heart activity.

Trainees who do not perceive their heart activity at any particular point in their body can use their pulse for orientation. With further training they will also experience the activity of the heart itself. If this help is not sufficient, a trainee may try to become aware of heart activity by other means. This can be done by lying flat on the back so that the right elbow is fully supported and lies at the same height as the chest. Now the right hand is placed in the heart area; the left arm's position remains unchanged. Now the trainee can go into the usual state of heaviness, warmth, and quietness and can concentrate on the sensations in the chest area just where the hand touches the skin. The pressure of the hand functions as a directional indicator. After a few exercises, the trainee is now likely to recognize heart activity, and with continuing repetition of the entire exercise the experience will become more obvious. The heart formula is "The heart is beating calmly and regularly"; this formula is repeated six times, and the word *quiet* is added once.

When the heart sensation has been learned (and in a sense "been discovered"), the hand does not need to be placed any longer in the area of the heart, but the exercise can be continued in the usual position. It should be strongly emphasized that the intent of the exercise is not to actively slow down the heartbeat, as this would prevent self-regulation. The emphasis of this exercise is on regular, even beats, but not on a reduction of the heartbeat frequency.

Fourth Exercise: Regulation of Breathing

Breathing is partially intentional and partially an autonomous activity. In AT the muscular, vascular, and heart relaxation become immediately integrated with the rhythm of breathing, much as heaviness and warmth automatically generalize from the trained arm to all the other extremities. In the AT procedure, however, any intentional influence on or modification of breathing is undesired, because an intentional change would be associated through a reflex-type mechanism with tension and voluntary activity. Again, the trainee is to enter all the other exercise levels before the new, fourth formula is added. "It breathes me" is repeated six times, and then the word *quiet* is added.

For many participants it is very seductive to attempt voluntary changes of breathing, as in a systematic breathing exercise (e.g., in yoga). This intentional modification needs to be prevented in AT, because breathing is supposed to function autonomously and in a self-regulatory system without any active adjustment. In order to prevent intentional change, the passive wording "it breathes me" has been chosen. This statement is intended to make it clear to the trainee that relaxation and the regulation of breathing will come by themselves—that the trainee will be carried by and is to give in to his or her natural breathing rhythm. It typically takes another week to make good progress with this exercise.

Fifth Exercise: Regulation of Visceral Organs ("Sun Rays")

For self-regulation of visceral organs, the trainee focuses on the area of the solar plexus, which is the most important nerve center for the inner organs. The image associated with this nerve center is that of a sun from which warm rays extend to all inner organs. The solar plexus is found halfway between the navel and the lower end of the sternum in the upper half of the body. The trainee now concentrates on the solar plexus area: The formula "Sun rays are streaming and warm" is repeated six times, and "quiet" is repeated once. This exercise also takes approximately 1 week for normal individuals to learn. The image of the breath streaming out of the body when the person breathes out can also help with this particular exercise.

Sixth Exercise: Regulation of the Head

The well-known relaxing effect of a cool cloth on the forehead forms the basis for the sixth exercise. In order to learn the sixth exercise, the trainee will engage in the first five exercises in the same careful and progressive manner as described and will then (initially only for a few seconds) proceed with the following formula: "The forehead is cool" (repeated six times). Just as warmth is associated with vasodilation, the experience of freshness on the forehead leads to a localized vasoconstriction and thereby to a reduced supply of blood, which in turn accounts for the cooling effect. During AT the concentrative relaxation will originate from the cortex as a central organ, which also possesses the capability of changing the distribution of blood within the body. The "cool forehead" exercise can be learned in about the same time as the other exercises, although up to a third of trainees fail to clearly acquire this formula response (Mensen, 1975).

Because most walls and windows are not entirely airtight, there will likely be a slight movement of air in any room. Therefore, the cool forehead may be sensed and described as a cool breeze.

Summary of Exercises

With these six formula-specific exercises, AT has been described in its basic but complete form. The entire exercise sequence can now be summarized as follows:

- "Arms and legs are heavy" six times; "quiet" once.
- "Arms and legs are pleasantly warm" six times; "quiet" once.
- "The heart is beating calmly and regularly" six times; "quiet" once.
- "It breathes me" six times; "quiet" once.
- "Sun rays are streaming and warm" six times; "quiet" once.
- "The forehead is cool" six times; "quiet" once.
- Now "taking back": "Make fists; bend arms; breathe deeply; open eyes."

After about 8 weeks of training, most individuals have acquired the complete set of sensations, and the emphasis can be placed on ease in achieving the described sensations reliably and rapidly. Daily training for another 4–6 months will lead to more profound and stronger sensations, and generalization of training to different environments can be targeted. It is important to go through the taking-back procedure after each session (except when the trainee has fallen asleep during AT). Thus the trainee will acquire a readily available mechanism for switching from active tension to deep relaxation and vice versa.

Monitoring Progress and Maximizing Compliance

Compliance and monitoring progress are intricately linked and are therefore discussed jointly in this section. Clearly, a trainee who does not see any progress despite twice-daily practice and weeks of training will quickly lose the motivation to continue. In some ways, this section could also be entitled "Maximizing Motivation," because this is the cornerstone of progress and compliance. Because progress is not immediately obvious, a trainee with high initial motivation is more likely to succeed, and it is extremely important that the therapist radiate confidence and a firmly anchored belief in the effectiveness of AT from the very beginning of training. It is recommended that the therapist give an optimistic but reasonable picture of the success to be expected: "I have trained x number of people or groups, and there is hardly anybody who has not benefited. Even after x number of years I still practice it myself. Within the first 2 weeks you can expect the first training effects, which will only become stronger and easier to bring about as you keep on practicing." It is important to reinforce compliance with daily practice, especially until the training effects themselves become apparent and take over as motivation enhancers. Even motivated patients, however, do not perfectly adhere to relaxation homework assignments (Taylor, Agras, Schneider, & Allen, 1983). Taylor et al. (1983) tested compliance with relaxation practice, using a special tape recorder that displayed instructions but also monitored unobtrusively the number of times it was actually used; they found that 71% of patients adhered to the instructions. Hoelscher, Lichstein, and Rosenthal (1986) similarly tested compliance with home practice instructions; they found that self-reported compliance exceeded monitored compliance by 91% and that only 32% of trainees averaged one practice a day. These results leave no doubt that poor compliance is a major problem and needs to be taken seriously. The implication for clinical researchers, then, is that compliance needs to be monitored carefully and that only those patients who comply should be included in statistical analyses of outcome.

On the basis of empirical findings on compliance and my own past experience with AT, I can recommend a number of concrete steps for monitoring progress and enhancing compliance.

Having Trainees Keep Diaries

Trainees should keep diaries in which they record their daily practices and particular success or failure experiences. Of course, trainees may cheat and record a practice that they actually skipped, but this does not happen often in my experience, and in fact the diary serves as a potent reminder to trainees. It is recommended that trainees rate the intensity of their perceived sensations in order to maximize the principle of the self-fulfilling prophecy. When trainees rate each practice after being told that the sensation will get stronger and stronger, they are likely to expect steady improvement, which will become even more obvious when they see the progressive ratings they have made. The diary is, of course, very useful for the review of the past week's training experiences, which should be undertaken at the beginning of a given therapy session. For maximum convenience and compliance, as well as to facilitate standardization, I actually supply all trainees with a preprinted diary that has a page for every training week. This prevents uneven record keeping and eliminates the excuse of "I could not find an appropriate booklet for a diary."

Emphasizing Regular Timing of Home Practice

Lack of compliance is a profound problem that plagues all behavioral prescriptions and treatments that require specific daily routines. Research on medication use (Haynes, Taylor, & Sackett, 1979) has revealed that taking medications at predetermined times of day, coupled with other already existing routines, is an important vehicle for enhancing compliance. In the same vein, I ask my trainees to think about and commit themselves to such practice times in the first training sessions. I would rather deal with their scheduling difficulties before they start practicing than find out a week later that they did not practice at all because they could not find the time. When I say "predetermined" times, I do not mean "6:47 P.M. every day" but "every time after I finish watching the evening news" or "when I am in bed before falling asleep." AT practice must become a routine that requires no thinking or planning; otherwise, it is much too vulnerable to daily mood fluctuations or outside disturbances.

Emphasizing the Need for Frequent Practice

AT trainees may find the rule of twice-daily practice for 2 months (or more) overly compulsive; when it is combined with other competition for their time, they may be tempted to cut down on practicing. My recommendation is to be understanding if one or two practices a week are skipped; however, trainees should be urged to stick to the rule. Frequent practicing is more likely to occur if trainees clearly understand the reason for this rule. In the first session it should be emphasized that relaxation is a skill that requires practice, just as is learning to talk or walk for a small child or reacquiring good balance for somebody with a complicated leg fracture and a cast. One can also compare AT practice with throwing a baseball or playing the backhand in tennis; any and all of these are skills that require practice, practice, practice.

Examining Reasons for Dropout

Although AT is popular, patients drop out for a variety of reasons: They move away; there is too much competition for their time; the training effects are too slow in coming; or a variety of other reasons. Even the most experienced therapist will have to face dropout and noncompliance rates of 20–25% in AT. If the dropout rates are noticeably higher than this, the therapist should question his or her own ability to motivate patients. Lack of trainer enthusiasm, poor communication skills, or poor session planning is sometimes the culprit. I have also seen—although rarely—that when AT is taught in groups, some groups never develop cohesion for no apparent reason or that one or more members are considered so obnoxious that other members stay away.

Highlighting Success

Nothing succeeds like success, as the old saying goes. The therapist can use this principle by regularly asking the trainees whether they have tried AT in acute stress situations (e.g., anticipating an exam or facing a confrontation with a superior) and highlighting their success stories. Trainees can be asked regularly whether they have noticed any generalizations of training effects, such as improvement in their ability to fall asleep or to relax after a hard day of work or a reduction in occasional tension headaches. Even if they have not personally experienced such benefits, hearing that somebody else has benefited from AT can serve as an extra motivator.

Also, the trainer should frequently praise the learners not only for apparent positive outcome but also for coming regularly to the training sessions and keeping up with the home practice.

Knowing Possible Problems and Potential Solutions

Anybody attempting to apply a standardized treatment such as AT will soon find out that clinical reality and full standardization are often incompatible: Trainees lose motivation, have unpredictable and confusing training experiences, have medical or psychological problems that may interfere with learning and/or practicing AT, or have other obligations that may prevent regular practice. Good general clinical skills are required to complement the training manual and still bring training to a fruitful end. Nevertheless, some problems are well known to experienced teachers of AT and are endemic either to specific exercises of AT or to the practice of relaxation at large. Although a full discussion is beyond the scope of this chapter, typical problems that can be anticipated and some suggested solutions are presented in the manual (Linden, 1990).

CLINICAL APPLICATIONS AND CASE STUDY

This section serves as a bridge between the prescriptive, standardized procedure described in the first part of this chapter and the recurrent need of practitioners to apply, modify, and adjust this procedure to the realities of the clinical situation. The practical approach taken in this section is of greatest value for the clinician who needs to make therapy plans on a case-by-case basis and who may have to make modifications to "classic" AT or to create a multicomponent therapy package. Modifications of the AT formulas to suit specific case needs, a case study, and a possible integration of an AT component into a stress management package are described next to illustrate the clinical applications of AT.

Modifications of Formulas to Suit Specific Clinical Needs

Modifications of the standard formulas typically fall into three types, in which (1) only a few of the formulas are taught (often the heaviness and warmth formulas only); (2) the standard set is taught, but one specific formula is left out or modified; (3) the standard formulas are taught and an additional, problem-specific formula is created and appended.

Teaching abbreviated AT would be cost-efficient if comparative effectiveness with the long version had been demonstrated empirically. Unfortunately, no such direct comparisons are available, although some abbreviated applications of AT have been found to produce therapeutic benefit (see Linden, 1994). Given the absence of clear comparative evaluations, I argue that teaching abbreviated AT methods (e.g., the heaviness and warmth formulas only) may be inadvisable if full therapeutic benefit is expected.

The need for elimination or modification of a certain formula from the standard set often results from an unanticipated difficulty. One possibility is that certain formulas trigger negative associations, images, and memories for a particular trainee. Another possibility is that of a rationale-application mismatch: For example, a cardiac patient may (at least initially) be hypersensitive to all cardiac sensations, and elimination of the heart regulation formula may be advisable.

Many other formula-specific patient problems are possible. I noted in one case that a trainee experienced searing heat sensations at the use of the words "very warm" in the warmth formula, and a toning down to "pleasantly warm" was judged more appropriate. The "sun rays" formula may be contraindicated for ulcer patients; a non-heat-related image may be preferable in order to set the desired sensation apart from the burning sensation of ulcer pain. Or the formula may be left out altogether in order not to direct even more attention to a potential pain site. Such decisions require clinical, on-the-spot judgment, and excessive standardization and prescription via a manual may be inappropriate.

A particularly appealing modification for many therapists and their patients is that of a person- or disorder-specific additional formula. Lindemann (1974) has provided a useful catalog of formulas for specific applications, from which I have selected a subset for demonstration here. There really are no limits to adapting such formulas (also called "intentional formulas") to idiosyncratic preferences in imagery and word choices or descriptions of desirable target behaviors. Characteristics of effective intentional formulas are brevity, a pleasant rhyme or rhythm, a positive choice of words, high relevance to the trainee, and a good match to his or her personality. Guidance for creating formulas with these characteristics can be drawn from Erickson and Rossi (1979).

Some of Lindemann's intentional formulas are as follows:

- "First work, then pleasure" to help against procrastination.
- "I am happy, relaxed, and free of hunger" to accompany a weight reduction program.
- "I sleep deeply, relaxed, and restfully" against insomnia.
- "I am calm and relaxed; my cheeks stay cool" against blushing.
- "I am completely relaxed and free; my stomach and bowels are working steadily and smoothly" against gastrointestinal complaints.
- "I am totally quiet and in peace; my joints are moving freely and without discomfort; they feel warm" against arthritis pain.

Case Study

Jane M was referred by her family physician because of elevated blood pressure. This 25-year-old woman had a 10-week-old baby at home and had developed high blood pressure during the pregnancy. Pregnancy-induced hypertension tends to disappear quickly after birth, but this was not apparent in her case.

The assessment consisted of a 1-hour interview in which Jane and I attempted to identify major sources of distress in her life. Throughout the interview, the patient's blood pressure was sampled at 2-minute intervals, using a fully automated blood pressure monitor with digital displays (Dinamap Model 850, Critikon Corp., Tampa, FL). I routinely use this procedure with all referrals for stress-related problems, because it may help identify emotion triggers that patients themselves may not be aware of (Lynch, 1985). The diagnosis of elevated blood pressure was confirmed, in that the 1-hour average reading was 138/95 mm Hg; these readings also supported her family physician's recommendation that drug treatment was not indicated for blood pressure at this level.

Jane remembered that at the age of 18 she had become aware of the family's positive history of high blood pressure, and she had been preoccupied with her own blood pressure ever since. Although I explained that this was probably not accurate, she claimed an awareness of sudden blood pressure changes and attributed subjective feelings of stress to excessive demands in her job as an administrative assistant. When she became pregnant and developed blood pressure problems, she had quit her job; she did not plan to return in the near future.

Neither Jane's verbal reports nor my attempts to link these reports with accompanying changes in her blood pressure identified specific stress triggers that could have become the targets for a stress management program. Instead, I chose to teach her AT, which appeared to hold credibility as an intervention for her.

Over an 8-week period with a total of seven 1-hour sessions, Jane learned the full AT package with six formulas. Using a daily diary system, she charted her practice times and successes, thus also documenting her compliance with the twice-daily home practice requirement. At the end of the seventh session, she was clearly comfortable with the full six-formula AT procedure. She continued to be puzzled that her subjective evaluations of her blood pressures as being high or low were as inaccurate at the end of training as they had been before. Her average blood pressure during the last session was 128/78 mm Hg, indicating a 10-point drop in systolic blood pressure and a 17-point drop in diastolic blood pressure from the readings in the first session. Although this averaging procedure is probably inferior to 24-hour ambulatory blood pressure monitoring, it is nevertheless better than determinations that are based on two or three readings only. The 1-hour averaging procedure at least captures the adaptation processes typical for repeated measurement (Linden & Frankish, 1988). At a 3-month follow-up, Jane reported that her blood pressure was still in the normal range (this was verified by her family physician). She continued to practice AT, although less often than during the acute training phase.

Autogenic Training in a Multicomponent Treatment Package

In the clinic patients often present with multiple complaints, and/or the therapist discovers during an individual assessment that a given problem is probably caused or exacerbated by a multiplicity of factors. This in turn calls for a program of therapy with multiple components. Although multicomponent therapy is the norm in everyday clinical work and is associated with better clinical outcome than single-component therapies (Shapiro & Shapiro, 1982), infinite numbers of such treatment combinations are possible; this fact makes extensive comparative outcome testing for each combination extraordinarily difficult. Clinical judgment, good training, experience, and an awareness of research findings are needed in order to judge the appropriateness of a treatment package for a given patient. The best packages tend to be those with strong individually tailored rationales and with components that have been shown to be efficacious when tested alone (Linden, 2004). Because there are so many possible combinations of treatment techniques, only a stress management combination that includes AT is described here.

A multicomponent package including AT has become the standard stress management approach in my own clinical work. First, the client is provided with a rationale that describes stress as a three-step process, involving (1) environmental stress triggers, (2) behavioral and cognitive responses to the challenge, and (3) the ultimately ensuing physiological stress response. For each of the three elements of the stress process, different intervention techniques are taught: (1) situational analysis for identification of stress triggers and use of stimulus control procedures to prevent these from triggering stress; (2) modification of the acute response to challenge via cognitive restructuring and assertiveness skill training; and (3) acquisition of a behavioral coping skill for reducing the physiological and subjective arousal via AT. Learning to relax via AT not only has desirable acute effects but also tends to generalize, insofar as patients typically learn to perceive themselves as being in control of their stress responses; this in turn has a positive impact on the way they perceive potential stress triggers and how they respond to them. The reader wanting to learn more about AT and its place within the scientific foundations of various stress management techniques is referred to Linden (2004).

REFLECTIONS ON THE CLINICAL OUTCOME OF AUTOGENIC TRAINING

Early clinical reports of AT are heavily dominated by case studies and uncontrolled research (Luthe, 1970a; Pikoff, 1984). If taken at face value, these clinical findings suggest that AT possesses treatment potential for almost every psychological and psychosomatic problem ever listed in a medical catalogue. Pikoff (1984) reviewed the available clinical studies published in English and found that the quality of published research was very uneven. Also, because most researchers used time-limited training programs and rarely trained participants in more than the heaviness and warmth formulas, he concluded that AT had never really been tested in this body of literature. Nevertheless, the overall evaluation of AT was quite promising; positive outcomes were reported for AT and insomnia, test anxiety, and migraine.

More recently, there have been two comprehensive reviews, one being a combination of narrative and meta-analytic review of outcomes (Linden, 1994), and the other solely a meta-analysis (Stetter & Kupper, 2002). Both reviews used similar search and inclusion criteria.

Results are reported here as effect sizes (d), which can be defined two ways. They can refer to raw means at posttest and pretest, respectively, when change within a group is determined. They can also reflect change scores or means obtained at posttest (but adjusted for pretest differences) for comparisons between treatment groups (e.g., AT vs. attention control groups). Quantitative meta-analytic findings indicated that autogenic training was associated with medium-sized pre- to posttreatment effects ranging from $d = -0.43$ for biological indices of change to $d = -0.58$ for psychological indices in the Linden (1994) review, and $d = -0.68$ (biological indices) and $d = -0.75$ (psychological outcomes) in the Stetter and Kupper review (2002). The pooled effect size estimates hide considerable variability in behavioral/psychological effects for individual target problems; moderately sized improvements were reported for tension headache and migraine, hypertension, coronary heart disease rehabilitation, asthma, somatoform pain disorder, Raynaud's disease, and anxiety and sleep disorders.

To place these observed outcomes of AT in context, one can compare the effect of AT with those reported for other psychophysiological arousal-reduction strategies and other psychotherapies (Linden, 2004). Data from six meta-analyses permitted aggregation and comparison of results (Eppley, 1989; Godfrey, Bonds, Kraus, Wiener, & Toth, 1990; Hyman, Feldman, Harns, Levin, & Malloy, 1989; Linden, 1994; Luebbert, Dahme, & Hasenbring, 2001; Stetter & Kupper, 2002). Effect sizes, when averaged for all types of arousal-reduction strategies and classes of endpoints, were:

- $d = -0.56$ for pre–post comparisons
- $d = -0.58$ for arousal reduction versus no treatment
- $d = -0.52$ for arousal reduction versus attention placebo
- $d = -0.15$ for arousal reduction versus other active psychotherapies

Interestingly, whereas effect sizes for self-reported distress weakened with increasing levels of nonspecific effects inherent in different controls, the effect sizes of AT for biological indices of stress remained at the same level. Overall, the effect sizes for AT fall clearly in the same range as those reported for other arousal-reduction methods, and all of these are slightly less effective than psychotherapy at large. In sum, a consistent picture of comparable, moderate effect sizes emerges; subgrouping for techniques produced no meaningful differences, and effect sizes for pre–post changes are essentially the same as for active treatment versus no-treatment controls. Biological indices were more robust than self-report indices to varying types of control comparison.

Given that the aggregation principle of meta-analyses means, at times, indiscriminate "lumping," there still remains the question of which technique is the best match for which problem. Note, however, that this literature is much broader than is needed for a discussion of AT effects. Lehrer and his collaborators (Lehrer, Carr, Sargunaraj, & Woolfolk, 1994, and also this volume) have presented a detailed review of effective technique for area-of-application matches for arousal-reduction strategies. These researchers classify techniques on the basis of their cognitive versus behavioral-autonomic emphasis, with meditation and mindfulness forming the more cognitive end of the spectrum, autogenic training possessing both a cognitive and autonomic rationale, and muscular relaxation and biofeedback being the most physiological, autonomically based techniques. Stress, anxiety, and phobias were considered most responsive to interventions with strong cognitive *and* behavioral elements.

Meta-analytic reviews, by definition, reveal nothing about design differences that could influence treatment outcomes. In this light, it is important to stress that the majority of AT studies have used less than ideal training programs (because of taped instructions, very brief treatments, and/or only a subset of the six-formula set). I suspect that comprehensive training and personal delivery are bound to make AT more effective. The effect sizes reported here may therefore underestimate the maximal effects possible with more appropriate training procedures.

Furthermore, the results of AT and similar self-regulation approaches can be evaluated with a variety of different endpoints. One such example is that of using AT to facilitate the reduction of prescription drug use as was done with headache patients (Zsombok, Juhasz, Budavari, Vitrai, & Bagdy, 2003). Within a 3-month training period, patients showed significant reductions in use of analgesics and anxiolytics, which was welcomed by patients and health care providers given the cost of drug treatment and lower risk of side effects with reduced medication intake.

CONCLUSIONS

AT deserves a place in the practice of clinicians working with psychophysiological disorders and in every stress management book, given its long history, its enthusiastic endorsement around the world (although somewhat less prominently in English-speaking countries), and the extensive database that is now available for critical evaluations of clinical outcome and for basic experimental effects of the AT formulas. However, it is also clear that there are still more remaining questions than available answers. There is tentative evidence that AT may be more useful than other self-regulation methods in certain disorders, whereas for others a different method (e.g., thermal biofeedback) may be better. Detecting specific effects will remain difficult, however, because the average effect associated with AT is of a medium size when AT's effects are tested in a pre–post manner or when they are compared with those of no-treatment controls. When different target problems are lumped together, the comparison with other active biobehavioral treatments generally reveals that these interventions tend to produce similarly medium-sized effects. It is safe to presume that shared nonspecific treatment elements account for a substantial portion of this effect. A more promising approach (at least in the clinical environment) is that of permitting clients to select their own treatment after a range of treatments and their rationales have been presented; clients who then choose AT may respond more strongly because of the *a priori* credibility that self-chosen methods embody.

At this time there is no evidence that full-length training (i.e., suggested to last at least 8 weeks) is superior to brief training with a selected subset of formulas. However, this question has never been subjected to a direct test in a single study that has targeted one clearly delineated clinical problem and in which trainees have been randomly assigned to either short or full-length training. The conclusion of no evidence for a difference between short and long training is based on comparisons of effect sizes from short versus long treatments across different studies. This also implies likely confounding of effect size with problem severity, in that less severe problems may have received shorter treatment, and quick recovery may have been attributable to lesser problem severity rather than shorter treatment length.

In summary, there is a strong research base supporting AT's rationale and clinical outcome, but it also seems true that AT is overall comparable in effect to other self-regulation interventions (such as meditation or muscular relaxation). Notwithstanding this observation of overall comparable outcomes, further research is welcomed and needed to test possible specificity effects; that is, some patients may benefit more from AT than others, and we need to know who they are. Also, some applications may favor AT for stronger outcomes than others. Resolving issues of ideal client-to-problem-to-technique matches is a laborious task because of the large number of possible comparisons that have to be tested (see Lehrer & Woolfolk, Chapter 26, this volume).

REFERENCES

Aivazyan, T. A., Zaitsev, V. P., & Yurenev, A. P. (1988). Autogenic training in the treatment and secondary prevention of essential hypertension: Five-year follow-up. *Health Psychology, 7*(Suppl.), 201–208.

Badura, H. O. (1977). Beitrag zur differentialdiagnostischen Validitaet des MMPI zur Prognose der Efflzienz des Autogenen Trainings [Contribution to the differential diagnostic validity of the MMPI for predicting the outcome of autogenic training]. *Archiv für Psychiatrie und Nervenkrankheiten, 224,* 389–394.

Benson, H. (1975). *The relaxation response.* New York: Morrow.

Bernstein, D. A., & Borkovec, T. D. (1973). *Progressive relaxation training: A manual for the helping professions.* Champaign, IL: Research Press.

Budzynski, T. H., Stoyva, J. M., & Pfeffer, K. E. (1980). Biofeedback techniques in psychosomatic disorders. In A. Goldstein & E. B. Foa (Eds.), *Handbook of behavioral interventions.* New York: Wiley.

Cannon, W. B. (1933). *The wisdom of the body.* New York: Norton.

Diehl, B. J. M., Meyer, H. K., Ulrich, P., & Meinig, G. (1989). Mean hemispheric blood perfusion during autogenic training and hypnosis. *Psychiatry Research, 29,* 317–381.

Dierks, T., Maurer, K., & Zacher, A. (1989). Brain mapping of EEG in autogenic training (AT). *Psychiatry Research, 29,* 433–434.

Dobeta, H., Sugano, H., & Ohno, Y. (1966). Circulatory changes during autogenic training. In J. J. Lopez Ibor (Ed.), *IV World Congress of Psychiatry, Madrid* (International Congress Series No. 117.48). Amsterdam: Excerpta Medica.

Eppley, K. R., Abrams, A. I., & Shear, J. (1989). Differential effects of relaxation techniques on trait anxiety: A meta-analysis. *Journal of Clinical Psychology, 45*, 957–974.

Erickson, M. H., & Rossi, E. L. (1979). *Hypnotherapy: An exploratory casebook*. New York: Irvington.

Fischel, W., & Mueller, V. P. (1962). Psychogalvanische Hautreaktionen im Autogenen Training und
waehrend der Hypnotherapie. *Zeitschrift für Psychologie, 167*, 80–106.

Godfrey, K. J., Bonds, A. S., Kraus, M. E., Wiener, M. R., & Toth, C. S. (1990). Freedom from stress: A
meta-analytic view of treatment and intervention programs. *Applied H.R.M. Research, 1*, 67–80.

Haynes, R. B., Taylor, D. W., & Sackett, D. L. (1979). *Compliance in health care*. Baltimore: Johns
Hopkins University Press.

Heide, F. J., & Borkovec, T. D. (1983). Relaxation-induced anxiety: Paradoxical anxiety enhancement
due to relaxation training. *Journal of Consulting and Clinical Psychology, 51*, 171–182.

Heide, F. J., & Borkovec, T. D. (1984). Relaxation-induced anxiety: Mechanisms and their theoretical
implications. *Behaviour Research and Therapy, 22*, 1–12.

Hoelscher, T. J., Lichstein, K. L., & Rosenthal, T. L. (1986). Home relaxation practice in hypertension
treatment: Objective assessment and compliance induction. *Journal of Consulting and Clinical Psychology, 54*, 217–221.

Hyman, R. B., Feldman, H. R., Harris, R. B., Levin, R. F., & Malloy, G. B. (1989). The effects of relaxation training on clinical symptoms: A meta-analysis. *Nursing Research, 38*, 216–220.

Ikemi, Y., Nakagawa, S., Kimura, M., Dobeta, H., Ono, Y., & Sugita, M. (1965). Blood flow change by
autogenic training—including observations in a case of gastric fistula. In W. Luthe (Ed.), *Autogenes
Training: Correlationes psychosomaticae* (pp. 64–68). Stuttgart, Germany: Thieme.

Israel, L., & Rohmer, F. (1958). Variations électroencéphalographiques au cours de la relaxation
autogène et hypnotique. In P. Aboulker, L. Chertok, & M. Sapir (Eds.), *La relaxation: Aspects
théoriques et pratiques*. Paris: Expansion Scientifique Française.

Jacob, R. G., Chesney, M. A., Williams, D. M., Ding, Y., & Shapiro, A. S. (1991). Relaxation therapy for
hypertension: Design effects and treatment effects. *Annals of Behavioral Medicine, 13*, 5–17.

Jacob, R. G., Kraemer, H. C., & Agras, W. S. (1977). Relaxation therapy in the treatment of hypertension: A review. *Archives of General Psychiatry, 34*, 1417–1427.

Jacobson, E. (1938). *Progressive relaxation* (2nd ed.). Chicago: University of Chicago Press.

Jacobson, N. S., Follette, W. L., & Revenstorf, D. (1984). Psychotherapy outcome research: Methods of
reporting variability and evaluating clinical significance. *Behavior Therapy, 75*, 336–352.

Jus, A., & Jus, K. (1968). Das Verhalten des Elektroencephalogramms waehrend des Autogenen
Trainings. In D. Langen (Ed.), *Der Weg des Autogenen Trainings* (pp. 359–375). Darmstadt, Germany: Wissenschaftliche Buchgesellschaft.

Katzenstein, A., Kriegel, E., & Gaefke, I. (1974). Erfolgsuntersuchung bei einer komplexen Psychotherapie essentieller Hypertoniker. *Psychiatrie, Neurologie, Medizinische Psychologie, 26*, 732–737.

Lang, P. J. (1979). A bio-informational theory of emotional imagery. *Psychophysiology, 16*, 495–512.

Lang, P. J., Kozak, M. J., Miller, G. A., Levin, D. N., & McLean, A., Jr. (1980). Emotional imagery: Conceptual structure and pattern of somato-visceral response. *Psychophysiology, 17*, 179–192.

Lang, P. J., Levin, D. N., Miller, G. A., & Kozak, M. J. (1983). Fear behavior, fear imagery, and the
psychophysiology of emotion: The problem of affective response integration. *Journal of Abnormal
Psychology, 92*, 276–300.

Lantzsch, W., & Drunkenmoelle, C. (1975). Studien der Durchblutung in Patienten mit Essentieller
Hypertonie [Studies of the circulation in patients with essential hypertension]. *Psychiatrica Clinica,
8*, 223–228.

Lehrer, P. M., Atthowe, J. M., & Weber, B. S. P. (1980). Effects of progressive relaxation and autogenic
training on anxiety and physiological measures, with some data on hypnotizability. In F. J.
McGuigan, W. E. Sime, & J. M. Wallace (Eds.), *Stress and tension control*. New York: Plenum
Press.

Lehrer, P. M., Carr, R., Sargunaraj, D., & Woolfolk, R. L. (1994). Stress management techniques: Are
they all equivalent, or do they have specific effects? *Biofeedback and Self-regulation, 19*, 353–401.

Ley, R. (1985). Blood, breath and fears: A hyperventilation theory of panic attacks and agoraphobia.
Clinical Psychology Review, 5, 271–285.

Lindemann, H. (1974). *Ueberleben im Stress: Autogenes Training*. Munich, Germany: Bertelsmann.

Linden, M. (1977). Verlaufsstudie des Wechsels der Atmung und des CO_2 Spiegels waehrend des Lernens
des Autogenen Trainings. *Psychotherapie und Medizinische Psychologie, 27*, 229–234.

Linden, W. (Ed.). (1988). *Biological barriers in behavioral medicine.* New York: Plenum Press.

Linden, W. (1990). *Autogenic training: A clinical guide.* New York: Guilford Press.

Linden, W. (1994). Autogenic training: A narrative and a meta-analytic review of outcome. *Biofeedback and Self-Regulation, 19,* 227–264.

Linden, W. (2004). *Stress management: From basic science to better practice.* Thousand Oaks, CA: Sage.

Linden, W., & Frankish, C. J. (1988). Expectancy and type of activity: Effects of prestress cardiovascular adaptation. *Biological Psychology, 27,* 227–235.

Linden, W., Lenz, J. W., & Con, A. H. (2001). Individualized stress management for primary hypertension: A controlled trial. *Archives of Internal Medicine, 161,* 1071–1080.

Linden, W., & Wen, F. (1990). Therapy outcome research, health care policy, and the continuing lack of accumulating knowledge. *Professional Psychology: Research and Practice, 21,* 482—488.

Luebbert, K., Dahme, B., & Hasenbring, M. (2001). The effectiveness of relaxation training in reducing treatment-related symptoms and improving emotional adjustment in acute non-surgical cancer treatment: A meta-analytical review. *Psycho-Oncology, 10,* 490–502.

Luthe, W. (1963). Autogenic training: Method, research and application in medicine. *American Journal of Psychotherapy, 17,* 174–195.

Luthe, W. (1970a). *Autogenic therapy: Vol. 4. Research and theory.* New York: Grune & Stratton.

Luthe, W. (1970b). *Autogenic therapy: Vol. 5. Dynamics of autogenic neutralization.* New York: Grune & Stratton.

Luthe, W. (1970c). *Autogenic therapy: Vol. 6. Treatment with autogenic neutralization.* New York: Grune & Stratton.

Luthe, W., & Schultz, J. H. (1969a). *Autogenic therapy: Vol. 2. Medical applications.* New York: Grune & Stratton.

Luthe, W., & Schultz, J. H. (1969b). *Autogenic therapy: Vol. 3. Applications in psychotherapy.* New York: Grune & Stratton.

Lynch, J. J. (1985). *The language of the heart.* New York: Basic Books.

Martin, A. R. (1951). The fear of relaxation and leisure. *American Journal of Psychoanalysis, 11,* 42–50.

Mensen, H. (1975). *ABC des Autogenen Trainings.* Munich, Germany: Goldmann

Ohno, Y. (1965). Studies on physiological effects of autosuggestion centered around autogenic training. *Fukuoka Acta Medica, 56,* 1102–1119.

Pelliccioni, R., & Liebner, K. H. (1980). Ultraschall-Doppler sonographische Messungen von Blutstroemungsaenderungen waehrend der Grunduebungen im Rahmen des Autogenen Trainings. *Psychiatrie, Neurologie, und Medizinische Psychologie, 32,* 290–297.

Pikoff, H. (1984). A critical review of autogenic training in America. *Clinical Psychology Review, 4,* 619–639.

Polzien, P. (1953). Versuche zur Normalisierung der S-T strecke und T-zacke im EKG von der Psyche her. *Zeitschrift für Kreislauf-Forschung, 42,* 9–10.

Sakakibara, M., Takeuchi, S., & Hayano, J. (1994). Effect of relaxation training on cardiac parasympathetic tone. *Psychophysiology, 31,* 223–228

Sapir, M., & Reverchon, F. (1965). Modifications objectives—circulatoires et digestives—au cours du Training Autogène. In W. Luthe (Ed.), *Autogenes Training: Correlationes psychosomaticae* (pp. 59–63). Stuttgart, Germany: Thieme.

Schaefgen, E. (1984). Lebensweg von J. H. Schultz nach seinem "Lebensbilderbuch eines Nervenarztes." In G. Iversen (Ed.), *Dem Wegbereiter Johann Heinrich Schultz.* Cologne, Germany: Deutscher Aerzte Verlag.

Schultz, J. H. (1932). *Das Autogene Training-Konzentrative Selbstentspannung.* Leipzig, Germany: Thieme.

Schultz, J. H. (1973). *Das Autogene Training-Konzentrative Selbstentspannung: Versuch einer Klinischpraktischen Darstellung.* Stuttgart, Germany: Thieme.

Schultz, J. H., & Luthe, W. (1969). *Autogenic therapy: Vol. 1. Autogenic methods.* New York: Grune & Stratton.

Schwartz, G. E. (1977). Psychosomatic disorders and biofeedback: A psychological model of dysregulation. In J. D. Maser & M. E. P. Seligman (Eds.), *Psychopathology: Experimental models.* San Francisco: Freeman.

Schwartz, M. S., & Andrasik, F. (2003). *Biofeedback: A practitioner's guide.* New York: Guilford Press.

Schwarz, G., & Langen, D. (1966). Gefaessreaktionen bei Autogenem Training und niedrigen Raumtemperaturen. In J. J. Lopez Ibor (Ed.), *IV World Congress of Psychiatry*, Madrid (International Congress Series No. 117.48). Amsterdam: Excerpta Medica.

Shapiro, D. A., & Shapiro, D. (1982). Meta-analysis of comparative therapy outcome studies: A replication and refinement. *Psychological Bulletin, 92*, 581–604.

Shapiro, S., & Lehrer, P. M. (1980). Psychophysiological effects of autogenic training and progressive relaxation. *Biofeedback and Self-Regulation, 5*, 249–255.

Stetter, F., & Kupper, S. (2002). Autogenic training: A meta-analysis of clinical outcome studies. *Applied Psychophysiology and Biofeedback, 27*, 45–98.

Taylor, C. B., Agras, W. S., Schneider, J. A., & Allen, R. A. (1983). Adherence to instructions to practice relaxation exercises. *Journal of Consulting and Clinical Psychology, 51*, 952–953.

Vinck, J., Arickx, M., & Hongenaert, M. (1987). Predicting interindividual differences in blood pressure response to relaxation training in normotensives. *Journal of Behavioral Medicine, 10*, 395–410.

von Siebenthal, W. (1952). Eine vereinfachte Schwereuebung des Schultz'schen Autogenen Trainings. *Zeitschrift für Psychotherapie und Medizinische Psychologie, 2*, 135–143.

Wallace, R. K. (1970). Physiological effects of transcendental meditation. *Science, 167*, 1751–1754.

Wallnoefer, H. (1972). *Seele ohne Angst-Hypnose, Autogenes Training, Entspannung*. Hamburg, Germany: Hoffmann & Campe.

Zsombok, T., Juhasz, G., Budavari, A., Vitrai, J., & Bagdy, G. (2003). Effect of autogenic training on drug consumption in patients with primary headache: An 8-month follow-up study. *Headache, 43*, 251–257.

CHAPTER 8

Autogenic Biofeedback Training in Psychophysiological Therapy and Stress Management

PATRICIA A. NORRIS
STEVEN L. FAHRION
LEO O. OIKAWA

HISTORY OF THE METHOD

Autogenic biofeedback training (ABT; Green, Green, Walters, Sargent, & Meyer, 1975) represents an integration of two distinct but well-established and documented self-regulatory techniques of the late 1960s and the early 1970s, autogenic training (AT) and biofeedback (BF); it provides a methodology that combines the best features of each.

ABT may be somewhat unusual compared with other psychophysiological therapies and stress management methods in that its goal, conscious acquisition of physiological self-regulation, was conceived of prior to the actual development of the specific methodology required to aid this training method for acquisition of self-regulatory skills.

To briefly summarize, AT is a system of psychosomatic self-regulation that was developed in Germany by Johannes H. Schultz, a psychiatrist and neurologist, early in the 20th century. This method permits the gradual acquisition of autonomic control through passive concentration on several standard repetitive verbal formulas (phrases) implying such subjective sensations as heaviness and warmth in the extremities (see Linden, Chapter 7, this volume).

BF, on the other hand, refers to a collection of different techniques developed by several independent researchers in the United States, largely during the 1950s and 1960s, each of which is useful in accelerating voluntary psychosomatic self-regulation. Although this basic concept of BF training was probably first formulated long ago by yogis learning to regulate the basal body metabolism rate, it is quite unique in that it was developed using modern electronic technology. With BF, exceedingly small electrophysiological activity is detected and monitored from the surface of the skin using electrodes, and information is presented (fed back), visually and/or auditorily, to show the client undergoing a BF session what is happening to his or her bodily functions that are normally too subtle to be sensed and unavailable to awareness. Control of a wide variety of physiological parameters—such as heart behavior, temperature, brain-wave activity, blood pressure, and muscle tension—using BF methodology has been demonstrated and seems limited only by the availability of opportunity to monitor the level of function in a physiological system consciously, by the possibility of providing continuous feedback on that level, and by the expectation of success on the part of the client (Leeb, Fahrion, & French, 1976).

Each of the three methods (ABT, AT, and BF) has wide-ranging applications not only in medicine but also in psychology and education.

The People Involved

We acknowledge the inspiration and aspiration of two individuals—Elmer Green, a physicist, and his wife, Alyce, a psychologist and counselor—who are the cofounders and developers of the ABT methods mentioned in this chapter. The Greens had always been interested in studying the development of human awareness and volition in order to develop ways of teaching people to become conscious of, and to learn voluntary control of, normally unconscious processes (both physiological and psychological). They were able to follow through with this idea in research work at the Menninger Foundation in the mid-1960s, through the influence of and support from the director of research at the foundation at the time, Gardner Murphy.

The Greens began their work at the Menninger Foundation by first measuring the physiological correlates of AT (Schultz & Luthe, 1969) without incorporating the use of feedback, to see, for example, the actual thermal consequences of repeating such a standard AT verbal formula or phrase as "My right hand is warm." While measuring the physiological correlates of autogenic phrases and finger temperature, Green and Green (1975) observed in one female client a strong relationship between symptomatic relief from a migraine headache and vasodilation in the hands (correlated with actual temperature increase in the hands of 10°F in 2 minutes, which suddenly occurred 9 minutes into the training). The discovery led directly to the first integration of AT and simultaneous feedback of the consequent psychophysiological changes and, hence, to the dawn of ABT.

After this observation, the first actual treatment with ABT took place in 1966. The wife of one of the Greens' colleagues in their research department, who suffered from migraine headaches, asked whether she could learn to eliminate them. Elmer Green explained the limbic–hypothalamic–pituitary rationale that had been constructed by that time (described later), gave her an autogenic biofeedback temperature training session, and loaned her one of the just-constructed temperature trainers, cautioning her that the treatment would be experimental. As so often happens in the development of a new treatment modality, the first patient was a great success. Although she had previously experienced an incapacitating headache almost every week, after a month of hand-temperature training she had the migraine under control, and she eliminated entirely her dependence on headache medication. She remained headache-free during 10 years of follow-up.

The Greens then developed a plan to study control of unconscious processes through their physiological correlates in autonomic nervous function. Gardner Murphy was open to and interested in this line of inquiry. With Murphy's encouragement, a proposal was prepared, and a government grant to fund this biofeedback research was obtained from the National Institute of Mental Health (NIMH) in 1967. The study, "Voluntary Control of Internal States" (Green, Ferguson, Green, & Walters, 1970; Green, Green, & Walters,

1970b), concerned the training of college students, with the aid of feedback, simultaneously to (1) reduce the level of muscle firing in the forearm as an indication of striate relaxation (Green, Walters, Green, & Murphy, 1969), (2) increase hand temperature as an indication of autonomic relaxation (Luthe, 1965) and (3) increase the density of alpha-wave rhythm in the electroencephalographic (EEG) record as an indication of central nervous system relaxation (Kamiya, 1968). From that project, the first BF research to be funded by the federal government, the Voluntary Controls Program at Menninger, was generated. (It needs to be mentioned, though, that the term *biofeedback* was actually not coined until the founding meeting of the Biofeedback Research Society in 1972).

Emergence of First Publications

A number of research reports and conceptual papers describing ABT began to emerge on a variety of topics, including deep relaxation (Green et al., 1969), voluntary control of internal psychological and physiological states (Green, Ferguson, et al., 1970; Green, Green, & Walters, 1970b), self-regulation and healing (Green, Green, & Walters, 1971a), creativity (Green, Green, & Walters, 1971b), migraine headaches (Sargent, Green, & Walters, 1972), and anxiety and tension reduction (Green, Green, & Walters, 1973). By the middle of the 1970s, other investigators began to use autogenic techniques combined with biofeedback, both clinically and experimentally, but few reports appeared until after 1975.

THEORETICAL FOUNDATIONS AND UNDERPINNINGS

Scope of Application

In considering theoretical foundations and underpinnings for ABT, it is well to examine the scope of application of the technique in order to assess the range of results for which that theory must account. Whereas a survey of the literature from 1975 to 1982 found papers on AT outnumbering papers on ABT by 15 to 1, during the period from 1983 to 1991 this ratio shrank to 1.7 to 1. The earlier period encompassed a total of 33 papers on ABT; 118 papers on this topic appeared in the latter period. During the latter period, 194 papers were published on AT.

An interesting difference was also seen in the languages and locations of publication for these two sets of papers. Papers on AT were predominantly published in English (59), German (55), Russian (31), Italian (15), French (11), and Spanish (7). Those on ABT were primarily published in English (93) and mainly in the United States, with 5 each in German and Russian and 4 each in Spanish and Japanese. AT maintains a strong European–Russian influence, whereas ABT has been more of a U.S. phenomenon.

These papers on ABT vary markedly in sophistication of design and conceptualization, in the use of experienced versus untrained therapists, in whether an adequate number of training sessions was used to obtain a clinical result, in the populations from which participants were drawn, and in the depth of physiological relaxation achieved. Such differences make comparison of results problematic at best. For that reason, we have not evaluated the level of efficacy of each reference mentioned in this chapter at this time.

The greatest number of ABT efficacy studies have examined cardiovascular applications (23 papers) and headache (28 papers). ABT has been used in the *treatment* of alcoholism (Peniston & Kulkosky, 1989; Fahrion, Walters, Coyne, & Allen, 1992; Sharp,

Hurford, Allison, Sparks, & Cameron, 1997), of test anxiety (Sun et al., 1986), of childhood disorders such as incontinence and hyperactivity (Barowsky, 1990), of fibrositis (Rouleau, Denver, Gauthier, & Biedermann, 1985), of collagen vascular disease (Keefe, Surwit, & Pilon, 1981), and of writer's cramp (Akagi, Yoshimura, & Ikemi, 1977); in the *management* of sickle cell crises (Cozzi, Tryon, & Sedlacek, 1987), of pain due to causalgia (Blanchard, 1979), of phantom limb pain (Sherman, Arena, Sherman, & Ernst, 1989; Tsushima, 1982), of dysmenorrhea (Dietvorst & Osborne, 1978), of tinnitus (Kirsch, Blanchard, & Parnes, 1987), of asthma (Meany, McNamara, Burks, Berger, & Sayle, 1988), and of angina pain (Hartman, 1979); and in the *prevention* of psychiatric treatment dropout (Hohne & Bohn, 1988) and of motion sickness (Dobie, May, Fischer, Elder, & Kubitz, 1987; Smirnov, Aizikov, & Kozlovskaia, 1988; Cowings & Toscanow, 2000; Jozsvai & Pigeau, 1995; Cowings et al., 1994; Toscano & Cowings, 1982).

Other studies, especially from Japan, describe treatments combining AT and BF, but without using the term *autogenic biofeedback training*. Applications have included chronic lumbar pain (Yamazaki, Hoshino, Ito, Matsuo, & Katsura, 1985), childhood migraine (Labbe, 1995), and chronic leg pain in arteriosclerosis obliterans (Oikawa et al., 1999). Although some reviews (Ikemi, 1979; Ishikawa & Robinson, 1981) have tried to introduce to English-language readers some of the methodologies of self-regulation and behavioral approaches used in Japan, the clinical-based research has mostly been printed and published in the Japanese language, thus never quite reaching international recognition.

In our experience, these diverse published reports represent only a small indication of the extent to which ABT is being utilized in clinical treatment. Clinical seminars in the use of these techniques began at the Menninger Foundation in 1971, and several thousand professionals have attended to date. Subsequently, many professionals have incorporated ABT into their clinical practice.

ABT has also had an impact on other than clinical areas. It has been used in educational settings with children with emotional disorders (Walton, 1979); with non-disordered children (Engelhardt, 1976); with incarcerated prisoners (Norris, 1976); in personal growth (Leeb et al., 1976); and in other health, physical exercise, and sports applications (Zaichkowsky & Fuchs, 1988; Blumenstein, Bar-Eli, & Tenenbaum, 1995). A study on airplane pilot performance (Cowings, Kellar, Folen, Toscano, & Burge, 2001) has been reported as well.

Mechanisms

Not all the neuromechanisms involved in voluntary self-regulation of the autonomic nervous system have been delineated, but the limbic–hypothalamic–pituitary axis is clearly an essential part. The classic article by Papez (1937), "A Proposed Mechanism of Emotion," laid the groundwork for an understanding of biopsychological factors, and additional work has elaborated Papez's position (Brady, 1958). The work of Penfield (1975) and of Heath and Becker (1954) in exploring tumor boundaries, in which brain areas were probed with depth electrodes in conscious patients, has demonstrated that limbic stimulation results in the experience of emotion and sensory perception. MacLean (1955) coined the phrase *visceral brain* for the limbic system, and others have referred to it as the *emotional brain*, but the important point is that emotional states are reflected in or correlated with electrophysiological activity in the limbic system. It seems that the limbic system is the major responder to psychological stress and that chronic psychological problems can manifest themselves in chronic somatic processes through numerous interconnections between the limbic system and autonomic and hormonal control centers in the hypothalamus and the pituitary gland.

It may be possible to bring under some degree of voluntary control any physiological process that can be continuously monitored, amplified, and displayed. This possibility is implied by the psychophysiological principle that, as the Greens postulated it, affirms: "Every change in the physiological state is accompanied by an appropriate change in the mental–emotional state, conscious or unconscious; and conversely, every change in the mental–emotional state, conscious or unconscious, is accompanied by an appropriate change in the physiological state" (Green, Green, & Walters, 1970b, p. 3). From a theoretical point of view, when coupled with volition, what is going on inside the skin that makes possible the self-regulation of what are usually "involuntary" physiological processes? A cybernetic model of the underlying neurological and psychological principles is described here (Green & Green, 1977).

Figure 8.1 is a highly simplified representation of processes that occur in the voluntary and involuntary neurological domain and simultaneously in the conscious and unconscious psychological domain. The upper half of the diagram represents the normal domain of conscious processes—that is, processes of which we normally have awareness when we wish it. The lower half of the diagram represents the normal domain of unconscious processes. The normal neurological locus for conscious processes seems to be the cerebral cortex and the craniospinal apparatus. The normal locus for unconscious processes appears to be the subcortical brain and the autonomic nervous system.

Electrophysiological studies show that every perception of outside-the-skin (OUTS) events (see the upper left box of Figure 8.1) has associated with it (arrow 1) electrical activity in both conscious and unconscious structures—those involved in emotional and mental responses. (The boxes labeled "emotional and mental response . . . " lie on the midline of the diagram, divided by the horizontal center line into conscious and unconscious parts in order to show their two-domain nature.) Arrow 2 leads to the box labeled "limbic response," which lies entirely in the "unconscious" section of the diagram, though some neural pathways lead from limbic structures directly to cortical regions, implying that "information" from limbic processes can reach consciousness.

Of major significance to a proper rationale is the fact that the limbic system is connected by many pathways, represented by arrow 3, to the central "control panel" of the brain, the hypothalamus. Though the hypothalamus weighs only about 4 grams, it regulates a large part of the body's autonomic neural machinery; in addition, it controls the pituitary gland. The pituitary, the so-called "king gland" of the body, is at the top of the hormonal hierarchy, and its action precipitates or triggers changes in other glandular structures. With these concepts in mind, it is easy to see how news from a telephone call could cause a person to faint or to have a sudden surge of high blood pressure. The perception of OUTS events leads to limbic–hypothalamic–glandular responses, and, of course, physiological changes are the inevitable consequence (arrow 4).

If a physiological change from the box at the lower right in Figure 8.1 is "picked up" by a sensitive electrical transducer and displayed to the person on a meter (arrow 5) or made audible by a tone in order to feed back physiological information, then there ensues (arrow 6) a "new" emotional response, a response to normally unconscious inside-the-skin (INS) information. The new emotional response is associated with a "new" limbic response (arrow 7). It combines with, replaces, or modifies the original limbic response (arrow 2). This new limbic response in turn develops a "new" pattern of hypothalamic firing and pituitary secretion, and a "new" physiological state ensues. Thus a biocybernetic control loop is completed as a result of providing the conscious cortex with in-

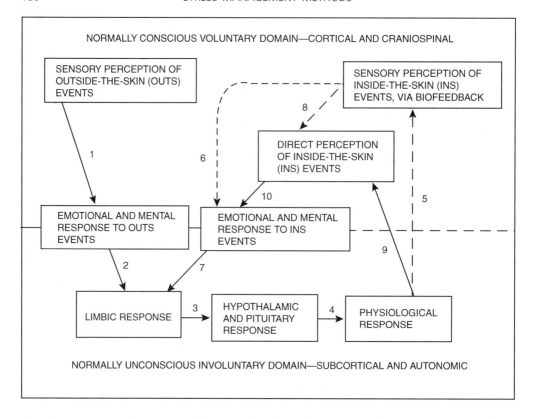

FIGURE 8.1. Simplified operational diagram of "self-regulation" of psychophysiological events and processes. Sensory perception of OUTS events, stressful or otherwise (upper left box), leads to a physiological response along arrows 1 to 4. If the physiological response is "picked up" and fed back (arrow 5) to a person who attempts to control the "behavior" of the feedback device, then arrows 6 and 7 come into being, resulting in a "new" limbic response. This response in turn makes a change in "signals" transmitted along arrows 3 and 4, modifying the original physiological response. A cybernetic loop is thus completed, and the dynamic equilibrium (homeostasis) of the system can be brought under voluntary control. Biofeedback practice, acting in the opposite way from drugs, increases a person's sensitivity to INS events, and arrow 8 develops, followed by the development of arrows 9 and 10. External feedback is eventually unnecessary, because direct perception of INS events becomes adequate for maintaining self-regulation skills. Physiological self-control through classical yoga develops along the route of arrows 7–3–4–9–10–7, but for control of specific physiological and psychosomatic problems, biofeedback training seems more efficient.

formation about normally unconscious INS processes. Closing the biocybernetic loop bridges the normal gap between conscious and unconscious processes and between voluntary and involuntary processes.

In learning voluntary control of normally unconscious processes, we do not become directly aware of the neural pathways and muscle fibers involved, any more than we become aware of what cerebral and subcerebral nerves are involved in hitting a golf ball. But, as in the case of hitting the golf ball, when we get external objective feedback, we can learn to modify the internal "setup" so as to bring about changes in the desired direction.

With the advent of biofeedback, certain previously existing distinctions between the voluntary and involuntary nervous system and between conscious and unconscious processes are being eroded. Conscious control of the autonomic nervous system (once conceptualized to be unconscious and involuntary) is as possible as conscious control of the muscular system is, and it takes place in much the same way. In picking up a pen, the intent is conscious, and visual and proprioceptive feedback are utilized to carry out the activity (consciously or unconsciously). The mechanism whereby the activity is carried out is unconscious; the cortical decision, the visual and motor coordination, and the messages from the visual and motor cortices to spinal ganglia, to motor neurons, and thus to contracting muscles are unconscious; and the result, the pen in hand, is conscious (at least to some extent) and is always available to consciousness.

In the same way, the intent to warm one's fingers is conscious, and visual feedback provided by a temperature trainer is utilized initially to carry out the activity. The mechanism whereby this vasodilation is accomplished (cortex to limbic system to hypothalamic–pituitary–adrenal axis, with accompanying neurohormonal changes in the autonomic nervous system) is unconscious; and the result, the change on the meter or the sensation of warmth, is once again conscious or available to consciousness, like the pen in hand. Initially, of course, the result is made conscious through the use of sensitive physiological monitoring and feedback. Through this process certain autonomic nervous system activity, as well as striate, craniospinal activity, can come under conscious, voluntary control.

It is useful to focus attention especially on arrows 5, 6, 7, 8, 9, and 10 of Figure 8.1. Biofeedback information, along arrow 5 and then arrow 6, is often not needed for more than a few weeks. Biofeedback is not addictive, it seems, because voluntary internal control is established instead of dependence on an external agency. In this respect, biofeedback differs considerably from drugs. Dosages of many drugs often need to be increased as time goes by in order to overcome the body's habituation. With biofeedback, however, sensitivity to subtle internal cues is increased rather than decreased. This increased sensitivity, indicated by arrow 8, is an essential step in closing the internal cybernetic loop, so that the need for feedback devices is only temporary. Eventually the ability to regulate autonomic activity without the aid of machinery can be developed (Green & Green, 1973).

Visualization, Awareness, and Choice

Visualization is an important part of autogenic feedback training. "Making mental contact with the part" (of the body to be regulated) is one of the most interesting concepts in AT. It is clear that "consciousness" is implicit in learning, and top athletes, musicians, and performers of all kinds have reported that conscious visualizations (which may be visual, auditory, and/or kinesthetic) are essential to correct learning and performing. Animal research has clearly demonstrated that perceptual stimuli may result in physiological and behavioral changes. There is, for example, the often-cited case of the stickleback fish that responds to an orange truck parked across the street from its aquarium with the same physiological changes (mating behavior) that would normally be elicited by the orange underbelly of a female fish nearby, because the truck subtends the same angle on the retina (Dobzhansky, 1951).

In humans, visualizing events or imagining sources of stimulation can create as great a physiological response as the actual experience of the event can. For many, the image of squeezing lemon juice onto the tongue produces increased salivation as effectively as actually doing so does; the physiological effects of sexual fantasies and visual stimulation are well known; advertisers are well aware of the connections between images created and eventual behavior. Whereas animals are regulated almost entirely by the environment, humans are regulated by the environment as "perceived by" themselves and by their own inner fantasies, visualizations, images, and expectancies; humans can thus regulate themselves by choosing appropriate visualizations and expectations of desired goals.

Many authors have focused on the nonspecific elements that all psychotherapies appear to share, including a confiding and emotionally charged relationship and a treatment rationale that is confidently conveyed and is accepted by both client and therapist. These are important in the process of ABT as well. There must be communication of new conceptual and experiential information through percept, example, and the process of self-discovery; a strengthening of the client's expectation of help; the provision of success experiences; and the facilitation of the arousal of emotions (Frank, 1971). Despite these commonalities, there are also striking contrasts among various therapies, especially when cross-cultural comparisons are made.

Even within the domain of relaxation-based therapies, quite different rationales appear to underlie the different procedures. Lehrer, Atthowe, and Weber (1980) have pointed out that with progressive relaxation, the focus is on achieving very deep levels of muscular relaxation, which may lower physiological activation in general; by contrast, the rationale of AT is to allow the body to reestablish a state of healthy homeostasis through states of deep relaxation and abreactive emotional discharges.

Karasu (1977) has classified the three predominating themes in the development of psychotherapies as "dynamic," "behavioral," and "experiential." This is very similar to the categorization of psychotherapies by Ikemi as "psychoanalytic," "behavioral," and "autogenic self-regulatory" (Ikemi & Aoki, 1976; Ikemi, Nakagawa, Suematsu, & Luthe, 1975). Indeed, Karasu (1977, p. 852) sees AT as experiential psychotherapy but places BF training as represented by the Greens in the behavioral category. His examples, among others, of the three therapeutic themes include the following: (1) dynamic—classical psychoanalysis (Freud), analytical psychology (Jung), character analysis (Horney), ego analysis (Klein), and biodynamic therapy (Masserman); (2) behavioral—reciprocal inhibition therapy (Wolpe), modeling therapy (Bandura), rational–emotive therapy (Ellis), reality therapy (Glasser), and BF training (the Greens); and (3) experiential—existential analysis (Binswanger), client-centered therapy (Rogers), psychoimagination therapy (Shorr), experiential therapy (Gendlin), and autogenic training (Luthe). An examination of Karasu's (1977, p. 853) description of the thematic dimensions of these psychotherapeutic categories suggests that operant conditioning biofeedback does fit the behavioral paradigm, whereas the Greens' ABT fits the experiential dimension most closely but combines features of both the behavioral and dynamic dimensions as well.

Behavioral therapies seek, as their primary concern, to reduce anxiety. Behaviorists see pathology as the product of maladaptive learned habits, and they conceive of health as an increased ability to take action or perform—a state enhanced by direct learning, conditioning, systematic desensitization, and shaping. Experiential therapies have as their primary concern a reduction in alienation. The source of pathology is seen as existential despair, fragmentation of self, and lack of congruence with one's experiences, and health is conceived of as actualization of potential, self-growth, authenticity, and spontaneity through immediate experiencing.

An examination of the research literature indicates that BF is used in both behavioral and experiential contexts. Furthermore, it is gradually becoming clear that when BF is applied in a conditioning context, the learning of self-regulatory skills proceeds less effectively than when BF is seen as a method to enhance awareness (Brown, 1978; Green & Green, 1977; Lynch, Thomas, Paskewitz, Malinow, & Long, 1982); this perhaps accounts for some of the marked variability in results reported in the BF research literature.

ABT as developed by the Greens is an experiential psychotherapy arising in the context of existentialism; it derives from the basic concept that humans have innate regulatory mechanisms that, if given the chance, can restore brain and body processes to optimal homeostatic conditions. Its concept of pathology derives both from experiential concepts of human loss of possibilities and of fragmentation of self and from the behavioral concept of learned maladaptive habits. Its concept of health emphasizes actualization of potential, self-growth, authenticity, and spontaneity (experiential); symptom removal and anxiety reduction (behavioral); and development of increased ego strength, a more positive self-image, and field independence (dynamic). The treatment model is educational, but treatment takes place in a partnership alliance, an egalitarian existential relationship between therapist and client. This therapy thus emphasizes self-regulation, self-actualization, choice as responsibility, an authentic client–therapist relationship, and awareness. Behavioral techniques such as symptom charting, shaping, and systematic desensitization are used as appropriate, but the therapeutic context is not primarily behavioral, because (1) the locus of control for improvement is seen to reside within the client, not with the dispenser of reinforcements; and (2) awareness is considered to be the prime requisite for higher levels of integration.

From this standpoint, it is important to emphasize that the therapeutic goal in ABT is to maintain and promote desirable levels of functional harmony, rather than simply to reduce anxiety by relaxing deeply. Along with improvements in physiological functioning, a higher order personality integration often does occur, together with increased empathy, creativity, and productivity.

What stands in the way of these therapeutic improvements is not just chronic, homeostasis-disturbing physiological activation of the autonomic and muscular systems as a result of stress but also habitual, functionally fragmented patterns of afferent and efferent corticolimbic activity. It is these disturbed psychophysiological patterns (*automatizations*, in psychoanalytic terminology) that are corrected (*deautomatized*) by the normalizing, self-repair functions and facilitated by autogenic discharge (*abreaction*), thereby overcoming the restricted capacity for self-regulation. This self-neutralizing process seems to be facilitated and stabilized by the client's insight into the previous antihomeostatic reaction patterns and distorted conditioning; such insight helps to avoid repetition of the same failures (Ikemi et al., 1975).

Luthe (1965) has contrasted the ergotropic nature of active concentration with trophotropic functional change resulting from passive concentration on autogenic formulas. He has also discussed the potential specificity of the physiological effect of visualization through the use of organ-specific formulas. These would seem essential features of the method, as embodied in the psychophysiological principle stated earlier: "Every change in the physiological state is accompanied by an appropriate change in the mental–emotional state, conscious or unconscious; and conversely, every change in the mental–emotional state, conscious or unconscious, is accompanied by an appropriate change in the physiological state" (Green, Green, & Walters, 1970b, p. 3).

Sympathetic Vasodilator System

It is worth noting that other mechanisms may be elicited during hand warming than those associated with the autogenic shift. A series of articles by Freedman and colleagues appeared in the early 1990s, purporting to provide evidence that feedback-induced vasodilation is mediated through a nonneural, beta-adrenergic mechanism (see Freedman, 1991). It remains unchallenged that blocking alpha-adrenergic vasoconstrictive responses (e.g., with clonidine) produces comparative vasodilation through a neural mechanism mediated by norepinephrine. Yet these articles have created some degree of confusion among treatment providers, largely because of a tendency to overgeneralize study results to procedures that have not been examined, including effective ABT.

Specifically, it has *not* been demonstrated that the results of these mechanism studies generalize (1) to hand temperatures above 90°F, including those in the maximally therapeutic range above 95°F; (2) to patients other than those with Raynaud's disease; or (3) to methods other than thermal biofeedback alone, such as ABT methods. The last point is notable, because clinicians have long observed that different mechanisms seem to be invoked by using thermal biofeedback alone (which results in increasingly localized response) and by using thermal biofeedback in combination with other relaxation techniques to promote a high thermal criterion (which produces an increasingly generalized, whole-body response). Limits of applicability of results obtained in these mechanism studies have not been explicitly explored in discussions of Freedman's work; more research is necessary to determine to which methodological domains his results apply.

ASSESSMENT

Clinical Indications for ABT

ABT, described in detail in the subsequent section, is widely useful in the treatment of stress-related disorders, including such problems as classical and common migraine headache (Sargent et al., 1972; Billings, Thomas, Rapp, Reyes, & Leith, 1984; Blanchard et al., 1985; Boller & Flom, 1979; Chapman, 1986; Daly, Donn, Galliher, & Zimmerman, 1983; Fahrion, 1977; Guarnieri & Blanchard, 1990), tension headache (Budzynski, Stoyva, & Adler, 1970), mixed tension–vascular headache (Fahrion, 1977), idiopathic essential hypertension (Fahrion, 1991; Green, Green, & Norris, 1979; McGrady, Yonker, Tan, Fine, & Woerner, 1981; Sedlacek, 1979), primary idiopathic Raynaud's disease (Taub & Stroebel, 1978; Freedman, 1987), irritable bowel syndrome (Blanchard, Radnitz, Schwarz, Neff, & Gerardi, 1987; Blanchard & Schwarz, 1987; Schwarz, Taylor, Scharff, & Blanchard, 1990), diabetic ulcer (Shulimson, Lawrence, & Iocono, 1986), and cardiac arrhythmias (Brody, Davison, & Brody, 1985).

ABT is also appropriate as an adjunctive treatment for other disorders in which stress may play a part in causing or exacerbating the problem. In neuromuscular rehabilitation with problems of paresis and spasticity following trauma or stroke, for example, ABT may be used to reduce the impact of the stresses associated with the disability, to improve circulation to damaged areas in the interests of healing, and to restore or improve function in areas affected by paresis. Autogenic biofeedback has also been found useful for self-regulation training in instances of tic, blepharospasm, Bell's palsy, and torticollis. Moreover, ABT may play an important adjunctive role in reducing symptoms and stress while potentiating other medical treatments in such illnesses as cancer, diabetes, and multiple sclerosis.

Psychological dysfunctions ameliorated by ABT include such stress-related disorders as agoraphobia, neurotic depression, impulse disorders (anger, acting out), and other generalized stress syndromes with no underlying organicity—for all of which, in nonpsychiatric medical settings, Valium or other palliatives are often prescribed. ABT and psychological monitoring also constitute a useful adjunct to desensitization psychotherapy.

Norris and Fahrion have found that ABT can be accommodated to any age group; they have treated people from ages 4 through 89 with equally good success. ABT can also be accommodated to a wide range of intelligence levels and has been used with positive results with retarded children (French, Leeb, & Fahrion, 1975).

At another level, assessment proceeds according to psychophysiological considerations, and the initial session as a whole may be seen as an opportunity for both therapist and client to assess the appropriateness of this treatment approach. Initial physiological levels for a typical client coming to a therapist's office for the first time provide a sample that represents some degree of the stress response. Then, as the client goes through the relaxation procedures of the first session, the therapist observes the client's levels and flexibility of response: To what extent is the client able to relax at the outset? Thus the initial evaluation and demonstration proceed simultaneously. With this information, the therapist can inform the client about the observed response and ask, on the basis of this sample of what the training will involve, whether the client wishes to proceed. This "self-selection" approach permits the client to provide truly informed consent for the treatment—an ideal that is all too often missing in practice in most medical treatment.

Side Effects, Limitations, and Contraindications

This treatment approach fails, when it does, primarily because of lack of motivation on the part of the client. Consistent (daily) effort is required to practice psychophysiological control until normal homeostatic functioning is restored. Thus, although observations show that most (90%) of our medicated clients with essential hypertension develop the ability to maintain normal blood pressures while eliminating most antihypertensive medications, those who fail are those who do not learn physiological control (indexed by objective criteria) or those who, having developed such control, do not practice the five to seven times per week required initially to make a significant change in their stress-related problems. Later, clients are able to maintain their gains with only infrequent formal practice, as average before-practice hand and foot temperatures increase through experience of the self-regulatory exercises.

There are no known contraindications to the application of these techniques in themselves. However, clients with psychosomatic and psychophysiological stress disorders—if they are taking medication with major systemic effects, such as antihypertensive drugs, thyroid medication, or insulin—may become overmedicated as they make progress in the acquisition of these self-regulatory skills with their consequent neurohormonal changes and physiological improvements. Close monitoring of such physiological changes in relation to medications is a necessity to prevent possible overmedication and its consequences and to be sure that medication levels are reduced when appropriate. This is always done in cooperation with, and at the direction of, such patients' managing physicians.

Individuals who have been highly stressed and who become very relaxed physiologically may also find themselves in much better touch with emotion-laden unconscious processes. This discharge phenomenon actually represents a part of the therapeutic action of ABT; however, if it should become temporarily overwhelming for a client, the therapist may wish to recommend that the client engage in several short sessions (5 minutes or less) during the day rather than in one or two longer sessions until this process resolves itself.

With some more severely disturbed clients, the therapist may find it necessary to conduct all the experiential processes with the clients in the office at first. We have observed that stress management therapy with more seriously disturbed clients often takes much longer, particularly in instances of high levels of psychoactive medications; that it may have definite but only limited beneficial effects; and that, in a few instances, improvement may not persist beyond the treatment period.

It is important to recognize in this regard that if a client is able to maintain a relaxed physiology in the face of this discharge of emotion-laden thoughts and images, a kind of naturalistic desensitization process ensues, and autogenic abreaction and neutralization are facilitated. At any rate, this phenomenon does not represent a contraindication for the experienced therapist so much as a technical problem to be dealt with in the psychotherapeutic process.

THE METHOD

Introducing the Method to the Client

Although considerable variability exists in the procedures used by various practitioners in teaching voluntary control of autonomic processes, those described here are fairly typical. At the beginning of psychophysiological therapy, each medically symptomatic client should have his or her medical records reviewed; if necessary, the client should have a further medical examination to establish the diagnosis and to ensure that any medical treatment that may be required in addition to the psychophysiological therapy will be recommended or provided.

That the variability in concepts among practitioners using BF contributes to a rather wide range of procedures and results can be seen from an examination of the literature. With respect to the role of awareness in BF, for example, the paradigms within which BF is used range from "biofeedback training has nothing to do with awareness" to "BF training is awareness training." The latter position is implicit in autogenic training, a procedure that mobilizes intention and volition; it is the position of the founders of ABT, as well as of clinicians who think of BF in terms of self-regulation and voluntary control rather than conditioning.

The philosophy under which autogenic biofeedback is used in treatment has an impact on all aspects of the method and is the determining factor in such aspects of treatment as the introduction of the method to the client and the nature of the client–therapist relationship. In our practice, we place great emphasis on engendering in the client a clear understanding of the basic mechanisms of stress and anxiety, of self-regulation concepts, of the principles underlying psychosomatic illness and psychosomatic health (Green, Green, & Walters, 1970b), and of the rationale for the methods to be employed. To this end, we frequently employ audiovisual aids (graphs, diagrams, films, and videotapes) and assigned readings, as well as a variety of experiential exercises to familiarize clients with their own mind–body coordination.

From the beginning of therapy, we make it clear to clients that the essence of self-regulation of any kind is proper visualization and that neither the machines nor the therapists are making anything "happen." This is true of all acquired skills, from executing a pole vault or a cartwheel to playing the piano, as well as in the learning of autonomic self-regulation.

The neurological rationale just described is provided to clients; every effort is made to "demystify" the topic of mind–body coordination and to foster a mental set within which physiological self-regulation is easier to learn. We hypothesize that understanding the rationale underlying treatment engages both hemispheres of a client's brain in the therapeutic process: The left cortex, appreciating the rational and practical nature of neurological self-regulation, enhances (or at least does not interfere with) the right cortex in creating appropriate visualizations. Each client participates in goal setting and in developing the treatment program and is in every sense a coparticipant in the treatment process.

The Physical Environment and Equipment

Training sessions typically occur in a standard office environment with, at a minimum, a reclining chair for the client, a nearby table for the equipment, and comfortable seating space for the therapist. The office setting should be pleasant and conducive to relaxation, rather than sterile and emotionally cold. Office temperatures will ideally be well stabilized and perhaps somewhat warmer than usual (72–74°F), and/or a light blanket should be available to cover the client during the early phases of training. The office should be quiet and softly lighted, without fluorescent lights to create electrical artifacts that are difficult to filter out. These ideal conditions facilitate early training, particularly with clients who are tense, anxious, and/or in pain. Later in training, it is important for clients to be able to accomplish relaxation in any environment.

Commercially available BF equipment is commonly used; this may vary markedly in complexity, from inexpensive thermometers to multiplex, multichannel microcomputers for data collection and display. Minimal equipment would include simple, stand-alone electronic thermal and electromyographic (EMG) BF units, plus a digital integrator to average data over variable time intervals. In general, the expense of equipment is largely determined by its sensitivity, by the complexity of its data processing, and by the variety of its feedback displays.

No comprehensive literature currently exists to compare the effects of these equipment parameters in training, but clinical observation suggests that individual clients may prefer one or another form of feedback display and that it is useful to follow these preferences insofar as this is possible. The fact that clients seem to learn self-regulation with many different feedback regimens suggests that these aspects of training are relatively unimportant as long as the feedback is immediate, continuous, and reasonably pleasant in character.

Some therapeutic advantage may actually accrue from the use of simpler, less expensive equipment, in that it is less likely to suggest to the client that the equipment itself will "do something to" the client rather than simply serving as an electronic mirror. This ensures that the mere presence of the equipment will be less likely to induce short-lived, counterproductive placebo effects that may produce initial confusion in the process of learning self-regulatory skills. Simpler equipment is also less subject to "downtime," an important consideration for the practicing clinician, as the expense of more complicated units may also inhibit acquisition of backup equipment. Thermal and EMG BF units, together with breathing exercises and other adjunctive strategies, can accomplish symptom alleviation or removal and can increase psychosomatic health in any and all of the clients seen. More specific training can often be facilitated with other feedback modalities, such as EEG, electrodermal response (EDR), electrocardiographic (EKG), sphygmomanometer, and goniometer feedback. These physiological measures may be used both for skills training and for objective measurement of other psychophysiological behaviors being treated.

The Therapist–Client Relationship

Because ABT emphasizes self-regulation, much importance is placed on the client's assuming and/or maintaining responsibility for his or her own stress responses, healing process, and state of wellness. This fact necessitates several strategies of approach, which differ from those of many other therapies. First, the relationship is not an authoritarian one; rather, it is a healing partnership in which the client participates fully. The client is not simply a passive receiver of health care but an active participant in a teamwork approach between therapist and client.

To this end, no information is withheld from any client. Clients are fully informed of their condition, their physiological parameters and measurements, and the nature of their progress through the treatment process. As part of increasing self-awareness, we encourage clients to know everything possible about themselves and their conditions. Blood pressure, EKG recordings, blood tests, X-rays, and other medical findings are shared with clients, and these may help form the basis of the visualizations employed.

Effective therapists are generally acute and objective observers. This is an invaluable skill for BF practitioners, as well, and is even more invaluable as a skill to pass on to clients. An ability to become an "observer of the self" maximizes choice and is a central part of self-regulation.

Description of the Method

In a typical case, a major portion of the initial appointment is spent by the therapist in developing rapport with the client, taking a full medical history from the client's point of view, and introducing the concept of BF training. Particular emphasis is placed on explaining the rationale, described earlier, for the way in which BF is applied to the client's specific disorder—that is, what body functions are being measured and how the normalization of these functions can help to alleviate the symptoms.

The client may be shown several graphs or other relevant data about successful training outcomes for similar clients, with the intent of inducing a sense of hopefulness and positive expectancy about the treatment process. Clients with psychophysiological disorders have typically undergone a variety of different treatments without successful results, and they often feel despondent or skeptical about the prospects of improving their condition. If appropriate, clinical data, including blood pressure, EKG, blood tests, and X-rays, are taken to rule out any contraindications.

At the onset of actual training, the client is monitored for baseline levels of skin temperature and forehead muscle tension, at least, and frequently EDR and other parameters are also evaluated. Because the initial training is usually performed with the client reclining in a chair, the baseline data are also taken in this position in our practice. Each physiological function is monitored and the data recorded, first over a few minutes of baseline and then during the relaxation experience, which together provide an index of the stress level. Some clinicians do initial diagnostic evaluations with stressors administered, as well. Although this procedure provides useful information for research and outcome measures, the advantages may be offset by the initial "message" to the client that is implicit in such a procedure.

In addition to the physiological assessment, our diagnostic evaluation includes psychological measures. Each client completes a Spielberger State–Trait Anxiety Inventory, a Cornell Medical Index, and a Personal Orientation Inventory at the beginning of treatment and again at termination. The test results are generally shared and discussed fully at the end of treatment. Occasionally other psychological measures may also be administered.

In a typical first training session, as soon as the baseline data are taken, the client-trainee is oriented to the training process with remarks such as the following:

> At this point I'm going to give you some autogenic training phrases, and I want you to say each phrase over and over to yourself. First, your attitude as you do this is quite important. This is the kind of thing where the more you try to relax, the less it will happen. So the best approach is to have the intention to warm and relax but to remain detached about your actual results. Everyone can learn voluntary control of these processes, and it is only a matter of time until you do, and therefore you can afford to be detached about the results. Second, saying the phrases is good because it keeps them in mind, but it is not enough. The part of the brain that controls these processes, called the limbic system, doesn't understand language well, so it is important to translate the content of the phrase into some kind of image. One of the phrases is "My hands are heavy and warm." If you can actually imagine what it would feel like if your hands did feel heavy or if they did feel warm, that helps to bring on the changes that we are looking for. Or use a visual image: Imagine that you are lying out on a beach in the sun, or that you are taking a warm and soothing bath, or that you are holding your hands over a campfire. Whatever works for you as a relaxing image or a warmth-inducing image is the thing to use, but the imaging itself is important. Finally, if you simply trust your body to do what you are visualizing it as doing, then you will discover that it will.

The modified autogenic training phrases adapted by Alyce Green, including the "mind-quieting" phrases she developed (see Figure 8.2), are then administered for approximately 20 minutes. Only verbal feedback is typically given during the first autogenic biofeedback experience, because direct instrument feedback may induce performance anxiety at this stage and because verbal feedback facilitates the focus of attention on internal awareness. The therapist observes the physiological response on the instrument and either provides verbal feedback for improvement in hand temperature between the autogenic phrases (if indicated) or records impressions for sharing at the conclusion of the experience. The client may be told, "You are beginning to get warmer," and "You're now warming more rapidly," as these events occur. The client is given encouragement and reinforcement. The therapist paces the phrases to correspond to the client's actual physiological changes; it is important for the client to be given sufficient time between phrases to be able to repeat each phrase slowly to himself or herself at least three times.

Toward the end of the first session, auditory or visual feedback may be introduced. Various instruments provide different forms of feedback, but the most widely used is either an analog or digital meter or a tone that decreases in pitch as the hands warm. Another sensitive and useful form of feedback is a tone that increases in pitch as the rate of warming increases.

In concluding the first training period, the therapist and client discuss the experience and the homework exercises to be practiced daily between office visits. The therapist informs the client that positive results are likely, provided that two criteria are met: (1) The client must perform hand-warming exercises every day until symptoms are overcome and must be able finally to sustain a hand temperature of at least 95.5°F for 10 minutes or more; and (2) the client must be able to increase hand temperature at a rate of at least 1°F per minute. (These criteria are perhaps somewhat more stringent than those currently used by most BF practitioners, but their achievement has been observed to be essential if the best clinical results are to be obtained and maintained over time.)

Menninger   **Temperature Feedback scoring sheet**

Trainee's initials _____   Date _____

Initial temperature _____

Temperature reading
(at the start of each phrase)   **Phrases**

_____   1. I feel quite quiet.

_____   2. I am beginning to feel quite relaxed.

_____   3. My feel feel heavy and relaxed.

_____   4. My ankles, my knees and my hips feel heavy, relaxed and comfortable.

_____   5. My solar plexus, and the whole central portion of my body, feel relaxed and quiet.

_____   6. My hands, my arms and my shoulders feel heavy, relaxed and comfortable.

_____   7. My neck, my jaws and my forehead feel relaxed. They feel comfortable and smooth.

_____   8. My whole body feels quiet, heavy, comfortable and relaxed.

_____   9. Continue alone for a minute.

_____   10. I am quite relaxed.

_____   11. My arms and hands are heavy and warm.

_____   12. I feel quite quiet.

_____   13. My whole body is relaxed and my hands are warm, relaxed and warm.

_____   14. My hands are warm.

_____   15. Warmth is flowing into my hands, they are warm, warm.

_____   16. I can feel the warmth flowing down my arms into my hands.

_____   17. My hands are warm, relaxed and warm.

_____   18. Continue alone for a minute.

_____   19. My whole body feels quiet, comfortable and relaxed.

_____   20. My mind is quiet.

_____   21. I withdraw my thoughts from the surroundings and I feel serene and still.

_____   22. My thoughts are turned inward and I am at ease.

_____   23. Deep within my mind I can visualize and experience myself as relaxed, comfortable and still.

_____   24. I am alert, but in an easy, quiet, inward-turned way.

_____   25. My mind is calm and quiet.

_____   26. I feel an inward quietness.

_____   27. Continue alone for a minute.

                           28. The relaxation and reverie is now concluded and the whole body is reactivated with a deep breath and the following phrases: "I feel life and energy flowing through my legs, hips, solar plexus, chest, arms and hands, neck and head . . . The energy makes me feel light and alive." Stretch.

_____

Final temperature _____

FIGURE 8.2. Autogenic biofeedback training phrases. Reprinted by permission of the Menninger Foundation.

In addition to the more formal practice, we also encourage our clients to experiment with the equipment. We may say something like this:

> This equipment is yours to use for the time being, so have fun with it; let the scientist within you come out. If you are watching TV, it is interesting to see what your hand temperature does during the news, during a comedy, or during tender or frightening moments. It may be enlightening to see what happens to your hand temperature if you have a difficult phone call to make . . . do your hands get cold? Can you keep them warm or make them warm? You may want to check this response during any opportunity to explore your own physiological functioning, so let your imagination be your guide.

A thorough description of all the specific training methods is beyond the scope of this chapter. A description of the aims of ABT will suffice to provide a guideline for clinical work and all its ramifications and applications. In autogenic therapy, as developed by Schultz and Luthe, the first four standard exercises are these:

1. Heaviness (associated with neuromuscular quietness)
2. Warmth (associated with autonomic quietness)
3. Cardiac regulation
4. Respiration

These exercises are considered mandatory to prepare the client for, and to optimize the effectiveness of, "organ-specific formulas" (Schultz & Luthe, 1969).

In the development of ABT, we have followed a similar paradigm. In order for visualization, intentional formulas, and specific physiological training to be most effective, the client first learns to achieve a quiet body, quiet emotions, and a quiet mind. To that end, the threefold ABT phrases (see Figure 8.2) were developed by the Greens to help initiate these states; they can be used with any or all of the training modalities, although they are customarily introduced at the outset with thermal training for vascular relaxation and sympathetic deactivation.

Also, to achieve these ends (quiet body, quiet emotions, quiet mind), training proceeds generally in the following order. First, emotional quietness is approached by thermal training, and it is considered to be achieved when criterion levels of hand warming are met. At the second or third session, breathing exercises are introduced, and corrective exercises are given if necessary to switch the client from thoracic to diaphragmatic breathing. The goals of the breathing exercises are for the client to do the following:

1. Establish deep diaphragmatic breathing.
2. Extend the breathing cycle until the breathing rate during relaxation is gradually reduced, over a period of weeks, to a maximum of three to four times per minute.
3. Develop awareness of gasping and holding of breath as a means of blocking feelings and awareness of rapid, shallow breathing at times of anxiety and/or daily life stress.
4. Learn to exhale, let go, and breathe slowly and deeply as an instant destressing technique.

Practice of both thermal training and breathing exercises is continued daily. Some attention must be paid to integrating the practice into the daily life of the client, and homework practice is considered imperative in facilitating a generalization of training skills.

Another technique we have found to be especially useful is one we have dubbed "constant-instance practice." When some mastery of physiological self-regulation is demonstrated (e.g., when a temperature of 95°F or more is reached in the hand a number of times, or a deeply relaxed EMG level is attained), the client is told to engage in the process of constant-instance practice for 1 week, with the following guidelines:

> Repeat to yourself as often as possible a brief phrase indicating the change you want to occur—for example, "My hands are warm and my muscles relaxed." The primary goal is to become relaxed, so if you forget for a while, don't be concerned; just think, "Good, I remembered now." But bear in mind that the more often you do it, the better—100 times is better than 50. So every time you come to a stop sign, every time you sit down, stand up, use the phone, or start or end any activity, simply think of the phrase and the accompanying sensation briefly, without interference in whatever you are doing, without performance anxiety, without checking to see whether anything is happening. Simply, over and over, generate the feeling and let go.

We have found with the majority of our clients that this practice consolidates the training, is especially facilitative of the transfer of training, and helps to establish a new homeostatic balance.

The client may practice briefly two or more times a day. Once a day, at the conclusion of a practice session, a short report of the training session is made (see Figure 8.3). This report is an invaluable part of the awareness enhancement, as the client tunes in to the physical sensations, emotions, and thoughts and fantasies that accompany relaxation. We have observed that psychotherapeutic gains are made by almost every individual learning peripheral temperature regulation. The realization on the part of a client that he or she can control some internal processes that were thought involuntary is always accompanied by a self-image change and an enhanced sense of self-mastery. Over a period of time, both physical and mental well-being are enhanced, as relaxation and self-regulatory skills are transferred to everyday life.

Third, a quiet body is further enhanced by EMG feedback (commonly introduced in the first or in an early session) and by general relaxation training until criterion levels of deep relaxation are reached and can be maintained for at least 10 minutes. Often these three steps are sufficient to produce a quiet mind, as well as physical and emotional quietness. If the "quiet mind" condition has not already been met, EEG alpha- and theta-wave training may reduce mental stress and aid in the achievement of mental quietness.

This training—the "core" of ABT and the sine qua non of our stress management training—precedes specific visualizations and training, whether the disorder being treated is agoraphobia, cancer, arthritis, multiple sclerosis, or any disorder in which stress is a complicating or etiological factor.

Maintenance of Treatment Results

Once clients' gains through daily deep relaxation have been achieved and consolidated, in many instances they may begin to taper off the daily practice. They may do this by warming only on days on which the hands are cool to begin with or only every other day. The symptoms are monitored during this process, and symptomatic regression is an indication of need to increase the daily practice once again; otherwise, practice may be reduced and eliminated, except for very stressful periods. The trainee continues to send the symptom report cards to the therapist for the next few months after treatment is concluded. If it appears from these reports that the trainee is experiencing difficulties, or if he or she does

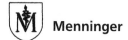 **Menninger**   **Temperature feedback training questionnaire**

Your name	Date	Time of day

Where did you practice?	Scarring skin temperature

Medication or medication changes	Highest temperature

Were you able to fed the following internal changes?

a. Warmth	Definitely	Moderately	Slightly	Not at all
b. Flushing	Definitely	Moderately	Slightly	Not at all
c. Throbbing/Pulsating	Definitely	Moderately	Slightly	Not at all

How did the training session seem?

Were you able to relax?   Yes   No   If not, what seemed to interfere?

Physical sensations mat occurred.

Emotional feelings that occurred.

Thoughts, fantasies, and imaginings.

Did your mind wander at all? Yes No   If so, A lot   Moderately   Slightly

Did you have any tendency to fall asleep (or get drowsy)?   Yes   No

Did you have any dream-like experiences or mental pictures?   Yes   No
a. If so, did these experiences occur in a particular way?   Visual Auditory Spatial Touch (pressure) Smell Taste
b. If so, were you aware of these experiences all of a sudden (very quickly) or in a gradual way? Sudden   Gradual

Was there anything that you particularly liked or did not like about this training session?

Further experiences you would like to share, or remarks you would like to make (if necessary, use reverse side of this sheet).

The Menninger Clinic

FIGURE 8.3. Daily report for enhancing psychophysiological self-awareness during home practice. Reprinted by permission of the Menninger Foundation.

not send in the cards, the therapist telephones the individual to inquire about progress and to recommend whatever modifications in training methodology seem appropriate. As a routine procedure, the therapist telephones each client-trainee after several months for a follow-up evaluation.

CASE EXAMPLE

The case example we present here has been chosen to illustrate several aspects of the technique and effect of ABT. We discuss a client treated for a major stress disorder: essential hypertension.

Although our treatment program is multifaceted, it is probably not possible or even useful to ascribe relative value to the various components, because of their synergistic nature. Yet in our clinical experience, the autonomic self-regulation gained through autogenic biofeedback procedures is the most synergistically powerful element of the entire package. ABT mediates stress reduction, aids visualization, enhances the psychotherapeutic process, and reduces the adversity and probably potentiates the effectiveness of the concurrent medical treatment (medications, diet, and exercise).

Autogenic biofeedback can thus play a significant role in the treatment of clients with essential hypertension (Fahrion, 1991). The major elements of the program are these:

1. Acquisition and daily practice of relaxation skills
2. Psychotherapy, including exploration of past and present stressors and self-image
3. Nutritional counseling
4. Exercise, including breathing exercises
5. Goal setting and play: participating as fully as possible in living, enjoyable activities, and productivity
6. Visualization and imagery of the specific healing process

A comprehensive wellness program, but also a straightforward stress management program based on BF-assisted relaxation, can have a significant impact on the lives and well-being of hypertensive clients. It is well to remember that there is often a triple stress associated with hypertension: the stress that may have contributed to developing high blood pressure in the first place, the stress of having a chronic illness such as hypertension, and the stress associated with taking medication and undergoing other aspects of medical treatment of this disease. The capacity to cope with stress through learned self-regulation can reduce blood pressure and the need for hypotensive medication; can ameliorate unpleasant side effects of treatment and potentiate its positive effects; and can enhance a sense of competence, self-esteem, and self-mastery. From a human perspective, self-regulation increases feelings of mastery and well-being, increases coping, and enhances the quality of life.

Patient B was a middle-management executive in his late 30s who was referred by his physician to a controlled research study of autogenic biofeedback and psychophysiological therapy for treatment of essential hypertension. He had been diagnosed as hypertensive 10 years prior to entering treatment on the basis of blood pressure readings taken in the physician's office, and he was placed on antihypertensive thiazide diuretic medication (methclothiazide; Enduron, 5 mg daily). His records indicated a normal blood chemistry profile and a normal treadmill EKG.

He entered treatment because of health concerns, stating, "I want to learn a technique that will allow me to better control my hypertension. I am frustrated by its controlling me, and disheartened by the need to medicate a response that I should and could control." His attitude, though cautious at first, soon became confident, and his expectations became positive.

Medication Washout and Pretreatment Condition

After signing informed-consent forms, B was instructed in the use of an aneroid sphygmomanometer with the dual-stethoscope equipment. He was then given a standard sphygmomanometer and asked to take his blood pressure daily. A stepwise medication washout was accomplished over a 2-week period. He was monitored weekly in the office with a random zero sphygmomanometer in order to remove some biases common in blood pressure measurement; the average of his first two weekly unmedicated office blood pressures was 156/107 mm Hg. One month later, his office blood pressures averaged 148/96 mm Hg. He was maintained in an unmedicated condition during cardiac reactivity evaluation.

Cardiac Reactivity Testing: Procedures and Initial Results

Cardiac reactivity testing consisted of a 1½-hour protocol during which the following measurements were taken: systolic and diastolic blood pressure; thoracic impedance (using a BOMED Noninvasive Continuous Cardiac Output Monitor); heart rate (HR); hand and foot temperatures (using a T-68 Temperature Monitor; J & J Electronics); and forehead and forearm muscle tension (using an M-57 EMG Monitor; J & J Electronics). Tasks began with a 20-minute self-relaxation baseline period with the examiner out of the room, followed by a 2-minute tilt-to-supine-position task. The remaining tasks included a 5-minute extemporaneous speech sample (Gottschalk, 1978, 1986), a 3-minute serial 7's subtraction task, a 2-minute hand dynamometer task, a video game, and a 90-second cold-pressor task. Each stressor was followed by a self-relaxation recovery period of 6 minutes. The session concluded with one additional 6-minute postbaseline recovery period with the examiner out of the room. During baseline and all recovery periods, the participant was encouraged to relax as much as possible, but without the aid of physiological feedback.

The reactivity test results are displayed according to the convention developed in 1988 by Dr. Robert Eliot (see Figure 8.4A). Normal hemodynamic functioning is represented by values in the white trapezoid at the lower right of Figure 8.4A, bounded on the top by a mean blood pressure of 107 mm Hg (equivalent to pressures of 140 mm Hg systolic and 90 mm Hg diastolic), and bounded on the left by a total systemic resistance of 1,400 (dynes/second/cm⁵). These values represent a situation of normal blood pressure and a relatively open arterial tree. Although this client's initial baseline level was in this normal range, his pressures became elevated with all of the stressors except the video game. The direction of the vectors indicates that his stress responses consisted predominantly of elevated beta-adrenergic drive, with the responses to the cold-pressor and speech tasks showing increased alpha-adrenergic drive, with increased systemic resistance and closing down of the arterial tree as well (Eliot, 1988). The video game task produced more beta-adrenergic response, with the vector moving more to the right, than was the case with the other tasks, indicating that the blood pressure increase observed here resulted primarily from an increase in cardiac output rather than in systemic resistance.

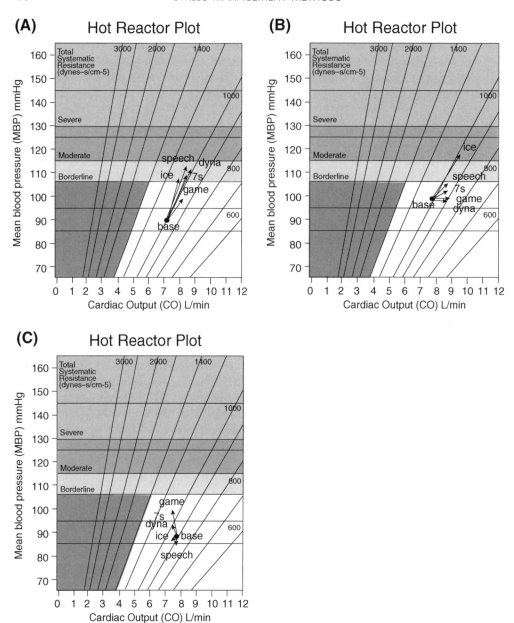

FIGURE 8.4. (A) B's pretreatment cardiac reactivity. Normal functioning is represented by values in the white trapezoid at the lower right. Abbreviations: base, baseline; speech, speech sample; 7s, serial 7's task; dyna, hand dynamometer task; game, video game; ice, cold-pressor task. (B) B's cardiac reactivity after attention placebo treatment. Despite higher baseline pressure, a reduction in alpha-adrenergic drive is apparent. Abbreviations as in A. (C) B's cardiac reactivity after autogenic BF training. Blood pressure is reduced both at baseline and under stress. An overall decrease in both alpha- and beta-adrenergic drive is evident. Abbreviations as in A.

Two very different adrenergically mediated hemodynamic stress responses underlie elevated blood pressure to different degrees in different individuals (Eliot, 1988; Fahrion, 1991). During stress, the alpha-adrenergic response first moves blood *out* of areas where it is *not* needed for fight or flight: out of the hands and feet, out of the lower abdominal area, and out of the kidney. Second, a beta-adrenergic response moves this available blood *into* the areas where it *is* needed for fight or flight: into the muscles and heart. Beta-adrenergic response includes increased cardiac output (CO) as a result of both increased HR and increased stroke volume (SV). Renin release into the plasma is simultaneously increased as part of this pattern.

Similarly, two basic types of hemodynamic response have been observed. The "hyperkinetic heart syndrome," which is similar to the beta-adrenergic pattern just described (with elevated CO, HR, and SV), is commonly seen in the early stages of essential hypertension. Total systemic resistance (TSR), which usually increases with stress, is usually observed to be normal at this point. We later describe how this is possible.

The second hemodynamic pattern, the "blood loss pattern," is similar to that seen when the body experiences hemorrhage and pulls the blood away from the periphery to maintain pressure and prevent blood loss. This pattern is commonly seen in the later stages of hypertension, when CO, HR, and SV have normalized but TSR has become elevated, increasing blood pressure.

In synthesizing these dynamic patterns, we see that in the first stage of stress, the alpha- and beta-adrenergic patterns occur together. TSR is normal because of increases in the diameter of arteries in muscle tissue (to prepare for fight or flight), providing a significant portion of open arterial tree (in the muscles) through which blood can readily flow, even though it is being squeezed out of other areas. If stress is sustained (i.e., impossible to terminate through physical activity), beta-adrenergic response normalizes, including arterial diameter in the muscles. CO also normalizes, as the body is no longer mobilized for action. Yet alpha-adrenergic response continues, squeezing blood out of the periphery, the kidneys, and the organs of digestion. TSR then becomes elevated, as the arterial tree as a whole is relatively constricted.

One implication of this model is that hypertension is also characterized by two quite different phenomenological stances, which may be observed singly or in combination. On the one hand, those with high systolic hypertension and elevated CO may be seen as evidencing "racehorse" hypertension; they commonly report that they have "too much to do and too little time." On the other hand, those with high diastolic hypertension and high TSR seem to be evidencing "turtle" hypertension; their reports are in concert with a need to have a shell around themselves to avoid emotional suffering, because of perceived vulnerability to others or fear that they will lose control and express their own emotions in an excessive fashion.

It is important for practitioners to recognize that when medications for hypertension are given, either or both of these psychophysiological stances may be affected, depending on the action of the medications prescribed. Simplistically, beta blockers reduce "racehorse" hypertension, whereas alpha blockers, calcium channel blockers, and angiotensin-converting enzyme inhibitors tend to reduce "turtle" hypertension.

In terms of this model, at initial testing the client in this case example was primarily responding with beta-adrenergic increases in CO, the hemodynamic pattern typically seen in early hypertension; yet in response to the cold-pressor stimulus, an alpha-adrenergic vasoconstrictive pattern was also activated. Thus specific hemodynamic response to stress may be seen to be a product of both client characteristics and stimulus "pull."

"Placebo" Treatment Results

B was next randomly assigned to a nondirective "self-exploration" (attention placebo) group conducted by a psychologist for 6 months. He took the self-exploration group very seriously and was an active and open participant in group discussions. Discussions focused on interpersonal stress both at work and in the family, financial stress, and stress related to beliefs and roles. The group members became sensitive to dynamic issues such as shame and guilt that related to present stress in their lives, and B developed and expressed greater awareness of how his emotions and his blood pressure interacted. During this time the group leader facilitated interaction between participants but did not provide suggestions, direction, or presentation of didactic material.

Following this treatment, B reported, "The group process helped me work through stressful situations and better developed my sense of stress, its source, and how better to deal with it. I have a more sensitive perception of reality and all of its imperfections." Despite these positive comments, at 150/91 mm Hg, his average office blood pressure was still hypertensive at the end of the 6-month self-exploration group.

The graph of B's cardiac reactivity testing at that point is presented in Figure 8.4B. It reveals that his baseline blood pressure, although still normal, was actually higher than during initial testing. His response to the speech, serial 7's, video game, and dynamometer tasks had normalized, and the direction of the vectors suggested some reduction in alpha-adrenergic response had occurred. His response to the cold-pressor task was somewhat higher than before but indicated more of a "racehorse" than a "turtle" pattern.

Self-Regulation Results

Next, B was treated with "self-regulation," a group autogenic biofeedback treatment, for 6 months. At the outset the client viewed a film on our work with essential hypertension (Hartley, 1981), which presents a rationale, describes the method of treatment, and presents the successful results, including the comments of a number of clients. B reported that he had believed there was little more he could do on his own behalf to make a difference in his health; however, seeing and hearing the previously successful clients describe their results awakened him to the possibility that he could be an active participant in the therapeutic processes.

B was then introduced to thermal biofeedback and breathing exercises and began daily home practice of these immediately, with the aid of a small electronic digital thermometer. These exercises began to help him with relaxing during the first week of practice, and by the end of the week he was able to achieve a hand temperature of 94.8°F, usually associated with deep autonomic relaxation. He reported practicing both autonomic relaxation and breathing during this time with good results, further reinforcing his sense of ability to control some psychophysiological processes.

After six weekly 1-hour sessions, B could usually warm his hands to 96–97°F and was ready to begin warming his feet. We regularly teach clients with essential hypertension to warm the feet, as this is associated with significant drops in blood pressure in our clinical experience.

Despite his good success with hand warming, B had difficulty reliably warming his feet to 93°F until the 24th week of the self-regulation group. To begin with, his feet would often start in the mid-80s (degrees Fahrenheit) and warm only 1–2°F. B was a runner, and we have observed with interest that other individuals who run extensively usually have more difficulty than most people in learning to warm their feet. It is worth noting, however, that he succeeded in raising his foot temperature effectively during the coldest part of winter.

Clients with essential hypertension are provided with a home blood pressure monitor and are asked to assume responsibility for taking their pressures every day. During the first week that B was taking his pressure daily in the home environment before and after relaxation, his weekly average before relaxing was 136/80 mm Hg, and readings ranged up to 144/94. During the last week of treatment his weekly home pressure before relaxing was 123/78 mm Hg, with his two highest pressures at 126/74 and 118/80.

During the course of treatment, B's first sessions with the therapist were spent in thermal training in developing awareness of related physical, emotional, and mental events correlated with autonomic relaxation, as well as awareness of associated imagery and insights. One session was spent in giving the breathing exercises and their rationale. Also during this time, transfer of training of these new autogenic skills was a focus in every session. B was found to have fairly high forehead muscle tension levels (3–4 µV), but within three sessions of EMG BF he was able to relax to criterion level (1 µV); he continued to practice with the EMG throughout the training process.

Emphasis on the psychotherapeutic process continued during the sessions and was frequently wide ranging, covering not only the imagery and insights that arose from the relaxation and visualization themselves but also past life events, present life stressors, present triumphs and accomplishments, and family concerns. Throughout the self-regulation group, clients were constantly reminded to use their new strategies when under stress. During the entire course of therapy, B continually experienced improvements in his blood pressure and in his ability to relax in the face of stressful events. He slept better, had a better appetite, and felt more trim and fit. His coworkers and his family both noticed that he was more relaxed and easygoing and was better able to cope with daily irritants, deadlines, and other stressors. At the end of treatment he reported, "Generally, I am more in touch with me and my environment, and seem to be more at peace with that relationship. I am more accepting of others and tend not to let them 'push my buttons.' "

The graph of the posttreatment cardiac reactivity evaluation is presented in Figure 8.4C. It demonstrates lowered mean blood pressure both at baseline and under stress compared with the previous testings; in fact, all readings fell within the "normal" range. Baseline TSR was also reduced compared with previous testings, suggesting lowered alpha-adrenergic drive. In contrast, the direction of the vectors suggests a trend of reacting to stressors, particularly the video game, with alpha-adrenergic mechanisms. No increase in beta-adrenergic response in relation to any of the stressors was observed.

Summary of Treatment

At 1-year follow-up, B had eliminated antihypertensive medication, and his blood pressures were normotensive, averaging 125/75 mm Hg off medication. On the basis of previous clinical experience, he was expected to maintain a normotensive stance off medications over the years, with only *ad libitum* practice of formal relaxation skills.

B is a person who is participating in life and in gaining health, who feels competent, who has eliminated hypertension and hypotensive medications, and who is enjoying an enhanced quality of life.

Reflections and Comments on Treatment

Although the initial training in ABT is oriented toward attaining states of deep relaxation, physiological studies of the passive concentration state of autogenic training have revealed an increased density of 15- to at least 20-cycle-per-second EEG activity, together with concurrent slow-wave activity density (Degossely & Bostem, 1977). Fischer (1978–1979) interprets these data as indicating that the passive concentration state represents not only a state of relaxation but also a state of arousal. Focused attention and the increased awareness of formerly unconscious events that occur during relaxed states are both part of the process of effective ABT. This unusual state, then, appears to share characteristics with both the vigilant rapid-eye-movement dreaming state and the hypoaroused relaxed-waking state. Therapeutically, it enables detached introspection concerning the exciting and possibly traumatic material emerging from the unconscious (Fischer, 1978–1979).

Similar observations were made in the Greens' studies of imagery and states of consciousness associated with creativity. Their first studies focused on normal, healthy participants and used BF methods to explore the relation between specific internal states, or states of consciousness, and specific brain wave patterns. They found theta waves to be associated with a deeply internalized (vigilant) state and with a quieting of the body, emotions, and thoughts, thus allowing usually "unheard or unseen things" to come to consciousness in the form of hypnogogic imagery (Green & Green, 1977).

There has been increasing interest in examining similar psychophysiological correlates of meditation. Fischer (1978–1979) likens the altered state of consciousness that accompanies autogenic training to Theraveda Buddhist meditation. In order to adapt the system for research in states of consciousness and to shorten the learning time associated with autogenic training, the Greens combined "the conscious self-regulation aspect of yoga and the psychological method of autogenic training with the modern instrumental technique called physiological feedback" (Green, Green, & Walters, 1970a, n.p.).

Benson, Beary, and Carol (1974), who adapted their methods for achieving the relaxation response from transcendental meditation, note that the physiological states thus achieved resemble those achieved through autogenic training, hypnosis, Zen, yoga, and other meditative techniques. Bostem and Degossely (1978) described, using spectral analysis of EEG data, the progressive spread of a dominant alpha band all over the scalp during autogenic training. These findings are very similar to those of Banquet (1973) in his spectral analysis of EEG during meditation. Fehmi (1978) has also observed a global high-amplitude, high-density alpha state brought about by a spatial-imagery meditative task and enhanced by EEG BF.

Levine (1976) developed a sophisticated method for analyzing EEG correlates of meditation-induced altered states of consciousness, which has not yet been comparatively applied to states associated with other meditative procedures and with ABT. Using this technique, Orme-Johnson, Clements, Haynes, and Badaoui (1977) found a significant correlation between the subjective experience of meditation and bilateral frontal lobe coherence. Frontal coherence in the alpha band was associated with increases or indices of creativity (ideational fluency on the Torrance Novel Uses Test), whereas frontal coherence in the theta band was associated with increased flexibility of concept formation. Interestingly, global coherence (all frequencies) increased with wakefulness and progressively decreased during sleep stages, with minimum coherence in stage 4 sleep. On the basis of these studies, we speculate that autogenic biofeedback produces the same global coherence associated with wakefulness, while inducing deep autonomic and muscular relaxation; this may provide a fruitful direction for future research.

Other cerebral changes have also been noted. Mathew et al. (1980) reported cerebral blood flow increases accompanying self-regulated hand warming. (This finding supports the Greens' original hypothesis regarding the mechanism of improvement in migraine headache activity with hand warming.) Because blood flow in the brain is correlated with increased metabolic activity, these results again substantiate the dual nature of the autogenic state—simultaneously concentrated and relaxed, creating ideal conditions for passive volition.

Recent improvements in measurement techniques, together with new paradigms encompassing expanded conceptual frameworks of human psychological functioning, are leading to new understandings of the commonalities underlying different healing and meditative states. The Greens' early observation (Hartley, 1974) that "if there is such a thing as psychosomatic illness, there must be such a thing as psychosomatic health," moves beyond the elimination of disease toward a greater actualization of human potential. Self-regulation for physical and emotional well-being etches a new image of the human being as volitional, well, and strong—self-affirmative and self-responsible.

SUMMARY AND CONCLUSION

Over three decades ago, Green, Green, and Walters (1971a) expressed the hope that

> with the resurgence of interest in self-exploration and in self-realization, it will be possible to develop a synthesis of old and new, East and West, pre-science and science, using both yoga and biofeedback training tools for the study of consciousness. . . . Much remains to be researched, and tried in application, but there is little doubt that in the lives of many people a penetration of consciousness into previously unconscious realms (of mind and brain) is making understandable and functional much that was previously obscure and inoperable. (p. 8)

The fusion and syntheses of concepts and techniques that derive from the diversity of different professional fields, countries, languages, and culture continues, all for the good of the clients and patients who need whatever treatment is available to them. At a practical level, many people have already begun to experience the healing and personally integrative consequences of unifying mind and body.

Although over a decade has passed since the second edition of this book, the basic etiology of ABT has not changed. So, as the reader can see, this chapter on ABT is mostly an exact replication of the original chapter as explicitly worded and organized by Norris and Fahrion in the previous edition. Oikawa's attempt in this edition was to update the contents merely by adding new references accumulated during the past decade. As mentioned before, although the etiology of ABT is the same, not all practitioners have used the same words (e.g., autogenic biofeedback) to describe the practice, and we were not able to extract and respect all the references that merit mentioning here. At this time, for that reason, we have not tried to evaluate and compare the extensive references mentioned in this chapter.

REFERENCES

Akagi, M., Yoshimura, M., & Ikemi, Y. (1977). A clinical study of the treatment of writer's cramp by biofeedback training. *Behavioral Engineering, 4,* 45–50.

Banquet, J. P. (1973). Spectral analysis of the EEG in meditation. *Electroencephalography and Clinical Neurophysiology, 35,* 143–151.

Barowsky, E. (1990). The use of biofeedback in the treatment of disorders of childhood. *Annals of the New York Academy of Sciences, 602,* 221–233.

Benson, H., Beary, J. F., & Carol, M. P. (1974). The relaxation response. *Psychiatry, 37*, 37–46.

Billings, R. F., Thomas, M. R., Rapp, M. S., Reyes, E., & Leith, M. (1984). Differential efficacy of biofeedback in headache. *Headache, 24*, 211–215.

Blanchard, E. B. (1979). The use of temperature biofeedback in the treatment of chronic pain due to causalgia. *Biofeedback and Self-Regulation, 4*, 183–188.

Blanchard, E. B., Andrasik, F., Evans, D. D., Ness, D. F., Appelbaum, K. A., & Rodichok, L. D. (1985). Behavioral treatment of 250 chronic headache patients: A clinical replication series. *Behavior Therapy, 16*, 308–327.

Blanchard, E. B., Radnitz, C., Schwarz, S. P., Neff, D. F., & Gerardi, M. A. (1987). Psychological changes associated with self-regulatory treatments of irritable bowel syndrome. *Biofeedback and Self-Regulation, 12*, 31–37.

Blanchard, E. B., & Schwarz, S. P. (1987). Adaptation of a multicomponent treatment for irritable bowel syndrome to a small group format. *Biofeedback and Self-Regulation, 12*, 63–69.

Blumenstein, B., Bar-Eli, M., & Tenenbaum, G. (1995). The augmenting role of biofeedback: Effects of autogenic, imagery and music training on physiological indices and athletic performance. *Journal of Sports Science, 13*(4), 343–354.

Boller, J. D., & Flom, R. P. (1979). Treatment of the common migraine: Systematic application of biofeedback and autogenic training. *American Journal of Clinical Biofeedback, 2*, 63–64.

Bostem, F., & Degossely, M. (1978). Spectral analysis of alpha rhythm during Schultz's autogenic training: A tentative approach to rapid visualization. *Electroencephalography and Clinical Neurophysiology, 34*(Suppl.), 181–190.

Brady, J. (1958). The paleocortex and behavioral motivation. In H. Harlow & C. N. Woolsey (Eds.), *The biological and biochemical bases of behavior.* Madison: University of Wisconsin Press.

Brody, C., Davison, E. T., & Brody, J. (1985). Self-regulation of a complex ventricular arrhythmia. *Psychosomatics, 26*, 754–756.

Brown, B. (1978). Critique of biofeedback concepts and methodologies. *American Journal of Clinical Biofeedback, 1*, 10–14.

Budzynski, T. H., Stoyva, J. M., & Adler, C. S. (1970). Feedback-induced muscle relaxation: Application to tension headache. *Journal of Behavior Therapy and Experimental Psychiatry, 1*, 205–211.

Chapman, S. L. (1986). A review and clinical perspective on the use of EMG and thermal biofeedback for chronic headaches. *Pain, 27*, 1–43.

Cowings, P. S., Kellar, M. A., Folen, R. A., Toscano, W. B., & Burge, J. D. (2001). Autogenic feedback training exercise and pilot performance: enhanced functioning under search-and-rescue flying conditions. *International Journal of Aviation Psychology, 11*, 303–315.

Cowings, P. S., & Toscanow, B. (2000). Autogenic-feedback training exercise is superior to promethazine for control of motion sickness symptoms. *Journal of Clinical Pharmacology, 40*, 1154–1165

Cowings, P. S., Toscano, W. B., Miller, N. E., Pickering, T. G., Shapiro, D., Stevenson, J., et al. (1994). Autogenic-feedback training: A potential treatment for orthostatic intolerance in aerospace crews. *Journal of Clinical Pharmacology, 34*, 599–608.

Cozzi, L., Tryon, W. W., & Sedlacek, K. (1987). The effectiveness of biofeedback assisted relaxation in modifying sickle cell crises. *Biofeedback and Self-Regulation, 12*, 51–61.

Daly, E. J., Donn, P. A., Galliher, M. J., & Zimmerman, J. S. (1983). Biofeedback applications of migraine and tension headaches: A double-blinded outcome study. *Biofeedback and Self-Regulation, 8*, 135–152.

Degossely, M., & Bostem, F. (1977). Autogenic training and states of consciousness: A few methodological problems. In W. Luthe & F. Antonelli (Eds.), *Proceedings of the 3rd World Congress, ICPM* (Vol. 4). Rome: Pozzi.

Dietvorst, T. F., & Osborne, D. (1978). Biofeedback-assisted relaxation training for primary dysmenorrhea: A case study. *Biofeedback and Self-Regulation, 3*, 301–305.

Dobie, T. G., May, J. G., Fischer, W. D., Elder, S. T., & Kubitz, K. A. (1987). A comparison of two methods of training resistance to visually induced motion sickness. *Aviation, Space, and Environmental Medicine, 58*, A34–A41.

Dobzhansky, T. (1951). *Genetics and the origin of species* (3rd ed.). New York: Columbia University Press.

Eliot, R. S. (1988). *Stress and the heart: Mechanisms, measurements and management.* Mount Kisco, NY: Futura.

Engelhardt, L. J. (1976, March). *The application of biofeedback techniques within a public school setting*. Paper presented at the annual meeting of the Biofeedback Society of America, Colorado Springs, CO.

Fahrion, S. L. (1977). Autogenic biofeedback for migraine. *Mayo Clinic Proceedings, 52*, 776–784.

Fahrion, S. L. (1991). Hypertension and biofeedback. *Primary Care, 18*, 663–682.

Fahrion, S. L., Walters, E. D., Coyne, L., & Allen, T. R. (1992). Alterations in EEG amplitude, personality factors and brain electrical mapping after alpha–theta brainwave training: A controlled case study of an alcoholic in recovery. *Alcoholism: Clinical and Experimental Research, 16*, 547–552.

Fehmi, L. (1978). EEG biofeedback, multi-channel synchrony training and attention. In A. A. Sugarman & R. E. Tarter (Eds.), *Expanding dimensions of consciousness*. New York: Springer.

Fischer, R. (1978–1979). Healing as a state of consciousness: Cartography of the passive concentration stage of autogenic training. *Journal of Altered States of Consciousness, 4*, 57–61.

Frank, J. (1971). Therapeutic factors in psychotherapy. *American Journal of Psychotherapy, 25*, 351–361.

Freedman, R. R. (1987). Long-term effectiveness of behavioral treatments for Raynaud's disease. *Behavior Therapy, 18*, 387–399.

Freedman, R. R. (1991). Physiological mechanisms of temperature biofeedback. *Biofeedback and Self-Regulation, 16*, 95–115.

French, D., Leeb, C. S., & Fahrion, S. L. (1975, March). *Biofeedback hand temperature training in the mentally retarded*. Paper presented at the annual meeting of the Biofeedback Society of America, Monterey, CA.

Gottschalk, L. A. (1978). Content analysis of speech in psychiatric research. *Comprehensive Psychiatry, 19*, 387–392.

Gottschalk, L. A. (1986). An objective method of measuring psychological states associated with changes in neural function: Content analysis of verbal behavior. In L. A. Gottschalk (Ed.), *Content analysis of verbal behavior*. New York: Springer-Verlag.

Green, A. M., & Green, E. E. (1975). Biofeedback: Research and therapy. In N. O. Jacobsen (Ed.), *New ways to health*. Stockholm: Naturock Kultur.

Green, E. E., Ferguson, D. W., Green, A. M., & Walters, E. D. (1970). *Preliminary report on the Voluntary Controls Program: Swami Rama* [Mimeograph]. Topeka, KS: Voluntary Controls Project, The Menninger Foundation.

Green, E. E., & Green, A. M. (1973, Winter). Regulating our mind–body processes. *Fields within Fields . . . within Fields*, pp. 16–24.

Green, E. E., & Green, A. M. (1977). *Beyond biofeedback*. New York: Delacorte Press.

Green, E. E., Green, A. M., & Norris, P. A. (1979). Preliminary observations on a new non-drug method for control of hypertension. *Journal of the South Carolina Medical Association, 75*, 575–586.

Green, E. E., Green, A. M., & Walters, E. D. (1970a, June). *Psychophysiological training for inner awareness*. Paper presented at the conference of the Association for Humanistic Psychology, Miami.

Green, E. E., Green, A. M., & Walters, E. D. (1970b). Voluntary control of internal states: Psychological and physiological. *Journal of Transpersonal Psychology, 2*, 1–26.

Green, E. E., Green, A. M., & Walters, E. D. (1971a, October). *Biofeedback for mind–body self-regulation: Healing and creativity*. Paper presented at the symposium "The Varieties of Healing Experience," De Anza College, Cupertino, CA.

Green, E. E., Green, A. M., & Walters, E. D. (1971b, September). *Psychophysiological training for creativity*. Paper presented at the meeting of the American Psychological Association, Washington, DC.

Green, E. E., Green, A. M., & Walters, E. D. (1973). Biofeedback training for anxiety tension reduction. *Annals of the New York Academy of Sciences, 233*, 157–161.

Green, E. E., Green, A. M., Walters, E. D., Sargent, J. D., & Meyer, R. G. (1975). Autogenic feedback training. *Psychotherapy and Psychosomatics, 25*, 88–98.

Green, E. E., Walters, E. D., Green, A. M., & Murphy, G. (1969). Feedback technique for deep relaxation. *Psychophysiology, 6*, 371–377.

Guarnieri, P., & Blanchard, E. B. (1990). Evaluation of home based thermal biofeedback treatment of pediatric migraine headache. *Biofeedback and Self-Regulation, 15*, 179–184.

Hartley, E. (1974). *Biofeedback: Yoga of the west* [Film]. Cos Cob, CT: Hartley Film Foundation.

Hartley, E. (1981). *Hypertension: The mind–body connection* [Film]. Cos Cob, CT: Hartley Film Foundation.

Hartman, C. H. (1979). Response of anginal pain to hand warming. *Biofeedback and Self-Regulation, 4,* 355–357.

Heath, R. G., & Becker, H. C. (1954). *Studies in schizophrenia.* Cambridge, MA: Harvard University Press.

Hohne, F., & Bohn, M. (1988). Biofeedback without a technical team—simple and cost effective. *Psychiatrie, Neurologie, und Medizinische Psychologie, Leipzig, 40,* 421–425.

Ikemi Y (1979). Eastern and Western approaches to self-regulation: Similarities and differences. *Canadian Journal of Psychiatry, 24,* 471–480.

Ikemi, Y., & Aoki, H. (1976). Comprehensive psychosomatic training for internists (at university level). *Dynamische Psychiatrie, 9,* 287–299.

Ikemi, Y., Nakagawa, T., Suematsu, H., & Luthe, W. (1975). The biologic wisdom of self-regulatory mechanism of normalization of autogenic and Oriental approaches to psychotherapy. *Psychotherapy and Psychosomatics, 25,* 99–108.

Ishikawa, H., & Robinson, A. (1981). Biofeedback and behavioral approaches in Japan. *Psychotherapy and Psychosomatics, 36,* 246–260.

Jozsvai, E. E., & Pigeau, R. A. (1995). The effect of autogenic training and biofeedback on motion sickness tolerance. *Aviation, Space, and Environmental Medicine, 66,* 631–634.

Kamiya, J. (1968, November). Conscious control of brain waves. *Psychology Today,* pp. 55–60.

Karasu, T. B. (1977). Psychotherapies: An overview. *American Journal of Psychiatry, 134,* 851–863.

Keefe, F. J., Surwit, R. S., & Pilon, R. N. (1981). Collagen vascular disease: Can behavioral therapy help? *Journal of Behavior Therapy and Experimental Psychiatry, 12,* 171–175.

Kirsch, C. A., Blanchard, E. B., & Parnes, S. M. (1987). A multiple baseline evaluation of the treatment of subjective tinnitus with relaxation training and biofeedback. *Biofeedback and Self-Regulation, 12,* 295–312.

Labbe, E. E. (1995). Treatment of childhood migraine with autogenic training and skin temperature biofeedback: A component analysis. *Headache, 35,* 10–13.

Leeb, C., Fahrion, S., & French, D. (1976). Instructional set, deep relaxation and growth enhancement: A pilot study. *Journal of Humanistic Psychology, 16,* 71–78.

Lehrer, P. M., Atthowe, J. M., & Weber, E. S. P. (1980). Effects of progressive relaxation and autogenic training on anxiety and physiological measures, with some data on hypnotizability. In F. J. McGuigan, W. E. Sime, & J. M. Wallace (Eds.), *Stress and tension control.* New York: Plenum Press.

Levine, P. H. (1976). The coherence spectral array (COSPAR) and its application to the study of spatial ordering in the EEG. *Proceedings of the San Diego Biomedical Symposium, 15,* 237–247.

Luthe, W. (1965). *Autogenic training.* New York: Grune & Stratton.

Lynch, J. J., Thomas, S. A., Paskewitz, D. A., Malinow, K. L., & Long, J. M. (1982). Interpersonal aspects of blood pressure control. *Journal of Nervous and Mental Disease, 170,* 143–153.

MacLean, P. D. (1955). The limbic system ("visceral brain") in relation to central gray and reticulum of brain stem. *Psychosomatic Medicine, 17,* 355–356.

Mathew, R. J., Largen, J. W., Dobbins, K., Meyer, J. S., Sakai, F., & Claghorn, J. L. (1980). Biofeedback control of skin temperature and cerebral blood flow in migraine. *Headache, 20,* 19–28.

McGrady, A. V., Yonker, R., Tan, S. Y., Fine, T. H., & Woerner, M. (1981). The effect of biofeedback-assisted relaxation training on blood pressure and selected biochemical parameters in patients with essential hypertension. *Biofeedback and Self-Regulation, 6,* 343–353.

Meany, J., McNamara, M., Burks, V., Berger, T. W., & Sayle, D. M. (1988). Psychological treatment of an asthmatic patient in crisis: Dreams, biofeedback, and pain behavior modification. *Journal of Asthma, 25,* 141–151.

Norris, P. A. (1976). *Working with prisoners, or, there's nobody else here* [Mimeograph]. Topeka, KS: Voluntary Controls Program, The Menninger Foundation.

Oikawa, O., Fujiki, N., Matsumoto, A., Tashiro, K., Igarashi, M., & Tsutsui, S. (1999). Combination therapy for chronic leg pain caused by arteriosclerosis obliterans (ASO): Autogenic training, EMG biofeedback and Kampo [in Japanese]. *Japanese Association of Oriental Psychosomatic Medicine, 14,* 68–75.

Orme-Johnson, D. W., Clements, G., Haynes, C. T., & Badaoui, K. (1977). Higher states of consciousness: EEG coherence, creativity, and experiences of the sidhis. In D. W. Orme-Johnson & J. T. Farrow (Eds.), *Scientific research on the transcendental meditation program: Collected papers* (Vol. 1). Rheinweiler, Germany: Maharishi European Research University Press.

Papez, J. W. (1937). A proposed mechanism of emotion. *Archives of Neurology and Psychiatry, 28,* 725–743.

Penfield, W. (1975). *The mystery of the mind: A critical study of consciousness and the human brain.* Princeton, NJ: Princeton University Press.

Peniston, E. G., & Kulkosky, P. J. (1989). Alpha–theta brainwave training and beta endorphin levels in alcoholics. *Alcoholism: Clinical and Experimental Research, 13,* 271–279.

Rouleau, J. L., Denver, D. R., Gauthier, J. G., & Biedermann, H. (1985). Le biofeedback électromyographique dans le traitement de la fibrosité: Evaluation d'une approche thérapeutique [Electromyographic biofeedback in the treatment of fibrositis: Evaluation of a therapeutic approach]. *Revue de Modification du Comportement, 15,* 7–19.

Sargent, J. D., Green, E. E., & Walters, E. D. (1972). The use of autogenic feedback in a pilot study of migraine and tension headaches. *Headache, 12,* 120–125.

Schultz, J. H., & Luthe, W. (1969). *Autogenic therapy: Vol. 1. Autogenic methods.* New York: Grune & Stratton.

Schwarz, S. P., Taylor, A. E., Scharff, L., & Blanchard, E. B. (1990). Behaviorally treated irritable bowel syndrome patients: A four-year follow-up. *Behaviour Research and Therapy, 28,* 331–335.

Sedlacek, K. (1979). Comparison between biofeedback and relaxation response in the treatment of hypertension. *Biofeedback and Self-Regulation, 4,* 259.

Sharp, C., Hurford, D. P., Allison, J., Sparks, R., & Cameron, B. P. (1997). Facilitation of internal locus of control in adolescent alcoholics through a brief biofeedback-assisted autogenic relaxation training procedure. *Journal of Substance Abuse Treatment, 14,* 55–60.

Sherman, R. A., Arena, J. G., Sherman, C. J., & Ernst, J. L. (1989). The mystery of phantom pain: Growing evidence for psychophysiological mechanisms. *Biofeedback and Self-Regulation, 14,* 267–280.

Shulimson, A. D., Lawrence, P. F., & Iacono, C. U. (1986). Diabetic ulcers: The effect of thermal biofeedback mediated relaxation training on healing. *Biofeedback and Self-Regulation, 11,* 311–319.

Smirnov, S. A., Aizikov, G. S., & Kozlovskaia, I. B. (1988). Effect of adaptive biofeedback on the severity of vestibulo-autonomic symptoms of experimental motion sickness. *Kosmicheskaya Biologiya i Aviakosmicheskaya Meditsina, 22,* 35–39.

Sun, Z., Zhao, J., Xia, M., Ren, R., Yan, H., Yang, L., et al. (1986). Comparative study on the efficiency of EMG and thermal biofeedback training and the combination of biofeedback and autogenic training in reducing test anxiety. *Acta Psychologica Sinica, 18,* 196–202.

Taub, E., & Stroebel, C. F. (1978). Biofeedback in treatment of vasoconstrictive syndromes. *Biofeedback and Self-Regulation, 3,* 363–373.

Toscano, W. B., & Cowings, P. S. (1982). Reducing motion sickness; a comparison of autogenic-feedback training and an alternative cognitive task. *Aviation, Space, and Environmental Medicine, 53,* 449–453.

Tsushima, W. T. (1982). Treatment of phantom limb pain with EMG and temperature biofeedback: A case study. *American Journal of Clinical Biofeedback, 5,* 150–153.

Walton, W. T. (1979). The use of a relaxation curriculum and biofeedback training in the classroom to reduce inappropriate behaviors of emotionally handicapped children. *Behavioral Disorders, 5,* 10–18.

Yamazaki, C., Hoshino, N., Ito, C., Matsuo, T., & Katsura, T. (1985). Nursing of a patient with chronic lumbar pain: Success with autogenic training combined with biofeedback [in Japanese]. *Kango Gijutsu, 31,* 628–634.

Zaichkowsky, L. D., & Fuchs, C. Z. (1988). Biofeedback applications in exercise and athletic performance. *Exercise and Sports Sciences Reviews, 16,* 381–421.

Biofeedback

CHAPTER 9

Psychophysiological Perspectives on Stress-Related and Anxiety Disorders

RICHARD N. GEVIRTZ

THEORETICAL FOUNDATIONS AND BACKGROUND

It is becoming increasingly accepted that individuals with so-called stress-related disorders represent a significant proportion of patients seeking medical care, that treating these patients is expensive and difficult, and that they are not generally satisfied with traditional Western medical care (Andrade, Walters, Gentil, & Laurenti, 2002; Cassidy et al., 2004; Cummings & VandenBos, 1981; Issakidis & Andrews, 2003; Katon, Von Korff, & Lin, 1992; Sharpe & Carson, 2001; Yates, 1984). Furthermore, many population studies have identified large numbers of these patients (including those with anxiety disorders) who have not sought, or have given up on, medical care (Drossman et al., 1999; Katon, 1996; Katon, Hart, & Montano, 1997)

This chapter lays out a heuristic model that integrates psychophysiological measures and biofeedback into a framework that may be useful in assessment and treatment planning. This approach is in sharp contrast to more psychodynamic models that assume that emotional factors operate through some central process to create symptom perceptions where no pathophysiology actually exists. Rather, "functional" symptoms are conceptualized as representing changes in physiology such that the symptoms are "real," that is, not "all in one's head." This approach has several advantages:

1. It is not in the least pejorative so as to be stigmatizing. As with any medical symptom, symptoms are presented in a scientific causal pathway with as neutral a value valence as possible. Thus patients can go public with their new "diagnosis" without shame or concealment.
2. It appears to produce symptom reduction over long-term follow-ups (DeGuire, Gevirtz, Hawkinson, & Dixon, 1996; DeGuire, Gevirtz, Kawahara, & Maguire, 1992; Humphreys & Gevirtz, 2000; Ryan, 2001; Sharpe & Carson, 2001).
3. It can be incorporated into medical settings, corporate stress management settings, or mental health settings with only small adjustments.

The model works by making a credible case for physiological mediators (between psychological factors and symptoms). For this reason the following sections describe a case for various autonomic, respiratory, and endocrine pathways that can be used to describe symptoms of many of these syndromes.

Potential Physiological Mediators

Four general physiological systems are candidates for most of the complaints or symptoms we encounter in this realm: the sympathetic branch of the autonomic nervous system (SNS), including the sympathetic adrenal medullary system; the parasympathetic branch of the autonomic nervous system (PNS); the respiratory system; and the hypothalamic–pituitary–adrenal system (HPA). Each has been described in many places (see Chapter 2, this volume; Gevirtz & Schwartz, 2003; Guyton & Hall, 1995), so I highlight only features that are often overlooked.

The perspective I am advocating involves first assessing the nature of the stress-related complaint, creating a "mediational model" based on multimodal, multimethod analyses, and thereby creating the basis for a treatment plan. To do this we must first review some physiology.

Sympathetic Branch of the Autonomic Nervous System

The SNS is a complex system, with multiple pathways synapsing on an intermediate ganglionic plexus and terminating at the target organs. Though named *sympathetic* by Cannon (1929) based on the belief that it operated as a mass action system, modern physiology has rejected this idea in favor of much more specificity (Porges, 1995a).

> With advances in experimental techniques, the early views of the sympathetic nervous system as a monolithic effector activated globally in situations requiring a rapid and aggressive response to life-threatening danger have been eclipsed by an organizational model featuring an extensive array of functionally specific output channels that can be simultaneously activated or inhibited in combinations that result in the patterns of autonomic activity supporting behavior and mediating homeostatic reflexes. With this perspective, the defense response is but one of the many activational states of the central autonomic network. (Morrison, 2001, p. 683)

From the earliest decades of the 20th century, physiologists have postulated the SNS as the primary mediator of the human stress response. "The neglect of these *(parasympathetic)* concepts and an emphasis on the global construct of *arousal* still abide within the sub-disciplines of psychology, psychiatry and physiology. This outdated view of arousal may restrict an understanding of how the autonomic nervous system interfaces with the environment and the contributions of the autonomic nervous system to psychological and behavioral processes" (Porges, 1995b, p. 302). Cannon's "fight or flight" concept (Cannon, 1929) has become a part of everyday language and has heavily influenced both medicine and psychology. This is certainly understandable, because the system seems to act to mobilize the organism for emergency situations. In everyday life, however, this mechanism becomes less clear. Most of us do not experience fight-or-flight types of challenges on an hourly or even daily basis. Rather, modern stress is more likely to stem from issues of social hierarchies, ruminative self-deprecating thoughts, general anxiety, worry, or boredom. Indeed, stress management training with firefighters or police officers almost always centers on issues of bureaucracy, paperwork, relationships, and so forth, not on the dangers of the job. Thus clients with stress-related symptoms cannot usually identify stressors that most would characterize as fight-or-flight triggers unless we move to meta-phorical models. This would seem to present a problem for models that postulate stress as primarily an SNS phenomenon.

Those readers familiar with clinical psychophysiological measurement know all too well that supposed indicators of SNS arousal (increased heart rate [HR], skin conductance [SC], and cooler fingertips) rarely cooperate in the clinic and work as a team. Rather, every combination of pattern is seen. This is in contrast to situations that do produce a dramatic response, such as parachuting out of a plane for the first time (Biondi & Picardi, 1999).

Nevertheless, subtler SNS pathways are undoubtedly involved in many disorders. These pathways may be unique to a specific organ system, but nonetheless they are potential mediators of symptoms when maintained for longer periods of time (as the stimuli mentioned earlier often are). For example, our group (Gevirtz, Hubbard, & Harpin, 1996; Hubbard, 1996, 1998; Hubbard & Berkoff, 1993; McNulty, Gevirtz, Hubbard, & Berkoff, 1994) has shown that nodules in muscles called *trigger points*, are (alpha) sympathetically mediated and are responsive to very mild stressors, such as worry, performance anxiety, and so forth. This is true even when SC or HR responses show only very subtle changes to the same stimuli. Similarly, a number of researchers (Adeyemi, Desai, Towsey, & Ghista, 1999; Waring, Chui, Japp, Nicol, & Ford, 2004) have shown that a high low-frequency (LF)–high-frequency (HF) ratio (thought to reflect SNS influence), calculated from sequential R–R intervals of the EKG, characterizes many patients with irritable bowel syndrome (IBS), a stress-related gastrointestinal disorder. Again, this finding is often not accompanied by other SNS indicators. As another example, Martinez-Lavin (Martinez-Lavin, 2001a, 2001b; Martinez-Lavin & Hermosillo, 2000; Martinez-Lavin et al., 1997; Martinez-Lavin, Hermosillo, Rosas, & Soto, 1998) has presented data that characterize fibromyalgia as at least partly stemming from SNS dominance.

Thus, despite the added complexity in the model, the SNS remains a key candidate for mediation of symptoms.

Parasympathetic Branch of the Autonomic Nervous System

Because the SNS has not been sufficient to explain many stress complaints, some physiologists have turned their attention to the PNS (Porges, 1995a, 1995b, 1997), and especially the 10th cranial nerve, the vagus nerve. The vagus presents a *yang* to the *yin* of the SNS for most target organs. The SNS accelerates the heart and increases stroke volume, while the PNS brakes the heart. The SNS bronchodilates, the vagus bronchoconstricts. Although this antagonistic relationship is roughly correct, in actuality the interactions between the systems are quite complex and nonlinear (Cacioppo, Uchino, & Berntson, 1994). For our purposes, however, it is useful to conceive of the vagus system as a brake that withdraws when the organism is in any situation that might call for increased attention, defensiveness, premobilization, and so forth. From an evolutionary point of view, it would make sense that the self-maintaining functions of the PNS be "put on hold" at the hint of danger.

Fluctuations in heart rate or interbeat interval (IBI) with inspiration and expiration often are used as an index of cardiovagal activity (see Lehrer, Chapter 10, this volume). The fluctuations can be divided into three clusters: (1) high frequency (HF), based on oscillations between 0.15 Hz and 0.4 Hz (almost totally produced by parasympathetic efferents), (2) low frequency (LF), reflecting baroreceptor feedback to the sinoatrial node based on blood pressure fluctuations (reflecting both sympathetic and parasympathetic pathways), and (3) very low frequency (VLF), probably reflecting vascular or temperature rhythms (Task Force of the European Society of Cardiology and the North American Society of Pacing and Electrophysiology, 1996; Pagani & Malliani, 2000). In this way, vagal withdrawal can be observed. Especially when prolonged, vagal withdrawal could be an active component of the mediation between symptoms and emotional factors.

Porges, nicely summarized by McEwen (2002), has written extensively about this topic and proposes a theory called the polyvagal theory, based on an evolutionary perspective. It proposes that for everyday human interactions, the PNS control of the ANS is dominant and regulates complex human interpersonal emotions (McEwen, 2002). Porges has labeled this the *vagal social engagement system*. If valid, this theory would have major consequences for stress management. The theory posits that humans have evolved to have three neural circuits involving the autonomic nervous system: immobilization, mobilization, and social communication/engagement. This last system involves mylenated vagal fibers originating in the nucleus ambiguous of the brainstem that control facial expressions, vocalizations, and listening. This system evolved to enable social bonding and attachment to be the foundation of effective human functioning. He believes, for example, that autism illustrates the limits of human function without this developmental stage.

Others (Grossman & Kollai, 1993) have criticized this perspective and have argued that "vagal tone" is a more complex phenomenon, only partially represented by respiratory sinus arrhythmia (RSA). However, researchers on both sides of the issue would agree that the PNS plays a crucial role in stress and stress management.

The implications are that by conceptualizing "stress" as primarily a vagal withdrawal phenomenon, we will shift our interventions and treatment models dramatically. For some disorders (i.e., IBS or recurrent abdominal pain [RAP]), this may provide a powerful tool for intervention in and of itself.

Respiratory Parameters as Potential Mediators

Another physiological system that has the potential to mediate stress-related symptoms is the respiratory system—more accurately, the acid-base regulation that occurs during relaxed breathing. This topic is covered extensively elsewhere (Chaitow, Bradley, & Gilbert, 2002; Fried, 1987; Fried, Fox, & Carlton, 1990; Gevirtz & Schwartz, 2003), but here we can note that subtle versions (e.g., sighing) of hyperventilation (producing more tidal flow than necessary to preserve the acid-base balance) can produce symptoms that are often characterized as stress related (i.e., dizziness, palpitations, dyspnea, panic, chest pain, anxiety, etc.). Therefore, in our search for links between "mind and body," respiration is often a very good place to start. To do this one must carefully observe breathing patterns, measure end-tidal carbon dioxide ($ETCO_2$), and note symptom clusters (Nijmegen test). No one measure is sufficient, but Nijmegen scores above 22, $ETCO_2$ below 32 mm HG, rapid respiration, and thoracic breathing, in combination, indicate that respiratory-based alkalosis is a prime candidate for symptoms such as those listed previously (Dixhoorn & Duivenvoorden, 1985). For some symptoms, simply correcting the overbreathing is quite effective (DeGuire et al., 1996; DeGuire et al., 1992). More often, respiratory factors play a contributory role, along with other mediational systems.

HPA Axis and the Sympathetic Adrenal Catacholamine System

Another potential pathway for mediation of psychological factors to physical states is based on endocrine responses to stress. The HPA axis functions as a systemic energy producer and anti-inflammatory system. When a stressor is detected by cortical and limbic brain systems, the hypothalamus can stimulate the pituitary to secrete adreno-corticotropic hormone (ACTH), which is picked up by adrenal receptor sites. The adrenal gland then secretes cortisol and other chemicals that produce effects in the brain and throughout the body. This is a relatively slow response, but it can have devastating effects if prolonged (McEwen, 2002). Similarly, the SNS stimulates the adrenal medulla to secrete epinephrine and norepinephrine (together called *catecholamines*), which reinforce SNS activation, especially to the cardiovascular system. Measurement of these "stress hormones" is commonplace in stress research. Thus these endocrine-based systems can also be considered as candidates for mediation. Modern analytic systems have brought the cost and invasiveness of these measures down, so clinicians may soon be able to use salivary cortisol (as one example) in clinical practice. Although the HPA and sympathoadrenal systems are quite complex, and although many methodological issues remain, reductions or increases in stress are usually reflected in comparable cortisol levels.

The preceding sections are meant to convey highlights of the current knowledge of autonomic, respiratory, and endocrine systems as they might apply to stress. This is, of course, a cursory description, and the reader is urged to seek other sources to expand his or her knowledge base. For the standard biofeedback modalities, an excellent source is Schwartz and Andrasik (2003). McEwen's (2002) book on stress is intended for the educated lay public but contains accurate and up-to-date material.

TREATMENT MANUAL

Based on the preceding I now present a biofeedback-based stress management manual. The model is based on a number of basic principles. This particular model is especially relevant to disorders that carry a stigma as being "psychosomatic," "somatoform," "neurotic," or "hysterical"—such as irritable bowel syndrome; many anxiety disorders, but especially panic and generalized anxiety disorder; chronic pain without obvious pathology; and similar complaints.

Before the Client Comes: The Trojan Horse Principle

The Trojan horse principle (Wickramasekera, 1994, 1995; Wickramasekera & Price, 1997) is based on the famous Greek myth related by Homer in *The Iliad*, in which the Greeks offered a hollow giant horse statue to Troy but filled it with invading troops. Here the Trojan horse is biofeedback, which appears to carry very little stigma or association with mental health procedures. When the clinician gives the client referral sources that emphasize the biomedical nature of the treatment, the client is less likely to think that the clinician believes the complaint is "all in my head." Thus the first principle is "medicalize, don't mentalize." Start treatment with a model that is as medical as possible and work slowly up to psychological or emotional factors over time.

Session 1: Symptoms

Take an elaborate oral history of symptoms, making sure to cover the *what*, *when*, *where*, and *how* of the complaint. Repeat back the history from your notes to obtain confirmation of accuracy. For example, if the complaint was headache, you would write a detailed description of the time course, the changes in severity, the precipitants, the attempts at self-treatment, and so forth. Symptom checklists can be used, but a face-to-face history is preferable. The Nijmegen Scale can be filled out with the client to clarify hyperventilation (HV) problems. The purpose of this procedure is twofold: to emphasize the legitimate nature of the symptoms and to begin building the mediational model, as described subsequently.

Session 2: Psychophysiological Stress Profile

After a clear picture of the symptoms is completed (including any questionnaires such as the Nijmegen), the clinician completes a psychophysiological stress profile (PSP). This procedure utilizes as many of the following modalities as possible: forehead EMG, skin conductance, respiration pattern and rate, $ETCO_2$, heart rate (EKG if possible), heart rate variability measures (see Lehrer, Chapter 10, this volume), pulse amplitude, and finger temperature. A simple model involves a 5-minute baseline, a mental arithmetic stressor, and a recovery period (2–5 minutes). Longer baselines are desirable, but often impractical. Additional stressors are often added, such as personally relevant images. Information obtained from the PSP should be fed back to the client as the beginning of the explanation for the mediational model.

Psychological or Environmental Factors

Finally, the clinician should attempt to assess environmental or ecological factors that might be contributing to the complaint. This should be done as casually as possible so as to keep the medical focus. It can be done by asking questions about the home and work environment, about any unusual recent events, and so forth. It is critical to be listening for hints as to where the critical path will be.

At this juncture, a preliminary mediational model is constructed. Figure 9.1 shows a generic version of a model. As can be seen, the model shows how physical symptoms develop from physiological mediators and psychological and/or emotional factors. The "hysteria" pathway should be saved for frank hypochondriasis or symptom phobia. For most problems, the other paths should be descriptive.

Some Common Configurations

A wide variety of combinations of physiological profiles exists. I now present some common themes that might appear. However, one must be prepared to individualize the profile for each client.

PNS Dominance I: An Exaggerated Freeze Response

In this extreme configuration, the behavior and physiology is consistent with an organism's exhibiting a shut-down or immobilization response. The behavior is withdrawal or lack of engagement, facial rigidity, and unexpressive voice production. The physiology is

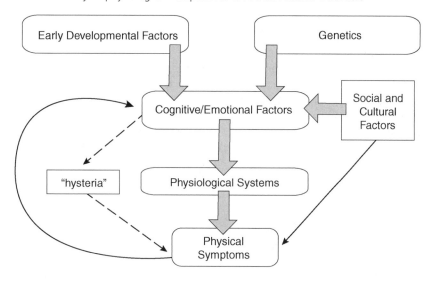

FIGURE 9.1. Mediational model of psychophysiological disorders.

characterized by high, flat heart-rate patterns consistent with the unmyelinated vagus taking over. This may occur without significant SNS involvement. Treatment strategies are complex and should build on the empirical work in trauma (Foa, 2000; Foa, Johnson, Feeny, & Treadwell, 2001; Foa & Meadows, 1997; Foa & Street, 2001; Rosen et al., 2004).

PNS Dominance II: Parasympathetic Rebound Response

Another variation that may be harder to spot is presumed to be involved in such disorders as asthma, vasovagal reactions, and perhaps some gastrointestinal problems. It is characterized by a strong parasympathetic response after a strong sympathetic surge. It can be seen when strong RSA occurs after a stressor (presumably a sympathetic surge). Careful observation and measurement may be needed to catch this response, but in cases in which the symptoms are bronchoconstriction, fainting, or constipation, this pattern should be considered (Lehrer, Feldman, Giardino, Song, & Schmaling, 2002).

SNS Dominance

The most obvious configuration (which dominated stress physiology for decades) is one in which the SNS dominates. The organism is in a fight-or-flight mode, and thus HR is elevated, the HR spectrum is solely in the low-frequency bands, SC is elevated, hands are cold, respiration is rapid and thoracic, some HV may be present (low $ETCO_2$), and facial muscle activity is high. During the stress, the levels are even higher, and they do not come down in recovery. The path model is obvious in that the client is in a "driven" state in which, over time, the autonomic and endocrine levels will cause a breakdown in some vulnerable organ system. You might think that this is a common configuration, but it is not. In fact we rarely see a pattern this obvious. Almost any cultivated low-arousal treatment modality should be helpful (Jacobson's progressive muscle relaxation, autogenic training, breathing retraining, EMG reduction, hand temperature increases, etc.).

PNS Dominance III: Vagal Withdrawal

Much more common is a configuration that is not nearly as obvious. Some traditional SNS pathways may be activated, but no consistent pattern exists. Instead, the profile is characterized by low HF–HR spectral data and episodes of HR that rise and become more monotonic or flat. This is important to notice, as it will greatly affect the way the clinician presents the mediational model to the client. Furthermore, it will guide the discussion toward subtler types of stress. One disorder usually presents in this way: generalized anxiety disorder (GAD). This is an anxiety disorder characterized by states of constant anxiety, inability to relax, and a general sense of dread. Several studies (Ballenger et al., 2001; Borkovec & Costello, 1993; Nutt, 2001; Nutt, Ballenger, Sheehan, & Wittchen, 2002; Thayer, Friedman, & Borkovec, 1996; Thayer, Friedman, Borkovec, Johnsen, & Molina, 2000) have shown that GAD patients have truncated vagal tone. Yet the patient and clinician usually conceive of the problem as SNS overdrive. McLeod and colleagues (McLeod, Hoehn-Saric, Porges, Kowalski, & Clark, 2000; McLeod, Hoehn-Saric, Porges, & Zimmerli, 1992) have shown that imipramine's antianxiety effect in GAD is moderated by the degree to which anticholinergic metabolites reduce cardiac vagal tone. The profile guides treatment and becomes a form of cognitive therapy in itself. Treatment strategies are discussed later.

Respiratory Configuration

Sometimes the respiratory factors are so strong that they trump the ANS–PNS profiles. This would occur when a Nijmegen is high (over 30), $ETCO_2$ is low (under 30), respiration is rapid (> 20 b/min), and the breathing pattern is predominantly thoracic. In these cases, breathing retraining or its equivalent should take precedence. This pattern can accompany many disorders and also can be secondary to severe chronic pain.

Vascular Configuration

A pattern of cold hands, fast HR, and low RSA may occur without other signs of SNS activation. Blood pressure should be checked. A pattern of low pulse amplitude may indicate vascular "clamping," with cold hands that are difficult to warm.

Mixed Configuration

Many other combinations are possible. In fact, most clients will be mixed in presentation. In these cases, the clinician should try to build a model that will be credible to the client For example, a client may present with warm hands and normal HR but with poor recovery and somewhat diminished RSA. This pattern may not present an exclusive path model, but there is sufficient patterning to justify an explanation and a treatment plan. Again, the change in attribution from vague psychological constructs to a "scientific" or medical type of explanation allows a fast start for cognitive-type therapies.

Other disorders, such as asthma and hypertension, are probably better characterized within an operant model, in which the treatment intervention aims at correcting a dysfunctional homeostatic loop but less stigma or mental focus is associated with the disorder (see Lehrer, Chapter 10, this volume). Educational materials are available on a disorder-by-disorder basis. For example, online information can easily be found for IBS (*www.ibsgroup.org*), fibromyalgia (National Fibromyalgia Association, *www.fmaware.org*), chronic fatigue syndrome (CFS), and anxiety disorders (Anxiety Disorders Association of America, *www.adaa.org*). Evidence for the psychoeducational approach can be found in the literature for brief interventions for many of the disorders listed.

Sessions 3–5: Biofeedback Training

Once the educational nature of the model is communicated and accepted by the client, intervention may begin. It is usually best to start with a psychophysiological intervention such as biofeedback. I explain that we are intervening at the path between physiology and symptoms to try and break the cycle. It is preferable to use a combination of heart-rate-variability (HRV) training (see Chapter 10, this volume), facial EMG feedback, and finger temperature as an indicator (watching for warming hands). Clients can usually master relaxing jaw, forehead, and other facial muscles fairly quickly. The rationale for this technique is based on the elaborate afferent network involved in the muscles used in emotional expression (Porges, 1995b). Clients must master voluntary relaxation of these muscles to move on to the HRV training. Lehrer (Chapter 10, this volume; Lehrer, Vaschillo, & Vaschillo, 2000) presents a complete manual for this biofeedback training. After initial mastery, the client must demonstrate a resonant peak without feedback.

Final Sessions

During subsequent sessions, work can proceed up the pathway to tackle emotional problems and dysfunctional cognitions. Most patients can benefit from five to eight sessions, depending on how quickly they master the biofeedback skills and how much cognitive-behavioral-type therapy is loaded on toward the end.

The most studied psychological intervention for most of the disorders I have mentioned is cognitive-behavioral therapy (CBT). A recent evolution and revision of CBT principles that is a very good fit with mediational models is acceptance and commitment therapy (ACT), introduced by Hayes, Strosahl, and Wilson (1999). To get to the more psychological aspects of treatment, one must first establish a credible physiological pathway and begin some training in a modality consistent with the model. For example, for GAD, once I have established that low vagal cardiac control is a likely mediator, I would initiate resonant frequency training (Gevirtz & Lehrer, 2003) with the stated purpose of restoring some vagal control. This might take five or six sessions of mostly biofeedback training, with only a hint of CBT or ACT present. As the symptoms diminish, the time is right to investigate the typical sources of irrational worry, of intolerance of uncertainty, of the usefulness of worry, and so forth. Similarly, many of the ACT strategies ("watching the parade," "deliteralizing language") are appropriate here. As another example, for chronic neck pain, the first stages would deal with elaborate psychoeducational explanations of how trigger points work, followed by resonant frequency training (RFT) and /or surface electromyography (sEMG) feedback, followed by an exploration of what environmental triggers are driving the sympathetically mediated trigger points and how to reduce the activation time to subpain threshold levels. Again CBT or ACT tools will be an obvious fit at this point.

As mentioned earlier, for some disorders, just the attribution shift and a few self-regulatory skills will be sufficient. For IBS, for example, a reformulation of brain–gut interconnection, together with RFT training and homework, often produces very rapid symptom reduction (especially when the problem is less chronic). It has been found (DeGuire et al., 1996; DeGuire et al., 1992) that eight sessions of breathing training alone greatly reduced chest pain in patients with functional cardiac pain, with continued improvement over 3 years. On the other hand, fibromyalgia will most often require more work in shifting perceptions, in establishing a shift in sympathovagal balance, in lifestyle changes (sleep, exercise, breathing, etc.) and in cognitive restructuring. Even here, however, the patients often label their treatment as "biofeedback" and tend to really value the objective physiological changes they see week to week.

INTERVENTIONS

Due to space limitations, treatment protocols for every stress-related disorder cannot be laid out here. Instead, I highlight ways in which the preceding presentations can be used for some disorders in various categories.

The model works very well for disorders that present with medical symptoms but that have a psychophysiological etiology. These are often labeled *somatoform*, or "medically unexplained," symptoms. Patients often pick up the disapproval or helplessness of medical personnel with regard to these disorders. For this reason the mediational model with an emphasis on biofeedback is often seen as a positive alternative to either traditional medical treatment (surgery or medications) or traditional psychotherapy.

Irritable Bowel Syndrome or Recurrent Abdominal Pain

Irritable bowel syndrome (IBS) is the most common gastrointestinal disorder in primary care settings. It occurs in 11–20% of the U.S. population (Drossman, 1993) and accounts for 12–19.5% of primary care visits (Longstreth & Wolde-Tsadik, 1993). It is estimated to cost over $30 billion in direct and indirect costs. In light of these numbers, a keen interest in managed care medical groups has developed in the quest to find a cost-effective way of treating these patients. Currently, most gastroenterologists accept that psychological factors such as stress play a key role in IBS. Therefore, presentation of the mediational model or of generic biofeedback is generally accepted. Within our framework, the main clinical task is to get the client to see his or her symptoms (usually abdominal pain, diarrhea, etc.) from the psychophysiological point of view. This means showing some pictures of the enteric nervous system and a simple explanation of how stress, worry, and anxiety, even at a low levels, could disrupt the way the gut processes food though the gastrointestinal track. In addition, several groups (Mayer, 1999, 2000; Mayer, Chang, & Lembo, 1998; Mayer, Derbyshire, & Naliboff, 2000; Mayer, Naliboff, & Chang, 2001; Mayer, Naliboff, Chang, & Coutinho, 2001; Naliboff, Chang, Munakata, & Mayer, 2000) have shown that this or other disruptions can lead to a growing visceral hypersensitivity. There is certainly a body of literature that supports ANS involvement in IBS and RAP (Gupta et al. 2002; Iovino et al., 1995; Waring, Chui, Japp, Nicol, & Ford, 2004; Jepson & Gevirtz, 2001). In some recent work of ours (Jepson & Gervitz, 2001) and Naliboff (2006), it is looking as if the physiological mediator might be prolonged vagal or parasympathetic withdrawal rather than excessive sympathetic drive. This type of information is used to convince the patient that his or her very physical symptoms could be related to long-term psychological states. Once that re-attribution is made, the interventions follow naturally.

Psychophysiological Interventions

Biofeedback-based relaxation training, HRV biofeedback, mindfulness meditation, and other techniques all make sense within this context. I prefer the HRV biofeedback (see Chapter 10, this volume) because it works to strengthen the autonomic reflexes that may be broken down with long-term stress or worry. The client is instructed to practice at least 10 minutes per day and to use the technique to interrupt prolonged rumination, anxiety, or worry. With children, have found that this intervention alone is usually sufficient to break the cycle of pain, stress, worry, more pain, and so forth. We presume, but have not yet shown, that the HRV practice restores enough vagal regulation to raise the threshold for abdominal pain.

CBT-Type Interventions

CBT, dialectical behavior therapy (DBT; Clarkin, Levy, Lenzenweger, & Kernberg, 2004; Linehan, 1995; Linehan, Heard, & Armstrong, 1993; Linehan et al., 1999), and ACT (Hayes, 2005; Hayes et al., 1999) are all applicable to IBS. In this case, though, the mediational model creates a nonthreatening and plausible lead-in to the modification of thoughts, attitudes, values, or emotions. Once a client sees that prolonged emotional states are contributing to the symptoms, it is not hard to motivate him or her to consider a cognitive-type intervention.

Case Example

James was a 38-year-old professional in a technical field. He had a PhD in computer sciences and was a linear thinker. He came to treatment with abdominal pain of moderate to severe intensity after exhausting a wide variety of traditional medical paths (in this field, one is sometimes tempted to put up a "Next Stop, Lourdes" sign on the door). He was skeptical about this "psychological stuff"and denied any unusual stress. His stress profile was unremarkable except that his RSA (peak valley HR differences during ordinary breathing in the range of 12–20 breaths per minute and during 6 breaths per–minute breathing) was low (4 beats/minute) for his age, and he had a prolonged peak in the VLF range of the HRV spectral analyses (see Chapter 10, this volume). I went through the results with him in great detail, showing slides of the ANS and other materials mentioned earlier. He was fascinated and asked many questions.

This case illustrates the Trojan horse approach. By medicalizing his symptoms, I removed the stigma associated with this "unexplained" condition and gave him a reasonable explanation without labeling it an anxiety disorder.

In the second session, we reviewed the hypothesis that his problems might be due to prolonged vagal withdrawal leading to gastrointestinal hyperalgesia. Again, using slides and poring over the physiological traces, he became convinced that this model made sense and began supplying information that was supportive. He was, indeed, a "worrier," spending many early mornings sleeplessly going over various concerns or plans in bed. When not distracted, he often found himself with a wandering mind and run-on thinking. Of course, his main worry was his health, so when a reasonable explanation appeared, he started feeling better immediately. We found his resonant frequency for HRV, set up a home practice schedule, had him buy an inexpensive temperature biofeedback unit as an indicator, and sent him off for 2 weeks of practice. In the next session we refined his breathing/RSA rate and focused on some ACT principles that seemed especially appropriate for his style of thinking (Hayes et al., 1999).

James reduced his symptom severity dramatically and managed to do so with few follow-up visits. At his 1-year follow-up, he was almost symptom-free, but when flares occurred, he would not catastrophize and could soon bring things back to normal. The same traits that made him quite resistant to traditional psychological interventions could be used to his advantage here. Linear thinking, suspicion of emotions, and fear of disclosing to a stranger were all easily used to help him manage his symptoms and, as a bonus, many other aspects of his life.

Fibromyalgia

Fibromyalgia (FM) may represent a somewhat different case, but a version of mediational modeling can also be used here. A case history illustrates how physiological data and biofeedback can be integrated into a mediational model.

Case Example

Beth was a 37-year-old attorney with three children and husband who was also an attorney. She had been very active in all phases of her life prior to the FM symptoms. She woke up early for a vigorous run each day before work, drove the children to soccer, water polo, and gymnastics, was active with their school and in her church, and was trying to achieve partner status in her law firm. Her husband was supportive but immersed in his own successfully emerging career. All was well until she contracted a cold that turned into a serious case of bronchitis. After a 6-week recovery, she thought she should be ready to resume her active life, but she was exhausted, in pain throughout her body, sleeping poorly, and unable to exercise at all. Again, after an exhaustive medical search, she was desperate enough to try biofeedback. In this case, the educational intervention was aimed at convincing her that her nervous system, both central and ANS, could be responsible for the symptoms, even without an occult viral infection, an autoimmune disorder, or some other "real" disease. I drew on materials from the scientific literature and tried to illustrate to her that her ANS, CNS, and perhaps enteric nervous system were operating in an idiosyncratic manner, consistent with the theories of several researchers (Martinez-Lavin, 2001a, 2001b; Martinez-Lavin, Amigo, Coindreau, & Canoso, 2000; Martinez-Lavin & Hermosillo, 2000; Martinez-Lavin et al., 1997; Martinez-Lavin et al., 1998; Moldofsky, 1993, 1994). Within these frameworks FM is seen as (1) a chronobiological disorder (Moldofsky, 1994) in which a disordered 24-hour body clock causes disturbed sleep, which in turn causes diffuse pain; (2) a CNS substance pain processing disorder (Russell, 1998, 2000) in which, due to physical or psychological trauma, the CNS gets stuck in a hyperalgesic or defensive stance with disturbance in a number of peptides and neurotransmitters; or (3) chronic sympathetic overdrive (Martinez-Lavin, 2001a, 2001b; Martinez-Lavin et al., 2000; Martinez-Lavin & Hermosillo, 2000; Martinez-Lavin et al., 1997; Martinez-Lavin et al., 1998), in which the CNS and ANS get stuck in a maladaptive high chronic level, flattening circadian rhythms, exhausting fight-or-flight mechanisms, and creating a subsequent HPA response. I used a number of graphs from the preceding material and compared them with Beth's psychophysiological profile. She, for example, had a predominant VLF wave in her HRV, a high LF/HF ratio (indicating sympathetic dominance), cold hands, and high skin conductance levels. Her HR was high for a seasoned athlete, and she was a rapid, shallow breather with slightly low $ETCO_2$. A circadian rhythm of LF/HF ratio has been shown to be flat in FM patients (Martinez-Lavin et al., 1998).

Over a few sessions, Beth became convinced that this explanation was at least reasonably correct, and she was willing to cooperate and practice the techniques and lifestyle changes that I suggested. In this case, that entailed my version of the SABRE protocol (Nixon, 1989; Nixon & Freeman, 1988):

Sleep: sleep hygiene with a detailed sleep log
Arousal: HRV biofeedback to restore autonomic reflexes and lower sympathetic arousal
Breathing: breathing retraining
Rest: activity management
Exercise: slow, gentle, graded exercise, starting with gentle yoga and slowly working up to aerobic exercise.

After 4 months of working this system, Beth was about 85% recovered and enjoying a fairly normal life. She never could return to her premorbid stressful life, but she is certainly doing much better. She recently joined a master swim class and is swimming competitively 3 days per week.

Other Stigmatized Disorders

Other disorders that could be classified in this category are chronic muscle pain, noncardiac chest pain (NCCP), GAD, and some types of panic disorder. In each case a mediational model can be created with varying degrees of empirical support. For muscle pain, our group (Gevirtz et al., 1996; Hubbard, 1996, 1998; Hubbard & Berkoff, 1993) has described a sympathetically mediated trigger point model for chronic pain. In another set of studies, DeGuire and colleagues (DeGuire et al., 1996; DeGuire et al., 1992) have shown that chronic respiratory factors such as hyperventilation may mediate symptoms of NCCP. Borkovec and Costello (1993) have postulated vagal withdrawal as a factor in GAD, and many research groups have emphasized the importance of breathing in panic disorder (Ley, 2005; Meuret, Ritz, Wilhelm, & Roth, 2005; Meuret, Wilhelm, Ritz, & Roth, 2003; Meuret, Wilhelm, & Roth, 2004; Roth, 2005; Roth, Wilhelm, & Trabert, 1998; Wilhelm, Gerlach, & Roth, 2001; Wilhelm, Gevirtz, & Roth, 2001; Wilhelm, Trabert, & Roth, 2001a, 2001b). As mentioned earlier (Ryan, 2001), an application of this model within a primary medical setting provided evidence for symptom reduction and cost savings (in FM, muscle pain, IBS, anxiety, and chest pain).

Negative Side Effects

No specific side effects have been reported from this approach. As is mentioned by Lehrer (Chapter 10, this volume), a relaxation-induced anxiety and some hyperventilation are possible during the initial stages of the cultivated low arousal or HRV training. Lehrer provides some useful ideas on how to handle these problems. Otherwise, the general approach usually provides a useful framework for the patient. If, however, the patient remains passive and skeptical, this approach is unlikely to be beneficial.

SUMMARY

This chapter has presented a heuristic model that I and my colleagues have found useful in stress management and treatment of a variety of disorders found commonly in primary care and in stress management groups. By using the physiological mediator model as a foundation, the trainer or therapist can gain acceptance from traditionally skeptical audiences, can introduce skills for specific purposes, and can transition into well-established therapies seamlessly. With some practice and knowledge of the various disorders, this method can greatly enhance the therapist's fulfillment, as well as helping patients find relief from the suffering that dominates their lives.

REFERENCES

Adeyemi, E. O., Desai, K. D., Towsey, M., & Ghista, D. (1999). Characterization of autonomic dysfunction in patients with irritable bowel syndrome by means of heart rate variability studies. *American Journal of Gastroenterology, 94*(3), 816–823.

Andrade, L., Walters, E. E., Gentil, V., & Laurenti, R. (2002). Prevalence of ICD-10 mental disorders in a catchment area in the city of Sao Paulo, Brazil. *Social Psychiatry and Psychiatric Epidemiology, 37*(7), 316–325.

Ballenger, J. C., Davidson, J. R., Lecrubier, Y., Nutt, D. J., Borkovec, T. D., Rickels, K., et al. (2001). Consensus statement on generalized anxiety disorder from the International Consensus Group on Depression and Anxiety. *Journal of Clinical Psychiatry, 62(Suppl. 11),* 53–58.

Biondi, M., & Picardi, A. (1999). Psychological stress and neuroendocrine function in humans: The last two decades of research. *Psychotherapy and Psychosomatics, 68*(3), 114–150.

Borkovec, T. D., & Costello, E. (1993). Efficacy of applied relaxation and cognitive-behavioral therapy in the treatment of generalized anxiety disorder. *Journal of Consulting and Clinical Psychology, 61*(4), 611–619.

Cacioppo, J. T., Uchino, B. N., & Berntson, G. G. (1994). Individual differences in the autonomic origins of heart rate reactivity: The psychometrics of respiratory sinus arrhythmia and preejection period. *Psychophysiology, 31*(4), 412–419.

Cannon, W. B. (1929). Organization for physiological homeostasis. *Physiological Reviews, 9,* 399–431.

Cassidy, K., Kotynia-English, R., Acres, J., Flicker, L., Lautenschlager, N. T., & Almeida, O. P. (2004). Association between lifestyle factors and mental health measures among community-dwelling older women. *Australian and New Zealand Journal of Psychiatry, 38*(11–12), 940–947.

Chaitow, L., Bradley, D., & Gilbert, C. (2002). *Multidisciplinary approaches to breathing pattern disorders.* London: Churchill Livingstone.

Clarkin, J. F., Levy, K. N., Lenzenweger, M. F., & Kernberg, O. F. (2004). The Personality Disorders Institute/Borderline Personality Disorder Research Foundation randomized control trial for borderline personality disorder: Rationale, methods, and patient characteristics. *Journal of Personality Disorders, 18*(1), 52–72.

Cummings, N. A., & VandenBos, G. R. (1981). The twenty year Kaiser-Permanente experience with psychotherapy and medical utilization: Implications for national health policy and national health insurance. *Health Policy Quarterly, 1*(2), 159–175.

DeGuire, S., Gevirtz, R., Hawkinson, D., & Dixon, K. (1996). Breathing retraining: A three-year follow-up study of treatment for hyperventilation syndrome and associated functional cardiac symptoms. *Biofeedback and Self-Regulation, 21*(2), 191–198.

DeGuire, S., Gevirtz, R., Kawahara, Y., & Maguire, W. (1992). Hyperventilation syndrome and the assessment of treatment for functional cardiac symptoms. *American Journal of Cardiology, 70*(6), 673–677.

Dixhoorn, J. v., & Duivenvoorden, H. J. (1985). Efficacy of Nijmegen Questionnaire in recognition of the hyperventilation syndrome. *Journal of Psychosomatic Research, 29*(2), 199–206.

Drossman, D. A., Creed, F. H., Olden, K. W., Svedlund, J., Toner, B. B., & Whitehead, W. E. (1999). Psychosocial aspects of the functional gastrointestinal disorders. *Gut, 45*(Suppl. 2), II25–30.

Drossman, D. A., Li, Z., Andruzzi, E., Temple, R. D., Talley, N. J., Thompson, W. G., et al. (1993). U.S. householder survey of functional gastroenterological disorders: Prevalence, sociodemography, and health impact. *Digestive Disease Science, 38*(9), 1569–1580.

Foa, E. B. (2000). Psychosocial treatment of posttraumatic stress disorder. *Journal of Clinical Psychiatry, 61*(Suppl. 5), 43–48.

Foa, E. B., Johnson, K. M., Feeny, N. C., & Treadwell, K. R. (2001). The child PTSD Symptom Scale: A preliminary examination of its psychometric properties. *Journal of Clinical Child Psychology, 30*(3), 376–384.

Foa, E. B., & Meadows, E. A. (1997). Psychosocial treatments for posttraumatic stress disorder: A critical review. *Annual Review of Psychology, 48,* 449–480.

Foa, E. B., & Street, G. P. (2001). Women and traumatic events. *Journal of Clinical Psychiatry, 62*(Suppl. 17), 29–34.

Fried, R. (1987). *The hyperventilation syndrome: Research and clinical treatment.* Baltimore: Johns Hopkins University Press.

Fried, R., Fox, M., & Carlton, R. (1990). Effect of diaphragmatic respiration with end-tidal CO_2 biofeedback on respiration, EEG, and seizure frequency in idiopathic epilepsy. *Annals of the New York Academy of Sciences, 602,* 67–96.

Gevirtz, R., Hubbard, D., & Harpin, E. (1996). Psychophysiologic treatment of chronic low back pain. *Professional Psychology: Research and Practice, 27*(6), 561–566.

Gevirtz, R., & Lehrer, P. (2003). Resonant frequency heart rate biofeedback. In M. S. Schwartz & F. Andrasik (Eds.), *Biofeedback: A practitioners guide* (3rd ed.). New York: Guilford Press.

Gevirtz, R., & Schwartz, M. S. (2003). The respiratory system in applied psychophysiology. In M. S. Schwartz & F. Andrasik (Eds.), *Biofeedback: A practitioners guide* (3rd ed., pp. 212–244). New York: Guilford Press.

Grossman, P., & Kollai, M. (1993). Respiratory sinus arrhythmia, cardiac vagal tone, and respiration: Within- and between-individual relations. *Psychophysiology, 30*(5), 486–495.

Gupta, V., Sheffield, D., & Verne, B. N. (2002). Evidence for autonomic dysregulation in the irritable bowel syndrome. *Digestive Disease Science, 47*(8), 1716–1722.

Guyton, A., & Hall, J. (1995). *Textbook of medical physiology* (9th ed.). Philadelphia: Saunders.

Hayes, S. (2005). *Get out of your mind and into your life.* Oakland, CA: New Harbinger Press.

Hayes, S. C., Strosahl, K. D., & Wilson, K.G. (1999). *Acceptance and commitment therapy.* New York: Guilford Press.

Hubbard, D. (1996). Chronic and recurrent muscle pain: Pathophysiology and treatment, a review of pharmocologic studies. *Journal of Musculoskeletal Pain, 4*(1–2), 123–143.

Hubbard, D. (1998). Persistent muscular pain: Approaches to relieving trigger points. *Journal of Musculoskeletal Medicine, 15*(5), 16–26.

Hubbard, D. R., & Berkoff, G. M. (1993). Myofascial trigger points show spontaneous needle EMG activity. *Spine, 18*(13), 1803–1807.

Humphreys, P. A., & Gevirtz, R. N. (2000). Treatment of recurrent abdominal pain: Components analysis of four treatment protocols. *Journal of Pediatric Gastroenterology and Nutrition, 31*(1), 47–51.

Iovino, P., Azpiroz, F., Domingo, E., & Malagelada, J. R. (1995). The sympathetic nervous system modulates perception and reflex responses to gut. *Gastroenterology, 108*(3), 680–686.

Issakidis, C., & Andrews, G. (2003). Rationing of health care: Clinical decision making in an outpatient clinic for anxiety disorders. *Journal of Anxiety Disorders, 17*(1), 59–74.

Jepson, N., & Gervitz, R. N. (2001). Cognitive-behavioral and biofeedback group treatments for irritable bowel syndrome. *Applied Psychophysiology and Biofeedback, 26,* 237.

Katon, W. (1996). Panic disorder: Relationship to high medical utilization, unexplained physical symptoms, and medical costs. *Journal of Clinical Psychiatry, 57*(Suppl. 10), 11–18.

Katon, W., Hart, R., & Montano, B. (1997). The effect of panic disorder in the managed care setting. *Managed Care Interface, 10*(11), 88–94, 98.

Katon, W. J., Von Korff, M., & Lin, E. (1992). Panic disorder: Relationship to high medical utilization. *American Journal of Medicine, 92*(1A), 7S–11S.

Lehrer, P., Feldman, J., Giardino, N., Song, H. S., & Schmaling, K. (2002). Psychological aspects of asthma. *Journal of Consulting and Clinical Psychology, 70*(3), 691–711.

Lehrer, P. M., Vaschillo, E., & Vaschillo, B. (2000). Resonant frequency biofeedback training to increase cardiac variability: Rationale and manual for training. *Applied Psychophysiology and Biofeedback*, *25*(3), 177–191.

Ley, R. (2005). Blood, breath, fears redux, and panic attacks: Comment on Roth, Wilhelm, and Pettit (2005). *Psychological Bulletin*, *131*(2), 193–198.

Linehan, M. M. (1995). Combining pharmacotherapy with psychotherapy for substance abusers with borderline personality disorder: Strategies for enhancing compliance. *NIDA Research Monograph*, *150*, 129–142.

Linehan, M. M., Heard, H. L., & Armstrong, H. E. (1993). Naturalistic follow-up of a behavioral treatment for chronically parasuicidal borderline patients. *Archives of General Psychiatry*, *50*(12), 971–974.

Linehan, M. M., Schmidt, H., III, Dimeff, L. A., Craft, J. C., Kanter, J., & Comtois, K. A. (1999). Dialectical behavior therapy for patients with borderline personality disorder and drug dependence. *American Journal on Addictions*, *8*(4), 279–292.

Martinez-Lavin, M. (2001a). Is fibromyalgia a generalized reflex sympathetic dystrophy? *Clinical and Experimental Rheumatology*, *19*(1), 1–3.

Martinez-Lavin, M. (2001b). Overlap of fibromyalgia with other medical conditions. *Current Pain and Headache Reports*, *5*(4), 347–350.

Martinez-Lavin, M., Amigo, M. C., Coindreau, J., & Canoso, J. (2000). Fibromyalgia in Frida Kahlo's life and art. *Arthritis and Rheumatism*, *43*(3), 708–709.

Martinez-Lavin, M., & Hermosillo, A. G. (2000). Autonomic nervous system dysfunction may explain the multisystem features of fibromyalgia. *Seminars in Arthritis and Rheumatism*, *29*(4), 197–199.

Martinez-Lavin, M., Hermosillo, A. G., Mendoza, C., Ortiz, R., Cajigas, J. C., Pineda, C., et al. (1997). Orthostatic sympathetic derangement in subjects with fibromyalgia. *Journal of Rheumatology*, *24*(4), 714–718.

Martinez-Lavin, M., Hermosillo, A. G., Rosas, M., & Soto, M. E. (1998). Circadian studies of autonomic nervous balance in patients with fibromyalgia: A heart rate variability analysis. *Arthritis and Rheumatism*, *41*(11), 1966–1971.

Mayer, E. A. (1999). Emerging disease model for functional gastrointestinal disorders. *American Journal of Medicine*, *107*(5A), 12S–19S.

Mayer, E. A. (2000). Spinal and supraspinal modulation of visceral sensation. *Gut*, *47*(Suppl. 4), iv69–72.

Mayer, E. A., Chang, L., & Lembo, T. (1998). Brain-gut interactions: implications for newer therapy. *European Journal of Surgery*, *582*(Suppl.), 50–55.

Mayer, E. A., Derbyshire, S., & Naliboff, B. D. (2000). Cerebral activation in irritable bowel syndrome. *Gastroenterology*, *119*(5), 1418–1420.

Mayer, E. A., Naliboff, B. D., & Chang, L. (2001). Basic pathophysiologic mechanisms in irritable bowel syndrome. *Digestive Diseases*, *19*(3), 212–218.

Mayer, E. A., Naliboff, B. D., Chang, L., & Coutinho, S. V. (2001). Stress and the gastrointestinal tract: V. Stress and irritable bowel syndrome. *American Journal of Physiology Gastrointestinal and Liver Physiology*, *280*(4), G519–524.

McEwen, B. L. (with Lasley, E. N.). (2002). *The end of stress as we know it*. Washington, DC: Joseph Henry Press.

McLeod, D. R., Hoehn-Saric, R., Porges, S. W., Kowalski, P. A., & Clark, C. M. (2000). Therapeutic effects of imipramine are counteracted by its metabolite, desipramine, in patients with generalized anxiety disorder. *Journal of Clinical Psychopharmacology*, *20*(6), 615–621.

McLeod, D. R., Hoehn-Saric, R., Porges, S. W., & Zimmerli, W. D. (1992). Effects of alprazolam and imipramine on parasympathetic cardiac control in patients with generalized anxiety disorder. *Psychopharmacology*, *107*(4), 535–540.

McNulty, W. H., Gevirtz, R. N., Hubbard, D. R., & Berkoff, G. M. (1994). Needle electromyographic evaluation of trigger point response to a psychological stressor. *Psychophysiology*, *31*(3), 313–316.

Meuret, A. E., Ritz, T., Wilhelm, F. H., & Roth, W. T. (2005). Voluntary hyperventilation in the treatment of panic disorder: Functions of hyperventilation, their implications for breathing training, and recommendations for standardization. *Clinical Psychology Review*, *25*(3), 285–306.

Meuret, A. E., Wilhelm, F. H., Ritz, T., & Roth, W. T. (2003). Breathing training for treating panic disorder: Useful intervention or impediment? *Behavior Modification*, *27*(5), 731–754.

Meuret, A. E., Wilhelm, F. H., & Roth, W. T. (2004). Respiratory feedback for treating panic disorder. *Journal of Clinical Psychology, 60*(2), 197–207.

Moldofsky, H. (1993). Fibromyalgia, sleep disorder and chronic fatigue syndrome. *Ciba Foundation Symposium, 173*, 262–271.

Moldofsky, H. (1994). Chronobiological influences on fibromyalgia syndrome: Theoretical and therapeutic implications. *Baillieres Clinical Rheumatology, 8*(4), 801–810.

Morrison, S. F. (2001). Differential control of sympathetic outflow. *American Journal of Physiology Regulatory, Integrative, and Comparative Physiology, 281*(3), R683–698.

Naliboff, B. D., Chang, L., Munakata, J., & Mayer, E. A. (2000). Towards an integrative model of irritable bowel syndrome. *Progress in Brain Research, 122*, 413–423.

Nixon, P. G. (1989). Human functions and the heart. In D. S. A. Cribb (Ed.), *Changing ideas in health care* (pp. 31–65). Chichester, UK: Wiley.

Nixon, P. G., & Freeman, L. J. (1988). The "think test": A further technique to elicit hyperventilation. *Journal of the Royal Society of Medicine, 81*(5), 277–279.

Nutt, D. J. (2001). Neurobiological mechanisms in generalized anxiety disorder. *Journal of Clinical Psychiatry, 62*(Suppl. 11), 22–27.

Nutt, D. J., Ballenger, J. C., Sheehan, D., & Wittchen, H. U. (2002). Generalized anxiety disorder: Comorbidity, comparative biology and treatment. *International Journal of Neuropsychopharmacology, 5*(4), 315–325.

Pagani, M., & Malliani, A. (2000). Interpreting oscillations of muscle sympathetic nerve activity and heart rate variability. *Journal of Hypertension, 18*(12), 1709–1719.

Porges, S. W. (1995a). Cardiac vagal tone: A physiological index of stress. *Neuroscience and Biobehavioral Reviews, 19*(2), 225–233.

Porges, S. W. (1995b). Orienting in a defensive world: Mammalian modifications of our evolutionary heritage: A polyvagal theory. *Psychophysiology, 32*(4), 301–318.

Porges, S. W. (1997). Emotion: An evolutionary by-product of the neural regulation of the autonomic nervous system. *Annals of the New York Academy of Sciences, 807*, 62–77.

Rosen, C. S., Chow, H. C., Finney, J. F., Greenbaum, M. A., Moos, R. H., Sheikh, J. I., et al. (2004). VA practice patterns and practice guidelines for treating posttraumatic stress disorder. *Journal of Traumatic Stress, 17*(3), 213–222.

Roth, W. T. (2005). Physiological markers for anxiety: Panic disorder and phobias. *International Journal of Psychophysiology, 58*(2–3), 190–198.

Roth, W. T., Wilhelm, F. H., & Trabert, W. (1998). Autonomic instability during relaxation in panic disorder. *Psychiatry Research, 80*(2), 155–164.

Russell, I. J. (1998). Advances in fibromyalgia: Possible role for central neurochemicals. *American Journal of the Medical Sciences, 315*(6), 377–384.

Russell, I. J. (2000). Fibromyalgia syndrome. In S. Mense, D. Simons, & I. J. Russell (Eds.), *Muscle pain: Understanding its nature, diagnosis and treatment* (pp. 289–337). New York: Lippincott, Williams & Wilkins.

Ryan, M. G., & Gervirtz, R. N. (2001). *The effects of biofeedback on cost effectiveness in primary care settings.* Paper presented at the Association for Applied Psychophysiology and Biofeedback, Raleigh-Durham, North Carolina.

Schwartz, M. S., & Andrasik, F. (Eds.). (2003). *Biofeedback: A practitioner's guide.* New York: Guilford Press.

Sharpe, M., & Carson, A. (2001). "Unexplained" somatic symptoms, functional syndromes, and somatization: Do we need a paradigm shift? *Annals of Internal Medicine, 134*(9, Pt. 2), 926–930.

Task Force of the European Society of Cardiology and the North American Society of Pacing and Electrophysiology. (1996). Heart rate variability: Standards of measurement, physiological interpretation, and clinical use. *European Heart Journal, 17*(3), 354–381.

Thayer, J. F., Friedman, B. H., & Borkovec, T. D. (1996). Autonomic characteristics of generalized anxiety disorder and worry. *Biological Psychiatry, 39*(4), 255–266.

Thayer, J. F., Friedman, B. H., Borkovec, T. D., Johnsen, B. H., & Molina, S. (2000). Phasic heart period reactions to cued threat and nonthreat stimuli in generalized anxiety disorder. *Psychophysiology, 37*(3), 361–368.

Waring, W. S., Chui, M., Japp, A., Nicol, E. F., & Ford, M. J. (2004). Autonomic cardiovascular responses are impaired in women with irritable bowel syndrome. *Journal of Clinical Gastro-enterology, 38*(8), 658–663.

Wickramasekera, I. (1994). Psychophysiological and clinical implications of the coincidence of high hypnotic ability and high neuroticism during threat perception in somatization disorders. *American Journal of Clinical Hypnosis, 37*(1), 22–33.

Wickramasekera, I., & Price, D. C. (1997). Morbid obesity, absorption, neuroticism, and the high risk model of threat perception. *American Journal of Clinical Hypnosis, 39*(4), 291–301.

Wickramasekera, I. E. (1995). Somatization: Concepts, data, and predictions from the high risk model of threat perception. *Journal of Nervous and Mental Disease, 183*(1), 15–23.

Wilhelm, F. H., Gerlach, A. L., & Roth, W. T. (2001). Slow recovery from voluntary hyperventilation in panic disorder. *Psychosomatic Medicine, 63*(4), 638–649.

Wilhelm, F. H., Gevirtz, R., & Roth, W. T. (2001). Respiratory dysregulation in anxiety, functional cardiac, and pain disorders: Assessment, phenomenology, and treatment. *Behavior Modification, 25*(4), 513–545.

Wilhelm, F. H., Trabert, W., & Roth, W. T. (2001a). Characteristics of sighing in panic disorder. *Biological Psychiatry, 49*(7), 606–614.

Wilhelm, F. H., Trabert, W., & Roth, W. T. (2001b). Physiologic instability in panic disorder and generalized anxiety disorder. *Biological Psychiatry, 49*(7), 596–605.

Yates, B. T. (1984). How psychology can improve effectiveness and reduce costs of health services. *Psychotherapy, 21*, 439–451.

CHAPTER 10

Biofeedback Training to Increase Heart Rate Variability

PAUL M. LEHRER

THEORETICAL FOUNDATIONS

One of the hallmarks of all stable systems, biological or otherwise, is a complex pattern of oscillation (Giardino, Lehrer, & Feldman, 2000). Our heart rate, blood pressure, body temperature, and energy level, along with our mood, relatedness, task orientation, and so forth are all constantly in motion and are never completely stable. The pattern of variability can be complex. It varies over months, weeks, days, hours, and even seconds—at all of these frequencies simultaneously. The closer we look, the more clearly we see the apparent chaos of variability as actually a complex pattern of overlapping oscillations.

For years, psychologists, biologists, and psychophysiologists have often looked at these oscillations as bothersome sources of noise that obscure the individual's "true" level of activity. We now know better. These oscillations represent the body's self-regulatory reflexes. When the body is well regulated, these oscillations have a complex pattern and are of relatively high amplitude. Reductions in either amplitude or complexity are a sign of vulnerability, indicating that the body's self-regulatory mechanisms are damaged or inefficient and unable to withstand the vicissitudes of stress, disease, injury, and so forth. When a biological variable rises, a regulatory reflex is triggered that makes it fall again; and, as it falls, a complementary reflex makes it rise. This sequence causes a pattern of continuing oscillation and also gives us a window to the body's processes for self-regulation and homeostasis. Any one physiological function is usually controlled by multiple reflexes. One could think of them as multiple backup systems for homeostatic control; hence the complexity of the oscillatory pattern, as well as the amplitude, reflects healthy adaptiveness.

In particular, decreased heart rate variability (HRV) is a marker of impaired cardiovascular regulation. It is associated with a wide variety of diseases and exposure to a variety of physical and emotional stressors. Cardiovascular disorders showing this pattern include hypertension, particularly when accompanied by left ventricular hypertrophy (Mancia, Ludbrook, Ferrari, Gregorini, & Zanchetti, 1978); sudden cardiac death (Goldberger, 1991; Goldberger & Rigney, 1990; Goldberger, Rigney, Mietus, Antman, &

Greenwald, 1988), particularly from arrhythmic events after myocardial infarction (Bigger, Fleiss, Rolnitzky, & Steinman, 1992; Farrell et al., 1991); ventricular arrhythmia (Matveev & Prokopova, 2002); presence and severity of ischemic heart disease (Huikuri & Makikallio, 2001); and risk of rejection after heart transplant (Izrailtyan et al., 2000). Patients with various other disorders that reflect autonomic dysregulation also tend to show decreased amplitude and complexity of HRV; such conditions include depression and anxiety disorders (Agelink, Boz, Ullrich, & Andrich, 2002; Gorman & Sloan, 2000; Kawachi, Sparrow, Vokonas, & Weiss, 1995; Yeragani, Balon, Phl, & Ramesh, 1995); asthma, when asthma symptoms are not active (Kazuma, Otsuka, Matsuoka, & Murata, 1997); and episodes of life-threatening events related to sudden infant death syndrome (Rother et al., 1987). HRV amplitude also is negatively correlated with age (Liao et al., 1995) and positively related to aerobic capacity in an adult population (Hedelin, Wiklund, Bjerle, & Henriksson-Larsen, 2000; Pardo et al., 2000). It increases among patients undertaking a program of cardiac rehabilitation (Lucini et al., 2002) that includes a relaxation intervention (Dixhoorn & White, 2005). One can think of HRV as a general measure of adaptability. Diminished HRV is a sign of vulnerability to stress, whether the decrease arises from psychological or physical stress or from the ravages of disease.

A New Biofeedback Method

Biofeedback is a widely used method for teaching voluntary control of various physiological functions by providing instantaneous "feedback" for variations in physiological activity (Schwartz & Andrasik, 2003). Feedback usually is given in the form of visual and/ or auditory signals derived from physiological recording devices. Most other biofeedback methods are designed to control *tonic* levels of various physiological functions (e.g., muscle tension, finger temperature, heart rate, blood pressure, etc.). Significant effects of these methods have been found for reducing blood pressure, although the magnitude and consistency have not been sufficient for the method to gain widespread acceptance. In this chapter, we describe a new biofeedback approach: that is, teaches control of *oscillatory variability* in heart rate and thus *directly* targets and exercises the body's own physiological control mechanisms, rather than affecting these mechanisms more indirectly by teaching control of tonic level of blood pressure, heart rate, skin temperature, and so forth—tasks that, in fact, are appreciably more difficult than learning to increase HRV.

Respiratory Sinus Arrhythmia, Vagus Nerve Function, and Autonomic Balance

Frequency characteristics of HRV have also been used to assess sympathetic–parasympathetic balance, as explained later. This property of HRV is sometimes confused with HRV as a measure of adaptability and health, probably because these decrease when sympathetic tuning increases in both psychological stress and cardiovascular disease. However, the two effects are not synonymous and may occur independently, as when the cardiovagal system becomes overactive in vasovagal syncope, in which patients tend to show elevated parasympathetic tuning (Piccirillo et al., 2004), but are sick nonetheless.

Respiratory sinus arrhythmia (RSA) is the variation in heart rate that accompanies breathing. Heart rate (HR) increases during inhalation and decreases during exhalation. RSA is sometimes used as index of parasympathetic tone (Porges, 1995). Respiratory-linked variations in HR usually occur in the frequency range of 0.15–0.4 Hz (9–24 breaths per minute) in the healthy human adult: the range of normal adult respiration rate. HR oscillations in this range are often referred to as "high-frequency" (HF) HR oscillations, and the spectral power within this range is often treated as synonymous with RSA and sometimes is denoted as "vagal tone." However, RSA is sometimes decoupled from the vagal pathways that affect tonic HR (Sargunaraj et al., 1996; Yasuma & Hayano, 2004), and people sometimes breathe at frequencies outside this range. Also some influences independent of vagal traffic may cause RSA to vary, such as rate of acetylcholine metabolism, which is a relatively slow process. Acetylcholine is released by vagus nerve activity during exhalation (causing RSA), but it may be metabolized more fully during slow than during fast respiration, in which the effects of inhalation may diminish the effect of vagus nerve output on HRV (Eckberg & Eckberg, 1982) and thus decouple amplitude of RSA from quantity of vagus nerve traffic. Under some circumstances, sympathetic activity may affect HF HRV (Taylor, Myers, Halliwill, Seidel, & Eckberg, 2001). Thus the imputation of vagal tone from RSA is complicated. At the very least, it is important to consider respiration rate while evaluating HRV as a measure of autonomic function. If increases in RSA occur *independently* of respiration rate and are coupled with decreases in HR, then one can confidently interpret these effects as reflecting increased vagal tone.

Slower oscillations in HR are not exclusively parasympathetically mediated. The low-frequency (LF) range (0.05–0.15 Hz) is closely associated with baroreflex function and is influenced by both the sympathetic and parasympathetic systems, whereas the very-low-frequency (VLF) range (0.005–0.05 Hz) is primarily influenced by the sympathetic system (Task Force of the European Society of Cardiology and the North American Society of Pacing and Electrophysiology, 1996; Berntson et al., 1997). Although some investigators use the LF:HF ratio as a measure of autonomic balance, there is some doubt about the validity of this use, particularly in the supine position (Eckberg, 2000), because there is evidence that the sympathetic system contributes only minimally to supine LF HRV (Myers, Cohen, Eckberg, & Taylor, 2001). In a controlled study of 54 healthy people, we found that HRV biofeedback differentially increased resting HF HRV independently of respiration rate (Lehrer et al., 2003), although changes in mean HR were minimal.

RSA and Respiratory Efficiency

Yasuma and Hayano (2004) have shown that RSA promotes respiratory efficiency by making more blood available when oxygen concentration in the alveoli is at a maximum, that is, during inhalation. Respiratory efficiency increases when people breathe at about six breaths per minute (Bernardi et al., 1998; Bernardi, Gabutti, Porta, & Spicuzza, 2001; Spicuzza, Gabutti, Porta, Montano, & Bernardi, 2000; Giardino et al., 2004). It is only at this frequency that RSA is completely in phase with breathing, so that HR rises simultaneously with inhalation and falls simultaneously with exhalation (Vaschillo & Lehrer, 2004). Thus, when people breathe at this rate, HR is highest when the oxygen concentration in the alveoli is highest (during inhalation), thus causing increased gas exchange efficiency. Bernardi and his colleagues have observed that yogis also tend to breathe at approximately the same frequency. Breathing at this frequency is accompanied by a decreased hypoxic ventilatory response, along with better oxygen saturation during the experimental challenge and better tolerance for exercise and altitude, with some advantage to people who have engaged in long-term practice of yoga (Bernardi, Passino, et al., 2001; Spicuzza et al., 2000). Saying the rosary prayers and yogic meditation are both associated with breathing at approximately six times per minute and produce predictably large increases in HRV at that frequency (Bernardi, Sleight, et al., 2001). Vaschillo et al. (2004) have shown that HRV biofeedback encourages the individual to breathe at the frequency at which HRV and respiration are exactly in phase with each other, a frequency that is usually near six breaths per minute, although not often exactly at this rate. HRV biofeedback thus should maximize respiratory efficiency.

The Baroreflexes and Low-Frequency HRV

Another contribution to HRV emanates from the baroreflexes (BRs). BRs are important mechanisms for control of blood pressure (Eckberg & Sleight, 1992). Baroreceptors are stretch receptors located in the aortic arch and carotid sinus that are very responsive to changes in blood pressure. When blood pressure increases, the BRs trigger decreases in HR and in vascular tone, thus producing subsequent mechanical homeostatic decreases in blood pressure. When blood pressure decreases, the BRs produce the opposite effects. Hypertension is often accompanied by BR dysfunction (Laitinen, Hartikainen, Niskanen, Geelen, & Länsimies, 1999; Pitzalis et al., 1999; Rau et al., 1994; Rau, Furedy, & Elbert, 1996; Robertson et al., 1993). The strength or gain of the BRs is measured in units of change in R–R interval (RRI) of the electrocardiogram (EKG; in milliseconds) per unit change in blood pressure (mm Hg). Eckberg (1979) found both a decrease in BR sensitivity and resetting of the BR among young men with hypertension (systolic blood pressure 140–165 mm Hg), compared with an age-matched sample of normotensive men, although only resetting occurred among individuals with high-normal blood pressure (135–140 mm Hg). Although the role of BR dysfunction in causing hypertension has not been definitively established, the strong modulatory effects of BR activity on blood pressure justify trying to increase BR gain as a treatment for hypertension, whether or not BR dysfunction is a major *cause* of the disorder. BR gain also is related to adaptiveness of the cardiovascular system—indeed, to survival. La Rovere, Bigger, Marcus, Mortara, and Schwartz (1998) showed that, among patients recovering from myocardial infarction, those with subnormal BR gain have high risk of fatal cardiac events, especially if the patient also has low HRV. The linkage between BR impairment and mortality may partially reflect patients' autonomic responses to cardiac rhythm changes. Ventricular tachycardia, a rapid rhythm that commonly precedes sudden death (Bayes de Luna, Doumel, & Leclercq, 1989), precipitously lowers arterial pressure, increases muscle–sympathetic nerve activity (Smith, Ellenbogen, Beightol, & Ekberg, 1991), and reduces vagal–cardiac nerve activity (Huikuri et al., 1989). During ventricular tachycardia, arterial perfusion pressures recover more rapidly in patients with stronger than weaker BRs (Hamdan et al., 1999). In an exercise/ischemia dog model of sudden cardiac death, ventricular fibrillation occurs when BRs are weak but does not occur when they are strong (Billman, Schwartz, & Stone, 1983).

BR gain can be reliably measured noninvasively by assessing the slope of increases in RRI against increases in systolic blood pressure and of decreases in RRI against decreases in blood pressure and by cross-spectral analysis of RRI and blood pressure. The last of these has been found to correlate highly with BR gain calculated from phenylephrine-induced blood pressure increases and with suction on the neck, which directly stimulates the carotid BR (James, Panerai, & Potter, 1998; Rudas et al., 1999). The cross-spectral and slope methods are particularly useful because they assess both aortic and carotid baroreflexes, without the unacceptable side effects often produced by phenylephrine.

Spectral BR gain is most sensitively measured in the low frequency (LF) range (0.05–0.15 Hz), suggesting that the HRV in the LF range is mediated, in part, by BR effects

(Robbe et al., 1987). A study from our laboratory (Vaschillo, Lehrer, Rishe, & Konstantinov, 2002) has confirmed that the latency of the HR BR is approximately 5 seconds, thus accounting for a source of HRV with a period of 10 seconds (i.e., the commonly observed HRV wave at ~0.1 Hz), a frequency that is at the center of the low-frequency range.

Mechanism by Which HRV Biofeedback Increases HRV

The cardiovascular system is known to have resonance characteristics, with a first resonant frequency of ~0.1 Hz (DeBoer, Karemaker, & Strackee, 1987; Vaschillo et al., 2002). The resonance characteristics appear to reflect BR influences on HRV. HRV biofeedback always influences the individual to breathe at his or her specific resonant HRV frequency. Breathing at resonant frequency augments oscillations in HR by stimulating it rhythmically at that frequency, as follows: We have found that the phase relationship between HR and blood pressure oscillations at the resonant frequency (and *only* at this frequency) is *exactly* 180°, that the phase relationship between HR oscillations and respiration is *exactly* 0° (Vaschillo et al., 2002; Vaschillo, Zingerman, Konstantinov, & Menitsky, 1983), with inhalation coinciding with HR accelerations, and that the highest amplitudes of biofeedback-produced HRV are achievable when people breathe at this frequency. Thus inhaling is associated with increases in HR (presumably driven by respiration—RSA) and decreases in blood pressure. The decreases in blood pressure then stimulates the BRs, so that they *also* produce increases in HR at this time, thus enhancing the respiratory-induced increases in HR. The same process happens in the reverse direction during exhalation. At the same time, respiratory activity also enhances oscillations produced by the BR. Thus, when people breathe at their resonant frequency, the amplitude of HRV is maximized, and the BR is greatly stimulated; and, conversely, when people try to maximize the amplitude of their HRV using biofeedback, they automatically breathe at their resonant frequency and thus also stimulate the BR. Frequent maximal stimulation of the BR, then, produces what exercise usually produces in reflexes: It makes them more efficient. Hence, daily practice of HRV biofeedback tends to increase BR gain (Lehrer et al., 2003) and to improve modulation of various autonomic functions that, directly or indirectly, are affected by the BR (Lehrer et al., 2003).

Looked at another way, the resonant characteristics of HRV ensure that oscillations at the resonant frequency persist after initial stimulation. Imagine striking an object without resonance characteristics (e.g., a tree trunk). What happens? *Thunk!* An auditory event that immediately disappears. Then imagine striking an object with resonance, such as a bell. You then produce a sound with a long decay: bo-o-o-o-o-ng. When *any* resonant system is *rhythmically* stimulated at its resonant frequency, the external stimulation magnifies the persistent oscillations, thus greatly increasing total variability. Imagine pushing a swing at its resonant frequency. If you push each time the swing starts going up (i.e., at its resonant frequency), the oscillations in the swing do not just persist and decay; they grow in amplitude. Figure 10.1 shows such an effect in a typical recording from our laboratory: *very* large oscillations in HR and blood pressure at approximately 0.1 Hz, 180° out of phase with each other, eclipsing all other sources of variability in either measure, and increasing average total amplitude of HR variability (summed across frequencies). In this case, the BR system is the analogue of the cord on the swing; it determines the resonant frequency. The repetitive "push" is then provided by rhythmic breathing at the resonant frequency.

Our research has found that resonant frequency differs among individuals, in our experience, between 4.5 and 7 cycles/minute among healthy people, replicating previous re-

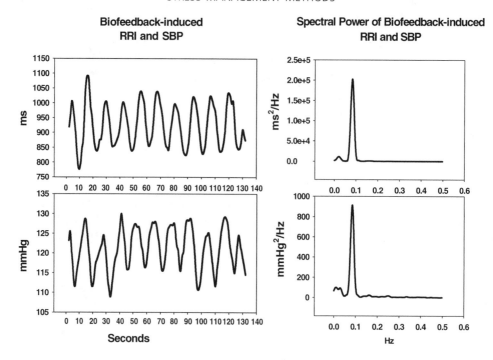

FIGURE 10.1. Typical HR and blood pressure patterns during HRV biofeedback. RRI, R–R interval; SBP, systolic blood pressure.

search by Vaschillo and colleagues (Vaschillo et al., 1983; Vaschillo et al., 2002). Each individual's resonant frequency is independently related to gender (higher in women) and inversely to height, but not to age or weight, suggesting that it may be related to the volume of the vasculature in each individual. (Note that the gender effects are independent of the effects of height.)

Effects of HRV Biofeedback on the BR

In a study of the method among healthy individuals (Lehrer et al., 2003), we found that BR gain was significantly increased, both acutely and chronically, and that LF HRV (0.05–0.15 Hz), in which BR effects are most clearly observed (Robbe et al., 1987), is acutely effectively doubled. Additionally, Vaschillo et al. (2002) showed that particularly great increases occur at the specific frequency that reflects BR activity in each individual.

Regular training of a reflex may be expected to produce chronic increases in reflex efficiency. This has been particularly well demonstrated for musculoskeletal reflexes (Bawa, 2002; Schalow, Blanc, Jeltsch, & Zach, 1996), and the process also has been demonstrated in the cardiovascular system (Zhao, Hintze, & Kaley, 1996). In HRV biofeedback, participants are instructed to practice the biofeedback for several periods each day. Thus, BR gain is greatly amplified *on a regular basis* by biofeedback practice. Recent data from our laboratory (Lehrer et al., 2003) show that this procedure produces *chronic* increases in BR gain among healthy people *at rest*. Slow breathing, such as occurs during HRV biofeedback, also has been shown to increase BR gain and sensitivity among patients with chronic heart failure (Bernardi et al., 2002).

Other Possible Mechanisms for HRV Biofeedback

In a recent clinical trial of HRV biofeedback as a treatment for asthma, an interesting pattern of results emerged. We studied 97 patients with asthma, approximately half of whom were given training in HRV biofeedback. The rest were divided into two control conditions: frontal EEG alpha biofeedback and a waiting-list condition (Lehrer et al., 2004). We titrated asthma controller medications (primarily inhaled steroids) based on patients' asthma symptoms and pulmonary function. We found that, compared with the control groups, participants given HRV biofeedback were able to decrease their consumption of controller medication to a clinically significant level while maintaining or improving their clinical condition (i.e., fewer asthma exacerbations, decreased respiratory resistance, greater compliance of airway tissue, less inhomogeneity of resistance in the airways, and fewer asthma symptoms). However, none of these results correlated with changes in HRV, BR gain, or any other autonomic measures we studied. Additionally, although the cardiovascular effects of HRV biofeedback were greater among younger people, the effects on respiratory resistance were greater in older people.

So what mediated the biofeedback effects on asthma? At the moment, we can only guess. Our forced oscillation pneumography findings suggested that tissues in the airways became more compliant, with less inhomogeneity in airway resistance among the various airway passages (Dubois, Brody, Lewis, & Burgess, 1956). These results suggest a decrease in airway inflammation, which causes generalized stiffness in the airways but tends to affect various air passages differentially. Another possibility may be an indirect effect of improved respiratory efficiency, as described earlier. Although a link between improved respiratory efficiency and improved asthma has not been established, one could speculate that muscular tone in the airways may be related in some way to the amount of effort required to breathe and maintain normal oxygenation. It will be up to future research to discover these links.

Why is there a need for special biofeedback technology, rather than simply telling people to breathe at six breaths per minute for 20 minutes twice daily? It is only at the resonant frequency that the baroreflex is specifically stimulated by respiration, because of the 180° phase relationship between HR and blood pressure when people breathe at this specific frequency. HRV biofeedback allows very sensitive assessment of the individual's resonant frequency. It is not known whether breathing at a standard rate of six breaths per minute (which, although close, is not the resonant frequency for everyone) produces clinical effects that are just as strong as those produced by HRV biofeedback. The more tenuous link with baroreflex stimulation at other frequencies suggests that HRV biofeedback may have more powerful effects, but this has not been proven. Indeed, a number of studies have found significant clinical effects for paced breathing at rates similar to those characteristic of typical resonant frequencies. It would be worthwhile to investigate whether results might be even stronger if people breathed at their *exact* resonant frequencies, at which respiratory and BR effects are strongest.

HISTORY OF THE METHOD

Diminished HRV as a predictor of cardiac mortality risk has been generally recognized for more than a decade (Dreifus et al., 1993), although well-documented reports appeared much earlier (Hon & Lee, 1965; Rudolph, Vallbona, & Desmond, 1965). We had found decreased HRV among alcoholics in an early study (Lehrer & Taylor, 1974), but we did not know how to interpret it at the time. Decreased HRV in diabetes also was recognized quite early (Morguet & Springer, 1981). Studies of HRV as a measure of autonomic nervous system function began to appear (e.g., Dalton, Dawes, & Patrick, 1983), and it was discovered that HRV decreases systematically with age in adults (O'Brien, O'Hare, & Corrall, 1986). Later in the 1980s, research on HRV began looking at the relationship between various frequencies of HRV and relative sympathetic and parasympathetic contributions to autonomic balance (Maayan, Axelrod, Akeslrod, Carley, & Shannon, 1988).

At the same time that this research was progressing in the West, Soviet scientists were studying HRV as a measure of autonomic function among cosmonauts. The first documented studies of HRV biofeedback were reported by Vaschillo et al. (1983). They initially used the technique to assess autonomic function and found that biofeedback could easily be used to teach cosmonauts to produce high amplitudes of HRV and blood pressure variability at various frequencies. Vaschillo et al. (1983) then performed transfer function analyses in order to examine specific frequency characteristics of biofeedback-induced HRV and found that participants uniformly produced the highest frequency-specific HRV oscillations only at certain frequencies, usually at about 0.1 Hz (10-second cycles). By examining the phase relationships between HR and blood pressure oscillations, the researchers discovered the relationships among BR activity, HRV biofeedback, and resonance characteristics in the cardiovascular system, described earlier. This work has more recently been reported in English (Vaschillo et al., 2002).

Because stimulation of an autonomic modulatory reflex was thought to have potentially important therapeutic implications, Vaschillo and his colleagues then began applying this biofeedback method to patients with various neurotic and psychosomatic problems (Chernigovskaya, Vaschillo, Petrash, & Rusanovsky, 1990). Smetankin founded the Biosvyaz company in St. Petersburg that manufactured a free-standing HRV biofeedback unit and operated a clinic devoted to treating pediatric asthma using this method (Lehrer, Smetankin, & Potapova, 2000). Influenced by this Russian research, Richard Gevirtz and I independently began programs of research in the United States to evaluate this method. The method has been adopted as part of standard biofeedback practice by many applied psychophysiologists.

However, the notion that salutary health effects can be obtained by breathing at particular rates has been with us for many centuries. Slow breathing underlies many of the Eastern meditative techniques, including yoga and Zen. HRV biofeedback systematizes these findings and makes them readily learnable in very little time.

ASSESSMENT

The level of empirical validation for HRV biofeedback in various applications is summarized in Table 10.1.

Asthma

Our research on asthma was introduced previously in this chapter in the subsection titled "Other Possible Mechanisms for HRV Biofeedback." Russian research on the topic was introduced in the preceding section. Indeed, asthma is the HRV biofeedback application that has been most systematically evaluated. Lehrer, Smetankin, and Potapova (2000) reported 20 consecutive cases of mild pediatric asthma treated with biofeedback but no

TABLE 10.1. Studies of HRV Biofeedback or Paced Breathing at Rates Similar to Those Obtained with HRV Biofeedback

Condition	Study	Design	Clinical significance	n	Level of evidence
Asthma	Lehrer et al. (2004)	RCT, PBO, WL, single blind	Significant	94	Efficacious and specific
	Lehrer et al. (2000)	Multiple case study, quantified outcome	n.a.	20	
	Lehrer et al. (1997)	RCT, WL, Tx equivalent design	n.a.	20	
	Lehrer et al. (2006)	Reanalysis of Lehrer et al. (2004) showing no age differences in effects.	Significant	36	
Hypertension	Del Pozo et al. (2004)	RCT, compared with WL	Significant	63	Efficacious and specific
	Herbs et al. (1993)	RCT, compared with thermal biofeedback	Significant	54	
	McCraty et al. (2003)	RCT, compared with no treatment	Significant	38	
	Joseph et al. (2005)	Within-subject comparison of 6/min with 15/min breathing	n.a. BP dropped more in 6/min	46	
	Elliot et al. (2004)	RCT, resp biofeedback machine only (no live training) vs. standard med care.	Significant	149	
Emphysema	Giardino et al. (2004)	Multiple case study combined with pulse oximetry biofeedback	Improvement in exercise tolerance, gas exchange efficiency, quality of life	20	Possibly efficacious
Depression	Karavidas et al. (2007)	Multiple case study	Clinically significant decrease	9 with major depression	Possibly efficacious
	Hassett et al. (2007)	Multiple case study	Clinically significant decrease in pain, depression, insomnia	12 with fibromyalgia	Possibly efficacious
Fibromyalgia	Hassett et al. (2007)	Multiple case study	Improvement in pain, sleep, and depression	12	Possibly efficacious
Heart disease	Cowan et al. (2001)	RCT (HRV biofeedback CBT vs. standard medical care)	Significant, fewer deaths	129 ventricular fibrillation or asystole survivors	Possibly efficacious
Unexplained abdominal pain	Humphreys & Gevirtz (2000)	RCT (HRV biofeedback + fiber vs. additional CBT and family therapy)	Equivalent or superior to effects of HRV biofeedback + fiber	64 children and adolescents	Possibly efficacious
Anxiety and various psycho-somatic problems	Chernigovskaya et al. (1990)	Anecdotal reports	n.a.	Not reported	Not systematically evaluated

Note. BP, blood pressure; CBT, cognitive-behavioral therapy; n.a., not applicable; PBO, placebo control; RCT, randomized controlled trial, compared with HRV biofeedback; WL, waiting list; Tx, treatment.

235

medicine. Significant improvements in pulmonary function were found. Similarly, a small, randomly controlled trial comparing HRV biofeedback with biofeedback-assisted muscle relaxation and a no-treatment control found significantly greater decreases in respiratory resistance among those receiving HRV biofeedback than among those in the other groups (Lehrer et al., 1997). In a larger, placebo-controlled trial with random assignment to treatments, we found that HRV biofeedback showed clinically significant improvement in asthma (Lehrer et al., 2004). Patients receiving HRV biofeedback took less asthma medication and had better pulmonary function, fewer asthma symptoms, and fewer asthma exacerbations. These findings were clinically significant. Patients receiving HRV biofeedback improved, on average, by one full level of asthma severity, based on the four-level classification scheme adopted by the National Heart, Lung, and Blood Institute (1997, 2002). In a later report, Lehrer et al. (2006) reanalyzed data from their randomized controlled trial (Lehrer et al., 2004) and found no age differences in clinical effects, despite the smaller change in HRV that occurs among older people. However, as caveats, it is important to mention that the method has not yet been tested by a "disinterested" clinical center with no involvement in development of the method, and no longer term follow-up studies have been done (of critical importance for studying asthma, which is inherently an episodic disease).

Hypertension

Another disorder with substantial though not as firm support from controlled clinical studies is hypertension. Gevirtz and colleagues recently completed a study of HRV biofeedback for hypertension using our protocol. They found that five of six participants with hypertension received biofeedback therapy became normotensive after treatment, whereas only four of eight participants in a no-biofeedback control group met this criterion (Del Pozo, Gevirtz, & Guanieri, 2004).

Also, Herbs, Gevirtz, and Jacobs (1993) compared the effects of HRV biofeedback with those of finger-temperature biofeedback in 91 patients with hypertension. Fifteen participants did not complete the training. The completers were well matched to the dropouts on all blood pressure and demographic variables except race (nonwhites were more likely to drop out). The groups were equivalent in blood pressure, age, gender, race, exercise, family history, medication use, major illnesses, and other demographic measures. Medication remained constant throughout the trial. Participants completed 16 sessions of either condition. The finger-temperature training followed the procedures of the Menninger Clinic trials (see Chapter 8, this volume). Participants were taught autogenic phrases and instructed to "make their fingers as warm as possible." During sessions, milestones were established, with the ultimate goal of reaching temperatures in the 90°F range. Peak–valley differences were greater for the HRV group during the first six sessions and continued to increase through the last sessions. The finger-temperature group maintained about a 7 beats-per-minute (BPM) peak–valley difference throughout, whereas the HRV group increased from 9.16 BPM to 10.9 BPM by the last sessions. Whereas the two groups started at equivalent finger temperatures, the finger-temperature (FT) training group increased maximum temperatures to 93.5°F compared with 91.7°F for the HRV group. In the 4 baseline measurement sessions, systolic blood pressure was stabilized at 156.5 ± 13/89.5 ±10) mm Hg for the HRV group and 152.8 ± 15/84 ± 10 for the FT group. Postpressures (the mean of blood pressure taken before last three biofeedback sessions) were 143 ± 12/85 ± 10 for the HRV group and 139 ± 17/76 ± 8 for the FT group. Each group individually showed a significant decrease in both systolic and diastolic blood pressure ($p < .001$). No significant interaction was found. A regression analysis showed that, in the HRV group, change in amplitude of RSA (peak–valley differences) was related to blood pressure reduction, with other factors held constant ($r = -.45$, $p < .01$), but this was not the case for the FT group ($r = -.21$, $p = .20$). Temperature increase was not related to the blood pressure decrease for the FT group. Neither race nor gender produced significant interactions as additional independent variables. These uncontrolled results suggest that both FT biofeedback and HRV biofeedback may be useful tools for treating hypertension, although only for HRV biofeedback did the specific biofeedback mechanism account for the blood pressure changes.

A recent study, done by the HeartMath Institute in a workplace (McCraty, Atkinson, & Tomasino, 2003), used a simple HRV biofeedback device as a home trainer with 18 patients with blood pressure in the range of 140–179/90–105. After a single day's training, decreases in blood pressure were found that averaged 10/6 mm Hg, without changes in medication. These changes were significantly different from those in a group of 14 individuals who were randomly assigned to the same protocol of medical monitoring but without biofeedback (McCarty et al., 2003).

Schein et al. (2001) have received FDA approval to market a biofeedback device for treating hypertension that helps to slow respiration to rates similar to those produced during HRV biofeedback. In their 2001 study, they reported that systolic pressure dropped by about 15 mm Hg, although respiration rate was higher than the average adult resonant frequency. In a study of 149 patients using this device alone (with no "live" training with a trainer or therapist), the same group (Elliot et al., 2004) found a decrease of approximately 15 mm Hg in systolic blood pressure among patients using the device more than 180 minutes in 8 weeks, but only approximately 9 mm Hg among other patients and among those randomly assigned to a control group. Joseph et al. (2005) trained 20 patients with hypertension to breathe at six breaths/minute (similar to the rate of breathing in HRV biofeedback) and compared the results with those of breathing at 15 times/minute (average normal respiration rate). They found that slow breathing decreased systolic and diastolic pressures in patients with hypertension (from 149.7+/–3.7 to 141.1+/–4 mm Hg, $p < .05$; and from 82.7+/–3 to 77.8+/–3.7 mm Hg, $p < .01$, respectively). Controlled breathing (15/minute) decreased systolic (to 142.8+/–3.9 mm Hg; $p < .05$) but not diastolic blood pressure and decreased RRI ($p < .05$) without altering the BR.

Unexplained Abdominal Pain

A preliminary study has also shown that HRV biofeedback is helpful as a component in biofeedback treatment of unexplained abdominal pain (Humphreys & Gevirtz, 2000), where effects were stronger for biofeedback alone than with no behavioral intervention or when combined with family therapy. All patients were advised to increase fiber in their diet.

Heart Disease

Because diminished HRV frequently occurs among patients who have had heart attacks and is a significant predictor of mortality in this population, it seems possible that training such people to increase HRV may actually improve survival. Some evidence for this idea was obtained in a study by Cowan, Pike, and Budzynski (2001). They studied 129 survivors of out-of-hospital ventricular fibrillation or asystole and provided 11 sessions of a treatment consisting of HRV biofeedback combined with cognitive behavioral therapy (CBT) aimed at self-management and coping strategies for depression, anxiety, and anger and cardiovascular health education and compared the treatment with a group who received only standard medical care. Risk of cardiovascular death was significantly reduced 86% by psychosocial therapy. Moreover, six of the seven cardiovascular deaths in the control group (of eight total deaths) were caused by ventricular arrhythmias, suggesting that the mechanism for the treatment effect was control of such arrhythmias. The single cardiovascular death in the therapy group (of three total deaths) was due to stroke. Cowan et al. (2001) concluded that this treatment significantly reduced the risk of cardiovascular death in survivors of sudden cardiac arrest. Although the cognitive components of their treatment could not be separated from HRV biofeedback, there is no other literature showing effects of cognitive therapy on cardiac arrhythmias. Del Pozo et al. (2004) found that the procedure increases resting HRV among patients with coronary artery disease, in which HRV is a strong predictor of survival.

Other

Karavidas et al. (2007) found decreases of over 50% in symptoms of major depression among 11 patients given HRV biofeedback. The effect size ($d = 3.6$) approximated that achieved by antidepressant medication. Hassett, Radvanski, and Lehrer (2007) found that HRV biofeedback improved sleep and decreased symptoms of depression among patients with fibromyalgia. Chernigovskaya et al. (1990) reported improvements in anxiety and in various psychosomatic symptoms. An uncontrolled study of 20 patients by Giardino, Chan, and Borson (2004) found an improvement in gas exchange efficiency and greater exercise tolerance among emphysema patients treated with HRV biofeedback.

SIDE EFFECTS AND CONTRAINDICATIONS

When people think about their breathing, they often tend to hyperventilate. This frequently happens during the first few sessions of HRV biofeedback. As a result, the training protocol guides the trainee to breathe shallowly, even if slowly, and to be sensitive to symptoms of hyperventilation. If available, monitoring end-tidal CO_2 with a capnometer during early sessions can be useful. Also, we have found that some patients with frequent extrasystolic heartbeats sometimes show an increase in these events during HRV biofeedback. We do not know the long-term effect or risk of the procedure in this population. Indeed, some Russian researchers have even used the method to *decrease* occurrence of certain cardiac arrhythmias (Chernigovskaya et al., 1990; Sidorov & Vasilevskii, 1994; Vasilevskii, Sidorov, & Suvorov, 1993). However, we suggest that the method be used with caution among people with an irregular pattern of heartbeat. Irregular and missed beats can easily be detected with software that displays a Poincaré plot (cf. Thayer, Yonezawa, & Sollers, 2000), in which each RRI is plotted against the previous one. It also can usually be easily observed from an instantaneous cardiotachometer output. Because irregular heartbeats increase the difficulty in following a cardiotachometer tracing in biofeedback, a Poincaré plot in the biofeedback display is recommended for clients having many irregular beats.

THE METHOD

A manual for HRV biofeedback training has been published by Lehrer, Vaschillo, and Vaschillo (2000). The materials presented in this section include some minor modifications of that procedure. A study by McCraty et al. (2003) shows that HRV biofeedback can be easily and economically used by most patients and that patients with hypertension tend to utilize the method at home sufficiently frequently and well to produce significant decreases in blood pressure after only a single session of training. The small investment in equipment (approximately $200 for a home trainer) should not be prohibitive, either for the physician or the patient, in ordinary clinical practice. In our experience, maximal control over HRV at the resonant frequency can be obtained in most people after approximately four sessions of training.

Manual for Training

Note: The therapist's interaction with the patient as a human being is just as important as following this manual. It is important that the patient feels that the therapist understands, sympathizes with, and respects his or her experiences, including demands that the treatment makes on the client's life (time, expense, travel, etc.). Respect, warmth, and caring on the part of the therapist can be just as important ingredients for success as proper use of specific biofeedback procedures.

Therefore, it is important and appropriate to chat a little at the beginning of each session about the client's experiences between sessions, difficulties faced (e.g., in taking measures, medications, etc.), or significant life experiences (births, deaths, illnesses, job or school changes or difficulties, etc.). Use an "active listening" approach: Ask the client to expand or clarify and repeat the patient's feeling statements, indicating that you understand how he or she feels. Try to avoid judgmental statements or giving advice, except regarding specific procedures in the training.

Try to be sensitive to changes in the client's mood. If the client appears to become sad, pessimistic, anxious, or fearful, or if he or she reports severe interpersonal or financial problems, discussing these may take precedence over biofeedback procedures.

Script for Introducing the Method

Your heart rate goes up and down with your breathing. When you breathe in, your heart rate tends to go up. When you breathe out. your heart rate tends to go down. These changes in heart rate are called "respiratory sinus arrhythmia," or RSA. RSA triggers very powerful reflexes in the body that help it to control the whole autonomic nervous system (including your heart rate, blood pressure, and breathing). We will train you to increase the size of these heart rate changes. Increasing the size of the heart rate changes will better exercise these important reflexes and help them to control your body.

As part of this treatment we will measure your RSA and give you information about the swings in heart rate that accompany breathing. That will be the RSA biofeedback. You will use the information that these machines provide to teach yourself to increase your RSA. If you practice the technique regularly at home, you will strengthen the reflexes that regulate the autonomic nervous system. This should help improve your health and ability to manage everyday stress.

Do you have any questions?

(Use a respiration pacer stimulus set to six breaths/minute. The stimulus may be visual [e.g., a bar rising and falling] or auditory [a tone rising or falling in pitch].)

Breathe at the rate of this bar, moving up and down. Breathe in as the bar goes up and out as it goes down. Try it. (*Give feedback about whether the client is accurately following instructions.*) . . .

Now continue to breathe at this rate. Do not breathe too deeply or you will hyperventilate. If this happens you may experience some lightheadedness or dizziness. You will be breathing slowly, so you will have to breathe a little more deeply than usual. If lightheadedness or dizziness occurs breathe more shallowly.

Breathe out longer than you breathe in. Provide prompts both for inhalation and exhalation.

In all breathing instructions exercises we will teach you here, the *most important thing* is to breathe in a *relaxed* way. Breathe easily and comfortably. *Do not try too hard.*

Determining Resonant Frequency

We will now find your "resonant frequency"—the speed of breathing at which your RSA is the highest. In this procedure we will ask you to breathe at various rates for periods of about 3 minutes each. You will breathe at rates of 6.5, 6, 5.5, 5, and 4.5 breaths per minute. You should not find this task difficult. However, if you feel uncomfortable at any time, you can simply stop the task. Do you have any questions?

Using prompts from a respiratory pacing program, have the client breathe for 2 minutes at each of five frequencies (6.5, 6, 5.5, 5, and 4.5 breaths/minute), as prompted. Set the pacing stimulus manually, as prompted by the screen. Ask the participant to breathe at each frequency for one minute before beginning the data acquisition part of the program. Record the height of the spectral frequency at the client's respiration rate for each frequency. Extend the measurement period if breathing or HRV patterns are unstable during the assessment period.

Ordinarily the resonant frequency is characterized by (1) the highest low-frequency peak; (2) the highest low-frequency power; and (3) respiration and HRV in phase with each other. If these measures are discrepant, this will usually be between two specific frequencies. Repeat the process at those frequencies. If the measures remain discrepant, choose the frequency that yields the highest low-frequency spectral peak. If there is capability for measuring beat-to-beat blood pressure, these measures will oscillate 180° out of phase with HR at the resonant frequency. Also, finger temperature usually rises quickly while breathing at the resonant frequency. HR oscillations are smooth and even.

If a respiratory frequency appears to meet all of these criteria (e.g., having a higher frequency power peak than adjacent higher and lower frequencies), it may not be necessary to test all of the other frequencies. However, repeat the frequency yielding the highest peak, along with adjacent frequencies, in order to confirm the finding.

Inform the client of his or her resonant frequency (i.e., the frequency of maximum amplitude).

If a capnometer is available, the therapist should monitor CO_2 values and instruct the participant to breathe less deeply if values fall below initial CO_2 levels.

Second Training Session

Inquire about the client's experiences with resonant-frequency breathing within the past week. If symptoms of hyperventilation occurred, remind the client to breathe more shallowly. Help the client to troubleshoot problems with scheduling and motivation. Then proceed to training in relaxed abdominal breathing, as follows.

RELAXED ABDOMINAL BREATHING

One of the things you will learn in biofeedback is relaxed breathing. When you are relaxed, your chest and your abdomen relax, and you begin to breathe more naturally, so that your abdomen expands when you inhale and contracts (goes back in) when you exhale. Let me show you what I mean. (*Place one hand on your own chest and the other on the abdomen and demonstrate abdominal breathing.*) When you breathe, your diaphragm moves down and seems to push out your abdomen, so it seems as though you are breathing from your abdomen. When your diaphragm moves down, a partial vacuum is created in your lungs, so your lungs fill up. Your lungs don't *do* anything during breathing. They are passive, like balloons. Movement of the diaphragm makes them fill, just like blowing into the balloon.

So your chest doesn't do anything in relaxed breathing. Your diaphragm does all the work. Your diaphragm is located here. (*Point to the position of the diaphragm in your own body.*) Usually, you seem to breathe from your chest only when muscles in your abdomen are tense. Then you breathe by using your chest muscles, because, when your diaphragm moves down, there is no place to go—so the diaphragm cannot force air into the lungs. In relaxed breathing, as you inhale and exhale, the bottom hand moves up and down and the top hand doesn't move much at all. (*Demonstrate with two or three inhalations.*) Do you see that? Why don't you try, just to get the feel of it? Relax and place one hand on your chest and the other on your abdomen.

(*Let the client try it a few times while you continue to model. If the client finds abdominal breathing too difficult, however, allow the client to breathe with some chest movement, and remind him or her to continue breathing slowly.*)

Practice at home for about five minutes each day. First try it lying down or standing in front of a mirror. You may find this easier than sitting. Then try doing it while sitting. Eventually you should be able to do abdominal breathing in all positions.

Now inhale through the nose and exhale through pursed lips, like this. (*Demonstrate. Give feedback to the client. Praise the client for doing it properly.*)

Now go back to breathing out for longer than you breathe in. Follow the pacing bar on the screen. Continue to do pursed-lips breathing when you exhale. Breathe abdominally. Combine all three styles of breathing, like this. (*Demonstrate. Give feedback. Praise the client for good attempts.*)

Remember: breathe easily and comfortably. Do not try too hard.

(*Answer questions about this procedure. Give feedback about abdominal pursed-lips breathing with longer exhalation than inhalation. Remind the client not to breathe too deeply.*) Remember: If you feel dizzy or lightheaded, you are breathing too deeply. You are hyperventilating. Breathe more shallowly and naturally. You will get the hang of it soon.

Instruct the client to practice relaxed abdominal pursed-lips breathing at the same resonant frequency as in the previous week.

Session 3

Review relaxed abdominal breathing and resonant frequency breathing. Troubleshoot problems with both procedures. Then have the client begin to breathe at resonant frequency while you show him or her a cardiotachometer display.

INSTRUCTION IN USING THE CARDIOTACHOMETER FOR BIOFEEDBACK

Instruct the client to maximize RSA using the cardiotachometer as biofeedback. Instruct the client to do this by breathing in phase with HR changes. Remind client not to breathe too deeply, particularly if experiencing dizziness or lightheadedness, and to continue breathing at a rate that is close to his or her resonant frequency.

Now breathe at your resonant frequency for about 30 seconds. Then shift to following your heart rate. Look at this red line. (*Point to cardiotachometer tracing.*) When your heart rate goes up, this line goes up. When it goes down, the line goes down. Breathe in phase with your heart rate. When your heart rate goes up, breathe in. When your heart rate goes down, breathe out.

But first, just continue breathing at your resonant frequency.

(After 30 seconds to 1 minute, depending on how well the client is doing the task, prompt the individual to follow his or her heart rate, using the cardiotachometer feedback signal. Turn the pacer signal off.)

Breathe in phase with your heart rate. When your heart rate goes up, inhale. When it goes down, exhale. Make your heart rate go up as far as possible and down as far as possible.

Breathe easily, without tension. Breathe naturally. Don't try too hard. It should just flow almost automatically. Don't think too much about how to do it. Maybe it won't work right away. It will improve with time.

Allow the client to practice for 10 minutes using biofeedback. Give praise and indicate when a correction in technique is necessary. Monitor end-tidal CO_2 if a capnometer is available, and coach the client to breathe more shallowly if hyperventilation occurs.

Session 4

Session 4 is similar to session 3. Here, the client may be encouraged to borrow or purchase a home trainer. Provide instructions to the client on the use of the particular hardware and software. Have the client practice with his or her own equipment in the office.

Subsequent Sessions

There are no specific changes from the fourth session. The primary task is to monitor progress and correct errors in technique.

CASE EXAMPLE

The client was a 34-year-old woman with a long-standing asthma condition, referred by her physician to a study evaluating the effect of HRV biofeedback as a treatment for asthma. Over a 2-month period, with weekly visits, a pulmonary specialist had attempted to maximize her clinical condition, using the minimum possible dose of steroid medication. At the time of her first session of training, she was taking a dose of asthma controller medication at the higher levels recommended for mild persistent asthma (National Heart, Lung, and Blood Institute, 2002): three puffs of triamcinolone acetonide (Azmacort) twice daily (600 micrograms/day). Her pulmonary function was slightly below the optimal value of 80% expected for FEV_1 (volume of air exhaled during the first second of a forced expiratory maneuver with maximum effort from full vital capacity): 73%. However, she reported frequent daytime and nighttime asthma symptoms at home, sufficient to be classified as severe asthma (National Heart Lung and Blood Institute, 2002). She took home measures of home expiratory flow twice daily. She received 10 weekly sessions of HRV biofeedback, according to the protocol previously described. Medication was titrated upward or downward biweekly by the pulmonary physician based on symptoms and pulmonary function.

As can be seen in Figure 10.2, measures of peak flow increased over weeks, and peak flow variability decreased. FEV_1 gradually increased across sessions, reaching 80% expected by the last treatment session, and her level of symptomatology decreased to the level of moderate asthma. These changes occurred despite a decrease in her level of controller medication to one puff of Azmacort twice daily (200 micrograms/day). At a 1-

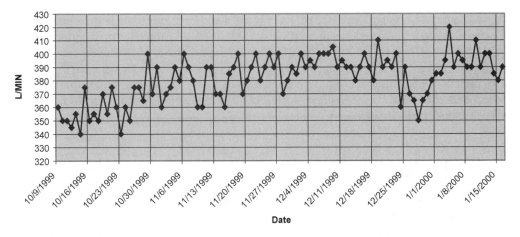

FIGURE 10.2. Home peak flow values in patient with asthma during HRV biofeedback training.

month follow-up visit, she had completely stopped taking Azmacort. Her home peak flow values remained stable during this period, with a brief dip during a respiratory infection. Because of the latter, her average symptomatology increased, although her pulmonary function values at the office remained stable. The patient's alpha BR gain also increased across sessions (Figure 10.3), as assessed by cross-spectral analysis of HR and beat-to-beat blood pressure (from a Finapres unit). It is not known whether the asthma improvement was related to improvement in baroreflex gain and consequent greater autonomic stability, although this is a distinct possibility.

The patient was informally followed up at 6 and 12 months. She continued practicing breathing at her resonant frequency, had not experienced any asthma flares, rarely used her bronchodilator, and had not returned to taking asthma controller medications.

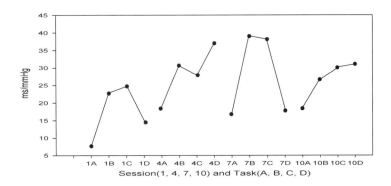

FIGURE 10.3. Spectral alpha low-frequency baroreflex gain in patient with asthma during HRV biofeedback training. Dots represent 5-minute tasks during biofeedback sessions. Task A was a rest period (without performing a biofeedback task) at the beginning of the session. Task B occurred at the beginning of a 20-minute biofeedback training session. Task C occurred at the end of the training period. Task D was a 5-minute rest period (without performing the biofeedback task) at the end of the session.

In summary, the patient showed a clinically significant improvement in pulmonary function, along with complete elimination of high doses of controller medication (an inhaled steroid). Her level of symptoms remained high, either because of overperception of symptoms or because the assessment metrics included periods in which she had a respiratory infection. BR gain increased both immediately, while performing biofeedback procedures, and chronically, as measured during the 5-minute pretraining periods in the 1st, 4th, 7th, and 10th sessions of training.

SUMMARY AND CONCLUSIONS

HRV biofeedback is a new approach to biofeedback therapy that, experimentally, produces effects that increase the gain of an important autonomic control reflex (the baroreflex) and increases respiratory efficiency. It is easy to learn, using inexpensive and friendly equipment with attractive displays. It appears to be useful as an adjunct treatment for a variety of respiratory and cardiovascular illnesses, with few and transient side effects.

REFERENCES

Agelink, M. W., Boz, C., Ullrich, H., & Andrich, J. (2002). Relationship between major depression and heart rate variability. Clinical consequences and implications for antidepressive treatment. *Psychiatry Research, 113*, 139–149.

Bawa, P. (2002). Neural control of motor output: Can training change it? *Exercise and Sport Sciences Reviews, 30*, 59–63.

Bayes de Luna, A., Coumel, P., & Leclercq, J.F. (1989). Ambulatory sudden cardiac death: Mechanisms of production of fatal arrhythmia on the basis of data from 157 cases. *American Heart Journal, 117*, 151–159.

Bernardi, L., Gabutti, A., Porta, C., & Spicuzza, L. (2001). Slow breathing reduces chemoreflex response to hypoxia and hypercapnia and increases baroreflex sensitivity. *Journal of Hypertension, 19*, 2221–2229.

Bernardi, L., Passino, C., Wilmerding, V., Dallam, G. M., Parker, D. L., Robergs, R. A., et al. (2001). Breathing patterns and cardiovascular autonomic modulation during hypoxia induced by simulated altitude. *Journal of Hypertension, 19*, 947–958.

Bernardi, L., Portta, C., Spicuzza, L., Bellwon, J., Spadacini, G., Frey, A. W., et al. (2002). Slow breathing increases the arterial baroreflex sensitivity in patients with chronic heart failure. *Circulation, 105*, 143–145.

Bernardi, L., Sleight, P., Bandinelli, G., Cencetti, S., Fattorini, L., Wdowczyc-Szulc, J., et al. (2001). Effect of rosary prayer and yoga mantras on autonomic cardiovascular rhythms: Comparative study. *British Medical Journal, 323*(7327), 1446–1449.

Bernardi, L., Spadacini, G., Bellwon, J., Hajric, R., Roskamm, H., & Frey, A. W. (1998). Influence of breathing frequency and pattern on oxygen saturation and exercise performance. *Lancet, 351*, 1308–1311.

Berntson, G. G., Bigger, J. T., Jr., Eckberg, D. L., Grossman, P., Kaufmann, P. G., Malik, M., et al. (1997). Heart rate variability: Origins, methods, and interpretive caveats. *Psychophysiology, 34*, 623–648.

Bigger, J. T., Fleiss, J. L., Rolnitzky, L. M., & Steinman, R. C. (1992). The ability of several short-term measures of RR variability to predict mortality after myocardial infarction. *Circulation, 88*, 927–934.

Billman, G. E., Schwartz, P. J., & Stone, H. L. (1983). Baroreceptor reflex control of heart rate: A predictor of sudden cardiac death. *Circulation, 66*, 874–880.

Chernigovskaya, N. V., Vaschillo, E. G., Petrash, V. V., & Rusanovsky, V. V. (1990). Voluntary regulation of the heart rate as a method of functional condition correction in neurotics. *Human Physiology, 16*, 58–64.

Cowan, M. J., Pike, K. C., & Budzynski, H. K. (2001). Psychosocial nursing therapy following sudden cardiac arrest: Impact on two-year survival. *Nursing Research, 50*, 68–76.

Dalton, K. J., Dawes, G. S., & Patrick, J. E. (1983). The autonomic nervous system and fetal heart rate variability. *American Journal of Obstetrics and Gynecology, 146*, 456–462.

DeBoer, R. W., Karemaker, J. M., & Strackee, J. (1987). Hemodynamic fluctuations and baroreflex sensitivity in humans: A beat-to-beat model. *American Journal of Physiology—Heart and Circulatory Physiology, 253*(22), H680–H689.

Del Pozo, J., Gevirtz, R., & Guanieri, M. (2004). Biofeedback treatment increases heart rate variability in patients with known coronary artery disease. *American Heart Journal, 147*, E11.

Dixhoorn, J. V., & White, A. (2005). Relaxation therapy for rehabilitation and prevention in ischaemic heart disease: A systematic review and meta-analysis. *European Journal of Cardiovascular Prevention and Rehabilitation, 12*, 193–202.

Dreifus, L. S., Agarwal, J. B., Botvinick, E. H., Ferdinand, K. C., Fisch, C., Fisher, J. D., et al. (1993). Heart rate variability for risk stratification of life-threatening arrhythmias. *Journal of the American College of Cardiology, 22*, 948–950.

Dubois, A., Brody, A., Lewis, D., & Burgess, B. (1956). Oscillation mechanics of lungs and chest in man. *Journal of Applied Physiology, 8*, 587–594.

Eckberg, D. L. (1979). Carotid baroreflex function in young men with borderline blood pressure elevation. *Circulation, 59*, 632–636.

Eckberg, D. L. (2000). Physiological basis for human autonomic rhythms. *Annals of Medicine, 32*, 341–349.

Eckberg, D. L., & Eckberg, M. J. (1982). Human sinus node responses to repetitive, ramped carotid baroreceptor stimuli. *American Journal of Physiology—Heart and Circulatory Physiology, 242*, H638–H644.

Eckberg, D. L., & Sleight, P. (1992). *Human baroreflexes in health and disease.* Oxford, UK: Clarendon Press.

Elliot, W. J., Izzo, J. L., Jr., White, W. B., Rosing, D. R., Snyder, C. S., Alter, A., et al. (2004). Graded blood pressure reduction in hypertensive outpatients associated with use of a device to assist with slow breathing. *Journal of Clinical Hypertension, 6*, 553–561.

Farrell, T. G., Bashir, Y., Cripps, T., Malik, M., Poloniecki, J., Bennett, E. D., et al. (1991). Risk stratification for arrhythmic events in postinfarction patients based on heart rate variability, ambulatory electrocardiographic variables and signal-averaged electrocardiogram. *Journal of the American College of Cardiology, 18*, 687–697.

Giardino, N., Lehrer, P. M., & Feldman, J. (2000). The role of oscillations in self-regulation: Their contribution to homeostasis. In D. Kenney & F. J. McGuigan (Eds.), *Stress and health: Research and clinical applications* (pp. 27–52). Newark: Harwood.

Giardino, N. D., Chan, L., & Borson, S. (2004). Combined heart rate variability and pulse oximetry biofeedback for chronic obstructive pulmonary disease: preliminary findings. *Applied Psychophysiology and Biofeedback, 29*, 121–133.

Goldberger, A. L. (1991). Is the normal heartbeat chaotic or homeostatic? *News in Physiological Science, 6*, 87–91.

Goldberger, A. L., & Rigney, D. R. (1990). Sudden death is not chaos. In S. Krasner (Ed.), *The ubiquity of chaos.* Washington, DC: American Association for the Advancement of Science.

Goldberger, A. L., Rigney, D. R., Mietus, J., Antman, E. M., & Greenwald, S. (1988). Nonlinear dynamics in sudden cardiac death syndrome: Heart rate oscillations and bifurcations. *Experientia, 44*, 983–987.

Gorman, J. M., & Sloan, R. P. (2000). Heart rate variability in anxiety and depressive disorders. *American Heart Journal, 140*, S77–S83.

Hamdan, M. H., Joglar, J. A., Page, R. L., Zagrodzky, J. D., Sheehan, C. J., Wasmund, S. L., et al. (1999). Baroreflex gain predicts blood pressure recovery during simulated ventricular tachycardia in humans. *Circulation, 100*, 381–386.

Hassett, A. L., Radvanski, D. C., Vaschillo, E. G., Vaschillo, B., Sigal, L. H., Karavidas, M. K., et al. (2007). A pilot study of heart rate variability (HRV) biofeedback in patients with fibromyalgia. *Applied Psychophysiology and Biofeedback, 32*, 1–10.

Hedelin, R., Wiklund, U., Bjerle, P., & Henriksson-Larsen, K. (2000). Pre- and post-season heart rate variability in adolescent cross-country skiers. *Scandinavian Journal of Medicine and Science in Sports*, 10, 298–303.

Herbs, D., Gevirtz, R. N., & Jacobs, D. (1993). The effect of heart rate pattern biofeedback for the treatment of essential hypertension [Abstract]. *Biofeedback and Self-Regulation*, 19, 281.

Hon, E. H., & Lee, S. T. (1965). Electronic evaluations of the fetal heart rate patterns preceding fetal death: Further observations. *American Journal of Obstetrics and Gynecology*, 87, 814–826.

Huikuri, H. V., & Makikallio, T. H. (2001). Heart rate variability in ischemic heart disease. *Autonomic Neuroscience: Basic and Clinical*, 90, 95–101.

Huikuri, H. V., Zaman, L., Castellanos, A., Kessler, K. M., Cox, M., Glicksman, F., et al. (1989). Changes in spontaneous sinus node rate as an estimate of cardiac autonomic tone during stable and unstable ventricular tachycardia. *Journal of the American College of Cardiology*, 13, 646–652.

Humphreys, P., & Gevirtz, R. (2000). Treatment of recurrent abdominal pain: Components analysis of four treatment protocols. *Journal of Pediatric Gastroenterology and Nutrition*, 31, 47–51.

Izrailtyan, I., Kresh, J. Y., Morris, R. J., Brozena, S. C., Kutalek, S. P., & Wechsler, A. S. (2000). Early detection of acute allograft rejection by linear and nonlinear analysis of heart rate variability. *Journal of Thoracic and Cardiovascular Surgery*, 120, 737–745.

James, M. A., Panerai, R. B., & Potter, J. F. (1998). Applicability of new techniques in the assessment of arterial baroreflex sensitivity in the elderly: A comparison with established pharmacological methods. *Clinical Science*, 94, 245–253.

Joseph, C. N., Porta, C., Casucci, G., Casiraghi, N., Maffeis, M., Rossi, M., et al. (2005). Slow breathing improves arterial baroreflex sensitivity and decreases blood pressure in essential hypertension. *Hypertension*, 46, 714–718.

Karavidas, M. K., Lehrer, P. M., Vaschillo, E. G., Vaschillo, B., Marin, H., Buyske, S., et al. (2007). Preliminary results of an open-label study of heart rate variability biofeedback for the treatment of major depression. *Applied Psychophysiology and Biofeedback*, 32, 19–30.

Kawachi, I., Sparrow, D., Vokonas, P. S., & Weiss, S. T. (1995). Decreased heart rate variability in men with phobic anxiety. *American Journal of Cardiology*, 75, 882–885.

Kazuma, N., Otsuka, K., Matsuoka, I., & Murata, M. (1997). Heart rate variability during 24 hours in asthmatic children. *Chronobiology International*, 14, 597–606.

La Rovere, M. T., Bigger, J. T., Jr., Marcus, F. I., Mortara, A., & Schwartz, P. J. (1998). Baroreflex sensitivity and heart-rate variability in prediction of total cardiac mortality after myocardial infarction. *Lancet*, 351(9101), 478–484.

Laitinen, T., Hartikainen, J., Niskanen, L., Geelen, G., & Länsimies, E. (1999). Sympathovagal balance is a major determinant of short-term blood pressure variability in healthy subjects. *American Journal of Physiology—Heart and Circulatory Physiology*, 276, H1245–H1252.

Lehrer, P. M., Carr, R. E., Smetankine, A., Vaschillo, E. G., Peper, E., Porges, S., et al. (1997). Respiratory sinus arrhythmia vs. neck/trapezius EMG and incentive inspirometry biofeedback for asthma: A pilot study. *Applied Psychophysiology and Biofeedback*, 22, 95–109.

Lehrer, P. M., Smetankin, A., & Potapova, T. (2000). Respiratory sinus arrhythmia biofeedback therapy for asthma: A report of 20 unmedicated pediatric cases using the Smetankin method. *Applied Psychophysiology and Biofeedback*, 25, 193–200.

Lehrer, P. M., & Taylor, G. (1974). The effects of alcohol on cardiac reactivity in alcoholics and normal subjects. *Quarterly Journal of Studies on Alcohol*, 35, 1044–1052.

Lehrer, P., Vaschillo, E., Lu, S.-E., Eckberg, D., Vaschillo, B., Scardella, A., et al. (2006). Heart rate variability biofeedback: Effects of age on heart rate variability, baroreflex gain, and asthma. *Chest*, 129, 278–284.

Lehrer, P. M., Vaschillo, E., & Vaschillo, B. (2000). Resonant frequency biofeedback training to increase cardiac variability: Rationale and manual for training. *Applied Psychophysiology and Biofeedback*, 25, 177–191.

Lehrer, P. M., Vaschillo, E., Vaschillo, B., Lu, S. E., Eckberg, D. L., Edelberg, R., et al. (2003). Heart rate variability biofeedback increases baroreflex gain and peak expiratory flow. *Psychosomatic Medicine*, *65*, 796–805.

Lehrer, P. M., Vaschillo, E., Vaschillo, B., Lu, S.-E., Scardella, A., Siddique, M., et al. (2004). Biofeedback as a treatment for asthma. *Chest*, *126*, 352–361.

Liao, D., Barnes, R. W., Chambless, L. E., Simpson, R. J., Sorlie, P., & Heiss, G. (1995). Age, race, and sex differences in autonomic cardiac function measured by spectral analysis of heart rate variability: The ARIC study. *American Journal of Cardiology*, *76*, 906–912.

Lucini, D., Milani, R. V., Costantino, G., Lavie, C. J., Porta, A., & Pagani, M. (2002). Effects of cardiac rehabilitation and exercise training on autonomic regulation in patients with coronary artery disease. *American Heart Journal*, *143*, 977–983.

Maayan, C., Axelrod, F. B., Akselrod, S., Carley, D. W., Shannon, D. C., & Shannon, C. D. (1987). Evaluation of autonomic dysfunction in familial dysautonomia by power spectral analysis. *Journal of the Autonomic Nervous System*, *21*, 51–58.

Mancia, G., Ludbrook, J., Ferrari, A., Gregorini, L., & Zanchetti, A. (1978). Baroreceptor reflexes in human hypertension. *Circulation Research*, *43*, 170–177.

Matveev, M., & Prokopova, R. (2002). Diagnostic value of the RR-variability indicators for mild hypertension. *Physiological Measurement*, *23*, 671–682.

McCraty, R., Atkinson, M., & Tomasino, D. (2003). Impact of a workplace stress reduction program on blood pressure and emotional health in hypertensive employees. *Journal of Complementary and Alternative Medicine*, *9*, 355–369.

Morguet, A., & Springer, H. J. (1981). Microcomputer-based measurement of beat-to-beat intervals and analysis of heart rate variability. *Medical Progress through Technology*, *8*, 77–82.

Myers, C. W., Cohen, M. A., Eckberg, D. L., & Taylor, J. A. (2001). A model for the genesis of arterial pressure Mayer waves from heart rate and sympathetic activity. *Autonomic Neuroscience: Basic and Clinical*, *91*, 62–75.

National Heart, Lung, and Blood Institute. (1997). *Expert panel report 2: Guidelines for the diagnosis and management of asthma*. Washington, DC: U.S. Department of Health and Human Services.

National Heart, Lung, and Blood Institute. (2002). *Expert panel report: Guidelines for the diagnosis and management of asthma: Update on selected topics*. Washington, DC: U.S. Department of Health and Human Services.

O'Brien, I. A., O'Hare, P., & Corrall, R. J. (1986). Heart rate variability in healthy subjects: Effect of age and the derivation of normal ranges for tests of autonomic function. *British Heart Journal*, *55*, 348–354.

Pardo, Y., Merz, C. N., Velasquez, I., Paul-Labrador, M., Agarwala, A., & Peter, C. T. (2000). Exercise conditioning and heart rate variability: Evidence of a threshold effect. *Clinical Cardiology*, *23*, 615–620.

Piccirillo, G., Naso, C., Moise, A., Lionetti, M., Nocco, M., Di Carlo, S., et al. (2004). Heart rate and blood pressure variability in subjects with vasovagal syncope. *Clinical Science*, *107*, 55–61.

Pitzalis, M. V., Passantino, A., Massari, F., Forleo, C., Balducci, C., Santoro, G., et al. (1999). Diastolic dysfunction and baroreflex sensitivity in hypertension. *Hypertension*, *33*, 1141–1145.

Porges, S. W. (1995). Cardiac vagal tone: A physiological index of stress. *Neuroscience and Biobehavioral Reviews*, *19*, 225–233.

Rau, H., Brody, S., Larbig, W., Pauli, P., Vohringer, M., Harsch, B., et al. (1994). Effects of PRES baroreceptor stimulation on thermal and mechanical pain threshold in borderline hypertensives and normotensives. *Psychophysiology*, *31*, 480–485.

Rau, H., Furedy, J. J., & Elbert, T. (1996). PRES- and orthostatic-induced heart rate changes as markers of labile hypertension: Magnitude and reliability measures. *Biological Psychology*, *42*, 105–115.

Robbe, H. W., Mulder, L. J., Ruddel, H., Langewitz, W. A., Veldman, J. B., & Mulder, G. (1987). Assessment of baroreceptor reflex sensitivity by means of spectral analysis. *Hypertension*, *10*, 538–543.

Robertson, D., Hollister, A. S., Biaggioni, I., Netterville, J. L., Mosqueda-Garcia, R., & Robertson, R. M. (1993). The diagnosis and treatment of baroreflex failure. *New England Journal of Medicine*, *329*, 1449–1455.

Rother, M., Zwiener, U., Eiselt, M., Witte, H., Zwacka, G., & Frenzel, J. (1987). Differentiation of healthy newborns and newborns-at-risk by spectral analysis of heart rate fluctuations and respiratory movements. *Early Human Development*, *15*, 349–363.

Rudas, L., Crossman, A. A., Morillo, C. A., Halliwill, J. R., Tahvanainen, K. U., Kuusela, T. A., et al. (1999). Human sympathetic and vagal baroreflex responses to sequential nitroprusside and phenylephrine. *American Journal of Physiology, 276,* H1691–H1698.

Rudolph, A. J., Vallbona, C., & Desmond, M. M. (1965). Cardiodynamic studies in the newborn: 3. Heart rate patterns in infants with idiopathic respiratory distress syndrome. *Pediatrics, 36,* 551–559.

Sargunaraj, D., Lehrer, P. M., Hochron, S. M., Rausch, L., Edelberg, R., & Porges, S. (1996). Cardiac rhythm effects of .125hz paced breathing through a resistive load: Implications for paced breathing therapy and Porges' poly-vagal theory. *Biofeedback and Self-Regulation, 21,* 131–147.

Schalow, G., Blanc, Y., Jeltsch, W., & Zach, G. A. (1996). Electromyographic identification of spinal oscillator patterns and recouplings in a patient with incomplete spinal cord lesion: Oscillator formation training as a method to improve motor activities. *General Physiology and Biophysics, 15*(Suppl. 1), 121–220.

Schein, M. H., Gavish, B., Herz, M., Rosner-Kahana, D., Naveh, P., Knishkowy, B., et al. (2001). Treating hypertension with a device that slows and regularizes breathing: A randomized, double-blind controlled study. *Journal of Human Hypertension, 15,* 271–278.

Schwartz, M. S., & Andrasik, F. (Eds.). (2003). *Biofeedback: A practitioner's guide* (3rd ed.). New York: Guilford Press.

Sidorov, Iu, A., & Vasilevskii, N. N. (1995). The physiological problems of biofeedback control by the pulse rate. *Neuroscience and Behavioral Physiology, 25,* 252–256.

Smith, M. L., Ellenbogen, K. A., Beightol, L. A., & Eckberg, D. L. (1991). Sympathetic neural responses to induced ventricular tachycardia. *Journal of the American College of Cardiology, 18,* 1015–1024.

Spicuzza, L., Gabutti, A., Porta, C., Montano, N., & Bernardi, L. (2000). Yoga and chemoreflex response to hypoxia and hypercapnia. *Lancet, 356,* 1495–1496.

Task Force of the European Society of Cardiology and the North American Society of Pacing and Electrophysiology. (1996). Heart rate variability: Standards of measurement, physiological interpretation and clinical use. *Circulation, 93,* 1043–1065.

Taylor, J. A., Myers, C. W., Halliwill, J. R., Seidel, H., & Eckberg, D. L. (2001). Sympathetic restraint of respiratory sinus arrhythmia: Implications for vagal–cardiac tone assessment in humans. *American Journal of Physiology—Heart and Circulatory Physiology, 280,* H2804–H2814.

Thayer, J. F., Yonezawa, Y., & Sollers, J. J., III. (2000). A system for the ambulatory recording and analysis of nonlinear heart rate dynamics. *Biomedical Sciences Instrumentation, 36,* 295–299.

Vaschillo, E., Lehrer, P., Rishe, N., & Konstantinov, M. (2002). Heart rate variability biofeedback as a method for assessing baroreflex function: A preliminary study of resonance in the cardiovascular system. *Applied Psychophysiology and Biofeedback, 27,* 1–27.

Vaschillo, E., Vaschillo, B., & Lehrer, P. (2004). Heartbeat synchronizes with respiratory rhythm only under specific circumstances. *Chest, 126,* 1385–1386.

Vaschillo, E. G., Zingerman, A. M., Konstantinov, M. A., & Menitsky, D. N. (1983). Research of the resonance characteristics for cardiovascular system. *Human Physiology, 9,* 257–265.

Vasilevskii, N. N., Sidorov, Iu. A., & Suvorov, N. B. (1993). [Role of biorhythmologic processes in adaptation mechanisms and correction of regulatory dysfunctions] [Russian]. *Fiziologii Cheloveka, 19,* 91–98.

Yasuma, F., & Hayano, J. (2004). Respiratory sinus arrhythmia: Why does the heartbeat synchronize with respiratory rhythm? *Chest, 125,* 683–690.

Yeragani, V. K., Balon, R., Pohl, R., & Ramesh, C. (1995). Depression and heart rate variability. *Biological Psychiatry, 38,* 768–770.

Zhao, G., Hintze, T. H., & Kaley, G. (1996). Neural regulation of coronary vascular resistance: Role of nitric oxide in reflex cholinergic coronary vasodilation in normal and pathophysiologic states. *EXS, 76,* 1–19.

CHAPTER 11

Neurofeedback for Stress Management

MICHAEL THOMPSON
LYNDA THOMPSON

HISTORY OF NEUROFEEDBACK

Neurofeedback (NFB) is a learning technique that leads to changes in brain wave patterns. As the electroencephalogram (EEG) changes, so does the client's behavior. Two lines of early research led to the development of NFB, one investigating consciousness and how the mind knows the brain (Kamiya, 1968, 1979) and the other applying operant conditioning techniques to the behavior of producing brain waves (Wyrwicka & Sterman, 1968).

Half a century ago, Joe Kamiya, at that time a young psychologist at the University of Chicago, demonstrated that participants could recognize when they were producing a mental state that related to particular brain wave frequencies. This work, begun in the mid-1950s, concerned alpha frequencies and eventually led to considerable research about this rhythmic, synchronized 8–12 Hz activity in the cortex. Most of the studies on alpha have concerned relaxed states, because alpha is an inverse indicator of activation; that is, when alpha is present in an area of the brain, that area is resting or in standby mode. This is easily seen when a person closes his or her eyes: There is a marked increase in alpha in the occipital regions in which visual processing is done. Studies concerning the treatment of anxiety using NFB have usually indicated successful outcomes when alpha was increased (Hardt & Kamiya, 1978; Rice, Blanchard & Purcell, 1993). Some participants, however, do not benefit from increasing alpha but do improve when alpha is decreased (Plotkin & Rice, 1981; Rice et al., 1993; Thomas & Sattlberger, 1997).

Research establishing that it was possible to train subjects to produce specific brain wave patterns was published a decade after Kamiya's experiments and came from an entirely different line of investigation being conducted with animals. A sleep researcher at the University of California at Los Angeles and the Sepulveda Veterans Administration Hospital, M. Barry Sterman, had noticed that cats, waiting for a signal before making a response that produced food, showed brain wave patterns that resembled sleep spindles. He set up experiments that rewarded the cats for producing bursts of that activity, which he named *sensorimotor rhythm* (SMR). (SMR refers to rhythmic, spindle-like EEG activity at frequencies between 12–15 Hz, the low end of the beta range, measured across the somatosensory and motor cortex of the brain, which is located across the top of the head going from ear to ear.)

Once it had been shown that operant conditioning techniques could be used to train cats to produce SMR, the learning technique known as neurofeedback, or EEG biofeedback, was ripe for further investigation. This kind of learning is based on Thorndike's law of effect: When a behavior is rewarded, it is more likely to recur. Sterman next discovered, while doing an unrelated series of experiments involving hydrazine-induced seizures, that the cats that had been rewarded with milk and chicken broth for increasing SMR were resistant to developing seizures. Sterman's research then shifted to include working with humans who had seizure disorders. Through his own studies and replications at other labs, it was established that EEG operant conditioning of particular brain wave frequencies in patients who had epilepsy could reduce the frequency, duration, and intensity of seizures in the majority of participants (about an 80% positive response rate across the various studies). A review of this work (Sterman, 2000b), as well as articles on other applications of NFB, such as for attention-deficit/hyperactivity disorder (ADHD), head injury, and depression, can be found in *Clinical Electroencephalography, 31*, published in January 2000.

In the 1970s Joel Lubar of the University of Tennessee, who was already investigating EEG in humans, took these techniques and applied them to the assessment and training of clients who exhibited symptoms of hyperactivity (Lubar & Shouse, 1976; Lubar, 1991, 2003; Lubar & Lubar, 1999). EEG changes, improved behavior, IQ increases, and improved academic performance have been reported in studies using NFB in clients with ADHD (Lubar, Swartwood, Swartwood, & O'Donnell, 1995; Linden, Habib, & Radojevic, 1996; Thompson & Thompson, 1998). Recent controlled research concerning children with ADHD, which used functional magnetic resonance imaging (fMRI) as the pre–post measure, has documented changes in specific brain areas (frontal lobes, basal ganglia, and anterior cingulate) after NFB training (Levesque, Beauregard, & Mensour, 2006). Though the precise mechanisms that produce change have not been identified, it is clear that NFB, properly applied, produces changes in neural circuits. These changes in the brain correlate with positive changes in behavior.

Applications of NFB to epilepsy and ADHD have been sufficiently studied at this point in time that NFB is deemed an efficacious treatment for these disorders (Yucha & Gilbert, 2004). Using NFB for other conditions, including stress management and optimal performance in athletes, would be considered experimental: that is to say, there is a lack of controlled studies. There are, however, promising clinical data that await corroboration through further research. NFB does have great face validity, because clients can see, by viewing feedback from a computer system that is monitoring their brain waves, how their EEG patterns correlate with their own perceptions of their mental states; for example, relaxed versus tense, focused versus daydreaming.

THEORETICAL FOUNDATIONS

Underlying Principles

In this chapter, a *stress* is defined as a circumstance that evokes in an individual a feeling that he or she cannot cope; in short, a *personally perceived potential adaptive incompetency* (Thompson, 1978). It usually involves a sense of crisis, and it is *personally* perceived in that it might not be considered a stress by other individuals; for example, some enjoy public speaking, and others find it stressful; one employee likes to keep busy with extra work, another feels an overload. Performance (*y*-axis) plotted against degree of stress (*x*-axis) produces an inverted-U-shaped curve: As stress rises, performance initially increases, then drops drastically as the stress gets higher. Hans Selye's concept of *eustress* (an optimal level of stress represented by the top of the inverted U) is relevant. Stress cannot be avoided in life, but people can be aware of what an appropriate level of stress is for them and can try to remain within that range. Being resilient and returning to a healthy baseline after a stress is the goal.

The effects of stress are seen in the individual's mental state, which can be inferred from the EEG pattern and other physiological variables (electromyography, heart rate, respiration, electrodermal response, skin temperature). Stress can be acute or chronic. It can be the result of external events (such as heavy workload, natural disasters, or loss), it can be generated internally (money worries, feelings of embarrassment or guilt, obsessive thoughts), or it can be physical (illness or chronic pain). In any case, there are typically two options for managing a stress: One takes action to change the situation that is stressful, or one changes one's response. The latter can be done through cognitive reframing (changing response in terms of attitude or cognitive set), through a different physiological response, or both. Both taking action and changing responses require appropriate, though different, mental states, as reflected in EEG patterns, and also an appropriate physiological state in order to be maximally effective. Training that includes NFB can give a person the mental edge he or she needs, with a flexible brain that can get into the appropriate state to respond to various kinds of stress. Note that this is not a static state; it changes with task demands as the stressful situation unfolds. Thus the emphasis is on a flexible brain that can activate and inhibit various mental states as needed. This is summed up in the motto of our ADD Centre: *You cannot change the wind, but you can adjust the sails.*

Another principle on which intervention for stress should be based comes from Roman times: *mens sana in corpore sano* (a sound mind in a sound body). This phrase exemplifies the idea of mind–body unity. With respect to stress management, this means that both mind and body must be flexible, that is, able to withstand stress, recover from stress, and return to a baseline characterized by a relaxed mind in tune with a relaxed body. Thus neurofeedback is not a stand-alone intervention; rather, a person trains the brain (NFB), the mind (using cognitive strategies), and the body (using regular biofeedback modalities) in order to be maximally effective and resilient.

Also keep systems theory in mind when planning intervention: When one alters any component in a system, all the other elements in the system will shift their functions in order to accomplish the goal, or function, of that system. In keeping with this principle, we often find on reassessment that functions that were not directly targeted have improved. A good example is improvement in social appropriateness in clients with ADD and in those with Asperger's syndrome after an intervention to encourage brain waves that reflect calm attentiveness to the outside world. In working with stress, when the client changes one variable, such as breathing, other variables usually adjust in the expected direction. Individual differences do occur; for example, some clients with yoga or meditation training can consciously control their breathing but without alteration in heart rate variability (HRV), skin temperature, muscle tension, or EEG variables. They still feel "stressed out," as reflected in those variables.

The final principle that underlies work with NFB is that operant conditioning of measurable neuronal variables (such as amplitude variations in various brain wave frequencies) can directly alter the biochemical and physiological underpinnings of a client's response to stress. This can result in a long-term change in one's response to stressors in daily living. To help the reader understand this better, we provide a summary of the body's stress response system.

Overview of the Neurophysiology of the Stress Response

The stress response is an adaptive biological mechanism that evolved because it was important for survival of the human species. In dangerous hunting situations, primitive man needed to have maximum energy in the large muscles of his shoulders and legs. This required an immediate increase in blood flow to these areas. He did not need to be digesting food, nor did he need much blood flow to his hands and feet. Thus blood vessels in the fingertips would constrict and heart rate would increase. Additionally, hands had to be moist so that his spear would not slip. The sympathetic nervous system is responsible for these fight-or-flight reactions (cool, moist palms with increased heart rate), and they occur in the acute phase of stress.

The stress response is controlled by interactions from the brain stem (especially the locus coeruleus) through to the frontal lobes. There is an amygdala–hypothalamus–pituitary–adrenal (AHPA) axis, with the frontal lobes and hippocampus having a major influence through connections to the amygdala and hypothalamus. This AHPA axis influences the sympathetic nervous system and thus the fight–flight response. An excellent overview of this process is given by Smith-Pellettier (2002), a detailed exposition of which is summarized in Thompson and Thompson (2003). Smith-Pellettier notes that, when overstressed, this AHPA system can become dysregulated. Hypoactivity may result in symptoms of anxiety, fibromyalgia, and chronic pain. Lower levels of the analgesic actions of hypothalamic corticotropin-releasing hormone (CRH) could contribute to the pain. Hyperactivity of this AHPA axis, with resultant increased CRH, has been implicated in depression. There is increased response sensitivity to noxious stimuli and decreased immune system response. The immune response is dampened by glucocorticoids (GC). Chronic stress increases GC, suppresses the immune response, and may even lead to a reduction in the size of the thymus and a reduction in circulating lymphocytes. The symptoms of overactivity in the AHPA axis are familiar to anyone in the mental health field. These clients exhibit a narrowing of their perspective that, in turn, produces a focus on their own preoccupations, ruminative thinking, and poor cognitive performance. Due to stress, their sleep is impaired, which further compounds their difficulties. There are male–female differences in this process, with the AHPA axis and CRH activity being generally higher in females. This might make females more susceptible to the negative effects of insomnia and stress. Aging is another factor; the elderly experience frequent awakening, decreased growth hormone secretion, and a decrease in deep or slow-wave sleep, with a concomitant decrease in immune regeneration and a reduction in the pain threshold.

The principle components of the APHA axis are all unconscious and automatic. However, the cortex has a major input to this axis. Perhaps the most central and clearest controlling influence comes from the anterior cingulate. The anterior cingulate is an area of the cortex that has major linkages to the frontal lobes (particularly the medial and orbital surfaces of the frontal lobes) and is linked to all areas of the APHA axis and to other key control areas, such as the thalamus.

Neurophysiologically, what appears to be common to the EEGs of clients who present with anxiety and/or panic and with whom we have done 19-channel EEG assessment is high-amplitude, high-frequency beta (> 20 Hz). When this is analyzed using LORETA (low-resolution electromagnetic tomographic assessment), the anterior cingulate and, in particular, Brodmann's area 24 is usually seen to be the source of this unusual EEG activity. (For a review of LORETA literature, see Pascual-Marqui, Esslen, Kochi, & Lehmann, 2002.)

The case example shown in Figures 11.1 and 11.2 was a 50-year-old woman who presented with a history of anxiety, occasionally panic; generally, her emotions were quite labile. She had very high ratios; for example, the 3-minute sample that the figures display showed 23–35 Hz/13–15 Hz = 2.52. (We find that > 1.55 correlates with ruminating or a very "busy brain.") The ratio 19–22 Hz/11–12 Hz was 3.05. (We find that > 1.0 usually correlates with anxiety or intensity.) In light of our previous discussion of the effects of drugs on the EEG, it is of interest that the patient reported that stimulants, benzodiazepines, and selective serotonin reuptake inhibitors (SSRIs) had all precipitated terrible panic attacks. The spindling beta may represent an irritable cortex, and benzodiazepines could increase the beta spindling. She was medication-free at the time of this recording.

The anterior cingulate is central to affect regulation and control, as well as having executive functions. Among the connections of the anterior cingulate are those to premotor areas, spinal cord, red nucleus, and locus coeruleus. It is said to have more connections with the thalamus than any other part of the brain. Through its connections to autonomic brainstem motor nuclei it exerts control over the sympathetic and parasympathetic portions of the autonomic nervous system. It also has a major influence over endocrine responses through its connections to all parts of the limbic system, including the amygdala, hypothalamus, and periaqueductal gray matter. Thus it has intimate connec-

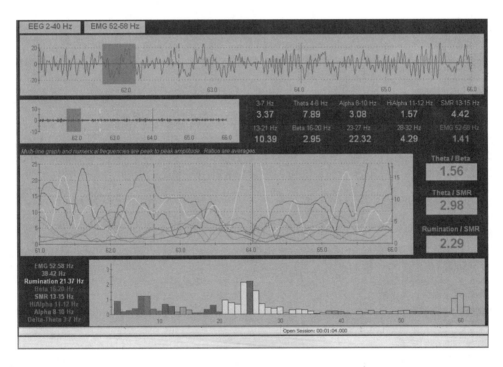

FIGURE 11.1. EEG beta spindling at FCz. This client presented with anxiety and panic. Beta spindles are seen at 63.8 seconds (frequency of 25 Hz) and at 65.5 seconds.

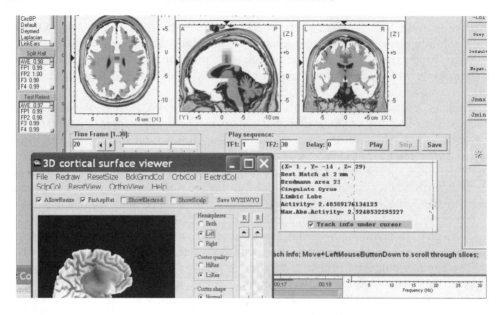

FIGURE 11.2. LORETA image. In this anxious client, high-amplitude beta activity at 20 Hz was observed. LORETA analysis suggested that the best fit for a source was in the anterior cingulate, Brodmann area 23 and 24. The activity was 2.5 *SD* greater than the database mean using Neuroguide (NG).

tions to the AHPA axis. The anterior cingulate can therefore be thought of as the neurological "hub" of our affective control system. It is central in discrimination tasks that concern the motivational content of internal and external stimuli. It is engaged in response selection, cognitively demanding information processing, and motor actions (Devinsky, Morrell, & Vogt, 1995).

From Theory to Practical Application

Stress, particularly chronic stress, is associated with a number of negative effects. Biofeedback has been demonstrated to be helpful in decreasing the symptoms caused by stress, as discussed in other chapters in this book. It is likely that future work will demonstrate that combining NFB with biofeedback may assist clients to even more effectively self-regulate their responses to stress in their daily lives.

　　The approach to applying this combination, as described in this chapter, has the goal of assisting the client to achieve a *state of physiological readiness*, followed by a *state of mental readiness*, and, finally, a *state of active mental work*. This approach is not about relaxation but, rather, about true management of stress for effective everyday functioning.

ASSESSMENT

Assessments should include all of the measures that are relevant to assisting your client in meeting his or her objectives, which means that you begin by taking a clinical history and discussing goals before doing measurements of both EEG and physiological parameters.

Listening to the clients' stories first is crucial, following the adage that they must know that you care before they care what you know. The approach used for stress management combines NFB (training the brain) with peripheral biofeedback. Using these measures, you can design and periodically evaluate a training program for stress management that is very similar to the training program used to help executives and athletes optimize their performance. The goal is to be able to achieve a mental state that is relaxed yet alert, calm, focused, and able to solve problems. Returning to this state of relaxed attentiveness after a period of stress is a sign of resiliency. The key to efficiently and effectively handling stress is the ability to self-regulate one's mental and physiological state throughout each day. NFB plus biofeedback provides the tools to do that.

Look at the raw EEG and also at quantitative EEG (QEEG); that is, mathematical calculations concerning the amount of activity across different bandwidths. The bandwidths are described in terms of frequency ranges, with frequencies measured according to cycles (complete waves) per second. The unit of measurement is Hertz (Hz). EEG frequencies are much slower than those used in EMG, often 2 to 45 Hz, with a higher range monitored to gauge whether EMG artifact is affecting the signal. Using a range of 2 to 62 Hz is helpful for the latter purpose. Table 11.1 gives both the frequency ranges and Greek letter designations commonly used.

How do you discern that a person is experiencing stress using the EEG? This topic has not yet received adequate research, and in this chapter we are sharing clinical observations, not established findings concerning this question. Our observation is that anxiety and emotional intensity usually correspond to an increase in 19–22 Hz activity found in conjunction with a decrease in 15–18 Hz activity measured with EEG recorded from a single electrode on top of the head (Cz). This is easily seen when the raw EEG, which is graphed as a line showing amplitude over time, is transformed into a spectral array that plots the amount of electrical activity, either magnitude (average amplitude) in microvolts (millionths of a volt) or power in picowatts (pW), across frequencies. Ruminating is also associated with higher beta frequencies. The specific frequency range that is elevated can be quite narrow and will be above 22 Hz, sometimes in a range as high as 32–37 Hz. This higher beta is often seen in conjunction with a decrease in SMR activity. The EEG of someone under stress usually corresponds to a decrease in both 11–12 Hz (alpha) and 13–15 Hz activity (SMR), and there may also be an increase in the amplitude of the EEG somewhere between 23 and 35 Hz (compared with activity immediately above and below that bandwidth). Bursts of increased high beta in the low 20s seem to be a state marker—the person reports feeling intense. The bursts of activity in frequencies in the mid-20s to low 30s may indicate that the person has what we term a "busy brain," which, in some, may correspond to worrying and ruminations. These patterns may be associated with clients who say they have trouble falling asleep because they cannot turn off their thinking.

EEG Assessment

Overview

The EEG acts like a "flag" that reflects brain functioning. Just as you infer from a flag's activity the wind's velocity and direction, you make inferences about the brain's activity by reading the EEG. One goal for assessment is to ascertain what is different from expected ("normal") patterns in your client's EEG so that you may decide on an EEG normalization training program. If you are in doubt about the pattern that you see when doing a 19-lead assessment, you can compare characteristics of the EEG in different frequency bands with expected age norms using databases. However, database norms for

TABLE 11.1. EEG Bandwidths and Correlation to Mental States

Frequency bands	Correlations at Cz and FCz
1–3 Hz; delta	Dominant activity in Stage IV sleep. Electrode movement, eye movement, or eye blink artifact all mimic delta. May be increased in awake EEG in those with brain damage and in learning disabilities.
4–5 Hz; low theta	Tuned out. Sleepy.
6–7 Hz; high theta	Internal orientation, may be creative but will not recall ideas for very long after emerging from this mental state. Not focused on external learning, such as reading or listening. Important in memory retrieval. Visualization is associated with 7 to 8 Hz activity.
8–10 Hz; low alpha	Internally oriented. Increased in some types of meditation. Around 9 Hz one may experience "dissociation."
11–12 Hz; high alpha	Correlates with a very alert, broad awareness state. Seen especially in high-level athletes when "in the zone." High intelligence associated with higher peak alpha frequency plus higher amplitude (at rest) and greater desynchronization when on task.
13–21 Hz; beta	Broad band of beta. Used in theta–beta power ratios for ADHD evaluations.
12–15 Hz; SMR when measured across the sensorimotor strip (C3, Cz, C4)	Correlates with inhibition of motor output and sensory input combined with a mental state that maintains alertness and focus. A calm state, with decreased anxiety and impulsivity, and improved immune function.
16–20 Hz; beta	Correlates with active problem solving and cognitive or motor activity. For most people, conscious thinking and problem solving are associated with 16–18 Hz activity. (Note: More beta is required when you are learning a task than after you have mastered it.)
19–22 Hz; high beta	Correlates with emotional "intensity" (which may, in some cases, be anxiety).
23–36 Hz; high beta	Correlates with a "busy brain." This can be related to work, or it may represent negative ruminating in some individuals. Elevated mid-20s activity may correlate with family history of alcoholism or addiction.
40 Hz ("Sheer rhythm"); gamma	Daniel Sheer (1977) related this to attention and cognitive function—a "binding" rhythm. Increasing it may help learning disabilities. A burst at 40 Hz occurs as you regain balance.
45–58 Hz	Range often monitored to reflect scalp, jaw, and neck muscle activity. "EMG inhibit" range. (Use inhibit at 53–59 Hz in Asia, Australia, Europe)
60 Hz (50 Hz in Europe, Asia, and Australia)	Usually electrical interference.

EEG in active tasks, such as reading and math, are very limited. They are available in the SKIL program from Sterman-Kaiser Imaging Labs (Sterman, 1999). Databases are available for eyes-closed EEG from a number of sources, such those created by Frank Duffy, E. Roy John, Robert Thatcher, or William Hudspeth (Duffy, Iyer, & Surwillo, 1989; Duffy, Hughes, Miranda, Bernod, & Cook, 1994; Lorensen & Dickson, 2003). If there is any concern about a primary medical condition, such as a seizure disorder, head injury, and so on, your client must be seen and assessed by a neurologist before undertaking EEG biofeedback. The QEEG that you are doing is typically being done to look at data concerning *normal* brain waves. Assessing, or even recognizing, abnormal waveforms or patterns is the task of a specially trained neurologist.

To assess your client's EEG, it is helpful to do an EEG assessment profile that plots the average power across frequencies during an artifacted sample as a histogram or graph. This can be done with data from a single active site, such as the vertex. A mathematical calculation (a fast Fourier transform, or FFT) changes the raw EEG information, which is displayed as amplitude over time, into the frequency domain, plotted as average power across the various frequencies (e.g., 2–62 Hz). This enables the practitioner to design EEG biofeedback intervention that is individualized for each client. Because the EEG can show different patterns depending on the conditions under which it is recorded, the gold standard for doing an assessment is to do four conditions: eyes closed, eyes open, reading, and math. A challenging mental math task constitutes a stress for most people, and you can use that to look at EEG changes with stress.

Method

Placement of electrodes follows a worldwide standardized arrangement called the International 10–20 Electrode Placement System (Jasper, 1958; see Figure 11.3). Note that newer references may use updated designations for some sites; namely, T3 becomes T7,

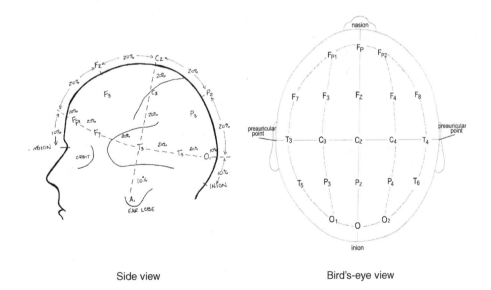

Side view   Bird's-eye view

FIGURE 11.3. International 10–20 Electrode Placement System. From Thompson and Thompson (2003). Copyright 2003 by Michael Thompson and Lynda Thompson. Reprinted by permission.

and T5 becomes P7 on the left. On the right, T4 becomes T8, and T6 becomes P8. New terminology is based on the modified combinatorial nomenclature of the American Clinical Neurophysiology Society (Fisch, 1999). There is also an expanded 10–20 system that has names for sites between these basic ones. EEG for research purposes is sometimes recorded with dense arrays, such as 256 leads, for greater spatial resolution.

CHOOSING ELECTRODE PLACEMENTS FOR ASSESSMENT

The initial assessment can use 1, 2, or 19 or more channels (*Full-Cap*). Your decision will depend on the complexity of the case being assessed, your equipment, and your experience. The most common placement for an initial single-channel recording is Cz, the vertex. This site is less influenced by artifact because it is far from the eyes (eye-blink and eye-movement artifacts) and from the jaws (a common source of muscle artifact). Cz is also furthest from the ear reference so that there is less common mode rejection and you can record higher amplitude activity than you would at sites closer to the earlobe. It provides information about activation (or lack of it) in the central region and across the sensorimotor strip. It also often picks up frontal beta spindling and other high-frequency beta activity that may correspond to the effects of stress on your client. If your client has ADHD, which is characterized by excess theta in frontal and central regions, this can also be readily seen at the Cz location. You will miss such things as differences between the hemispheres.

   For clinicians who do not have 19-channel equipment, a second channel or a second assessment can usefully be carried out at FCz (halfway between Fz and Cz), F3 and/or F4. This will sometimes pick up either high-amplitude "thalpha" (6–10 Hz) or high-amplitude higher frequency beta (19–36 Hz) activity that had not been seen at Cz. This can be very helpful with clients who present due to difficulties coping with stress. A two-channel assessment, one channel at F3 and a second channel at F4, with either a Cz or a linked-ears common reference, can be helpful in assessing dysphoria or depression that may underlie a susceptibility to stress. Less activation in the left frontal lobe, as compared with the right frontal lobe, has been identified by Richard Davidson as a pattern associated with a focus on negative thoughts and avoidance behavior (Davidson, 1995). It may also indicate overactivation of the right frontal lobe, a pattern observed in some clients who present with anxiety and panic (Weidmann et al., 1999). Anxiety and vulnerability to stress is characteristic of clients who exhibit symptoms associated with Asperger syndrome (AS). A two-channel assessment comparing P3 with P4 activity or T5 with T6 activity in those with AS may demonstrate high-amplitude slow waves in the right parietal and temporal areas at P4 and T6. This corresponds to the difficulties those with AS have with spatial reasoning and with interpreting emotion and innuendo. They have brilliant vocabularies, yet they take things very literally, corresponding to their stronger left hemisphere's logical, analytic processing.

CAUTIONS REGARDING INTERPRETATION OF FINDINGS

If one does not carefully remove artifacts, the data may be distorted in a way that makes either normal theta or beta to appear abnormally high. For example, 4–8 Hz activity may be high due to electrode movement, eye movement, or eye blinks that affect not just delta but also lower theta frequencies. This would give a false impression of a high theta–beta ratio, the latter being indicative of ADHD. Beta activity may appear high due to muscle tension, giving a false impression of a low theta–beta ratio or of high amplitude, high-frequency beta, which might be misinterpreted as reflecting stress with anxiety or ruminating.

Medications may also distort EEG findings. Even supposedly nonsedating antihistamines (commonly used by clients for allergy relief) may cause high-amplitude theta waves. In the example of Diane, later in the chapter, her 4–8/16–20 ratio moved from 2.1 to 3.4 when she took a small dose of over-the-counter antihistamine medication. Your client might be on a benzodiazepine for anxiety or an antidepressant for a mood disorder. Benzodiazepines and SSRIs may increase beta activity—particularly beta over 20 Hz. They may also decrease alpha. Tricyclic antidepressants may increase asynchronous slow waves and may even result in some spike and wave activity. Lithium can increase asynchronous slow waves. If you are working with teenagers and young adults, you may find that some self-medicating activity is taking place to try to relieve stress. Marijuana will increase alpha, and this may be observed in the EEG even 1–2 days after use. People with alcohol problems can show increased beta above 20 Hz and decreased theta and alpha as a baseline, but the alpha increases when they have a drink. Medication effects on the EEG is a complex topic, but the message is that many clients who come wanting to relieve stress may also have tried prescription and nonprescription drugs. Although these drug influences may seem disconcerting, they are usually easily seen, and the practitioner may, to a large extent, decrease their influence on the 19-channel EEG assessment by using an assessment program such as Neuroguide that allows one to switch to a Laplacian montage in which the electrode is compared with those electrodes that surround it, thus cancelling out effects that are in common to all sites. However, you do need to know what the client is taking and recognize that it may have an effect on your EEG assessment. Always ask what medications a client is taking.

You can also misinterpret data if you do not look at the raw EEG and pay adequate attention to the morphology of the waveforms. For example, alpha is usually a relatively high-amplitude, sinusoidal wave. Mu waves occur in the same frequency range, but the morphology differs because one end of the wave (either peak or trough) will be pointed rather than both ends being rounded. Location and reactivity also help distinguish waveforms. If you do not look carefully at the entire raw EEG, you may also miss other very important EEG changes. For example, a quantitative analysis of EEG that contained a brief absence seizure (spike and after-following slow-wave activity that occurs at 3 cycles per second) would give the false impression of very high delta activity (the slow waves) and some increase in high-frequency beta activity (due to the spikes). There is simply no substitute for a careful analysis of the raw, dynamic EEG. Being able to see a mathematically derived spectrum, plotting frequencies by power, is helpful in discerning a client's patterns, but only after you have carefully looked at and artifacted the raw EEG.

DECIDING ON REWARD AND INHIBIT FREQUENCY BANDS: USING THE DECISION PYRAMID

The decision pyramid (Figure 11.4) covers the components of an assessment. These include client goals and the assessment of EEG amplitudes at different frequencies. It suggests that with some clients you may additionally wish to do a *psychophysiological stress profile* to glean information about the autonomic nervous system and EMG changes with stress. It requires that we use the assessment information in conjunction with knowledge of neurophysiology and anatomy in order to derive appropriate placements of sensors for training. The top of the pyramid, regarding communication between areas of the cortex, is relevant when 19 lead assessments are done and the data are compared with a normal database. The triangle at the base of the pyramid applies to all NFB work.

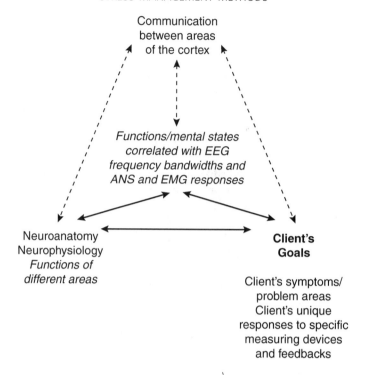

FIGURE 11.4. Decision-making pyramid for neurofeedback parameters. From Thompson and Thompson (2003). Copyright 2003 by Michael Thompson and Lynda Thompson. Reprinted by permission.

OVERVIEW OF INTERPRETATION OF FINDINGS USING DIFFERENT TYPES OF ASSESSMENT

Single-Channel Findings. When dealing with stress management in a person who does not have any suspected brain pathology, a single-channel assessment is usually adequate to guide training. You are checking to see which frequencies need to be enhanced (those that are deemed to be too low) and which need to be decreased (those that are initially too high). With a referential montage, with the active electrode placed at Fz, Cz, or Pz and referenced to one ear with the ground on the other ear, you can be reasonably certain that the electrical activity recorded reflects the cortical activity under the electrode placed on the scalp. It is unlikely that you will have a false positive result. On the other hand, you may have a false negative, because significant activity (either too high or too low) may be occurring at a different site in the cortex (e.g., F3 or F4). An example would be a client who experiences panic when subjected to stress who shows overactivation and beta spindling only in the right frontal area. This might not be seen at a midline location.

With a *sequential* (formerly called *bipolar*) montage, in which both electrodes are on the scalp (for example, Fz and Cz) with a ground on an ear, you will not know which of the two electrodes on the scalp has the higher amplitude electrical activity under it. One only knows only that a potential difference exists, without knowing which is higher. Indeed, it could be that there is no difference between the two waves at the two sites in terms of type of activity but a potential difference (voltage) is being recorded because they are not in phase. Amplitudes will be lower than with a referential montage because of common mode rejection done by the differential amplifier in the electroencephalograph.

(Activity that is common at the two sites is not amplified, whereas that which is different is amplified.) In some cases you may want to use sequential placement to reduce unwanted artifact that is common to both sites, such as cardiac or EMG artifact.

Two-Channel Findings. Two-channel results may clarify differences between two different areas of the brain. However, special caution must be exerted to ensure that impedances are the same for all electrode placements before findings at different sites are compared. Again, many areas of the brain are ignored, and findings are therefore still quite limited. As another caution, be sure that the influence of muscle tension artifact is approximately the same for both sites. This can be very subtle and can make beta activity for the site at which there is more EMG influence appear (falsely) high compared with the other site. It is easier and better to compare two sites using two channels with a common reference using a special linked ear reference electrode. Alternatively, do a 19-channel assessment, in which the whole picture can be seen.

Full-Cap (19-or-More-Channel) Findings. These findings are obviously more complex and complete. Different sites may be compared and thus communication between areas of the brain elucidated. However, as previously noted, it takes many years of experience to accurately interpret the findings. Each way of referencing the electrodes will yield slightly different information. Unusual sites of high- or low-amplitude activity at different frequencies can be distinguished. Hyper- or hypocommunication between areas of the brain can be evaluated and compared with normal databases. All of these findings will provide additional suggestions for NFB training.

Low-Resolution Electromagnetic Tomographic Assessment. This method of EEG analysis is a mathematical program that uses the surface EEG to infer which structures deeper in the cortex are the source of the electrical activity being measured. LORETA's ability to pinpoint the origins of EEG activity that stems from deeper structures of the brain is still being investigated. LORETA was developed by Roberto Pascual-Marqui of the Key Institute in Zurich. It can be obtained free of charge over the Internet. Programs such as Neuroguide(NG) allow the user to move directly into LORETA analysis. The Neuroguide database also offers z-scores for LORETA and enables the practitioner to correlate surface EEG magnitude and z-score findings with the hypothesized ("best fit") source of these EEG differences and see how they differ from the normal database.

Advantages of Doing Assessments with a Spectrum Going to 62 Hz. Negative ruminating may be reflected in high-amplitude activity between 23 and 36 Hz (infrequently, this may be at a slightly higher frequency), as discussed earlier. Constructive cognitive activity, on the other hand, may be reflected in activity both between 16 and 19 Hz and also around 40 Hz (Sheer rhythm), which is considered by some to be a "binding" rhythm. The problem is that beta frequencies are prone to the effects of EMG (muscle) artifact. The influence of muscle can usually be distinguished from beta and gamma bursts by examining the effect of EMG on the activity across all the higher frequencies going right up to 62 Hz. Electrical interference at 60 Hz (50 Hz in Asia, Australia, and Europe) can also be evaluated. If you look only at activity going up to 32 Hz (and some databases for full-cap assessments go up only to the mid-20s), then you will have more trouble distinguishing EMG artifact from elevations in higher beta frequencies that are due to true cortical activity.

Quality Data Collection. The following tips apply to data acquisition, whether it is done through 1 channel or 19. They also apply whether one is doing an assessment or running a training session. Training outcomes are going to be influenced by the quality of the feedback, which depends first and foremost on the quality of the EEG information. So it is good to make it a habit to be careful about site preparation (abrade gently with an EEG prep material, such as NuPrep, to remove such things as surface skin cells or hair spray that could act as insulators, and then use a conductive gel or paste, such as 10–20 Conductive Paste, for each of your electrodes). Aim to meet research standards of impedance readings that are all below 5 Kohms and, if possible, within 1 Kohm of each other. Checking impedance is very important if you want to do good quality work, and you cannot just slap on electrodes without prepping when using most equipment for NFB. (There are special saline electrodes used in research using dense arrays of > 100 electrodes that do not require the same kind of prepping, but that is quite different equipment than is generally used for NFB.)

Autonomic Nervous System and Muscle Tension Assessment

Goal of the Stress Assessment

In addition to the EEG changes, differences are also observed in physiological variables. It is very simple to show how even a small stress can result in a decrease in peripheral skin temperature, an increase in skin conduction, muscle tension, and heart rate, and a respiratory pattern that is shallow, rapid, and irregular. HRV is not in synchrony with respiration. The client can then see that, with appropriate diaphragmatic breathing and a relaxed mental state, he or she can rapidly shift these variables to produce a healthier pattern.

The goal of the EEG and stress assessment (autonomic nervous system and EMG assessment) is to discover how a particular client responds to and recovers from mental stress. These findings may then be used to set up both neurofeedback and biofeedback interventions to help that client self-regulate, that is, control his or her own mental and physiological responses even under stressful circumstances. In addition, practicing this control may produce an automatic, unconscious, beneficial change in that client's response to stress in the future. The objective is to help your client produce an optimal state of mental and physiological functioning at will. In this state the client is both relaxed and alert. This will broaden associative capabilities and perspective, decrease fatigue, allow calm reflection on alternative approaches to tasks, and, when combined with high levels of alertness, improve reaction time and increase response accuracy. The individual will be flexible in terms of mental state and resilient in terms of physiology.

In the first or second interview, after EEG parameters have been set, we use a structured interview process with the client to fill out a single-page questionnaire. The format is an assessment profile called the TOPS evaluation (Tools for Optimal Performance States), and it outlines the variables that we can measure and use to give feedback. (This form is found in Figure 11.7 on page 273, in which the method of intervention is outlined.)

Description of a Quick Stress Test

This is not a research assessment protocol, and you can modify it to suit your needs. It is a practical, clinical approach to clarify what general biofeedback modalities, if any, are going to be important, in addition to NFB, in training a particular client. We want to observe changes in respiration, including rate, depth, and regularity. We like to be able to see the same types of changes in heart rate: regularity, rate, and extent of variability in heart rate. To do this requires a computer feedback screen that shows respiration and the heart rate variations that occur with inspiration and expiration as line graphs. It is desirable, with the client, to be able to correlate these changes visually with changes in peripheral skin temperature, electrodermal response (EDR, a measure of arousal dependent on sweat), and muscle tension (EMG). The psychophysiological feedback screen illustrated in Figure 11.5 is a helpful way to display the data and monitor responses during the stress assessment. The practitioner can watch this screen while the client is watching a neutral spot. The screen can be used to give the client feedback during the final portion of the assessment, when the practitioner is guiding relaxation with paced breathing.

In the stress assessment, we want the client to begin in as relaxed a manner as possible to establish a baseline. We explain that we are going to ask him or her to carry out two tasks that are meant to be stressful, that is, emotionally uncomfortable. After each task, he or she will sit for 2 minutes and just relax and think of something pleasurable (recovery period). The first stressor is to think about and, if possible, mentally experience a very stressful event. This can be done with eyes open or closed, whichever is more comfortable for the client. (If imagining a stress seems unsuitable for your client for any reason, then use the Stroop color test as the first stressor—which, of course, would be done with eyes open.) Next, the client rests (recovery) for 2 minutes. This is followed by a sec-

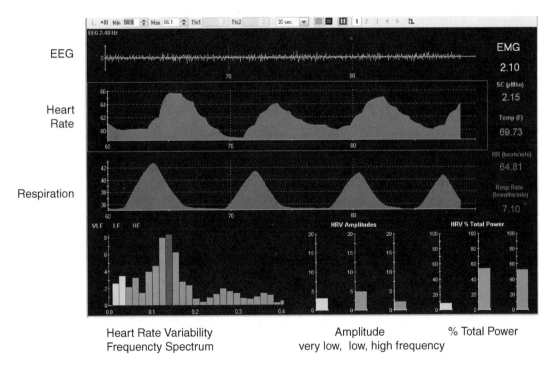

FIGURE 11.5. Example of screen for psychophysiological feedback. The figure shows a client early in training. As training progresses, the client will try to shift heart rate variability, in the spectrum shown, to 0.1 cycles/second. Skin temperature will rise to somewhere between 90 and 95 degrees, and the EMG will drop to less than 1.5.

ond stressor, a mental math problem that you make challenging. The client then rests again for 2 minutes. Then the client is asked to open his or her eyes (if they had been closed) and to work on some relaxation techniques with guidance regarding how to breathe. Pace the client to breathe diaphragmatically at about six breaths per minute. Also include instructions to relax the muscles and feel warmth in the hands. Your aim is for the client to achieve a degree of synchrony between HRV and breathing, known as respiratory sinus arrhythmia (RSA). Then the summary graph of the whole time period (Figure 11.6) is reviewed with the client to show him or her how his or her body's physiology responded to each phase of the test. The trainer must be careful to help the client distinguish between overbreathing and relaxed, "effortless" breathing. Overbreathing (hyperventilation) is a potentially serious side effect that may be avoided by emphasizing that breathing should be effortless and comfortable and that the next breath should be only taken when the "need" is felt. If you are doing this work with clients, you would be well advised to review the literature on this subject.

Figure 11.6 illustrates a classic stress response and then a relaxation response. This client's response to stress included increased heart rate and fast, irregular, and shallow respiration. Her skin conduction rose, and peripheral skin temperature fell. This client was able to demonstrate quick control of these variables after being reassured and asked to breathe along with the trainer at six breaths per minute in the last 2 minutes of the test. She was able to see the synchrony between her HRV and her breathing on the feedback screen shown in Figure 11.5.

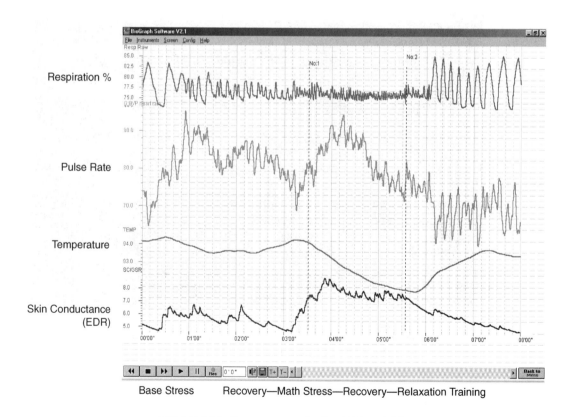

FIGURE 11.6. Summary graphs for ANS variables.

SIDE EFFECTS AND CONTRAINDICATIONS TO INTERVENTION
Neurofeedback Side Effects

In general, it appears that NFB is a safe, noninvasive intervention that rarely produces negative side effects. Out of approximately 2,000 clients and more than 80,000 hours of training over the past decade, we can relate one incident of a side effect in an adult that might have been related to NFB training. In this case, a senior executive who had recently started training for optimal performance felt "spaced out" and was unable to chair a meeting with his usual intensity. He had abruptly left his training session when he recalled the meeting time. On reviewing the incident later, we felt he might have trained too hard to lower his very high 21 Hz activity and inadvertently raised alpha, especially 9 Hz activity, and put himself into a dissociated state.

As to other potential side effects, it is theoretically possible that, if you are encouraging theta increases, as is done, for example, in alpha–theta work with alcoholics, you might precipitate a seizure in a vulnerable client as that client becomes drowsy. With alpha–theta work, you must also be able to handle abreactions, as theta is a state in which the unconscious becomes more accessible. This could be considered a side effect, though in some instances it is actually encouraged as part of therapy. There are, for example, analysts who use EEG feedback to help their patients get into a hypnagogic state between sleep and wakefulness, a mental state in which the person in analysis can access free associations and dreamlike states. This state allows memories and fantasies to emerge, and therein lies its potential for use in psychotherapy and work with positive replacement imaging (Peniston & Kulkosky, 1990) as well as its danger. The danger is that any suggestion occurring in this state can solidify the mixture of fantasy and memory, with the unfortunate production of "false memories." (Alpha–theta work is not usually done in our ADD Centre, as we characterize our NFB work as educational—learning self-regulation skills—rather than as therapy.) People doing "neurotherapy" and adding other potentially helpful techniques, such as audiovisual stimulation or brain-blood-flow biofeedback (HEG), might see more side effects with patients than we do with our clients, who are primarily learning to reduce slow-wave activity, especially theta, while increasing calm attentiveness that is associated with increased SMR and/or beta in the 13–19 Hz range.

Some people who use NFB say that a client can become overactive after a session in which they have been training beta. With respect to side effects, one must be aware of the power of suggestion, and this is particularly true in clients with ADHD who have, generally speaking, higher hypnotizability in line with their excess theta activity. It is possible that a therapist could unwittingly impart expectations to clients by asking the clients to tell him or her whether the training makes them agitated or more excitable. Increased excitability has not been our experience with beta training in the 15–18 Hz range, except on a single occasion, when a student whose prescribed training was for SMR enhancement was inadvertently trained on a screen for beta enhancement. The client's mother reported that her daughter was much bouncier than usual on the car trip home. One experienced clinician has reported that training to increase beta over the left hemisphere in children with reactive attachment disorder can worsen their behavior (Budzynski, personal communication, 1998).

It is true that NFB training is frequency specific and site specific, so, theoretically, if one were to train the wrong frequencies at a particular site, then one could get negative results or side effects. When cats, in Sterman's early experiments, were trained to decrease SMR activity rather than to increase it, they became twitchy. Two early research studies employing an A-B-A design, one with hyperkinetic children and one with adults who had epilepsy, showed improvement during the treatment phase, worsening when the contingencies were reversed, and improvement when the correct treatment was again given. Training the wrong frequencies should not, of course, happen if you have assessed your client and individualized his or her training.

A kind of side effect—which could be either positive or negative depending on circumstances—is that family relationships and interpersonal relationships will change as a person's behavior changes in response to NFB.

With respect to contraindications, it has been the experience of many clinicians that children in families that are dysfunctional are not good candidates for NFB training. NFB is a kind of learning, and a person must have emotional energy for learning. This energy may not be available if a child is preoccupied with a difficult situation at home. Money might be better spent on family therapy. The same principles would apply to working with adult clients.

Biofeedback Side Effects

Biofeedback actually has more side effects than NFB, especially when it is used in conjunction with relaxation training. As mentioned earlier, there is, for example, the danger of "overbreathing" (hyperventilation) with resultant hypocapnea (decreased partial pressure of carbon dioxide in the bloodstream). When some clients are asked to breathe diaphragmatically, they may, in their eagerness to follow the trainer's instructions, breathe too deeply. This may also occur with anxiety.

Hypocapnea may have a number of negative effects. The increased bonding of oxygen to hemoglobin in red blood cells results in a poor release of oxygen (Bhor effect) to the brain and heart. Cerebral vasoconstriction occurs. The increased alkalinity from pH of 7.4 to 7.5 (normal is 7.38–7.4) can decrease blood flow by 50%, and the alkalosis can result in hyperexcitability and a compromise of the blood buffering system and, therefore, impaired ability to regulate acidosis. The overall result is cerebral hypoxia and cerebral glucose deficit. Thus the combined effect of these factors is to lower oxygenation of the brain and change the mineral balance. Calcium, potassium, and magnesium tend to move into the cells, resulting in irritability of nerves and muscles. There may be metabolic effects with sustained overbreathing, including an increased release of adrenaline and noradrenaline that will, in turn, result in increased blood glucose, fatty acids, low-density lipoprotein (LDL) cholesterol, and insulin release. These changes can result in coronary artery spasms and a rise in blood pressure.

Unfortunately, the chemical changes can occur in minutes, and your client may be unaware that anything is wrong. The early signs of overbreathing include: lightheadedness, tingling skin, tightness of the chest, sweaty hands, breathlessness, a restless mind, and memory loss; ordinary lights appear brighter, and sounds may seem louder than usual. The client may startle more easily and even display muscle twitching. These symptoms may, in themselves, arouse apprehension, anxiety, fear, panic, emotional lability (disinhibition), anger, and fear of losing control. Thus, if diaphragmatic breathing results in hyperventilation, it can exacerbate the very condition you are attempting to relieve. If the client persists in overbreathing outside of your office situation, it may result in impairment of cognition, decision-making skills, memory, focus, and concentration. There may also be some impairment of perceptual–motor skills and an increase in fatigue. The effect on the EEG is an increase in theta activity. Overbreathing could also precipitate a seizure or migraine headache. Other rare possible effects of overbreathing are a constriction of smooth muscles with an exacerbation of asthma or irritable bowel syndrome. Although this side effect of overbreathing is a very rare one, it is important to watch your clients carefully and ensure that they are breathing comfortably. A small number of practitioners measure CO_2. However, most practitioners find that they do not have a problem if they warn their clients about the early signs of overbreathing and make sure that the client takes the next breath only when he or she feels the need to breathe.

Relaxation training can result in a client experiencing discomfort while relaxing if he or she is not used to that experience. A less often discussed side effect of biofeedback training for relaxation is a loss of alertness. In our work with clients who complain of the effects of stress, we emphasize how the client can optimize his or her performance despite the frequent stressors found in everyday life. Traditional relaxation training is an excellent way to help a client fall asleep. This is not the goal, however, in the athletic, academic, or job situation. The client needs to be able to relax physically while still maintaining a highly alert mental state.

METHOD OF INTERVENTION

Principles on Which Intervention Is Based

Individual differences dictate that we must be flexible in terms of how we deal with similar appearing clinical entities. How a specific individual responds with respect to different biofeedback modalities will help determine the best approach for that client. Assessment measurements are tools that help us decide which feedback modalities to use. Therefore, we do not advocate using specific protocols in the usual way that term is used. Instead, we employ a model to determine what and where to train using the decision-making pyramid presented earlier (Figure 11.4). The premise is that our knowledge base is continually updated and that each client is unique in his or her responses, both to our measurements and to our feedback techniques. The model also allows for change in the way we practice over the years, as we learn more about neurophysiology and as our biofeedback instruments improve.

The client's goal is more than just to reduce stress. Reduction of stress implies a change in stressors, but this is usually outside of the client's control, or he or she would have altered the situation long ago. If it is within the individual's power to alter the external stressors but, for unconscious reasons, he or she has not done so, then one of the appropriate initial interventions should be psychotherapy. Psychotherapy can be combined with NFB, biofeedback, and cognitive strategies. In this chapter our assumption is that, from his or her own point of view, the client is under realistic stress and has not found a way to productively deal with the effects that this stressor has on his or her ability to function. A client like Diane, who is described later, needs to find a means of dealing with stress in a manner that allows her to move ahead despite the stress.

Stress can change a client's entire physiology, including altering his or her brain wave patterns. The result can be akin to a kind of paralysis of efficient mental functioning. The mind may jump from one topic to another, ruminating on insoluble problems, or bounce from thought to thought and never stay with one long enough to produce constructive problem solving. Some people may show a combination of both patterns.

Whatever the specifics of their original reasons for coming, most clients want to optimize conscious, task-oriented performance. The goal to optimize performance can be expanded as being to help a client to achieve self-regulation of his or her mental state, to develop mental flexibility, and to become able to produce a self-defined optimal mental state. This is usually a state of relaxed, alert, aware, calm, focused, problem-solving concentration. Different aspects will be emphasized with different clients and at different times with specific clients, so every client's training is individualized. The individual training plans are variations on a theme, because each of these states, such as being relaxed, alert, and so on, can be rewarded as an enabling objective. To achieve each enabling objective, you can use one or more biofeedback or NFB procedures that are designed to assist the client in learning self-regulation. The next sections provide a brief overview of these enabling objectives and of some of the biofeedback methods that can be used to improve them. The process is summarized in the form of a structured interview questionnaire called TOPS, our acronym for Tools for Optimal Performance States. In what follows, we recognize that complex multichannel training is not done by the majority of trainers. Only further research will be able to discern whether the emphasis here on flexibility of attention states and the linkage to increasing high-frequency alpha with relaxed, broad, open awareness may obtain similar results to those of Les Fehmi's attention and neurotherapy synchrony training (McKnight & Fehmi, 2001). Those techniques emphasize the importance of the client being able to voluntarily increase and decrease brain-phase synchrony, and they teach the patient attentional flexibility. Similarly, the conscious changing of mental states is a learning process that is emphasized in all our work. Self-regulation is the goal. In the long term, we want the client to move from changing attentional processes consciously to an automatic process doing so automatically.

Note in the following discussion that EEG work is absolutely entwined and enmeshed with regular biofeedback when working with adults. For this reason EEG is not described in isolation in most of the following, though it is the core modality being trained.

Combining EEG and General Biofeedback Modalities

As previously described, mental states are correlated with particular EEG bandwidths. Trainers should help their clients discover this for themselves. Later in this chapter we show how Diane was able to confirm correlations between EEG patterns and mental states for herself using EEG biofeedback screens, purposefully altering her mental state and noting the changes in the EEG. The following 7-step overview is adapted from Thompson and Thompson (2003). In the following the electrode site is usually FCz (halfway between Fz and Cz). Brodmann's area 24 of the anterior cingulate cortex is best represented at this site. Training up high alpha (11–12 Hz) may be done at Pz.

To Achieve a Relaxed Mental and Physical State

To help the client achieve a relaxed state, we most often have him or her increase EEG activity between 11–12 Hz (high alpha) and 13–15 Hz (SMR) and teach him or her to breathe diaphragmatically at a rate of about six breaths per minute (BrPM), to relax his or her muscles, and to raise peripheral skin temperature. The 11–12 Hz bandwidth may be associated, in most adults, with an open external awareness state (our measurements have been mainly at FCz). In this mental state the individual can have a peaceful awareness of the whole of his or her environment. The individual may feel that he or she is one with what is being observed. The competent archer or competitive shooter may go into this mental state immediately prior to releasing the arrow or shooting the gun. The martial artist is in this "readiness" state when he or she is totally alert and ready to spar. The client doing NFB may feel he or she is "in" the picture on the wall. However, a caution: In our experience, although training up high alpha is, for the most part, associated with a relaxed state of open awareness, it appears that it may be an inverted-U-shaped phenomenon. The occasional person may, instead of being externally openly aware, go into a mental state of being "spaced out." Rarely, as previously noted, a client may report feeling brittle and overanxious. The later phenomena seem rare, but they should be recognized.

The 13–15 Hz state is associated with a mentally calm readiness without muscle tension or movement. For most adult clients, the 6 BrPM diaphragmatic breathing results in breathing in synchrony with heart rate (RSA). In children, the respiration rate will be a little faster than in adults. Trained athletes may have slower rates. Find the comfortable rate for your client. It should seem effortless. The heart rate will increase with inspiration and decrease with expiration (RSA). At the same time, the client is taught to warm his or her hands and relax his or her muscles. The client is taught to gradually relax the forehead, followed by the neck, shoulders, arms, and hands. Relaxing often corresponds to a decrease in anxiety. Anxiety may correlate with a high or labile EDR. Chronic stress, on the other hand, may result in an abnormal response to a new stress. The EDR may appear flat rather than showing an increase and finger temperature may actually increase, rather than decrease.

An exception to this general rule of raising high alpha (11–12 Hz) concerns those infrequent clients for whom alpha 8–12 Hz (which includes the high alpha) is already very high amplitude in the eyes-open state when feeling anxious. In these instances, increasing alpha may not have the expected relaxing effect. The correct procedure in these cases is to down-train the overly high amplitude alpha (Thomas & Sattlberger, 2001). This is a good example of how results from a careful assessment dictate intervention settings.

In addition, the expected good outcomes from up-training SMR (13–15 Hz) may, like the preceding high-alpha example, be confounded in those very rare circumstances in which you have a client whose impulsive–hyperactive behavior correlates with sudden bursts of high-amplitude spindling beta at 14 or 15 Hz. In these complex cases, intervention must both enhance the low-amplitude SMR and simultaneously inhibit the sudden bursts of high-amplitude beta spindling. The SMR and the spindling beta appear to have quite different origins. LORETA can help to clarify this. This needs to be the subject of future research.

Anxiety and/or emotional intensity may also be reflected in the EEG. It usually corresponds to an increase in 19–22 Hz activity relative to 15–18 Hz beta. A relaxed frame of mind implies that the individual is not negatively ruminating and worrying about aspects of his or her life. This type of unproductive mental activity may be found in conjunction with an increase in the amplitude of the EEG somewhere between 23 and 36 Hz, as compared with beta activity immediately above and below that bandwidth. Relative percentage of total EEG power may be a useful way to quantify these differences.

Note that you adjust these general guidelines for individual clients. Depending on the EEG findings in assessment, one may, for example, train 14–15 Hz rather than 13–15 Hz if alpha extends into the 12–13 Hz range. A few cautions must be registered at this juncture. As noted earlier, if high-amplitude alpha correlates with anxiety, it must be decreased, not increased. Bursts of spindling beta in the usual range of SMR must be *down-*trained. On the other hand, high-amplitude high-frequency beta that does *not* correspond to beta spindling or to negative circular thinking (ruminating) but rather to complex problem solving and cognitive processing must *not* be down-trained, whereas beta spindling in the same frequency range should be decreased.

Given the foregoing, it should be becoming quite clear that the use of standard protocols should be strongly discouraged. Rather, the competent trainer should base training strategies on a careful assessment of the symptoms and goals of the client in light of the EEG and psychophysiological stress test findings and his or her knowledge of functional neuroanatomy and neurophysiology.

To Achieve an Alert Mental State

To accomplish this objective, we encourage the client to maintain his or her EDR at a level that corresponds to alertness. The level should, however, not be as extreme as it could be with anxiety (too high) or with a drop in mental alertness (too low). EDR is measured between two electrodes placed across the palm or on two fingers. The EDR corresponds to sweat gland activity, which is controlled by the sympathetic nervous system. For most young children, being alert corresponds to a level between 12 and 16 micromhos (µMhos); for adolescents, 10–15 µMhos; for middle-aged adults, 8–12 µMhos; and for older client, as low as 3–7 µMhos. (As always there are exceptions to this general outline.) It is usually desirable to see the client's EDR constantly shifting but not fluctuating wildly between extremes.

To Be Aware of the Environment

As noted earlier, in athletics awareness corresponds to the ability to respond rapidly to changing conditions. For example, a goalie in hockey must be aware of every player's position around the net. In this mental state, the EEG can show a clear increase in 11–12 Hz. The athlete moves rapidly in and out of this state depending on the task. An archer, shooter, or golfer may be in *narrow focus* (beta, 16–18 Hz activity) when judging the wind and the distance. He or she is then likely to move to this state of calm, *open awareness* (11–12 Hz) just prior to releasing the arrow, pulling the trigger, or putting the ball.

However, nothing is ever as simple as it first appears. It should be recognized that quite specific work in sports with high-frequency alpha has been done by such authors as Kerick, Douglass, and Hatfield (2004) and Landers et al. (1991). The phenomenon looked at in these investigations appears to be quite different from the open awareness that we have been discussing in stress reduction. The work with athletes thus far has focused, for the most part, on specific sites and on the measurement of alpha as an inverse marker of a specific site's (e.g., T3 or T4) degree of activation (more alpha = less activation). In shooting, with practice and improvement, this high alpha may be recorded at T3, where it is related to a decreased reliance on working memory and on conscious regulation during aiming. For the skilled performer, the task becomes more automatic. As Kerick and colleagues (2004) have pointed out, although the air-pistol shooter usually is seen to increase the 11–13 Hz Alpha at T3 with practice (not at T4), it is not always true. It is, quite possibly, an inverted U-shaped curve, in which one can raise this alpha activity too much and decrease performance (Kerick et al., 2004).

Flexibility is important in terms of moving appropriately between different states, and small changes between different ranges within alpha appear to be important in performance. As implied earlier, the alpha rhythm appears to be associated with a number of functional states. Some authors have said that low alpha (approximately 8–10 Hz) is associated with general or global attention. We find that this is more often global in the sense of internal rather than external attention. People with good (vs. poor) memories desynchronize (show desynchronized beta activity) and 8–12 Hz alpha drops in amplitude during the encoding and retrieval of memory while a brief rise in 6 Hz synchronous theta is observed (Klimesch, 1999). A high alpha band (approximately 11–12 or 13 Hz) may be associated with task specific attention (Klimesch, Pfurtscheller, & Schilmke, 1992; Barry Sterman, personal communication, 2002). In this case the words *task specific* may actually refer to what we term *broad total awareness*, which is a state of intense focus and readiness, without tension, that is seen in the high-level athlete and that may turn into a singular focus on the target (being one with the target).

To Be Appropriately Reflective

This mental state may correspond to a temporary increase in the amplitude of high alpha, around 11–12 or 13 Hz and SMR 13–15 Hz followed by desynchronization (production of beta). A task such as scanning text, organizing the important facts and registering them in one's memory, requires that an individual move from broad to narrow external focus on the material, then back to internal reflection. Moving flexibly and continually between states is characteristic of effective learning.

To Remain Calm Even under Stress

This mental state is also associated with being both *aware* and *reflective*. As noted previously, it may be attained by increasing 11–12 Hz high alpha and 13–15 Hz SMR and by decreasing 19–22 Hz and 23–35 Hz. The broadband area between 11 and 15 Hz corresponds to the production of high alpha both for open external awareness and for reflection plus SMR for a sense of *calm*. As discussed earlier, increases in 19–35 Hz are often found to correspond to moments when a person is anxious and worrying or ruminating (usually negatively). This kind of "busy brain" with ruminating mental state is the opposite of being calm. It is not usually conducive to efficient action or to the breadth of associations that would be necessary for creative thinking. In a calm mental state a person may also be physically relaxed. This state may, therefore, be associated with diaphragmatic breathing, good RSA, warm hands, and relaxed musculature. One can also be calm mentally while carrying out a physically strenuous task. In this instance breathing and muscle tension would vary with the task.

To Be Capable of Sustaining a Narrow Focus

Being capable of sustaining a *narrow focus* for the required length of time for a specific task is a key to efficient academics and to optimal athletic performance. The student who is continually distracted by either internal or external stimuli will not achieve at the level of his or her intellectual potential. The athlete who loses focus in the middle of a golf swing will not win that round. Most of us produce bursts of waves either in the theta or the alpha range (somewhere between 3 and 10 Hz) when we are *internally* distracted. However, some adults produce high-amplitude high-frequency beta activity when they are distracted by internal ruminations. The latter, high-amplitude high-beta state, appears to be particularly evident in persons who feel under stress.

To Be Able to Turn On and Remain
in a State of Problem-Solving Concentration

Clients need to be able to turn on and remain in a state of *problem-solving concentration* until a task is complete or a problem is solved. This sustaining of focused concentration is a key to success both in school and in business. This state is usually associated with 16–

18 Hz activity. It is also said to be associated with activity in the 39–41 Hz range known as Sheer rhythm, or a "binding" rhythm.

Generalization

Most clients can learn reasonable control of general biofeedback modalities in 10 to 20 sessions, although the NFB results, to ensure lasting changes, typically take about 40 sessions. The two kinds of training are done concurrently. The real challenge is helping clients generalize what they have learned in your office to their everyday lives. This requires that, from day 1, the trainer assist the client to find ways to integrate what he or she is learning into the routine of daily living. The techniques for doing this include attaching a new habit, such as relaxing with diaphragmatic breathing, to old habits or routines. The latter are simply regular daily activities, such as getting out of bed, brushing your teeth, eating meals, driving, or answering the phone. The new learning, which combines both NFB and biofeedback, must become an integral part of daily living. Most clients are able to pair relaxed diaphragmatic breathing with control of the other biofeedback and NFB variables. Thus, through classical conditioning, a client who begins to breathe at 6 BrPM in different situations automatically enters a relaxed, open external awareness state with faster reflexes. When driving, for example, he or she is relatively free of internal distracters and is ready for contingencies that may occur on the road.

Goal Setting with the Client

Clients deserve to have a full understanding of the what, why, and how of the steps they will be taking to alter their everyday living. After all, you are not changing them; indeed, you cannot even tell them how to make the variables on feedback screens change. They are working to change themselves, with you as a coach, and the more knowledge they have about the process, the more they will feel in control. Because people subjectively feel less stressed when they have control in a situation, this approach is a logical part of setting up for success in stress management. Each client should understand the correspondence of EEG bandwidths and mental states in addition to knowing about the fundamental physiology of the autonomic nervous system. This allows the setting of operational definitions of goals, as outlined in the TOPS sheet in the following section. (An operational definition is an objective measure of a variable used in an experiment; for example, an operational definition of *intelligence* is "what an IQ test measures"; the experimenter might use scores on the Wechsler Adult Intelligence Scale. The operational definition is not the same as the meaning of the word in everyday usage.) The TOPS is a handy reference for both the trainer and the client. Its purpose is to help the client to formulate his or her goals in operational terms that can be achieved using NFB + biofeedback + metacognitive strategies rather than vague terms. *Metacognition* goes beyond the concept of cognition and refers to awareness of how you learn and remember things. It is sometimes defined as "thinking about thinking" or "what you know about what you know."

The TOPS Self-Assessment Structured Interview Questionnaire

The TOPS questionnaire (Figure 11.7) has been designed to be discussed with your clients so that, with the trainer, they can do self-ratings of various components necessary for successful stress management. It can be used initially and then repeated at various points

(*Describe* beneath or in the margin *times when you are exactly the opposite* of the problem area you are working on during your training sessions (e.g., "I'm a calm leader in catastrophic situations, but I worry a lot about little things").   (Score 1–10)

A. State of Physiological Readiness

1. Relaxed
   - Objective: To broaden associative capabilities and perspective, increase reaction time, and decrease fatigue, tension, and stress
   - Measurement: ↑peripheral temperature, stabilize EDR, ↓pulse, ↓respiration rate, ↓EMG
2. Alert
   - Objective: To efficiently respond to new information (state of eustress—*eu* as in *euphoria* is a positive, so a zone of positive stress)
   - Measurement: moderate increase in EDR (arousal and performance relate in a U-shaped curve), plus increases in 11–12 Hz and low beta (15–18 Hz)

B. State of Mental Readiness

3. Calm
   - Objective: To allow reflection and consideration of alternative approaches
   - Measurement: ↑SMR (13–15 Hz), ↓high beta (19–35 Hz); ↑peripheral skin temperature, respiration (diaphragmatic about 6 BrPM), ↓EMG, EDR (control), ↓pulse , ↑RSA (synchrony), ↑HRV
4. Aware
   - Objective: To broaden input range—a state of calm readiness (e.g., sports: goalie, martial arts, golf, archery) and increase creativity
   - Measurement: 11 Hz and 12 Hz↑
5. Reflective
   - Objective: To increase accuracy, breadth and completeness of responses
   - Measurement: bursts of alpha 11–13 Hz, SMR 13–15 Hz, and beta 15–18 Hz
6. Optimistic in Attitude
   - Track your number of positive versus negative comments

C. State of Active Mental Work

7. Focused
   - Objective: To maintain attention to work area
   - Measurement: decreased slow waves (theta and low-frequency alpha); increased fast waves (beta) 16–18 Hz
8. Concentrating and Creative
   - Objective:
     a. To problem solve, elaborate on ideas, and make decisions (↑beta 16–18 Hz); beta is interspersed with theta and high-frequency alpha as one shifts between narrow focus and broad open awareness
     b. To have "fluency of ideas" and be flexible and creative (↑ bursts of both theta and 11–13 Hz alpha activity)
   - Measurement: beta: controlled increase of 15–21 Hz (39–42 Hz) + shifts to high alpha
9. (a) Strategic Goal-Oriented Approach with (b) Openness to New Innovation and a Commitment to Objectives and Time Management
   - Objective: To work efficiently and effectively without constricting response possibilities—that is, active learning techniques and SMIRB (*Stop My Irritating Ruminations Book*)
   - Measurement: cognitive and metacognitive strategies, goals, techniques for handling stress, such as cognitive reframing or imagery of successful coping
10. Flexible Yet Decisive
    - Objective: To respond with openness and thoughtfulness and appropriate flexibility to new ideas while remaining able to make decisions and commit to a goal
    - Measurement: Find and weigh the positives in each new presentation and decide on direction and actions

ULTIMATE GOAL: Self-regulate to achieve "flow."

Flow is as easy as ABC:
A and B Setting the stage
C Performing and producing

Put it all together, automatically, in order to be Efficient–Effective–Productive

FIGURE 11.7. Tools for Optimal Performance States (TOPS) Program Evaluation.

during training, such as once a month or after every 8–10 sessions, in order to gauge progress and determine where the training emphasis needs to be for upcoming sessions. It represents, of course, a simplification of the complex processes involved in self-regulation for stress management, but it is quite comprehensive and it has been field tested with our own clients. There are no set norms for scores, and it is meant to be used like a structured interview.

Notes Concerning the TOPS Structured Interview

1. It is noted that to sustain external focus one may wish to control the production of theta. However, one should also note that cognitive tasks require encoding and that memory retrieval (episodic memories) and semantic processing require brief bursts of theta. Theta may be associated with tuning out from the external environment, but it is also apparently necessary for encoding and for *memory recall*. It may be that this is hippocampal theta (Klimesch, 1999). By asking the client to recall information, you can observe the frequency of theta and the waveform produced for that individual. It will be different from the theta produced when that client is in a rather dreamy, *tuned-out* state. Often a lower frequency theta is evident in the tuned-out state. This theta, which appears to correspond to a tuned-out state, is more likely produced by a thalamocortical circuit. Alpha–theta training in very accomplished music students (people who probably quite readily produced a lot of beta) was found to enhance aspects of their musical performance (Gruzelier & Egner, 2003). In addition, semantic processing with eyes open has been observed to be associated with a decrease in synchronous high alpha (Klimesch, 1999). The best performers have higher high-frequency alpha amplitudes at rest and greater desynchronization of both low- and high-frequency alpha on task (alpha attenuates and beta is produced). Clearly one does not just shift into beta (15–18 Hz) and stay there to solve problems. There is a constant shifting among frequencies as one actively receives and processes information.

2. When working, studying, or being involved in athletic events, the efficient individual is constantly shifting between the beta of narrow problem-solving focus, high-amplitude alpha for inner reflection, and autopilot states, along with brief bursts of theta for encoding and memory retrieval. Sterman, Mann, and Kaiser (1994) have also noted that there is a brief burst of alpha activity after the successful completion of a task that required sustained concentration. In the research he conducted with top-gun pilots, an alpha burst was observed when the wheels touched down during landing. These bursts are sometimes referred to as *event-related synchronization*. This seems to be a way in which the brain rewards itself with a brief rest.

3. Self-regulation combined with mental flexibility is the final goal.

Normalization of the EEG

Some clients who present for stress management turn out to have other associated specific disorders and needs. In these cases, the goal of training will include the reduction of a defined symptom or problem, such as a learning disability, seizure disorder, movement disorder, stroke, speech disorder, depression, Asperger traits, and so on. Although the client has requested your services in order to decrease the effects of stress and optimize his or her academic and workplace performance, you may find that one or more other conditions are interfering with your client's performance. ADHD or a mild learning disability are two fairly common coexisting conditions (Thompson, 2003). In Diane's case (see the next section), a different syndrome was present, albeit in a mild form. She displayed many features of Asperger syndrome. In some ways this accelerated her learning, because she was very compliant concerning concrete suggestions and would follow the trainer's prescriptions concretely and perfectly. She also had symptoms of attention-deficit disorder, which included a tendency to fall asleep when studying, a degree of dysphoria (not a clinical depression), and a clinically significant panic disorder.

Normalization includes such factors as bringing the amplitudes of frequency bands and the communication between areas of the brain (called *coherence* or *comodulation*, depending on what instrument and database you are using) into the ranges found in normal databases.

We distinguish between educational goals and clinical goals. Trainers who have purely a clinical background may not have the experiential base to work with and train clients who have educational, business, athletic, and peak performance goals. The converse may also be true. Those with an educational or coaching background may not have the experience and training to make a clinical diagnosis and provide a therapeutic intervention to a client who has a clinical disorder such as obsessive–compulsive disorder. Know your own limitations and ask for help or refer to other colleagues as appropriate.

CASE EXAMPLE

Mental states correspond to specific frequency bandwidths, but they vary slightly from one individual to the next. The responsible trainer has the client experiment with making relevant brain wave frequency bands rise and fall by changing his or her mental state. Then the client knows what those frequencies represent in terms of his or her own mental state. The particular frequencies trained in Diane's case would not be appropriate for all clients. We do not advocate a set protocol; we want you to tailor your intervention to your client's patterns.

The EEG Patterns

Diane was unable to pass her doctoral-level practice examinations due to anxiety. In addition, she had been diagnosed with attention-deficit disorder (ADD). She also had social anxiety and had always found relating in both personal and professional situations very stressful. She conquered the stress of written examinations by withdrawing from other activities and overlearning the subject matter, and she had already earned two graduate degrees before doing professional training. She could not effectively use this overlearning formula for practical and oral examinations, however, due to the addition of interpersonal stress. Panic attacks, anxiety, and tension had led to her failing the practical examination in her chosen profession. She had attempted to deal with her anxiety and ADD through appropriate use of medications prescribed by her physician. She was participating in ongoing psychotherapy with a psychologist. She had also tried relaxation techniques, dietary approaches, and chiropractic interventions. She faithfully followed the prescriptions of her practitioners, but the panic attacks, rumination, and general anxiety had not subsided. She constantly felt "stressed out" and feared that, after years of study, she would never be able to practice.

First Interview: EEG Assessment

After taking a thorough history and measuring attentional variables using questionnaires and continuous performance tests (Diane scored in the bottom 2% for females her age), we did a single-channel EEG assessment. The active electrode was at FCz (halfway between the vertex, Cz, and Fz) referenced to A2 (the right ear) with ground on the left ear (A1). The findings indicated differences from the EEG pattern that would normally be expected in terms of excess slow-wave activity and, even more pronounced, excess high beta (beta frequencies > 20 Hz). Figure 11.8 shows 1½ seconds of activity. It is representative of what was observed in Diane's EEG in general when she was feeling stressed. In a normal woman of the same age, we would see a different picture, namely an eyes-open recording of EEG with no high-frequency (31 Hz), high-amplitude beta spindling. A normal spectral pattern would usually show a low voltage and a relatively flat histogram with a gradual reduction in power as frequencies get higher; that is, alpha 10–12 Hz, SMR 13–15 Hz, and productive problem-solving beta 15–18 Hz activity would be higher than 19–36 Hz (high beta). Without EMG interference the higher beta frequencies are typically very low.

Diane's EEG demonstrated a contrasting picture. It showed an unusual form of beta at FCz and F2, namely spindling beta. The spectrum that quantifies the 1-second sample in Figure 11.8 shows extremely high 31 Hz activity in conjunction with very low 13–15 Hz (SMR) activity. High amplitude 19–21 Hz activity can also be observed. Throughout the remainder of the record, this pattern of a rise of around 31 Hz would repeatedly correspond to low amplitude at 11–12 and/or 13–15 Hz. Diane was able to report that this pattern corresponded to her feeling tense, anxious, and worrying.

Diane also showed spindling beta at Cz. These spindles were at 23 Hz. The brain map (Figure 11.9) shows this 23 Hz at Cz on the surface EEG. LORETA (Figure 11.10)

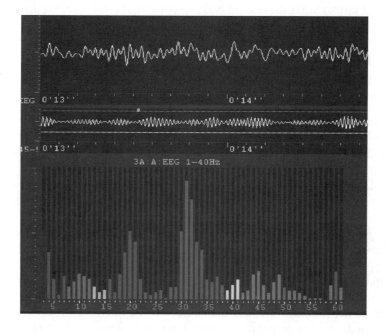

FIGURE 11.8. Example of raw EEG, EMG indicator, and EEG frequency spectrum.

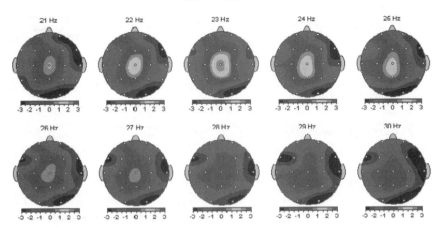

FIGURE 11.9. Neuroguide brain map: Z-scored relative power. This eyes-closed, Laplacian-montage, relative-power brain map shows that the amplitude of beta at 23 Hz is > 3 *SD* above the NG database mean at Cz. This corresponds to the beta spindling seen at this frequency in the raw EEG.

shows that the origin of this 23 Hz activity is the anterior cingulate, Brodmann area 24 (immediately anterior to area 23). The anterior cingulate often appears to be the origin of activity and is found to correspond to anxiety and the syndromes related to anxiety.

Second Interview: Stress Assessment

In addition to Diane's EEG differences, which indicated vulnerability to stress and high anxiety, characteristic alterations appeared in autonomic nervous system variables (see Figure 11.11). With stress, her heart rate increased and respiration became fast, irregular, and shallow.

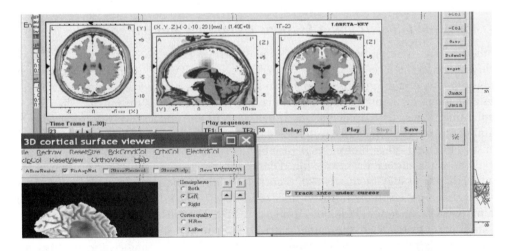

FIGURE 11.10. LORETA image. LORETA shows that this high-amplitude 23-Hz beta activity may be originating in the anterior cingulate. In this figure it is 1.6 *SD* greater than the NG database mean.

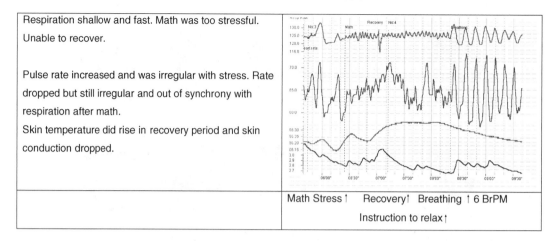

Respiration shallow and fast. Math was too stressful. Unable to recover.	
Pulse rate increased and was irregular with stress. Rate dropped but still irregular and out of synchrony with respiration after math. Skin temperature did rise in recovery period and skin conduction dropped.	
	Math Stress ↑ Recovery↑ Breathing ↑ 6 BrPM Instruction to relax↑

FIGURE 11.11. Graph of respiration, pulse, temperature and ERD during stress and recovery.

Diane's initial stress assessment demonstrated some less common responses due to the chronic nature of her stress. Instead of a decrease in peripheral skin temperature with the math stress, Diane initially demonstrated a rise in temperature. Skin temperature was in the mid-80s and skin conductance was below 3 μMhos. Being very conscientious, Diane followed instructions for breathing at 6 BrPM but was anxious and worried about how well she was doing. This performance anxiety is reflected in the drop in skin temperature and the slight rise in EDR. Her forehead EMG was 13–22 microvolts. We concluded, while discussing the profile with her, that breathing, EMG (not shown in Figure 11.11), and skin temperature could all be used as indicators of stress. We further agreed that skin conduction might be a useful measure of alertness and that it was valuable to maintain alertness, along with being calm and relaxed.

Sessions 3–6: Initial Training Sessions Using NFB and Biofeedback

In the first few training sessions, the goal was to train Diane to control variables in the following order: (1) Breathing diaphragmatically at 6 BrPM; (2) decreasing her forehead EMG while continuing the breathing at 6 BrPM; (3) in her words, "empty her mind" while maintaining diaphragmatic breathing and low EMG. This meant that she stopped ruminating. When that occurred, she noted that 23–34 Hz activity was reduced. One training screen that helped her to follow changes in a number of EEG variables in addition to HRV and other biofeedback variables is shown in Figure 11.12.

Even when surface EMG was low, Diane still might experience the sensation of tension. Perhaps this may be thought of as corresponding to the findings of Gevirtz and colleagues that muscle spindle fusiform fiber tension can exist without surface EMG abnormality (Gevirtz, Shannon, Hong & Hubbard, 1997). The muscle spindle tension appears, in large part, to relate to sympathetic drive. Sympathetic drive may be effectively decreased through training of respiration and HRV. The muscle spindle fusiform fiber tension may also be related to gamma motor efferent overactivity. The effects of decreasing this by increasing SMR and thus decreasing the firing of the red nucleus have been documented by Sterman (2000). Feedback that emphasizes both EEG and autonomic nervous

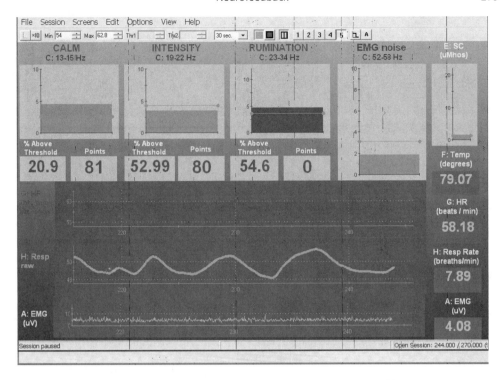

FIGURE 11.12. Feedback screen for EEG, breathing, heart rate, electrodermal responses, skin temperature, and EMG. This screen is from the Infiniti program, which allows the client to observe heart rate variability (HRV) beginning to synchronize with diaphragmatic breathing. At this juncture Diane had not quite achieved this, but she did so when she began to breathe at a rate of 6 breaths per minute. When this occurred, the HRV increased. This screen also allowed her to observe skin temperature, EDR and skin conduction while she increased her 13–15 Hz and decreased her high beta 19–22 Hz and 23–35 Hz. Diane's skin temperature was normally higher than shown in the figure and it was not necessary to have it or the EDR on most feedback screens after the first few sessions. Forehead EMG was sometimes included on feedback screens but it did drop to < 2 μV.

system biofeedback appear to have a place in working with stress. This combination of biofeedback and NFB was highly effective for Diane.

By her sixth session, Diane was trying to combine this breathing and maintain an external focus with a technique of looking at old paintings and her favorite dog pictures (she loves animals) while at the same time opening her awareness to the gestalt of these pictures. She experienced her hands getting warm, her forehead and shoulder muscles relaxing, and a sense of calm. She said that when she truly sensed this peaceful, open, external awareness, everything seemed to fall into place. In addition to control of breathing and raising peripheral skin temperature to 93° and skin conduction to 5–7 μMhos, shifts occurred in her EEG pattern: 19–21 Hz, 24–32 Hz, and 4–7 Hz all dropped markedly, while 11–15 Hz and 17 Hz rose. She could get into this state for only a few minutes at a time near the end of the session, but she was elated at how this corresponded to feeling peaceful and calm, yet alert.

In her initial training sessions, Diane was having difficulty getting her breathing to remain relaxed and comfortable at about 6 BrPM. This is shown in Figure 11.13.

	13–15 Hz Forehead EMG
Diane tries to move the ball on the balance beams to the right and hold it to the right as long as possible. Note that respiration is irregular and about 2 breaths in a 10-second frame. The muscle inhibit will stop the ball rolling and stop sound feedback and changes in % and point values.	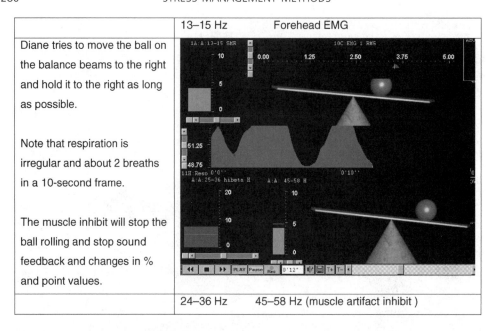
	24–36 Hz 45–58 Hz (muscle artifact inhibit)

FIGURE 11.13. Feedback screen for EEG, breathing, and EMG.

Sessions 7–9

At this juncture some cognitive-behavioral work was added to augment the feedback, which was continued. Diane was given two strategies to help her generalize what she was learning in her sessions to her everyday life. The first method is called "Attach a Habit to a Habit" (previously described). She was asked to practice her diaphragmatic breathing with hand warming and relaxation of her forehead, neck, and shoulders, combined with feeling calm and emptying her mind before (and later during) each activity that she listed as being a habit or a daily routine, such as while brushing her teeth and while driving.

The second strategy was called SMIRB: "Stop My Irritating Ruminations Book." It is a method for compartmentalizing negative thoughts. The book was a pocket-sized daily calendar with a blank telephone number booklet inserted at the end. The front pages were for her positive goals in each key area of her life. The back pages were set aside to be her SMIRB. Diane wrote one "worry" heading at the top of the left-hand page and listed below it the repetitive thought or thoughts that kept coming into her head. She then put the second worry area on the next left-hand page, working her way from the back toward the middle of the book. She was surprised to discover that she had only a small number of worry areas and only a few repetitive thoughts under each area. The problem for her was that they were continually repeated in her head and were preventing her from getting on with important activities. She agreed that she would worry about these things at one, and only one, preset time each day. She also agreed that if she woke up in the middle of the night she would ask herself, before opening her eyes, whether the thing she was ruminating about was in her SMIRB. If it was, she would not open her eyes but would think of a repetitive pleasant activity, do her breathing, and relax so that she fell back to sleep. If, however, the thought was not in her SMIRB, then she would open her eyes, turn on her light, write it in her SMIRB, and then leave that thought and go back to sleep. If she ever did think of a solution to one of these worries, she would enter it on the right-hand page opposite the negative thought.

Diane carried out these two strategies faithfully. The speed with which she began to take control of her mental states, as reflected in her EEG changes, physiological shifts, and her self-report of controlling her negative thinking, was probably associated with her practicing what she was learning every day. By her 10th training session she was feeling some control over a number of variables. The screen shown in Figure 11.14 was one of Diane's favorites. She could now, by the end of a session, sometimes manage to keep 24–32 Hz and 19–23 Hz very low and 11–13 Hz up for a short while (1 to 2 minutes) . The percentage-over-threshold computations on this screen were originally set at 50% for her. Thus 25%, 36%, and 57% are very good values. Note also that forehead EMG is at 3 microvolts (down from > 13) and that she is keeping her breathing at one breath every 10 seconds. At this stage she could not hold this state for more than about 2 minutes, but her comment was, "It feels wonderful."

Sessions 10–20: Intermediate Sessions Using NFB and Biofeedback

At this stage, Diane had sufficient self-control to experiment with making and breaking specific mental states. She was able to demonstrate to herself precisely what frequencies correlated with several mental states: (1) feeling emotionally intense and anxious versus feeling calm and relaxed; (2) feeling worried, with negative, circular, nonproductive ruminations versus a mind "empty" of distracting thoughts and focused on the problem at hand; (3) being focused on one intrusive thought after another versus an open focus that could concentrate flexibly on a single target in a calm mental state.

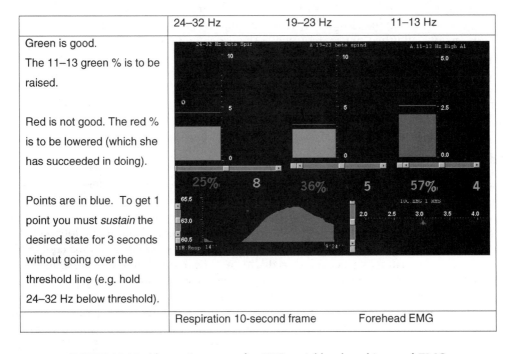

FIGURE 11.14. Alternative screen for EEG variables, breathing, and EMG.

	Sailboat disappears 23–32 Hz high
Diane said that, if she *"emptied her mind"* of negative, circular thinking and felt calm and externally oriented, then she could maintain a low bar-graph and an intact sailboat. The moment she started worrying, the music would stop and the sailboat would disappear as is shown opposite. This occurred because EEG amplitude for 23–32 Hz is above the threshold. Note that the 45–58 Hz is low. It would reflect the effect of muscle activity on the EEG.	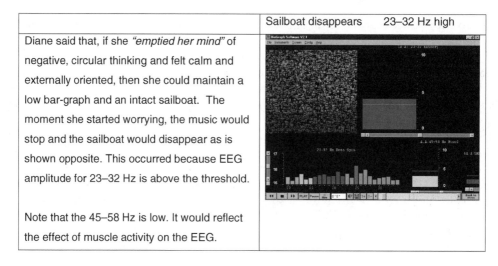

FIGURE 11.15. Sailboat screen to gain control of ruminating.

To accomplish this practice of being in and out of specific mental states, she used a sailboat screen (Figure 11.15). We altered the screen so that the bar graph represented different frequency bandwidths. Initially, we did not label the bar graph, and we tried not to suggest to her what she might do in order to make the picture of the boat appear, or make it disappear. Our goal was to make the feedback clear so that Diane could feel confident that what she experienced was being consistently reflected on the computer monitor. We let her discover which frequencies were related to which mental states.

Diane noted that if she felt as though she was going into a panic at home, she could calm herself by breathing at 6 BrPM while she emptied her mind. She said that practicing this in sessions and then practicing it while she drove home meant that she could attain the desired state, and no panic attack ensued.

We do not doubt that different mental states do correspond to different bandwidths, but note that there may be different frequencies for different individuals. (Age also plays a role, with frequencies moving higher with age. Pediatric alpha may be at 7 Hz, but in adults the peak alpha frequency is around 10 Hz.)

Sessions 20–35

Diane interspersed one or more of the "sailboat" exercises (using different frequency bands) with more general screens that gave her the opportunity to work on biofeedback goals (such as respiration, forehead or trapezius EMG, or peripheral skin temperature) while controlling one or more of the following: high-frequency beta, high alpha (11–12 Hz), SMR, and theta. The goal was self-regulation. After 30 sessions, when she could voluntarily combine emptying her mind (reduced high beta spindling) and breathing at 6 BrPM, she reported that for the first time in as long as she could remember she had not experienced a panic attack all week. Diane's training for the high-beta bandwidth was done at F2 (frontally and just to the right of the midline) and, at other times, at FCz, where beta spindling had been observed. (FCz is usually the site at which activity originating from the anterior cingulate, Brodmann's area 24, is observed.) The right frontal area is overactive in panic disorder, and these findings suggest that Diane had achieved some control of this episodic overactivity in the right frontal area. For Diane, the specific goal was the ability to sustain a mental state wherein she was feeling relaxed and calm yet alert, completely free of unwanted thoughts and ruminations, and able to switch appropriately from broad external awareness to narrow focus on a problem-solving task.

Sessions 36–40

At this juncture Diane was working to make control of all variables automatic and achievable, even under conditions in which she was being asked questions similar to those that she had previously experienced in stress-producing situations such as oral examinations. In the screen shown in Figure 11.16, she has gone from the usual starting point for percentage-over-threshold calculations of 50–55% to 79% for 11–15 Hz and dropped the 25–36 Hz band to a remarkable 17%. Her forehead EMG had originally been above 12 and had dropped to 2.6. She was keeping her breathing steady at 6 BrPM. She was starting (note the second breath after 10'11") to learn to increase the time of expiration compared with inspiration.

After 40 sessions a reassessment was done, and Diane demonstrated shifts in her EEG patterns, improved performance on the continuous performance test (from 2nd percentile to 37th percentile for attention), and decreased symptoms on the self-report questionnaires. Most important, Diane retook her practical examinations shortly thereafter and achieved passing grades, so that she could practice in her profession. Her demeanor

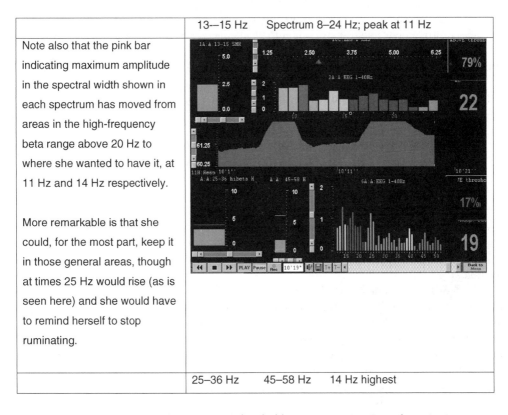

	13—15 Hz Spectrum 8–24 Hz; peak at 11 Hz
Note also that the pink bar indicating maximum amplitude in the spectral width shown in each spectrum has moved from areas in the high-frequency beta range above 20 Hz to where she wanted to have it, at 11 Hz and 14 Hz respectively. More remarkable is that she could, for the most part, keep it in those general areas, though at times 25 Hz would rise (as is seen here) and she would have to remind herself to stop ruminating.	
	25–36 Hz 45–58 Hz 14 Hz highest

FIGURE 11.16. Screen showing EEG thresholds, spectrum, EMG, and respiration.

has also changed, with the old anxiety that was evidenced by averted gaze and stooped shoulders replaced by direct looks, smiles, and posture that reflects confidence.

SUMMARY AND CONCLUSIONS

Both the brain and the body react to stress. A certain amount of stress can actually improve performance, with this amount of stress termed *eustress*. Chronic stress can produce pathological alterations in normal brain and physiological–biochemical functioning.

Individuals are capable of identifying mental states that correlate to EEG frequency bands, as Joe Kamiya had originally demonstrated with identification of alpha states (Kamiya, 1968). With appropriate EEG feedback using EEG operant conditioning techniques first developed by Sterman, a person can train his or her brain to shift the EEG patterns, becoming more flexible in his or her ability to find the correct mental state to fit the task demands of the moment. Individuals can also identify mental states that correlate to physiological changes that include heart and respiratory rate, skin conduction and temperature, and muscle tension. Using biofeedback of the EEG and other physiological variables, people can shift their responses to stressors and optimize their performance in academic, work, athletic, and social situations. The relative importance of particular variables will differ between people and according to underlying strengths or pathologies.

Although it is reasonable to propose that a combined NFB and biofeedback approach is helpful in assisting individuals to deal with stress and optimize their performance, it should be recognized that this approach still requires more research. It should also be emphasized that NFB and biofeedback are only a part of an overall approach to lifestyle improvement. Such factors as nutrition, sleep, exercise, and evoking constructive patterns of viewing oneself and relating to others are adjunctive components of a training program.

The ability to self-regulate, in particular the ability to gain the mental edge, is achievable through NFB training and leads to effective management of the stresses of everyday life.

APPENDIX 11.1. STEPS TO OPTIMIZE PERFORMANCE

1. Decide which mental state the client wishes to encourage and/or discourage. This investigation is facilitated by the intake interview and history. Goals may be clarified by psychological and performance testing, as is appropriate for your client. Goals should be realistic and put in writing. After the EEG, ANS (autonomic nervous system), and EMG assessments, these goals will be linked to specific objectives for NFB combined with biofeedback.

2. Assess the client's central nervous system (CNS) state by means of the EEG. Delineate how the client's quantitative electroencephalogram (QEEG) differs from expected age values. If you are not using a database, you can look at the pattern, both watching the dynamic EEG and looking at average values in different frequency ranges for the time period. Some programs produce a histogram and statistics; others provide values from which you can create your own graph.

3. Place electrodes at the sites you decide on based on EEG data, client's goals and history, and your knowledge of neuroanatomy and brain function (see the decision-making pyramid in Figure 11.4.) You want to inhibit the frequencies prone to EMG arti-

fact in order to provide accurate feedback. Encourage the client to decrease the appropriate slow-wave frequency band(s) while simultaneously increasing the appropriate fast-wave frequency band. (*Appropriate* here means appropriate for that client's EEG pattern, symptom picture, and goals.) Remember, the EEG acts like a "flag" that reflects brain functioning. You can infer from a flag's activity the wind's velocity (amplitude) and direction. You make inferences about the brain's activity by reading the EEG. You are now ready to set up display screen instruments to assist the client in self-regulating his or her mental state using EEG biofeedback or NFB.

4. Decide on the training screen you wish to use. The selection will depend on the EEG equipment you are using. Some allow you to customize the visual and audio feedback, and nearly all instruments offer a range of feedback screens. It is helpful if there are methods for measuring achievement. These may include percentage of time over or under threshold and a measurement that gives the client a sense of how often he or she is able to hold a mental state for 1 or more seconds (*decrease variability*). It is also helpful if the raw EEG is available for viewing. Children, in particular, become very good at pattern recognition quite quickly.

5. Assist those clients who demonstrate anxiety and tension to relax in order to facilitate their work on self-regulation of their mental state. Both you and the client can see how he or she is doing if you set up the equipment for electromyogram ANS/EMG feedback. If you do not have general biofeedback capabilities, you can still work on diaphragmatic breathing, imagery, and other relaxation techniques. Remember, however, that you are usually not trying to achieve the kind of relaxation associated with being in a hammock. *You want to maintain mental alertness but be free of tension.* Use the example of the top-gun pilots (Sterman et al., 1994) to epitomize being alert yet physically relaxed (not tense).

6. Do the training until the client has mastered an appropriate degree of self-regulation and achieved the goals that were set out initially.

7. Help the client develop techniques for generalizing the learned relaxed, calm, open focus readiness state to his or her activities of daily living.

REFERENCES

Davidson, R. J. (1995). Cerebral asymmetry, emotion and affective style. In R. J. Davidson & K. Hugdahl (Eds.), *Brain asymmetry* (pp. 369–388). Cambridge, MA: MIT Press.

Devinsky, O., Morrell, M., & Vogt, B. (1995). Contributions of anterior cingulate cortex to behaviour. *Brain, 118,* 279–306.

Duffy, F. H., Hughes, J. R., Miranda, F., Bernad, P., & Cook, P. (1994). Status of quantitative EEG (QEEG) in clinical practice. *Clinical Electroencephalography, 25,* vi–xxii.

Duffy, F. H., Iyer, V. G., & Surwillo, W. W. (1989). *Clinical electroencephalography and topographic brain mapping: Technology and practice.* New York: Springer-Verlag.

Fisch, B. J. (1999). *Fisch and Spehlmann's EEG primer: Basic principles of digital and analog EEG* (3rd rev. ed.). New York: Elsevier.

Gevirtz, R., Shannon, S., Hong, D., & Hubbard, D. (1997). Myofacial trigger points show spontaneous needle EMG activity. *Pain, 69,* 65–73.

Gruzelier, J. H., & Egner, T. (2003). Ecological validity of neurofeedback modulation of slow wave EEG enhances musical performance. *NeuroReport, 14*(9), 1221–1224.

Hardt, J. V., & Kamiya, J. (1978). Anxiety change through electroencephalographic alpha feedback seen only in high anxiety subjects. *Science, 201,* 79–81.

Jasper, H. (1958). Report of the committee on methods of clinical examination in electroencephalography. *EEG and Clinical Neurophysiology, 10,* 374.

Kamiya, J. (1968, April). Conscious control of brainwaves. *Psychology Today, 1*, 57–60.

Kamiya, J. (1979). Autoregulation of the EEG alpha rhythm: A program for the study of consciousness. In E. Peper, S. Ancoli, & M. Quinn (Eds.), *Mind body integration: Essential readings in biofeedback* (pp. 289–298). New York: Plenum Press.

Kerick, S. E., Douglass, L. W., & Hatfield, B. D. (2004). Cerebral cortical adaptations associated with visuomotor practice. *Medicine and Science in Sports and Exercise, 36*(1), 118–129.

Klimesch, W. (1999). EEG alpha and theta oscillations reflect cognitive and memory performance: A review and analysis. *Brain Research Reviews, 29*, 169–195.

Klimesch, W., Pfurtscheller, G., & Schimke, H. (1992). Pre- and post-stimulus processes in category judgement tasks as measured by event-related desynchronization (ERD). *Journal of Psychophysiology, 6*, 185–203.

Landers, D. M., Petruzzello, S. J., Salazar, W., Crews, D. J., Kubitz, K. A., Gannon, T. L., et al. (1991). The influence of electrocortical biofeedback on performance in pre-elite archers. *Medicine and Science in Sports and Exercise, 23*(1), 123–128.

Levesque, J., Beauregard, M., & Mensur, B. (2006). Effect of neurofeedback training on the neural substrates of selective attention on children with attention-deficit/hypearctivity disorder: A functional mangnetic resonance imaging study. *Neuroscience Letters, 394*, 216–221.

Linden, M., Habib, T., & Radojevic, V. (1996). A controlled study of the effects of EEG biofeedback on cognition and behavior of children with attention deficit disorder and learning disabilities. *Biofeedback and Self Regulation, 21*(1), 106–111.

Lorensen, T. D., & Dickson, P. (2003). Quantitative EEG normative databases: A comparative investigation. *Journal of Neurotherapy, 7*(3), 53–68.

Lubar, J. (2003). Low resolution electromagnetic tomography (LORETA) of cerebral activities in chronic depressive disorder. *International Journal of Psychophysiology, 49*(3), 175–185.

Lubar, J. F. (1991). Discourse on the development of EEG diagnostics and biofeedback treatment for attention deficit/hyperactivity disorders. *Biofeedback and Self-Regulation, 16*(3), 201–225.

Lubar, J. F., & Lubar, J. (1999). Neurofeedback assessment and treatment for ADD/hyperactivity disorder. In J. R. Evans & A. Abarbanel (Eds.), *Introduction to quantitative EEG and neurofeedback*. San Diego: Academic Press.

Lubar, J. F., & Shouse, M. N. (1976). EEG and behavioral changes in a hyperkinetic child concurrent with training of the sensorimotor rhythm (SMR): A preliminary report. *Biofeedback and Self-Regulation, 3*, 293–306.

Lubar, J. F., Swartwood, M. O., Swartwood, J. N., & O'Donnell, P. H. (1995). Evaluation of the effectiveness of EEG neurofeedback training for ADHD in a clinical setting as measured by changes in TOVA scores, behavioural ratings, and WISC-R performance. *Biofeedback and Self Regulation, 21*(1), 83–99.

McKnight, J. T., & Fehmi, L. T. (2001). Attention and neurofeedback synchrony training clinical results and their significance. *Journal of Neurotherapy, 5*(1/2), 45–62.

Pascual-Marqui, R. D., Esslen, M., Kochi, K., & Lehmann, D. (2002). Functional imaging with low resolution electromagnetic tomography (LORETA): A review. *Methods and Findings in Experimental and Clinical Pharmacology, 24C*, 91–95.

Peniston, E. G., & Kulkosky, P. J. (1990). Alcoholic personality and alpha-theta brainwave training. *Medical Psychotherapy, 3*, 37–55.

Plotkin, W. B., & Rice, K. M. (1981). Biofeedback as a placebo: Anxiety reduction facilitated by training in either suppression or enhancement of brain waves. *Journal of Consulting and Clinical Psychology, 49*, 590–96.

Rice, K. M., Blanchard, E. B., & Purcell, M., (1993). Biofeedback of generalized anxiety disorder: Preliminary results. *Biofeedback and Self-Regulation, 18*(2), 93–105.

Sheer, D. E. (1997). Biofeedback training of 40 Hz EEG and behavior. In I. N. Burch & H. I. Altshuler (Eds.), *Behavior and brain electrical activity* (pp. 501–512). New York: Plenum Press.

Sterman, M. B. (1999). *An atlas of topometric clinical displays*. Los Angeles: Sterman-Kaiser Imaging Labs.

Sterman, M. B. (2000). Basic concepts and clinical findings in the treatment of seizure disorders with EEG operant conditioning. *Clinical Electroencephalography, 31*(1), 45–55.

Sterman, M. B., Mann, C. A., & Kaiser, D. A. (1994). Topographic analysis of a simulated visual–motor task. *International Journal of Psychophysiology, 16*, 49–56.

Thomas, J. E., & Sattlberger, E. (1997). Treatment of chronic anxiety disorder with neurotherapy: A case study. *Journal of Neurotherapy, 2*(2), 14–19.

Thompson, L., & Thompson, M. (1998). Neurofeedback combined with training in metacognitive strategies: Effectiveness in students with ADD. *Applied Psychophysiology and Biofeedback, 23*(4), 243–263.

Thompson, M. (1978). *A resident's guide to psychiatric education.* New York: Plenum Press.

Thompson, M., & Thompson, L. (2003). *The neurofeedback book: An introduction to basic concepts in applied psychophysiology.* Wheat Ridge, CO: Association for Applied Psychophysiology and Biofeedback.

Weidmann, G., Pauli, P., Dengler, W., Lutzenburger, W., Birbaumer, N., & Buckkremer, G. (1999). Frontal brain asymmetry as a biological substrate of emotions in patients with panic disorders. *Archives of General Psychiatry, 56*, 78–84.

Wyrwicka, W., & Sterman, M. B. (1968). Instrumental conditioning of sensorimotor cortex EEG spindles in the waking cat. *Physiology and Behavior, 3*, 703–707.

Yucha, C., & Gilbert, C. (2004). *Evidence–based practice in biofeedback and neurofeedback.* Wheat Ridge, CO: Association for Applied Psychophysiology and Biofeedback.

Breathing Retraining and Exercise

CHAPTER 12

Whole-Body Breathing
A Systems Perspective on Respiratory Retraining

JAN VAN DIXHOORN

HISTORY

This chapter describes a breathing method that has been developed over the past 50 years in Europe. It includes elements of direct respiratory retraining, as well as indirect approaches to modify respiration by way of its connections to the whole body. It is combined with a systems perspective by taking mental and physical tension states into account.

One of the roots of the method is the work of voice teachers in Germany and the Netherlands. Gerard Meyer imported the techniques of audible inhalation through the lips, developed by the German laryngologist Ulrich (1928) into the Netherlands. The main focus was to achieve an optimal inhalation at high speed and well distributed along the whole of the trunk. It implied full relaxation of exhalatory tension and contraction, which could remain after previous exhalatory effort, in singing a phrase. Inhaling through pursed lips was meant to open the throat and allow a full column of air to flow in. It was combined with body movements, such as swinging a leg, flexing the spine, or moving the head forward and back, to facilitate coordination through the whole body.

Although the purpose was to increase voice production among students of singing, it appeared that breathing and vocal problems responded well. One of Meyer's pupils, Bram Balfoort, was a voice teacher as well as a therapist. He had a private practice and worked in an academic hospital, where he successfully treated lung patients with "relaxed breathing therapy" from the early 1950s to the late 1970s. At the end of his career, he started treating patients with hyperventilation syndrome and was one of the first to have success. He found that many had the tendency for high exhalatory residual tension, which led to difficulty inhaling and a sense of dyspnea. Another of the pupils of Gerard Meyer developed a method for treatment of stuttering based on the breathing techniques in the same time period.

I cooperated with Balfoort for several years. This resulted in a popular book (Balfoort & Dixhoorn, 1979) and further development of the techniques. By applying them in the context of cardiac rehabilitation and studying the effects of various procedures using biofeedback, I shifted the emphasis from breathing technique to a wider perspective of relaxation, body awareness, and tension regulation. An initial treatment protocol was the basis of a clinical trial of breathing therapy in the early 1980s on patients who had experienced a myocardial infarction. Clear benefits appeared from adding relaxation to exercise training (Dixhoorn & Duivenvoorden, 1989; Dixhoorn, Duivenvoorden, Staal, & Pool, 1989). This outcome had far-reaching effects on cardiac rehabilitation practice in the Netherlands. Now most hospitals conduct a cardiac rehabilitation program that includes relaxation therapy using the present method.

I applied the concepts of Edmund Jacobson (see McGuigan & Lehrer, Chapter 4, this volume) to systematically reduce residual, unnecessary muscle tension and effort associated with breathing. This was supplemented by elements from the dynamic system of Feldenkrais (Feldenkrais, 1972), who defined effort as muscle tension that is in excess relative to its function in moving the bony structure of the body. As a result, I developed a model for breathing patterns in relation to skeletal movement, particularly the spinal column. Instructions were designed that influence breathing movement throughout the body, from the head to the feet, in a way that is accessible to everyone. Finally, a systems perspective was applied. Breathing was seen in continuous interaction with mental and physical tension states. The main function of therapy is the self-regulation of tension. The method has been described in a manual (Dixhoorn, 1998a) that became the basis of a 3-year part-time education in breathing therapy for professionals, who apply it to a wide range of problems.

THEORETICAL FOUNDATIONS

Basics of Respiration

Respiration is a rhythmic contraction and expansion of the body, as a result of which air flows in and out of the lungs. It can be represented as a curve, going up as the air flows in with inhalation and down as the air flows out with exhalation (Figure 12.1). Normal inhalation time is about 40% of total cycle length, and exhalation is about 60%. There are slight pauses or breath holds at the end of inhalation (about 3–5%) and at the end of exhalation (5–10%), when the flow reverses. However, there is great variation in the timing of respiration. Total cycle length determines the rate of respiration per minute, or cycles per minute (CPM), which also shows great variation, and can be anywhere between very low frequencies of 3–6 CPM and higher frequencies of 16–24 CPM, or even higher. The amount of air that flows in and out of the lungs is another variable that determines

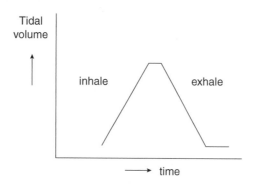

FIGURE 12.1. Respiration curve.

breathing pattern. It is called tidal volume, V_t, and varies greatly as well. In resting situations it is normally between 0.3–0.5 liters. The minute volume (MV) is the total amount of air that passes in and out of the lungs per minute. It is the product of V_t and CPM.

The action of air passing in and out of the lungs is called *ventilation*. The outside air that comes in supplies fresh oxygen, and the air that is expelled from the lungs contains carbon dioxide (CO_2). Both gases are essential for (aerobic) metabolism, which provides the energy that the living system requires. Oxygen combines with nutrient substances to produce energy and leaves water and CO_2 as waste products. Thus the metabolism in living tissues produces CO_2, which is passed to venous blood and carried to the lungs. In the small air sacs, or *alveoli*, the blood capillaries allow diffusion of the gases between the blood and the air. The high concentration of CO_2 in the blood creates diffusion to the alveoli, which contain the outside air with much lower concentration of CO_2. At the end of expiration, the concentration of CO_2 in the expired air almost equals the venous concentration. This end-tidal CO_2 ranges between 37 and 43 mm Hg. Carbon dioxide is important for many reasons, including its determination of the acidity of the blood, or pH. The pH is vital for homeostasis and needs to be regulated within a strictly delimited range. When CO_2 drops, the blood becomes less acidic; when CO_2 rises, the blood becomes more acidic.

By contrast, oxygen concentration is higher in inspired air than in venous blood, and oxygen diffuses in the alveoli into the capillary blood vessels. The oxygenated blood circulates back into the heart and from there throughout the body. Almost all of the oxygen is bound to hemoglobin molecules in the blood, which carry and store it. A small percentage is dissolved in the blood and has sufficient pressure to allow it to pass to the tissues that need it. Under normal conditions the hemoglobin in arterial blood is almost 100% saturated with oxygen. When the pressure of the dissolved oxygen (pO_2) drops, the saturation decreases slowly but leaves sufficient oxygen in storage. However, when the acidity of the blood decreases because of low CO_2 levels, oxygen is bound here tightly to the hemoglobin and passes less easily to the tissues. This is called the *Bohr effect* (Lumb, 2000).

Normally, minute ventilation is regulated automatically on the basis of the requirements for gas exchange. When the body becomes more active and requires more energy, metabolism increases, more oxygen is required, and more CO_2 is produced. Mostly on the basis of CO_2 levels, the body increases ventilation. Hypoventilation can occur when the lungs function insufficiently because of lung disease—for instance, chronic obstructive pulmonary disease (COPD). In that situation, oxygen levels can drop (hypoxemia), CO_2 levels rise, and the need for ventilation cannot be met, which results in dyspnea or the sense of air hunger or laborious breathing. In patients who are prone to hypoxemia, it is recommended therefore to increase physical effort in exercise training only on the basis of regular measurement of the pO_2 in the blood. This can be done quite easily by way of an oximeter through thin skin, for instance, of an earlobe (Tiep, Burns, Kao, Madison, & Herrera, 1986). By contrast, hyperventilation occurs when ventilation is too large for the metabolic requirements of the moment. As a result, CO_2 pressure drops, resulting in hypocapnia, and the blood becomes less acid. Although the pO_2 may rise in acute hyperventilation, after some time the pH increases, which causes the oxygen to be bound tighter to the hemoglobin, which results, paradoxically, in less tissue oxygenation. Thus hyperventilation is primarily characterized by hypocapnia. Hypocapnia can be measured by capnography of the expired air, either exhaled through a mouthpiece or sampled from a tube in the nostrils. It may also be measured transcutaneously, but that is less accurate. Hypocapnia can lead to many complaints (see Table 12.2 later in the chapter), but it does not cause dyspnea. When there is no physical cause for hyperventilation, the excess ventilation is thought to be a problem of tension, anxiety, or faulty breathing.

The same ventilation can be achieved through many combinations of CPM and V_t: Many small breaths per minute move the same amount of air in and out of the lungs as a few large breaths. Although mechanical constraints limit the number of possible combinations without extra work in breathing, the remaining range is large. So far, no optimal breathing pattern has been established. The actual choice of V_t and CPM, made in the breathing regulatory centers in the brain, depends much on the state of the organism as a whole and reflects its condition.

The effect of ventilation is that outside air, which is high in oxygen and low in CO_2, comes into contact with capillary venous blood, which is low in oxygen and high in CO_2, so that diffusion occurs. An important factor, therefore, is the space between the opening for air (mouth and nose) and the lung alveoli. It is called "dead air space" because the air passes through it without actual diffusion. It consists of the throat, trachea, and bronchi. The size depends on the structure of the body, but it averages about 0.15 L. It can be enlarged by breathing through a tube, which decreases effective ventilation. When the tube is so large that the volume of the dead-air space equals tidal volume, there is no effective ventilation: No outside fresh air comes into the lung alveoli. Similarly, high-frequency breathing with very small breaths leads to very little effective ventilation, because the size of V_t approaches dead-air space. Its main use is to cool the body by the flow of air: inhaling cool outside air, which is heated inside the body and flows outside by exhalation. By contrast, when the body becomes more active and metabolism increases, ventilation increases first by an increase of V_t (Wientjes, 1993). The deeper breaths lead directly to more effective ventilation because the dead-air space becomes a smaller part of tidal volume.

The combination of time and volume results in flow: The amount of air that flows in during inhalation time represents inhalatory force or drive. When more air is inhaled in a shorter time, the inhalatory drive is high. This may occur when the person is dyspneic, for instance, if COPD is present, or when a novice diver breathes through a gas mask for the first time under water. It may lead to a breathing pattern of "gasping," that is, making great effort to inhale air.

The contraction and expansion of the body is performed by the respiratory muscles, which change the volume of the trunk. When the volume of the trunk increases, the interior pressure decreases relative to the atmospheric pressure. When the airways are open, the air flows inside the lungs. However, the movement of expansion is made in the trunk as a whole, reaching from the first rib to the pelvic floor. Under resting conditions, about two-thirds of the volume changes are achieved by the diaphragm. This is a double dome-like muscle that separates the chest from the abdominal cavity. When it contracts, it increases the size of the chest cavity in three directions. It moves downward, pressing on the abdominal cavity, and it lifts the lower ribs, which elevate sideways and in anterior direction (Kapandji, 1974). Other respiratory muscles include the intercostal muscles, some of which elevate the ribs for inhalation while others bring them down for exhalation. The scalene muscles elevate the upper ribs toward the neck. The abdominal muscles compress the abdominal cavity and help the diaphragm to move upward for exhalation. The pelvic floor muscles resist the downward pressure of the diaphragm and help with exhalation.

A Systems Perspective

Breathing is dependent on many factors, both physical and mental, that influence its rate, depth, and shape. Within psychophysiology, respiratory measures function mainly as dependent variables, reflecting the state of the individual. Within *applied* psychophysiology, however, respiration also functions as an independent variable, a potential influence on one's state. Breathing is the only vital function that is open to conscious awareness and modification (Ley, 1994). The individual may voluntary modify breathing patterns in order to change mental or physical tension states. A study by Umezawa found that such modification was the most popular maneuver for managing stress (Umezawa, 2001). Thus there is a double relationship between breathing and the state of the system, represented in Figure 12.2, which makes matters rather complicated. The arrows that lead from respiration toward physical or mental tension state represent the regulatory role of breathing; the arrows that lead toward respiration represent its role as indicator. The distinction is important to avoid confusion, but it tends to be overlooked. For instance, breathing may respond to relaxation of the system, indicated by longer exhalation pauses or participation of the abdomen in breathing movement. These characteristics are then taken as a guide for regulation by practicing exhalation pauses or abdominal breathing. It does not follow however, that the system automatically relaxes when these characteristics are imitated. Voluntary breath modification in a high-tension state may give a sense of control but may also disturb respiration even more. This explains why some individuals do not respond favorably to simple breathing advice or instruction. The model further shows that measuring breathing to estimate the individual's state (indicator role) can be complicated by voluntary changes in breathing or control of breathing by the individual who is aware that breathing is being measured. Focusing attention on breathing may modify it. It is, therefore, not easy to measure "spontaneous" breathing. Conversely, any breathing maneuver involves both respiratory changes and changes in mental and physical state. Thus, although its effects may be attributed to respiration, they also may be caused by concomitant changes in the entire body system that affect both respiration and the outcome parameter.

Paced breathing, for example, consists of modification of respiration rate but also involves focusing of attention and often a stabilization of posture, which have widespread effects as well. It is therefore important in studies of breathing therapies that respiratory measures be included to see whether breathing actually changes, although even in such cases the effects may also be attributed to other factors. For instance, Meuret, Wilhelm, and Roth (2005) studied the effect of six sessions of clear-cut breathing regulation, assisted by capnography feedback, for patients with panic disorder. Panic attacks decreased, and pCO_2 rose. These effects were correlated, leading to the conclusion that the anxiety decreased as a result of ventilation decrease. However, the sessions equally taught the participants to focus their minds and sit still for an extended period of time, which may have resulted in a relaxation response that led to lower anxiety and reduced ventilation (Benson, Beary, & Carol, 1974). Alternatively, participants in the study may have

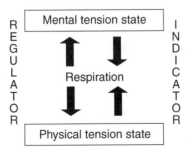

FIGURE 12.2. Model of double relationship between respiration and individual system.

concluded from the sessions that their anxiety attacks were not due to an impending catastrophic event but simply related to breathing. This process of cognitive reattribution of their attacks to an innocent and controllable factor may have reduced their anxiety and, as a result, reduced ventilation. The researcher who wants to disentangle these factors must measure all of them. For clinical practice, it is recommended that the complexity of the interrelationships be taken as a starting point.

This model represents a systems view of respiration. It underlines the complexity of breathing instruction, which always includes both mental and physical components and effects. One consequence of the model is that breathing instruction consists of two parts—one in which breathing is consciously modified or regulated and one in which this regulation is consciously stopped. This is comparable to Jacobson's procedure of consciously tensing a muscle in order to learn to consciously stop muscle tension. One cannot ask the participant to stop breathing, but it is possible to stop a conscious regulatory practice. The purpose is to observe how the system responds to the regulation and whether there is a durable and stable effect on breathing after regulation has stopped. The instruction that regulates breathing is more like an invitation to the system to respond favorably than a dominant influence. To underline this, it is important to teach a specific skill to practice, but it is equally important to have the participant stop practicing.

Another consequence of the model is that breathing instruction may consist of instructions for posture, body movement, or attention, not even mentioning breathing explicitly, but influencing it indirectly. The list of practical strategies shows this clearly (see the "Instructions" in the Treatment Manual later in this chapter). A good example is an intervention that helps lung cancer patients deal with dyspnea (Bredin et al., 1999) of which direct respiratory regulation is only a part. Once breathing has changed, this may spontaneously draw the attention of the patient, or the patient may be asked to pay attention to it. In scientific studies the complexity is often overlooked or ignored to reduce the treatment to a reproducible protocol. However, the model specifies that such a reduction may be costly when the context of an instruction is as important as the instruction itself. For instance, many participants, particularly novice ones, have trouble performing a breathing instruction and use too much effort initially. This may lead to an overshoot and production of opposite effects. Such effects probably occur less often when sufficient attention is paid to the physical and mental tension state. For instance, Choliz (1995) reported on a highly effective breathing instruction for insomnia, in which underventilation gradually led to a state of drowsiness. He simply described the respiratory protocol without mentioning any strategy to make the system accept the instruction and facilitate a favorable response. The protocol was replicated (Hout & Kroeze, 1995) and led, in many participants, to *hyper*ventilation! On the basis of this, the treatment and its supposed mechanism were rejected.

A further consequence of the systems view is that it is very difficult to define "good" and "bad" or "functional" and "dysfunctional" breathing. A particular breathing pattern may look irregular or effortful but actually result from a specific factor within the system to which breathing responds. A good example is the breathing pattern of patients with COPD whose lungs are hyperinflated and whose diaphragms are maximally active. Their breathing is clearly upper thoracic and effortful, involving auxiliary respiratory muscles, and they are often told or taught to breathe more abdominally. In that condition, however, upper thoracic breathing may be a functional way of elevating the chest to inhale air, and "abdominal" breathing may not be functional at all and may even worsen their already insufficient ventilation (Cahalin, Braga, Matsuo, & Hernandez, 2002;

Gosselink, Wagenaar, Rijswijk, Sargeant, & Decramer, 1995). However, upper thoracic breathing may also be a dysfunctional exaggeration of a functional adaptation. The sense of dyspnea, for instance, leads to a quick inhalation (Noseda, Carpiaux, Schmerber, Valente, & Yernault, 1994), which may result in insufficient time for adequate distribution of inhalation and thus to excess ventilatory effort. It is difficult, therefore, to differentiate between functional and dysfunctional breathing. A good way is to observe whether instructions that aim to reduce unnecessary effort in breathing are successful in changing the breathing pattern and whether the sense of dyspnea responds to that (Dixhoorn, 1997b; Thomas, McKinley, Freeman, & Foy, 2001). It is important to include time for the response to occur after instruction. When a particular breathing pattern changes and remains visibly less effortful after instruction, the pattern was probably dysfunctional to some extent. This formulation refers to the first consequence of the model: that breathing instruction entails that regulation is also stopped. If that condition is not fulfilled, the observed change in breathing pattern may be simply the result of conscious practice while being monitored or observed.

Definitions of Breathing

Breathing instruction and the sense of laborious breathing, or dyspnea, can be viewed from various perspectives, depending on the definition of breathing. The most common definition of breathing refers to the *passage of air* that serves for *lung function and ventilation*. Breathing is measured by way of lung function parameters such as rate, inhalation time, exhalation time, pauses, tidal volume, minute volume, flow (duty cycle), O_2 saturation, and end-tidal CO_2. The mechanics by which the air is moved in and out of the lungs are of secondary importance, because they hardly influence lung function. Dyspnea is a common complaint in lung disease, and the medical point of view is to objectify its basis in lung function. This is partly successful. Also, lung function does not account for the function of air passage in communication. Without air movement, there is no voice or sound, and the person cannot smell. The regulation of air passage to ensure speech and communication is highly complex and represents a different process from ventilation (Conrad, Thalacker, & Schonle, 1983). The behavioral demands contingent on communication mostly overrule the ventilatory requirements (Phillipson, McClean, Sullivan, & Zamel, 1978). Thus air passage has an important expressive function that is often neglected. The implication is that breathing difficulties may signify difficulties in social interaction and experience rather than ventilatory problems.

A second definition refers to the *rhythmic expansion and contraction* of the body. This breathing motion serves, of course, to bring the air in and out of the lungs, but it has other functions as well. Breathing is a central pump, or oscillator, in the body that moves various organs and the fluids; for example, it acts to move venous blood, lymph fluid, and the cerebrospinal fluid. In addition to these hydraulic effects throughout the body, there is a clear oscillatory relationship with heart rate and heart rate variability that affects the autonomic nervous system (see Lehrer, Chapter 10, this volume). Next, the mechanical properties of volume changes have a dynamic of their own. The coordination of breathing movement determines, to a large extent, the effort of the pump and the sense of dyspnea but also affects movement and posture. The components of the breathing apparatus play a role in posture, weight bearing, walking, and lifting objects, as well as in moving air in and out of the lungs. The qualities that apply here have to do with smoothness of movement, fluency, effortlessness, and coordination throughout the whole system, from head to feet.

A third definition of breathing refers to its role in *self-perception*. Like any movement, breathing is a sensory motor activity that serves to provide important feedback to the conscious individual about his or her state. The sense of freedom of movement or restriction in space, the sense of tension or relaxation within oneself, the sense of safety or danger within the environment, all have much to do with the quality of internal feedback. Thus a person may feel free and at ease or restricted and even dyspneic because of changes in self-perception. An important aspect of breathing is, therefore, to what degree its sensation is accessible to conscious awareness without this awareness leading to disruption of the natural rhythm. For instance, patients with lung disease can be "non perceivers," which means that they do not notice changes in lung function (Noseda, Schmerber, Prigogine, & Yernault, 1993). This is a risk because it prevents them taking adequate measures in time, but it also appears that the response to medication is greater in "perceivers." Poor perceivers of respiratory sensations, for example, have more "near death" experiences from asthma (Kikuchi et al., 1994). In clinical practice it appears that many individuals have little awareness of the quality of breathing and lack this sort of feedback. The purpose of breathing therapy is to enhance this awareness by inducing a marked improvement in perceived quality. At the same time, overconsciousness needs to be avoided. Breathing is a natural and automatic function that does better without constant conscious attention. For that reason, the indirect strategies are extremely useful.

These three perspectives are complementary; they represent three ways of looking at dyspnea and breathing difficulties, and they lead to different measurements and treatment strategies. Ideally, breathing therapy should take all three into account. It is interesting what the result of a dysfunction is in the latter two viewpoints—when the quality of breathing movement is low and effortful but at the same time self-perception is also limited. What will a person with these characteristics report? Clearly, nothing special. Although internal tension may be high, it does not enter conscious awareness. This is a quite common situation and may explain why breathing instructions can be met with mixed feelings. An increased ease in breathing may feel pleasant, but the increased awareness of the tension is unpleasant. It all depends on which one dominates.

Strategies for Breathing Regulation

In this section strategies are described to modify breathing that are either direct or indirect, that often consist of combinations of breathing instruction with attentional and/or movement instruction, and that aim at either breath or tension regulation or both.

Timing

Counting breathing is a common procedure that consists of coupling attention to breathing. In Benson's Respiration One Method (Benson, 1993) breathing is counted '1, 1, 1,' and so on because the person may lose count, which gives rise to unrest. Breathing may also be counted from 1 to 10, or the inhalation and exhalation may be mentally followed with such words as *in, out, in, out*. Attention can also be coupled to breathing without counting; the instruction may be to mentally follow inhalation and exhalation. *Pacing breathing* is used mostly to slow down breathing and may consist of the instruction to breathe at fixed rates: "in, 2, 3, out, 2, 3," or "1, 2, 3, 4" during inhalation and "5, 6, 7, 8, 9" during exhalation. There may be protocols for this, gradually increasing length, and it may be prescribed in a directive fashion or may be more open and free. The rationale is mostly that slower breathing leads to relaxation or that it increases CO_2 and reduces hyperventilation or both. Sometimes a device is constructed that indicates by a tone of varying pitch how long to inhale and how long to exhale. Again, this may be a fixed preset rate, or the instruction may depend on the actual breathing rate of the individual, in which case the instrument contains a sensor to measure that rate (Schein et al., 2005). Sometimes the rate is subsequently adapted to breathing measured during sessions (Grossman, Swart, & Defares, 1985) to achieve a feasible lengthening.

Focusing on *exhalation pauses* is a good way to lengthen breathing, because pauses naturally appear under relaxation conditions (Umezawa, 1992). Instructions that can help achieve this state are "in, out, stop" or "pause" or "in, 2, 3, out, 2, 3, pause 2, 3." In the Buteyko method, these pauses are gradually lengthened to approach almost one minute (Bowler, Green, & Mitchell, 1998). During transcendental meditation they are observed to occur spontaneously for about 30 seconds, particularly during EEG changes (Badawi, Wallace, Orme-Johnson, & Rouzere, 1984). In hyperventilation treatment, the focus on exhalation pause serves to increase CO_2. By contrast, pacing may also be used to increase respiration rate and decrease depth. An example is to count "in, out, stop" at such a pace that it results in a ratio of respiration to heart rate of approximately 1:4. Such short and shallow breathing helps to break an overconscious pattern of slow breathing or to induce shallow breathing, which is useful when there is a persistent unproductive cough. The therapist should warn the client not to breathe deeply. This pattern fits a situation of high tension or challenge, for instance, during delivery of a child, but it is also useful to show that, during rest, reduced ventilation is sufficient.

Interestingly, short and shallow breathing during rest may lead to effortless breathing, whose movement is perceptible throughout the whole trunk. The reason is that a low volume requires little effort and leads to relaxation of respiratory muscles. Another variation is to pay attention to the *transitions* between inhalation and exhalation and exhalation and inhalation. The breathing cycle is divided into four parts: in, pause, out, pause. Attention is brought to the period when breathing reverses direction and stops for a brief moment. This is a natural control strategy that helps to focus and calm the mind and make breathing less hurried. It is useful when someone is dyspneic from lung disease, because it provides a small margin of control. It may be a starting point for gradually increasing the time period of the transitions.

Coupling to Movement

An indirect and natural way of pacing breathing is through *coupling to movement*. Any movement that has a periodicity similar to breathing tends to synchronize with it. Walking, cycling, or running tend to go easier when the rate of repetition has a whole number ratio to the rate of breathing. When coupling has occurred, slowing down the movement tends to slow down breathing. For example, walking slowly for some time may gradually lead to slower and deeper breathing. At the same time, inhibition of habitual speed leads to increased mental focus and attention, which, in turn, favors slower breathing. When the goal is too slow, however, the effort to do it creates unrest and distraction and thus quickens respiration.

Small, repetitive movements are easy to couple to breathing: rolling the hands or arms in and out, moving the head up and down, pressing the fingers together and relaxing them, flexing and extending the feet. Single tense–release cycles can also be coupled to breathing, as is done in the abbreviated version of progressive relaxation (see Chapter 5, this volume), in which tensing a muscle is coupled to inhaling. This is a natural combination, but in the present method it is reversed: tensing is coupled to exhaling (see "Instructions" section in Treatment Manual). This combination requires attention and, therefore, acts as a focus of attention. Movements that flex and extend the spine play a special role, because this tends to couple mechanically with inhaling and exhaling. When running, animals such as dogs and horses tend to inhale when the four legs are spread out and breathe out when the legs are together. Similarly, the yoga exercise series, "sun greeting," consists of an alternation of flexing the whole body (exhaling) and extending it (inhaling). On a smaller scale, in the sitting position, bending forward or sitting upright tends to extend the spine and couples with inhaling, whereas sitting backward in a slump tends to flex the spine and couples with exhaling (see "Instructions"). Using these combinations facilitates breathing instruction, but it may also be used with reverse coupling. The reason to *reverse coupling* is to break the habitual combination and thereby increase the flexibility and the area of breathing movement. For instance, sitting slumped or with head down helps the body to breathe in while the spine is flexed. Once this is possible, the movement to sit back and round the spine can be combined with inhalation and sitting upright with exhalation. This facilitates "width breathing," which may feel unfamiliar and strange. When someone gets the knack of it, however, the range of breathing movement increases, the diaphragmatic motion is stimulated (Cahalin et al., 2002), and dyspnea may decrease. Another option is to reverse the habitual combination of raising the shoulders while inhaling (see "Instructions"). These kinds of instructions may extend to ones in which movement and breathing are *uncoupled*. This increases flexibility of breathing. Also, breathing serves as an indicator of the effort involved in the movement. Thus, in Feldenkrais's method, a fully functional movement implies that it is carried out with undisturbed breathing. A simple example is rolling the head in the supine position, which tends to interfere with breathing until breathing has become more flexible and/or the rolling movement has become more effortless.

Air Passage

The *passage of air* is a good way to modify respiration, which is done naturally by patients with COPD who use *pursed-lips breathing* to lengthen exhalation when dyspnea occurs. The added resistance to the air by the lips helps to keep the airways open and postpones airway collapse, thus enhancing ventilation. Similarly, audible exhalation through the lips (see "Instructions") lengthens it; in this method, however, it is done with less force than in pursed-lips breathing and is combined with slow inhalation. After a longer exhalation, one tends to inhale hurriedly, and a fast inhalation tends to be an upper-thoracic movement with auxiliary breathing muscles, particularly when one has gotten out of breath. The resulting "gasping" inhalation confirms the sense of dyspnea. Gasping is prevented by the instruction to exhale gently and slowly. It results in generally larger tidal volumes and should be done a few times (5–6), after which normal nose breathing is resumed. This is to prevent hyperventilation.

Slow inhalation tends to improve the distribution of breathing movement, because all the components are allowed more time to become involved. It results in a larger volume, more involvement of the whole body, and less risk of hyperventilation, particularly when breathing though the nose. A good example is the idea of smelling a nice fragrance, such as a flower. The image of enjoying the inhalation of the air slowly into the body adds to this effect. It may be combined with imagery of the airways and of the air passing from the tip of the nose through the inside of the nose and throat, down into the lungs and chest, and even further down the body. By contrast, mouth breathing tends to result in shorter inhalation times.

Resistance training is a technique for strengthening the power of inhalatory muscles, such as the diaphragm. It can be done by breathing through a mouthpiece with a varying opening width, thus increasing the resistance and providing a training impulse to the muscles (Dekhuijzen, 1989). This is useful for patients with lung disease, but a recent study showed a good effect on exercise capacity and dyspnea in patients with heart failure (Laoutaris et al., 2004). A similar method of resistance training comes from voice training and is used by singers to open the upper airways. They breathe in through the lips, making a sound like "fff" from the lips, in order to increase resistance (Ulrich, 1928; Balfoort & Dixhoorn, 1979). This trains rapid and full inhalation, which is important for performance. Generally, inhaling through a mouthpiece tends to increase ventilation (Han et al., 1997). This effect counteracts the effect of breathing through a tube, which is used for hyperventilation complaints to increase dead-air space.

Distribution of Breathing

The shape or form of the volume changes with breathing can vary considerably, because the potential volume change in the trunk is much larger than is possible for the lungs. Thus the same ventilation can be achieved by different parts of the trunk, which ensures that ventilation can be maintained in very different postures. This leaves a large margin of flexibility and also allows conscious control and modification. Before practicing voluntary control of the location and form of breathing movement, however, it is important to realize that the areas of the body that are actively involved in breathing movement largely depend on posture, on mental state (focused or passive), on emotional or expressive state, and on physical tension state (energy and ventilation requirement, nervous tension). When a person is resting, mentally and physically, tidal volume is relatively low, primarily achieved by the diaphragmatic pump, and the muscles of the trunk are relatively relaxed. In this situation visible breathing is mainly costoabdominal: the lower ribs widen, and the abdomen expands with inhalation. The upper ribs and so-called auxiliary muscles, such as the scalenes, nevertheless also contract with each inhalation. This is necessary to prevent a slight collapse of the rib cage under the increased negative pressure inside that leads to the inflow of air (Decramer & Macklem, 1985). It is hardly visible, but its absence is not functional, and maintaining upper chest immobility should not be taken as a sign of functional breathing. When the activity and tension levels rise, volume increases and involves more movement of the rib cage, and the muscles around the abdomen may tighten a little. As a result, breathing becomes "higher." From this natural response, many strategies advocate that breathing remain "low" in the body while under stress or during greater activity.

Thus *abdominal breathing*, diaphragmatic breathing, and slow deep breathing are common practices, probably the most common (Gevirtz & Schwartz, 2005). This strategy is quite effective in remaining or becoming quiet and calm and in reducing stress (Peper & Tibbets, 1994; Czapszys, McBride, Ozawa, Gibney, & Peper, 2000). The person is taught to put the hands on the abdomen (or the therapist may do so) or to put a weight, such as a book (Lum, 1977), on the abdomen in the reclining position and make it move up and down with breathing. Lum reported 75% success among more than 1,000 patients with anxiety and hyperventilation (Lum, 1981). It is particularly useful in individuals who demonstrate an exaggerated response to the rise of tension, which is dysfunctional and dysponetic (Whatmore & Kohli, 1974) and which can be reduced in this way. This makes breathing a quick and easy tool for handling stress.

However, two points need to be considered. First, the effect of this strategy may not be due to breathing itself but to the concomitant shift in attention, which is directed to the center of the body. This is the area of the center of gravity, and, as such, it represents a neutral ground for attention, less threatening or challenging than the visual perspective in front or in one's mind. This reduces the mental tension state. Attention in the center also implies that body movement tends to become more functional and less effortful. This reduces the physical tension state. Thus breathing may simply be the tool to induce these shifts. A second point is that the emphasis on abdominal movement may lead to the mistaken notion that the (upper) chest should be immobile. As stated earlier, reducing exaggerated upper thoracic breathing does not imply that the upper ribs should not move at all. Functional inhalation requires the rib cage to change its shape as a whole (Parow, 1980; Bergsmann & Eder, 1977; Balfoort & Dixhoorn, 1979).

Functional upper chest movement is important for breathing and, in particular, for emotional freedom of expression, as well as for voice production. It is intimately linked to an adequate use of the upper back. In the best singers, the upper chest rises simultaneously, with a slight lengthening of the upper spine, thereby increasing the length of the scalene muscles and making their contraction more effective. The head is tilted slightly forward, relative to the neck, which moves slightly backward. Thus the head remains still. This pattern is evoked by the beginning of a yawn (Xu, Ikeda, & Komiyama, 1991), whereby the throat and vocal cords descend. This favors voice production. It is the basis for the instruction "looking up and down" (see "Instructions"). The opposite pattern is seen in a dyspneic person, whose head is tilted backward relative to the neck, increasing lordosis of the neck during inhalation. This moves the head frontally and up, which appears as a movement of gasping for air. Instructions that promote functional upper chest breathing are also important for neck problems.

Another aspect of location of breathing movement is the *pelvic floor*. This lower diaphragm is a natural antagonist of the middle respiratory diaphragm, and their functions support each other. When the respiratory diaphragm contracts during inhalation, the pelvic diaphragm relaxes, and vice versa. Adequate contraction of the pelvic floor is necessary to carry the weight of the internal organs and to counteract the force of breath holding when lifting or carrying a weight. Thus pelvic floor dysfunction tends to compromise breathing, as well as posture. The instruction "sitting, standing" aims to facilitate pelvic floor contraction when getting up because of its coupling to exhalation. This helps to prevent urine leakage in women who suffer from this problem. Another option is the Muslim prayer posture, in which relaxation of the pelvic floor during inhalation can be observed.

Focus of Attention

Providing a *single focus of attention* is the most common way to relax and reduce tension (Benson, 1993), and it also tends to quiet and regulate breathing. Its effect on breathing does not require a focus on respiration. For some, it is best not to focus on breathing directly, as that tends to disturb it and to cause overconsciousness and dysregulation. The object of attention may be breathing movement anywhere in the body, sound or sensation of air passage, or respiratory feedback signals, but also the sense of body weight in sitting, standing, or lying quietly or during movement, the sense of touch by the therapist or oneself, words that are repeated to oneself, or any visual or auditory focus. Another dimension of attention is active versus passive concentration. *Passive attention, or receptivity,* is a hallmark of relaxation (Smith, 1988) and can be seen as a prerequisite for self-regulation of tension (Peper, 1979). It is in particular present when the indicator role of breathing is emphasized. In an older study, Burrow (1941) found that during "cotention," which is like an unfocused gaze in the distance, respiration rate drops greatly. He associated this with a state of mind in which the individual is in more direct contact with the whole organic system of the body. In a more recent study, passive attention, or mindfulness, was found to be associated with a different pattern of EEG activity than was focused attention (Dunn, Hartigan, & Mikulas, 1999). Thus the very attitude of passivity and not being goal directed may induce a change, including a respiratory response.

An intriguing aspect is a relationship between the *object of attention* and *distribution of breathing*. Respiratory movement follows the direction and content of attention. For instance, Peper (1996) found that the image of standing on a hard concrete floor resulted in breathing that was shallower and higher in the body than the image of natural grass. Calling attention to the supporting ground for the body on the backside and also emphasizing the width of the body may help distribute an evenness of breathing in the body. In the instruction "circling knees," the repetitive movement of rolling over the sitting bones draws attention to the supporting ground in a passive way. Awareness of the width of the eyes and the distance between the outer corners of the eyes or of the corners of the mouth and slightly increasing their distance induces the beginning of a smile, as well as a sense of breathing very easily (Dixhoorn, 1998a). This relationship is also present in the influence of attention on the *direction of inhalation*. Although the diaphragm moves downward as it contracts, a common image of inhalation is a movement upward, as if drawing in the air from above. This is strengthened when experiencing dyspnea. By contrast, the image of inhalation as a downward movement helps to let the air flow in easily and reduces dyspnea.

Feedback Devices

Various measurements of respiration can be used as a source of biological or instrumental feedback. A detailed description is given by Gevirtz and Schwartz (2005). An obvious parameter is CO_2 feedback, using capnographic measurements (Doorn, Folgering, & Colla, 1982; Fried, 1984; Meuret, Wilhelm, & Roth, 2001; Terai & Umezawa, 2004). The patient may or may not receive instructions for breathing. The main purpose is for CO_2 to reach normal levels. CO_2 biofeedback is particularly useful when hypocapnia is present. Similarly, feedback of oxygen tension is useful when PO_2 is low (Tiep et al., 1986). Another parameter is feedback for respiration rate. In contrast to paced respiration, in which a specific frequency is given, respiration rate feedback does not impose a frequency but only provides feedback of actual respiration rate. It appears to have a soothing influence, and respiration rate gradually slows down (Zeier, 1984; Schein et al., 2005; Leuner, 1984). A more directive approach is to use measurement of muscle tension and to teach a specific way of breathing that does or does not involve these muscles (Reybrouck, Wertelaers, Bertrand, & Demedts, 1987; Johnston & Lee, 1976; Kotses et al., 1991; Peper & Tibbets, 1992; Tiep, 1995). In these approaches the breathing strategy is the prime intervention, and the feedback device serves as an aid for teaching it. Another intervention is to give feedback for tidal volume in order to make patients aware that they tend to hold their breath when under stress. This may or may not be accompanied by teaching strategies for inhaling more effectively (MacHose & Peper, 1991; Peper, Smith, & Waddell, 1987; Peper & Tibbets, 1992; Roland & Peper, 1987). An overview of biofeedback techniques for lung patients is given by Tiep (1995). Finally, a more recent form of biofeedback is resonance feedback, in which the parameter consists of heart rate variability that increases with slow breathing (Del Pozo, Gevirtz, Scher, & Guarneri, 2004; Lehrer et al., 2004; see also Chapter 10, this volume).

Whole-Body and Spinal Column Involvement

Given the many interdependencies of respiration that follow from the system's perspective, the method on the one hand seeks orientation in specifying attention and posture and on the other hand follows the skeletal structure of the body. A model was developed during the 1980s that specified the relationship of the spinal column, the core structure of the skeleton, to respiratory movement (Dixhoorn, 1997a). The spinal column connects the rib cage with the head and the pelvis. When it is extended, standing upright or in the supine position, respiration involves a minute wave-like motion in the spine, which is more like a preference for motion than an actual visible movement. It originates from the rib cage, which makes a rolling movement during respiration. Inhalation involves an upward rolling movement of the chest, which is accompanied by a preference for slight lumbar lordosis and flattening of the cervico–thoracic junction. The opposite preference is present during exhalation. Therefore, small movements, initiated from the legs, arms, or head, are able to influence respiration indirectly. This is the first pattern of interaction between spinal column and respiration. The coupling of inhalation to extension is called "length" breathing. It is complemented by the opposite pattern of "width" breathing. When the spinal column is flexed, for instance in a slightly slumped sitting posture, the connections of the first pattern are blocked. This is also the case when a person lies prone. In that situation, the rib cage cannot roll upward, and the cervico–thoracic junction cannot flatten during inhalation. Instead, the costoabdominal circumference expands and lumbar lordosis flattens during inhalation. Because of the emphasis on sideways expansion, it is called *width breathing*. Breathing in both directions, horizontally and vertically, allows the body to respond flexibly to various postures. Therefore, the degree to which both patterns can be utilized is an important indicator of functional breathing and serves as a parameter of the success of breathing therapy (Dixhoorn, 1997b).

These connections are the background for many instructions of the method. They also help to deal with the issue of attention and of conscious control of breathing in several ways. First, the perception of "whole body involvement" invites a more passive concentration than attention that is actively focused on one particular area or movement. The instruction starts with one area or movement and then invites the individual to notice connected movements all over the body. Second, the periphery (arms and legs) and the back are, for most individuals, not consciously related to breathing. Thus facilitation of breathing through the instructions happens unwittingly and does not elicit conscious control. Third, the skeletal connections promote a functional use of the muscles, which tends to lead to a greater ease of movement and of breathing. The patterns may not be fully habitual, and the instructions may feel strange at first, but they tend to remain present after the period of conscious practice. Thus the instructions tend to generalize and become part of automatic movement.

Flexibility and Variability

In the 1990s the Dutch branch of what later became the International Society for the Advancement of Respiratory Psychophysiology (ISARP) set up a series of meetings to discuss the criteria for what constitutes a proper breathing pattern. It was also a theme at the international meetings (Ley, Timmons, Kotses, Harver, & Wientjes, 1996). In the end, not a single characteristic could be validated to serve as such a criterion. This conclusion supported the assumption of this method that a key characteristic of functional breathing is its variability. The manual (Dixhoorn, 1998a) stated that, rather than working toward a particular pattern of breathing, the main goal is that breathing should be flexible and should adapt to changing demands without causing a sense of effort. From this goal several implications may be derived.

1. Functional breathing responds to changes in the environment. For example, a respiratory response to imagery cues, touch, speech, posture, or movement is likely to be noticeable. Many instructions from the method have as their purpose to test and promote this responsiveness.

2. Variability in breathing is a sign of healthy function. Donaldson (1992) found irregularity in all respiratory parameters: lowest for CO_2, highest for expiratory time. He concluded "that the chaotic nature of resting human respiration allows for fast and flexible responses to sudden changes" (p. 313), which strengthens the stability of the system as a whole. In some studies variability was associated with a positive emotional state (Boiten, 1998; Wittenboer, Wolf, & Dixhoorn, 2003). The power spectrum of variations is probably complex, because many determinants exist.

3. High irregularity is not always healthy; for instance, when it is the result of two conflicting determinants. Highly anxious people tend to have a high standard deviation around the mean respiration rate because of an alternation between relatively fast regular breathing and deep sighs (Wilhelm, Trabert, & Roth, 2001b). The power spectrum is probably less complex.

4. Healthy variability includes adequate recovery from a stimulus, which includes the response to hyperventilation provocation. A delayed recovery of CO_2 after fast, deep breathing or a single deep breath can be taken, therefore, as a sign of reduced flexibility (Wilhelm, Trabert, & Roth, 2001a).

5. The criterion of flexibility also includes the possibility of slow, deep breathing. Although there is increasing evidence that periodic slow, deep breathing is healthy (see Chapter 10, this volume), it cannot be stated that one should always breathe that way. Flexibility entails that slow, deep breathing should occur or be possible under proper conditions and without giving rise to a sense of dyspnea.

To summarize, an individual with an erratic, highly irregular breathing pattern may benefit from measures to introduce rhythm and stabilize breathing. However, a too-regular pattern is not optimal, and the person may benefit from measures that require variable respiratory responses.

ASSESSMENT OF EFFECTS

Respiratory and Physiological Effects

The method has been tested so far in one clinical trial in which 156 patients with myocardial infarction were randomly assigned to exercise rehabilitation only or to exercise plus six individual sessions for breathing and relaxation therapy. Although the breathing method did not focus on teaching a particular form of breathing and utilizes mainly an indirect approach to respiration, respiratory changes did occur and figured prominently among the physiological effects. Respiration was measured in a protocol of 20 minutes' duration, consisting of standing, lying down, slow breathing, lying still for 6 minutes, and slow breathing. Care was taken that the patients did not practice any technique. Average respiration rate at pretest was about 15 cycles per minute (CPM) in both groups. It remained at this frequency in the control group but dropped in the treatment group to 12 CPM at posttreatment and at follow-up (Dixhoorn & Duivenvoorden, 1989). The difference was small but statistically highly significant. Figure 12.3 shows that a small but consistent reduction occurred across all measurements of spontaneous respiration (time periods 1, 2, 4, 5) but not during slow, controlled breathing (time periods 3 and 6). Thus the responsiveness of respiration to standing, lying down, and quietness remained intact. The small increase during quietness (4 → 5) indicates that patients were not practicing or controlling breathing. During the 20-minute testing period, estimated minute volume decreased in both groups, before and after rehabilitation, indicating lowered arousal from lying down and quietness. In the experimental group significantly more patients reported pleasant body sensations during testing after rehabilitation.

The effect on respiration rate was evident even at 2-year follow-up, when respiration was measured in 38 patients. Two patients from the treatment group appeared to practice the breathing technique during measurement. Their respiration rate was about 7 CPM, and they were excluded from analysis. The control group was still breathing at a rate of 15 CPM, and the treatment group continued to show a reduction to 11 CPM. Further analysis showed that all of the time components lengthened somewhat but that the reduction was mainly due to an increase in exhalation pause time (Dixhoorn, 1994a). This indicates that the patients were breathing in a more relaxed way. Another aspect was the distribution of inhalation movement, assessed in the sitting position (see the section on "Assessment of Breathing" in the Treatment Manual, later in this chapter). The distribution of breathing in the treatment group was lower in the body and remained lower during deep breathing. This indicates that the participants in the treatment group were sitting in a more relaxed way, less upright, and, as a result, were breathing a little more slowly and abdominally. This supports the conclusion that the reduction of respiration rate was not the result of training aimed at this particular goal but more likely represented an increased restfulness in breathing, which probably coincided with, and at least did not conflict with, physical and mental tension state.

Heart rate and heart rate variability (HRV) data were available for 76 patients before, after, and at 3 months' follow-up (Dixhoorn, 1998b). Heart rate was reduced in both groups, which is to be expected, as both underwent physical training. Surprisingly, it was more pronounced in the relaxation group, particularly at 3-month follow-up, when heart rate rose a little in the control group but continued to decline in the treatment group. This indicates a stable reduction in physical tension state. However, this reduction was associated with the lower respiration rate, and the effect disappeared when respiration was controlled for. Thus a lower respiration rate may have contributed to a state of

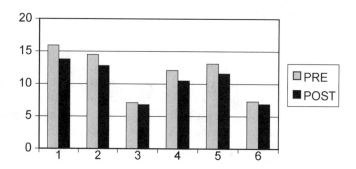

FIGURE 12.3. Respiration rate before and after breathing therapy in patients with myocardial infarction. 1, standing; 2, after lying down; 3, 6, slow, deep breathing through mouthpiece; 4, 5, beginning and end of 6 minutes of lying quietly.

lower arousal (regulator role), or it may have reflected a state of lower arousal (indicator role), or both may have been the case. The same held true for HRV. It remained unchanged in the control group but steadily increased with time in the treatment group. The difference was statistically highly significant but again was associated with respiration rate. When controlling for respiration rate, statistical significance disappeared, except when comparing HRV at the end of the 20-minute testing period. The latter fact may mean that spending 20 minutes in the supine position was more restful and resulted in greater relaxation for the treatment group. Mental relaxation is known to result in increased HRV (Sakakibara, Takeuchi, & Hayano, 1994). Two years after treatment, there no longer were effects on heart rate or HRV. Thus the effect on breathing pattern appears to be a rather specific result of treatment, not only a reflection of lowered arousal.

Evidence of Clinical Effects

The effects of the trial with patients with myocardial infarction on clinical parameters are summarized here and discussed in the light of other studies. It appeared that breathing therapy had multiple effects on psychological, social, and physical states and on prognosis. It clearly increased a sense of well-being. Patients felt more at ease and more relaxed (Dixhoorn, Duivenvoorden, Pool, & Verhage, 1990). Interestingly, patients who improved in well-being in the treatment group were breathing more slowly than at baseline, whereas patients who did not improve or patients in the control group did not change in respiration rate (Dixhoorn & Duivenvoorden, 1989). Data on exercise testing showed that breathing therapy improved the effect of exercise training. It significantly reduced, by half, the occurrence of myocardial ischemia (ST-depression; Dixhoorn et al., 1989). This unexpected effect could not be accounted for by heart rate reduction. It was confirmed in three other studies (Dixhoorn & White, 2005). Also, the outcome of exercise training was assessed by a composite criterion of all parameters of exercise testing, which divided patients into those groups with a clear benefit, those with no change, and those with clear deterioration. It appeared that the occurrence of training failure was reduced by half when relaxation was added to exercise training. The outcome was not associated with respiration rate. There was no effect on blood pressure.

In the longer term, breathing therapy improved return to work to a moderate degree, an effect that was confirmed in two other studies (Dixhoorn & White, 2005). The effect was particularly apparent in patients who did not become more fit after exercise training (Dixhoorn, 1994b). In the longer term, the occurrence of cardiac events (cardiac death, reinfarction, coronary artery bypass graft [CABG]) was reduced by half over a 5-year period (Dixhoorn & Duivenvoorden, 1999). This long-term clinical effect was confirmed in several other studies over varying time periods (Dixhoorn & White, 2005).

From these outcomes it may be concluded that relaxation and breathing therapy is effective but also that stress and tension play an important role in the condition of cardiac patients and that its management is beneficial to them in many respects. This study boosted the application of relaxation and breathing therapy in the field of cardiac rehabilitation, and the method has been included in the Dutch guidelines for cardiac rehabilitation (Commissie Voor de Revalidatie van Hartpatienten, 1996).

The same composite criterion for training outcome was later assessed in 138 patients with myocardial infarction or coronary surgery, all of whom attended one group session of relaxation therapy alongside regular exercise training. In addition, 54 of them were referred for individual relaxed breathing therapy. The percentage of patients with clear benefit was larger in those who had participated in individual therapy (67%) than in those who had not (48%). This confirmed the previous finding that relaxed breathing therapy improves the effect of exercise training.

In three studies, the application to hyperventilation patients was investigated on the basis of changes in their main complaints and the Nijmegen Questionnaire (NQ; Doorn, Colla, & Folgering, 1983). In one study, 12 patients, diagnosed as having hyperventilation syndrome, were compared with 13 patients with nonspecific pain, mainly in head, neck, and back, and also with elevated scores (> 20) on the Nijmegen hyperventilation questionnaire (Dixhoorn & Hoefman, 1987). It appeared that NQ scores were reduced in both groups and that the main complaint improved in both groups equally. Thus breathing therapy is useful when hyperventilation complaints are present, irrespective of the diagnosis of hyperventilation syndrome.

In a second, unpublished study, the outcome was assessed in 51 patients referred for breathing therapy because of tension problems diagnosed as hyperventilation syndrome, 30 of whom also had a medical condition (mainly heart or lung disease). Outcome was determined as the degree to which the patients could manage their tension problems and by NQ scores. A total of 26 patients (51%) had greatly reduced tension problems or were able to manage them satisfactorily. In this group, the elevated scores on NQ (about 25) normalized after treatment (to about 15). Their occurrence did not differ between patients with (47%) and without (57%) medical conditions. The reasons for no response or insufficient response to treatment were: aggravation of medical condition (16%), need for psychological treatment (12%), and lack of motivation (21%). In these patients, scores on the NQ did not change. It was concluded that breathing therapy was useful, irrespective of the presence of a medical condition. Thus the presence of an organic condition is no reason to exclude patients from treatment. However, breathing therapy appears to be an adequate and sufficient treatment for about half of the patients with hyperventilation syndrome. This outcome is in agreement with one of the few studies that did not report average change as outcome but divided patients into those with clear benefit, with small benefit, and with no benefit (Han, Stegen, DeValck, Clement, & Woestijne, 1996). Han et al. (1996) studied 92 patients with anxiety and hyperventilation syndrome and found that 22% had no benefit and 35% had clear benefit.

In a third, also unpublished, study, 55 hyperventilation patients were followed up for 3 years after breathing therapy, 16 of whom (29%) had additional psychological therapy (Leeuwen, 1993). The average decrease in the NQ, from 29 to 24, was highly significant. This is in agreement with two other long-term follow-up studies of breathing intervention (DeGuire, Gevirtz, Hawkinson, & Dixon, 1996; Peper & Tibbets, 1992). However, only 31 (58%) reported major and stable improvement of the main complaints for which they were treated. These treatment responders showed high reductions in the NQ. Treatment responders who did not receive psychotherapy changed from an elevated score of 26 to a normal, average score of 18, whereas those who received psychotherapy had higher scores (about 30), which were reduced but still elevated after 3 years (about 22). Interestingly, nonresponders had high initial scores on the NQ (about 30), which did not change. An important finding was that very few patients (8%) needed a second or third round of treatment sessions with breathing therapy. It seems, therefore, that patients with hyperventilation who respond to breathing therapy have lasting and sufficient benefit but that almost half of them do not respond or need additional psychological treatment.

These studies demonstrate that many patients with hyperventilation symptoms respond to breathing therapy, in which case it is an adequate treatment. Also, the NQ is suitable for selecting patients with other diagnoses for treatment and for evaluating treatment success. However, high scores on the NQ may also signify a more complicated situation, in which case breathing therapy by itself may not be sufficient.

Successful Application

Before beginning treatment, it is important to verify whether a given problem is suitable for this method, that is, that it is at least partly caused by dysfunctional tension and/or dysfunctional breathing. The list of diseases, complaints, or problems that are, at least in part, due to dysfunctional tension is obviously quite long, and there is much anecdotal evidence for positive effect on a wide variety of conditions. The website *www.methodevandixhoorn.com* offers case histories from students of breathing therapy in which they specified the degree to which the problems responded to treatment and probably were due to tension and the degree to which other factors were the cause. Each year a survey is done in which practitioners of the method report conditions in which treatment success occurred and in which the problems were due to tension (Bestuur AOS, 2004). These conditions are listed in Table 12.1, divided into four categories. In each category the conditions are sorted according to the number of practitioners who mention them. They resemble the list of conditions for breathing therapy in Germany (Buchholz, 1994). Treatment of patients with specific somatic causes often occurs in specialized settings such as a rehabilitation clinic, but all conditions are also mentioned by therapists in private practice.

SIDE EFFECTS AND CONTRAINDICATIONS

Although very few side effects have been reported in the literature, clinical experience affirms that they do occur and are reason for caution. Some of them are nonspecific; others are specific for breathing.

Hyperventilation

The most common and specific side effect of breathing interventions is hyperventilation. Individuals use too much effort, breathe too deeply, leave postexhalation or postinhalation pauses that are too short, or perform regulated breathing exercises for too long a time. When attention is brought to breathing, a person tends to breathe deeper, particularly if he or she is tense, anxious, or dyspneic. Tidal volume increases, and respiration rate decreases, as well, because larger inhalation volumes take more time. These

---

TABLE 12.1. List of Conditions for Which Breathing Therapy Has Been Applied Successfully

Tension-related problems without specific cause
- Feelings of tension
- Hyperventilation complaints
- Burnout
- Headache
- Chronic fatigue
- Sleeping problems
- Concentration problems

Psychological problems
- Anxiety and phobia
- Panic disorder
- Depression

Functional problems of musculoskeletal nature and breathing
- Lower back, shoulder, and neck complaints
- Shortness of breath
- Chronic pain (repetitive strain injury, whiplash, fibromyalgia)
- Functional voice disorders, dysphonia, stuttering

Tension problems with a specific, somatic cause
- Lung disease (asthma, COPD)
- Heart disease (myocardial infarction, arrhythmia, CABG)
- Neurological disease (hemiplegia, Parkinson disease)

two effects counteract each other. However, when volume increases more than frequency drops, the result is minute ventilation increases and, after some time, hypocapnia. The inverse relationship between volume and rate may not be sufficient to prevent hyperventilation. For instance, when V_t increases from 0.3 L to 0.6 L and frequency drops from 16 to 8 CPM, the resulting minute volume remains the same: 4.8 L. However, effective ventilation is ventilation minus the dead-air space. Thus effective ventilation actually increases from $(0.3 - 0.15$ L$) \times 16 = 2.4$ L to $(0.6 - 0.15$ L$) \times 8 = 3.6$ L. When one maintains such slow, controlled breathing for some time, hypocapnia is the result. Although it is quite common, few authors have reported it (Hout & Kroeze, 1995; Terai & Umezawa, 2004). It occurred, for instance, in cardiac patients, particularly when they breathed relatively quickly, and techniques to improve the coordination of breathing led to larger tidal volumes with an equal amount of effort. In our experience, some participants mention feeling lightheaded, but no one panics. This experience has led to the explicit instruction to stop any breathing technique after a short time and to let normal breathing resume. Hyperventilation is relatively harmless. The body adapts to it, and in most healthy, resting individuals, the experiences of hypocapnia decrease in time (Hout, Jong, Zandbergen, & Merckelbach, 1990). However, when one is under strain, is shocked by a negative experience, or has an illness, hypocapnia may cause lasting symptoms and even be harmful. Thus it is better to avoid it, and at least to be aware that it may occur. According to Lum (1976), hypocapnia causes vasoconstriction and decreased dissociation of oxygen from hemoglobin in the blood. Both lead to hypoxia, which can trigger angina pectoris (Neill, Pantley, & Makornchai, 1981), dizziness, or an epileptic insult. Hypocapnia also leads to bronchoconstriction, which adds to the dyspnea in lung patients (Varray, Mercier, & Prefaut, 1995). It may impair psychomotor abilities, which are important in high-stress situations, such as for airplane pilots (Gibson, 1978). Generally, hypocapnia leads to increased irritability of the nervous system, which may result in many symptoms, such as tingling sensations, blurred vision, and muscle cramps (Macefield & Burke, 1991).

Thus voluntary hyperventilation results in many symptoms, in people with and without panic disorder. Performing a hyperventilation provocation test with measurement of the ventilated air to ensure that hypocapnia occurs is a common way to establish hyperventilation as a cause of symptoms. In order to distinguish between the effect of hypocapnia per se and the effect of deep, fast breathing of the testing situation, Hornsveld and Garssen (1996) compared such a test with the same test but adding CO_2 to the inhaled air in order to prevent hypocapnia. Many symptoms occur more frequently during the hypocapnic test compared with the isocapnic test, in particular those that are associated with the hyperventilation syndrome (Table 12.2). Interestingly, respiratory symptoms and dyspnea were not among them.

Increased Unpleasant Awareness

A second common side effect of breathing therapy is the unpleasant confrontation with bodily functions that hitherto have remained unconscious. Breathing is largely automatic, but breath regulation leads necessarily to an awareness that helps to deal with tension but that may also be disturbing. This unpleasant awareness may be characterized by an increasing sense of dyspnea or may extend to feelings and sensations in general. Such unpleasant experiences were assessed by a checklist that contained six pleasant and six unpleasant experiences of breath regulation; for instance, more quiet versus less quiet, more tired versus less tired (Dixhoorn, 1992; also available from *www.methodevandixhoorn.com*). It was completed by 181 students in a professional course in breathing therapy and by 144 patients with hyperventilation complaints. It appeared that the two scales were

TABLE 12.2. Symptoms of True Hypocapnic Hyperventilation Compared with Isocapnic Hyperventilation

General symptoms

- Dizziness (NQ)
- Paresthesias (NQ)
- Faintness
- Muscle stiffness (NQ)
- Cold hands or feet (NQ)
- Shivering
- Muscle cramps
- Fatigue

- Hot flashes
- Headache
- Muscle weakness
- Stiffness around the mouth (NQ)
- Warm feeling in the head
- Sweating
- Blurred vision (NQ)
- Rapid heartbeat (NQ)

Respiratory symptoms

- Tightness in the chest (NQ)

Psychological symptoms

- Unrest/tension (NQ)
- Anxiety/panic (NQ)
- Feelings of unreality (NQ)

Note. (NQ), items from the Nijmegen Questionnaire.

unrelated; that is, unpleasant sensations occurred independently of pleasant experiences. The students had six times more pleasant than unpleasant experiences. Only in 4% of responses were the unpleasant experiences as large as the pleasant experiences. However, students with relatively high scores on the Dyspnea subscale of the NQ (Dixhoorn & Duivenvoorden, 1985) had more unpleasant and fewer pleasant experiences. The experiences were not related to anxiety. This confirms that negative awareness of breathing (dyspnea) is a specific reason for unpleasant sensations in general after breathing therapy.

In the patients with hyperventilation complaints, the unpleasant experiences were, on average, more frequent and the pleasant experiences less frequent than in the students (Dixhoorn, 2002). Still, pleasant experiences outweighed the unpleasant ones, and they were three times as frequent. However, the experience greatly differed between those who achieved a good or moderate clinical success and those who experienced no clinical effect on their main complaints. The latter group tended to stop treatment early and not to complete the checklist; nevertheless, 14 checklists were available. These listed as many unpleasant experiences as pleasant ones. By contrast, patients with good clinical success reported the same number of positive experiences as the students and just as few unpleasant experiences.

It is important, therefore, in evaluating the experiences with breathing instructions to include unpleasant ones and name them specifically. This needs to be done in addition to evaluating clinical effect on the main complaints. Moreover, evaluation needs to be done individually. The group that shows no benefit is probably rather small, and their presence will be masked when only average outcome scores are reported. The presence of unpleasant awareness has been a major reason to use instructions with an indirect approach to breathing, thereby offering the option of avoiding direct confrontation with breathing.

Relaxation Overdose

Like any relaxation instruction, breathing therapy may lead to a decrease in sympathetic tone. The normal relaxed state consists of a decrease in ergotropic tuning and lessened sympathetic activity. However, the resulting effect may, on occasion, turn out to be too big. This may happen when getting up from a reclining position or when practicing in the upright position, sitting or standing. The person may feel dizzy or lightheaded or may want to lie or sit down again. When blood pressure drops too much, fainting may occur, and the person's face becomes pale. It is important, therefore, always to get up slowly and not to practice too long in the standing position at first. Usually, faintness is temporary and passes in a few minutes, but sometimes it takes a while for the person to recover. It may happen more frequently after an illness or when one is tired. Usually the individual does not feel bad, only tired, or sometimes even refreshed. Faintness or fainting is promoted by concentrating too long or too intensely on the supporting surface when sitting or standing upright, without moving the body.

Relaxation-Induced Anxiety

The fear of losing control may result in a higher anxiety state after relaxation instruction than before. This is most frequently described when the instructions are suggestive, as in autogenic training (Heide & Borkovec, 1983). It rarely seems to occur during instructions that focus on movement and muscle tension. It is a reason to choose primarily movement instructions to influence breathing and not to have the patient sit or lie still for too long a time. When signs of unrest appear, one option is to modify the instruction and introduce some kind of movement. When that rule is observed, panic or anxiety attacks rarely occur during breathing therapy. However, during any kind of relaxation instruction, panic may be caused by unintentional hyperventilation (Ley, 1988).

Cathartic Responses

An intriguing possibility is that, during relaxation, spontaneous movements or emotions occur that are like a discharge of pent-up emotional energy. They are described in autogenic training as the result of homeostatic processes in the brain (Luthe, 1965; Linden, 1993). Someone may start shivering or yawning, legs or arms may move, or sudden movements may occur along the whole body. It is like sneezing or sobbing heavily, an involuntary bodily response. When this happens, first ask what the person notices and how it feels. Do not try to stop it right away, because it may feel natural or good. When that is the case, the impulses may simply run their course and leave the person refreshed and relieved afterward. If they are too disturbing for the individual or in a group session, ask the person to start moving voluntarily or to inhale deeply and hold the breath for a few seconds. This usually stops it.

Sometimes the responses are emotionally charged and include experiencing past traumatic events, with associated sadness, shock, or anger. This is not a bad thing, either, but the situation should be appropriate for it. If that is the case, they may feel beneficial.

Another form of spontaneous self-regulation is a positive side effect on memory. During the passive attentional state ideas, images, memories, and mental pictures may arise, which may have specific meaning for a problem at hand. An unexpected solution or a new perspective on a problem may be helpful. Somehow, hidden resources may come to the front, a development that can only be welcomed.

Cardiac Arrhythmia

In over 30 years of working with breathing therapy with cardiac patients, it has struck me that cardiac arrhythmias sometimes are accompanied by specific breathing patterns that may provoke them. Arrhythmias increase under the influence of sympathetic activity, and relaxation may be helpful (Benson, Alexander, & Feldman, 1975). Similarly, breathing slowly and more abdominally may be helpful. However, this may also be counterproductive. It seems that sometimes breathing is too slow and exhalation pauses too long in comparison with the state of agitation of the whole system. Also, exhalation constricts the intrathoracic space and may stimulate the heart mechanically. The heart responds with extra beats, mostly supraventricular; but also premature ventricular contractions (PVCs) or even ventricular tachycardia may occur.

The association with breathing is confirmed when the frequency of abnormal beats decreases or disappears on altering breathing and a more shallow and functional upper thoracic breathing pattern is elicited. Inhaling to the upper chest and not exhaling too strongly or for too long helps to create more space in the chest, and this respiratory pattern matches the state of the organism as a whole. Similarly, sitting more upright and elevating the chest may be helpful in that situation. When the heart has calmed down, respiration may be changed to a more slow and abdominal pattern that does not evoke arrhythmia.

TREATMENT MANUAL

The method utilizes a relatively large number of instructions, as well as manual techniques, 50 of which are described in detail in a Dutch handbook (Dixhoorn, 1998a). A few instructions are available in English through the internet (*www.methodevandixhoorn.com*). In this chapter, seven techniques are described for use with the client mainly in the sitting position. A chair with a flat, horizontal surface is required, preferably a stool without back support. The techniques are described in a sequence that may actually take place during several sessions, although you should evaluate each step and may decide to change the sequence. First, decide whether you want to start with manual assessment of breathing pattern or with an instruction. For manual assessment, you take a position behind the client and place both hands on his or her lower back. If either you or the client does not feel comfortable doing this, it can be skipped or postponed.

Assessment of Breathing

Distribution of Breathing Movement

Have the client sit comfortably on a stool and sit behind it on a lower stool. Pass your hand along the spinal column, feel the curvature of the back and whether posture is erect or slumped. Put the palms of both hands alongside the lumbar spinal column, with the thumbs in a vertical direction, parallel to each other, with the top at about the level of the lower thoracic vertebra and the fingers spread out. The second and third fingers should touch the lower ribs, and the fourth and fifth fingers should touch the area below the ribs. The full surface of the hands should touch the body. Do not squeeze the ribs together but lightly touch the middle of the body. When the client is sitting erect, this area is tight. In that case, ask the client to sit "at ease"; support the body with your hands. When the client is slumping too much, this part is round. In that case, ask the client to sit up a bit more and push the body a bit forward. Ask the client to move forward and backward a few times and find the middle position, sitting fully on the sitting bones.

You may notice the breathing movement under your hands. Do not try to change, guide, improve, or amplify it. Simply let your hands notice the direction of movement at inhalation, and mentally try to form a picture of the area in which respiratory movement

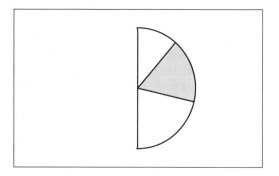
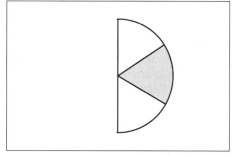

FIGURES 12.4 and 12.5. Graphic description of distribution of breathing movement. Figure 12.4: sitting upright; Figure 12.5: sitting easy. Data from 6 participants.

is present. The fingers on the ribs may notice a sideways movement, a lateral expansion. This is the result of both the elevation of the rib cage and the diaphragmatic pull on the ribs (Kapandji, 1974). Try to feel to what degree there is upward movement and to imagine how much the upward movement extends to the top of the rib cage. When the elevation of the rib cage dominates, there is largely an upward movement and little lateral expansion. When the diaphragmatic down-pull dominates, there is a large sideways movement that spreads upward only a little and is particularly present at the fourth and fifth fingers below the ribs and in the palm of the hands. Try to form an image of the degree to which there is an outside push. This originates from the diaphragm, which descends with inhalation and pushes the abdominal content outward. Then release your touch, get up, and graphically describe the area by drawing two lines to form a slice of a pie chart (see Figures 12.4 and 12.5). The center of the pie corresponds with the thoraco–lumbar junction. The size of the slice, the distance between the upper and lower lines, corresponds with the *area* in which inhalation movement is present, in your estimation. The place of the slice in the pie corresponds with the location of breathing: upper half corresponds to chest, lower half to abdomen. Together, they represent *distribution of breathing movement*. Interrater reliability of the procedure has shown satisfactory values (Dixhoorn, 2004).

Further Observations

During this assessment, you have an opportunity to observe other qualities, which may be noted on an observation sheet (Figure 12.6). You get an impression of respiratory speed, and you may count the exact frequency per minute. Although it may be expected that a small area of distribution coincides with a small and rapid respiration, the correlation between size of the area and respiration rate is relatively low. Next, you may notice other time-domain qualities, including the transitions between inhaling and exhaling and irregularities. Transitions may be clearly present as a momentary "pause" at the end of a movement, which is a natural phenomenon and represents proper coordination of the breathing movement. They may be marked or take longer time, in particular after exhalation, and may be noted as such (e.g., marked, long). They may also be clearly absent, in which case breathing is hurried, coordination is not smooth, and the process of reversing breathing from inhalatory to exhalatory movement and vice versa is abrupt and choppy.

Irregularity of rhythm is to some extent a natural phenomenon, reflecting a relaxed state of the individual and prepared for environmental changes. It indicates that breathing is responsive, and it should occur when the person is asked to move, for instance, turning the head left or right or shifting the body. Marked irregularities, however, consist mostly of deep sighs, which are a sign of dyspnea, shortage of breath, or anxiety. They should be noted, particularly when they are frequent.

Tidal volume is impossible to estimate manually. Size of area cannot be taken as a proxy measure of tidal volume. It also correlates poorly with measurements of circumference changes of the abdominal and thoracic compartments, which do provide a good estimate of tidal volume once they are properly calibrated. Thus it is quite possible to breathe a large volume with little sideways expansion or to have a wide distribution along a large area with relatively small volume. A wide distribution reflects the involvement of the ribs, their ease of movement, and coordination with the diaphragm. However, within one individual, changes in area probably correlate highly with changes in volume. Having someone take a deep breath results in a marked increase in area. From this, the tendency to hyperventilate can be estimated from the time it takes to return to normal breathing after a deep breath. Also, the degree that breathing shifts upward can be assessed and noted graphically.

An important aspect of functionality is smoothness of movement and ease of breathing. Manual assessment is the best way to judge this, because the hands are sensitive to the amount of effort or strength employed by the intercostal muscles to breathe. Also, notice the occurrence of extra "pushes" during inhalation or exhalation, which diminish smoothness and indicate some form of voluntary or habitual controlled breathing pattern. Manual assessment is the best way to find asymmetry between the left and right sides of the chest. In addition to visual inspection, the hands may find that one side is moving more than the other. This can be represented graphically by drawing both sides in the pie chart. Asymmetry may be a cause of dyspnea or breathing difficulty of which the person is often unaware. It may coincide with scoliosis of the spinal column, which is also assessed at the beginning but which requires more attention when the rib cage shows asymmetry. The degree of the convexity should be described, its direction (left/right), and its location along the spine. In general, the shape of the spinal column deserves attention.

Pace and respiratory frequency:	Rapid, slow, cycles per minute
Pauses:	Natural, marked, long, inhalatory or exhalatory, or absent
Irregularity:	Normal, absent, marked, frequent
Response to breathing deeply:	Normal return, slow return, area, location
Smoothness:	Normal, absent
Symmetry:	Present, absent, degree and location of curve
Scoliosis (lateral curves):	Absent, present, degree and location of curve
Spinal (sagittal) curves:	Normal, marked, diminished, lordosis/kyphosis
Sounds:	Absent, marked, origin, inhalatory or exhalatory
Awareness of "width" breathing:	Normal, pleasant or absent, disturbs breathing

FIGURE 12.6. Breathing observation sheet for sitting.

Pronounced kyphosis or pronounced lordosis of the lumbar or cervical parts is important, as well as a marked absence of the natural curves, for instance, in the lumbar or upper thoracic area.

Finally, the observer may pay attention to the sounds of air passage. During quiet
breathing, clearly audible sounds reflect turbulence in the airways, which deserves attention because they reflect marked effort in passing the air and great pressure gradients.
Sounds may occur during inhalation or exhalation and may originate from the chest,
throat, mouth, or nose. Individuals who habitually breathe through their mouths should
be asked to close them and try breathing through their noses. Sounds that originate from
the chest usually reflect lung problems.

Observe Breathing Awareness

An essential quality of functional breathing is that it is open to and accessible for conscious attention. Although awareness always influences function somewhat, it should not
disturb breathing nor lead to marked changes or to a particular voluntary breathing pattern. This happens frequently when attention is drawn to breathing in the chest or abdomen. Because few people are conscious of their backs or of breathing in their backs, this
procedure is well suited to assess openness of awareness of breathing.

Ask the client to pay attention to your hands on the back and ask how it feels. Then
ask whether the client is aware of any respiratory movement in the back at the location of
your hands. If the client notices respiratory movement and breathing does not change
much, then ask in what direction movement is felt during inhalation: upward, forward,
backward, or sideways. Next, ask the client to focus on the movement sideways and to
describe it: the ribs or back broaden during inhalation and become smaller during exhalation. Then ask how it feels to mentally follow this breathing pattern. The normal response is a feeling of pleasant, natural breathing, which does not require much effort or
control. However, some people do not notice any movement in their backs, although it is
obvious to the observer; or the movement may be absent or may disappear when the person pays attention, to be replaced by inhalations upward and extending the back to lift
the chest. Others are unable to passively notice respiration and try to actively control it,
which often is accompanied by a decrease in smoothness and increase in effort. These responses constitute disturbances in breathing awareness.

Instructions

Seven instructions are described. The texts of the instructions themselves are numbered
and can be read verbatim to the patient. (In these enumerations, *you* refers to the patient,
whereas in the rest of the text, *you* refers to the reader). Each row consists of several sentences. Do not read all the sentences one after another, but pace the reading to the client.
Pause and observe after each sentence and determine whether continuing is appropriate.
Each instruction consists of several steps in which the instruction evolves. You must observe the response of the patient before deciding to proceed. You may also stay at a step
and repeat it.

A good way to start is in the sitting position, because it easily transfers to daily life.
After each sitting instruction, it is a good idea for the client to stand up in order to notice
any changes in habitual posture. It is also a good idea for the client to lie down for a few
minutes, when the occasion allows it, in order to let the spine relax. Instructions in the su-

pine position are indicated when the client seems a little tired or in need of a rest, or when you want to emphasize passive relaxation.

The first instruction in the sitting position can be "circle knees" or "forward, backward." "Circle knees" takes more time and requires an undisturbed situation for the person to practice. "Forward, backward" can be done in between activities and is less conspicuous. "Sitting, standing" teaches a specific way of standing up, which the client can apply each time he or she gets up without doing the exercise itself. "Shoulders up" improves coordination of the breathing movement of the chest. "Exhale audibly" is a direct instruction to change breathing and can be done in any posture. In the supine position, "pulling up the feet" is a good way to start, because it is easy to do and gradually involves breathing. "Looking up and down" is more difficult. When the client has trouble doing it, it is better to stop the exercise. Generally it is recommended to first do the easy instructions, which prepare the way for direct breathing regulation. Then proceed with the more difficult instructions.

Start with . . . Circle knees . . .   Forward, backward . . . Pulling up the feet
Next . . .   Audible exhaling
End . . .   Shoulders up . . .   Sitting, standing . . .   Looking up and down

Instruction: Sit, Circle Knees

Position yourself on a chair at right angles to the client, so that you see each other obliquely and do the instruction while giving it in order to model it.

1. Place the feet a little beyond the knees. Put the hands on the knees, palm downward, and notice how you sit.
2. Move the hands around the knees, circling the knees, downward at the outside, upward at the inside, about 20 or 25 times. Do it unhurriedly, as easily as you can, somewhat carelessly, without counting.
   Notice that the body moves forward when the hands go down and backward when the hands go upward. You may feel this movement in the sitting bones.
   Stop the movement, look straight ahead, and notice how the body feels.
3. Repeat the movement, about 20 to 25 times. This time pay attention to the shifting of weight between the sitting bones and feet. When you move back, the weight on the sitting bones increases until you sit fully on top of them. When you move forward, there is more weight or pressure on the feet.
   Stop the exercise, look straight ahead, and notice how the body feels.
4. Do the same movement for the third time, again 20 to 25 times. Is there a difference in the way your body moves? This time notice that, each time when you come back, with the weight fully on the sitting bones, you look straight ahead.
   Stop the exercise, look straight ahead, and notice how the body feels.
   Stand up. Notice what you feel.

Check whether the body really moves back and forth and that the client does not limit the movement to the arms and hands circling the knees. The continuous shifting or rolling of weight on the sitting bones tends to draw attention in a passive way. Afterward, most clients are more aware of the fact that they are sitting; they feel their weight more clearly when asked. This attentional shift tends to facilitate a less erect sitting posture, a sense of relaxation, both physical and mental, and thus a more quiet respiration. Also, the movement tends to become slower during subsequent steps. The awareness of the supporting surface, including the feet, is emphasized in steps 3 and 4. When leaning more forward, one notices the weight on the feet more. This helps to enlarge the movement in a natural way, which also occurs as a result of repetition and increasing ease of movement.

You may manually assess breathing movement after each step or at the end, or simply ask or observe. An optimal response is that breathing becomes easy and almost automatic, undisturbed by one's perception. Emphasis on the position of the head, in the step 4, facilitates involvement of the spine: straightening a little when going forward, flexing when going backward. Observe to what degree this actually occurs. When it does, the sensation of standing on both feet at the end is much more clear and the body is more erect, but without effort.

Sitting Forward, Backward

You may join this instruction but may also visually observe the movement from the side or from the back, with both hands on the body of the client, to check whether the spine really changes shape and to encourage it, when necessary.

1. Lean the body forward and backward a few times. Then go backward, stay there, and notice the back. Go forward, stay there, and feel the back. Repeat this a few times and notice the change in the form of the back: becoming a bit rounder when leaning backward and straightening up when leaning forward. Do not tilt the pelvis intentionally.

   Stop the movement, sit in the middle, and notice how you are sitting.

2. Move back and forth slowly and pay attention to the change in the shape of the back. Go backward, stay there, breathe in and out a few times, and notice the place of breathing movement. Go forward, stay there, breathe, and notice the place of breathing. Repeat this until you notice that respiration responds to the position. Be aware of this response and follow the way breathing changes with posture.

   Stop the movement, sit in the middle, notice how you sit, and breathe.

3. Move back and forth, and do it in a rhythm similar to your breathing. Continue and notice whether a connection appears. Are you breathing in when moving forward or when moving backward? Continue this a while until the connection becomes easy.

   Then try and change the connection. If you inhaled when moving forward, now move forward during exhalation, and vice versa. Continue this and notice how it feels. Both options are equally possible.

   Stop the movement, sit in the middle, notice how you sit, and breathe.

   Stand up and notice what you feel.

This instruction is essential for awareness of the relationship between posture and breathing. When the spinal column really changes in shape, breathing responds. When the spine is extended, respiration follows the pattern of "length" breathing. When the spine is flexed, respiration follows the pattern of "width" breathing. So moving forward and backward can both be connected to inhalation. When both patterns can be present, flexibility of both posture and breathing is increased. It demonstrates that there is not one pattern of "good" breathing. This may require explanation and discussion in order to restructure the client's cognitions.

Sitting, Standing

This instruction facilitates standing up from a chair with less effort by using the strength of the feet and legs economically. You may join the instruction or you may observe from the side.

1. While sitting in a chair, place the feet a little behind the knees, flat on the floor. Move the body slowly forward and backward, and notice the pressure changes in the feet.

    Continue, and, when going forward, press the feet more toward the floor a few times.

    Continue, and, when going forward, look straight ahead. Notice the effect on your back.

    Stop and feel how you are sitting.

2. Lean backward, inhale, move forward and exhale, again backward and inhale. Repeat this a few times until it is easy.

    Then go forward, press the feet, exhale, look ahead, and go further until the buttocks lift off the chair a little. Return, lean backward, and inhale. Do this a few times.

    Stop and feel how you are sitting.

3. Finally, move forward, exhale, and stand up, remain standing, and inhale, exhale, and sit down. Do this a few times, then remain standing and notice how you stand. Sit down and notice how you sit.

When one leans forward, presses the feet on the floor, and looks ahead, the spine tends to extend. Continue with the instruction only when spinal extension actually occurs in the first step. Observe that the hands are lying loosely on the upper legs and slide forward and backward with the body. They should not press on the legs or be held stiff.

In the second step, respiration is coupled to the movement in a way that is contrary to what is done habitually by most people. Inhaling when leaning backward promotes "width" breathing and sideways expansion of the ribs. As a result, the lower ribs in the back are in an optimal position to contract with exhalation while moving forward, and this facilitates extension of the spine. Moreover, exhaling when starting to lift off the chair helps to contract the pelvic floor muscles and to withstand the rise in abdominal pressure. This prevents urine leakage, particularly for people who have urinary incontinence problems. Also, it prevents the tendency to "brace" when making effort, which is coupled to inhalation and excessive muscular effort. The hands may move forward and extend beyond the knees to help the shifting of weight. At the end of step 2, the client may sit differently, often more active and erect but without much effort.

In step 3 the client actually stands up and sits down again, both with exhalation. When successful, standing up requires less effort, although the procedure may still feel somewhat strange. It is important to have the client remain standing for a while and to observe any differences from habitual posture. Usually, the person stands more firmly on both feet and is aware of the weight in the feet. The client is encouraged to notice this many times during the day.

Exhale Audibly

This instruction can be done in any position, preferably when respiration is not disturbed by conscious awareness. Therefore, preparatory instructions are appropriate. In the supine position the client may be asked to let a hand rest on the abdomen and notice the respiratory movement. In the sitting position it is sufficient to ask the client to notice respiration, or he or she may be asked to observe the sides of the body.

1. Take some time to notice your breathing, pay attention to the breathing movement without changing it by breathing more deeply or more abdominally. Form a mental picture of the breathing curve, with inhalation going up and exhalation going down. Notice the steepness of the rise and fall and the pauses in between.

    Inhale slowly through the nose and exhale through slightly pursed lips, making the sound of "fff" at the lips. Inhale again, slowly, through the nose and exhale audibly, softly.

Do it five to six times, then stop and take time to notice your breathing until it has resumed its natural rhythm.

Compare the breathing pattern with the beginning of this step: depth, speed, volume, location, pauses.

2. Repeat this two to three times.

What changes in respiration do you notice? Is there any other change that you observe? In mental state, in the head, or in the way the body feels, sits, lies, stands?

The instruction results in a temporarily larger tidal volume that involves more parts of the respiratory apparatus, particularly the ribs. It is essential that respiration resume its natural rhythm after exhaling audibly and that deeper breathing stop. Some clients have trouble in stopping the controlled breathing, and they continue breathing steadily deeper, often at a fixed pace. This may result in hyperventilation. It is important to have the client understand the necessity of stopping the direct control of breathing and then to observe any changes in spontaneous breathing. These are usually rather small changes in breathing pattern: slightly longer and/or deeper but, more important, more easy and unhurried, with more smooth transitions from inhaling to exhaling and from exhaling to inhaling, and with an increased sense of "space" for breathing in the body. Breathing involves more parts, is more evenly distributed, and can be perceived all over the trunk. When asked, clients may notice that their mental state is changed as if the head is more empty or more clear, with fewer thoughts. Also, because the instruction involves modest training of the respiratory muscles, the coordination of respiratory muscles may have improved, as well as their role in posture. This results in a more balanced and stable erect posture or in sitting more firmly (Czapszys et al., 2000).

The instruction differs from pursed-lips breathing, which is a familiar technique for emphysema patients, in some respects: Inhalation is slower, and exhalation is not as strong, but with a moderate, even sound. Although it may reduce dyspnea, it is not meant to be done continuously but only a few times, then stopped and the changes observed.

Sit, Shoulders Up

This instruction helps to improve movement of the ribs and chest with breathing and is feasible when respiration is not disturbed by conscious awareness. It is helpful to assist by having manual contact with the lower ribs in the back during instruction, but you may also do the movement while teaching it. It can be done standing as well.

1. Notice the breathing movement in the chest. The lower ribs expand sideways when you inhale, and the chest bone lifts a little upward. Continue until breathing is clearly perceptible but no longer disturbed by your attention. Stop if it becomes disturbed. Raise the shoulders toward the ears, then keep them there and continue breathing. Notice the ribs and chest. Let the shoulders sink down. Compare the breathing with the beginning of this step.

   Repeat this until the breathing movement in ribs and chest is hardly influenced anymore by raising the shoulders.

   Stop the movement, feel how you are sitting (standing), how your body is breathing, and how you are.

2. When you succeed easily with the first step, raise the shoulders about halfway to the ears and keep them there. Then try raising the shoulders a little during exhalation and let them sink down a little during inhalation. Do this a number of times, then let the shoulders sink fully during an inhalation and leave them there.

   Stop the movement, feel how you are sitting (standing), how your body is breathing, and how you are. Repeat this two times.

Although the bony connection between shoulders and rib cage is limited to the clavicle, the muscular interconnection is so tight and the habitual association so strong that raising the shoulders is usually closely coupled to inhalation and elevation of the ribs. This instruction helps to disengage the tight association, thereby improving mobility of both the shoulders and the rib cage.

First, respiratory movement in the chest must be felt and allowed to happen. Sometimes the mistaken idea that respiration should happen only in the abdomen needs to be discussed. When the movement of the ribs, in particular the lateral expansion of the lower ribs and the elevation of the chest bone, is perceived clearly, then the instruction is to raise the shoulders to the ears and to continue this movement as much as possible. Say "Let the position of the shoulders not bother you or interfere with breathing, just continue breathing in and out." This requires some repetition. Each time, ask whether any differences occurred after the instruction, in comparison to before the instruction. Although clients differ in the degree to which they tolerate new or strange actions, most feel afterward that breathing is easier and better distributed and includes the chest but is equally present in the abdomen. The body feels more relaxed and more open to breathing. It is important to explain that improved mobility of the ribs facilitates diaphragmatic action and improves its downward motion. Also, when the chest bone quietly elevates, this helps diaphragmatic descent and thus promotes lower abdominal breathing. Breathing is a natural 'whole body' movement, and this instruction can make the point clear. It may give a sense of relief, both somatic with respect to breathing sensation in the chest and relief of dyspnea and cognitive with respect to the mental picture that breathing can simply be allowed to happen along the whole of the trunk.

When the first step is successful, the second step increases the difficulty. Its aim is to reverse the association between raising the shoulders and inhalation by asking the client to do the opposite: Raise the shoulders a little during exhalation. This creates two opposing movements. The shoulders go up, the ribs go down. As a result, when during inhalation the shoulders sink a little, there is a very clear sensation of lateral expansion and elevation of the ribs. This creates an unusually large space for inhalation. Also, the shoulders relax even more. As a side effect, this instruction opposes the habit of bracing or forceful, upper thoracic inhalation during stress.

Supine Position

For instructions in the supine position, a flat, horizontal surface is required, such as a treatment couch or a mat on the floor. A reclining chair or "relaxation" chair will not work, particularly for "looking up and down."

Be sure that the client's head is supported well. Instruction may include having the client try several layers of support under the head, for instance, in the form of a large towel that you may fold several times to increase its thickness. Offer various layers of support and ask the client how each feels. When the client reports feeling all right, offer even more variations, and observe the position of the head until it is clear that one level of support is optimal. Usually the face is horizontal and parallel to the surface. It may not be the habitual position of the head, but it actually feels comfortable. It is worthwhile to take some time with this procedure, because it contains several messages. First, the client may answer "I am okay" when asked how he or she feels, but this may be a social answer, and it does not mean that the position of the head is optimal. However, the awareness of differences in tension and the sensation of optimal comfort is essential for success with these breathing instructions. Second, the care taken to find an optimal position for the client demonstrates your intention that the client's comfort is the prime concern. You should not challenge or put the client to a test to find out about his or her level of tension. Finally, the procedure clarifies that support for the head should be just that: an elevated surface for the head to rest on, while maintaining its mobility. It is not a cushion stuffed behind the neck that blocks motion.

Pulling Up the Feet

This instruction is very easy and can be done by almost everybody, particularly the first part. It is a good way to start in the supine position. It attracts attention to the feet, away from the location of most tension problems.

1. Pull your toes toward you while the legs remain straight, and notice where the tension increases in the legs. Stop the exercise and take time to notice the tension slowly disappearing. Repeat this 2 or 3 times.

    Then stop the movement and notice how your legs and body are lying.

2. Do it again, and this time pay attention to the difference in tension in the legs, and to the difference in breathing with the legs relaxed and tense. When is inhaling easier? Then stop and notice how the legs and body are lying.

3. Do it a third time, now coupling it to breathing. When you exhale, and while exhaling, slowly and gradually pull up the feet. When exhalation is complete, release the feet and relax the legs completely. Then inhale. Continue this until it feels natural and easy.

    Then stop, and notice how your legs and body are lying. How do you feel?

4. Get up slowly. First, sit up and notice how you feel. Take your time. Then get to your feet, stand, and notice how you stand.

This instruction starts as a tense–release instruction in Jacobson's manner, but it does not focus on the source of tension, the tibialis muscle. Instead, all signals are accepted—the stretch sensation in the calf, the joint movement in the ankle, the tensing of the quadriceps muscle. During instruction you may discuss the client's observations. With repetition, tension signals are felt in the whole of the leg and even in the lower half of the body. That is, the abdomen tightens a little, making inhalation more difficult. Inhalation becomes easier when the legs are relaxed. This is the experience to emphasize in the second step. Some clients fail to notice this, and any attention to breathing disturbs it. In that case, continue with tense–release cycles until the legs are lying more relaxed, and stop there. For some clients, the experience of easy inhalation when the legs are relaxed is sufficiently new and impressive. In that case, stop there and ask the client to repeat the exercise at home.

When the second step is clear and easy, the third step of the instruction introduces an unusual coupling of tension increase with exhalation. Our system is programmed for the association of inhalation with tension increase. This is easy to do and is utilized in the abbreviated form of progressive relaxation (see Chapter 5, this volume). In this instruction, the reverse is done. This requires conscious attention and therefore stimulates distraction of attention away from the tension; that is, when the tension problem is not in the legs. Coupling breathing to a small movement also tends to slow down respiration. Also, making an effort during exhalation implies that inhalation becomes associated with less or no effort. This favors natural breathing, that is, letting the body inhale and not adding extra effort. Pulling up the feet is mechanically coupled to exhalation, as the abdomen tightens and the pelvis tilts backward. Thus relaxing the legs helps to relax the abdomen, which allows the diaphragm to descend. Also, the pelvic tilt pushes the spinal column upward, which facilitates exhalation according to the pattern of "length" breathing: the ribs flatten, the head tilts upward, and the chest bone descends. This reverse coupling may take a while to get used to, but once the client gets the knack of it, it feels very easy. Altogether it makes the instruction a good way to introduce very slow breathing, as in resonant breathing. Afterward, most clients stand surprisingly stable and full on both feet.

Looking Up and Down with Breathing

This instruction is somewhat difficult because it influences rather directly the position of the head, as well as respiration. Clients with severe tension problems in the head, neck, or jaw or clients with severe dyspnea may benefit from it, but it may also be unsuccessful and even cause problems. It is important, therefore, to observe carefully and to inquire of the client how the response feels during each step. It can be done in the supine, sitting, or standing position, but it is best to start with the client lying down.

1. Look comfortably straight ahead. Focus on a point in front of you. Then slowly look up, stay there, breathe in and out a few times, and look back again. Repeat this a few times and notice that there is a tendency for the head to tilt a little upward when you look up. Allow this to happen. Also, the jaw may tend to open a little. Allow this.
   Stop the movement, and notice what you feel.
2. Feel your breathing going in and out a few times, and then, while exhaling, look slowly up. When inhaling, look ahead again. Do it in such a way that the exhalation and the shift of your gaze coincide. As long as you exhale, continue looking upward. Repeat a few times. Stop, and notice how you are breathing. Do it again, until the coupling feels easy and the result feels comfortable.

The instruction directly appeals to the pattern of length breathing in the upper body. Exhalation implies a slight sinking of the chest bone. This downward motion of the upper ribs in the front results in and is facilitated by a small bending forward movement of the upper back. When this is accompanied by a small increase of cervical lordosis, the position of the head remains stable, and breathing movement is functional. Thus breathing deeper in and out is accompanied by and facilitated by a small motion at the cervico–thoracic junction: going forward with exhaling and backward with inhaling. The eye movement tends to enhance and emphasize this pattern of coordination. When looking up with the eyes, the head tends to tilt backward a little, and the reverse occurs when looking down.

Another aspect of the instruction is that respiration responds synchronously to any stimulus that occurs. Thus the very fact of coupling a movement to inhaling or exhaling tends to lengthen and consequently deepen respiration. Because in this instruction respiration is coupled to a movement that is matched mechanically, the effect tends to be longer lasting.

CASE EXAMPLE: REPETITIVE STRAIN INJURY

A 40-year-old woman, married, without children, had a hectic job in an international company that involved much computer work. Four years ago she developed pains in the right shoulder, hand, and fingers. The arm felt stiff, tired, and painful. Physiotherapy and yoga had no success. After 1 year she eventually changed her job for a less demanding one with less computer work, but the pain remained, even when she took days off. After

3 years she finally found a treatment, manipulation therapy, that greatly diminished the complaints. However, the pains returned fully when she was under stress. It became clear that she had difficulty relaxing. She was referred for relaxation therapy.

First Session

The client's pain in her right arm was present daily. She had trouble relaxing. Her score on the NQ was high—35.

Assessment of breathing in the sitting position showed a small area of movement, located high in the chest, with almost no lateral expansion (Figure 12.7). The lower back was rather tight, the right shoulder was a bit lower than the left, the head was bending forward a bit, and she was looking downward. There were no marked irregularities, no air sounds, and no asymmetry in breathing.

The instruction "circle knees" was done and went well. The client was sitting more stably, her lower back was a bit rounder, and she felt more relaxed. Respiration responded only slightly (Figure 12.8); the distribution shifted a little downward, it increased a little in area, and long postexhalation pauses appeared. She was standing more firmly on her feet and found it easier to look straight ahead. In the supine position, her legs were lying rather close together and turned inward. The instruction was given to roll the legs inward a bit more, to notice the tension and stop it. After a few times, her legs were lying more open, and this felt more comfortable for her. In the standing position, her feet were also rather close together and pointing straight ahead. The instruction to try to put a bit more distance between the feet and to point them more toward the outside resulted in a pleasant and more stable posture, with knees slightly bent. She was asked to practice all three instructions.

Second Session

Two weeks later the client had practiced "sit, circle knees" regularly and felt that it was relaxing, but she could not specify concrete changes. The instruction to stand with feet further apart was very helpful; she practiced it often during the day and stood more stably, and she felt the weight more in the feet, which decreased the tension in her shoulders. The instruction in the supine position did not work; she felt no effect. Generally she had become more aware of a high level of tension. I explained that treatment is not aimed

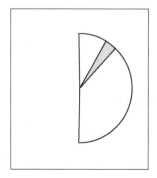 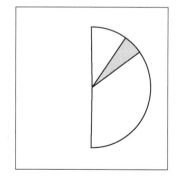

FIGURES 12.7 and 12.8. Distribution of breathing at the beginning and end of the first session.

at reduction of complaints but at increasing relaxation and that focusing on tension areas usually increases tension, whereas focusing on relaxed states does not. This helped her to understand and accept the purpose of the treatment. The instruction "sit, circle knees" was repeated and went quite well. Next the instruction "sitting, standing" was given, and she became aware that she usually used her arms too much to stand up. After she rested awhile in the supine position, her legs were lying more open and relaxed. In the standing position, she felt a variety of changes but could not specify them.

Third Session

Two weeks later the client had continued to practice "sit, circle knees" and had become more aware of changes in the whole body afterward. She also noticed that the effects were greater when she moved more from the trunk than from the arms. The explanation that the primary aim was to increase moments of relaxation rather than fighting the tension was a very new perspective that helped her to find such moments. She had also become aware that her breathing was often short and erratic. The pain was less; pain episodes occurred now every other day instead of daily and were of shorter duration. The NQ showed a reduction to a score of 28. This time only techniques in the supine position were selected to emphasize passive rest. First, the therapist employed manual techniques (not described here) by holding both feet and influencing breathing from there. There was a good response: Respiration became deeper and felt freer. Also, long postexhalation pauses became apparent. Next the instruction "pulling up the feet" was done, which helped to deepen breathing. Standing straight afterward, her shoulders felt more relaxed and her arms were hanging more loosely.

Fourth Session

Three weeks later the client had practiced all instructions occasionally and had noticed that, when awareness of the lower body increased, this helped to decrease tension in the upper body. The instruction "pulling feet up" helped to relax her legs. The instruction "sitting, standing" was quite difficult. The pain had continued improving. The pain episodes occurred only 2 days per week, particularly after she worked too long or watched a thrilling movie. Her NQ score had dropped further, to 19, which is just within the normal range. The instruction "sitting, standing" was repeated, and her attention was brought to the fact that she tended to close the knees when trying to get up. The movement became much easier when she opened her knees a little in getting up. In the sitting position, breathing was assessed and used to bring her attention to the movement of lateral expansion during inhalation. She was asked to pay attention to this movement regularly. Finally, the instruction "sit, shoulders up" was done to enhance the whole body involvement of the respiratory movement. The first step went well, but the second step did not. Raising the shoulders during exhaling was too difficult for her and too contrary to her habit.

Fifth Session

One month later the client occasionally practiced the sitting instructions "circle knees" and "sitting, standing." "Shoulders up" was too difficult, and the combination with breathing was contrary to what she was instructed to do in fitness classes. However, she had become increasingly attentive to moments of rest during the working day, and she

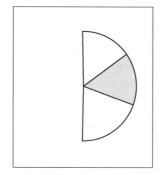

FIGURE 12.9. Distribution of breathing at the end of therapy.

noticed quickly when tension started to rise too high. She liked this a lot, and this awareness helped her to gain a more relaxed style of working. The sensation of "width breathing" was not very clear to her. The pain continued to improve; it occurred now once a week, was less intense, and involved fewer body parts. She had no more pain in her arms.

The instruction "sit forward, backward" was chosen in order to clarify the concept of "width breathing," to demonstrate that proper sitting can be done in more than one way and that it involves alternation of posture. The movement went well, and breathing felt quiet and easy for her, as if the body were breathing by itself. This corresponded with the assessment (Figure 12.9). Because her conscious attention did not disturb respiration, the instruction "exhaling audibly" was added. This went well, and afterward breathing became even fuller and slower. Then, standing straight, she felt very heavy in the lower body and light in the upper body. It was emphasized to her that the purpose of the exercises was to learn to enjoy and recognize moments of relaxation rather than to think "I have to relax in order to combat the tension signs."

Sixth Session

After 6 weeks the client came for the final session. The pain was better; she had only one episode per 3 weeks. Her NQ score had dropped to a low level of 7. She felt the rise of tension much earlier; signs included shoulders and arms tensing up, breathing becoming shorter and less free. She frequently practiced the breathing instruction "slow inhaling, exhaling audibly," as well as the instruction "sitting, standing," and she attended to opening her knees when getting up. She also made plenty of alterations in posture and movement during the day. When watching a thrilling movie, she was less involved and could take more distance, which resulted in smaller increases in tension.

Because her right shoulder remained a bit lower than her left, an instruction from the Feldenkrais method was done to regain better balance in the rib movement on the left and right side. We stopped the treatment with the agreement that she would phone if the complaints returned.

Discussion

This is clearly a case of high and dysfunctional muscle tension, which remains present but without awareness during rest. Thus resting is not helpful, and tension flares up immediately under challenge. This pattern is a good indication for relaxation therapy, but it does not explain the effects of treatment. One mediator may have been the client's increasing awareness of her own tension state. This was the direct result of the success of the instructions to lower her tension, which she reported. As relaxation grew stronger, she became increasingly aware of early warning signals of rising tension. Thus tension reduction and body awareness went hand in hand. This was supported by an important cognitive change: her understanding that increasing relaxation is more helpful than fighting tension. She gradually developed a more positive perspective on her complaints. However, these discussions followed her experiences and clarified them rather than preceding them, as would be the case in cognitive therapy, in which the cognitive intervention is primary.

There was little indication of a mental shift, or mental relaxation. She did not feel more mentally calm or quiet, but she had no trouble in sleeping and did not worry much. Also, restorative processes were not clearly present. She was not tired, and thus she did not feel more refreshed or more energetic. Interestingly, the complaints in her upper body decreased to the degree that she became more aware of her legs and lower body and of receiving support for posture from the ground rather than from her shoulders and arms. Instructions for the position of her feet were particularly helpful and practical in daily life, as was the idea of slightly opening the knees rather than closing them when getting up. The instruction "sit, circle knees" was helpful from the beginning to the end. Initially, it helped to shift her focus on the sitting bones, which made her sit in a more relaxed and less effortful way. Gradually she noticed that the effect was greater and involved the whole body, as the quality of movement improved and became more functional. Thus awareness of and making a better use of the bony structure seems to have been an important mediator.

This case was chosen because it clearly illustrates the indicator role of breathing and the utility of indirect breathing instructions. The breathing pattern seemed obviously dysfunctional: small tidal volume, high frequency, and a predominance of upper thoracic breathing movement. I could have confronted this breathing pattern and tried to correct it directly. Instead, I observed it and waited for the response of the client. Distribution of breathing movement responded slightly in the first session, and long postexhalation pauses appeared, without her awareness. This indicated a functional respiratory response to a change in the tension state to which breathing should respond without drawing attention to itself. The postexhalation pauses, which also appeared in the third session, indicated a functional compensation to increased tidal volume, thus preventing hyperventilation that may occur when trying to improve breathing. Instead, the dominant subjective response was a sense of increased weight on the feet and ease in standing up. This process of functional movement guided the choice for movement instructions instead of direct breathing instructions in subsequent sessions. In the third session, the client had noted that her breathing was often short and erratic. This guided the choice for the instruction "pulling feet up," which helps to relax the legs and connects relaxation to inhaling. In the fourth session, she reported only the effect of relaxation of the legs and did not mention any effect on breathing. Thus the indirect approach to breathing was confirmed. I followed up by bringing her attention to the pattern of breathing that naturally occurs when sitting comfortably, that is, "width" breathing with sideways expansion. This did not have great effect. The instruction to combine exhaling with raising the shoulders was too difficult and too different from her habitual pattern. Only in the fifth session, when breathing had clearly responded to her increasingly relaxed state and showed a normal pattern and distribution, was a direct breathing instruction given: exhaling audibly. She was able to perform the instruction; it enhanced both breathing and the relaxed state. She felt very heavy in the lower body and very light in the upper body. In the final session, she reported having used the breathing instruction quite a lot. Thus respiration could finally play its role as an instrument for self-regulation of tension effectively.

To conclude, although no capnographic measurements were done, the client's seemingly dysfunctional breathing pattern, as well as her high score on the NQ, indicated an important role of respiration in the etiology of her complaints. Nevertheless, following the process model, instructions were chosen that matched the response of the individual. These did not include direct breathing regulation but focused on reduction and awareness of physical tension. It appeared that when the physical tension state had decreased, the breathing pattern and the complaints score on the NQ became normal. From that moment, direct breathing instructions could be used effectively for self-regulation of tension.

Four years later, the client's condition still remained stable, and she is able to self-regulate tension. She becomes aware at an early stage when tension starts to increase. The complaints may return a little, but when she takes appropriate action to find and change their cause, the complaints remain absent. She is satisfied and functions normally.

REFERENCES

Badawi, K., Wallace, R. K., Orme-Johnson, D., & Rouzere, A. M. (1984). Electrophysiologic characteristics of respiratory suspension periods occurring during the practice of the transcendental meditation program. *Psychosomatic Medicine, 46*(3), 267–276.

Balfoort, B., & Dixhoorn, J. v. (1979). *Ademen wij vanzelf* [Are we breathing naturally]? Baarn, the Netherlands: Bosch en Keuning.

Benson, H. (1993). The relaxation response. In D. J. Goleman & J. Gurin (Eds.), *Mind body medicine* (pp. 233–257). Yonkers, NY: Consumer Reports Book.

Benson, H., Alexander, S., & Feldman, C. L. (1975). Decreased premature ventricular contractions through the use of the relaxation response in patients with stable ischaemic heart disease. *Lancet, 2,* 380–381.

Benson, H., Beary, J. F., & Carol, M. (1974). The relaxation response. *Psychiatry, 37,* 37–45.

Bergsmann, O., & Eder, M. (1977). *Thorakale Funktionsstorungen [Thoracic dysfunctions].* Heidelberg, Germany: Haug Verlag.

Bestuur AOS. (2004). *Jaarverslag 2003 [Annual Report 2003].* Amersfoort, The Netherlands: Adem- en Ontspanningstherapie Stichting.

Boiten, F. A. (1998). The effects of emotional behaviour on components of the respiratory cycle. *Biological Psychology, 49,* 29–51.

Bowler, S. D., Green, A., & Mitchell, C. A. (1998). Buteyko breathing techniques in asthma: A blinded randomised controlled trial. *Medical Journal of Australia, 169,* 575–578.

Bredin, M., Corner, J., Krishnasamy, M., Plant, H., Bailey, C., & A'Hern, R. (1999). Multicentre randomised controlled trial of nursing intervention for breathlessness in patients with lung cancer. *British Medical Journal, 318,* 901–904.

Buchholz, I. (1994). Breathing, voice and movement therapy: Applications to breathing disorders. *Biofeedback and Self-Regulation, 19,* 141–153.

Burrow, T. (1941). Kymograph records of neuromuscular (respiratory) patterns in relation to behavior disorders. *Psychosomatic Medicine, 3*(2), 174–186.

Cahalin, L. P., Braga, M., Matsuo, Y., & Hernandez, E. D. (2002). Efficacy of diaphragmatic breathing in persons with chronic obstructive pulmonary disease: A review of the literature. *Journal of Cardiopulmonary Rehabilitation, 22,* 7–21.

Choliz, M. (1995). A breathing-retraining procedure in treatment of sleep-onset insomnia: Theoretical basis and experimental findings. *Perceptual and Motor Skills, 80,* 507–513.

Commissie Voor de Revalidatie van Hartpatienten. (1996). *Richtlijnen Hartrevalidatie [Guidelines for cardiac rehabilitation] 12995/1996.* Den Haag, The Netherlands: Nederlandse Hartstichting/Ned Ver Cardiologie.

Conrad, B., Thalacker, S., & Schonle, P. W. (1983). Speech respiration as an indicator of integrative contextual processing. *Folia Phoniatrica, 35,* 220–225.

Czapszys, R., McBride, N., Ozawa, H., Gibney, K. H., & Peper, E. (2000). Effect of breath patterns on
balance: Breathe diaphragmatically to prevent falling. *Proceedings of the Thirty-First Annual Meeting of the Association for Applied Psychophysiology and Biofeedback,* 18–19.

Decramer, M., & Macklem, P. T. (1985). Action of inspiratory muscles and its modification with hyper-
inflation. *Airways, 4,* 19–21.

DeGuire, S., Gevirtz, R., Hawkinson, D., & Dixon, K. (1996). Breathing retraining: A three-year follow-
up study of treatment for hyperventilation syndrome and associated functional cardiac symptoms.
Biofeedback and Self-Regulation, 21, 191–198.

Dekhuijzen, P. N. R. (1989). *Target-flow inspiratory muscle training and pulmonary rehabilitation in patients with chronic obstructive pulmonary disease.* Nijmegen, The Netherlands: Academisch
proefschrift Nijmegen University.

Del Pozo, J. M., Gevirtz, R. N., Scher, B., & Guarneri, E. (2004). Biofeedback treatment increases heart
rate variability in patients with known coronary artery disease. *American Heart Journal, 147,* E11.

Dixhoorn, J. J. v. (1998a). *Ontspanningsinstructie: Principes en oefeningen [Relaxation instruction: Principles and practice].* Maarssen, The Netherlands: Elsevier/Bunge.

Dixhoorn, J. J. v. (2004). A method for assessment of one dimension of dysfunctional breathing: Distribution of breathing movement [abstract]. *Biological Psychology, 67,* 415–416.

Dixhoorn, J. J. v., & Duivenvoorden, H. J. (1999). Effect of relaxation therapy on cardiac events after
myocardial infarction: A 5-year follow-up study. *Journal of Cardiopulmonary Rehabilitation, 19,*
178–185.

Dixhoorn, J. J. v., & White, A. R. (2005). Relaxation therapy for rehabilitation and prevention in
ischaemic heart disease: A systematic review and meta-analysis. *European Journal of Cardiovascular Prevention and Rehabilitation, 12,* 193–202.

Dixhoorn, J. v. (1992). Voordelen en nadelen van adembewustwording bij therapeuten [Advantages and
disadvantages of breathing awareness in therapists]. *Bewegen and Hulpverlening, 9,* 40–51.

Dixhoorn, J. v. (1994a). Breath relaxation: Two-year follow-up of breathing pattern in cardiac patients.
In *Proceedings 25th annual meeting* Wheat Ridge, CO: Association for Applied Psychophysiology
and Biofeedback.

Dixhoorn, J. v. (1994b). Significance of breathing awareness and exercise training for recovery after myocardial infarction. In J. G. Carlson, A. R. Seifert, & N. Birbaumer (Eds.), *Clinical applied
psychophysiology* (pp. 113–132). New York: Plenum Press.

Dixhoorn, J. v. (1997a). Functional breathing is "whole-body" breathing. *Biological Psychology, 46,* 89–
90.

Dixhoorn, J. v. (1997b). Hyperventilation and dysfunctional breathing. *Biological Psychology, 46,* 90–
91.

Dixhoorn, J. v. (1998b). Cardiorespiratory effects of breathing and relaxation instruction in myocardial
infarction patients. *Biological Psychology, 49,* 123–135.

Dixhoorn, J. v. (2002). Experiences of breathing therapy for patients with "hyperventilation" complaints
and healthy students. *Biological Psychology, 59,* 234–235.

Dixhoorn, J. v., & Duivenvoorden, H. J. (1985). Efficacy of Nijmegen Questionnaire in recognition of
the hyperventilation syndrome. *Journal of Psychosomatic Research, 29*(2), 199–206.

Dixhoorn, J. v., & Duivenvoorden, H. J. (1989). Breathing awareness as a relaxation method in cardiac
rehabilitation. In F. J. McGuigan, W. E. Sime, & W. J. Macdonald (Eds.), *Stress and Tension Control* (Vol. 3, pp. 19–36). New York: Plenum Press.

Dixhoorn, J. v., Duivenvoorden, H. J., Pool, J., & Verhage, F. (1990). Psychic effects of physical training
and relaxation therapy after myocardial infarction. *Journal of Psychosomatic Research, 34*(3), 327–
337.

Dixhoorn, J. v., Duivenvoorden, H. J., Staal, J. A., & Pool, J. (1989). Physical training and relaxation
therapy in cardiac rehabilitation assessed through a composite criterion for training outcome.
American Heart Journal, 118(3), 545–552.

Dixhoorn, J. v., & Hoefman, J. D. (1987). Registratie van behandelings resultaat van ademtherapie
[Treatment outcome after breathing therapy]. *Nederlands Tijdschrift Fysiotherapie, 96*(1), 10–15.

Donaldson, G. C. (1992). The chaotic behaviour of resting human respiration. *Respiratory Physiology,
88,* 313–321.

Doorn, P. v., Colla, P., & Folgering, H. Th. M. (1983). Een vragenlijst voor hyperventilatieklachten [A questionnaire for hyperventilation complaints]. *De Psycholoog, 18*, 573–577.

Doorn, P. v., Folgering, H. Th. M., & Colla, P. (1982). Control of the end-tidal PCO2 in the hyperventilation syndrome: Effects of biofeedback and breathing instructions compared. *Bulletin Européen de Physiopathologie Respiratoire, 18*, 829–836.

Dunn, B. R., Hartigan, J. A., & Mikulas, W. L. (1999). Concentration and mindfulness meditations: Unique forms of consciousness? *Applied Psychophysiology and Biofeedback, 24*, 147–165.

Feldenkrais, M. (1972). *Awareness through movement*. New York: Harper & Row.

Fried, R. (1984). The use of end-tidal carbon dioxide feedback in the treatment of idiopathic epilepsy. *Biofeedback and Self-Regulation, 9*(1), 111.

Gevirtz, R., & Schwartz, M. S. (2005). The respiratory system in applied psychophysiology. In M. S. Schwartz & F. Andrasik (Eds.), *Biofeedback: A practitioner's guide* (pp. 212–244). New York: Guilford Press.

Gibson, T. M. (1978). Effects of hypocapnia on psychomotor and intellectual performance. *Aviation Space and Environmental Medicine, 49*, 943–946.

Gosselink, H. A. A. M., Wagenaar, R. C., Rijswijk, H., Sargeant, A. J., & Decramer, M. L. A. (1995). Diaphragmatic breathing reduces efficiency of breathing in patients with chronic obstructive pulmonary disease. *American Journal of Respiratory and Critical Care Medicine, 151*, 1136–1142.

Grossman, P., Swart, J. C. G. d., & Defares, P. B. (1985). A controlled study of a breathing therapy for treatment of hyperventilation syndrome. *Journal of Psychosomatic Research, 29*(1), 49–58.

Han, J. N., Stegen, K., DeValck, C., Clement, J., & Woestijne, K. P. v. d. (1996). Influence of breathing therapy on complaints, anxiety and breathing pattern in patients with hyperventilation syndrome and anxiety disorders. *Journal of Psychosomatic Research, 41*, 481–493.

Han, J. N., Stegen, K., Simkens, K., Cauberghs, M., Schepers, R., Bergh, O. v. d., et al. (1997). Unsteadiness of breathing in patients with hyperventilation syndrome and anxiety disorders. *European Respiratory Journal, 10*, 167–176.

Heide, F. J., & Borkovec, T. D. (1983). Relaxation-induced anxiety: Paradoxical anxiety enhancement due to relaxation training. *Journal of Consulting and Clinical Psychology, 51*, 171–182.

Hornsveld, H., & Garssen, B. (1996). The low specificity of the Hyperventilation Provocation Test. *Journal of Psychosomatic Research, 41*, 435–449.

Hout, M. A. v. d., Jong, P. d., Zandbergen, J., & Merckelbach, H. (1990). Waning of panic sensations during prolonged hyperventilation. *Behaviour Research and Therapy, 28*, 445–448.

Hout, M. A. v. d., & Kroeze, S. (1995). An untenable rationale for treating insomnia. *Perceptual and Motor Skills, 81*, 316–318.

Johnston, R., & Lee, K.-H. (1976). Myofeedback. A new method of teaching breathing exercises in emphysematous patients. *Physical Therapy, 56*, 826–829.

Kapandji, I. A. (1974). *The physiology of the joints: III*. London: Churchill Livingstone.

Kikuchi, Y., Okabe, S., Tamura, G., Hida, W., Homma, M., Shirato, K., et al. (1994). Chemosensitivity and perception of dyspnea inpatients with a history of near-fatal asthma. *New England Journal of Medicine, 330*, 1329–1334.

Kotses, H., Harver, A., Segreto, J., Glaus, K. D., Creer, T. L., & Young, G. A. (1991). Long-term effects of biofeedback-induced facial relaxation on measures of asthma severity in children. *Biofeedback and Self-Regulation, 16*, 1–21.

Laoutaris, I., Dritsas, A., Brown, M. D., Manginas, A., Alivizatos, P. A., & Cokkinos, D. V. (2004). Inspiratory muscle training using an incremental endurance test alleviates dyspnea and improves functional status in patients with chronic heart failure. *European Journal of Cardiovascular Prevention and Rehabilitation, 11*, 489–496.

Leeuwen, J. G. v. (1993). *Adembewustwordingstherapie Verslag keuzecoschap huisartsen geneeskunde [Breathing awareness therapy: Report from family medicine apprenticeship]*. Rotterdam, The Netherlands: Erasmus Universiteit.

Lehrer, P. M., Vaschillo, E., Vaschillo, B., Shou-en, L., Scardella, A., Siddique, M., et al. (2004). Biofeedback treatment for asthma. *Chest, 126*, 352–361.

Leuner, H. (1984). Indications and scientific basis of respiratory feedback. *General Practitioner, 6*, 344–354.

Ley, R. (1988). Panic attacks during relaxation and relaxation-induced anxiety: A hyperventilation interpretation. *Journal of Behavior Therapy and Experimental Psychiatry, 19*, 253–259.

Ley, R. (1994). An introduction to the psychophysiology of breathing. *Biofeedback and Self-Regulation*, *19*, 95–96.

Ley, R., Timmons, B. H., Kotses, H., Harver, A., & Wientjes, C. J. E. (1996). Highlights of the annual meeting of the International Society for the Advancement of Respiratory Psychophysiology and the 14th International Symposium on Respiratory Psychophysiology. *Biofeedback and Self-Regulation*, *21*, 241–260.

Linden, W. (1993). The autogenic training method of J. H. Schultz. In P. M. Lehrer & R. L. Woolfolk (Eds.), *Principles and practice of stress management* (2nd ed., pp. 205–229). New York: Guilford Press.

Lum, L. C. (1976). The syndrome of chronic habitual hyperventilation. In O. Hill (Ed.), *Modern trends in psychosomatic medicine* (pp. 196–230). London: Butterworth.

Lum, L. C. (1977). Breathing exercises in the treatment of hyperventilation and chronic anxiety states. *The Chest, Heart and Stroke Journal*, *2*, 6–11.

Lum, L. C. (1981). Hyperventilation and anxiety state. *Journal of the Royal Society of Medicine*, *74*, 1–4.

Lumb, A. B. (2000). *Nunn's applied respiratory physiology*. Oxford, UK: Butterworth, Heineman.

Luthe, W. (1965). Autogene entladungen wahrend der Unterstufenubungen [Autogenic discharges during basic exercises]. In W. Luthe (Ed.), *Autogenes training correlationes psychosomaticae* (pp. 22–52). Stuttgart, Germany: Thieme.

Macefield, G., & Burke, D. (1991). Paraesthesiae and tetany induced voluntary hyperventilation. *Brain*, *114*, 527–540.

MacHose, M., & Peper, E. (1991). The effect of clothing on inhalation volume. *Biofeedback and Self-Regulation*, *16*, 261–265.

Meuret, A. E., Wilhelm, F. H., & Roth, W. T. (2001). Respiratory biofeedback-assisted therapy in panic disorder. *Behavior Modification*, *25*, 584–605.

Meuret, A. E., Wilhelm, F. H., & Roth, W. T. (2007). *Effects of capnometry-assisted breathing therapy on symptoms and respiration in panic disorder*. Manuscript under review.

Neill, W. A., Pantley, G. A., & Makornchai, V. (1981). Respiratory alkalemia during exercise reduces angina threshold. *Chest*, *80*(2), 149–153.

Noseda, A., Carpiaux, J. P., Schmerber, J., Valente, F., & Yernault, J. C. (1994). Dyspnoea and flow-volume curve during exercise in COPD patients. *European Respiratory Journal*, *7*, 279–285.

Noseda, A., Schmerber, J., Prigogine, T., & Yernault, J. C. (1993). How do patients with either asthma or COPD perceive acute bronchodilation? *European Respiratory Journal*, *6*, 636–644.

Parow, J. (1980). *Funktionelle Atmungstherapie* [Functional breathing therapy]. Heidelberg, Germany: Haug Verlag.

Peper, E. (1979). Passive attention: The gateway to consciousness and autonomic control. In E. Peper, S. Ancoli, & M. Quinn (Eds.), *Mind–body integration: Essential readings in biofeedback* (pp. 119–124). New York: Plenum Press.

Peper, E., Smith, K., & Waddell, D. (1987). Voluntary wheezing versus diaphragmatic breathing with inhalation (Voldyne) feedback: A clinical intervention in the treatment of asthma. *Clinical Biofeedback and Health*, *10*(2), 83–88.

Peper, E., & Tibbets, V. (1992). Fifteen month follow-up with asthmatics utilizing EMG/incentive inspirometer feedback. *Biofeedback and Self-Regulation*, *17*, 143–151.

Peper, E., & Tibbets, V. (1994). Effortless diaphragmatic breathing. *Physical Therapy Products*, *6*, 67–71.

Peper, E., & Tibbets, V. (1996). *Changes in breathing pattern by meadows and concrete images: Implications for health*. Paper presented at the Third Annual Conference of the International Society for the Advancement of Respiratory Psychophysiology, Nijmegen, the Netherlands.

Phillipson, E. A., McClean, P. A., Sullivan, C. E., & Zamel, N. (1978). Interaction of metabolic and behavioral respiratory control during hypercapnia and speech. *American Review of Respiratory Disease*, *117*, 903–909.

Reybrouck, T., Wertelaers, A., Bertrand, P., & Demedts, M. (1987). Myofeedback training of the respiratory muscles in patients with chronic obstructive pulmonary disease. *Journal of Cardiopulmonary Rehabilitation*, *7*, 18–22.

Roland, M., & Peper, E. (1987). Inhalation volume changes with inspirometer feedback and diaphragmatic breathing coaching. *Clinical Biofeedback and Health*, *10*(2), 89–97.

Sakakibara, M., Takeuchi, S., & Hayano, J. (1994). Effect of relaxation training on cardiac parasympathetic tone. *Psychophysiology, 31*, 223–228.

Schein, M. H., Gavish, B., Herz, M., Rosner-Kahana, D., Naveh, P., Knishkowsky, B., et al. (2005). Treating hypertension with a device that slows and regularises breathing: A randomised, double-blind controlled study. *Journal of Human Hypertension, 15*, 271–278.

Smith, J. C. (1988). Steps toward a cognitive-behavioral model of relaxation. *Biofeedback and Self-Regulation, 13*(4), 307–329.

Terai, K., & Umezawa, A. (2004). Effects of respiratory self-control on psychophysiological relaxation using biofeedback involving the partial pressure of end-tidal carbon dioxide. *Japanese Society of Biofeedback Research, 30*, 31–37.

Thomas, M., McKinley, R. K., Freeman, E., & Foy, C. (2001). Prevalence of dysfunctional breathing in patients treated for asthma in primary care: Cross-sectional survey. *British Medical Journal, 322*, 1098.

Tiep, B. L. (1995). Biofeedback and ventilatory muscle training. In T. Kikuchi, H. Sakuma, I. Saito, & K. Tsuboi (Eds.), *Biobehavioral self-regulation* (pp. 398–406). Tokyo: Springer.

Tiep, B. L., Burns, M., Kao, D., Madison, R., & Herrera, J. (1986). Pursed lips breathing training using ear oximetry. *Chest, 90*, 218–221.

Ulrich, B. (1928). *Die Sängeratmung [Singers' breathing]*. Leipzig, Germany: Dörffling & Franke Verlag.

Umezawa, A. (1992). Effects of stress on post expiration pause time and minute ventilation volume. In K. Shirakura, I. Saito, & S. Tsutsui (Eds.), *Current biofeedback research in Japan* (pp. 125–132). Tokyo: Shinkoh Igaku Shuppan.

Umezawa, A. (2001). Facilitation and inhibition of breathing during changes of emotion. In Y. Haruki, I. Homma, A. Umezawa, & Y. Masaoka (Eds.), *Respiration and emotion* (pp. 139–148). Tokyo: Springer Verlag.

Varray, A. L., Mercier, J. G., & Prefaut, C. G. (1995). Individualized training reduces excessive exercise hyperventilation in asthmatics. *International Journal of Rehabilitation Research, 18*, 297–312.

Whatmore, G. B., & Kohli, D. R. (1974). *The physiopathology and treatment of functional disorders.* New York: Grune & Stratton.

Wientjes, C. J. E. (1993). *Psychological influences upon breathing: situational and dispositional aspects.* Doctoral dissertation, Tilburg University, Tilburg, The Netherlands.

Wilhelm, F. H., Trabert, W., & Roth, W. T. (2001a). Characteristics of sighing in panic disorder. *Biological Psychiatry, 49*, 606–614.

Wilhelm, F. H., Trabert, W., & Roth, W. T. (2001b). Physiological instability in panic disorder and generalized anxiety disorder. *Biological Psychiatry, 49*, 596–605.

Wittenboer, G. v. d., Wolf, K. v. d., & Dixhoorn, J. J. v. (2003). Respiratory variability and psychological well-being in schoolchildren. *Behavior Modification, 27*, 653–670.

Xu, J. H., Ikeda, Y., & Komiyama, S. (1991). Biofeedback and the yawning breath pattern in voice therapy: A clinical trial. *Auris Nasus Larynx, 18*, 67–77.

Zeier, H. (1984). Arousal reduction with biofeedback-supported respiratory meditation. *Biofeedback and Self-Regulation, 9*, 497–508.

CHAPTER 13

Exercise Therapy for Stress Management

WESLEY E. SIME

THEORETICAL FOUNDATIONS

A growing body of scientific evidence shows that exercise is a potent stress-relieving strategy, as well as a healthy, preventive measure to ward off the impending symptoms of emotional distress well in advance of provocation (Petruzzello, Landers, & Salazar, 1993; Skrinar, Unger, Hutchinson, & Faigenbaum, 1992; Dixhoorn, Duivenvoorden, Pool, & Verhage, 1990; Blumenthal et al., 2002). The acute effects of exercise serve to relieve stress and tension symptoms, and the long-term metabolic and biochemical effects serve to buffer against the onslaught of day-to-day challenges (Dua & Hargreaves, 1992; Motl & Dishman, 2004; Sime, 2002; Sime & Hellweg, 2001). By contrast, it is also well known that any form of physical activity can be a major stressor to the body when taken to excess, especially if it precipitates overuse injury (Gordon, 1991; Clarkson & Hubal, 2002). Muscle strain and joint pain are common side effects among individuals who become dependent on exercise to relieve psychological effects of emotional stress. Overuse injury is a paradoxical by-product of negative addiction, that is, an "exercise dependence" syndrome (Furst & Germone, 1993). This syndrome is not easily identified and usually appears in association with forced withdrawal from long-term habitual exercise patterns. In particular, those individuals who are accustomed to a regular regimen of voluntary exercise but are suddenly precluded from exercise by family emergencies, work commitments, overseas travel, injury, or surgery will often experience addiction-like withdrawal symptoms (tension, irritability, depression, and anger) until they are able to become active once again (Cockbrill & Riddington, 1996).

With this wide range of positive and negative affect linked to habitual exercise or deprivation thereof as a foundation, the epidemiology of exercise habit patterns across divergent populations becomes of interest. This chapter provides a comprehensive overview of exercise therapy and how it has been used effectively. It also provides an analysis of the physiological relationship between exercise levels and stress coping and between relaxation and optimum mental health, while noting side effects and contraindications for exercise. Finally, the chapter offers a detailed manual for a 10-step approach, with practical guidelines, to conducting exercise therapy, along with a case study analysis of two clients at different stages in the clinical application of exercise therapy.

Although physical activity has been associated with reduction in numerous emotional and behavioral disorders related to stress among adults and children (Weyerer, 1992), many questions remain to be answered. I evaluate how to determine whether or not the accumulated evidence meets criteria for stating definitively that exercise therapy is effective in stress management, in accordance with the guidelines set forth by the Association for Applied Psychophysiology and Biofeedback (LaVaque et al., 2002). Evaluative categories ranging from highest to lowest are employed in this review: (1) efficacious and specific, (2) efficacious, (3) possibly efficacious, and (4) further research needed to establish efficacy.

Origin of the Exercise and Health Concept

Exercise has been described as one of the elements of the "healing power of nature," along with diet, rest, fresh air, massage, and baths since the time of Hippocrates. Medical philosophers, including Hippocrates, declared the virtues of exercise without necessarily having a rational scientific explanation of the mechanisms by which it was effective. Exercise was not recognized as a credible scientific issue so long as most people spent their lives doing some form of moderate to intense physical labor to sustain their livelihoods. Technological advancements since the Industrial Revolution, however, have eliminated much of the physical work in agriculture, as well as in most industrial, blue-collar jobs (Paffenbarger, Lee, & Leung, 1994). Furthermore, with one or more televisions in every household (during the last two to three decades), habits of sedentary living have grown dramatically. Workers often come home "stressed out," because most people who work in service or production jobs are required to stand but do not move actively as they are attending to customers or operating machines. Mechanization is designed to minimize the labor fatigue of physical work, but the machines are sometimes dangerous and simply create mental strain because of the risk of making mistakes and/or causing an accident. The constant vigilance required to monitor and manipulate a powerful machine (or an automobile in traffic) has been shown to be very fatiguing due to mental stress and strain (Johansson, Evans, Rydstedt, & Carrere, 1998).

Throughout the 20th century, the sociocultural shift from hard physical labor to sedentary living has been associated with both physical and mental health complications some of which are related to emotional stress (Paffenbarger et al., 1994). In the 21st century, very few occupations include a healthy level of daily exercise without the risk of overload strain or repetitive-motion injury. Farming during the mid-1900s (most familiar to me) included a variety of ergonomically healthy physical demands (shoveling, pulling or hoeing weeds, etc.) and a great deal less of the emotional stress of handling financial debts than it has during the past two or three decades. More recently, the use of powerful machinery and chemical weed and pest controls eliminated much of the vigorous physical effort in exchange for increased financial strain and worry about creating a toxic environment.

Numerous scientific studies have documented the association between habitual exercise and positive mood and affect (Acevedo, Dzewaltowski, Gill, & Noble, 1992; Kavussanu & McAuley, 1995; Oman & Haskel, 1993). Specifically, individuals who are accustomed to a regular routine of physical labor on the job or to moderately intense leisure exercise or competitive games (recreational basketball, racquetball, jogging, etc.) report that they feel better when they exercise (Leith & Taylor, 1990). Furthermore, in most cases individuals who are accustomed to a regular regimen of physical activity experience mild withdrawal symptoms if they stop due to injury or if they fail to maintain a regular schedule of exercise. Engaging in some form of physical activity at least once every 2–3 days is the minimum threshold for gaining physiological and psychological benefit for most individuals (Furst & Germone, 1993; Cockbrill & Riddington, 1996). Unfortunately, most of those early studies were not well controlled, and some lacked large population sampling, so the evidence shows only that exercise is *possibly efficacious*.

What Is Exercise Therapy?

Exercise therapy (also known as *walk/talk therapy*) is the practice of combining a program of exercise with traditional psychotherapy. Unique to psychotropic exercise therapy is the fact that walking is done during a counseling session under the guidance of an experienced exercise therapist. In addition to the walk/talk therapy sessions, the client is encouraged to establish a regular program of daily exercise that he or she can continue as a lifestyle habit pattern (unsupervised) long after the therapy has concluded (Wankel, 1993). Exercise habits usually continue because of the inherent satisfaction (enjoying movement or play), in addition to the psychological benefits.

Therapeutically, brisk activity (such as walking side by side with the client) is helpful in breaking down barriers and subtly helping clients engage in difficult topics of conversation. In addition, the walk/talk approach appears to be highly therapeutic and cathartic (i.e., it aids in "getting it all out") when the issues are complicated or entangled (Hays, 1999).

The walking helps to stimulate both the client and the therapist to be alert and creative in the problem-solving process. In addition, there is also the advantage of the constantly changing scenery, which seems to be refreshing for most clients. When client and therapist are walking side by side, there is less face-to-face interaction, which can be beneficial in allowing the therapist to pose difficult questions or to make confrontations without the pressure of continuous eye contact (Hays, 1999). Similarly, if the client is having difficulty formulating responses, having the option to gaze at a point of scenery or to focus on pace or rhythm of the walking stride seems to help create an informal atmosphere, thus allowing more spontaneous responses. *Obviously, these are empirical observations, not yet tested by formal research methodology.*

Adding exercise to psychotherapy can be beneficial for people suffering from a wide variety of mental health issues and interpersonal problems, it has been described by some as the "neglected intervention" (Callaghan, 2004). Because exercise has risks as well as benefits, it is important to be cautious and to make sure that the client has gotten clearance from a physician. For those under the age of 40 who do not have medical complications (neurological disorders, orthopedic limitations, back injuries, chest pain, or an endocrine disorder such as diabetes), a moderately intense, progressively increasing program of exercise is usually safe (Shephard, 1991). Enjoyment of the activity is more important than the intensity or vigor.

HISTORY OF EXERCISE AS A STRESS COPING METHOD

The first documented use of exercise (walk/talk) therapy for stress management and enhancing mental health was conducted by Thaddeus Kostrubala, a psychiatrist in San

Diego, California, who took many of his patients walking or running on the beach (Sime, 1981). Kostrubala demonstrated that the metabolic effects of physical exertion pertain also to psychological catharsis such that expression of emotionally charged descriptions of past stressful trauma comes forth more freely and can be processed in therapy. Subsequently, many other health care professionals began to recommend exercise for their clients, and some clinical researchers documented the objective benefits of using an exercise prescription for two major stress symptoms, depression and anxiety (Johnsgard, 1989). Johnsgard reported that exercise participants loosen up and become less inhibited and less self-conscious and more in touch with their immediate feelings (anger, irritability). As a result, clients who tended to repress their anger and to defer to others became more assertive about their needs and were more willing to talk about what they felt at a deeper level. Walk/talk therapy is a relatively convenient and safe method of conducting exercise during psychotherapy, although other forms, such as talking while riding stationary bicycles, also can be functional.

Epidemiological Research on the Effects of Exercise

There is a significant association between exercise and several psychological measures of mental health based on research with large populations. The most significant evidence linking exercise to emotional stress coping lies in epidemiological studies on coronary heart disease on more than 5,000 men (Nicholson, Fuhrer, & Marmot, 2005) and other studies showing that level of fitness was inversely related to depression (Pelham, Campagna, Ritvo, & Birnie, 1993). Subsequently, other medical research studies revealed that depression is a common outcome following myocardial infarction (Frasure-Smith, Lesperance, & Talajic, 1993). Even more compelling was the evidence of a strong correlation between depression and incidence of heart disease that came from epidemiological studies on exercise as part of cardiac rehabilitation that were well controlled for other clinical variables (Achat, Kawachi, Spiro, DeMolles, & Sparrow, 2000; Kavussanu & McAuley, 1995). As an extension of this research, exercise as a stress management intervention became even more viable given the fact that exercise and stress coping are now considered essential components of cardiac rehabilitation therapy. Those patients who participated regularly also showed improved mood changes, along with increases in cardiopulmonary function (Froelicher, 1990; Sime, Buell, & Eliot, 1979). More definitive evidence on the psychological benefits of exercise came to light when studies appeared showing that depression is a predictor of reinfarction in this population and that a side benefit of exercise for cardiac rehabilitation was reduction in depressed affect (Denollet, 1993; Herrmann, Buss, Buecker, Gonska, & Kreuzer, 1994).

It should be noted that severe anxiety is also a major risk factor for heart disease (Kawachi, Colditz, & Ascherio, 1994) and that it is treatable with exercise. The correlation is very high between regular exercise habits and anxiety reduction (Emery, Hauck, & Blumenthal, 1992; Ruuskanen & Parkatti, 1994). Even among adolescents, level of exercise was inversely related to anxiety, as well as to depression, hostility, and stress (Camacho, Roberts, Lazarus, Kaplan, & Cohen, 1991; Norris, Carroll, & Cochrane, 1992).

The influence of exercise habits on the incidence of overall anxiety and depression rates in younger patients without chronic heart disease is particularly intriguing. Given that exercise is associated with healthier and more stable mood, it also reduces the rate of suicide, which is the worst possible psychological outcome of depression (Paffenbarger et al., 1994). These results reach the level of being efficacious.

Clinical Effects of Exercise Therapy

Substantial improvements in mood and affect following organized exercise programs have occurred in part because patients found exercise particularly enjoyable, challenging, and satisfying on completion (Bosscher, 1993; Brown, Welsh, Labbe, Gitulli, & Kulkarni, 1992; Martinsen, 1993, 1994). Others have found that the combination of exercise and talk therapy was more effective than an equivalent experience in cognitive therapy alone (McNeil, LeBlanc, & Joyner, 1991; Sime, 1987).

In general, the psychiatric community has come to view exercise as a valuable adjunct to mental health therapy (Steptoe, Kearsley, & Walters, 1993), especially in the reduction of anxiety in nonclinical populations (Brown, Morgan, & Raglin, 1993) and in treatment for depression (Lehofer, Klebel, Gersdorf, & Zapotoczke, 1992). A number of review articles using meta-analyses also support the effectiveness of exercise as a part of a comprehensive treatment program (Byrne & Byrne, 1993; Hinkle, 1992; North, McCullaugh, & Tran, 1990; Petruzzello, Landers, Hatfield, Kubitz, & Salazar, 1991; Rabins, 1992). Because of limitations in experimental design and lack of control for expectancy, the conclusion is that these treatments are only *possibly efficacious*.

However, one very well-controlled intervention study, a cognitive-behavioral stress management program, was instigated while clients were in the midst of a heavy training program (rowing), with very encouraging results (Perna, Antoni, Kumar, Cruess, & Schneiderman, 1998). There was a significant reduction in depression, fatigue, and cortisol, together with an increase in adaptation to heavy training, among those getting psychological (cognitive-behavioral) intervention along with exercise.

Exercise Modalities

A variety of different forms of exercise, including functional activities of daily living (ADL) such as walking, lifting, pushing, or climbing stairs, can be beneficial. Aerobic exercise (walking, jogging, bicycling, and/or swimming) of moderate intensity carried out for 30–60 minutes (at minimum) at least 3–5 days per week was effective in altering mood and fitness levels. Anaerobic exercise (weight lifting and isometrics) that includes intense, short bouts of activity with an occasional valsalva maneuver (breath holding) effort can also be beneficial (Hansen, Stevens, & Coast, 2001). A wide variety of enjoyable recreational or leisure activities, such as hiking, biking, snowshoeing, and cross-country skiing, are particularly effective when conducted in moderately adverse weather conditions, in part because of psychological hardiness and mood-enhancement side benefits that develop accordingly (Dienstbier, 1991; Dienstbier, LaGuardia, & Wilcox, 1987; Rejeski, Thompson, Brubaker, & Miller, 1992). In addition, the competitive games (e.g., basketball, racquetball, soccer, etc.) have also been shown to have positive benefits for mood and affect (Steptoe et al., 1993). This evidence is *well documented that these activities are efficacious*.

Prescription Dose–Response and Type of Exercise for Effectiveness

Although aerobic exercise (walking, running, bicycling, and swimming) is preferred over anaerobic (strength training) exercise (Berger & Owen, 1992; Folkins & Sime, 1981; Norvell & Belles, 1993) because of rhythm and continuity therein, the benefits from strength training in reducing anxiety, depression, and hostility are surprisingly high (Johnston, Petlichkoff, & Hoeger, 1993). Although running is popular among populations of "macho" young and middle-aged mildly depressed adults (Bosscher, 1993; McMurdo & Rennie, 1993), there appear to be equivalent benefits from other types of exercise. Personal preference and enjoyment of the activity may be most important for mental health benefits rather than any single modality of exertion (Wankel, 1993). Recent studies suggest that high-intensity aerobic activity is not necessary to achieve the mental health benefits of exercise (Doyne, Schambless, & Beutler, 1983; Martinsen, 1993; Blumenthal et al., 2002). Ironically, nonaerobic exercise was superior to the aerobic methods in enhancing self-concept in at least one study (Stein & Motta, 1992). Similarly, in a comparison of aerobic swimming with low-intensity yoga in college students, the yoga produced greater reductions in tension, fatigue, and anger than did the more intensive swimming intervention (Berger & Owen, 1992).

In a definitive series of studies, the dose–response and duration factors were examined in regard to the treatment of mild to moderate major depressive disorder. Well- controlled experimental trials (Dunn, Trivedi, Kampert, Clark, & Chambliss, 2002) were conducted to determine the minimum level of aerobic exercise dosage that was effective in reducing the clinical manifestation of depression. A moderate level of exercise was just as effective an antidepressant as intense activity, and the low-dosage (duration) exercise was comparable to the placebo effect (Dunn, Trivedi, Kampert, Clark, & Chambliss, 2005; Dunn, Trivedi, & O'Neal, 2001). Even stair climbing was shown to be moderately efficacious and cost-effective in managing negative mood states. However, in regard to specific duration of exercise, there were no significant differences in effects on mood for the range of 20- to 60-minute bouts of exercise (Daley & Welch, 2004). Further study of dose and duration effects are needed, because few studies have shown rigor in titrating and monitoring dosages of exercise prescription.

PHYSIOLOGICAL MECHANISMS LINKING EXERCISE AND MENTAL HEALTH

Several possible physiological mechanisms that may account for the psychological benefits of exercise include endorphin release, hardiness effects, sleep quality, and changes in several neurotransmitters and/or receptors in the autonomic nervous system (Hays, 1999; Johnsgard, 2004; Leith & Taylor, 1990; Seraganian, 1993).

Hardiness and Relaxation Theory

Exercise has been shown to increase heat tolerance and cold tolerance, thereby instilling a degree of physical and emotional hardiness and stability (Dienstbier et al., 1987). When core temperature rises during and after moderate to intense exercise, a simultaneous reduction in muscle tension occurs (DeVries, Beckman, Huber, & Dieckmeir, 1968; Sime & Hellweg, 2001). The physiological process of adapting to variations in core temperature also modulates emotions substantially (Koltyn & Morgan, 1993). In addition, there is a reduction in gamma motor activity that accounts for the reductions in muscle tension and state anxiety following exercise and passive heating (Morgan, 1988). Last, improvements in brain wave laterality are associated with a reduction in anxiety when core temperature increases after an intense bout of exercise (Petruzzello et al., 1993; Robbins, 2000). Although the thermogenic hardiness hypothesis appears appropriate to account for some relaxation effects and a reduction in anxiety, there are no data available regarding the linkage to depression.

Anaesthetic Pain Relief Theory

Vigorous exercise (running, jumping, lifting, etc.) generates minor trauma to the tissues of the body, which in turn causes a release of endorphins and endocannabinoids (Lobstein & Rasmussen, 1991; Dietrich & McDaniel, 2004). As a result, positive mood changes appear in the form of analgesia, sedation, anxiolysis, and a sense of well-being. This outcome is particularly common when intense endurance training elevates resting plasma beta-endorphins and the enhanced sense of well-being among healthy middle-aged men. Testing this theory under experimental conditions, naltrexone, the opiate receptor antagonist, was used to block the effects of endorphins, in contrast to a placebo, in a randomized double-blind crossover design using two levels of exercise therapy. The results showed unequivocally that high-intensity exercise improved mood state more than did low-intensity or placebo-control conditions (Daniels, Martin, & Carter, 1992).

Increase in the endorphin levels has other positive psychological effects as well. For example, a reduction in the stress reactivity effects (McCubbin, Cheung, Montgomery, Bulbulian, & Wilson, 1992) and reduced sensitivity to pain (Haier, Quaid, & Mills, 1981) are linked to higher levels of endorphins following exercise. Most avid exercise enthusiasts report universally the feeling of an "exercise high" following an intense workout. These euphoric sensations are likely associated with a surge in serum endorphin levels in the bloodstream and in the brain (Dietrich & McDaniel, 2004). Interestingly, the use of naltrexone (given before a bout of exercise to neutralize the anesthetic effects of endorphins) has been so effective in experimental assessment that we can draw strong conclusions. It would appear that the effects of endorphins is a highly efficacious and specific mechanism associated with a positive sense of well-being and a relief from discomfort due to the effects of low- to high-intensity exercise, depending on individual specificity.

Stress and Relaxation Hormone Theory

It is common knowledge that deficiencies in norepinephrine and serotonin are concordant with the onset of depression, and evidence now exists that exercise increases levels of both hormones (Guszkowska, 2004; Johnsgard, 2004). It is also clear that adaptive changes in these receptor sites occur as part of the metabolic action of various antidepressant medications. Furthermore, exercise increases the sensitivity of serotonin receptors, making these naturally produced chemicals more potent in the process of reducing depression (Dey, 1994; Dey, Singh, & Dey, 1992). Because antidepressant medications also produce a neurotransmitter receptor effect, it is assumed that the serotonin reuptake theory is one of the more important mechanisms linking exercise to stress coping. Last, it appears that the role of exercise in decreasing sympathetic and increasing parasympathetic activity is also associated with simultaneous improvement in emotional stability (Kubitz & Landers, 1993; Perna et al., 1998). These exercise effects (reducing stress and enhancing relaxation) are possibly efficacious given the fact that the hormonal changes described here can be replicated and validated.

Rebound Restorative High-Quality Sleep Theory

Stress affects the quality and quantity of sleep negatively. Especially regarding work stress, there is clear evidence that higher levels of stress on alternate weeks (among the same employees in an A–B–A design) showed a close correlation with the level of impaired sleep at night and "sleepiness" during daytime hours (Dahlgren, Kecklund, & Akerstedt, 2005). In addition, levels of stress reported by employees each week (low or high) were highly correlated with cortisol levels obtained at the end of each work period. These results are particularly relevant because exercise has been shown to be a very effective intervention to improve quality of sleep (Youngstedt, 1997) even in the face of high caffeine intake (Youngstedt, O'Conner, Crabbe, & Dishman, 2000).

The link between exercise, stress, sleep, and depression was further supported in a study in which both high- and low-intensity exercise were randomly assigned to individuals in a population of mature, elderly (over 60 years of age) individuals whose depression levels were high (Singh et al., 2005). Reports of enhanced quality of life, in addition to increased self-efficacy and locus of control, were found among those assigned to higher levels of exercise intensity. Greater reductions in depression and increased quality of sleep were found among the high-intensity exercisers compared with the low-intensity exercisers and those who got no exercise in the control condition. Because high-quality sleep and sufficient quantity thereof are essential to maintaining a mood state that is resistant to stress, the effects of vigorous exercise are very helpful in fatiguing (and relaxing) the body and mind, leading to sleep onset. Normal sleep keeps the hypophyseal–pituitary–adrenal (HPA) axis efficient and responsive. Acute sleep loss, however, alters the cortisol secretion profile such that negative feedback loops (so important to maintaining homeostasis) are impaired (see McGrady, Chapter 2, this volume).

Summary of Psychological Benefits and Mechanisms

It would appear that a preponderance of the available literature *supports the efficacy* of exercise therapy for psychological benefits related to stress management and relaxation among clinical populations. Although the majority of studies are encouraging, it is of concern that a substantial number of patients (up to 50% or more) are not able or willing to continue exercise on a long-term basis (Dishman, 1991). Further understanding of the acute and long-term mechanisms whereby exercise provides stress management benefits may ultimately aid in the creative design of programs to facilitate initiative and adherence to exercise treatment in the future (Dixhoorn et al., 1990).

Rather than trying to isolate single mechanisms (physiological or cognitive) associated with stress coping outcomes, it is important to consider the obvious and most logical explanation for the effects of exercise, that is, the "interaction effect." For example, temperature elevation may influence the release, synthesis, or uptake of certain brain monoamines, or they might interact in a synergistic manner (Morgan, 1988). Further, it has been suggested that there may be an interaction between endorphins and monoamines (Hamachek, 1987; Perna et al., 1998). Interactive cognitive effects are also likely. For example, exercise has been shown to produce a "hardiness effect," overlapping with an increase in report of positive self-worth brought about by the social support inherent in group physical activity (Oman & Haskel, 1993). It is also possible that both physiological and cognitive interactions are present, as exercise has been shown to develop overall hardiness by attenuating sympathetic nervous system responses (Dienstbier, 1991). Regardless of the exact mechanism or the statistical proof of benefits therein, the use of clinical exercise therapy appears to merit consideration in therapy.

SPECIFIC EFFECTS OF EXERCISE ON DEPRESSION

The prevalence of depression among apparently healthy, middle-aged individuals is higher than previously recognized (Rajala, Uusimaki, Keinanen-Kiukaanniemi, & Kivela,

1994; Sime & Hellweg, 2001). Thus it is not surprising that a systematic public health appeal for increasing activity with advancing age has been instigated and pursued vigorously (Rooney, 1993).

Anecdotally and in survey research, many individuals report a "feeling good" effect, especially in the immediate postexercise period, as long as the duration and the dosage do not exceed the exercise tolerance of the individual (Folkins & Sime, 1981; Hassmen, Koivula, & Uutela, 2000). Given that exercise is definitely efficacious in the prevention of some diseases and somatic disorders and that it is advocated to promote psychological health and well-being, it is disturbing to note that exercise therapy (as described herein) is a badly neglected intervention among mental health professionals (Callaghan, 2004). That depression symptoms are potent and affect other medical conditions is documented by the data that link depression to angina and overall coronary artery disease. As a result, more opportunities are becoming available in the relatively new specialty of behavioral medicine, wherein mental health professionals collaborate regularly with private practice physicians and other health care professionals (personal trainers, stress management specialists, etc.; Krittayaphong, Light, Golden, Finkel, & Sheps, 1996).

Moderate exercise has been shown to combat stress-related symptoms such as depression as effectively as pharmaceutical intervention when it is maintained as a regular, ongoing lifestyle activity (Kugler, Seelbach, & Kruskemper, 1994; Babyak et al., 2000). The use of exercise, alone and in combination with antidepressant medication, showed a significant reduction in symptoms. At 6-month follow-up, the benefits persisted, especially for the exercise group that maintained their habits. However, long-term improvements in mood were significantly greater for the group that received exercise only than for either of the groups on antidepressants (whether alone or in combination with exercise). Ironically, it appears that in some cases, the concurrent use of medication with exercise (Alonso, Castellano, Quintero, & Navarro, 1999; Babyak et al., 2000; Martinsen & Stanghelle, 1997) may actually undermine the psychological benefits of exercise alone. The exhilaration associated with physical activity (designed to combat the depression) makes it a preferred intervention for most patients who dislike the feeling of being medicated back to health on pills.

Unfortunately, most physicians recommend antidepressant medication first and only consider other lifestyle variables (e.g., stress management, counseling, or exercise) if the patient complains of side effects of the medications. In light of the fact that stress and depression bring on a sense of hopelessness and despair, it is not surprising how difficult it is to initiate exercise therapy without simultaneous use of antidepressant treatment (Alonso et al., 1999).

SPECIFIC EFFECTS OF EXERCISE ON ANXIETY

Levels of anxiety and panic associated with perceived threat are related to both acute and chronic effects of exercise. Well-controlled experimental studies on animals have shown unequivocally that physical exercise reduces both anxiety and impulsiveness in social environmental challenges with field and maze tasks (Binder, Droste, Ohl, & Reul, 2004; Fulk et al., 2004). In humans, exercise has been an effective intervention for posttraumatic stress disorder (PTSD) over the course of 12 sessions, showing significant reductions in anxiety (as well as depression); the effects persisted at 1-month follow-up (Manger & Motta, 2005).

It is remarkable to note that panic disorder has been shown to occur frequently as a comorbid factor with coronary artery disease (Lavoie et al., 2004). Heart rate variability biofeedback appears to be helpful for a variety of emotional, respiratory, and cardiovascular diseases (see Lehrer, Chapter 10, this volume). Because anxiety and physical inactivity are both known to be implicated as risk factors for heart disease (Bonnet et al., 2005), it would appear that the aggressive use of exercise therapy in dealing with anxiety may have a side benefit (in a collective manner) in treating or preventing heart disease.

Exercise therapy has been compared with other stress management techniques (e.g., relaxation, bibliotherapy, etc.) in a review of 34 medical and homeopathic remedies, wherein the differential treatment effects were quite compelling (Jorm et al., 2004). Exercise showed specific benefits for generalized anxiety disorder (GAD), whereas relaxation therapy was associated with significant effectiveness across the board for GAD, panic, dental phobia, and test anxiety. In regard to experimental significance, for both anxiety and depression there appears to be sufficient information to show the efficacy of treatment when the exercise therapy can be instigated effectively and perpetuated without recidivism.

OTHER CLINICAL EFFECTS OF EXERCISE THERAPY

Cognitive Functioning and Aging

With the deteriorating functions that are associated with aging, concerns about cognitive function and menopause become relevant. Aerobic exercise has been associated with higher cognitive functions, such as executive control (Kubesch et al., 2003). Measures of quick recognition and reaction to the Stroop task and several other neuropsychological paradigms were notably improved following moderate- versus low-intensity exercise efforts of 30 minutes' duration. At the other extreme, women who were experiencing climacteric symptoms of menopause were shown to have improved quality of life and reduced paresthesia, nervousness, and other psychosomatic symptoms following a 12-week program of moderate exercise at least three times per week (Ueda, 2004). Finally, other studies on the effects of exercise on aging and declining cognitive function have shown similar results, indicating positive affect and feelings of well-being and revitalization among women, more so than men (Goldstein et al., 1999; Rejeski, Gauvin, Hobson, & Norris, 1995). These are encouraging results that suggest the need for more research to establish efficacy.

Diabetes and Metabolic Problems

The role of emotional stress in pathophysiology (especially diabetes) has been demonstrated unequivocally (see McGrady, Chapter 2, this volume). Complications are often observed during the cycle of exercise and hypoglycemia among patients with type 1 diabetes (Ertl & Davis, 2004). Although exercise has been shown to be the cornerstone in the management of diabetes (because it aids in glycemic control), weight management and quality of life are also important outcomes for the diabetic patient. An acute episode of emotional stress prior to exercise can triple the metabolic reactions to exercise, causing severe hypoglycemia (Araki & Ito, 1999). Thus it is critical to maintain careful monitoring and prudent prescription of exercise procedures, especially among older patients with diabetes.

By contrast, patients who suffer with Crohn's disease and other inflammatory bowel disorders often have severe emotional adjustments due to the pain and altered lifestyle complications. In a study of sedentary patients with Crohn's disease, the benefits of low-intensity exercise of moderate duration were demonstrated for psychological stress coping (including reduction in depression) without causing any exacerbation of the symptoms (Loudon, Corroll, Butcher, Rawsthorne, & Bernstein, 1999).

Cancer

Compromises in immune function associated with emotional stress are also associated with some types of cancer (Huang, Hara, Homma, Yonekawa, & Ohgaki, 2005). On the other hand, exercise increases immune function (Hutnick et al., 2005) and has been effective as an adjunctive coping strategy for dealing with the side effects of various chemical and radiological treatments. Specifically, one study demonstrated the efficacy of a combination of relaxed breathing together with physical exercise in reducing anxiety, depression, and leukocyte activity during stem-cell transplantation and during chemical and radiological treatments (Kim & Kim, 2005). Similarly, another study has shown that physical activity, together with the subsequent quality-of-sleep outcomes associated with exercise training, was effective in reducing the anticipatory distress and anxiety preceding breast cancer surgery (Tatrow, Montgomery, Avellino, & Bovbjerg, 2004). In regard to cancer treatment, the use of home-based physical activity training programs was found to increase cardiorespiratory fitness levels (shortly after chemotherapy) significantly and simultaneously produced lower depression and anxiety (Thorsen et al., 2005). Unfortunately, the results of this research on exercise did not show reductions in fatigue or mental distress, nor increases in the quality-of-life measure, as had been hypothesized. Clearly, exercise is a potent, though little-used, technique (in clinical practice) for cancer-related problems, though more research is needed to establish the efficacy of it.

Heart Disease

Heart disease is the single most deadly and complex pathological condition of modern society (Sime & Hellweg, 2001). The role of emotional stress as an etiological factor has been considered controversial, as the evidence to document a pathophysiological mechanism is elusive at best (Sime, Buell, & Eliot, 1980). In addition to other evidence discussed earlier that shows that exercise has a significant impact on symptoms of depression among those with cardiac disease, exercise programs in cardiac rehabilitation are associated with a decrease in anger and hostility (Tennant et al., 1994). Others have also found a combined effect of lessened anger and depression as an outcome of exercise training (Hassmen et al., 2000).

Exercise training has also been associated with decreased cardiovascular reactivity as an integral outcome of cardiac rehabilitation (de Geus, van Doornen, & Orlebeke, 1993). These results provide support for the overall psychological, as well as physiological, benefits of exercise, especially when presented as part of a prudent and conservative treatment plan (Dixhoorn et al., 1990; Sime & Hellweg, 2001). One particular study demonstrated that the link between depression and angina pectoris pain in patients with coronary artery disease turns out to be related to beta-endorphin levels (Krittayaphong et al., 1996). That is, depressed patients had more exercise-induced angina pain and higher levels of endorphins. However, when actual ischemic measures (indicative of coronary obstruction) were analyzed, it was interesting to note that the depressed patients simply had a lower threshold for pain than those without depression. Thus the impact of exercise therapy (as an antidepressant factor) has the potential to reduce clinical angina symptoms, as well.

Infectious Disease (Flu, Herpes)

The plethora of recent evidence in psychoneuroimmunology shows that emotional stress is associated with increased risk of infectious disease (see McGrady, Chapter 2, this volume), especially with increasing age. Specifically, significantly greater immune response following influenza vaccination was observed in older adults who exercised regularly than among those who were sedentary (Kohut, Cooper, Nickolaus, Russell, & Cunnick, 2002). Exercise is one of several lifestyle factors (in addition to diet and other stress management efforts) that offset the immunosenescence of aging and onset of depression (Fuchs & Hahn, 1992). However, caution is in order with regard to excess in exercise intensity or duration, as both acute and chronic overexertion actually compromise immune function (Shephard & Shek, 1998). Obviously, more research is needed to demonstrate the efficacy herein, especially when noting gender differences that favor women for some of the psychoneuroimmunological effects of exercise (Brown et al., 2004).

Eating Disorders

One of the most important life-threatening health problems associated with emotional stress involves the eating disorders complex. The role of stress, exercise, and eating in maintaining caloric balance is inextricably interwoven, such that healthy weight loss among overweight individuals generally requires carefully prescribed exercise. In addition, athletes sometimes struggle with critical mass and difficulty mobilizing body weight in sports such as gymnastics and diving (among others) such that they develop eating disorders (Yates, Edman, Crago, & Crowell, 2003). In dealing with the stress of competition in sport, those with anorexic and/or bulimic symptoms sometimes use exercise to excess as a means of purging unwanted calories (Holtkamp, Hebebrand, & Herpertz-Dahlmann, 2004). Excessive exercise appears in 40–80% of anorexia patients. Ironically, when anxiety is present among these patients, the voluntary food restriction derails the homeostatic mechanisms for maintaining healthy appetite. As a result, appetite control governed by a negative feedback loop fails.

Even among apparently healthy college students (females = 235, males = 86) who were polled in a survey of exercise, stress coping, eating attitudes, self-esteem, depression, and anxiety, a high correlation appeared between exercise and negative affect (Thome & Espelage, 2004). That is, exercise habits were associated with higher levels of depression and anxiety. One interpretation is that exercise served as an important coping mechanism among those with negative affect. Similarly, obese patients with binge-eating habits who were following an exercise prescription in addition to traditional cognitive-behavioral and nutrition education showed significantly greater reductions in anxiety than those in traditional treatment without exercise (Fossati et al., 2004). Last, it is disturbing to note that those seriously affected by anorexia nervosa also were found to be exhibiting exercise dependence and characteristics of "addiction" (Klein et al., 2004). This particular study leads us into further discussion in the next section about contra indication issues for exercise therapy to follow.

The evidence supporting the benefits of exercise for prevention of heart disease and cognitive decline due to aging is clear in showing that it is *efficacious and specific*. On the other hand, the evidence on the possible benefits of exercise for preventing diabetes, cancer, eating disorders, and some infectious diseases (e.g., flu and herpes) are only *possibly efficacious*.

SIDE EFFECTS, CONTRAINDICATIONS, AND PRESCRIPTIONS IN EXERCISE THERAPY

In some circumstances, exercise is not the most appropriate and efficacious intervention for stress management, either because improvements in mood state are not coincidental with physiological changes in fitness levels (Gronningsaeter, Hyten, Skauli, & Christensen, 1992) or because life-threatening suicidal ideation precludes the immediate application of nonclinical psychiatric interventions (Paffenbarger et al., 1994). Exercise may not be indicated in the acute phase of infectious illness, in which overexertion may depress immune function or when sleep deprivation is a critical factor (Shepard & Shek, 1998). In addition, not all studies have found lower levels of negative affect or depression among community studies on previously sedentary participants (Szabo & Gauvin, 1992). In these studies, it was noted that adherence was usually poor and that many of the earlier studies were not well designed with experimental controls (Dishman, Farquhar, & Cureton, 1994). Therefore, caution must be used in drawing conclusions, either positively or negatively, from the accumulated data that are available.

Even though it appears that more potential benefits than risks (as in eating disorders or with diabetic hypoglycemia) are associated with exercise therapy, it is not likely that benefits from exercise are universal (Ertl & Davis, 2004; Klein et al., 2004). Clearly there are many very happy, healthy, functioning individuals who are not exercising regularly. In fact, some individuals seem to be allergic to activity and may never develop an appreciation for the potential benefits of exercise. In addition, the risk of falling or being struck by an automobile in the course of walking or jogging in a public area may outweigh any potential psychological benefits. Those who choose not to exercise regularly may have had discouraging experiences with exercise at work or in the military under adverse conditions (heat, cold), or they may have old injuries that cause pain in muscles or on weight-bearing joints (Clarkson & Hubal, 2002). Difficulties in initiating and maintaining the exercise therapy may be prevalent.

The antianxiety and antidepressant effects of exercise are relatively short term, lasting not much longer than 1–2 days. Thus it is recommended that exercise (of shorter duration and lower intensity) be conducted at frequent intervals throughout the day for anxiolytic effects. For depression, exercising at daily intervals but with somewhat greater intensity is more likely to be effective. Still, some clients may overdo the exercise habit in the same way they have become workaholics or alcoholics—by taking the exercise prescription to excess due to poor perception of appropriate exercise intensity or misguided efforts to achieve the "exercise high" (Hassmen, Stähl, & Borg, 1993). Caution should be taken in the use of exercise for clients with eating disorders, as described previously. Exercise may produce more opiate-like endorphins than the client can handle, which eventually can become addictive. Some depressed patients are bulimic and may use exercise as a means of purging (Prussin & Harvey, 1991), thus neglecting the need to deal with the cause of the depression. Even though clients who exercise regularly are less depressed, they still may be victims of exertional bulimia and therefore need careful supervision, together with psychological evaluation during therapy.

The exercise prescription should not override the need for traditional psychotherapy in circumstances in which the client may tend to avoid the real problem and use exercise as a risky substitute for dealing with deeper issues in counseling (Sime, 1987). Exercise, like medication, is a method of getting immediate (though temporary) stress reduction and symptom relief. As such, medication and exercise are similar in that they allow the person to get through a particularly difficult period of pain or discomfort (either physical or emotional), after which time insight-oriented counseling may be appropriate for prevention of escalating problems. Once again, the preponderance of evidence shows that more research is needed in this area to show efficacy related to exercise prescription and for treatment of these mental health issues.

All therapy is fraught with similar problems of poor adherence and compliance and recidivism. Because exercise incurs a certain degree of accommodation, strain, and/or physical discomfort, it is not surprising that exercise programs in healthy as well as clinical populations show a 50% recidivism rate after 6 months (Dishman, 1991; Dishman et al., 1994). On the other hand, patient compliance with other psychological treatments (psychotherapy and drug therapy) can be equally compromised by client resistance to therapy or by the side effects of drug therapy (Martinsen & Stanghelle, 1997). Even exercise prescriptions given in physical therapy for rehabilitation of injury are poorly adhered to (Sluijs, Kok, & van der Zee, 1993). By following proper guidelines for clinical applications of walk/talk (exercise) therapy, the therapist can improve on the recidivism rate to achieve the desired psychological benefits. A manual for training in this therapy follows.

MANUAL FOR TRAINING IN EXERCISE (WALK/TALK) THERAPY

Background and Introduction

Walk/talk therapy is an adjunctive therapeutic technique most commonly used as an alternative among other traditional therapies. Only rarely is it indicated during the initial session with a new client unless he or she presents with either a great deal of nervous energy (being tense and fidgety) or with anger and resistance. In most cases, walk/talk therapy should be considered only after intake and testing have been completed and perhaps only after other standard counseling approaches have been exploited fully. It is most likely to be effective when both the client and the therapist eagerly welcome the opportunity to move about freely and yet carefully while talking candidly.

There is potential for a verbal cathartic effect that occurs when most clients are engaged in casual walking with a defined purpose in psychotherapy. Spontaneous questions, as well as insightful discoveries, often come out naturally in the process of moving while talking. The rhythm of "left–right" patterned walking, together with the effort of vocal expression, does, in fact, also accelerate respiratory demands. At the outset, it is important to explore past experiences with physical activity (both good and bad reactions) given the fact that previous research shows that finding an "enjoyable" exercise is critical to the long-term continuity of an exercise program (Wankel, 1993).

Presentation to the Client

Hopefully, you and the client can identify some positive past experiences associated with either hard work or vigorous game-like activity that may date back to high school or college years. Most clients can recall having had a sense of satisfaction in completing a hard physical task or the enjoyment of having accomplished a significant achievement (in sport or recreation). Interview the client to obtain answers to the questions listed in Table 13.1.

When it feels timely to explore the walk/talk therapy option, give the client some advance warning for appropriate preparations, such as wearing comfortable shoes, warm coat, gloves, and so forth. One way to introduce the concept is to ask the client, "Do you feel that you might enjoy walking a little while we talk in our next session?" If the client

TABLE 13.1. Interview Questions for Exercise (Walk/Talk) Therapy Candidate

1. How much physical exercise do you get right now, either at work or in recreational activities? Options: none; yard work only; walk to work 1–2 miles daily; tennis once a week, etc.
2. Do you recall a time in your life when you might have been active in sports or work such that you were physically fit? Options: sports in school; biking; working construction, etc.
3. Do you recall feeling a sense of relief on getting into a soothing and invigorating shower (or bath) immediately after vigorous work or exercise?
4. Do you recall enjoying the good taste of a cold drink and a healthy meal sometime after either sport or physical work?
5. Do you recall a time in your life when you may have slept better and felt better in association with having been involved in a regular program of vigorous activity?
6. Do you recall a time in your life when you felt exceptionally happy, stress-free, and/or particularly tolerant of stressful circumstances? If so, were you more or less active physically at that time of your life?
7. Is there a particular sport or recreational activity (hiking, gardening, etc.) that you enjoy a great deal but have not been engaged in during the past few years? If so, would you consider starting up once again? What obstacles stand in your way?
8. Do you have the opportunity to get more activity either by commuting to work (walking/bicycling) or at work by taking on more effort (e.g., using stairs instead of elevator)?
9. Do you have a friend or relative (spouse) with whom you would enjoy walking or engaging in other forms of exercise? If so, please explore that option.
10. Do you have any injuries or physical limitations in which exercise might cause aggravating symptoms? Options: ankle, foot, knee, hip or back pain, and/or arthritis.

responds positively, suggest also that you intend to pick a route that seems desirable given the weather and other conditions (minimal traffic, access to an aesthetically appealing environment such as a park or garden). For inclement weather conditions, a local mall or a stairwell can be a suitable alternative, with some caution taken to maintain confidentiality when privacy is required.

Session 1

Encourage the client to help set the pace of walking. There is no need to hurry, especially at the beginning, but eventually you would like to pick up the pace to make it reasonably challenging without risking injury or discomfort. Suggest that the client find a secure place for personal belongings (purse or briefcase locked in the trunk of his or her car or in a locked cabinet in your office) so that the client does not have to lug it along or worry about having something stolen.

If you know how to monitor heart rate, teach the client to take a resting rate before starting the walk and then stop periodically during the walk to find out how much intensity this session of exercise elicits. Resting heart rate (HR) may be 50–80 beats per minute (BPM). During a walking session, HR might be 15–30 BPM higher than at rest; thus during the walk/talk session HR = 80–110 BPM would likely be both safe and effective. Your purpose is to facilitate walking at a pace that can be maintained comfortably while talking and also can be maintained for 20–40 minutes continuously during home sessions (nonclinic time) in order to achieve reduction in stress-related symptoms. In the first session of walk/talk therapy, it would be prudent to limit the duration to no more than 10–20 minutes and to stay close to the vicinity of office resources and ancillary help in case of any difficulties, particularly with older clients or those with marginal disabilities. Safety and relative comfort are paramount so as to avoid health risks such as straining muscles, falling, or causing chest pain due to cardiac ischemia (angina).

Session 2

At the outset of this session, inform the client that you have options, depending on how he or she responded to the first exercise session. That is, you can repeat it and perhaps extend the distance and duration. However, it is important to know how the client felt after the first session and whether he or she did, in fact, embark on any exercise at home since that session. Depending on how the client responds, it may be appropriate to either repeat the session or modify it in some way regarding location or distance for the comfort of the client. If walking served to enable the client's verbal interaction, then consider extending the duration by 5–10 minutes. However, if the walk ever tends to be a strain for the client, then you should return to the counseling office immediately to process the effects of the exercise, in addition to the specific content of the session. Talking while engaged in walking is slightly more demanding metabolically than just walking.

Monitor the client's exercise HR compared with your own, to be sure that he or she is not exerting too vigorously. If HR = 70 BPM at rest (standing) before starting, then exercise HR = 90–110 BPM could be reasonable while walking. In this session, explore with the client whether the walk/talk experience is pleasant and invigorating (or aversive) and whether he or she discovers some degree of refreshing aftereffects during recovery from exercise. Share with the client several explanations (theories) for the potential benefits of exercise that most people experience. For example, both aesthetic and kinesthetic experiences are associated with movement (e.g., appreciation of nature and tactile sense of control, as well as the synergistic achievement effects of having walked a considerable distance—a half-mile, a mile, or more). If this experience is satisfying, then encourage him or her to repeat it at home daily or every other day. After several days of walking the same distance, the client should feel that there is less effort, and that will indicate that he or she is developing higher fitness (tolerance) for the physical work involved in the exercise.

Session 3

During this session the goal is to have the client engage in the walking experience with a mind open to exploring the cognitive catharsis. That is, we want the exercise to be a catalyst to help clear out worry and anxiety, to free associate, and to embrace some creative thinking. This can be an opportunity for introspection and the development of more lucid thinking. Acknowledge that both you and the client may come up with spontaneous questions and comments in the midst of engaging in walk/talk conversation. For some clients, the side-by-side conversation (in contrast to face-to-face therapy) seems to elicit more candor, as though the movement, together with the informal nature of the activity, tends to break down barriers and to facilitate greater emotional release (Kendzierski & Johnson, 1993).

Session 4

During this session, consider exploring the array of environmental conditions—such as water, beach, hills, wooded areas, stairs, streets, malls (in cold weather), and the home exercise environment (e.g., walking in a scenic neighborhood)—to increase the potential aesthetic pleasure of the exercise and, ultimately, to eliminate excuses for not being active. Dealing with motivation to participate is a critical issue in all health behavior change, but especially so with exercise (Kendzierski & Johnson, 1993). Eliminating barriers and establishing exercise as a habit is critically important (Fahlberg, Fahlberg, & Gates, 1992). Having amenities, such as comfortable and attractive clothing (shorts, warm-up clothes, shoes), should be encouraged as rewards or added incentives for accomplishment. Clients may benefit from personal role model anecdotes, such as, "Regular exercise was much easier to maintain when I was younger and did not have the luxury of a car (or second car for the family) because I chose to commute to work on a bicycle, thus saving substantially in bus and train fare. Do you have any similar opportunity for functional commuter exercise?" Other options to make exercise functional include walking to the store for milk, mowing the lawn, raking leaves, or gardening, all of which could raise a sense of satisfaction when the task is completed. Be cautious about dangerous physical work (shoveling snow or lifting boxes) depending on age, health, and physical ability.

Session 5

After several weeks of walk/talk therapy, evaluate progress with the client. Breathing should be monitored periodically and especially after more intense segments (e.g., climbing a hill or flight of stairs) to observe whether the client uses chest muscles more than the diaphragm to take in the air. HR biofeedback appears to be helpful for a variety of emotional, respiratory, and cardiovascular diseases. Refer to chapters in this volume on biofeedback training and HRV (Lehrer, Chapter 10) and respiratory retraining (Dixhoorn, Chapter 12) to review efficient breathing techniques.

For some clients, walking and/or stair climbing may be uncomfortable because of joint strain associated with past injuries or simply being overweight. If so, consider switching to multiple-station workouts (e.g., stationary bicycle, rowing machine, or low-impact exercise machines). If boredom is a problem with home exercise sessions, consider using radio, television, or audiotapes for entertainment. Some clients enjoy dancing, which provides a healthy and refreshing alternative mode of activity while gradually building up fitness and tolerance for the exertion.

Standards for exercise prescription are based on the client's age, fitness level, and medical condition. Use caution and seek assistance from a personal trainer or rehabilitation specialist to establish reasonable goals and appropriate adjustment of the workload (duration, intensity, and frequency).

Session 6

It is always important to evaluate the influence of family and friends on the daily habits of exercise. If the client received little or no support from his or her spouse, or, worse yet, if family members show disdain for exercise, the client will have a bigger hurdle to overcome in maintaining exercise habits. Initially, try to facilitate activities that bring the client into positive interaction with others while also enjoying the exercise. Also consider encouraging the client to exercise regularly to set a good example for his or her children or some other family member. Exercising with a friend or family member while engaged in pleasant conversation becomes an extension of the walk/talk therapy. Reinforcing the benefits of voluntary physical activity independent of therapy is important for the long-term impact of exercise therapy.

Session 7

Help the client set up structured behavior modification strategies to reinforce the activity. For example, clients might make a pact whereby they will watch television only while simultaneously exercising on a bicycle ergometer, mini-tramp on-line, stair-stepper, cardio-glide or elliptical machine, or treadmill. Alternatively, the client might agree not to watch more than 1 hour of television without engaging in at least 10–20 minutes of exercise. The TV becomes the reinforcement for the exercise behavior. Set up a log and a system of accountability for the client, such that he or she can review his or her progress in accomplishments (distanced walked; consecutive days; change in mood, alertness, sleep quality; appetite regulation and reduced fatigue; relief from nagging joint or muscle pain). A system of record keeping may ensure greater compliance and continuity in the training regimen to obtain the desired stress management and the resulting psychological changes that should occur.

Session 8

Recognize individual differences in ability, motivation, and preferences. Some clients may be unwilling to try the approaches described here. Some are endowed with the burning desire to stay involved in exercise, and others may have lethargy built into their genetic makeup. Kenneth Cooper, the author of *Aerobics* (1968), tells the story of a man with heart disease who was so despondent that he wanted to die. Because his heart was weak, he logically thought that the best way to commit suicide without embarrassing his family was to run around the block as fast as he could until he killed himself. After several futile attempts at causing a fatal heart attack in this manner, he discovered to his surprise that he began to feel better (after exercising), and eventually he chose to live instead of to die. It is important to note that very intense exercise (e.g., marathon running) is, in fact, associated with much greater candor and catharsis and more dramatic changes in cognitive orientation than we would ordinarily see in walk/talk therapy (Acevedo et al., 1992). However, most therapists and most clients are not prepared for such vigorous activity during therapy.

Session 9

Anticipate the first bout of recidivism, as nearly every client will have occasional lapses, that is, reverting to sedentary living due to job pressures, family emergencies, illness, injury, and so forth. Planning ahead to counter the feeling of failure serves to defuse negative emotions (i.e., guilt, remorse, low self-esteem). Help your client anticipate the problem, plan for the adjustment, and welcome the return to activity following a lapse. To prevent future relapse, seek to identify the client's immediate rewards for exercise, which may include (1) the break from the hassles of the day, (2) an opportunity to enjoy the fresh air out of doors, (3) the chance to talk with you, or with a friend, about problems while walking, (4) the refreshing sensation of the cool air or warm shower, depending on the existing weather conditions, and (5) the pleasant culinary satisfaction of a good meal or fluid replacement with a favorite nonalcoholic drink immediately after the exercise session.

Session 10

Consider the difficulties during inclement weather. In northern regions especially there are periods of time in which cold and wind make it difficult to enjoy being outdoors. Under these conditions, it is important to dress warmly and to stay relatively close to indoor access to warm up periodically. Public buildings and shopping malls can be good locations for dealing with the inclement weather, if accessible. In addition, after nine or more session some clients may be ready to advance to running. This obviously challenges the therapist to be fit enough to keep up. For those clients who seek to transition from walking to running, the best advice is to run as slowly as possible at first until becoming fatigued or short of breath, slow to a walk until recovered, then return to running as soon as possible. Running for 1–2 minutes followed by a 1-minute walk is a good ratio to target in the initial sessions. Obviously, running vigorously compromises the ability to talk somewhat, but it is still feasible when you run at a slow speed. A rule of thumb about running (in moderation) is that it should never compromise one's ability to carry on a conversation.

Conclusion of 10-Session Exercise Manual

Evaluate progress using one or more well-accepted, standardized psychological tests. Examples of tests for several of the important domains include the Profile of Mood States (McNair, Lorr, & Droppleman, 1971), the Beck Depression Inventory (Beck, Ward, Mendelson, Mock, & Erbaugh, 1961), the State–Trait Anxiety Scale (Spielberger, 1983), and the Tennessee Self-Concept Scale (Fitts, 1964). Also evaluate sleep habits and appetite control. It is possible that a client will notice serendipitously that he or she has more rapid sleep onset and more restful sleep patterns with continuous sleep maintenance (Bliwise, King, Harris, & Haskell, 1992). Healthy foods such as fruits and vegetables taste much better following a vigorous bout of exercise, together with a shower and an extended recovery period. These aesthetic rewards of exercise can be very powerful, immediate reinforcers. Plan to revise the exercise program based on client feedback at 2–4 week intervals.

The aspiring exercise (walk/talk) therapist should follow ethical practices involving responsibility to and communication with other health care professionals. It is important to get medical approval for the exercise and to regularly communicate with other professionals, such as the client's primary care physician, physical therapist, psychiatrist, social worker, or counselor, regarding progress, concerns, and so forth. Observe other ethical guidelines and medical or psychological licensing requirements. Maintain clearly established boundaries. During the walk/talk counseling session, maintain strict ethical boundaries and only cautiously cite the potential benefits of exercise, being careful not to overstate the claims (Sime, 1987). The therapist should not feel personally responsible for the client's motivation or personal accomplishments. Be prepared to articulate your purpose and your methods to the psychology licensing board should a disgruntled client or a concerned community member express concern.

CASE EXAMPLES: SOCIAL AND PERFORMANCE ANXIETY

Amy and Becky (both pseudonyms) are Caucasian females in their early 60s who were seen for mild depression and panic disorder. Amy had started therapy 15 years previously (at age 50), and Becky had started therapy only 4 to 6 months earlier in the clinic. Both reported ego-threatening experiences at work (fear of failure) and had long histories of nervous, tense, type-A behaviors. Both had been prescribed a combination of tranquilizers and antidepressant medications to get them through the rough stages of panic. Becky, in particular, wanted to get off the medications as soon as possible.

Initial therapy consisted of 3–4 weeks of traditional relaxation training and cognitive-behavioral intervention, followed by exercise walk/talk therapy that was con-

ducted by the therapist for 20- to 30-minute periods. The exercise was sandwiched between 10–15 minutes of office-based orientation, and 5–10 minutes of closure. Each subsequent clinical session consisted of gradually increasing the time and distance traveled.

Amy's goal in therapy included treatment of her primary medical concern, elevated
blood pressure. Average blood pressure of 165/105 mm Hg was treated with relaxation
and counseling with only modest success (posttreatment = 158/98 mm Hg). With the addition of exercise therapy, her average values decreased to 150/90 mm Hg, results that coincide with those found in traditional cardiac rehabilitation research studies (Blumenthal
et al., 2002; Sime & Hellweg, 2001).

Both Amy and Becky had a strong work ethic, and their jobs were exceptionally satisfying elements in their lives. It seemed logical to both that the physical demands of
walking fit well with their occupational work ethic, and, as a bonus, they loved the outdoors and enjoyed the walk/talk mode of our therapy sessions. In essence, the walk/talk
therapy opened new dimensions to therapy not possible in the confines of a cramped clinical office with a traditional face-to-face counseling session.

Fifteen-Year Follow-Up with Amy

Amy moved to another city but maintained communication about once a year to report
long-term follow-up. On one occasion she returned specifically to engage in another
walk/talk session, but for the most part, she got along well on her own. In recent e-mail
correspondence for this case analysis, the client reported that she has retired from her job
but that she has exercised regularly at a health club since moving away. In addition, her
husband exercises four times a week indoors, while she extends her workouts to walk
outside for a mile or two every day. She averages five exercise sessions per week. She has
learned the importance of anaerobic work and uses an elastic band for resistance to
strengthen her arms and back muscles. In addition, she reports doing stretching exercises
before and after her walking to maintain flexibility as she ages. She reports candidly, "My
exercise has kept me feeling so much better all these years."

Immediate Follow-Up with Becky

Becky completed 6 months of combined counseling and stress management with walk/
talk therapy. Over this time period, her physician very slowly reduced the medication, until she was off all medications and returned to limited part-time work that served her
needs for affiliation and accomplishment without concern for financial gain. She continued to exercise on a daily basis and practiced with her relaxation tape as needed to
achieve the trophotropic anxiety-free state that she has come to appreciate. She agreed to
check in with the therapist at the clinic at 6- to 12-month intervals, much like the common practice of periodic dental visits for preventive maintenance.

CONCLUSION

In this chapter, exercise has been considered as a viable, adjunctive stress management
treatment for anxiety and depression, as well as for several other medical disorders with
underlying psychophysiological etiology. Evidence has been presented supporting the effectiveness of various modalities of exercise treatment among numerous divergent populations across a wide range of disorders. However, not all available evidence fits the high-

est standards for experimental design in research conditions. Although most of the evidence is positive in regard to exercise, the exact mechanisms that underlie the benefits (cognitive or physiological) are not yet fully understood. The dosage of exercise needed to achieve benefits may differ greatly across individuals, and the type of exercise prescribed should be based on personal preference and accessibility. It appears that the optimal benefits of exercise appear when clients become actively involved in vigorous yet enjoyable movement three to five times per week. In addition, less recidivism occurs if the exercise program is functional and rewarding (commuting to work, chopping wood, dancing, hiking in a scenic area, etc.; Marcus et al., 1998). Numerous guidelines, contraindications, and pitfalls have been provided in this chapter. The exercise therapist is encouraged to be bold in the use of innovative strategies but cautious in the presence of extenuating circumstances that might be risky for the client. Exercise can be effective independent of other conjoint counseling with many cases of emotional stress, anxiety, and depression, but the judicious use of exercise together with counseling appears to be exceptional powerful therapeutically. Thus it is disconcerting that the number of therapists who are utilizing exercise (walk/talk) therapy is so very small (McEntee & Halgin, 1996). In spite of the resurgence of exercise as a recreational activity, many adults choose not to engage in any form of regular exercise training. Complicating the issue further, it is common for some stressed and depressed individuals to feel guilty because they are sedentary, and the added negative affect intensifies the impact of clinical depression itself (Martin, Sinden, & Fleming, 2000). The use of exercise in this therapeutic manner is still in the pioneering stage and must be subject to a great deal more research and many clinical trials.

REFERENCES

Acevedo, E., Dzewaltowski, D., Gill, D., & Noble, J. (1992). Cognitive orientations of ultramarathoners. *The Sport Psychologist, 6,* 242–252.

Achat, H., Kawachi, I., Spiro, A., DeMolles, D., & Sparrow, D. (2000). Optimism and depression as predictors of physical and mental health functioning: Aging study. *Annals of Behavioral Medicine, 22*(2), 127–130.

Alonso, S., Castellano, M., Quintero, M., & Navarro, E. (1999). Action of antidepressant drugs on maternal stress-induced hypoactivity in female rats. *Experimental and Clinical Pharmacology, 21*(4), 291–295.

Araki, A., & Ito, H. (1999). Perspective of dietary management and exercise therapy in diabetes mellitus. *Nippon Rinsho, 57*(3), 650–656.

Babyak, M., Blumenthal, J., Khatri, P., Doraiswamy, M., Moore, K., Craighead, W., et al. (2000, September–October). Exercise treatment for major depression: Maintenance of therapeutic benefit at ten months. *Psychosomatic Medicine, 62*(5), 633–638.

Beck, A. T., Ward, C. H., Mendelson, M., Mock, J., & Erbaugh, J. (1961). An inventory for measuring depression. *Archives of General Psychiatry, 4,* 561–571.

Berger, B., & Owen, D. (1992). Mood alteration with yoga and swimming: Aerobic exercise may not be necessary. *Perceptual and Motor Skills, 75,* 1331–1343.

Binder, E., Droste, S. K., Ohl, F., & Reul, J. M. (2004). Regular voluntary exercise reduces anxiety-related behavior and impulsiveness in mice. *Behavior and Brain Research, 155*(2), 197–206.

Bliwise, D., King, A., Harris, R., & Haskell, W. (1992). Prevalence of self-reported parsleep in a healthy population aged 50 to 65. *Social Science in Medicine, 34,* 49–55.

Blumenthal, J. A., Babyak, M., Wei, J., O'Connor, C., Waugh, R., Eisenstein, E., et al. (2002). Usefulness of psychosocial treatment of mental stress-induced myocardial ischemia in men. *American Journal of Cardiology, 89*(2), 164–168.

Bonnet, F., Irving, K., Terra, J., Nony, P., Berthexend, F., & Moulin, P. (2005). Anxiety and depression are associated with unhealthy lifestyle in patients at risk of cardiovascular disease. *Atherosclerosis, 178*(2), 339–344.

Bosscher, R. J. (1993). Running and mixed physical exercises with depressed psychiatric patients: Exercise and psychological well-being. *International Journal of Sport Psychology, 24*, 170–184.

Brown, A. S., Davis, J. M., Murphy, E. A., Carmichael, M. D., Ghaffar, A., & Mayer, E. P. (2004). Gender differences in viral infection after repeated exercise stress. *Medicine and Science in Sports and Exercise, 36*(8), 1290–1295.

Brown, D., Morgan, W., & Raglin, J. (1993). Effects of exercise and rest on the state anxiety and blood pressure of physically challenged college students. *Journal of Sports Medicine and Physical Fitness, 33*, 300–305.

Brown, S., Welsh, M., Labbe, E., Gitulli, W., & Kulkarni, P. (1992). Aerobic exercise and the psychological treatment of adolescents. *Perceptual and Motor Skills, 74*, 555–560.

Byrne, A., & Byrne, D. (1993). The effect of exercise on depression, anxiety and other mood states: A review. *Journal of Psychosomatic Research, 37*, 565–574.

Callaghan, P. (2004). Exercise: A neglected intervention in mental health care? *Journal of Psychiatric Mental Health Nursing, 11*(4), 476–483.

Camacho, T. C., Roberts, R. E., Lazarus, N. B., Kaplan, G. A., & Cohen, R. D. (1991). Physical activity and depression: Evidence from the Alameda County study. *American Journal of Epidemiology, 134*, 220–231.

Clarkson, P. M., & Hubal, M. J. (2002). Exercise-induced muscle damage in humans. *American Journal of Physical Medicine and Rehabilitation, 81*(11), S52–69.

Cockbrill, I., & Riddington, M. (1996). Exercise dependence and associated disorders. *Counseling Psychology Quarterly, 9*(2), 119–129.

Cooper, K. H. (1968). *Aerobics*. New York: Evans.

Dahlgren, A., Kecklund, G., & Akerstedt, T. (2005). Different levels of work-related stress and the effects on sleep, fatigue and cortisol. *Scandinavian Journal of Work and Environmental Health, 31*(4), 277–285.

Daley, A., & Welch, A. (2004). The effects of 15 min and 30 min of exercise on affective responses both during and after exercise. *Journal of Sports Science, 22*(7), 621–628.

Daniels, M., Martin, A., & Carter, J. (1992). Opiate receptor blockade by naltrexone and mood state after acute physical activity. *British Journal of Sports Medicine, 26*, 111–115.

de Geus, E. J. C., van Doornen, L. J. P., & Orlebeke, J. F. (1993). Regular exercise and aerobic fitness in relation to psychological make-up. *Physiological Stress Reactivity, 55*, 347–363.

Denollet, J. (1993). Emotional distress and fatigue in coronary heart disease: The Global Mood Scale (GMS). *Psychological Medicine, 23*, 111–121.

DeVries, H., Beckman, P., Huber, H., & Dieckmeir, L. (1968). Electromyographic evaluation of the effects of sauna on the neuromuscular system. *Journal of Sports Medicine and Physical Fitness, 8*, 61–69.

Dey, S. (1994). Physical exercise as novel antidepressant agent: Possible role of serotonin receptor subtypes. *Psychological Behavior, 55*, 323–329.

Dey, S., Singh, R., & Dey, P. (1992). Exercise training: Significance of regional alterations in serotonin metabolism of rat brain in relation to antidepressant effect of exercise. *Psychological Behavior, 52*, 1095–1099.

Dienstbier, R. (1991). Behavioral correlates of sympathoadrenal reactivity: The toughness model. *Medicine and Science in Sports and Exercise, 23*, 846–852.

Dienstbier, R. A., LaGuardia, R. L., & Wilcox, N. S. (1987). The relationship of temperament to tolerance of cold and heat: Beyond "cold hands–warm heart." *Motivation and Emotion, 11*, 269–295.

Dietrich, A., & McDaniel, W. (2004). Endocannabinoids and exercise. *British Journal of Sports Medicine, 38*(5), 536–541.

Dishman, R., Farquhar, R., & Cureton, K. (1994). Responses to preferred intensities of exertion in men differing in activity levels. *Medicine and Science in Sports and Exercise, 26*(6), 783–790.

Dishman, R. K. (1991). Increasing and maintaining exercise and physical activity. *Behavior Therapy, 22*, 345–378.

Dixhoorn, J. v., Duivenvoorden, H. J., Pool, J., & Verhage, F. (1990). Psychic effects of physical training and relaxation therapy after myocardial infarction. *Journal of Psychosomatic Research, 34*(3), 327–337.

Doyne, E., Schambless, D., & Beutler, L. (1983). Aerobic exercise as a treatment for depression in women. *Behavior Therapy, 41*, 434–440.

Dua, J., & Hargreaves, L. (1992). Effects of aerobic exercise on negative affect, positive affect, stress, and depression. *Perceptual and Motor Skills, 75*, 355–361.

Dunn, A. L., Trivedi, M. H., Kampert, J. B., Clark, C. G., & Chambliss, H. O. (2002). The DOSE study: A clinical trial to examine efficacy and dose response of exercise as treatment for depression. *Controlled Clinical Trials, 3*(5), 584–603.

Dunn, A. L., Trivedi, M. H., Kampert, J. B., Clark, C. G., & Chambliss, H. O. (2005). Exercise treatment for depression: Efficacy and dose response. *American Journal of Preventive Medicine, 28*(1), 1–8.

Dunn, A. L., Trivedi, M. H., & O'Neal, H. A. (2001). Physical activity dose–response effects on outcomes of depression and anxiety. *Medicine and Science in Sports and Exercise, 33*(6), S587–597.

Emery, C., Hauck, E., & Blumenthal, J. (1992). Exercise adherence and maintenance among older adults: One year follow-up study. *Psychology and Aging, 7*, 466–470.

Ertl, A. C., & Davis, S. N. (2004). Evidence for a vicious cycle of exercise and hypoglycemia in type 1 diabetes mellitus. *Diabetes Metabolism Research Review, 20*(2), 124–130.

Fahlberg, L. L., Fahlberg, L. A., & Gates, W. K. (1992). Exercise and existence: Exercise behavior from an existential–phenomenological perspective. *The Sport Psychologist, 6*, 172–191.

Fitts, P. M. (1964). Perceptual–motor skill learning. In W. A. Melton (Ed.), *Categories of human learning.* New York: Wiley.

Folkins, C. H., & Sime, W. E. (1981). Physical fitness training and mental health. *American Psychologist, 36*, 373–389.

Fossati, M., Amati, F., Painot, D., Reiner, M., Haenni, C., & Golay, A. (2004). Cognitive-behavioral therapy with simultaneous nutritional and physical activity education in obese patients with binge eating disorder. *Eating and Weight Disorders, 9*(2), 134–138.

Frasure-Smith, N., Lesperance, F., & Talajic, M. (1993). Depression following myocardio infarction: Impact on six-month survival. *Journal of the American Medical Association, 270*(15), 1819–1825.

Froelicher, V. (1990). Exercise, fitness, and coronary heart disease. In C. Bouchard, R. Shephard, T. Stephens, J. Sutton, & B. McPherson (Eds.), *Exercise, fitness and health* (pp. 429–450). Champaign, IL: Human Kinetics.

Fuchs, R., & Hahn, A. (1992). Physical exercise and anxiety as moderators of the stress–illness relationship. *Anxiety, Stress and Coping, 5*, 139–149.

Fulk, L., Stock, H., Lynn, A., Marshall, J., Wilson, M. A., & Hand, G. (2004). Chronic physical exercise reduces anxiety-like behavior in rats. *International Journal of Sports Medicine, 25*(1), 78–82.

Furst, D., & Germone, K. (1993). Negative addiction in male and female runners and exercisers. *Perceptual and Motor Skills, 77*, 192–194.

Goldstein, M., Pinto, B., Marcus, B., Lyn, H., Jett, A., Rakowski, W., et al. (1999). Position-based physical activity counseling for middle-aged and older adults: A randomized trial. *Annals of Behavioral Medicine, 21*(1), 40–47.

Gordon, G. A. (1991). Stress reactions in connective tissues: A molecular hypothesis. *Medical Hypotheses, 36*(3), 289–294.

Gronningsaeter, H., Hyten, K., Skauli, G., & Christensen, C. (1992). Improved health and coping by physical exercise or cognitive behavioral stress management training in a work environment. *Psychology and Health, 7*, 147–163.

Guszkowska, M. (2004). Effects of exercise on anxiety, depression and mood. *Psychiatry Policy, 38*(4), 611–620.

Haier, R. J., Quaid, B. A., & Mills, J. S. (1981). Naloxone alters pain perceptions after jogging. *Psychiatric Research, 5*, 231–232.

Hamachek, D. E. (1987). *Encounters with the self.* New York: Holt, Rinehart, & Winston.

Hansen, C. J., Stevens, L. C., & Coast, J. R. (2001). Exercise duration and mood state: How much is enough to feel better? *Health Psychology, 20*(4), 267–275.

Hassmen, P., Koivula, N., & Uutela, A. (2000). Physical exercise and psychological well being: A population study in Finland. *Preventive Medicine, 30*, 17–25.

Hassmen, P., Stähl, R., & Borg, G. (1993). Psychophysiological responses to exercise in type A/B men. *Psychosomatic Medicine, 55*, 178–184.

Hays, K. F. (1999). *Working it out: Using exercise in psychotherapy.* Washington, DC: American Psychological Association.

Herrmann, C., Buss, U., Buecker, A., Gonska, B., & Kreuzer, H. (1994). Relationship of cardiologic findings and standardized psychological scales to clinical symptoms in 3,705 ergometrically studied patients. *Zeitschrift für Kardiologie, 83,* 264–272.

Hinkle, J. (1992). Aerobic running behavior and psychoteutics: Implications for sport counseling and
psychology. *Journal of Sport Behavior, 15,* 163–177.

Holtkamp, K., Hebebrand, J., & Herpertz-Dahlmann, B. (2004). The contribution of anxiety and food
restriction on physical activity levels in acute anorexia nervosa. *International Journal of Eating Disorders, 36*(2), 163–171.

Huang, H., Hara, A., Homma, T., Yonekawa, Y., & Ohgaki, H. (2005, October). Altered expression of
immune defense genes in pilocytic astrocytomas. *Journal of Neuropathology and Experimental
Neurology, 64*(10), 891–901.

Hutnick, N. A., Williams, N. I., Kraemer, W. J., Orsega-Smith, E., Dixon, R. H., Bleznak, A. D., et al.
(2005, November). Exercise and lymphocyte activation following chemotherapy for breast cancer.
Medicine and Science in Sports and Exercise, 37(11), 1827–1835.

Johansson, G., Evans, G., Rydstedt, L., & Carrere, S. (1998). Hassles and cardiovascular reaction patterns among urban bus drivers. *International Journal of Behavioral Medicine, 5*(4), 267–280.

Johnsgard, K. (2004). *Conquering depression and anxiety through exercise.* New York: Prometheus
Books.

Johnsgard, K. W. (1989). *The exercise prescription for depression and anxiety.* New York: Plenum Press.

Johnston, J. N. L., Petlichkoff, L. M., & Hoeger, W. (1993). Effects of aerobic and strength training exercise participation on depression. *Medicine and Science in Sports and Exercise, 25,* S-135.

Jorm, A., Christensen, H., Griffiths, K., Parslow, R., Rodgers, B., & Blewitt, K. (2004). Effectiveness of
complementary and self-help treatments for anxiety disorders. *Medical Journal of Australia, 181*(7),
S29–46.

Kavussanu, M., & McAuley, E. (1995). Exercise and optimism: Are highly active individuals more optimistic? *Journal of Sport and Exercise Psychology, 17,* 246–258.

Kawachi, I., Colditz, G. A., & Ascherio, A. (1994). Prospective study of phobic anxiety and list of coronary disease in men. *Circulation, 89,* 1992–1997.

Kendzierski, D., & Johnson, W. (1993). Excuses, excuses, excuses: A cognitive behavioral approach to
exercise implementation. *Journal of Sport and Exercise Psychology, 15,* 207–219.

Kim, S. D., & Kim, H. S. (2005). Effects of a relaxation breathing exercise on anxiety, depression, and
leukocyte in hemopoietic stem cell transplantation patients. *Cancer Nursing, 28*(1), 79–83.

Klein, D. A., Bennett, A. S., Schebendach, J., Foltin, R. W., Devlin, M. J., & Walsh, B. T. (2004). Exercise
"addiction" in anorexia nervosa: Model development and pilot data. *CNS Spectrum, 9*(7), 531–
537.

Kohut, M. L., Cooper, M. M., Nickolaus, M. S., Russell, D. R., & Cunnick, J. E. (2002). Exercise and
psychosocial factors modulate immunity to influenza vaccine in elderly individuals. *Journal of Gerontology, 57*(9), M557–562.

Koltyn, K., & Morgan, W. P. (1993). The influence of wearing a wet suit on core temperature and anxiety responses during underwater exercise. *Medicine and Science in Sports and Exercise, 25,* S-45.

Krittayaphong, R., Light, K. C., Golden, R. N., Finkel, J. B., & Sheps, D. S. (1996). Relationship among
depression scores, beta-endorphin, and angina pectoris during exercise in patients with coronary artery disease. *Clinical Journal of Pain, 12*(2), 126–133.

Kubesch, S., Bretschneider, V., Freudenmann, R., Weidenhammer, N., Lehmann, M., Spitzer, M., et al.
(2003). Aerobic endurance exercise improves executive functions in depressed patients. *Journal of
Clinical Psychiatry, 64*(9), 1005–1012.

Kubitz, K., & Landers, D. (1993). The effects of aerobic training on cardiovascular responses to mental
stress: An examination of underlying mechanisms. *Journal of Sport and Exercise Psychology, 15,*
326–337.

Kugler, J., Seelbach, H., & Kruskemper, G. (1994). Effects of rehabilitation exercise programmes on exercise and depression in coronary patients: A meta-analysis. *British Journal of Clinical Psychology,
33,* 401–410.

LaVaque, T., Hammond, D., Trudeau, D., Monastra, V., Perry, J., Lehrer, P., et al. (2002). Template for
developing guidelines for the evaluation of the clinical efficacy of psychophysiological evaluations.
Applied Psychophysiology and Biofeedback, 27(4), 273–281.

Lavoie, K., Fleet, R., Laurin, C., Arsenault, A., Miller, S., & Bacon, S. (2004). Heart rate variability in coronary artery disease patients with and without panic disorder. *Psychiatry Research, 128*(3), 289–299.

Lehofer, M., Klebel, H., Gersdorf, C. H., & Zapotoczke, H. G. (1992). Running in motion therapy for depression. *Psychiatria II Danubina, 4,* 149–152.

Leith, L., & Taylor, A. (1990). Psychological aspects of exercise: A decade literature review. *Journal of Sport Behavior, 13,* 122.

Lobstein, D., & Rasmussen, C. (1991). Decreases in resting plasma beta-endorphine and depression scores after endurance training. *Journal of Sports Medicine and Physical Fitness, 31,* 543–551.

Loudon, C. P., Corroll, V., Butcher, J., Rawsthorne, P., & Bernstein, C. N. (1999). The effects of physical exercise on patients with Crohn's disease. *American Journal of Gastroenterology, 4*(3), 697–703.

Manger, T., & Motta, R. (2005). The impact of an exercise program on posttraumatic stress disorder, anxiety, and depression. *International Journal of Emergency Mental Health, 7*(1), 49–57.

Marcus, B., Bock, B., Pinto, B., Forsyth, L., Roberts, M., & Traficante, R. (1998). Efficacy of an individualized, motivationally-tailored physical activity intervention. *Annuals of Behavioral Medicine, 20*(3), 174–180.

Martin, K., Sinden, A., & Fleming, J. (2000). Inactivity may be hazardous to your image: The effects of exercise participation on impression formation. *Journal of Sport and Exercise Psychology, 22,* 283–291.

Martinsen, E. (1994). Physical activity and depression: Clinical experience. *Acta Psychiatrica Scandinavica Supplement, 377,* 23–27.

Martinsen, E. W. (1993). Therapeutic implications of exercise for clinically anxious and depressed patients: Exercise and psychological well-being. *International Journal of Sport Psychology, 24,* 185–199.

Martinsen, E. W., & Stanghelle, J. K. (1997). Drug therapy and physical activity. In W. P. Morgan (Ed.), *Physical activity and mental health* (pp. 81–90). Washington, DC: Taylor & Francis.

McCubbin, J. A., Cheung, R., Montgomery, T. B., Bulbulian, R., & Wilson, J. F. (1992). Aerobic fitness and opiodergic inhibition of cardiovascular stress reactivity. *Psychophysiology, 19,* 687–697.

McEntee, D., & Halgin, R. (1996). Therapists' attitudes about addressing the world of exercise in psychotherapy. *Journal of Clinical Psychology, 52,* 48–60.

McMurdo, M., & Rennie, L. (1993). A controlled trial of exercise by residents of old people's homes. *Age and Ageing, 22*(1), 11–15.

McNair, D. M., Lorr, N., & Droppleman, L. F. (1971). *Manual for the profile of mood states.* San Diego, CA: Educational and Industrial Testing Service.

McNeil, J., LeBlanc, E., & Joyner, M. (1991). The effect of exercise on depressive symptoms in the moderately depressed elderly. *Psychology and Aging, 6,* 487–488.

Morgan, W. P. (1988). Exercise and mental health. In R. K. Dishman (Ed.), *Exercise adherence: Its impact on public health* (pp. 91–121). Champaign, IL: Human Kinetics.

Motl, R., & Dishman, R. (2004). Effects of acute exercise on the soleus H-reflex and self-reported anxiety after caffeine ingestion. *Physiology and Behavior, 80*(4), 577–585.

Nicholson, A., Fuhrer, R., & Marmot, M. (2005). Psychological distress as a predictor of CHD events in men: The effect of persistence and components of risk. *Psychosomatic Medicine, 67*(4), 522–530.

Norris, R., Carroll, D., & Cochrane, R. (1992). The effects of physical activity and exercise training on psychological stress and well-being in an adolescent population. *Journal of Psychosomatic Research, 36,* 55–65.

North, T. C., McCullaugh, P., & Tran, Z. V. (1990). Effect of exercise on depression. *Exercise and Sports Sciences Review, 18,* 379–415.

Norvell, N., & Belles, D. (1993). Psychological and physical benefits of circuit weight training and law enforcement personnel. *Journal of Consulting and Clinical Psychology, 61,* 520–527.

Oman, R. F., & Haskel, W. L. (1993). The relationships among heartiness, efficacy, cognition, social support and exercise behavior. *Medicine and Science in Sports and Exercise, 25,* S135.

Paffenbarger, R., Jr., Lee, I., & Leung, R. (1994). Physical activity and personal characteristics associated with depression and suicide in American college men. *Acta Psychiatrica Scandinavica Supplement, 377,* 16–22.

Pelham, T. W., Campagna, P. D., Ritvo, P. G., & Birnie, W. A. (1993). The effects of exercise therapy on clients in a psychiatric rehabilitation program. *Psychosocial Rehabilitation Journal, 16,* 75–84.

Perna, F., Antoni, M., Kumar, M., Cruess, D., & Schneiderman, N. (1998). Cognitive-behavioral intervention effects on mood and cortisol during exercise training. *Annals of Behavioral Medicine, 20*(2), 92–98.

Petruzzello, S., Landers, D., Hatfield, P., Kubitz, K., & Salazar, W. (1991). A meta-analysis on the anxiety-reducing effects of acute and chronic exercise: Outcomes and mechanisms. *Sports Medicine, 11,* 143–182.

Petruzzello, S. J., Landers, D. M., & Salazar, W. (1993). Exercise and anxiety reduction: Examination of temperature as an explanation for effective change. *Journal of Sport and Exercise Psychology, 15,* 63–76.

Prussin, R., & Harvey, P. (1991). Depression, dietary restraint, and binge eating in female runners. *Addictive Behaviors, 16,* 295–301.

Rabins, P. (1992). Prevention of mental disorder in the elderly: Current perspective and future prospects. *Journal of the American Geriatrics Society, 70,* 727–733.

Rajala, U., Uusimaki, A., Keinanen-Kiukaanniemi, F., & Kivela, F. (1994). Prevalence of depression in a 55-year-old Finnish population. *Social Psychiatry and Psychiatric Epidemiology, 29,* 126–130.

Rejeski, W., Thompson, A., Brubaker, P., & Miller, H. (1992). Acute exercise: Buffering psychosocial stress responses in women. *Health Psychology, 11,* 355–362.

Rejeski, W. J., Gauvin, L., Hobson, M. L., & Norris, J. L. (1995). Effects of baseline responses, in-task feelings, and duration of activity on exercise-induced feeling states in women. *Health Psychology, 14*(4), 350–359.

Robbins, J. (2000). *A symphony of the brain.* New York: Grove Press.

Rooney, E. M. (1993). Exercise for older patients: Why it's worth your effort. *Geriatrics, 48,* 68–77.

Ruuskanen, J., & Parkatti, T. (1994). Physical activity and related factors among nursing home residents. *Journal of the American Geriatric Society, 42,* 987–991.

Seraganian, P. (1993). Current status and future directions in the field of exercise psychology. In P. Seraganian (Ed.), *Exercise psychology: The influence of physical exercise on psychological processes* (pp. 383–390). New York: Wiley.

Shephard, R. (1991). Benefits of sports and physical activity for the disabled: Implications for the individual and for society. *Scandinavian Journal of Rehabilitation Medicine, 23*(2), 51–59.

Shephard, R. J., & Shek, P. N. (1998). Acute and chronic overexertion: Do depressed immune responses provide useful markers? *International Journal of Sports Medicine, 19*(3), 159–171.

Sime, W. (1981). Role of exercise and relaxation in coping with acute emotional stress. In S. Fuenning & R. Rose (Eds.), *Physical fitness and mental health: Proceedings of the first research seminar* (pp. 92–95). Lincoln: University of Nebraska.

Sime, W. (1987). Exercise in the prevention and treatment of depression. In W. P. Morgan & S. E. Goldston (Eds.), *Exercise and mental health* (pp. 145–152). Washington, DC: Hemisphere.

Sime, W. (2002). Guidelines for clinical application of exercise therapy for mental health. In J. van Roalte & B. Brewer (Eds.), *Exploring sport and exercise psychology* (pp. 159–187). Washington, DC: American Psychological Association.

Sime, W., & Hellweg, K. (2001). Stress and coping. In J. Roitman, M. Herridge, M. Kelsey, T. LaRontaine, L. Miller, M. Wegner, M. Williams, & T. York (Eds.), *ACSM'S resource manual for guidelines for exercise testing and prescription* (4th ed., pp. 541–548). Philadelphia: Lippincott Williams & Wilkins.

Sime, W. E., Buell, J. C., & Eliot, R. S. (1979). Psychophysiological (emotional) stress testing: A potential means of detecting the early reinfarction victim [Abstract]. *Circulation Supplement: II, 60,* 56.

Sime, W. E., Buell, J. C., & Eliot, R. S. (1980). Cardiovascular responses to emotional stress (quiz interview) in postmyocardial infarction patients and matched control subjects. *Journal of Human Stress, 6,* 39–46.

Singh, N., Stavrinos, T., Scarbek, Y., Galambos, G., Liber, C., & Fiatarone-Singh, M. (2005). A randomized controlled trial of high- versus low-intensity weight training versus general practitioner care for clinical depression in older adults. *Journal of Gerontology, 60*(6), 768–776.

Skrinar, G., Unger, K., Hutchinson, D., & Faigenbaum, A. (1992). Effects of exercise training in young adults with psychiatric disabilities. *Canadian Journal of Rehabilitation, 5,* 151–157.

Sluijs, E., Kok, G., & van der Zee, J. J. (1993). Correlates of exercise compliance in physical therapy. *Physical Therapy, 73*, 41–53.

Spielberger, C. D. (1983). *Manual for the state–trait anxiety inventory (Form Y)*. Palo Alto, CA: Consulting Psychologists Press.

Stein, P., & Motta, R. (1992). Effects of aerobic and nonaerobic exercise on depression and self-concept. *Perceptual and Motor Skills, 74*, 79–89.

Steptoe, A., Kearsley, M., & Walters, N. (1993). Acute mood responses to maximal and submaximal exercise in active and inactive men. *Psychology and Health, 8*, 89–99.

Szabo, A., & Gauvin, L. (1992). Reactivity to written mental arithmetic: Effects of exercise lay-off and habituation. *Physiological Behavior, 51*(3), 501–506.

Tatrow, K., Montgomery, G. H., Avellino, M., & Bovbjerg, D. H. (2004). Activity and sleep contribute to levels of anticipatory distress in breast surgery patients. *Behavioral Medicine, 30*(2), 85–91.

Tennant, C., Mihailidou, A., Scott, A., Smith, R., Kellow, J., Jones, M., et al. (1994). Psychological symptom profiles in patients with chest pain. *Journal of Psychosomatic Research, 38*, 365–371.

Thome, J., & Espelage, D. L. (2004). Relations among exercise, coping, disordered eating, and psychological health among college students. *Eating Behavior, 5*(4), 337–351.

Thorsen, L., Skovlund, E., Stromme, S. B., Hornslien, K., Dahl, A. A., & Fossa, S. D. (2005). Effectiveness of physical activity on cardiorespiratory fitness and health-related quality of life in young and middle-aged cancer patients shortly after chemotherapy. *Journal of Clinical Oncology, 23*(10), 2378–2388.

Ueda, M. (2004). A 12-week structured education and exercise program improved climacteric symptoms in middle-aged women. *Journal of Physiological Anthropology and Applied Human Science, 23*(5), 143–148.

Wankel, L. (1993). The importance of enjoyment to adherence and psychological benefits from physical activity. *International Journal of Sports Psychology, 24*, 151–169.

Weyerer, S. (1992). Physical inactivity and depression in the community: Evidence from the Upper Bavaria Field Study. *International Journal of Sports Medicine, 13*, 492–496.

Yates, A., Edman, J. D., Crago, M., & Crowell, D. (2003). Eating disorder symptoms in runners, cyclists, and paddlers. *Addictive Behavior, 28*(8), 1473–1480.

Youngstedt, S. (1997). Does exercise truly enhance sleep? *Physician and Sports Medicine, 25*, 72–82.

Youngstedt, S., O'Conner, R. J., Crabbe, B., & Dishman, R. (2000). The influence of acute exercise on sleep following high caffeine intake. *Physiology and Behavior, 68*, 563–570.

Methods Based on Eastern Meditative and Therapeutic Disciplines

CHAPTER 14

Modern Forms of Mantra Meditation

PATRICIA CARRINGTON

HISTORY OF THE METHOD

Modern forms of mantra meditation, simplified and divested of esoteric trappings and religious overtones, possess some outstanding therapeutic properties. This chapter presents ways in which these new, noncultic techniques can be applied in clinical practice.

Mantra meditation is distinguished by the use of a repeated sound (mantra) as the focus of meditation. In this respect it differs from those meditation methods that direct the person's attention to the breath or the contents of the mind or to contemplation of some other meditational object. Mantra meditation differs from these other forms in the protocol followed, in the type of client it appeals to, and in its clinical applications. It is therefore discussed separately from mindfulness meditation, which is discussed by Kristeller in Chapter 15, this volume.

Technically, meditation can be classified as "concentrative" or "nonconcentrative" in nature. A concentrative technique limits stimulus input by directing attention to a single unchanging or repetitive stimulus (e.g., a mantra, a candle flame). The directives of mantra meditation are concentrative in nature. A nonconcentrative technique expands the meditator's field of attention to include as much of his or her conscious mental activity as possible (e.g., the directives of mindfulness meditation as here defined are nonconcentrative in nature).

The modern forms of mantra meditation discussed in this chapter are simple to learn. These techniques are typically practiced while the person is seated in a quiet environment, with the object of the meditator's attention being a mentally repeated sound. When the meditator's attention wanders, he or she is directed to bring it back to this attentional object in an easy, unforcing manner.

Although mantra meditation is basically a simple procedure, various forms of it have been used by numerous societies throughout recorded history to alter consciousness in a way that has been perceived as deeply beneficial. Traditionally, its benefits have been defined as spiritual in nature, and meditation has constituted a part of many religious practices. Recently, however, simple forms of mantra meditation have been used for stress management, with excellent results. Contributing to the rising interest in these meditative techniques is the fact that they are related to the biofeedback techniques (which also emphasize a delicately attuned awareness of inner processes) and to muscle relaxation and visualization techniques used in the behavior therapies.

In addition to providing deep relaxation, however, the majority of the meditative disciplines appear to assist the client in an area peripheral to many other therapeutic interventions: the fostering of a new kind of communication between the client and his or her own self, apart from his or her interpersonal environment. In a world in which inner enrichment from any source is a rare commodity, many people hunger for a more profound sense of self than is implicit in merely "getting along with others." Such people seek an awareness of their identity as "being" (as distinct from their identity as "doing"). The inner communion of meditation offers a means of fulfilling this need, thus promising to heal an aspect of the psyche that may be as needful as any other presently identified. The use of meditation, along with other forms of therapy, may therefore be an inevitable accompaniment to the trend currently seen in the behavioral sciences toward encompassing more and varied aspects of life.

Noncultic Methods

Of all the Westernized forms of mantra meditation, transcendental meditation (TM) has been up until now the most widely known and extensively studied. More accurately described as "transitional" rather than modern, because it retains certain cultic features such as the *puja* (Hindu religious ceremony), TM is taught by transcendental meditation teachers who do not permit mental health practitioners to assume an active role in its clinical management, unless they are also TM teachers. Despite its popularity with segments of the general public, therefore, the TM method has been less widely used in clinical settings than might be expected in light of the extensive research available on this technique.

Among the clinically oriented mantra meditation techniques, *clinically standardized meditation* (CSM; Carrington, 1978) and the *respiratory one method* (ROM), most commonly known as the *relaxation response* technique (Benson, 1975), have been the most widely studied to date. Benson no longer formally uses ROM today but uses a mantra-like prayer or the repetition of secular phrases, coupled with attention to the breath, to induce relaxation, he does not advocate any standardized approach (Benson & Stark, 1996). However, his original method is still studied experimentally and is therefore considered in this chapter. CSM is currently in use, with training available in its clinical application (see Carrington, 1978).

These techniques were devised with clinical objectives in mind and are strictly noncultic. The two methods differ from each other in several important respects, however. A trainee learning CSM selects a sound from a standard list of sounds (or creates one according to directions) and then repeats this sound mentally, without intentionally linking the sound to the breathing pattern or pacing it in any structured manner. CSM is thus a permissive meditation technique and may be subjectively experienced as almost "effortless." By contrast, when practicing ROM, the trainee repeats the word *one* (or another word or phrase) to himself or herself mentally, while at the same time intentionally linking this word with each exhalation. ROM is thus a relatively disciplined form of meditation, with the attention placed on two meditational objects—the chosen word and the breath. Accordingly, ROM requires more mental effort than CSM and may appeal to a different type of person.

Some nonconcentrative methods of meditation have also been used in certain clinical settings. Mindfulness meditation is probably the most commonly used of the nonconcentrative methods for this purpose (see Chapter 15). It is somewhat more difficult to learn than the modern forms of mantra meditation, however, because it requires handling one's spontaneous train of thought in a manner that is foreign to most people. By contrast, repeating a sound mentally over and over again, as in mantra meditation, is a relatively simple act that requires little preparation to be executed successfully. The student's success in learning a simple form of mantra meditation actually depends more heavily on the individual expertise and personality of the instructor. Other, nonstandardized forms of meditation are not discussed here, although their usefulness in the proper hands is not to be negated.

The Physiology of Mantra Meditation

All of the simplified mantra meditation techniques—including the transitional form, TM—have in common the fact that they can rapidly bring about a deeply restful state that possesses certain well-defined characteristics. Although mantra meditation is not the only intervention that can create such a state, it is clearly one of the most effective for this purpose. An extensive series of psychophysiological studies in this area established the nature of the meditative state in the 1970s and 1980s. Because its basic characteristics were established in that period, only a handful of studies have been conducted in this area following that time. For the most part these newer studies simply confirm the earlier ones and add some refinements. I report here on the full research to date, with a necessary emphasis on the earlier studies.

Much research has shown that during mantra meditation, body and mind typically enter a state of profound rest. Oxygen consumption can be lowered during 20–30 minutes of meditation to a degree ordinarily reached only after 6–7 hours of sleep (Wallace, Benson, & Wilson, 1971), and heart and respiration rates typically decrease during meditation (Allison, 1970; Wallace, 1970). However, the heart rate can also speed up during meditation in response to the introduction of stimuli perceived as stressful (Goleman & Schwartz, 1976), a finding that these researchers interpret as showing heightened alertness. The latter researchers' findings also indicated faster physiological recovery—a stress-protective effect that the authors suggest may reflect the fact that an adaptive organism should be prepared to respond to threatening stimuli but also should recover quickly so that there are no ill effects of long-term stress.

In addition, electrical resistance of the skin tends to increase during meditation (Wallace, 1970), suggesting a lowering of anxiety at this time, and a sharp decline in the concentration of blood lactate may occur (Wallace et al., 1971). Although some studies have failed to show such clear-cut indications of decreased physiological arousal or heightened recoverability during meditation as the preceding, subjective reports of meditators typically describe marked anxiety reduction during this state, and clinical reports generally confirm the anxiety-reducing properties of meditation (Delmonte, 1987).

During the meditative state, the electroencephalogram (EEG) shows an alert–drowsy pattern with high alpha and occasional theta wave patterns, as well as an unusual pattern of swift shifts from alpha to slower (more sleep-like) frequencies and then back again (Das & Gastaut, 1957; Wallace et al., 1971). These findings suggest that meditation may be an unusually fluid state of consciousness, partaking of qualities of both sleep and wakefulness, and possibly resembling the hypnogogic or "falling asleep" state more than any other state of consciousness. A number of studies have also shown that the physiology of meditation differs from that of ordinary rest with eyes closed and from that of most hypnotic states (Brown, Stewart, & Blodgett, 1971; Travis & Wallace, 1999;

Wallace, 1970; Wallace et al., 1971). Other studies, however, have shown that true unin-terrupted "rest," as induced in the laboratory, shares many of the same features.

In summary, the research suggests that during meditation deep physiological relax-ation, somewhat similar to that occurring in the "deepest" non-rapid-eye-movement (NREM) sleep phase, occurs in a context of wakefulness. Wallace et al. (1971) have thus characterized meditation as being a "wakeful, hypometabolic physiologic state" (p. 79), and Gellhorn and Kiely (1972) consider it a state of trophotropic dominance compatible with full awareness. When practiced regularly, meditation also appears to alter behavior occurring outside of the meditative state itself, with both clinical and research evidence suggesting that a number of beneficial changes may take place in people who meditate. These changes are described later, when clinical indications for meditation are discussed.

THEORETICAL FOUNDATIONS

Several theories have been proposed concerning the manner in which mantra meditation operates to effect change. Four of the most widely accepted are presented next.

Global Desensitization

There is an interesting similarity between the situation that occurs during a meditation session and that which occurs during the technique of systematic desensitization used in behavior therapy (Carrington & Ephron, 1975; Goleman, 1971). In the latter process, in-creasingly greater increments of anxiety (prepared in a graded hierarchy) are systemati-cally "counterconditioned" by being paired with an induced state of deep relaxation. If the treatment is successful, presentation of the originally disturbing stimulus ceases to produce anxiety. In mantra meditation, awareness of the meditative "focus" (the mantra) becomes a signal for turning inward and experiencing a state of deep relaxation. Simulta-neously, the meditator maintains a permissive attitude with respect to thoughts, images, or sensations experienced during meditation. Without rejecting or unduly holding onto these thoughts, he or she lets them "flow through the mind" while continuing to direct attention to the focal point of the meditation—the mantra.

This dual process—free-flowing thoughts occurring simultaneously with a repetitive stimulus that induces a state of calm—sets up a subjective state in which deep relaxation is paired with a rapid, self-initiated review of an exceedingly wide variety of mental con-tents and areas of tension, both verbal and nonverbal. As thoughts, images, sensations, and amorphous impressions drift through the mind during meditation, the soothing effect of the mantra appears to neutralize the disturbing thoughts. No matter how unsettling a meditation session may feel, a frequent response of meditators is that they discover that, on emerging from meditation, the "charge" has been taken off their current concerns or problems.

Do the modern forms of mantra meditation "work," then, merely because they are a form of systematic desensitization? Such a reductionist point of view would seem to over-look certain important differences between these approaches. In systematic desensitiza-tion, therapist and patient work together to identify specific areas of anxiety and then proceed to deal with a series of single isolated problems in a sequential, highly organized fashion. During meditation, the areas of anxiety to be "desensitized" are selected by the responding organism (the meditating person) in an entirely automatic manner. At this time, the brain of the meditator might be said to act like a computer programmed to run certain material through "demagnetizing" circuits capable of handling large amounts of data at one time. We might conceptualize subsystems within the brain scanning vast memory stores at lightning speed during the meditative state, with the aim of selecting those contents of the mind that are most likely to be currently tolerated without undue anxiety. For these reasons, meditation would seem to operate with a considerably wider scope than systematic desensitization, although, for exactly this reason, it may lack the clinical precision of the latter.

Blank-Out

Ornstein (1972) has proposed that mantra meditation (or other forms of concentrative meditation in which stimulus input is intentionally limited) may create a situation similar to that occurring when the eye is prevented from continuously moving over the surface of the visual field but is instead forced to view a constant fixed image without recourse to scanning. When an image is projected onto a contact lens placed over the retina, the lens can follow the movement of the eye, so that the image becomes stabilized in the center of the visual field. Under such conditions, the image soon becomes invisible; without constantly shifting his or her eyes to different parts of the perceived image, the person apparently cannot register the object mentally. At this point, which Ornstein refers to as "blank-out," prolonged bursts of alpha waves may be recorded in the occipital cortex.

It may be, therefore, that the central nervous system is so constructed that if awareness of any sort is restricted to one unchanging source of stimulation, then consciousness of the external world may be turned off or greatly attenuated, and the individual may achieve a form of mental blank-out. Because mantra meditation involves continuously recycling the same input over and over, it may result in a blank-out effect, which in turn has the effect of temporarily clearing the mind of all thoughts. The aftereffect of blank-out may be an opening up of awareness and a renewed sensitivity to stimuli. After meditation, some meditators seem to experience an innocence of perception similar to that of the young child who is maximally receptive to all stimuli.

Although Ornstein (1972) does not address the therapeutic implications of the blank-out effect, it is evident that, at the least, such a phenomenon may break up an unproductive mental set, thus giving the meditator the opportunity to restructure his or her thoughts along more productive lines. This could result in a fresh point of view on emotional problems, as well as on other aspects of life. Also, becoming more open to direct sensory experience may in itself be valuable in a world beset by problems that derive from overemphasis on cognitive activity. The enlivened experiencing that follows meditation (often described by meditators as "seeing colors more clearly," "hearing sounds more sharply," or "sensing the world more vividly") may in fact be a prime reason for the antidepressive effects of meditation.

Effects of Rhythm

In mantra meditation, in which a lilting sound is continuously repeated, rhythm is an obvious component. But rhythm also plays a role in all other forms of meditation, as the inner stillness involved allows the meditator to become profoundly aware of his or her own bodily rhythms. In the unaccustomed quiet of the meditative state, one's own breathing may be intimately sensed, the pulse rate may be perceived, and even such subtle sensations as the flow of blood through the veins are sometimes described as emerging into awareness. Some meditative techniques even use bodily rhythms as their object of focus, as when the Zen meditator is instructed to concentrate on his or her own natural, uninfluenced breathing.

This rhythmic component of mantra meditation may be a major factor in inducing calm. Rhythm has universally been used as a natural tranquilizer; virtually all known societies use repeated sounds or rhythmic movements to quiet agitated infants, for example. The world over, parents have rocked children gently, hummed lullabies to them, recited nursery rhymes, repeated affectionate sounds in a lilting fashion, or bounced the children rhythmically on their laps, with an intuitive awareness of the soothing effects of such rhythmic activities on the children's moods. Similarly, in the psychological laboratory, Salk (1973) demonstrated that neonates responded to a recorded normal heartbeat sound (played to them without interruption day and night) by greatly lessening their crying, as compared with a control group of infants who were not exposed to the sounds, and also by gaining more weight than the controls. If contacting deep biological rhythms in oneself is a prominent component of meditation, then regular meditation might be expected to exert a deeply soothing effect. One might, so to speak, gain considerable stabilization from returning periodically to a source of well-being (in meditation) from which one could draw strength in order to deal more effectively with an outer environment whose rhythms are, more often than not, out of phase with one's own.

Balance between Cerebral Hemispheres

Research suggests that during mantra meditation a greater equalization in the workload of the two cerebral hemispheres may occur (Banquet, 1973). Verbal, linear, time-linked thinking (processed through the left hemisphere in the right-handed person) seems to be lessened during meditation as compared with the role it plays in everyday life, whereas holistic, intuitive, wordless thinking (usually processed through the right hemisphere) comes more to the fore. The therapeutic effects derived from meditation may reflect this relative shift in balance between the two hemispheres.

During the early stages of meditation practice, when the technique is relatively new to the meditator, the left-hemispheric activity of the brain—which predominates during waking life in our modern world, often almost to the exclusion of "right-hemispheric" activity—has been shown to take a lesser role during meditation, with a shift toward right-hemisphere dominance occurring (Davidson, Goleman, & Schwartz, 1976). During the more advanced types of meditation, however, EEG records of experienced meditators frequently display an unusual balancing of the activity of the two cerebral hemispheres during meditation (Earle, 1981). In terms of the clinical applications of mantra meditation considered here, this distinction is relatively unimportant, because the "early" stages of a meditation practice constitute the entire meditative experience for the vast majority of those who take up modern forms of mantra meditation. An occasional client in psychotherapy does advance beyond these beginning stages, but such a person is likely to be using meditation to explore altered states of consciousness or to further spiritual development rather than for therapeutic purposes. More advanced practices of meditation are, of course, valid in their own right, but a discussion of them is beyond the scope of this chapter.

Because restrictive moral systems are for the most part transmitted verbally, with much role modeling dependent on verbal imitation, ameliorative effects of meditation on self-blame—a clinically relevant benefit of this technique—might be explained by this basic shift away from the verbal left-hemispheric mode during meditation. Minimizing verbal–conceptual experience (yet still remaining awake) may afford the individual temporary relief from self-derogatory thoughts, as well as from excessive demands on the self that have been formulated through internal verbalizations. Having obtained a degree of relief from these verbal injunctions during the meditative state, the meditator may find himself or herself less self-critical when returning to active life. The reduction in the strength of self-criticism may have generalized from the meditative state to the life of action.

There are, therefore, a number of theoretical reasons why a simple form of meditation may be of benefit in clinical practice. I now turn to the identification of those clinical conditions that have been shown to respond to the mantra meditation techniques.

ASSESSMENT

Clinical Conditions Responding to Mantra Meditation

Based on research and clinical reports, a substantial body of knowledge has accumulated on the usefulness of meditation in clinical practice. As in most areas of research, however, not everyone agrees in interpretation of the findings. Holmes (1984), for example, considers meditation to be no more effective in lowering arousal or providing therapeutic benefit than is resting with eyes closed, whereas other researchers (Benson & Friedman, 1985; Shapiro, 1985; Suler, 1985; Travis & Wallace, 1999; West, 1985) cite compelling evidence to support the concept that meditation possesses some special therapeutic properties distinct from those of rest. Because many of the more clinically relevant effects of meditation are not readily identifiable by standard psychometric measures, it is probably necessary for the clinician to note only that the conditions of a meditation experiment tend to create a type of uninterrupted "guilt-free" rest that is atypical of our society. Such rest can occur in the laboratory because the experimenter has carefully set up the conditions for it: Rest has become a "demand characteristic" of the experiment. Laboratory-induced rest may well possess some special therapeutic properties, particularly if, while "resting," the subject experiences what I have called the "meditative mood"[1] (Carrington, 1977).

Most people in our fast-paced society find it difficult, if not impossible, to truly rest during the day, and therefore a practice of meditation may supply a highly structured, especially effective form of enforced rest each day—one that is easier for the average person to observe than are vague therapeutic prescriptions to "take it easy and get more rest." In fact, meditation may be particularly effective in this respect because it is a novel, out-of-the ordinary activity.

Such practical considerations as these constitute the focus of indications for mantra meditation in clinical practice. The discussion that follows summarizes the major clinical findings in this area.

Reduction in Tension/Anxiety

In research in which the effects of mantra meditation on anxiety have been measured, results have consistently shown anxiety to be sharply reduced in a majority of participants after they commenced the practice of meditation (Carrington, 1998; Pearl & Carlozzi, 1994; Zuroff & Schwarz, 1978). There is also some evidence suggesting that the regular practice of meditation may facilitate a reduction in anxiety for individuals with clinically elevated (i.e., high or average) anxiety levels, but that it shows a "floor" effect (i.e., not much change) in those with low anxiety (Delmonte, 1987). In addition, meditation may be less effective for some patients with long-term severe anxiety neurosis or those who suffer from panic disorder, because such patients can easily be overwhelmed by their symptoms and drop out of the practice. Glueck (1973), however, in a study conducted with a group of psychiatric inpatients, found that dosages of psychotropic drugs could be greatly reduced after these patients had been meditating for several weeks; in a majority of cases, the use of sedatives could also be reduced or eliminated in these patients. Meditation has also successfully been used to lower the anxiety experienced by patients preparing for cardiac surgery (Leserman, Stuart, Mamish, & Benson, 1989) and for ambulatory surgery (Domar, Noe, & Benson, 1987).

The quieting effects of mantra meditation differ, however, from the effects brought about by psychotropic drugs. Whereas the relaxation brought about by drugs may slow the person down and cause grogginess, the relaxation resulting from meditation does not bring with it any loss of alertness. On the contrary, meditation seems, if anything, to sharpen alertness. Groups of meditators have been shown to have faster reaction times (Appelle & Oswald, 1974), to have better refined auditory perception (Pirot, 1978), to show increased vigor (Kirsten, 2001), and to perform more rapidly and accurately on perceptual–motor tasks (Rimol, 1978) than nonmeditating controls. Mantra meditation may therefore be indicated in cases in which anxiety is a problem, and it can often be used productively in place of tranquilizers or as a supplement to drug treatment.

Attenuated Stress Responses

Several studies have shown psychophysiological indicators of stress to be sharply reduced in persons who practice mantra meditation. Credidio (1982) found that CSM meditators showed significantly greater frontalis electromyographic (EMG) decreases and peripheral skin temperature increases than did a group practicing biofeedback. Lehrer, Schoicket, Carrington, and Woolfolk (1980) showed that participants practicing CSM meditation, compared with those practicing progressive relaxation or with controls, displayed greater cardiac deceleration, more frontal alpha, and fewer symptoms of cognitive anxiety than those in the other groups. These researchers concluded that meditation may prepare people to cope better with stress. Similarly, a study by Maclean et al. (1997) showed positive changes in neuroendocrine responses to laboratory stress in participants practicing transcendental meditation. These and similar studies confirm a number of clinical findings that suggest that mantra meditation can be a highly effective intervention when a person is under high stress.

Improvement in Stress-Related Illnesses

Many stress-related illnesses have proven responsive to meditation. Research has shown mantra meditation to be correlated with improvement in the breathing patterns of patients with bronchial asthma (Honsberger & Wilson, 1973); with decreased blood pressure in both pharmacologically treated and untreated hypertensive patients (Benson, 1977; Friskey, 1984; Hafner, 1982; Kondwani, 1998; Patel, 1973, 1975); with reduced premature ventricular contractions in patients with ischemic heart disease (Benson, Alexander, & Feldman, 1975); with reduced symptoms of angina pectoris (Tulpule, 1971; Zamarra, Besseghini, & Wittenberg, 1978); with reduced cardiovascular and all-cause mortality (Barnes, 1997); with reduced serum cholesterol levels in hypercholesterolemic patients (Cooper & Aygen, 1979); with reduced sleep-onset insomnia (Miskiman, 1978; Woolfolk, Carr-Kaffashan, McNulty, & Lehrer, 1976); with amelioration of stuttering

(McIntyre, Silverman, & Trotter, 1974); with lowered blood sugar levels in diabetic patients (Heriberto, 1988); with amelioration of psoriasis (Gaston, 1988–1989); with reduced pain and bloating in irritable bowel syndrome (Keefer & Blanchard, 2002); and with reductions in the symptoms of psychiatric illness (Glueck & Stroebel, 1975). Studies have also shown that meditation may reduce salivary bacteria and thus be useful in treating dental caries (Morse, 1982) and may decrease periodontal inflammation (Klemons, 1978). It may also reduce some coronary-prone behavior patterns (Muskatel, Woolfolk, Carrington, Lehrer, & McCann, 1984) and may be beneficial in lowering central nervous system responsivity to norepinephrine (Benson, 1989). Mantra meditation can thus be a useful intervention in a wide variety of stress-related illnesses.

Increased Productivity

Mantra meditation may bring out increased efficiency by eliminating unnecessary expenditures of energy; a beneficial surge of energy is often noted in persons who have commenced the practice (e.g., Kirsten, 2001). This energy can manifest itself variously as a lessened need for daytime naps, increased physical stamina, increased productivity on the job, increased ideational fluency, the dissolution of writer's or artist's "block," or the release of hitherto unsuspected creative potential. Mantra meditation may therefore be useful when it is desirable to increase a client's available energy and/or when a client is experiencing a block to productivity.

Improvement in Cognitive Functioning

Several studies have shown improved cognitive functioning among those who meditate regularly. A study by Yucel (2001) showed the beneficial effects of meditation on memory in elderly persons. Benson, Wilcher, Greenberg, Huggins, and Ennis (2000) found that students who meditate tend to achieve higher grade-point averages, and Kirsten (2001), studying a group of secondary school teachers who were taught CSM, found that these meditators scored significantly lower on the Confusion–Bewilderment scale of the Profile of Mood States (POMs) than did nonmeditating teachers. These and similar studies suggest that mantra meditation can be used productively in the educational system.

Lessening of Self-Blame

A useful by-product of mantra meditation may be increased self-acceptance, often evidenced in clients as a lessening of unproductive self-blame. A spontaneous change in the nature of a meditator's self-statements—from self-castigating to self-accepting—suggests that the noncritical state experienced during the meditation session itself can generalize to daily life. Along with the tendency to be less self-critical, the meditator may show a simultaneous increase in tolerance for the human frailties of others, and concomitant improvement often occurs in interpersonal relationships. Mantra meditation may therefore be indicated when a tendency toward self-blame is excessive or when irrational blame of others has become a problem.

Antiaddictive Effects

Several studies (Benson & Wallace, 1971; Hawkins, 2003; Shafii, Lavely, & Jaffe, 1974, 1975) have shown that, at least in persons who continue meditating for long periods of time (usually for a year or more), a marked decrease may occur in the use of nonprescription drugs, such as marijuana, amphetamines, barbiturates, and psychedelic substances (e.g., LSD). Many long-term meditators, in fact, appear to have discontinued use of such drugs entirely. Similar antiaddictive trends have been reported in ordinary cigarette smokers and abusers of alcohol, as well (Murphy, Pagano, & Marlatt, 1986; Royer, 1994; Shafii et al., 1976). Mantra meditation may therefore be useful for a patient suffering from an addiction problem, particularly if that problem is in its incipient stage.

Mood Elevation

Both research and clinical evidence suggest that people suffering from mild chronic depression or from reactive depression may experience distinct elevation of mood after commencing mantra meditation (Carrington et al., 1980; Kirsten, 2001). People with acute depressive reactions do not generally respond well to meditation, however, and are likely to discontinue practicing it (Carrington & Ephron, 1975). Meditation, therefore, appears indicated in mild or chronic depressive reactions but not in acute depressions.

Increase in Available Affect

Those who have commenced meditating frequently report experiencing pleasure, sadness, anger, love, or other emotions more easily than before. Sometimes they experience emotions that have previously been unavailable to them. Release of such emotions may occur during a meditation session or between sessions and may be associated with the recovery of memories that are highly emotionally charged (Carrington, 1977, 1998). Meditation is therefore indicated when affect is flat, when the client tends toward overintellectualization, or when access to memories of an emotional nature is desired for therapeutic purposes.

Increased Sense of Identity

Meditating clients frequently report that they have become more aware of their own opinions since commencing meditation; that they are not as easily influenced by others as they were previously; and that they can arrive at decisions more quickly and easily. They may also be able to sense their own needs better and thus may become more outspoken and self-assertive and more able to stand up for their own rights effectively. Such effects may not be easily measurable by any existing tests, although it is possible that the trait known as "field independence" may be relevant to some of the effects noted. Several studies (Hines, 1970, cited in Carrington, 1977; Pelletier, 1978; Sridevi & Krishna, 2003) have shown changes in the direction of greater field independence (or "inner-directedness") following the commencement of the practice of mantra meditation, whereas other researchers have found no such changes. The clinically important observation that there tends to be an increased sense of identity in meditators may not as yet have been validly tested in an experimental setting.

One result of the increased sense of identity noted by clinicians may be marked improvement in the ability of a meditator to separate from significant others when such separation is called for. Meditation can thus be extremely useful in pathological bereavement reactions or in cases in which an impending separation (threatened death of a loved one, contemplated divorce, upcoming separation from growing children, etc.) presents a problem. Meditation is therefore indicated in cases in which separation anxiety is a problem.

Because it is particularly useful in bolstering the inner sense of self that is necessary for effective self-assertion, it may also be helpful as an adjunct to assertiveness training.

Lowered Irritability

The meditating person may become markedly less irritable and impulsive in his or her interpersonal relationships within a relatively short period of time (Carrington et al., 1980). Kirsten (2001), for example, found that a group of teachers practicing CSM scored significantly lower on the Anger–Hostility and Hostility scales in the POMS and the Symptom Checklist 90 (SCL-90) after commencing meditation than did matched controls. A similar reduction in irritability and impulsivity could well be related to the lowered recidivism noted in prisoners practicing mantra meditation (Alexander, Walton & Goodman, 2003; Anklesaria & King, 2003; Hawkins, 2003; Rainworth, Alexander, & Cavanaugh, 2003). Meditation thus appears indicated in cases in which impulsive outbursts or chronic irritability is a symptom. This recommendation includes cases of organic irritability, as preliminary observations have shown meditation to be useful in increasing overall adjustment in several cases of brain injury (Glueck, 1973).

How to Assess for Use of the Method

A few attempts have been made to identify personality characteristics of the meditation-responsive person. Most of these have led to inconclusive results, with the possible exception of the research on "absorption," a component of hypnotic susceptibility. Absorption refers to the disposition to display episodes of total attention "during which the available representational apparatus seems to be entirely dedicated to experiencing and modeling the attentional object, be it a landscape, a human being, a sound, a remembered incident, or an aspect of one's self" (Tellegen & Atkinson, 1974, p. 274). Meditative skills such as focusing and receptivity may be reflected in items on the Tellegen Absorption Scale. For example, "When I listen to music I can get so caught up in it that I don't notice anything else" may reflect the focusing ability that Smith (1987) considers an essential meditative skill. In the same manner, the statement "I sometimes 'step outside' my usual self and experience an entirely different state of being" may reflect a receptivity to altered states of consciousness useful for meditation. Some evidence (Davidson & Goleman, 1977; Tjoa, 1975; Warrenburg & Pagano, 1982–1983) suggests that the absorption trait may predict a positive response to meditation, although this possibility has not been tested in clinical settings.

The majority of the studies attempting to predict what kind of person responds positively to meditation or stays with the practice over time have used nonclinical populations, and their criteria for "responsiveness to meditation" have generally not been relevant to problems involved in clinical assessment. One of the only measures of clinical improvement that has been experimentally addressed in meditation research in an attempt to identify a correlation with personality factors is improvement in anxiety. Beiman, Johnson, Puente, Majestic, and Graham (1980) noted that the more "internal locus of control" participants reported prior to learning meditation, the greater were their reductions in anxiety as measured by the Fear Survey Schedule; and Smith (1978) found that reductions in trait anxiety following mantra meditation training were moderately correlated with two of Cattell's Sixteen Personality Factor Inventory (16-PF) factors: *autia* (preoccupation with inner ideas and emotions) and *schizothymia* (steadiness of purpose, withdrawal, emotional flatness, and "coolness"). However, when my colleagues and I (Carrington et al., 1980) studied employee stress in a large corporation, we found no significant correlations between any of the 16-PF factors (including anxiety) measured at pretest and subsequent drops in symptomatology as measured by the Symptom Checklist 90—Revised (SCL-90-R; Derogatis, Rickels, & Rock, 1976), a validated self-report inventory.

At this point, therefore, the research is too inconclusive to permit us to predict which clients will respond to meditation by means of standard personality tests. There has, however, been an attempt to identify predictive personality variables correlated with successful meditation practice on a theoretical basis. Davidson and Schwartz (1976) have suggested that relaxation techniques have varied effects, depending on the system at which they are most directly aimed. They categorize progressive relaxation as a "somatically oriented technique," because it involves learning to pay closer attention to physiological sensations, particularly muscle tension; they categorize forms of meditation in which a word or sound is internally repeated as "cognitively oriented techniques," as repeating a word (i.e., the mantra) presumably blocks other ongoing cognitive activity. In support of this idea, Schwartz, Davidson, and Goleman (1978) report questionnaire data that show that meditation produces greater decreases in cognitive symptoms of anxiety than does physical exercise, whereas exercise appears to produce greater decreases in somatic anxiety symptoms.

On the basis of the Davidson–Schwartz hypothesis, some clinicians have felt justified in advising meditation for clients who show symptoms of cognitive anxiety and in advising physiologically oriented techniques, such as progressive relaxation or autogenic training, for those who show symptoms of somatic anxiety. Although this criterion has the advantage of offering the therapist clear-cut guidelines, the empirical support for cognitive-versus-somatic specialization remains at best insubstantial. Given the absence of any solid predictive measures at present and the fact that even those that show promise (such as the Tellegen Absorption Scale) are not readily available in the clinic, a clinician attempting to assess the suitability of meditation for a particular client will do well to determine whether this client shows one or more of the meditation-responsive symptoms or difficulties.

Indicators for Use of Meditation to Manage Stress

Table 14.1 lists 14 disorders that are frequently reported in the literature as having been effectively treated with mantra meditation. It then evaluates their treatment efficacy in terms of the guidelines of the Association for Applied Psychophysiology and Biofeedback (AAPB). Because the clinical utility of mantra meditation is intrinsically high—the method is usually readily available in a clinically effective form at very low or no cost—the criterion of clinical utility is not included. Anecdotal reports and/or case studies are included in the evaluation, but only when these have been strongly advocated by clinicians experienced in this technique on the basis of relatively large (i.e., N = more than 50 cases) samples. Because quite an extensive body of research on mantra meditation exists, I have referenced in the table only those studies referred to in this chapter or in *The Book of Meditation* (Carrington, 1998). Anyone wishing to delve further into the subject will find the book a useful starting point.

If the therapist determines that the client possesses the requisite pathology for use of meditation, he or she should recognize that other modalities may also be used for treating these same symptoms. At this point, therefore, the decision to employ meditation becomes a practical one. The following are some of the factors that may guide this decision:

TABLE 14.1. Evaluation of Treatment Efficacy of Mantra Meditation for 14 Disorders

Reference[a]	Disorder	Treatment efficacy
1	Anxiety	Efficacious
2	Psychophysiological stress response	Efficacious
3	Stress-related illness	Probably efficacious, differs with clinical condition
4	Low energy level	Possibly efficacious, further research needed"
5	Insomnia or hypersomnia	Efficacious
6	Abuse of "soft" drugs, alcohol, or tobacco	Efficacious
7	Excessive self-blame	Looking up and down
8	Chronic low-grade depression	Possibly efficacious, further research needed
9	Pathological bereavement reaction	Anecdotal reports or case studies, research needed
10	Anger–hostility/irritability	Efficacious
11	Difficulty with self-assertion/poor sense of identity	Possibly efficacious, further research needed
12	Separation anxiety	Anecdotal reports or case studies, research needed
13	Blocked productivity/creativity	Possibly efficacious, further research needed
14	Inadequate contact with affect Anecdotal reports or case studies, research needed	

[a] The following references refer to pages in the present chapter or in Carrington (1998): (1) pp. 365, 369–370, and Carrington (1998, Ch. 12); (2) pp. 370–371; (3) pp. 370–371 and Carrington (1998, Ch. 12); (4) p. 370; (5) p. 371 and Carrington (1998, Ch. 12); (6) pp. 371–372 and Carrington (1998, Ch. 12); (7) p. 371 and Carrington (1998, Ch. 13); (8) p. 372 and Carrington (1998, Ch. 12); (9) Carrington (1998, Ch. 14); (10) p. 373; (11) pp. 372–373 and Carrington (1998, Ch. 13); (12) Carrington (1998, Ch. 14); (13) p. 371 and Carrington (1998, Ch. 14); (14) Carrington (1998, Ch. 14).

1. *Self-discipline.* The degree to which the client has a disciplined lifestyle may be an important factor to consider when deciding on mantra meditation as a stress management technique. This form of meditation requires less self-discipline than do most other methods currently used for stress control. The technique itself can usually be taught in a single session, with the remainder of the instruction consisting of training in practical management of the method. Unlike some other techniques, mantra meditation does not require memorizing and carrying out any sequential procedures. It does not even require the mental effort involved in visualizing muscle groups and their relaxation or in constructing "calm scenes" or other images. The modern forms of mantra meditation are simple one-step operations that soon become quite automatic. They are therefore particularly useful for those clients who may not be willing to make a heavy commitment in terms of time or effort or in situations in which relatively rapid results are desired. By contrast, mindfulness meditation often requires more commitment and self-discipline on the part of the learner.

2. *Self-reinforcing properties.* For many clients, the peaceful, drifting mental state of meditation is experienced as unusually pleasurable, a "vacation" from all cares. This self-reinforcing property of meditation makes it especially appealing to many clients. Other things being equal, a modern form of mantra meditation is more likely to be continued, once experienced, than are the more focused relaxation procedures. Therefore, when motivation to continue with a program for stress management is minimal, mantra mediation may be an especially useful strategy.

3. *Meditative skills*. Smith (1985, 1986) postulates three meditative skills: *focusing* (the ability to attend to a restricted stimulus for an extended period), *letting be* (the ability to put aside unnecessary goal-directed analytical activity), and *receptivity* (the willingness to tolerate and accept subjective experiences that may be uncertain, unfamiliar, and paradoxical). He suggests a skills-focused approach to meditation, which can both teach such skills in an organized manner and help select prospective meditators on the basis of whether or not they already possess some components of these skills. This is a promising approach, but one that awaits a test battery to measure "meditation readiness" before it can be applied in the clinic. Informal assessment of an individual as to whether or not he or she may possess meditative skills is a possibility, however.

Side Effects and Contraindictions

Side Effects of Tension Release

Like all techniques used to effect personality change, mantra meditation has its limitations. One of these is the stress-release component of meditation, which must be understood if this technique is to be used effectively. Particularly in the new meditator, physiological and/or psychological symptoms of a temporary nature may appear during or following any form of meditation. These have been described elsewhere (Carrington, 1977, 1998) and appear to be caused by the release of deep-seated nonverbal tensions. Their occurrence can be therapeutically useful, provided that the therapist is trained in handling them properly; however, too rapid a release of tension during or following meditation can cause difficulties and discouragement in a new meditator and may result in a client's backing off from meditation or even abandoning the practice altogether. For this reason, careful adjustments of meditation time and other key aspects of the technique must be made if this modality is to be used successfully. Such adjustments can usually eliminate problems of tension release in short order; accordingly, adjustment of the meditation to suit each practicer's individual needs is central to such modern forms of mantra meditation as CSM.

Rapid Behavior Change

Another potential problem in the use of meditation stems from the rapidity with which certain alterations in behavior may occur. Some of these changes may be incompatible with the lifestyle or defensive system of the client. Should positive behavioral change occur before the groundwork for it has been laid (i.e., before the client's value system has readjusted through therapy), an impasse can occur, which must then be resolved in one of two ways: (1) The pathological value system must be altered to incorporate the new attitude brought about by the meditation or (2) the practice of meditation must be abandoned. If the meditator facing such an impasse has recourse to psychotherapy to work through the difficulties involved, this usually allows the individual to continue productively with meditation and make use of it to effect a basic change in lifestyle.

Some of the ways in which meditation-related behavioral changes may threaten a client's pathological lifestyle are as follows:

1. Meditation may foster a form of self-assertion that conflicts with an already established neurotic "solution" of being overly self-effacing. The tendency toward self-effacement must then be modified before meditation can be accepted into the person's life as a permanent and beneficial practice.

2. Meditation tends to bring about feelings of well-being and optimism, which may threaten the playing out of a depressive role that may have served an important function in the client's psychic economy.

3. The deeply pleasurable feelings that can accompany or follow a meditation session may cause anxiety. For example, clients with masturbation guilt may unconsciously equate meditation (an experience in which one is alone and gives oneself pleasure) to masturbation and thus may characterize it as a "forbidden" activity.

4. Meditation can result in an easing of life pace, which may threaten to alter a fast-paced, high-pressured lifestyle that is used neurotically as a defense or in the service of drives for power, achievement, or control. Clients who sense that this may happen may refuse to start meditating in the first place—or, if they start, may quickly discontinue the practice—unless these personality problems are treated.

5. A client may develop negative reactions to the meditation process or to a meditational object of focus, such as a mantra. Some individuals initially view meditation as being almost "magical." When they are inevitably forced to recognize that the technique varies in its effectiveness according to external circumstances or according to their own moods or states of health, they may then become angry and quit the practice unless the clinician can help them modify their irrational demands.

Fortunately, such complications as these do not occur in all meditating patients. Often meditation assists the course of therapy in such a straightforward fashion that there is little necessity to be overly concerned with the client's reaction to it.

Contraindication for Clients with Excessive Need to Control

Clients who fear loss of control may equate meditation with hypnosis or forms of mind control and may thus be wary of learning the technique. If they do learn it, they may experience the meditation as a form of punishment, a surrender, a loss of dominance, or a threat to a need on their part to manipulate others. These people may soon discontinue the practice unless therapeutic intervention brings about a sufficient change in attitude. Such overly controlling clients may prefer a more "objective" technique that they can manage through conscious effort (e.g., by tensing and relaxing muscles, dealing with biofeedback hardware). The response of a client to the clinician's initial suggestion that he or she learn meditation will often be the deciding factor: Those clients who fear loss of control during meditation will usually indicate this and will respond negatively to the suggestion that they learn the technique.

Cautions

1. An occasional person may be hypersensitive to meditation, so that he or she needs much shorter sessions than the average. Such a person may not be able to tolerate the usual 15- to 20-minute sessions prescribed in many forms of modern mantra meditation and may require drastic reductions in meditation time before benefiting from the technique. Most problems of this sort can be successfully overcome by adjusting the meditation time to suit the individual's needs.

2. Overmeditation can be dangerous. On the theory that "If one pill makes me feel better, taking the whole bottle should make me feel exceptionally well," some clients may, on their own, decide to meditate 3 or 4 hours (or more) per day instead of the prescribed 15–20 minutes only once or twice a day. Like a tonic or medicine, meditation may cease

to have beneficial effects if it is taken in too-heavy doses and may become detrimental instead. Release of emotional material that is difficult to handle may occur with prolonged meditation; in a person with an adverse psychiatric history, the commencement of meditation training has been known to precipitate psychotic episodes (Carrington, 1977; Glueck & Stroebel, 1975; Lazarus, 1976; Sethi & Bhargava, 2003). Although it is not certain that overmeditation will lead to such serious results in relatively stable people, it is probably unwise for any person to enter into prolonged meditation sessions except in special settings (such as a retreat) where careful supervision is available.

3. The fact that meditation may be a tonic and facilitator when taken in short, well-spaced dosages but may have an antitherapeutic effect when taken in unduly prolonged sessions is thus essential to consider when reviewing a psychiatric case history in which any form of meditation has previously been practiced by a client. Certain forms of meditation currently promoted by "cults" demand up to 4 hours of daily meditation from their followers—an important factor to note when assessing some of the "brainwashing" effects frequently reported by ex-members of these cults.

4. Meditation may enhance the action of certain drugs in some clients. Requirements for antianxiety and antidepressive drugs, as well as antihypertensive and thyroid-regulating medications, should therefore be monitored in patients who are practicing meditation. Sometimes the continued practice of meditation may permit a desirable low-dosage treatment of such drugs over more prolonged periods and occasionally may permit the discontinuance of drug therapy altogether.

To avoid such difficulties as these, meditation should be practiced in moderation, with the meditator following instructions in a reliable meditation training program. Full training in the management and adjustment of the technique, not just instruction in how to meditate, is essential for the clinical use of meditation.

THE METHOD

Optimal use of mantra meditation in a clinical setting depends on teaching the client to manage the technique successfully—a consideration that can all too easily be overlooked. Unless routine problems that arise during the practice of meditation are handled, the likelihood of obtaining satisfactory compliance is poor. If the technique is regulated to meet the needs of the particular client, however, compliance is often excellent.

It is doubtful whether meditation can ever be taught effectively through written instructions, as correct learning of the technique relies on the communication of the "meditative mood"—a subtle atmosphere of tranquility best transferred through nuances of voice and tonal quality. Meditation can be taught successfully by means of tape recordings, however, provided that the latter effectively convey this elusive meditative mood (i.e., that they are not "cold" or "mechanical" in nature) and that the recorded teaching system is sufficiently detailed in terms of the information it conveys, so that the trainee is instructed in handling minor problems that may arise before the technique becomes truly workable.

The CSM method (which incorporates ROM as an alternative form of meditation) teaches meditation through CDs and a programmed instruction text and comprises a total training program in the management of meditation. Because of these advantages, the following discussion on method is confined to CSM. Some of the points made, however, can be applied to any of the mantra meditation methods. The following discussion covers some of the ways in which CSM may be introduced to a client.

Introduction of the Method

Clinicians are in a strategic position to introduce the idea of learning CSM to their clients. This is best done by referring to specific difficulties or symptoms that a client has previously identified. Simply mentioning research that suggests that meditation may be useful for these problems is often all that is needed to motivate the client to learn the technique. To forestall misunderstandings, however, several aspects of the CSM method are useful to mention when the subject of meditation is first introduced.

The clinician will want to emphasize that this form of meditation is strictly noncultic in nature. Clients with religious convictions will not want their beliefs violated by competitive belief systems, and they can be relieved to learn that CSM is a "scientifically developed" form of meditation. In addition, clients who are uncomfortable with seemingly unconventional interventions will also benefit from being reassured about the noncultic nature of the method. The clinician will also want to emphasize that the technique is easily learned, because one of the most prevalent misconceptions about meditation is the notion that it requires intense mental concentration. Most people are reassured by the knowledge that a modern mantra meditation technique such as CSM does not require forced "concentration" at all but actually proceeds automatically once it has been mastered. The clinician should also routinely check on the client's knowledge about and/or previous experience with meditation in order to clear up any further questions about the method.

The preliminary discussion between therapist and client is typically brief, but certain clients may need to be introduced to meditation in a more planned manner. "Type A" clients, for example, may resist learning meditation (or any other relaxation technique) because the idea of "slowing down" threatens their lifestyle, which is often hectic and high-pressured. When a clinician is recommending CSM to a Type A person, therefore, a useful strategy is to indicate that the time that this person will take out of his or her day for meditation practice is likely to result in increased efficiency. Much research suggests that this is so, and Type A individuals are typically achievement-oriented.

Type A or extremely active people can also be helped to accept meditation by being informed that they can break up their practice into a series of what have been termed "minimeditations" (Carrington, 1978, 1998). These are short meditations of 2 or 3 minutes (sometimes only 30 seconds) in duration, which can be scattered throughout the day. Frequent minimeditations may be much more acceptable to an impatient, driven sort of person than longer periods of meditation may be (although these can be used, too), and they have the advantage of helping the client reduce transient elevations in stress levels as these occur.

A final strategy useful when recommending meditation to Type A or exceedingly active persons can be to inform them that they can use CSM while simultaneously engaged in some solitary sport that they may already practice and enjoy. Meditation can be successfully combined with solitary, repetitive physical activities such as jogging, walking, bicycling, or swimming, and this practice may be a salutary one. Benson, Dryer, and Hartley (1978) have shown, for example, that repeating a mantra mentally while exercising on a stationary bicycle can lead to increased cardiovascular efficiency.

The Physical Environment and Equipment

CSM is usually taught by means of four CDs and a programmed instruction workbook (see *www.masteringeft.com* for information), but instruction in the technique can also be carried out in person when indicated.

With the recorded training, the client is introduced to the principles of meditation by an introductory tape played before instruction per se is undertaken. Later (usually on another day), the client listens to the actual instruction recording under quiet conditions in a room arranged to certain specifications. During the instruction session, the trainee repeats his or her mantra out loud in imitation of the instructor on the tape and meditates silently "along with" the instructor. Subsequently, the client fills out a postinstruction questionnaire and completes the instruction session by listening to the other side of the tape, which directs meditation practice for the next 24 hours. On the following day, the trainee listens to still another tape, which discusses potential problems involved in meditation practice, and plays the final tape of the series 1 week later. This last tape prepares the trainee for a permanent practice of meditation. During the week's training period, the trainee works with the programmed instruction text to master the details of his or her meditation practice and to adjust the technique to suit his or her personal needs. The clinician may assist at this point by making clinically relevant adjustments of the technique.

Most clients learn CSM in their homes (or hospital or dormitory rooms) and make their own arrangements for a suitable instruction environment. When clients are taught on the premises of the clinician (usually so that the latter can advise immediately on adjustment of the technique), a quiet, uncluttered room in which the client can be alone while learning should be made available. This room typically contains a comfortable straight-backed chair and some visually pleasant object, such as a plant or vase, on which the trainee can gaze when entering and exiting from meditation. The arrangements are simple, but they must be carefully observed for maximum effect.

Therapist–Client Relationship

Once a clinician has selected mantra meditation as the intervention of choice, he or she must then decide whether to teach CSM by means of the recordings or in person. Factors influencing this decision typically center on special requirements of the client. When the clinician is weighing the factors involved, the following advantages of recorded instruction should be noted:

1. Learning the technique in his or her home or room facilitates the client's generalization of the meditative response to the living situation; this helps to prevent problems that can occur when instruction is given in person in a setting outside the home. In the latter instance, trainees frequently complain that their subsequent meditation sessions are never "the same as" or "as good as" their initial learning session—a factor that may adversely affect compliance.

2. Learning the technique alone, through his or her own efforts, fosters the client's reliance on him- or herself as an initiator of the practice.

3. Replaying the recordings at intervals reinforces the meditation practice. The recordings may also be used to reestablish the meditation routine if the client has temporarily ceased to practice it.

4. The client's family or friends can also learn to meditate from the recordings. Their subsequent involvement in the practice (plus the fact that on occasion they may meditate together with the client) can substantially improve compliance.

5. Certain clients are embarrassed at the idea of speaking a mantra out loud or sitting with eyes closed in anyone else's presence. Such clients prefer learning by tape.

There are some situations in which tape-recorded instruction is not suitable, however. Clients experiencing severe thought disturbances or other clinical symptoms that make it difficult for them to learn from a recording require personal instruction in the technique. Similarly, non-English-speaking clients, clients who belong to a subculture that uses highly idiomatic speech, clients who are too physically ill to concentrate on a recording, or clients who may have a natural antipathy to learning from recordings also need to be instructed in person. There is a standardized procedure for teaching CSM by means of personal instruction. People who have successfully used other meditation techniques often make excellent instructors of CSM, as almost all meditation techniques have a number of points in common. Even those trained in some of the more disciplined forms of meditation have been able to teach the permissive approach of CSM after first learning the technique themselves and practicing it for several months prior to teaching it. Personal experience with CSM is essential, in order for the prospective instructor to understand the basic permissiveness of the technique.

Procedure

Trainees receiving personal instruction first select a mantra from a list of 16 mantras in the workbook. They are instructed to choose the one that sounds most pleasant and soothing to them or to make up a mantra according to simple instructions. The mantras used in this method are resonant sounds (often ending in the nasal consonants *m* or *n*) that have no meaning in the English language but that, in pretesting, have been shown to have a calming effect on many people. Such sounds as *ahnam*, *shi-rim*, and *ra-mah* are among those used. After the trainee has selected a mantra, training is conducted in a peaceful setting removed from any disturbances that may detract from the meditative mood. The instructor walks quietly, speaks in low tones, and typically conveys by his or her behavior a respect for the occasion of learning meditation.

When teaching meditation, the instructor repeats the trainee's mantra out loud in a rhythmical manner to demonstrate how this is done. The trainee then repeats the mantra in unison with the instructor, and finally alone. He or she is next asked to "whisper it" and then simply to "think it to yourself" silently, with eyes closed. Instructor and trainee then meditate together for a period of 10 minutes, after which the trainee remains seated for a minute or two with eyes closed, allowing the mind to return to "everyday thoughts." The trainee is then asked to open his or her eyes very slowly. At this point the instructor answers any questions the trainee may have about the technique and corrects any misconceptions; he or she then leaves the room so that the trainee can meditate alone for a stated period of time (usually 20 minutes). The experience of meditating on one's own is included in order to wean the trainee as soon as possible from dependency on the instructor's presence when meditating.

Immediately following the first meditation session, the trainee completes a post-instruction questionnaire and reviews his or her responses with the instructor. In the postinstruction interview, procedures for a home meditation practice are clarified, and instructions are given for the trainee's meditation program for the following week. The trainee is then apprised of possible side effects of tension release (Carrington, 1998) and is taught how to handle these should they occur.

Individual follow-up interviews are later held at intervals, or group meetings are scheduled in which new meditators can gather to share meditation experiences, meditate in a group, or pick up new pointers on handling any problems that may arise in their practice. These trainees then learn to adjust their techniques to suit their own individual needs and lifestyles. Whatever the method of instruction (recorded or in person), close clinical supervision of the meditation practice is strongly advised. A careful follow-up program insures much greater participation in a continued program of meditation. (For information on the CSM training materials, see *www.eftupdate.com/products*)

Resistance, Compliance, and Maintenance of Behavior Change

Problems of resistance have been discussed in the section titled "Side Effects and Contraindications." Compliance and maintenance of behavior change are now considered.

Compliance

Researchers have found compliance with the modern forms of mantra meditation to be about 50% among adults in a typical community, with about half of those who learn to meditate discontinuing the practice within 3 years of having learned it and an even larger number cutting down to once instead of twice a day or to only occasional use of the practice (Carrington, 1998). Several problems emerge when we try to evaluate the existing compliance figures, however. The trend has been to define *compliance* as "regular daily practice" of the meditation technique in question, a viewpoint undoubtedly influenced by TM's founder, Maharishi Mahesh Yogi's firm conviction that twice-daily practice is necessary in order to obtain benefits from meditation. Some recent findings cast doubt on the necessity of daily meditation for all people, however, and suggest that the degree of compliance that is necessary to produce benefits may be an individual matter.

When my colleagues and I (Carrington et al., 1980) studied the use of two mantra meditation techniques (CSM and ROM) in a working population self-selected for symptoms of stress, we found that after 5½ months of practicing meditation, these participants showed highly significant reductions in symptoms of stress as measured by the SCL-90-R in comparison with controls. However, when the groups were broken down into (1) "frequent practicers" (individuals who practiced their technique several times a week or more), (2) "occasional practicers" (individuals who practiced it once a week or less), and (3) "stopped practicers" (individuals who no longer practiced their technique), the results were unexpected. Although SCL-90-R improvement scores for stopped practicers and controls did not differ (as might be expected), no differences in degree of symptom improvement were found between frequent and occasional practicers when the scores for these two groups were compared, contrary to our expectation. Nevertheless, when frequent and occasional practicers were collapsed into a single "practicers" group, and stopped practicers and controls into a single "nonpracticers" group, the difference in degree of symptom reduction between these two groups was highly significant. As long as participants practiced at all, they were likely to show improvement in symptoms of stress. When they did not practice, they were unlikely to improve more than controls.

The finding in this study—that frequent practice appears unnecessary to produce symptomatic improvement—disagrees with those in several studies using the TM technique. The latter studies have reported positive effects of frequent (as opposed to occasional) practice of meditation on neuroticism (Ross, 1978; Tjoa, 1978; Williams, Francis, & Durham, 1976), trait anxiety (Davies, 1978), autonomic instability (Orme-Johnson, Kiehlbauch, Moore, & Bristol, 1978), intelligence test scores (Tjoa, 1975), and measures of self-actualization (Ross, 1978). However, our findings (Carrington et al., 1980) are in agreement with research that has reported no differences between frequent and occasional practicers with respect to anxiety reduction (Lazar, Farwell, & Farrow, 1978; Ross, 1978; Zuroff & Schwarz, 1978).

It should be noted that there were several differences between our study with the employee group and those studies using the TM technique that did not show effects for frequency of practice. All but one of the TM investigations were conducted with participants who had signed up to learn TM at TM training centers. These participants were not selected for high initial stress levels (although in some cases perceived stress may have played a role in their decision to learn meditation). It is therefore unlikely that they were under the same degree of stress as the employees in the Carrington et al. (1980) study, who had been self-selected for this variable and whose initial SCL-90-R scores fell at the edge of the clinical range. Possibly when stress symptoms approach clinical levels, even a moderate amount of meditation, or the use of meditation when needed, is sufficient to achieve sharp reductions in symptomatology. When the initial stress levels are close to the norm, however, it may be necessary to practice meditation more frequently in order to reduce symptoms to a still lower level.

Another factor differentiating the employee study from the TM studies is that teachers of the TM technique prohibit the use of minimeditations, which they consider harmful to proper meditation practice. In the employee study, however, strong emphasis was laid on the use of minimeditations in addition to full meditation sessions, and the effectiveness of this teaching was demonstrated by the fact that at the end of 54 months, 88% of the employees who had learned meditation reported that they were using minimeditations. Minimeditations may therefore have exerted a leveling effect, causing a blurring of expected distinctions between frequent and occasional practicers.

Although frequency of practice could not predict stress reduction in the employee study, this should not be taken to mean that frequent practice of a meditation technique is not valuable. For *some* participants in the study, regular daily practice may have been necessary to acquire noticeable benefits. Realizing this, such people may have developed the habit of meditating frequently. Other participants, however, may have found it unnecessary to practice their technique more than a few times a week to obtain noticeable symptom improvement. It is also not presently known whether frequent practice will in time produce beneficial changes in some practicers who do not report benefits from frequent practice during the first 6 months; whether physiological (as opposed to psychological) measures respond to occasional practice as well as they do to frequent practice; or whether effective control of a maladaptive form of behavior (e.g., drug addiction) requires the frequent practice of meditation in order to alter this behavior. Research findings such as those described herein, coupled with clinical reports on the benefits of using meditation on a contingency basis (and/or of using frequent minimeditations), suggest the wisdom of reconsidering our present criteria for compliance. This might serve to lessen some of the current confusion in the field. For example, in the Carrington et al. (1980) study, when "practicing at all" (whether frequent or occasional) was used as the criterion for compliance, 81% of the participants using CSM and 76% of the participants using ROM were still "practicing" their respective techniques at the end of 5½ months. However, when "frequent practice only" was used as the criterion for compliance, 50% of the CSM participants and 30% of the ROM participants were "practicing" their techniques by the end of this time. Which figures are the "true" ones?

Spontaneous comments offered by participants in this study (on a postexperimental questionnaire) may offer some clues. When these comments were examined in relation to frequency of practice, analysis revealed that more occasional practicers than frequent practicers were using their techniques for strategic purposes (i.e., as needed); that more frequent practicers than occasional practicers made strong positive statements about the benefits derived from their technique; and that only occasional practicers qualified their statements about their benefits (e.g., "Under extreme pressure in my department, I don't feel as tensed up, but don't find meditation as beneficial as I had hoped" or "I think there has been some possible effect"). The tentative statements of many of the occasional practicers attest to the "in-between" quality of their evaluative statements, as opposed to the certainty that characterized those of the frequent practicers.

We might summarize the findings to date, then, by saying that the effects of frequency of practice are only partially known. Frequency may not play a major role in symptom reduction per se for certain patients (although it may for others), but it may be positively related to perceived benefits in other areas, such as personal growth and job performance, and it seems clearly related to the degree of enthusiasm that participants express for their technique. In a practical sense, therefore, it would seem wise to encourage regularity of practice for a client whenever possible, without being unduly alarmed if that client should shift from meditating regularly to using the technique for strategic purposes only or to relying mainly on minimeditations. The deciding factor should be the degree of benefit that the client is deriving from the practice. If this factor remains satisfactory in the estimation of the clinician, then even if the client meditates only occasionally or uses only minimeditations, his or her decision to employ the technique in this manner should be supported.

Also relevant to compliance is the manner in which meditators stop practicing. In the Carrington et al. (1980) study, the timetable for quitting in the stopped practicers was revealing. The practice of meditation appears to have stabilized markedly within the first 3 months. One-third of the stopped practicers reported that they had abandoned their technique within the first 2 weeks after having learned it; another 27% reported that they abandoned it between 2 and 6 weeks; and still another 37% reported having abandoned it between 6 weeks and 3 months. Only one participant had abandoned the technique between 3 and 5½ months (during the final 2½ months of the study). It would seem, therefore, that during the first 3 months of their practice, a more or less permanent stand was taken by these trainees with respect to continuation of their meditation practice. Thereafter, although a trainee might shift from frequent to occasional practice (or back again), he or she was extremely unlikely to stop practicing entirely. This timetable of attrition strongly suggests that once meditation has been successfully adopted and practiced for several months, it may become a permanent coping strategy that can then be called on by a trainee when he or she has need for it—in short, that the *strategic* use of meditation is not likely to be abandoned.

It has also been observed that meditators may stop practicing meditation temporarily for a variety of reasons. These "vacations" from meditation appear to be a normal part of the practice for many people and are not evidence of noncompliance. It is important, therefore, that the clinician not label a cessation of meditation practice as "dropping out" until such a fact has been proven correct. The client should be helped instead to understand that such "vacations" can be normal occurrences and that meditators frequently return to their regular practice later on with renewed enthusiasm. In CSM, use of a special renewal-of-practice recording by the client is recommended as a useful means of reinstating the meditation practice after having taken a break from it.

The clinician should also be aware that even if a client eventually abandons his or her technique, this is not necessarily a negative sign. Recent reports from a corporate program using CSM at New York Telephone (G. H. Collings, personal communication, 1982) suggest that after an extended period (e.g., 1 year or more) of successful meditation practice, some people may no longer need to practice meditation on a formal basis, because its benefits have been incorporated into their lifestyles. One telephone company employee reported that he no longer needed to meditate, because he had begun to spend his lunch hour eating by the fountain in the courtyard where he worked, just watching the water rise and fall. He described this as so peaceful that afterward I feel better for the rest of the day. He typically spent 20 minutes watching the fountain, but he said that before he learned to meditate (approximately a year earlier). He stated that he would never have thought of such a thing, because then he was always in a hurry, even when he had a lunch break. When asked whether his experience of gazing into the fountain had any features in common with meditation, he replied that although this had not occurred to him before, actually the two processes seemed exactly the same to him, except that he didn't think the mantra when he watched the fountain.

Similar reports from other long-term meditators, collected at New York Telephone, suggest that formal meditation may be phased out by some clients as a meditative approach to life is phased in. Such people appear to have substituted their own meditation equivalents for formal meditation sessions. This is by no means the case with all meditators, however. A sizable number of people need to continue with the formal practice of meditation indefinitely in order to maintain the beneficial changes brought about by the use of the technique.

Maintenance of Behavioral Change

As noted, the maintenance of behavioral change is substantial and may be closely linked with compliance in some, but not necessarily in all, instances. However, cases have occasionally been reported in which, after several years of mantra meditation, meditators have ceased to notice any more benefits accruing from their practice. Because these have all been anecdotal reports, it is unclear whether the people involved were actually no longer benefiting from their meditation practice or whether benefits were still occurring but were not perceived because the meditators' tension levels had been reduced for so long a time. In clinical practice, an empirical test can be applied in the event of reports of diminished benefits. The client can be asked to stop practicing meditation for a stated period of time; if cessation of meditation brings no change in the clinical condition, or if it results in a beneficial change, then meditation (at least as originally learned and practiced) may have outgrown its usefulness for the client. Substitution of another variant of meditation, if this is desired, is sometimes useful at this point and can result in a revival of beneficial effects in some cases. The reasons for these occasional apparent habituations to the method are unclear, as are the causes of reports of certain meditators' having experienced adverse effects after having practiced their techniques for prolonged periods of time. Although the latter problem can usually be brought under control by proper readjustment of the meditation routine, discontinuance of the practice is in order when it cannot.

CASE EXAMPLE

Training in meditation was recommended for a middle-aged female client because her chronic tension headaches had consistently resisted all forms of intervention, even though her other psychosomatic symptoms (e.g., gastric ulcer and colitis) had abated with psychotherapy. After she commenced meditation, this client's headaches worsened for about a week (temporary symptom acceleration is not unusual following commencement of meditation) and then abruptly disappeared; the patient remained entirely free of headaches for 4 months (for the first time in many years).

During this period, however, she noticed personality changes that disturbed her and that she attributed to meditation. Formerly self-sacrificing and playing the role of a "martyr" to her children, husband, and parents, she now began to find herself increasingly aware of her own rights and impelled to stand up for them, sometimes so forcefully that it alarmed her and her family. Although she was apparently effective in this new self-assertion (her adolescent sons began to treat her more gently, making far fewer scathing comments), other members of her family commented that she was no longer the "sweet person" that she used to be, and the client soon complained that "meditation is making me a hateful person."

At the same time, this client also noticed that she was no longer talking compulsively—a change for which she received favorable comments from others but that bothered her because she was now able to sense the social uneasiness that had been hidden beneath her compulsive chatter. She related this tendency to remain quieter in social situations directly to meditation, as it was more apt to occur soon after a meditation session. Unable to assimilate the personality changes she was noticing, the client stopped meditating, despite the fact that her tension headaches then returned.

It was necessary at this point in therapy to trace the origins of this client's need to be self-effacing before she could consider reinstating the practice of meditation. In doing so, it was discovered that her competition with an older sister was at the root of much of her difficulty in this respect. This sister had been considered a "saint" by their parents, whereas the client had always been considered a troublesome, irritating child. During her childhood she had despaired at this state of affairs; however, in her adolescence she developed an intense compulsion to become more "saintly" than her exalted sister, although this often meant total sacrifice of her own wishes or needs to those of others. Even the simple pleasure of a total meditation session seemed to this client to be a self-indulgence out of character for so "self-sacrificing" a person.

After working on these problems in therapy, and after some role-playing with respect to positive forms of self-assertion, the client finally agreed to resume daily meditation. It was soon discovered, however, that the meditative process was once again pushing her toward self-assertion at too rapid a rate for her to handle. The therapist then suggested that she reduce her meditation to once weekly. Her meditation session was to take place only at the start of each therapy session, and the therapist was to meditate with the client at these times, giving tacit support to the client's right to independence and self-assertion and serving as a role model in terms of acceptance of a meditation practice in one's life.

These weekly joint meditative sessions proved extremely productive; the client described her sessions with her therapist as being "deeply restful," pleasurable, and constructive. Because her emotional responses to each meditation session could be promptly dealt with in the discussion that followed, guilt over self-indulgence was prevented from occurring. With this approach, the client's headaches again disappeared, and she began to experience personality changes typical of regular daily meditators, such as marked enrichment of a previously impoverished fantasy life. She repeatedly stated, however, that this weekly meditation session was all she could "take" of meditation at one time without feeling "pounded" by it. In this moderate dose, the client appeared well able to assimilate the changes in self-concept brought about by meditation, and the client–therapist relationship was used to enhance the effectiveness of the meditation through the joint meditation sessions.

As this case illustrates, the use of psychotherapy along with meditation can be crucial in certain instances to the success of the technique. In most cases, however, meditation contributes to the patient's therapeutic progress with few, if any, complications.

SUMMARY AND CONCLUSIONS

A note of caution seems appropriate at this point. Although it is clearly desirable to be clinically oriented in one's approach to meditation training, this need not be defined as making the instruction of the technique impersonal in nature. The clinician should be aware that in his or her zeal for objectivity, he or she could inadvertently "throw the baby out with the bathwater." The attitude of quiet respect and the peaceful surroundings that have traditionally accompanied the teaching of meditation may have something important to teach us. They cannot, it seems, be lightly dispensed with without losing something essential to the meditative process. Properly taught, meditation can be a compelling subjective experience. To hand a client a sheet of instructions and tell him or her to "go home and meditate" is therefore likely to result in a serious decrease in the importance the client will attach to learning the meditation, as well as to deprive him or her of a role model to demonstrate the subtle meditative mood.

Following the old adage "easy come, easy go," clients who are taught meditation in an abbreviated fashion and without attention to the conveying of the delicate mood inherent in this practice are apt to treat meditation casually and may soon discontinue its practice. When field-testing versions of the CSM recorded instructions, I discovered, for example, that clients' compliance increased in direct proportion to the inclusion in later versions of informal, "personal," mood-setting recordings. Similarly, when giving personal instruction in meditation, clinicians are advised to give careful attention to the setting and the mood that accompany the teaching of meditation. The instruction need not reflect any belief system, but it should be pleasant, peaceful, and in some sense rather special in nature. Learning meditation is an important moment in an individual's life. If it is treated as such, the entire practice takes on a new and deeper meaning.

A somewhat related issue is the tendency of some clinicians to view meditation as so "simple" that it can be taught in one session merely by imparting the technique itself and that the client can then be left to his or her own devices. As Smith (1987) has pointed out, many therapists and researchers tend to use truncated versions, or "analogues," of authentic meditation training on the assumption that these are equivalent to the full training. In fact, the analogues merely supply components of meditation that have been isolated from their context. For proper training in meditation, *context* is extremely important. Although the actual techniques of meditation can often be taught in a single, carefully structured session, this does not mean that a successful practice of meditation has been established by doing this. The latter requires that a number of changes be made in the trainee's daily routine, that individual regulation of the technique be provided, and that knowledge of ways to handle problems that may arise in meditation practice be taught. Without full training in the management of meditation, in fact, learning the technique alone can be detrimental in that it may lead a trainee to believe that he or she is not a likely candidate for meditation (because he or she may have run into some problems with its practice), when, in fact, this may not be the case at all.

The clinician who recommends meditation to a client must, therefore, be careful to supply complete training in all the practical aspects of the technique. Only in this manner can the method have the best opportunity to be successful.

In summary, present experimental and clinical evidence supports the conclusion that, if it is imparted with full respect for both its inherent ease and the potential problems involved in learning it, meditation can be a potent tool for personality change—one that greatly extends the clinician's repertoire.

NOTE

1. The meditative mood has been defined as a special, drifting sort of consciousness quite similar in its subjective features to hypnogogic (presleep) mentation. It is familiar to most people, as it typically occurs at intervals during waking life when the individual is especially relaxed and quiet. Presence of the meditative mood during a control procedure can thus render comparisons between meditation and "control" conditions misleading.

REFERENCES

Alexander, C. N., Walton, K. G., & Goodman, R. S. (2003). Walpole study of the transcendental meditation program in maximum security prisoners: 1. Cross-sectional differences in development and psychopathology. *Journal of Offender Rehabilitation, 36*(1–4), 97–125.

Allison, J. (1970). Respiratory changes during the practice of transcendental meditation. *Lancet, 7651*, 833–834.

Anklesaria, F. K., & King, M. S. (2003). The transcendental meditation program in the Senegalese penitentiary system. *Journal of Offender Rehabilitation, 36*(1–4), 303–318.

Appelle, S., & Oswald, L. E. (1974). Simple reaction time as a function of alertness and prior mental activity. *Perceptual and Motor Skills, 38*, 1263–1268.

Banquet, J. (1973). Spectral analysis of the EEG in meditation. *Electroencephalography and Clinical Neurophysiology, 35*, 143–151.

Barnes, V. A. (1997). Reduced cardiovascular and all-cause mortality in older African-Americans practicing the transcendental meditation program. Unpublished doctoral dissertation. *Dissertation Abstracts International, 57*(8B), 4999.

Beiman, I. H., Johnson, S. A., Puente, A. E., Majestic, H. W., & Graham, L. E. (1980). Client characteristics and success in TM. In D. H. Shapiro & R. N. Walsh (Eds.), *The science of meditation* (pp. 283–296). Chicago: Aldine.

Benson, H. (1975). *The relaxation response.* New York: Morrow.

Benson, H. (1977). Systemic hypertension and the relaxation response. *New England Journal of Medicine, 296*, 1152–1156.

Benson, H. (1989). The relaxation response and norepinephrine: A new study illuminates mechanisms. *Australian Journal of Clinical Hypnotherapy and Hypnosis, 10*(2), 91–96.

Benson, H., Alexander, S., & Feldman, C. L. (1975). Decreased premature ventricular contractions through use of the relaxation response in patients with stable ischaemic heart disease. *Lancet, 2*, 380.

Benson, H., Dryer, T., & Hartley, H. L. (1978). Decreased CO_2 consumption during exercise with elicitation of the relaxation response. *Journal of Human Stress, 4*, 38–42.

Benson, H., & Friedman, R. (1985). A rebuttal to the conclusions of David S. Holmes's article: "Meditation and somatic arousal reduction." *American Psychologist, 40*(6), 725–728.

Benson, H., & Stark, M. (1996). *Timeless healing: The power and biology of life.* New York: Scribner.

Benson, H., & Wallace, R. K. (1971). Decreased drug abuse with transcendental meditation: A study of 1,862 subjects. *Congressional Record*, 92nd Cong., 1st Session, Serial No. 92–1.

Benson, H., Wilcher, M., Greenberg, B., Huggins, E., & Ennis, M. (2000). Academic performance among middle-school students after exposure to a relaxation response curriculum. *Journal of Research and Development in Education, 33*(3), 156–165.

Brown, F. M., Stewart, W. S., & Blodgett, J. I. (1971, November). *EEG kappa rhythms during transcendental meditation and possible threshold changes following.* Paper presented to the Kentucky Academy of Science, Lexington.

Carrington, P. (1977). *Freedom in meditation.* Garden City, NY: Doubleday/Anchor.

Carrington, P. (1978). *Clinically standardized meditation (CSM) professional pack.* Kendall Park, NJ: Pace Educational Systems.

Carrington, P. (1998). *The book of meditation.* Kendall Park, NJ: Pace Educational Systems.

Carrington, P., Collings, G. H., Benson, H., Robinson, H., Wood, L. W., Lehrer, P. M., et al. (1980). The use of meditation–relaxation techniques for the management of stress in a working population. *Journal of Occupational Medicine, 22*, 221–231.

Carrington, P., & Ephron, H. S. (1975). Meditation as an adjunct to psychotherapy. In S. Arieti (Ed.), *New dimensions in psychiatry: A world view.* New York: Wiley.

Cooper, M. J., & Aygen, M. M. (1979). A relaxation technique in the management of hypercholesterolemia. *Journal of Human Stress, 5,* 24–27.

Credidio, S. G. (1982). Comparative effectiveness of patterned biofeedback vs. meditation training on EMG and skin temperature changes. *Behaviour Research and Therapy, 20*(3), 233–241.

Das, N. N., & Gastaut, H. (1957). Variations de l'activité électrique du cerveau, du coeur, et des muscles squelletiques au cours de la méditation et de l'extase yogique. *Electroencephalography and Clinical Neurophysiology, 6*(Suppl.), 211–219.

Davidson, R., & Goleman, D. (1977). The role of attention in meditation and hypnosis: A psychobiological perspective on transformation of consciousness. *International Journal of Clinical and Experimental Hypnosis, 25,* 291–308.

Davidson, R., Goleman, D., & Schwartz, G. (1976). Attentional and affective concomitants of meditation: A cross-sectional study. *Journal of Abnormal Psychology, 85,* 235–238.

Davidson, R., & Schwartz, G. (1976). The psychobiology of relaxation and related states: A multiprocess theory. In D. I. Mostofsky (Ed.), *Behavior control and the modification of physiological activity* (pp. 364–392). Englewood Cliffs, NJ: Prentice Hall.

Davies, J. (1978). The transcendental meditation program and progressive relaxation: Comparative effects on trait anxiety and self-actualization. In D. W. Orme-Johnson & J. T. Farrow (Eds.), *Scientific research on the transcendental meditation program: Collected papers* (Vol. 1, pp. 449–452). Livingston Manor, NY: Maharishi European Research University Press.

Delmonte, M. M. (1987). Personality and meditation. In M. West (Ed.), *The psychology of meditation* (pp. 118–132). New York: Oxford University Press.

Derogatis, L. R., Rickels, K., & Rock, A. F. (1976). The SCL-90 and the MMPI: A step in the validation of a new self-report scale. *British Journal of Psychiatry, 128,* 280–290.

Domar, A. D., Noe, J. M., & Benson, H. (1987). The preoperative use of the relaxation response with ambulatory surgery patients. *Journal of Human Stress, 13*(3), 101–107.

Earle, J. B. (1981). Cerebral laterality and meditation: A review of the literature. *Journal of Transpersonal Psychology, 13,* 155–173.

Friskey, L. M. (1984). *Effects of a combined relaxation and meditation training program on hypertensive patients.* Unpublished doctoral dissertation, University of Arizona.

Gaston, L. (1988–1989). Efficacy of imagery and meditation techniques in treating psoriasis. *Imagination, Cognition and Personality, 8*(1), 25–38.

Gellhorn, E., & Kiely, W. F. (1972). Mystical states of consciousness: Neurophysiological and clinical aspects. *Journal of Nervous and Mental Disease, 154,* 399–405.

Glueck, B. C. (1973, March). *Current research on transcendental meditation.* Paper presented at the Transcendental Meditation Conference, Rensselaer Polytechnic Institute, Hartford Graduate Center, Hartford, CT.

Glueck, B. C., & Stroebel, C. F. (1975). Biofeedback and meditation in the treatment of psychiatric illness. *Comprehensive Psychiatry, 16,* 302–321.

Goleman, D. (1971). Meditation as a meta-therapy: Hypothesis toward a proposed fifth state of consciousness. *Journal of Transpersonal Psychology, 3,* 1–25.

Goleman, D. J., & Schwartz, G. E. (1976). Meditation as an intervention in stress reactivity. *Journal of Consulting and Clinical Psychology, 44,* 456–466.

Hafner, R. J. (1982). Psychological treatment of essential hypertension: A controlled comparison of meditation and meditation plus biofeedback. *Biofeedback and Self-Regulation, 7,* 305–316.

Hawkins, M. A. (2003). Effectiveness of the transcendental meditation program in criminal rehabilitation and substance abuse recovery: A review of the research. *Journal of Offender Rehabilitation, 36* (1–4), 47–65.

Heriberto, C. (1988). *The effects of clinically standardized meditation (CSM) on type II diabetics.* Unpublished doctoral dissertation, Adelphi University, Institute of Advanced Psychological Studies.

Holmes, D. S. (1984). Meditation and somatic arousal reduction: A review of the experimental evidence. *American Psychologist, 39,* 1–10.

Honsberger, R. W., & Wilson, A. F. (1973). Transcendental meditation in treating asthma. *Respiratory Therapy: The Journal of Inhalation Technology, 3,* 79–80.

Kanellakos, D. (Ed.). (1974). *The psychobiology of transcendental meditation.* Menlo Park, CA: Benjamin.

Keefer, L., & Blanchard, E. B. (2002). A one-year follow-up of relaxation response meditation as a treatment for irritable bowel syndrome. *Behaviour Research and Therapy, 40*(5), 541–546.

Kirsten, G. J. V. (2001). *The use of meditation as a strategy for stress management and the promotion of wellness in teachers: An educational psychology study.* Unpublished doctoral dissertation, Potchefstroom University for Christian Higher Education, Potchefstroom, South Africa.

Klemons, I. M. (1978). Changes in inflammation in persons practicing the transcendental meditation technique. In D. W. Orme-Johnson & J. T. Farrow (Eds.), *Scientific research on the transcendental meditation program: Collected papers* (Vol. 1, pp. 287–291). Livingston Manor, NY: Maharishi European Research University Press.

Kondwani, K. A. (1998). Nonpharmacologic treatment of hypertensive heart disease in African-Americans: A trial of the transcendental meditation program and a health education program. *Dissertation Abstracts International, 59*(6B), 3114.

Lazar, Z., Farwell, L., & Farrow, J. T. (1978). The effects of the transcendental meditation program on anxiety, drug abuse, cigarette smoking, and alcohol consumption. In D. W. Orme-Johnson & J. T. Farrow (Eds.), *Scientific research on the transcendental meditation program: Collected papers* (Vol. 1, pp. 524–535). Livingston Manor, NY: Maharishi European Research University Press.

Lazarus, A. A. (1976). Psychiatric problems precipitated by transcendental meditation. *Psychological Reports, 10,* 39–74.

Lehrer, P., Schoicket, S., Carrington, P., & Woolfolk, R. L. (1980). Psychophysiological and cognitive responses to stressful stimuli in subjects practicing progressive relaxation and clinically standardized meditation. *Behaviour Research and Therapy, 18*(4), 293–303.

Leserman, J., Stuart, E. M., Mamish, M. E., & Benson, H. (1989). The efficacy of the relaxation response in preparing for cardiac surgery. *Behavioral Medicine, 15*(3), 111–117.

Maclean, C. R. K., Walton, K. G., Wenneberg, S. R., Debra, K., et al. (1997). Effects of the transcendental meditation program on adaptive mechanisms: Changes in hormone levels and responses to stress after 4 months of practice. *Psychoneuroendocrinology, 22*(4), 277–295.

McIntyre, M. E., Silverman, F. H., & Trotter, W. D. (1974). Transcendental meditation and stuttering: A preliminary report. *Perceptual and Motor Skills, 39,* 294.

Miskiman, D. E. (1978). Long-term effects of the transcendental meditation program in the treatment of insomnia. In D. W. Orme-Johnson & J. T. Farrow (Eds.), *Scientific research on the transcendental meditation program: Collected papers* (Vol. 1, pp. 299–306). Livingston Manor, NY: Maharishi European Research University Press.

Morse, D. R. (1982). The effect of stress and meditation on salivary protein and bacteria: A review and pilot study. *Journal of Human Stress, 8*(4), 31–39.

Murphy, T. J., Pagano, R. R., & Marlatt, G. A. (1986). Lifestyle modification with heavy alcohol drinkers: Effects of aerobic exercise and meditation. *Addictive Behaviors, 11*(2), 175–186.

Muskatel, N., Woolfolk, R. L., Carrington, P., Lehrer, P. M., & McCann, B. S. (1984). Effect of meditation training on aspects of coronary-prone behavior. *Perceptual and Motor Skills, 58,* 515–518.

Orme-Johnson, D. W., Kiehlbauch, J., Moore, R., & Bristol, J. (1978). Personality and autonomic changes in prisoners practicing the transcendental meditation technique. In D. W. Orme-Johnson & J. T. Farrow (Eds.), *Scientific research on the transcendental meditation program: Collected papers* (Vol. 1, pp. 556–561). Livingston Manor, NY: Maharishi European Research University Press.

Ornstein, R. (1972). *The psychology of consciousness.* San Francisco: W. H. Freeman.

Patel, C. H. (1973). Yoga and bio-feedback in the management of hypertension. *Lancet, 2,* 1053–1055.

Patel, C. H. (1975). 12-month follow-up of yoga and bio-feedback in the management of hypertension. *Lancet, 1,* 62–64.

Pearl, J. H., & Carlozzi, A. F. (1994). Effect of meditation on empathy and anxiety. *Perceptual and Motor Skills, 78*(1), 297–298.

Pelletier, K. R. (1978). Effects of the transcendental meditation program on perceptual style: Increased field independence. In D. W. Orme-Johnson & J. T. Farrow (Eds.), *Scientific research on the transcendental meditation program: Collected papers* (Vol. 1, pp. 337–345). Livingston Manor, NY: Maharishi European Research University Press.

Pirot, M. (1978). The effects of the transcendental meditation technique upon auditory discrimination. In D. W. Orme-Johnson & J. T. Farrow (Eds.), *Scientific research on the transcendental meditation program: Collected papers* (Vol. 1, pp. 331–334). Livingston Manor, NY: Maharishi European Research University Press.

Rainworth, M. V., Alexander, C. N., & Cavanaugh, K. L. (2003). Effects of the transcendental meditation program on recidivism among former inmates of Folsom Prison: Survival analysis of 15-year follow-up data. *Journal of Offender Rehabilitation, 36*(104), 181–203.

Rimol, A. G. P. (1978). The transcendental meditation technique and its effects on sensory-motor performance. In D. W. Orme-Johnson & J. T. Farrow (Eds.), *Scientific research on the transcendental meditation program: Collected papers* (Vol. 1, pp. 326–330). Livingston Manor, NY: Maharishi European Research University Press.

Ross, J. (1978). The effects of the transcendental meditation program on anxiety, neuroticism, and psychoticism. In D. W. Orme-Johnson & J. T. Farrow (Eds.), *Scientific research on the transcendental meditation program: Collected papers* (Vol. 1, pp. 594–596). Livingston Manor, NY: Maharishi European Research University Press.

Royer, A. (1994). The role of the transcendental meditation technique in promoting smoking cessation: A longitudinal study. *Alcoholism Treatment Quarterly, 11*(1–2), 221–239.

Salk, L. (1973). The role of the heartbeat in the relations between mother and infant. *Scientific American, 228*, 24–29.

Schwartz, G., Davidson, R., & Goleman, D. (1978). Patterning of cognitive and somatic processes in the self-regulation of anxiety: Effects of meditation versus exercise. *Psychosomatic Medicine, 40*, 321–328.

Sethi, S., & Bhargava, S. C. (2003). Relationship of meditation and psychosis: Case studies. *Australian and New Zealand Journal of Psychiatry, 37*(3), 382.

Shafii, M., Lavely, R. A., & Jaffe, R. D. (1974). Meditation and marijuana. *American Journal of Psychiatry, 131*, 60–63.

Shafii, M., Lavely, R. A., & Jaffe, R. D. (1975). Meditation and the prevention of alcohol abuse. *American Journal of Psychiatry, 132*, 942–945.

Shafii, M., Lavely, R. A., & Jaffe, R. D. (1976). Verminderung von zigarettenrauchen also folgc transzendentaler meditation [Decrease of smoking following meditation]. *Maharishi European Research University Journal, 24*, 29.

Shapiro, D. H. (1985). Clinical use of meditation as a self-regulation strategy: Comments on Holmes's conclusion and implications. *American Psychologist, 40*(6), 719–722.

Smith, J. C. (1978). Personality correlates of continuation and outcome in meditation and erect sitting control treatments. *Journal of Consulting and Clinical Psychology, 46*, 272–279.

Smith, J. C. (1985). *Relaxation dynamics: Nine world approaches to self-relaxation.* Champaign, IL: Research Press.

Smith, J. C. (1986). *Meditation: A sensible guide to a timeless discipline.* Champaign, IL: Research Press.

Smith, J. C. (1987). Meditation as psychotherapy: A new look at the evidence. In M. A. West (Ed.), *The psychology of meditation* (pp. 136–149). New York: Oxford University Press.

Sridevi, K., & Krishna, P. V. (2003). Temporal effects of meditation on cognitive style. *Journal of Indian Psychology, 21*(1), 38–51.

Suler, J. R. (1985). Meditation and somatic arousal: A comment on Holmes's review. *American Psychologist, 40*(6), 717.

Tellegen, A., & Atkinson, G. (1974). Openness to absorbing and self-altering experiences ("absorption"), a trait related to hypnotic susceptibility. *Journal of Abnormal Psychology, 83*, 268–277.

Tjoa, A. (1975). Increased intelligence and reduced neuroticism through the transcendental meditation program. *Gedrag: Tijdschrift voor Psychologie, 3*, 167–182.

Tjoa, A. (1978). Some evidence that the transcendental meditation program increases intelligence and reduces neuroticism as measured by psychological tests. In D. W. Orme-Johnson & J. T. Farrow (Eds.), *Scientific research on the transcendental meditation program: Collected papers* (Vol. 1, pp. 363–367). Livingston Manor, NY: Maharishi European Research University Press.

Travis, F., & Wallace, R. K. (1999). Autonomic and EEG patterns during eyes-closed rest and transcendental meditation practice: The basis for a neural model of TM practice. *Consciousness and Cognition: An International Journal, 8*(3), 302–318.

Tulpule, T. (1971). Yogic exercises in the management of ischemic heart disease. *Indian Heart Journal, 23*, 259–264.

Wallace, R. K. (1970). Physiological effects of transcendental meditation. *Science, 167*, 1751–1754.

Wallace, R. K., Benson, H., & Wilson, A. F. (1971). A wakeful hypometabolic state. *American Journal of Physiology*, 221, 795–799.

Walton, K. G., & Levitsky, D. K. (2003). Effects of the transcendental meditation program on neuroendocrine abnormalities associated with aggression and crime. *Journal of Offender Rehabilitation*, 35 (1–4), 67–87.

Warrenburg, S., & Pagano, R. R. (1982–1983). Meditation and hemispheric specialization: Absorbed attention in long-term adherents. *Imagination, Cognition and Personality*, 211–229.

West, M. A. (1985). Meditation and somatic arousal reduction. *American Psychologist*, 40(6), 717–719.

Williams, P., Francis, A., & Durham, R. (1976). Personality and meditation. *Perceptual and Motor Skills*, 43, 787–792.

Woolfolk, R. L., Carr-Kaffashan, K., McNulty, T. F., & Lehrer, P. M. (1976). Meditation training as a treatment for insomnia. *Behavior Therapy*, 7, 359–365.

Yucel, H. G. (2001). The effects of the practice of the transcendental meditation technique and exercise on cognitive and psychophysiological measures in the elderly. *Dissertation Abstracts International*, 62(4B), 2100.

Zamarra, J. W., Besseghini, I., & Wittenberg, S. (1978). The effects of the transcendental meditation program on the exercise performance of patients with angina pectoris. In D. W. Orme-Johnson & J. T. Farrow (Eds.), *Scientific research on the transcendental meditation program: Collected papers* (Vol. 1, pp. 270–278). Livingston Manor, NY: Maharishi European Research University Press.

Zuroff, D. C., & Schwarz, J. C. (1978). Effects of transcendental meditation and muscle relaxation on trait anxiety, maladjustment, locus of control, and drug use. *Journal of Consulting and Clinical Psychology*, 46, 264–271.

CHAPTER 15

Mindfulness Meditation

JEAN L. KRISTELLER

Mindfulness meditation is one of the two traditionally identified forms of meditative practice, along with concentrative meditation (Goleman, 1988). Mindfulness meditation, also referred to as "insight meditation" or "Vipassana practice," is playing an increasingly large role in defining how meditation can contribute to therapeutic growth and personal development. Although all meditation techniques cultivate the ability to focus and manage attention, mindfulness meditation primarily cultivates an ability to bring a nonjudgmental sustained awareness to the object of attention rather than cultivating focused awareness of a single object, such as a word or mantra, as occurs in concentrative meditation (see Carrington, Chapter 14, this volume). Virtually all meditative approaches combine elements of both concentrative and mindfulness practice, but for therapeutic purposes, there are important differences in technique and application. In mindfulness meditation, attention is purposefully kept broader, utilizing a more open and fluid focus but without engaging analytical thought or analysis. Mindfulness meditation may utilize any object of attention—whether an emotion, the breath, a physical feeling, an image, or an external object—such that there is more flexibility in the object of awareness than there is in concentrative meditation and such that the object may shift from moment to moment.

HISTORY OF MINDFULNESS MEDITATION: FROM TRADITIONAL PRACTICE TO CONTEMPORARY THEORIES

Although the therapeutic use of mindfulness meditation is often associated with the Mindfulness-Based Stress Reduction group program developed by Jon Kabat-Zinn (Kabat-Zinn, 1990, 2005) or a variant of it, there is a substantial and growing clinical literature on integrating mindfulness meditation into individual therapy (Brach, 2003; Delmonte, 1990a, 1990b, 1990c; Forester, Kornfeld, Fleiss, & Thompson, 1993; Fulton, 2005; Germer, Siegel, & Fulton, 2005; Kornfield, 1993; Rubin, 1985, 1996). Mindfulness techniques, including brief meditation, are also used in dialectical behavior therapy (Linehan, 1993a, 1993b). Concepts of mindfulness are also central to Hayes's work on acceptance and commitment therapy (ACT; Hayes, Strosahl, & Wilson, 1999), although ACT does not utilize formal meditation practice. Other therapeutic uses of mindfulness meditation practices include very traditional retreat-based programs (Hart, 1987) and, alternatively, use of meditation-type practices primarily within individual therapy sessions (Emmons, 1978; Emmons & Emmons, 2000; Germer et al., 2005).

All of these approaches have been informed in various ways by traditional mindfulness meditation practices, mostly based in Buddhism. However, meditative practices exist in virtually all religious traditions (Walsh & Shapiro, 2006). Buddhism contains a wide range of traditions with distinct practices. Mindfulness meditation is most commonly associated with the contributions of Americans who entered monastic training in Asia, particularly in the Thai Theravadan tradition, most notably psychologist Jack Kornfield (1993) and Sharon Salzburg (1999), who were central in founding the Insight Meditation Society in 1976. Burmese traditions have influenced Brown and Engler's work (1984) and are reflected in the 10-day retreat programs of Goenka (Hart, 1987). Mindfulness elements are also strongly represented in Tibetan meditation. Tibetan meditation was first introduced in the early 1970s by Chogyam Trungpa Rinpoche, who founded the Naropa Institute in Boulder, Colorado, dedicated to teaching Tibetan and Buddhist studies and psychology. Interest in Tibetan meditation practices has been growing rapidly in the past decade due to the influence of the Dalai Lama and through continued efforts by psychologists to investigate the impact of traditional Tibetan meditation practices on emotional and physical self-regulation (Davidson et al., 2003; Goleman, 2003). Another influential Asian teacher is Thich Nhat Hanh (Hanh, 1975), a Vietnamese monk who has resided for many years in France and whose lineage is influenced by both Theravadan and Chinese Zen (Ch'an) Buddhism. His prolific and approachable writings both universalize (Hanh, 1995) and broaden mindfulness approaches; he is particularly associated with using loving kindness meditation (Hanh, 1997) and contemplative walking meditation (Hanh, 1991) as central practices. Although Zen meditation is not always considered as one of the mindfulness meditation traditions, many aspects of Zen practice, such as *shinkantaza* ("just sitting"), are essentially mindfulness practices and had early influence on the incorporation of meditation and Buddhist perspectives into psychotherapy (Fromm, 1994; Horney, 1945, 1987; Stunkard, 1951, 2004). The Zen tradition continues to influence therapeutic practices through the work of Marsha Linehan (Linehan, 1993a, 1993b), Jeffrey Rubin (Rubin, 1996, 1999), and others (Germer et al., 2005; Mruk & Hartzell, 2003; Rosenbaum, 1998). Zen practice in the United States also draws on Korean traditions (Coleman, 2001), which influenced Kabat-Zinn's work, among others.

THEORETICAL FOUNDATIONS:
MEDITATION AS A COGNITIVE PROCESS

Hundreds of studies on a wide range of meditation effects have been conducted, both on concentrative and, increasingly, on mindfulness-based techniques (Baer, 2003; Delmonte, 1985; Murphy, Donovan, & Taylor, 1999; D. H. Shapiro & Walsh, 1984; S. L. Shapiro & Walsh, 2003, 2004). The stress management effects of meditation practice have most commonly been construed as a function of physical relaxation (Benson, 1975; Ghoncheh & Smith, 2004; Smith & Novak, 2003; Smith, 2003, 2004; Smith & Joyce, 2004), but it can be argued that meditation effects are better conceptualized as a function of the cognitive–attentional processes that are engaged (Austin, 2006; Bishop et al., 2004; Boals, 1978; Gifford-May & Thompson, 1994; Kristeller, 2004; Teasdale, Segal, & Wil-

liams, 1995; Wallace, 2006; Walsh & Shapiro, 2006). Furthermore, as a function of cultivating such processes, the effects of meditation are well understood to develop in stages,
with practice (Austin, 2006; Brown & Engler, 1980), consistent with the model presented
here.

Mindfulness meditation involves the cultivation of moment-to-moment, nonjudgmental awareness of one's present experience, whether narrowly or more broadly focused. The goal of these practices is to cultivate a stable and nonreactive awareness of
one's internal (e.g., cognitive–affective–sensory) and external (social–environmental) experiences. Therefore, it can be argued that it is the development of stable attention and
nonjudgmental awareness that mediates the much wider range of effects, including physical relaxation, emotional balance, behavioral regulation, and changes in self-judgment,
self-awareness, and relationship to others. Improvements in each of these areas of functioning may then decrease the experience of stress. Although other mediating processes
may also be involved, including direct effects on physiological aspects of stress and relaxation, meditation practice is better conceptualized as a way of changing usual processes
of attention, awareness, and cognition. These attentional skills enable one to disengage
from or limit usual emotional or analytical reactivity to the object of attention and to respond to life more mindfully. Suspending these habitual patterns of reactivity may then
facilitate the emergence of self-regulatory functions that are experienced as healthier,
more balanced, or somehow "wiser," in an enduring way, and reflective of sustained
neurophysiological change (Davidson et al., 2003; Lazar et al., 2000; Lutz, Greischar,
Rawlings, Ricard, & Davidson, 2004).

Meditation may not be unique in its ability to facilitate this type of processing, but
evidence suggests that the adaptation of these tools from their traditional roots to a therapeutic context is promising. Although concentrative techniques also cultivate attentional
stability, with a wide range of documented effects, mindfulness practices may more
quickly engage nonreactive awareness and growth within particular areas of functioning.
The very limited evidence to date (Dunn, Hartigan, & Mikulas, 1999) suggests that
somewhat different neuropsychological processes are engaged in concentrative versus
mindfulness practices.

The question remains: How do changes in the processes of attention and awareness
create the wide range of effects observed with meditative practice? Our perceptual processes are inherently designed to constantly scan our external environment for sources of
danger, for sources of gratification, and for novelty—or the unknown. We now understand that such scanning includes our internal world as much as the external; in Buddhist
psychology, thoughts are considered one of the "senses," comparable to sight, hearing,
touch, taste, and smell. Thoughts and emotional responses arise and are then observed
and responded to as if they were "real." Not only are these responses the result of imposed meaning on the stimuli that impinge on our brains, but they also engender further
reactions, thoughts, feelings, and behavior. In fact, cognitive psychotherapy is largely
based on the premise that we construct much of our reality through this imposed meaning. The body then responds as though the external or internal experiences were actual
danger signals; a physiological preparedness occurs that is marked by changes in blood
pressure, heart rate, muscle tension, and so forth. Cognitive therapy acts directly on these
meaning experiences by directing us to substitute alternative content—by substituting optimistic thoughts for pessimistic thoughts or by reframing the meaning of particular experiences. Behavioral therapy works by repeatedly changing the pairing of actual triggers
and responses through extinction or by practice. Meditation acts somewhat differently,
although it can readily be integrated into cognitive or behavioral treatments.

First, meditation provides a way to passively disengage attention from whatever signal is impinging on the mind, whether threatening or engaging. It does this in several ways. The most basic is by resting attention on relatively meaningless repetitive stimuli, such as the mantra in concentrative meditation or the breath in mindfulness meditation; this process may have stress-reducing effects similar to those resulting from use of any distracter, but it is different in that the mind is not then caught up in some alternative source of attention. Linked to this process, but heightened in mindfulness meditation, is the means to observe the occurrence of patterns of conditioned reacting, a type of reflective self-monitoring. In this way, mindfulness meditation involves the cultivation of bare attention, of training the process of attention in and of itself, rather than as a function of the level of engagement with the object. Learning to attend without engaging in the usual train of thinking creates the possibility of suspension of reactivity. This process may share similarities with systematic desensitization in that a deconditioning process occurs. In mindfulness meditation, rather than using a mantra to distract oneself, one simply observes the object of attention without reacting, responding, or imposing further meaning or judgment on it. Doing this has several effects. First, at the conscious level, one becomes aware that most physical or emotional experiences are unstable; they rise and fall, rather than being constant. Second, by disengaging the stimulus from the response over and over again, the mind creates different patterns of responding, much as is recognized to occur in contemporary learning theory. Third, one becomes aware of an increased ability to purposefully disengage from the usual chatter of the conscious mind; this is often experienced as a sense of liberation and freedom, a release from operating on "automatic."

A final step can then occur. The process of suspending reactivity also appears to create the opportunity for more integrated responses to occur. With the suspension of our usual, conditioned, or overly determined responses, we may experience an increased emergence of more novel, creative, or "wiser" perspectives on life challenges. Once the overdetermined conditioned, reactive (and dysfunctional) response is suspended, a new reintegration or synchronization of other neural networks becomes possible. The process of deconditioning, of disengaging the most immediate associative responses, allows a broader range of connections and perspectives. Patients often report that they observe their alternative choices as fresh and in some way unexpected yet emerging from their own capabilities rather than being directed or prescribed from the outside, often experienced as a growing sense of insight and wisdom. One of the challenges to understanding the neuropsychological processes underlying these effects of meditation is determining how or why these emergent realizations generally appear to be positive or "wise" in quality rather than simply random or novel. Spiritual growth as a function of meditation practice may also occur as a function of disengagement of more immediate "survival" needs; although examination of the neurophysiological processes underlying spiritual or mystical experience is at an exploratory stage (Austin, 1998, 2006; D'Aquili & Newburg, 1998), meditation practice is almost universally used to cultivate such experiences, and the processes appear to involve a disengagement and then most likely a potentiation of neurological functions specific to spiritual experience.

To review, meditation can affect the stress response in four separate stages: First, it provides a way to free the senses from whatever is pulling at them. Second, with somewhat more practice, mindfulness meditation provides a way to observe patterns of responding or reacting, as they occur. Third, with yet more practice, conditioned reactions and responses to these sense objects gradually disengage and weaken. Finally, in the course of this uncoupling, meditation allows more integrative, "wiser," or distinct levels of processing to emerge, contributing to more effective responses. In conceptualizing meditation practice as operating through these general principles, it becomes clearer how such a relatively simple process can have such wide-ranging impact, from physiological relaxation to spiritual awakening. Specific therapeutic goals may be facilitated by directing meditation awareness toward the target of concern, such as anxiety symptoms or ruminative thinking. As appreciation grows for the unique ways in which meditative practices may cultivate these powerful regulatory processes, investigation of meditation effects may contribute in an integral and substantive way to a fuller understanding of human capacity for self-regulation, rather than simply being viewed as a way of documenting the value of an esoteric but useful therapeutic technique (Walsh & Shapiro, 2006).

CLINICAL EFFECTS OF MINDFULNESS MEDITATION: APPLICATION OF THE MULTIDOMAIN MODEL

Because meditation practice affects basic processes by which we encode and respond to meaning in our perceptual and internal experience, effects of meditation practice can appear across all areas of functioning. Based on contemporary psychological theory, clinical application, and research to date, the following six domains are posited as heuristically useful in framing meditation effects: cognitive, physiological, emotional, behavioral, relation to self, relation to others, and spiritual (Kristeller, 2004; see Figure 15.1). The order of the columns in Figure 15.1 is not arbitrary. Cognition is placed first, as both the primary mediating process and as an object of practice, in that thought content, ability to focus, and levels of awareness are all cognitive processes. Physiological effects are next; most clients, on first experiencing meditation, note how physically relaxing it feels. Emotional effects represent the next domain to be accessed, generally as positive experiences but occasionally as flooding by traumatic memories that may be uncovered. Behavioral change is somewhat more challenging and may benefit from guided meditation experience. Shifts in relation to self and to others proceed as experience with practice develops. Finally, cultivation of spiritual well-being ande experience is a virtually universal goal of meditative practice, but how spirituality can be defined or cultivated is only beginning to be systematically investigated.

The dashed vertical lines in Figure 15.1 reflect that, although effects may develop within each domain, the domains interact with each other. The dashed horizontal line is intended to indicate that initial effects (below the line) are most likely to be experienced after relatively little practice, sometimes within the first introduction to meditation. The level above the line represents effects that follow with more extended practice; evidence suggests that there may be considerable individual variability in how readily such effects are experienced. Practice within a particular domain—for example, by using guided meditations—may cultivate more rapid growth within that domain. More advanced effects such as spiritual reawakening, as generally beyond the goals of therapeutic work, but are depicted in Figure 15.1 for heuristic purposes. One of the hallmarks of this level is the sustainability of effects, despite life challenges; the other is cultivation of certain exceptional capacities. Because the traditional literature on meditation is replete with references to extraordinary states of experience, insight, and spiritual enlightenment, it is not uncommon for beginning meditators to be confused about what to expect, leading either to anxiety or to unrealistic expectations. Fleeting experiences with unusual states of clarity, insight, or spiritual awareness may occur very early in practice for some, contributing to this confusion and possibly a lack of appreciation for more readily accessible effects.

Integration of Effects/Exceptional Capacities/Sustained Insight and Spiritual Wisdom

Stage of Development	Attentional/Cognitive	Physical	Emotional	Behavioral	Relation to Self/Others	Spiritual
Advanced						Altered states ↑ Mystical experiences Awareness of "transcendence" ↑ Compassion ↑ Unselfish love Heightened sense of inner peace/calm
Intermediate	Altered states ↑ Attentional flexibility ↓ Ruminative thinking ↑ Mindfulness	Pain reduction ↑ Pain control Change in physiologic processes Breath control	↑ Sustained equanimity ↑ Positive emotion ↑ Engagement in the moment ↓ Anxiety/anger/depression	↑ Compassionate behavior ↓ Addictive behavior ↑ Adaptive behavior Deconditioning	Dissolving attachment to sense of self ↑ Connectedness to others ↑ Empathy Self-integration ↓ Narcissism	
Initial	↑ Ability to focus ↑ Awareness of mind/thoughts	↑ Awareness of Breath ↑ Awareness of Body Relaxation Response	↓ Reactivity ↑ Awareness of emotional patterns	↑ Impulse control ↑ Awareness of behavior patterns	↑ Self-acceptance ↑ Sense of self	↑ Spiritual engagement ↑ Awe

FIGURE 15.1. A multidomain model of meditation effects in stress management. The order of effects within the intermediate stage may vary considerably across individuals. The dashed lines between domains reflect that these domains interact with each other.

ASSESSMENT: MINDFULNESS MEDITATION
AND EMPIRICAL EVIDENCE

The research and clinical literature supports a wide range of use of mindfulness meditation, and it is summarized here drawing on the multidomain model outlined above. Table 15.1 provides an overview of research in relation to demonstrated efficacy. However, the systematic investigation of mindfulness meditation is still at an early stage; even though well-designed randomized trials have been conducted, typically only one or two have been published to date that use a given population and symptom area, other than in regard to general adjustment or quality of life. Furthermore, the sample sizes in randomized studies have generally been small. At the same time, a formal meta-analysis of 20 mindfulness-based stress reduction studies (Grossman, Niemann, Schmidt, & Walach, 2004) showed consistent effect sizes of approximately 0.5 ($p < .0001$) across target areas. Whether mindfulness meditation is appropriate for particular individuals or is contraindicated for certain types of presenting issues remains to be investigated. Furthermore, virtually no studies have been conducted that compare the therapeutic impact of different types of meditation practice.

Meditation and Cognition

As noted earlier, meditation is fundamentally a cognitive process that involves learning to shift and focus the attention at will onto an object of choice, such as bodily feelings or an emotional experience, while disengaging from usual conditioned reactivity or elaborative processing. Mindfulness meditation also facilitates metacognitive processing, in which thoughts are observed as "just thoughts" (Bishop et al., 2004). One of the initial effects of meditation is acute awareness of the "monkey mind," the continuous jumping of thought from one point to another; this is one of the metaphors often brought into contemporary usage from the classical texts (Bodhi, 2000). In mindfulness or insight meditation, cultivating "bare attention" may be one of the most powerful aspects of meditation practice for individuals whose conscious minds are habitually caught up in thoughts and in reactions to those thoughts. Unlike concentrative techniques, mindfulness meditation is not designed to "block out" conscious thinking but rather to cultivate the ability to relate to conscious awareness in a nonreactive way. Whereas concentrative approaches may be more effective in producing trance-like states, particularly with extended practice, mindfulness meditation may be more effective in cultivating an ability to maintain awareness of experience without engaging habitual reactions to such experience.

The mind is designed to construct meaning out of experience, and that constructed meaning is encapsulated by conscious thoughts (Mahoney, 2003). A central tenet of Buddhist psychology is that conditioned desires distort perception, create an illusionary sense of self, and, to the extent that conditioning produces craving and attachment, are the primary source of distress. It is well recognized that compulsions and obsessions such as those that occur in eating disorders or addictions are powerfully directed by constructed thoughts and conditioned reactions, which the individual experiences both as uncontrollable and as an integral aspect of "self." Similar to some aspects of cognitive therapy, a goal is to disengage the identity of the "self" from the content of one's thought (Kwee & Ellis, 1998). The recognition that mindfulness meditation practice can heighten objective self-awareness and disengage ruminative thinking patterns has been utilized effectively by Teasdale and his colleagues within Mindfulness-Based Cognitive Therapy (MBCT) (Segal, Williams, & Teasdale, 2002). Although the goal for that treatment is to ameliorate re-

TABLE 15.1. Outcome Research in Mindfulness Meditation

Target area/ condition	Representative studies	Design	Clinical significance	Level of evidence
Cognitive				
Thought disorders	Chadwick et al. (2005)	Pre–post (N = 11)	Exploratory	Possibly efficacious
Attention	Linden (1973) Semple et al. (2006)	Randomized	Suggestive	Possibly efficacious
ADHD	Hesslinger et al. (2002)	Single group (N = 8)	Suggestive	Possibly efficacious
Physical				
Chronic pain	Kabat-Zinn et al. (1985, 1987)	Large sample; extended follow-up	Adjustment to pain improved	Possibly efficacious
	Plews-Ogan et al. (2005)	Randomized	Improved mood	
Fibromyalgia	Goldenburg et al. (1994) Astin et al. (2003)	Randomized	Mixed effects	Possibly efficacious
Psoriasis	Bernhard et al. (1988)	Randomized	Clinically significant (N = 19)	Probably efficacious
	Kabat-Zinn, Wheeler, et al. (1998)	Randomized		
Immune function	Davidson et al. (2003) Carlson et al. (2003)	Randomized	Mixed effects	Possibly efficacious
Emotional				
Depression—relapse prevention	Teasdale et al. (2000)	Randomized	Effects limited to those with 3 or more episodes of depression	Probably efficacious
Anxiety disorders	Kabat-Zinn et al. (1992) Miller et al. (1995) Kabat-Zinn, Chapman, & Salmon (1997)	Single group Extended baseline/follow-up (6 years)	Clinically significant	Probably efficacious
Emotional regulation	Kutz et al. (1985)	Single group	Clinically significant	Possibly efficacious
Mood—General	Multiple studies	See Grossman et al. (2004)	Clinically significant	Probably efficacious
Adjustment to Illness	Mutliple studies	See Grossman et al. (2004)	Clinically significant	Probably efficacious
Anger	Woolfolk (1984)	A–B–A design case study	Clinically significant	Possibly efficacious
Behavioral				
Eating disorders/ obesity	Kristeller & Hallett (1999)	Single group, extended baseline	Clinically significant	Probably efficacious
	Kristeller et al. (2006)	Randomized		
Alcohol and drug abuse/dependence	Marlatt et al. (in press)	Nonrandomized	Suggestive	Possibly efficacious

(continued)

TABLE 15.1. *(continued)*

Target area/ condition	Representative studies	Design	Clinical significance	Level of evidence
Relationship to self/others				
Personal growth	Lesh (1970) Shapiro et al. (2005) Weissbecker et al. (2002)	Nonrandomized Randomized	Suggestive	Probably efficacious
Marital adjustment	Carson et al. (2004)	Randomized	Normal sample	Possibly efficacious
Spiritual				
Spiritual well-being	Carmody et al. (in press) Shapiro, Schwartz, & Boumer (1998)	Anecdotal Single group Randomized	Normal samples	Possibly efficacious

lapse in chronic depression (discussed below), the underlying rationale links cognitive therapy to cognitive science at a fundamental level. Teasdale (1999a) differentiates between metacognitive *knowledge* (*knowing* that thoughts are not always accurate reflections of reality) and metacognitive *insight* (*experiencing* thoughts as events, rather than as being necessarily reflective of reality). Teasdale further differentiates between the experience of thoughts and feelings as transient events in conscious awareness and the ability to engage a metacognitive perspective "to particular thoughts and feelings *as they are being processed*" (Teasdale, 1999b). In our work, we introduce a model of meditation practice in which the first step is heightening awareness of the "cluttering mind," followed by awareness of usual and often automatic patterns of thoughts, habits, and emotions, and finally moving to experience of the "wise mind," which emerges in the suspension of everyday preoccupations and activities.

Bach and Hayes (2002), in a large randomized study, have used mindful awareness and acceptance approaches, although without meditation per se, with psychiatric inpatients with active auditory and visual hallucinations and delusions and found significant decreases in the patients' likelihood of interpreting these experiences as real, along with decreased rehospitalization. A study (Chadwick, Taylor, & Abba, 2005) on a small sample of patients (N = 11) with active psychosis found that group treatment that included training in mindful awareness of the breath and observing unpleasant experiences without judgment was well tolerated and led to significant improvement in psychotic thinking.

I observed similar responses in a young woman I saw in brief group treatment using various meditation techniques; she had had several hospitalizations for paranoid psychosis, although she was otherwise relatively highly functioning, was married, and worked in a responsible position. During treatment, she became aware that under stress she tended to construe even mild criticism, particularly at work, as very harsh; she would then ruminate on this and experience increasingly paranoid ideation. First, using a mantra meditation, she was able to disengage the emotional reactivity; she was then able to simply observe milder levels of negative thoughts rather than reacting to them, thereby interrupting the escalating course of paranoid ideation. Experiencing thoughts as "just" thoughts—that can be separated from the reactions they normally trigger and that need not be responded to—can be extremely powerful in returning a sense of control to the individual, regardless of the nature and content of the cognitions.

A distinct clinical application lies in the cultivation of sustained attention. The use of meditation-based interventions for training attentional processes in attention-deficit/hyperactivity disorder (ADHD) has only been explored to a limited degree (Arnold, 2001). A German study (Hesslinger et al., 2002) adapted Linehan's dialectical behavior therapy, including mindfulness exercises, to treat eight individuals with adult ADHD; pre–post effects were statistically significant. Research on nonclinical samples is also suggestive. An early study (Linden, 1973) showed increased field independence in third-grade children randomly assigned to a mindfulness-type meditation practice for 20-minute twice-weekly sessions over 18 weeks. Semple, Lee, and Miller (2006) summarize their recent work, including results of a randomized study with 9- to 12-year-olds who showed significant improvement on an attention measure. Lazar and her colleagues (Lazar et al., 2005) have shown thickening in parts of the right prefrontal cortex in experienced meditators, which they interpret as indicating heightened cognitive capacity.

Physiological and Health Effects

Even the most basic instruction in meditation techniques elicits a sense of physical relaxation for most people. Sitting quietly, letting the breath slow down, and disengaging the mind from active thinking generally leads to a sense of substantial relaxation. Meditation, through the process of disengaging reactive attention, appears to influence the balance between sympathetic arousal and parasympathetic relaxation, slowing heart rate (Cuthbert et al., 1981) and decreasing blood pressure (Benson, 1975). This shift is essentially the "relaxation response" and has been well documented, primarily through research on mantra-based meditation. Other peripheral physiological effects include changes in endocrine and immune system functioning (Davidson et al., 2003). There may also be primary physiological effects not mediated by attentional processes, such as shifts in physiological balance and increases in well-being that accompany slower, paced breathing (Grossman et al., 2004; Lehrer, 1983).

Effects of meditation on the central nervous system have also been a focus of research for many decades. Early studies (Glueck & Stroebel, 1975) primarily focused on changes in alpha and theta rhythm dominance during meditation practice. Recent work investigating synchronization of brain activity (Singer, 2001) is finding heightened signs of this during meditation in highly experienced meditators (Lutz et al., 2004). Brain imaging technology has allowed increasingly sophisticated work on changes in localization of brain activity during meditative practice, with intriguing evidence emerging regarding brain responses during spiritual experience in highly trained meditators (D'Aquili & Newburg, 1998). Lazar and colleagues (2005) found that the thickening of cortical structure in highly experienced meditators was correlated with slowing of respiration, both of which were related to years of meditation practice.

Health benefits have been a primary goal of the Mindfulness-Based Stress Reduction (MBSR) program developed by Kabat-Zinn (1990) and now available across the country and around the world. Benefits to chronic pain patients have been documented both short term and long term (Kabat-Zinn, Lipworth, & Burney, 1985; Kabat-Zinn, Lipworth, Burney, & Sellers, 1986) in nonrandomized samples, although others have found a lack of impact on pain experience with chronic pain patients in comparison with massage therapy (Plews-Ogan, Owens, Goodman, Wolfe, & Schorling, 2005). A randomized clinical trial (Goldenberg et al., 1994) of patients with fibromyalgia found greater improvement symptoms in patients enrolled in a 10-week meditation-based program as compared with controls, but Astin and his colleagues (Astin et al., 2003) failed to find differential effects using an education control group. In patients with psoriasis, a disease that involves immune system disregulation and overproliferation of cell growth resulting in scaly, itchy patches of skin, guided mindfulness meditation, delivered by tape recorder, has proved highly effective as an adjunctive treatment (Bernhard, Kristeller, & Kabat-Zinn, 1988; Kabat-Zinn, Wheeler, et al., 1998), significantly improving the rate of clearing.

MBSR may also improve immune function in cancer patients, although evidence is still limited (Speca, Carlson, Mackenzie, & Angen, 2006). Carlson and her colleagues (Carlson, Speca, Patel, & Goodey, 2003) found that several indicators of immune response improved in breast and prostate cancer patients, with interleuken (IL)-4 increasing threefold. They also found, in the same study, improved diurnal profiles in salivary cortisol, which has also been associated with survival time. Other research by this group (Carlson et al., 2004) has found improvement in sleep quality and duration, a common concern among cancer patients.

Meditation and Emotion

Improvement in mood, anxiety, and general well-being has been documented in a wide range of individuals enrolled in MBSR and in other mindfulness-based practices. Much of the value of using meditation-based interventions with medical patients lies in relieving emotional distress related to the challenges of treatment and natural fears of disability or mortality (e.g., Reibel, Greeson, Brainard, & Rosenzweig, 2001; Sagula & Rice, 2004; Tacon, McComb, Caldera, & Randolph, 2003). Mindfulness meditation may be particularly powerful for patients dealing with cancer (Kabat-Zinn, Massion, et al., 1998; Rosenbaum & Rosenbaum, 2005; Speca, Carlson, Goodey, & Angen, 2000). Mindfulness meditation is also documented to contribute to better coping in individuals in high-stress work environments, such as medical students (Rosenzweig, Reibel, Greeson, Brainard, & Hajat, 2003; Shapiro, Schwartz, & Bonner, 1998) or business executives (Davidson et al., 2003), and community members enrolled in a wellness program (Williams, Kolar, Reger, & Pearson, 2001). Meditation can be considered one of the few tools for systematic cultivation of emotional equanimity, an advanced level of stress and affect tolerance (Walsh & Shapiro, 2006), although even beginner meditators may experience decreased reactivity and growing ability to "let things be." Cultivation of positive emotion may be a distinct process that has played a central role in Tibetan Buddhism (Ricard, 2006). Davidson has been able to document that meditation practice enhances activity in areas of the left prefrontal cortex that underlie positive emotion, to a limited degree in novice meditators (Davidson et al., 2003) and to a striking amount in highly adept (> 10,000 hours of meditation practice) Buddhist monks and other practitioners (Goleman, 2003).

Within the psychiatric setting, mindfulness techniques, including brief meditation practice, play a central role in dialectical behavior therapy in treating the emotionally chaotic inner lives of individuals diagnosed with borderline personality disorder and related disorders (Linehan, 1993a; Lynch & Bronner, 2006; Welch, Rizvi, & Dimidjian, 2006). Meditation practice may be particularly powerful in the treatment of anxiety disorders. Kabat-Zinn and his associates (1992) demonstrated the effectiveness of an 8-week mindfulness meditation program in significantly lowering anxiety, panic symptoms, and general dysphoria of individuals with documented anxiety disorders, benefits that remained 3 years later (Miller, Fletcher, & Kabat-Zinn, 1995). The effects appeared to be particularly enduring for those with panic attacks and agoraphobia, declining gradually for those with generalized anxiety disorder (Carmody, personal communication, July 2004). A second study (Kabat-Zinn, Chapman, & Salmon, 1997) documented substantial decreases in both cognitive and somatic anxiety following MBSR treatment.

The MBCT program (Teasdale, Segal, & Williams, 2003; Teasdale et al., 2000), an adaptation of MBSR for treating major depression, has been shown to be effective by Teasdale and his colleagues (Ma & Teasdale, 2004; Teasdale et al., 2000) in randomized clinical trials for substantially reduced relapse in individuals with a history of three or more episodes of major clinical depression. Mindfulness meditation appears to interrupt cascades of negative thinking that otherwise contribute to psychobiological disregulation and relapse into major depression.

One of the most systematic evaluations of a mindfulness-based intervention as an adjunct to psychotherapy was done by Kutz and his colleagues (Kutz, 1985; Kutz, Borysenko, & Benson, 1985). Twenty patients, who had been in individual psychodynamic–explorative therapy for an average of about 4 years, participated in adjunctive treatment largely modeled after the MBSR program. Participants improved significantly on most subscales of the Symptom Checklist 90 (SCL-90) and on the Profile of Mood States (POMS). Ratings by the primary therapists identified substantial change in most patients on anxiety and anxiety tolerance, optimism about the future, and overall enjoyment of life. Of participants, 80% indicated that the daily meditation experience was the most valuable part of the intervention; in particular, they noted using meditation practice to cultivate a sense of relaxation that generalized to other aspects of their lives.

Anger management may be particularly well suited to mindfulness meditation approaches in that awareness, acceptance, and the ability to suspend immediate reaction are core to disengaging anger responses. Woolfolk (1984) used a single-case reversal design to assess meditation training in a 26-year-old construction worker with substantial problems in managing anger. The client had lost several jobs, and his long-term relationship was at risk. The client was trained to use mantra meditation, separately and in combination with brief Zen-based mindful-awareness meditations, at times he identified as typical precursors to his angry outbursts during a 4-week active intervention period. The results were clear: It was only the combination of meditations, rather than the mantra meditation alone, that affected experience and expression of anger. Improvement in both client ratings and those of others was maintained at 3 months. This case is notable for several reasons: It illustrates the value of single-case design for investigating meditation practice, it shows how readily meditation techniques can be learned in the face of a clinically meaningful problem, and it distinguishes the effects of different types of practice. Bankart (2006) elaborates a wide range of mindfulness exercises related to anger management, most based on guided meditation practice, that he integrates with basic cognitive behavioral approaches within a broader framework of Buddhist psychology. His book, written for the layperson, would be an excellent accompaniment to anger-management therapy.

Meditation and Behavior

Improved behavioral regulation in response to meditation practice may be the result of several factors: improving emotional regulation, slowing the chain of behavioral reactions as awareness is cultivated, increasing receptivity to behavioral and lifestyle recommendations, or learning to tolerate and "ride out" waves of craving rather than respond impulsively (Breslin, Zack, & McMain, 2002; Marlatt & Kristeller, 1999). Initial effects include increased awareness of behavioral patterns, followed by decreases in impulsive and compulsive behavior. There may be a sense of a general "deconditioning," of being somehow "freed" from the power of earlier patterns of avoidance or compulsions. This sense of freedom may be accompanied by increases in purposeful, focused or "wise" action. The degree to which behavioral changes occur spontaneously as a function of meditation practice is not clear; for behavioral change to occur, the meditation may need to focus on the behavioral goals explicitly.

Eating behavior and food choices appear particularly responsive to mindfulness practice. A nonrandomized explorative study of men who had been treated for prostate cancer (the Stanford Group; Saxe et al., 2001) successfully combined the MBSR program with a 4-month nutritional education program. Overall diet and weight improved, along with prostate specific antigens (PSA). A number of eating-disorder and weight-control programs are beginning to incorporate meditation and mindfulness components (Kristeller, Baer, & Quillian-Wolever, 2006). In our Mindfulness-Based Eating Awareness Treatment (MB-EAT) program for binge eaters (Kristeller, Hallett, & Wolever, 2003; Kristeller & Hallett, 1999), we begin to train the skills of mindful eating immediately, first by having participants eat a single raisin mindfully, an exercise adopted from the MBSR program, and then by using more complex and challenging foods in later sessions, including a buffet meal. There are also guided meditations on awareness of hunger, satiety, and emotional eating. After only a few weeks of practice, participants in the MB-EAT program report increased awareness of habitual triggers for overeating and experience an increasing ability to sustain moments of detached observation, realizing that they do not need to respond to every impulse that arises. The MB-EAT intervention showed comparable effects to a psychoeducational intervention in decreasing bingeing, but with greater improvement on measures of internalization of change. The degree of improvement, including weight loss, was directly related to the amount of meditation practice reported (Kristeller, Wolever, & Sheets, 2007).

Some studies have shown a reduction in drug and alcohol use among prisoners as a result of practicing Vipassana meditation. A recent study by Marlatt and his associates (2004; Bowen et al., 2006) examined the effectiveness of a 10-day traditional Vipassana retreat, as created by Goenka (Hart, 1987), on drug relapse and recidivism in men and women incarcerated at the North Rehabilitation Facility (NRF), a short-term minimum-security jail in the Seattle area. Individuals who volunteered for the Vipassana retreat and who were available at 3-month follow-up ($N = 57$) were compared with those who chose not to participate ($N = 116$). The Vipassana course participants were significantly more likely to have decreased their reported marijuana, crack cocaine, and alcohol use, and few reported any worsening of problems, unlike the comparison group. The participants also showed improvement on impulse control, psychiatric symptoms, optimism, and locus of control relative to the comparison group. Investigations on the effects of mindfulness meditation on smoking cessation are currently under way; given the role of paced inhalation, the compelling nature of craving for nicotine, and the highly conditioned associations with smoking, this application seems particularly suitable.

Improved Self-Acceptance and Relation to Others

Harsh self-judgment is a chronic source of stress, and lack of social connectedness is increasingly recognized as contributing to poor adjustment. A traditional goal of mindfulness meditation is to improve self-concept and self-acceptance. Although this outcome is generally associated with advanced levels of practice, Shapiro and colleagues (Shapiro,

Astin, Bishop, & Cordova, 2005) found a consistent improvement in self-compassion in eight health professionals enrolled in an MBSR program, a change that was also related to improvement in perceived stress. A large study (Weissbecker et al., 2002) of women with fibromyalgia also found that sense of coherence (finding life meaningful and manageable) improved significantly after participation in an MBSR program.

Walsh and Shapiro (2006) suggest that a core process in meditation is *disidentification*, in which experiences can be observed without investing them with a sense of self. Disidentification might be considered a subtype of the process of disengagement referred to earlier, specific to neuroprocesses related to self-identity. Suspending this identification of self with either positive or negative experience promotes self-growth and may allow engagement of inner sources of strength and higher capacities. Such processes may also be involved in the transformative experiences that occur following the intensive 1-week retreats being offered in prison environments, as noted earlier, or may be evident in individuals with severe levels of personality disorder and psychopathology when mindfulness practice is taught in the context of ongoing psychotherapy (Segall, 2005).

Easterlin and Cardena (1998) found that more experienced meditators in the Vipassana tradition reported a higher sense of "self-acceptance" when under stress than did less experienced meditators. Haimerl and Valentine (2001) drew on Cloninger's theory of self-concept (Cloninger, Svrakic, & Przybeck, 1993) and investigated the relationship between amount of meditation practice (prospective meditators vs. those with less than 2 years' practice vs. greater than 2 years) and a measure of personality that taps into three dimensions: intrapersonal (e.g., self-acceptance vs. self-striving), interpersonal (e.g., empathy vs. social disinterest), and transpersonal (transpersonal identification vs. self-isolation and spiritual acceptance vs. rational materialism) development. Each dimension improved with practice, with the linear effect clearest for the intrapersonal and transpersonal dimensions. For interpersonal growth, increases appeared only after 2 years of practice.

Lesh (1970) explored the effect of 4 weeks of Zazen training on development of empathy in 16 master's-level student therapists compared to a waiting-list nonrandomized comparison group and to a group of students with no interest in the meditation. Only the Zazen group showed increases in empathy, but the changes were not related to their index of meditation experience. This study was hampered by lack of randomization and a small sample size, but it suggests relatively rapid effects and possible value within the therapy training environment. Carson and his colleagues (Carson, Carson, Gil, & Baucom, 2004), in a randomized intervention study, found that a loving kindness meditation therapy program improved relationships between married couples, even when the quality of the relationship was already high.

Tibetan practices (Davidson & Harrington, 2002; Wallace, 2006) incorporate a strong focus on cultivation of compassion, both for others and for the self. Kornfield (1993) has written eloquently of meditation as a path to loving kindness and to opening the heart, as has Sharon Salzberg (1999). Thich Nhat Hanh's brief meditations on loving kindness (Hanh, 1997) are particularly powerful and easily incorporated into psychotherapy. A paradox of meditation practice is how an apparently inner-focused and even self-preoccupied undertaking can cultivate empathic and altruistic orientation (Engler, 1998); the answer may lie within the process of decreasing self-protective reactivity but may also be a function of guided meditations that access and cultivate caring for others (Kristeller & Johnson, 2005). This aspect of meditation practice links to spiritual experience and is widely recognized as such within religious traditions. Yet because individuals who do not consider themselves spiritually inclined may still claim a deep sense of compassion, it can be placed within both domains in the current model.

Meditation and Spiritual Well-Being

Spiritual well-being has, until relatively recently, received little attention within the context of stress management, but it is increasingly being recognized as an important component of optimal coping (Kristeller, Rhodes, Cripe, & Sheets, 2006; Pargament, 1997) in the face of significant life stressors, such as cancer (Peterman, Fitchett, Brady, Hernandez, & Cella, 2002). Traditionally, meditation practices have developed as part of religious training, and spiritual growth is an explicit goal of virtually all meditative traditions (Walsh, 1999b). Spiritual effects cover a wide range of experiences, but there is little agreement as to whether relatively accessible experiences such as a general sense of inner peace or transcendence share underlying psychoneurological mechanisms with altered states or mystical experiences often associated with meditative experience. For the novice meditator, such experiences may occur on occasion, and may be profound, frightening, or puzzling, depending partly on the cultural context in which they occur. Despite the long-standing association between meditation and cultivation of spiritual experience, most contemporary research on meditation, at least in the United States, has attempted to secularize meditation practice. However, as attention to spirituality as an appropriate and meaningful focus for therapeutic engagement has been growing (Marlatt & Kristeller, 1999; Sperry, 2001), research is beginning to document effects of meditation and related practice on spiritual well-being, even within secular programs. For example, a large questionnaire study (Cox, 2000) found that meditation and contemplative prayer were related to greater well-being in comparison with other types of prayers. A recent randomized study (Shapiro et al., 1998) with medical and premedical students showed substantial and consistent changes across all measures of well-being, including increased spirituality, in those participating in a 7-week mindfulness meditation program, as did a randomized MBSR study (Astin, 1997) with undergraduates. Similar effects have been documented with medical populations, with improvement in a sense of meaning and peace highly related to improvement in physical well-being (Carmody, Reed, Kristeller, & Merriam, in press).

MEASUREMENT OF MINDFULNESS MEDITATION

Approaches to assessing the use of mindfulness meditation in therapy have focused primarily on four aspects: (1) use of different aspects of meditation (i.e., sitting meditation vs. walking meditation); (2) the quality of experience during practice; (3) the construct of mindfulness in everyday life; and (4) general or specific therapeutic impact. When using meditation practice with a client, it is important to assess how much sitting meditation the individual is actually doing during the week, their experiences of it, and problems that may be arising. This can be done informally or by using a simple self-monitoring scale that can be modified to suit the needs of the individual client. I use one that has five columns: time of day, type of practice (e.g., sitting vs. mini-meditation), length of practice, benefits, and problems that arose.

The Toronto Mindfulness Scale (TMS; Bishop et al., 2004) is designed for use immediately after a sitting, whether in a group or individually, to assess the quality of experience during the meditation itself. The TMS was developed by a group of therapists and meditation instructors to reflect those experiences that they felt best reflected high qualities of practice. The Freiburg Mindfulness Inventory (Walach, Buchheld, & Buttenmüler, 2006) was also designed for use with experienced meditators and assesses nonjudgmental present-moment observation and openness to negative experience; items include "I watch my feelings without becoming lost in them" and "I am open to the experience of the present moment," but it can be used independently from meditation practice to measure mindfulness (Leigh, Bowen, & Marlatt, 2005).

Several other scales have been developed to tap into mindfulness during daily activities. These include the Mindful Attention Awareness Scale (MAAS) (Brown & Ryan, 2004; Brown & Ryan, 2003) that assesses experiences of acting on automatic pilot, being preoccupied, and not paying attention to the present moment; the Cognitive and Affective Mindfulness Scale (CAMS) (Hayes & Feldman, 2004; Feldman, Hayes, Kumar, Greeson, & Larenceau, in press) designed to measure attention, awareness, present focus, and acceptance/nonjudgment; and the Mindfulness Questionnaire (Chadwick, Mead, & Lilley, 2004), which assesses a mindful approach to distressing thoughts and images. Finally, the Kentucky Inventory of Mindfulness Skills (KIMS; Baer, Smith, & Allen, 2004) was designed to measure four elements of mindfulness: observing, describing experience, acting with awareness, and accepting without judgment. A factor analytic study (Baer, Smith, Hopkins, Krietemeyer, & Toney, 2006) administered these scales (except for the TMS), identifying five factors: Nonreactivity, Observing, Acting with Awareness, Describing, and Nonjudging. Baer's final 39-item Five-Factor Mindfulness Questionnaire draws from all scales, which load somewhat differentially on separate factors. In an assessment of criterion validity, Nonreactivity, Acting with Awareness, and Nonjudging were most associated with indicators of psychological well-being. A limitation of this research is that it was conducted on undergraduates with little or no meditation experience; further work is being done to assess the value of these scales as measures of meditation practice effects, both in the general and clinical populations.

THE METHOD: BASIC ELEMENTS OF MINDFULNESS MEDITATION

Innumerable meditation techniques exist, as developed not only within the Buddhist traditions but also within other contemplative traditions, including Hinduism, Christianity, and Judaism. However mindfulness practices, as generally used in the therapeutic context in the United States, can be divided into three aspects: breath awareness, open-focus mindfulness techniques, and guided mindfulness meditation practices.

Breath Awareness

Vipassana practice, or insight meditation, the Southeast Asian school of mindfulness meditation popularized by Kornfield, Salzberg, and others, often uses a focus on the breath as a way to both cultivate and reengage the attention when it becomes caught up with analytical thinking. This use of the breath is arguably the element of mindfulness meditation that most overlaps with concentrative techniques. The breath is a particularly potent focus of attention, in that it is always present, is highly sensitive to stress reactions, and is inherently rhythmic in nature. Learning to shift one's attention to the breath mindfully at times of stress may not only serve to disengage reactivity but may also cultivate a positive physiological feedback system that brings sympathetic and parasympathetic responses into better balance. Training the mind to hold attention on the breath is an important element of mindfulness traditions, yet unlike the concentrative use of the mantra, emphasis is generally placed on cultivating awareness of the complexity and richness of something as simple as the process of breathing (Hanh, 1996). See Table 15.2 for brief instructions in breath awareness meditation. Purposefully slowing the breath is an aspect of several meditation traditions, including Zen Rinzai practice (Lehrer, Sasaki, & Saito,

1999) and Tibetan practices. Slowing the breath has been shown to reliably produce unconditioned relaxation effects (Lehrer & Woolfolk, 1994); very low respiration rates (2–6 cycles/minute) trigger powerful relaxation effects and raise body temperature substantially (Benson, 1982; Lehrer et al., 1999).

Open Awareness

Open awareness is generally considered the core of mindfulness meditation. Table 15.2 contains elements of open awareness, although with instructions to bring awareness back to the breath frequently as an anchor. As noted earlier, cultivating "bare hovering attention" has several goals: (1) to bring awareness to experience both in the body and the mind; (2) to disengage the reactive and analytical mind, in regard to both behavioral impulses and to tendencies to "think about" content of thought rather than simply observing it; (3) to train the ability to engage mindfulness more easily and fully during daily activities. In open awareness, one gently rests attention on whatever has risen to the realm of consciousness; as that fades, one moves one's attention to the next object of awareness. A useful teaching metaphor is to imagine oneself sitting on the banks of a river and observing what comes floating by: leaves, branches, perhaps a piece of trash. Our usual analytical way of observing might

---

TABLE 15.2. Basic Instructions in Breath Awareness and Mindfulness Meditation

1. Find a quiet place and time. If you prefer, set a timer for 20 to 40 minutes. Become comfortable in your chair, sitting with a relaxed but straight, erect posture that is balanced but not straining. Allow your hands to rest comfortably in your lap. Loosen any tight clothing that will restrict your stomach. Gently close your eyes.

2. Simply allow your body to become still. Allow your shoulders, chest, and stomach to relax. Focus your attention on the feeling of your breathing. Begin by taking two or three deeper breaths from your diaphragm, letting the air flow all the way into your stomach, without any push or strain, and then flow gently back out again. Repeat these two or three deep breaths, noticing an increased sense of calm and relaxation as you breath in the clean, fresh air and breath out any sense of tension or stress.

3. Now let your breathing find its own natural, comfortable rhythm and depth. Focus your attention on the feeling of your breath as it comes in at the tip of your nose, moves through the back of your throat, into your lower diaphragm, and back out again, letting your stomach rise and fall naturally with each breath.

4. Allow your attention to stay focused on your breath and away from the noise, the thoughts, the feelings, the concerns that may usually fill your mind.

5. As you continue, you will notice that the mind will become caught up in thoughts and feelings. It may become attached to noises or bodily sensations. You may find yourself remembering something from your past or thinking about the future. This is to be expected. This is the nature of the mind. If the thought or experience is particularly powerful, without self-judgment, simply observe the process of the mind. You might note to yourself the nature of the thought or experience: "worry," "planning," "pain," "sound." Then gently return your attention to the breath.

6. And again, as you notice your mind wandering off, do not be critical of yourself. Understand that this is the nature of the mind—to become attached to daily concerns, to become attached to feelings, memories. If you find your mind becoming preoccupied with a thought, simply notice it, rather than pursuing it at this moment. Understand, without judging, that it is the habit of your mind to pursue the thought. When you notice this happening, simply return your attention to your breathing. See the thought as simply a thought, an activity that your mind is engaging in.

7. When you are ready, gently bring your attention back just to the breath. Now bring your attention back into the space of your body and into the space of the room. Move around gently in the space of the chair. When you are ready, open your eyes and gently stretch out.

be to think about, analyze, or judge each object—"What type of leaf is that? . . . Where did it fall into the river? . . . When did that branch fall in? . . . When will it sink? . . . Oh, who threw that trash in? . . . Isn't that terrible." In contrast, mindfulness involves simply observing: "leaf . . . branch . . . trash . . ." without letting the mind be carried along. A more contemporary metaphor, offered by one of my clients, is the difference between "mall walking" for exercise and window shopping. When window shopping in the mall, one may stop to chat with friends or enter a store to browse. When mall walking, stopping to do these things would defeat the purpose of steadily moving for exercise, but one might still acknowledge friends or make a mental "note" of something displayed in a store window to return to later. This type of "noting" is often used during mindfulness practice, particularly when first learning to meditate—silently naming the type of thought or experience one is having, such as "analyzing," "pain," "desire to move," or "impatience"—and then moving back to the breath or to bare attention, without following the thought or experience further. This technique helps train attention to be aware of, rather than "grab" onto, the content of a thought. Many individuals find mindfulness training very powerful because they are not aware that they have this capacity simply to observe, rather than to analyze or judge. "Noting" is also useful when some type of insight has arisen; by making a mental note of it and reminding oneself that if it is important, it is more likely be recalled later, without interrupting the sitting to pursue it.

Guided Awareness

In guided meditation practice, the content carries significance and is intended to engage a particular aspect of self but in a mindful, rather than analytical or judgmental, way. In traditional meditation practices, the focus may be a particular chant, the symbolic *mandala* of Tibetan tantric practices, a Zen *koan*, complex universal experiences such as images of death or suffering, or feelings of compassion (as in loving kindness meditations). In contemporary therapeutic practice, the focus may be on physical sensations such as hunger (Kristeller, Baer, & Quillian-Wolever, 2006) or stress (Kabat-Zinn et al., 1992), on depressive thoughts (Segal, Williams, & Teasdale, 2002), or on interpersonal connectedness (Carson et al., 2004), with the goal of first increasing awareness in relation to the targeted issue and then modifying the nature of cognitive, behavioral, or emotional response and reactivity to these experiences. Guided meditations can be incorporated into therapeutic approaches in many ways, whether as elements of general mindfulness practice, such as occurs in the MBSR program in relation to symptoms such as pain or anxiety or as fully "scripted" meditations. Such scripted meditations may be as brief as a loving kindness meditation or as structured as the instructions used in the treatment meditation tapes for psoriasis (Bernhard et al., 1988; Kabat-Zinn, Wheeler, et al., 1998), or they may make up a substantial part of an entire treatment program, such as for depression in the MBCT program (Segal et al., 2002) or aspects of eating in the MB-EAT program (Kristeller et al., 2003). Guided meditation may also form an important aspect of mindfulness approaches in individual therapy, as in treatments described by Emmons and Emmons (2000), Rubin (1996a), or in couples work (Carson et al., 2004; Surrey, 2005).

The question is sometimes raised how such focused or guided meditations differ from imagery work or hypnosis. There is, of course, overlap (Holroyd, 2003; Otani, 2003) in the use of focused attention and disengagement of usual thought processes. The distinctions are nevertheless evident: Hypnosis more generally cultivates mental processing of images and experience, both spontaneous and suggested, whereas mindfulness practice cultivates "bare awareness." Furthermore, mindfulness emphasizes awareness of internal experience that the individual discovers for him- or herself. In my experience, individuals often experience hypnosis as something that is "done to them," whereas mind-fulness meditation cultivates a greater sense of internalization of awareness and self-control. However, there has been long-standing interest in combining these approaches clinically (Brown, Forte, Rich, & Epstein, 1982; Brown & Fromm, 1988); for example, Marriott (1989) describes brief treatment of a woman with panic attacks in which hypnotic induction and guided meditation were used jointly to deepen access and processing of memories and trauma.

It is also useful to consider body-focused practices as a distinct type of guided or targeted meditation. The word *yoga* comes from the Sanskrit term *yuj*, meaning "to yoke," as in yoking the mind and body (Budilovsky & Adamson, 2002). Most meditative traditions recommend use of particular body postures to facilitate practice. Other body practices include walking meditation, body scanning, and guided meditations on the senses or interoceptive experience. From a therapeutic perspective, the type and degree of emphasis on body work should be adjusted to therapeutic goals and the needs (or limitations) of a particular client or population.

Length of Practice

Formal mindfulness meditation practice, similar to concentrative meditation, involves putting aside a certain length of time, such as 20 or 40 minutes, once or twice per day. Daily practice is emphasized as a way of training the mind most effectively to shift into a mindful state. Shorter periods of time, such as 5–10 minutes, may be helpful in teaching children meditation (Fontana & Slack, 1997; Rozman, 1994) or in using meditation in special settings, but it may not allow the mind enough time to shift into an absorptive state, particularly early in practice. At the same time, gradual integration of the meditative experience through moment-to-moment awareness in daily life, whether by training the mind to be focused or to remain mindful and nonreactive, is the goal of all practice. Such "mini-meditations" (Carrington, 1998), whether of 3–5 minutes' or 3–5 seconds' duration, may become a very powerful part of practice.

When integrating meditation into daily activities, a person may be instructed to shift attention to the breath or to simply stop and attend mindfully to whatever he or she is doing. One effective way to use "mini-meditations" is with a regularly occurring signal, such as a clock chiming or the telephone ringing, to bring oneself into a moment of mindful awareness rather than responding reactively or being on "automatic." In our MB-EAT program, we emphasize using mini-meditations just before meals or while eating to facilitate bringing mindful awareness to the food, counteracting "automatic eating." A client of mine was struggling with almost incapacitating anger and anxiety in her work environment. She had practiced TM but had a difficult time using her mantra in daily activities without "zoning out," as she put it. After a weekend retreat spent learning mindfulness meditation and further work in individual treatment, we discussed how to use "mini-meditations" in her work setting. She stuck small red dots in various places in her office (her computer monitor, on the side of the door, on her telephone, etc.) as reminders to attend to her experience and then if she was feeling agitated to shift her attention briefly to her breath. She returned the next week noting that this had been very helpful—and that she had also imagined sticking a red dot on the forehead of the person whom she found most difficult to work with.

Far more intensive training in a retreat environment is an aspect of virtually all meditative traditions. Such retreats may last from several days to several months. Such experiences are understood to be particularly valuable for more complete control over various aspects of mind and body and as a path of entry into what could be considered altered states or spiritual enlightenment (Austin, 1998; Dass, 1987; Welwood, 2000). Such retreats may serve as a complement to therapeutic work and will generally be supervised by a highly experienced meditation teacher.

GROUP PROGRAMS

Mindfulness-Based Stress Reduction

Perhaps the best known and most fully researched mindfulness approach is the MBSR group program developed by Jon Kabat-Zinn (Kabat-Zinn, 1990). The basic structure includes eight weekly sessions of 2½–3 hours each, with a full-day (7½ hours) silent retreat after session 6. Typically, about 25 individuals attend, and group sharing is an important aspect of the program. Participants are first taught breath awareness and body scan meditations and then continue with formal sitting mindfulness meditation. Yoga is introduced in session 3 and walking meditation by session 4. Participants are provided with audiotapes of 45 minutes in length and are expected to practice once per day. Substantial didactic material is provided on stress management and managing a healthy lifestyle. Although the program is informed by Buddhist practice, presentation of material is strictly secular. Individual or group orientation sessions occur prior to the program; assessment includes medical and psychiatric symptom checklists. Elevated responses are noted, but individuals are rarely screened out based on their responses. It is not uncommon for individuals to experience highly charged emotional responses during the program, but rarely (less than 1%) are these at a level that require withdrawal from the program (Kabat-Zinn, personal communication, June 2004). A structured program for training and certification of MBSR leaders is available through the Center for Mindfulness (*www.umassmed.edu/cfm*).

Other Group Therapeutic Programs

Mindfulness-Based Cognitive Therapy (MBCT) adapts the MBSR program specifically to address the downward spiral of negative thinking and emotion that contribute to relapse in clinical depression (Segal et al., 2002; Teasdale et al., 1995). MBCT is structured in a very similar way to MBSR; the first few sessions are almost identical, with gradual engagement of awareness of mood states. Sessions 4 to 6 introduce the importance of observing negative automatic thoughts, cultivating acceptance, and seeing thoughts as "just thoughts." The last two sessions focus on engaging in positive self-care, creating mastery, and relapse prevention. Development of Mindfulness-Based Relapse Prevention for drug and alcohol treatment is underway (Witkeiwitz, Marlatt, & Walker, 2005).

Mindfulness-Based Eating Awareness Therapy (MB-EAT) diverges somewhat further from the MBSR program in that a more substantial portion of the sessions use guided meditations that focus explicitly on cultivating awareness of hunger signals, satiety signals, and triggers for eating. In addition to guided meditations focused on eating behavior and emotional triggers for overeating, other meditation practices include the body scan, chair yoga, and walking meditation to increase comfort with the body, and forgiveness meditation and wisdom meditation to address negative self-judgment and to heighten a sense of meaning and purpose. Weekly sitting meditation tapes use 20-minute sessions. The number of sessions has been expanded from seven (Kristeller & Hallett, 1999) to nine (Kristeller, Baer, & Quillian-Wolever, 2006); a version under current evaluation adds more focus on weight loss across 10 weekly sessions, with 2 monthly follow-up meetings.

A very traditional form of Vipassana meditation is gaining more attention within the United States. The program, which follows a traditional 10-day retreat model, was developed by Goenka, a Burmese businessman who became a highly regarded lay leader in India of Vipassana retreats about 20 years ago (Hart, 1987). In this program, silence is maintained for the entire period, except for instruction, with approximately 10 hours per day spent in meditation. For the first 3 days, the focus is on breath awareness. This shifts to mindful observation of physical and mental experiences during the remaining days. Each evening a videotaped discourse by Goenka presents a secular Buddhist perspective on suffering and stress and on the value of meditative practice. This 10-day program has been used extensively in prisons in India; the transformative impact on participants is documented in the film *Doing Time, Doing Vipassana* (Menahemi & Ariel, 1997). The program has been evaluated in the U.S. prison system for preventing drug and alcohol relapse following release (Bowen et al., 2006).

INDIVIDUAL THERAPY AND MINDFULNESS MEDITATION

Integrating mindfulness meditation practice into individual therapy has been discussed by a number of practitioners, although with little empirical investigation. There is an increasing number of very valuable accounts of the use of mindfulness-based meditation within psychotherapeutic contexts from the perspective of both Theravadan mindfulness practice (e.g., Brach, 2003; Walsh, 2004) and Zen practice (Epstein, 1995, 2001; Mruk & Hartzell, 2003; Rosenbaum, 1998; Rubin, 1996). Integration can range from using meditation as a primary component of individual treatment, taught within the therapeutic setting, to drawing on clients' own personal meditation practice experience to complement and facilitate more traditional psychotherapy.

Emmons and Emmons (Emmons, 1978; Emmons & Emmons, 2000) have developed a technique that they call Meditative Therapy (MT), which they describe as "a synthesis between meditation and inner-oriented psychotherapy." In MT the therapy session is used as a meditative space; the client, with eyes closed and in a relaxed posture, is directed by the therapist to verbalize everything that comes to mind, regardless of content. Emmons compares this to a verbalized mindfulness meditation practice. However, unlike most meditative approaches, there is no home or individual practice, no use of the breath as a focus, and no training in formal meditation practice. The instruction focuses on directing the client to be aware of inner experiences: " . . . close your eyes and allow your awareness to shift inward. . . . Now allow yourself to ask for help from your Inner Source." Although a light trance state may occur, this is not the intention of the process, unlike in hypnosis. Emmons recommends use of MT as a component of more extended therapeutic work, ranging from traditional insight-oriented therapy to cognitive-behavioral techniques.

USE OF MINDFULNESS MEDITATION: OTHER CLINICAL AND PRACTICAL ISSUES

How to deliver mindfulness meditation instruction most effectively in the therapeutic environment is a key question, both in terms of clinical impact and in regard to patient receptivity, patient burden, and cost. Mindfulness meditation practice is more complex than is concentrative meditation in that there is no single focus, such as a mantra. For therapeutic value, most of the approaches either make use of group multisession programs or incorporate practice into ongoing psychotherapy. Taped programs (e.g., Salzberg & Goldstein, 2002) are also available for home use; other creative adaptations include the psoriasis treatment program developed by Jon Kabat-Zinn that delivered all instructions on brief audiotapes during medically standard phototherapy sessions.

Preference for Types of Practice

Individuals may have a preference for different types of practice. A group of MBSR participants (N = 135) were asked to rate different aspects of the program (sitting meditation, body scan, and yoga) on a 1–100 visual analogue scale (Kabat-Zinn, Chapman, & Salmon,1997). Although average scores did not differ much (sitting meditation: 64.5 [SD = 29.4]; body scan: 56.4 [SD = 33.1]; yoga: 62.4 [SD = 30.1]), there was considerable variability, with 44% of participants reporting at least a 20-point difference in preference between types of practice. This study also sought to confirm the hypothesis that differences in preference relate to underlying patterns of experiencing anxiety in that individuals higher in somatic anxiety prefer body-based interventions, whereas those with higher cognitive anxiety prefer more cognitive interventions, such as sitting meditation (Davidson, Goleman, & Schwartz, 1976; Schwartz, Davidson, & Goleman, 1978). Contrary to previous results, the opposite was found: Individuals high on cognitive anxiety and low on somatic anxiety (n = 9) had a stronger preference for hatha yoga practice (sitting meditation: 44.6; body scan: 55.8; yoga: 72.7), whereas the low cognitive anxiety–high somatic anxiety participants (n = 20) showed the opposite (sitting meditation: 72.5; body scan: 66.0; yoga: 53.9). However, correlations between anxiety ratings and preferences were low to nonexistent. Several implications for treatment can be considered. First, for those few individuals with high cognitive and low somatic anxiety (only 6.7% of this treatment group), adding a somatic component to treatment may be helpful. Because they may also poorly tolerate the experience of racing thoughts, such individuals may also benefit from adding a mantra component to the meditation practice, while gradually working toward use of mindfulness meditation. Individual variability in preference is poorly understood, so experimenting with different techniques with an individual client seems a viable approach.

Combining with Other Techniques

As noted earlier, mindfulness meditation can be readily combined with other therapeutic approaches, whether as adjunctive treatment or within ongoing individual or group therapy. For example, Kutz's work (Kutz, 1985) demonstrates the use of an MBSR-based treatment as an adjunct to insight-oriented therapy, whereas Linehan's work (Dimidjian & Linehan, 2003; Robins, 2002) with borderline personality disorder incorporates more limited meditation practice as a way to cultivate skills in mindfulness. Mindfulness meditation is strikingly compatible with a range of theoretically distinct approaches. The MBSR and MBSR-related programs (such as MBCT and MB-EAT) incorporate substantial amounts of cognitive-behavioral and educational components. The value of mindfulness practice for helping someone move beyond surface reactions and become more aware of subtle or complex feelings is compatible with insight-oriented psychodynamic approaches (Epstein, 1995; Rubin, 1985). The presumption—and evidence—that mindfulness meditation helps access higher levels of wisdom or spiritual experience in the face of stress or anxiety makes it compatible with transpersonal/humanistic approaches to therapy (Walsh, 1992, 1999a).

As noted earlier, virtually all meditation practices are combinations of concentrative and mindfulness techniques (Goleman, 1988). For example, use of a mantra during daily activities may help to disengage reactivity while engaging a sense of calm and wise awareness or mindfulness (Easwaren, 1991; Keating, 1997). Although most mindfulness practices being taught within therapeutic contexts avoid use of a mantra, some individuals may benefit from combining brief mantra-based practice with mindfulness meditation, particularly if they experience persistent intrusion of "racing" thoughts or experience increased agitation while practicing, as noted earlier in relation to individuals with high cognitive anxiety. Because a mantra engages the language center of the brain, it may be more effective than is a non-language-based focus (such as the breath) in interrupting intrusive or ruminative thinking.

Compliance and Adherence

Not all individuals will enjoy meditation practice or find it compelling. Completion rates of the MBSR program speak to this consideration. Within one 2-year period, of 784 individuals enrolled, 598 (76.3%) completed the program, with completion rates somewhat higher for individuals with stress-related syndromes (79%) than with chronic pain patterns (70%; Kabat-Zinn & Chapman-Waldrop, 1988). Considerable attention has been given to maintaining high levels of involvement in the MBSR program (Salmon, Santorelli, & Kabat-Zinn, 1998). The standard MBSR training and the MBCT therapy includes 45-minute meditation sessions, delivered by tapes, once per day. This length is modeled on the length of practice in traditional Vipassana and Zen settings. Briefer lengths have been used in adaptations of the MBSR with some groups, such as medical students. One concern with the 45-minute period is compliance, although evidence suggests that more practice occurs when longer sessions are used (Kabat-Zinn, personal communication, June 2004). Other adaptations of the MBSR program, such as MB-EAT, may use shorter tapes. Many teachers emphasize the regularity of practice over the length of practice. Sitting for even 10 minutes per day may be preferable to skipping days—or weeks. In the mindfulness tradition, even 3 minutes may reinforce the value of bringing a meditative or mindful perspective to a range of daily activities or tasks (Harp, 1996). In my experience working with students, brief but regular periods help them move toward valuing the transformative elements of meditation. Although it may be more important to transmit the importance of the mindful/aware experience than it is to focus on the length of time required, during initial periods of learning meditation, 20 minutes is probably an appropriate minimal goal for most individuals. Otherwise, it is less likely that the person will experience a shift in ability to focus attention and then to manage awareness. Offering the analogy of learning a musical instrument or a new sport can be helpful; patients understand that regular practice heightens the skills needed under the more challenging circumstances of a concert or a game.

As noted earlier, an important issue in clinical use of meditation is the degree to which practice, particularly of mindfulness, is carried over into everyday activities. Although there is artificiality in distinguishing between formal meditative practice and integrating the lessons or results of that practice into daily life, it is an issue particularly important to consider in the therapeutic context. Although continued formal practice (sitting every day or most days) unquestionably deepens and sustains the effects achieved, it is the transfer of mindfulness to everyday life that is particularly important.

Other Challenges to Practice

Gunaratana, a Sri Lanka Buddhist monk and meditation teacher, in his useful small book *Mindfulness in Plain English* (Gunaratana, 1991), outlines 11 problems that arise when meditating, including physical pain, "odd" sensations, drowsiness, inability to concentrate, boredom, fear, agitation, and trying too hard. He addresses each one, with the common thread being encouragement simply to observe each of these experiences as aspects of the mind and the self that may arise even for experienced meditators. It is also useful to realize that if these states arise during meditation practice, they may be present in the background of other activities and represent issues to be dealt with. Typically, most individuals are able to find enough calm in the midst of these experiences to be encouraged to continue to practice. Occasionally, someone reports that his or her mind is racing so much that he or she is unable to find any type of relaxation at all during the initial experiences. This may occur regardless of whether the content of the thoughts is distressing. Reassurance that such agitation reflects a common aspect of the mind, that he or she is not "going crazy," that with 1–2 weeks of practice this should improve, and that such experience reflects an ever-greater potential value of meditation can help increase someone's willingness to stay with developing a practice. More active approaches to working with such experiences can include using a mantra, the technique of "noting," meditating with eyes open with a low unfocused gaze (as in Zen meditation), or using shorter time periods. As practice advances, the person may be able to more easily simply "watch" the rush of thoughts as they arise, but this remains difficult until there has been at least some successful experience of relaxation.

Another pitfall may occur in more advanced meditators who misunderstand Buddhist-based teachings as requiring that one give up the ego or any sense of self. Rather than cultivating mindful awareness of the natural fluctuations of human experience, they suppress the presence of craving or desire to try to meet a goal of psychological growth or spiritual attainment that is unrealistic, particularly at their level of practice. Epstein (1995) discusses this as confusion between "egolessness" as direct realization that desires or aversions do not define the "self," versus a steady state that can rarely be sustained. Although this issue seldom arises in therapeutic use of meditation in beginners, it may be a concern in individuals who pursue substantial reading in traditional teachings or who attend meditation retreats without understanding the broader context of the teaching.

Uncovering Memories, Dissociation, and Trance Experiences

Mindfulness meditation is often characterized as cultivating the ability to "fall awake," but all meditative approaches have the potential to induce trance states, access hidden memories, or create dissociative experiences (Walsh & Shapiro, 2006). Kutz and his colleagues (Kutz, 1985), in the study described earlier that investigated a mindfulness-based meditation program as an adjunct to traditional psychotherapy, also carefully assessed the occurrence of untoward or unpleasant reactions; they found that 4 of the 20 patients recovered memories of a past traumatic event. Others described increases in feelings of "defenselessness," leading to emotionality, anger, fear, and despair. These experiences were, however, balanced by an enhanced sense of self and inner centeredness. For example, one of the therapists noted that a hypochondriacal patient, in dealing with the increased sadness experienced during meditation, finally understood that her excessive concern with physical health had functioned as a defense. This insight almost immediately lessened her preoccupations with somatic symptoms and health problems.

As noted earlier, the prevalence of traumatic reactions within the MBSR program, which draws from a general medical population, has tended to be very low, generally under 1%. Within a psychiatric setting, such experiences may be far more prevalent. Within my own therapy practice, they have covered a range: a woman who found the mild dissociation she could induce so appealing that she began to "zone out" to avoid engaging with her husband ("I could be right there, and he didn't even know I was somewhere else"); an older man who recovered memories of childhood sexual abuse within 1 week of practice; and a woman who, on trying meditation for treatment for smoking, immediately (within 5 minutes) became flooded with images related to severe sexual abuse. In the case of the first woman, we reviewed appropriate use of meditation practice and explored the need for marital counseling; in the second case, the client decided he wished to continue meditating but followed it with journaling so we could more readily use recovered material in therapy; in the third case, the woman became aware that she had been using her smoking as a way to suppress these memories of abuse, and therefore she decided to return to her previous therapist for more in-depth work. There are also individuals who, for reasons that are not well understood, will experience extremely vivid and even bizarre imagery while meditating, without this necessarily signifying a history of significant abuse or psychiatric problems. Such individuals may need to work to modulating the depth or type of meditation used, to consult with senior meditation teachers, or to further explore the significance of the imagery in other therapeutic contexts.

Therapist Training and Practice

It is very important that a therapist have substantive personal experience with meditation practice before using it professionally. As in hypnotherapy, internal experiences are being cultivated, and it is difficult, if not impossible, to understand the reports of the client in regard to such experiences if one has not practiced it oneself. The certification programs developed for the MBSR program assume that individuals who begin the certification program already have a personal sitting practice. At the same time, it is increasingly recognized that practicing at the level of a meditation "master" is not necessary for incorporating basic techniques into a therapeutic context or for teaching such techniques to others. Personal practice is best started, if available, with a local sitting group or meditation center, where ongoing support is more readily available, or at one of the several Vipassana or insight meditation retreat centers around the country. As Lesh (1970) noted, cultivating mindful awareness may also benefit the clinician in maintaining focus and cultivating empathic concern. Karen Horney (1945, 1987), who was exposed to Zen practice through contact with D. T. Suzuki, found that it allowed her to cultivate "wholehearted attention," a capacity that contributes to high-quality therapy.

Maintenance of Practice

One question often raised regarding the value of meditation training is whether individuals will continue to practice on their own once formal instruction or involvement with a meditation group has ceased, the implication being that there is little value in learning meditation if it is not practiced on an extended basis. This is a valid question within contemporary clinical practice, and it has been frequently addressed within the traditional literature. It is also a more complicated question than it seems and one that is grappled with in a number of areas of therapeutic practice and behavioral change. For example, there is no question that improving diet or exercise has value; maintaining such improvements is well recognized to be a separate issue.

Mindfulness meditation training might be considered as analogous to certain types of therapeutic interventions, such as cognitive restructuring, in that it is cultivating a set of skills in addition to inducing a particular state of being. The individual who has participated in a substantial meditation experience learns how to better shift attention at will, to focus more easily, to use the breath to facilitate physical relaxation, to recognize emotional reactivity more quickly, and to return to a state of equanimity. Such abilities exist independent of meditation practice, but they are rarely as systematically cultivated.

In the long-term follow-up of Kabat-Zinn's study of individuals with anxiety and panic attacks (Miller, Fletcher, & Kabat-Zinn, 1997; Miller et al., 1995) effects were maintained up to 5 years, yet only about half of the participants reported any continued use of meditation practice, and most of that was irregular. Long-term follow-up of chronic pain patients (Kabat-Zinn, Lipworth, Burney, & Sellers, 1986) revealed similar patterns; about half of participants available for follow-up reported continued use of breath awareness up through 4 years, with 30–40% reporting regular sitting practice (at least 3 times/week for 15 minutes or more). A practice effect on pain experience was evident, but it failed to reach statistical significance due to sample size limitations. Much like any skill (playing a musical instrument, learning a sport), basic capacities are retained to a substantial degree, but regular practice will deepen and expand them.

Continued sitting practice appeals to many individuals and undoubtedly deepens the experience, contributing to an ability to handle difficult situations with equanimity and to maintaining the likelihood of drawing on mindfulness under a range of circumstances. Many individuals maintain regular sitting, coupled with occasional longer retreats, feeling that this combination allows them to deepen their stress management skills and to access an inner wisdom and insight more readily and that it cultivates spiritual growth, self-acceptance, and compassion for others.

RESOURCE MATERIAL

Several types of resources can be considered in introducing clients to mindfulness meditation practice, including reading materials and referral to meditation sitting groups or retreats. Many communities have ongoing sitting groups, which may help a client deepen a personal practice and provide group support, particularly if he or she is otherwise learning meditation within an individual therapy context. Whether a client is encouraged to attend a retreat, for a weekend or longer, should probably depend on the client's enthusiasm for practice. Most sitting groups and retreat environments are focused on a particular tradition (i.e., Zen, Tibetan, or Vipassana), so that should be investigated either by the therapist or the client and preferably considered in relation both to therapeutic goals and to the specific training or spiritual messages that might be conveyed. The programs offered at the Omega Institute in Rhinebeck, New York, tend to be wide ranging in focus (*www.omega.com*).

A substantial amount of available resource material is appropriate for helping beginning meditators understand and appreciate the potential value of practice. One consideration in suggesting material is whether a client is interested in the spiritual context of meditative traditions. Clients who are unfamiliar with the literature available may be put off by the religious or spiritually oriented material shelved with other books on meditation in a typical large bookstore. The list of suggested resources at the end of the chapter contains several highly readable guides that present meditation practice from a secular perspective. *Meditation for Dummies* (Bodian, 1999) is a particularly well-balanced overview of different meditation approaches at an introductory level. I generally ask clients whether they have read material or used meditation tapes. If I am unfamiliar with the material, I ask the client to bring it in to show me; this often helps identify sources of misunderstanding or clarify the type of previous experience they have had.

CASE EXAMPLE

Choosing a case example to illustrate use of mindfulness meditation in a therapeutic context is challenging. The applications have been quite varied and are becoming increasingly so; furthermore, much of the empirically validated use is within a group context, presenting distinct challenges for identifying a single typical case. In regard to the MBSR program, *Full Catastrophe Living* (Kabat-Zinn, 1990) presents substantial case material, much of it related to chronic pain management. Segal and his colleagues (Segal et al., 2002), in their manual on Mindfulness-Based Cognitive Therapy for depression, also present useful case material. In relation to use of mindfulness meditation in individual therapy, Germer and his colleagues (Germer et al., 2005) illustrate a range of applications of varying types of mindfulness practice in psychotherapy. Jeffrey Rubin (1996) and Tara Brach (2003) also draw on rich case material to illustrate their applications of mindfulness-based approaches in therapy.

The case presented here is that of a 40-year-old woman who participated in our MB-EAT program and then continued in individual therapy under my supervision. This case illustrates how someone can draw substantial benefit from a highly structured group experience that utilizes both general sitting practice and guided meditations; that benefit can then be deepened by integrating meditation work into individual treatment. M.W. entered our treatment program for binge-eating disorder. She weighed more than 300 pounds, was married, and worked as a master's-level therapist. She was vivacious, very intelligent, and extremely articulate, and she acknowledged turning to food primarily to manage stress. She had tried many diets, often losing substantial amounts of weight and then gaining it back. She had grown up in a professional family that placed substantial importance on physical fitness and weight, but she had struggled with weight since childhood and admitted having binge-eat problems since age 15. Aside from meeting criteria for binge eating disorder, she had no other notable psychiatric symptoms, but she had a history of sexual abuse in childhood. She acknowledged that although she projected a confident persona, she was in reality extremely hard on herself, with much of the negative self-judgment focused on her inability to control her weight and eating.

During the MB-EAT program, she responded very positively to the meditation practice, reporting high levels of compliance with sitting, and noting how valuable the mindfulness exercises were in staying away from automatic eating. Unlike most of the group participants who found the meditation practice particularly valuable, she lost little or no weight during the group treatment. However, she noted that her relationship to food changed markedly. She said that she had learned to "honor my hunger," became aware of satiety, and came to "care about what I put in my body," and her eating patterns continued to improve during the 4-month follow-up. When being interviewed almost 3 years later, she recalled the last meal that she ate with the group (a buffet prepared by group members) as "one of the best meals I've ever eaten in my life."

Several months after the end of the group, she began individual therapy with one of her group coleaders, with the focus primarily on interpersonal relations and some other long-standing issues. Two and a half years later, she had begun to focus on weight issues again, enrolling first in a commercial high-protein weight-loss program and then in Weight Watchers, and had lost over 50 pounds. At that time, she acknowledged binge eating only a few times a year; when she did, she said she was always mindful of the circumstances and used the episode to examine why her stress levels were high enough to trigger the binge. She also noted that although she was no longer as hungry for rich foods, she actually enjoyed food more and that it played a better role in her life. She also noted that she was now able to tolerate "slips" in her dieting efforts, without these triggering binges. Although she was rarely practicing formal meditation, she frequently used mindfulness and breath awareness and continued to attribute much of her self-growth, not only in regard to eating but also in relation to other areas of her life, to the meditation training and practice, saying "it helps me hook into my inner wisdom. Meditation slows you down enough to be in touch with God . . . and God lives in all of us."

COMMENTS AND REFLECTIONS

I have tried to convey the potential value of mindfulness meditation within the therapy context. There is a growing appreciation of mindfulness as a cognitive process that is powerful in its potential for heightening self-regulation and for disengaging the type of automatic reactivity, whether emotional or behavioral, that leads to suffering. Meditation practice, although not the only path to cultivating an ability to bring mindfulness into moment-to-moment activity, is certainly a powerful one. Over the past 25 years, the range and complexity of mindfulness meditation practices is being increasingly recognized and appreciated. The empirical foundation for understanding the value of mindfulness-based approaches is growing rapidly, both within the framework of "stress management" and more broadly as a means to understanding how optimal functioning may require optimal management of stress-inducing situations. As with a number of other stress management approaches outlined in this volume, it is important to keep in mind that many of these approaches go far beyond relatively simple "relaxation" effects in their value to individuals. Mindfulness meditation may, in particular, provide clients with tools to engage the full range of their capabilities without becoming caught up in patterns of overdetermined emotional and behavioral reactions to stress situations.

REFERENCES

Arnold, L. E. (2001). Alternative treatments for adults with attention-deficit hyperactivity disorder (ADHD). *Annals of the New York Academy of Sciences, 931*, 310–341.

Astin, J. A. (1997). Stress reduction through mindfulness meditation: Effects on psychological symptomatology, sense of control, and spiritual experiences. *Psychotherapy and Psychosomatics, 66*(2), 97–106.

Astin, J. A., Berman, B. M., Bausell, B., Lee, W.-L., Hochberg, M., & Forys, K. L. (2003). The efficacy of mindfulness meditation plus qigong movement therapy in the treatment of fibromyalgia: A randomized controlled trial. *Journal Of Rheumatology, 30*(10), 2257–2262.

Austin, J. H. (1998). *Zen and the brain: Toward an understanding of meditation and consciousness.* Cambridge, MA: MIT Press.

Austin, J. H. (2006). *Zen-brain reflections: Reviewing recent developments in meditation and states of consciousness.* Cambridge, MA: MIT Press.

Bach, P., & Hayes, S. C. (2002). The use of acceptance and commitment therapy to prevent the rehospitalization of psychotic patients: A randomized controlled trial. *Journal of Consulting and Clinical Psychology, 70*(5), 1129–1139.

Baer, R. A. (2003). Mindfulness training as a clinical intervention: A conceptual and empirical review. *Clinical Psychology: Science and Practice, 10*(2), 125–143.

Baer, R. A., Smith, G. T., & Allen, K. B. (2004). Assessment of mindfulness by self-report: The Kentucky Inventory of Mindfulness Skills. *Assessment, 11*, 191–204.

Baer, R. A., Smith, G. T., Hopkins, J., Krietemeyer, J., & Toney, L. (2006). Using self-report assessment methods to explore facets of mindfulness. *Assessment, 13*(1), 27–45.

Bankart, C. P. (2006). *Freeing the angry mind.* Oakland, CA: New Harbinger Press.

Benson, H. (1975). *The relaxation response.* New York: Morrow.

Benson, H. (1982). Body temperature changes during the practice of g Tum-mo yoga. *Nature, 295*(5846), 234–236.

Bernhard, J. D., Kristeller, J., & Kabat-Zinn, J. (1988). Effectiveness of relaxation and visualization techniques as an adjunct to phototherapy and photochemotherapy of psoriasis. *Journal of the American Academy of Dermatology, 19*(3), 572–574.

Bishop, S. R., Lau, M., Shapiro, S., Carlson, L., Anderson, N. D., Carmody, J., et al. (2004). Mindfulness: A proposed operational definition. *Clinical Psychology: Science and Practice, 11*(3), 230–241.

Boals, G. F. (1978). Toward a cognitive reconceptualization of meditation. *Journal of Transpersonal Psychology, 10*(2), 143–182.

Bodhi, B. (2000). *The connected discourses of the Buddha: A new translation of the Samyutta nikaya* (Vol. 2). Boston: Wisdom.

Bodian, S. (1999). *Meditation for dummies.* Foster City, CA: IDG Books Worldwide.

Bowen, S., Witkeiwitz, K., Dillworth, T., Chawla, N., Simpson, T., Ostafin, B., et al. (2006). Mindfulness meditation and substance use in an incarcerated population. *Psychology of Addictive Behaviors, 20*(3), 343–347.

Brach, T. (2003). *Radical acceptance: Embracing your life with the heart of a buddha.* New York: Bantam Books.

Breslin, F. C., Zack, M., & McMain, S. (2002). An information-processing analysis of mindfulness: Implications for relapse prevention in the treatment of substance abuse. *Clinical Psychology, 9,* 275–299.

Brown, D., & Engler, J. (1984). A Rorschach study of the stages of mindfulness meditation. In D. Shapiro & R. N. Walsh (Eds.), *Meditation: Classic and contemporary perspectives* (pp. 232–262). New York: Aldine.

Brown, D., Forte, M., Rich, P., & Epstein, G. (1982). Phenomenological differences among self hypnosis, mindfulness meditation, and imaging. *Imagination, Cognition and Personality, 2*(4), 291–309.

Brown, D. P., & Fromm, E. (1988). Hypnotic treatment of asthma. *Advances, 5*(2), 15–27.

Brown, K. W., & Ryan, R. M. (2003). The benefits of being present: Mindfulness and its role in psychological well-being. *Journal of Personality and Social Psychology, 84*(4), 822–848.

Brown, K. W., & Ryan, R. M. (2004). Perils and promise in defining and measuring mindfulness: Observations from experience. *Clinical Psychology: Science and Practice, 11*(3), 242–248.

Buchheld, N., & Walach, H. (2002). Achtsamkeit in vipassana-meditation und psychotherapie: Die entwicklung des 'freiburger fragebogens zur achtsamkeit.' *Zeitschrift für Klinische Psychologie, Psychiatrie und Psychotherapie, 50*(2), 153–172.

Budilovsky, J., & Adamson, E. (2002). *The complete idiot's guide to meditation* (2nd ed.). New York: Alpha.

Carlson, L. E., Speca, M., Patel, K. D., & Goodey, E. (2003). Mindfulness-based stress reduction in relation to quality of life, mood, symptoms of stress, and immune parameters in breast and prostate cancer outpatients. *Psychosomatic Medicine, 65*(4), 571–581.

Carlson, L. E., Speca, M., Patel, K. D., & Goodey, E. (2004). Mindfulness-based stress reduction in relation to quality of life, mood, symptoms of stress and levels of cortisol, dehydroepiandrosterone sulfate (dheas) and melatonin in breast and prostate cancer outpatients. *Psychoneuroendocrinology, 29*(4), 448–474.

Carmody, J., Reed, G., Kristeller, J. L., & Merriam, P. (in press). Mindfulness, spirituality, and health-related symptoms. *Journal of Psychosomatic Research.*

Carrington, P. (1998). *The book of meditation.* Boston: Element Press.

Carson, J. W., Carson, K. M., Gil, K. M., & Baucom, D. H. (2004). Mindfulness-based relationship enhancement. *Behavior Therapy, 35*(3), 471–494.

Chadwick, P., Mead, S., & Lilley, B. (2004). *Responding mindfully to unpleasant thoughts and images: Reliability and validity of the mindfulness questionnaire.* Manuscript in preparation.

Chadwick, P., Taylor, K. N., & Abba, N. (2005). Mindfulness groups for people with psychosis. *Behavioural and Cognitive Psychotherapy, 33*(3), 351–359.

Cloninger, C. R., Svrakic, D. M., & Przybeck, T. R. (1993). A psychobiological model of temperament and character. *Archives of General Psychiatry, 50*(12), 975–990.

Coleman, J. W. (2001). *The new Buddhism.* New York: Oxford University Press.

Cox, R. J. (2000). Relating different types of Christian prayer to religious and psychological measures of well-being. *Dissertation Abstracts International, 61*(2), 1075.

Cuthbert, B., Kristeller, J., Simons, R., Hodes, R., & Lang, P. J. (1981). Strategies of arousal control: Biofeedback, meditation, and motivation. *Journal of Experimental Psychology: General, 110*(4), 518–546.

D'Aquili, E. G., & Newburg, A. B. (1998). The neuropsychological basis of religions, or why God won't go away. *Zygon: Journal of Religion and Science, 33*(2), 187–201.

Dass, R. (1987). A ten-year perspective. In D. Anthony & B. Ecker (Eds.), *Spiritual choices: The problems of recognizing authentic paths to inner transformation* (pp. 139–152). St. Paul, MN: Paragon House.

Davidson, R. J., Goleman, D. J., & Schwartz, G. E. (1976). Attentional and affective concomitants of meditation: A cross-sectional study. *Journal of Abnormal Psychology, 85*(2), 235–238.

Davidson, R. J., & Harrington, A. (Eds.). (2002). *Visions of compassion: Western scientists and Tibetan Buddhists examine human nature.* New York: Oxford University Press.

Davidson, R. J., Kabat-Zinn, J., Schumacher, J., Rosenkranz, M., Muller, D., Santorelli, S. F., et al. (2003). Alterations in brain and immune function produced by mindfulness meditation. *Psychosomatic Medicine, 65*(4), 564–570.

Delmonte, M. M. (1985). Meditation and anxiety reduction: A literature review. *Clinical Psychology Review, 5*(2), 91–102.

Delmonte, M. M. (1990a). George Kelly's personal construct theory: Some comparisons with Freudian theory. *Psychologia: An International Journal of Psychology in the Orient, 33*(2), 73–83.

Delmonte, M. M. (1990b). Meditation and change: Mindfulness versus repression. *Australian Journal of Clinical Hypnotherapy and Hypnosis, 11*(2), 57–63.

Delmonte, M. M. (1990c). Repression and somatization: A case history of hemodynamic activation. *International Journal of Psychosomatics, 37*(1), 37–39.

Dimidjian, S., & Linehan, M. M. (2003). Defining an agenda for future research on the clinical application of mindfulness practice. *Clinical Psychology: Science and Practice, 10*(2), 166–171.

Dunn, B. R., Hartigan, J. A., & Mikulas, W. L. (1999). Concentration and mindfulness meditations: Unique forms of consciousness? *Applied Psychophysiology and Biofeedback, 24*(3), 147–165.

Easterlin, B. L., & Cardena, E. (1998). Cognitive and emotional differences between short- and long-term vipassana meditators. *Imagination, Cognition and Personality, 18*(1), 69–81.

Easwaren, E. (1991). *Meditation: A simple 8-point path for translating spiritual ideals into daily life.* Tomales, CA: Nilgiri Press.

Emmons, M. L. (1978). *The inner source: A guide to meditative therapy.* San Luis Obispo, CA: Impact.

Emmons, M. L., & Emmons, J. (2000). *Meditative therapy.* Atascadero, CA: Impact.

Engler, J. (1998). Buddhist psychology: Contributions to Western psychological theory. In A. Molino (Ed.), *The couch and the tree: Dialogues in psychoanalysis and Buddhism* (pp. 111–118). New York: North Point Press.

Epstein, M. (1995). *Thoughts without a thinker: Psychotherapy from a Buddhist perspective.* New York: Basic Books.

Epstein, M. (2001). *Going on being: Buddhism and the way of change, a positive psychology for the West.* New York: Broadway Books.

Feldman, G. C., Hayes, A. M., Kumar, S. M., Greeson, J. M., & Larenceau, J. P. (in press). Development, factor structure, and initial validation of the cognitive and affective mindfulness scale. *Journal of Psychopathology and Behavioral Assessment.*

Fontana, D., & Slack, I. (1997). *Teaching meditation to children.* Boston: Element Books.

Forester, B., Kornfeld, D. S., Fleiss, J. L., & Thompson, S. (1993). Group psychotherapy during radiotherapy: Effects on emotional and physical distress. *American Journal of Psychiatry, 150*(11), 1700–1706.

Fromm, E. (1994). *The art of being.* London: Continuum International.

Fulton, P. R. (2005). Mindfulness as clinical training. In C. K. Germer, R. D. Siegel, & P. R. Fulton (Eds.), *Mindfulness and psychotherapy* (pp. 55–72). New York: Guilford Press.

Germer, C. K., Siegel, R. D., & Fulton, P. R. (Eds.). (2005). *Mindfulness and psychotherapy.* New York: Guilford Press.

Ghoncheh, S., & Smith, J. C. (2004). Progressive muscle relaxation, yoga stretching, and ABC relaxation theory. *Journal of Clinical Psychology, 60*(1), 131–136.

Gifford-May, D., & Thompson, N. L. (1994). "Deep states" of meditation: Phenomenological reports of experience. *Journal of Transpersonal Psychology, 26*(2), 117–138.

Glueck, B., & Stroebel, C. (1975). Biofeedback and meditation in the treatment of psychiatric illness. *Comprehensive Psychiatry, 16*(4), 303–321.

Goldenberg, D. L., Kaplan, K. H., Nadeau, M. G., Brodeur, C., Smith, S., & Schmid, C. H. (1994). A controlled study of a stress-reduction, cognitive-behavioral treatment program in fibromyalgia. *Journal of Musculoskeletal Pain, 2*(2), 53–66.

Goleman, D. (1988). *The meditative mind: The varieties of meditative experience.* New York: Putnam.

Goleman, D. (2003). *Destructive emotions: How can we overcome them? A scientific dialogue with the Dalai Lama.* New York: Bantam Books.

Grossman, P., Niemann, L., Schmidt, S., & Walach, H. (2004). Mindfulness-based stress reduction and health benefits: A meta-analysis. *Journal of Psychosomatic Research, 57*(1), 35–43.

Gunaratana, H. (1991). *Mindfulness in plain English.* Boston: Wisdom.

Haimerl, C. J., & Valentine, E. R. (2001). The effect of contemplative practice of intrapersonal, interpersonal, and transpersonal dimensions of the self-concept. *Journal of Transpersonal Psychology, 33*(1), 37–52.

Hanh, T. N. (1975). *The miracle of mindfulness.* Boston: Beacon Press.

Hanh, T. N. (1991). *Peace is every step.* Berkeley, CA: Parallax Press.

Hanh, T. N. (1995). *Living Buddha, living Christ.* New York: Riverhead Books.

Hanh, T. N. (1996). *Breathe! You are alive.* New York: Bantam Books.

Hanh, T. N. (1997). *Teachings on love.* Berkeley, CA: Parallax Press.

Harp, D. (1996). *The three minute meditator* (3rd ed.). Oakland, CA: New Harbinger.

Hart, W. (1987). *The art of living: Vipassana meditation as taught by S. N. Goenka.* San Francisco: HarperCollins.

Hayes, A. M., & Feldman, G. (2004). Clarifying the construct of mindfulness in the context of emotion regulation and the process of change in therapy. *Clinical Psychology: Science and Practice, 11*(3), 255–262.

Hayes, S. C., Strosahl, K. D., & Wilson, K. G. (1999). *Acceptance and commitment therapy: An experiential approach to behavior change.* New York: Guilford Press.

Hesslinger, B., van Elst, L. T., Nyberg, E., Dykierek, P., Richter, H., Berner, M., et al. (2002). Psychotherapy of attention deficit hyperactivity disorder in adults: A pilot study using a structured skills training program. *European Archives of Psychiatry and Clinical Neuroscience, 252*(4), 177–184.

Holroyd, J. (2003). The science of meditation and the state of hypnosis. *American Journal of Clinical Hypnosis, 46*(2), 109–128.

Horney, K. (1945). *Our inner conflicts.* New York: Norton.

Horney, K. (1987). *Final lectures.* New York: Norton.

Kabat-Zinn, J. (1990). *Full catastrophe living.* New York: Delacorte Press.

Kabat-Zinn, J. (2005). *Coming to our senses: Healing ourselves and the world through mindfulness.* New York: Hyperion.

Kabat-Zinn, J., Chapman, A., & Salmon, P. (1997). The relationship of cognitive and somatic components of anxiety to patient preference for alternative relaxation techniques. *Mind/Body Medicine, 2,* 101–109.

Kabat-Zinn, J., & Chapman-Waldrop, A. (1988). Compliance with an outpatient stress reduction program: Rates and predictors of program completion. *Journal of Behavioral Medicine, 11*(4), 333–352.

Kabat-Zinn, J., Lipworth, L., & Burney, R. (1985). The clinical use of mindfulness meditation for the self-regulation of chronic pain. *Journal of Behavioral Medicine, 8*(2), 163–190.

Kabat-Zinn, J., Lipworth, L., Burney, R., & Sellers, W. (1986). Four-year follow-up of a meditation-based program for the self-regulation of chronic pain: Treatment outcomes and compliance. *Clinical Journal of Pain, 2,* 159–173.

Kabat-Zinn, J., Massion, A., Hebert, J., & Rosenbaum, E. (1998). Meditation. In J. Holland (Ed.), *Psycho-oncology* (pp. 767–779). Oxford, UK: Oxford University Press.

Kabat-Zinn, J., Massion, A. O., Kristeller, J., Peterson, L. G., Fletcher, K. E., Pbert, L., et al. (1992). Effectiveness of a meditation-based stress reduction program in the treatment of anxiety disorders. *American Journal of Psychiatry, 149*(7), 936–943.

Kabat-Zinn, J., Wheeler, E., Light, T., Skillings, A., Scharf, M. J., Cropley, T. G., et al. (1998). Influence of a mindfulness meditation–based stress reduction intervention on rates of skin clearing in patients with moderate to severe psoriasis undergoing phototherapy (uvb) and photochemotherapy (puva). *Psychosomatic Medicine, 60*(5), 625–632.

Keating, T. (1997). *Active meditations for contemplative prayer.* New York: Continuum.

Kornfield, J. (1993). *A path with heart.* New York: Bantam Books.

Kristeller, J. (2004). Meditation: Multiple effects, a unitary process? In M. Blows, S. Srinivasan, J. Blows, C. P. Bankart, M. M. Delmonte, & Y. Haruki (Eds.), *The relevance of the wisdom traditions in contemporary society: The challenge to psychology* (pp. 21–37). Delft, the Netherlands: Eburon.

Kristeller, J., Hallett, B., & Wolever, R. Q. (2003). *A mindfulness meditation–based treatment for binge eating disorder: Treatment manual.* Unpublished manuscript.

Kristeller, J., & Johnson, T. (2005). Cultivating loving kindness: A two-stage model of the effects of meditation on empathy, compassion, and altruism. *Zygon, 40,* 391–407.

Kristeller, J. L., Baer, R. A., & Quillian-Wolever, R. (2006). Mindfulness-based approaches to eating disorders. In R. A. Baer (Ed.), *Mindfulness-based treatment approaches* (pp. 75–93). Burlington, MA: Academic Press.

Kristeller, J. L., & Hallett, C. B. (1999). An exploratory study of a meditation-based intervention for binge eating disorder. *Journal of Health Psychology, 4*(3), 357–363.

Kristeller, J. L., Rhodes, M., Cripe, L., & Sheets, V. (2006). Exploring spiritual and religious concerns with cancer patients improves quality of life and relationship with physician. *International Journal of Psychiatry in Medicine, 35,* 329–347.

Kutz, I. (1985). Meditation as an adjunct to psychotherapy: An outcome study. *Psychotherapy and Psychosomatics, 43*(4), 209–218.

Kutz, I., Borysenko, J. Z., & Benson, H. (1985). Meditation and psychotherapy: A rationale for the integration of dynamic psychotherapy, the relaxation response, and mindfulness meditation. *American Journal of Psychiatry, 142*(1), 1–8.

Kwee, M., & Ellis, A. (1998). The interface between rational emotive behavior therapy (REBT) and Zen. *Journal of Rational-Emotive and Cognitive Behavior Therapy, 16*(1), 5–43.

Lazar, S. W., Bush, G., Gollub, R. L., Fricchione, G. L., Khalsa, G., & Benson, H. (2000). Functional brain mapping of the relaxation response and meditation. *NeuroReport, 11*(7), 1581–1585.

Lazar, S. W., Kerr, C., Wasserman, R. H., Gray, J. R., Greve, D., Treadway, M. T., et al. (2005). Meditation experience is associated with increased cortical thickness. *NeuroReport, 16,* 1893–1897.

Lehrer, P. M. (1983). Progressive relaxation and meditation: A study of psychophysiological and therapeutic differences between two techniques. *Behaviour Research and Therapy, 21*(6), 651–662.

Lehrer, P. M., Sasaki, Y., & Saito, Y. (1999). Zazen and cardiac variability. *Psychosomatic Medicine, 61*(6), 812–821.

Lehrer, P. M., & Woolfolk, R. L. (1994). Respiratory system involvement in Western relaxation and self-regulation. In B. H. Timmons & R. Ley (Eds.), *Behavioral and Psychological Approaches to Breathing Disorders* (pp. 191–203). New York: Plenum Press.

Leigh, J., Bowen, S., & Marlatt, G. A. (2005). Spirituality, mindfulness and substance abuse. *Addictive Behaviors, 30*(7), 1335–1341.

Lesh, T. V. (1970). Zen meditation and the development of empathy in counselors. *Journal of Humanistic Psychology, 10*(1), 39–74.

Linden, W. (1973). Practicing of meditation by school children and their levels of field dependence–independence, test anxiety, and reading achievement. *Journal of Consulting and Clinical Psychology, 41*(1), 139–143.

Linehan, M. M. (1993a). *Cognitive-behavioral treatment of borderline personality disorder.* New York: Guilford Press.

Linehan, M. M. (1993b). *Skills training manual for treating borderline personality disorder.* New York: Guilford Press.

Lutz, A., Greischar, L. L., Rawlings, N. B., Ricard, M., & Davidson, R. J. (2004). Long-term meditators self-induce high-amplitude gamma synchrony during mental practice. *Proceedings of the National Academy of Sciences of the U.S.A., 101*(46), 16369–16373.

Lynch, T. R., & Bronner, L. (2006). Mindfulness and dialectical behavior therapy: Application with depressed older adults with personality disorders. In R. A. Baer (Ed.), *Mindfulness and acceptance-based interventions: Conceptualization, application and empirical support* (pp. 217–236). Burlington, MA: Academic Press.

Ma, S. H., & Teasdale, J. D. (2004). Mindfulness-based cognitive therapy for depression: Replication and exploration of differential relapse prevention effects. *Journal of Consulting and Clinical Psychology, 72*(1), 31–40.

Mahoney, M. J. (2003). *Constructive psychotherapy: A practical guide.* New York: Guilford Press.

Marlatt, G. A., & Kristeller, J. L. (1999). Mindfulness and meditation. In W. R. Miller (Ed.), *Integrating spirituality into treatment: Resources for practitioners* (pp. 67–84). Washington, DC: American Psychological Association.

Marlatt, G. A., Witkiewitz, K., Dillworth, T. M., Bowen, S. W., Parks, G. A., Macpherson, L. M., et al. (2004). Vipassana meditation as a treatment for alcohol and drug use disorders. In S. C. Hayes, V. M. Follette, & M. M. Linehan (Eds.), *Mindfulness and acceptance: Expanding the cognitive-behavioral tradition* (pp. 261–287). New York: Guilford Press.

Marriott, J. A. (1989). The "cord" component in panic attack syndrome: Five case studies. *Australian Journal of Clinical Hypnotherapy and Hypnosis, 10*(1), 17–24.

Menahemi, A. (Director), & Ariel, E. (Writer). (1997). *Doing time, doing vipassana* [DVD]. Karuna Films.

Miller, J., Fletcher, K., & Kabat-Zinn, J. (1997). Three-year follow-up and clinical implications of a mindfulness meditation–based stress reduction intervention in the treatment of anxiety disorders. *Mind/Body Medicine, 2*(3), 101–109.

Miller, J. J., Fletcher, K., & Kabat-Zinn, J. (1995). Three-year follow-up and clinical implications of a mindfulness meditation–based stress reduction intervention in the treatment of anxiety disorders. *General Hospital Psychiatry, 17*(3), 192–200.

Mruk, C. J., & Hartzell, J. (2003). *Zen and psychotherapy: Integrating traditional and nontraditional approaches.* New York: Springer.

Murphy, M., Donovan, S., & Taylor, E. (1999). *The physical and psychological effects of meditation: A review of contemporary research with a comprehensive bibliography, 1981–1996.* Sausalito, CA: Institute of Noetic Science.

Otani, A. (2003). Eastern meditative techniques and hypnosis: A new synthesis. *American Journal of Clinical Hypnosis, 46*(2), 97–108.

Pargament, K. I. (1997). *The psychology of religion and coping: Theory, research, practice.* New York: Guilford Press.

Peterman, A. H., Fitchett, G., Brady, M. J., Hernandez, L., & Cella, D. (2002). Measuring spiritual well-being in people with cancer: The Functional Assessment of Chronic Illness Therapy–Spiritual Well-Being Scale (FACIT-SP). *Annals of Behavioral Medicine, 24*(1), 49–58.

Plews-Ogan, M., Owens, J. E., Goodman, M., Wolfe, P., & Schorling, J. (2005). A pilot study evaluating mindfulness-based stress reduction and massage for the management of chronic pain [Electronic version]. *Journal Of General Internal Medicine, 20*(12), 1136–1138.

Reibel, D. K., Greeson, J. M., Brainard, G. C., & Rosenzweig, S. (2001). Mindfulness-based stress reduction and health-related quality of life in a heterogeneous patient population. *General Hospital Psychiatry, 23*(4), 183–192.

Ricard, M. (2006). *Happiness: A guide to developing life's most important skill.* New York: Little, Brown.

Robins, C. J. (2002). Zen principles and mindfulness practice in dialectical behavior therapy. *Cognitive and Behavioral Practice, 9*(1), 50–57.

Rosenbaum, E. H., & Rosenbaum, I. (2005). *Everyone's guide to cancer supportive care: A comprehensive handbook for patients and their families.* Kansas City, MO: Andrews McMeel.

Rosenbaum, R. (1998). *Zen and the heart of psychotherapy.* Philadelphia: Brunner/Mazel.

Rosenzweig, S., Reibel, D. K., Greeson, J. M., Brainard, G. C., & Hojat, M. (2003). Mindfulness-based stress reduction lowers psychological distress in medical students. *Teaching and Learning in Medicine, 15*(2), 88–92.

Rozman, D. (1994). *Meditating with children.* Boulder Creek, CA: Planetary Publications.

Rubin, J. B. (1985). Meditation and psychoanalytic listening. *Psychoanalytic Review, 72*(4), 599–613.

Rubin, J. B. (1996). *Psychotherapy and Buddhism: Toward an integration.* New York: Plenum Press.

Rubin, J. B. (1999). Close encounters of a new kind: Toward an integration of psychoanalysis and Buddhism. In R. Segall (Ed.), *Encountering Buddhism* (pp. 31–60). Albany: State University of New York Press.

Sagula, D., & Rice, K. G. (2004). The effectiveness of mindfulness training on the grieving process and emotional well-being of chronic pain patients. *Journal of Clinical Psychology in Medical Settings, 11*(4), 333–342.

Salmon, P., Santorelli, S., & Kabat-Zinn, J. (1998). Intervention elements promoting adherence to mindfulness-based stress reduction programs in the clinical behavioral medicine setting. In S. A. Shumaker, E. B. Schron, J. K. Ockene, & W. L. McBee (Eds.), *Handbook of health and behavior change* (2nd ed., pp. 239–266): New York: Springer.

Salzberg, S. (1999). *Voices of insight.* Boston: Shambhala.

Salzberg, S., & Goldstein, J. (2002). *Insight meditation: A step-by-step course on how to meditate.* Boulder, CO: Sounds True.

Saxe, G. A., Hebert, J. R., Carmody, J. F., Kabat-Zinn, J., Rosenzweig, P. H., Jarzobski, D., et al. (2001). Can diet in conjunction with stress reduction affect the rate of increase in prostate specific antigen after biochemical recurrence of prostate cancer? *Journal of Urology, 166*(6), 2202–2207.

Schwartz, G. E., Davidson, R. J., & Goleman, D. J. (1978). Patterning of cognitive and somatic processes in the self-regulation of anxiety: Effects of meditation versus exercise. *Psychosomatic Medicine, 40*(4), 321–328.

Segal, Z. V., Williams, J. M. G., & Teasdale, J. D. (2002). *Mindfulness-based cognitive therapy for depression: A new approach to preventing relapse.* New York: Guilford Press.

Segall, S. R. (2005). Mindfulness and self-development in psychotherapy. *Journal of Transpersonal Psychology, 37*(2), 143–163.

Semple, R. J., Lee, J., & Miller, L. F. (2006). Mindfulness-based cognitive therapy for children. In R. A. Baer (Ed.), *Mindfulness and acceptance-based interventions: Conceptualization, application and empirical support* (pp. 143–166). Burlington, MA: Academic Press.

Shapiro, D. H., & Walsh, R. N. (Eds.). (1984). *Meditation: Classic and contemporary perspectives.* New York: Aldine.

Shapiro, S. L., Astin, J., Bishop, S., & Cordova, M. (2005). Mindfulness-based stress reduction for health care professionals: Results from a randomized trial. *International Journal of Stress Management, 12*(2), 164–176.

Shapiro, S. L., Schwartz, G. E., & Bonner, G. (1998). Effects of mindfulness-based stress reduction on medical and premedical students. *Journal of Behavioral Medicine, 21*(6), 581–599.

Shapiro, S. L., & Walsh, R. (2003). An analysis of recent meditation research and suggestions for future directions. *Humanistic Psychologist, 31*(2), 86–114.

Shapiro, S. L., & Walsh, R. (2004). An analysis of recent meditation research and suggestions for future directions: Correction. *Humanistic Psychologist, 32*(1), 2.

Singer, W. (2001). Consciousness and the binding problem. *Annals of the New York Academy of Sciences, 929*, 123–146.

Smith, H., & Novak, P. (2003). *Buddhism: A concise introduction.* New York: HarperCollins.

Smith, J. C. (2003). "How sturdy is the empirical groundwork of clinical relaxation?" A reply. *PsycCRITIQUES, 48*(4), p. 530.

Smith, J. C. (2004). Alterations in brain and immune function produced by mindfulness meditation: Three caveats. *Psychosomatic Medicine, 66*(1), 148–149.

Smith, J. C., & Joyce, C. A. (2004). Mozart versus new age music: Relaxation states, stress, and ABC relaxation theory. *Journal of Music Therapy, 41*(3), 215–224.

Speca, M., Carlson, L. E., Goodey, E., & Angen, M. (2000). A randomized, wait-list controlled clinical trial: The effect of a mindfulness meditation–based stress reduction program on mood and symptoms of stress in cancer outpatients. *Psychosomatic Medicine, 62*(5), 613–622.

Speca, M., Carlson, L. E., Mackenzie, M. J., & Angen, M. (2006). Mindfulness-based stress reduction as an intervention for cancer patients. In R. A. Baer (Ed.), *Mindfulness and acceptance-based interventions: Conceptualization, application and empirical support* (pp. 239–261). Burlington, MA: Academic Press.

Sperry, L. (2001). *Spirituality in clinical practice: Incorporating the spiritual dimension in psychotherapy and counseling.* Philadelphia: Brunner-Routledge.

Stunkard, A. J. (1951). Some interpersonal aspects of an Oriental religion. *Psychiatry, 14*, 419–431.

Stunkard, A. J. (2004). Suzuki Daisetz: An appreciation. *The Eastern Buddhist, 36*, 192–228.

Surrey, J. L. (2005). Relational psychotherapy, relational mindfulness. In C. K. Germer, R. D. Siegel, & P. R. Fulton (Eds.), *Mindfulness and psychotherapy* (pp. 91–110). New York: Guilford Press.

Tacon, A. M., McComb, J., Caldera, Y., & Randolph, P. (2003). Mindfulness meditation, anxiety reduction, and heart disease: A pilot study. *Family and Community Health, 26*(1), 25–33.

Teasdale, J. D. (1999a). Emotional processing, three modes of mind and the prevention of relapse in depression. *Behaviour Research and Therapy*, 37(1), S53–S77.

Teasdale, J. D. (1999b). Metacognition, mindfulness, and the modification of mood disorders. *Clinical Psychology and Psychotherapy*, 6, 146–155.

Teasdale, J. D., Segal, Z., & Williams, J. M. (1995). How does cognitive therapy prevent depressive relapse and why should attentional control (mindfulness) training help? *Behaviour Research and Therapy*, 33(1), 25–39.

Teasdale, J. D., Segal, Z. V., & Williams, J. M. G. (2003). Mindfulness training and problem formulation. *Clinical Psychology: Science and Practice*, 10(2), 157–160.

Teasdale, J. D., Segal, Z. V., Williams, J. M. G., Ridgeway, V. A., Soulsby, J. M., & Lau, M. A. (2000). Prevention of relapse/recurrence in major depression by mindfulness-based cognitive therapy. *Journal of Consulting and Clinical Psychology*, 68(4), 615–623.

Walach, H., Buchheld, N., & Buttenmüller, V. (2006) Measuring mindfulness: The Freiburg Mindfulness Inventory. *Personality and Individual Differences*, 40(8), 1543–1555.

Wallace, B. A. (2006). *The attention revolution: Unlocking the power of the focused mind*. Ithaca, NY: Snow Lion.

Walsh, R. (1992). The search for synthesis: Transpersonal psychology and the meeting of east and west, psychology and religion, personal and transpersonal. *Journal of Humanistic Psychology*, 32(1), 19–45.

Walsh, R. (1999a). Asian contemplative disciplines: Common practices, clinical applications, and research findings. *Journal of Transpersonal Psychology*, 31(2), 83–107.

Walsh, R. (1999b). *Essential spirituality*. New York: Wiley.

Walsh, R. (2004). Asian psychotherapies. In R. J. Corsini & D. Wedding (Eds.), *Current psychotherapies* (7th ed., pp. 547–559). Belmont, CA: Wadsworth.

Walsh, R., & Shapiro, S. (2006). The meeting of meditative disciplines and Western psychology. *American Psychologist*, 61(3), 1–13.

Weissbecker, I., Salmon, P., Studts, J. L., Floyd, A. R., Dedert, E. A., & Sephton, E. (2002). Mindfulness-based stress reduction and sense of coherence among women with fibromyalgia. *Journal of Clinical Psychology*, 9, 297–307.

Welch, S. S., Rizvi, S. L., & Dimidjian, S. (2006). Mindfulness in dialectical behavior therapy. In R. A. Baer (Ed.), *Mindfulness and acceptance-based interventions: Conceptualization, application and empirical support* (pp. 117–139). Burlington, MA: Academic Press.

Welwood, J. (2000). *Toward a psychology of awakening: Buddhism, psychotherapy, and the path of personal and spiritual transformation*. Boston: Shambala Press.

Williams, K. A., Kolar, M. M., Reger, B. E., & Pearson, J. C. (2001). Evaluation of a wellness-based mindfulness stress reduction intervention: A controlled trial. *American Journal of Health Promotion*, 15(6), 422–432.

Witkieiwitz, K., Marlatt, G. A., & Walker, D. (2005). Mindfulness-Based Relapse Prevention for alcohol and substance use disorders. *Journal of Cognitive Psychotherapy*, 19(3), 211–228.

Woolfolk, R. L. (1984). Self-control meditation and the treatment of chronic anger. In Shapiro, D. H., & Walsh, R. N. (Eds.), *Meditation: Classic and contemporary perspectives* (pp. 550–554). New York: Aldine.

SUGGESTED RESOURCES

Bodian, S. (1999). *Meditation for dummies*. Foster City, CA: IDG Books Worldwide.

Borysenko, J. (1987). *Minding the body, mending the mind*. New York: Bantam.

Harp, D. (1996). *The three minute meditator* (3rd ed.). Oakland, CA: New Harbinger.

Kabat-Zinn, J. (1990). *Full catastrophe living*. New York: Dell.

Kabat-Zinn, J. (2005). *Coming to our senses: Healing ourselves and the world through mindfulness*. New York: Hyperion.

Segal, Z. V., Williams, J. M. G., & Teasdale, J. D. (2002). *Mindfulness-based cognitive therapy for depression: A new approach for preventing relapse*. New York: Guilford Press.

CHAPTER 16

Qigong Therapy for Stress Management

KEVIN CHEN

HISTORY OF THE METHOD

The Term

Qigong (pronounced "chi kung") is a general term for a variety of traditional Chinese energy exercises and healing practices. The word *Qigong* is a combination of two Chinese ideograms: *qi*, meaning "vital energy," and *gong*, meaning "skill," "work," and "achievement." So *Qigong* refers to integrated mind–body exercise for mastering vital energy, or cultivation of vital energy. Only with the accumulation of time and effort can the cultivation of vital energy be developed.

Like acupuncture, herbal medicine, massage, and cupping, Qigong forms an integral component of traditional Chinese medicine. Traditional Chinese medicine (TCM) posits the existence of a subtle energy (*qi*) circulating throughout the entire human mind and body. When it is strengthened or balanced, it can improve health and ward off or slow down the progress of disease. The concept of bioenergy can also be found in other cultures, such as *ki* in Japan, *prana* in India, and *mana* in Hawaii and the Philippines.

There are more than 1,000 registered Qigong schools or forms in contemporary China, and many more have existed throughout history. As a result, there is no consistent definition of Qigong within the Qigong or health communities. According to the textbook used in colleges of Chinese medicine, Qigong is a self-training technique or process that integrates the body posture, breathing, and mentality into oneness to achieve the optimal state for both body and mind (Liu et al., 2005).

As Qigong gains popularity, it is very important for beginners to learn how to determine the authenticity and applicability of a form of Qigong to meet their individual needs and goals. In addition, there are, unavoidably, less qualified Qigong practitioners who pose as Qigong masters or teachers but who have not mastered the science and art of qi cultivation. It is important for the beginner to be able to differentiate those who are qualified to teach Qigong from those who are not.

A Long History

Qigong is the key component of TCM. It has a history longer than that of Chinese medicine itself. *Qigong* has existed as a term for a long time, but it did not become popular until the 1950s, when scientists and doctors started researching its effectiveness in health maintenance. At that time, *Qigong* gained public acceptance over other traditional and more abstruse terms such as *daoyin* ("conduction"), *tuina* ("taking out the stale energy and putting in the fresh energy"), *yangxiou* ("health maintenance and cultivation"), *Xiounian* ("cultivation and practice"), and *Yangsheng* ("health maintenance and improvement"). References to Qigong can be found throughout more than 3,000 years' worth of written records, which can be divided approximately into four major periods of development (Yang, 1991), as follows.

   1. The period of *united heaven, earth, and man* (before 206 B.C.). This period was marked in history by the famous book *Yi Jing* ("Book of Changes"), introduced in 1122 B.C. It presented qi as the concepts of natural energies and the integration of heaven, earth, and man. The first step in Qigong development involved the study of the relationship between these three natural powers. Ancient Chinese practiced Qigong to better understand the relationship between humans and nature. Some developed an inner vision through Qigong meditation that enabled them to view and draw accurately the body meridian system (the channel of qi flow) 3,000 years ago. Acupuncturists still use this system today.
   During the Zhou dynasty (1122–934 B.C.), Lao Zi's *Dao De Jing* mentioned certain breathing techniques and established the philosophical foundation for Qigong and Daoism. He stressed that the way to obtain health was "to concentrate on qi and achieve softness." Later, the historical record *Shi Ji* (770–221 B.C.) contained a more complete description of methods of breath training.
   The most detailed description of Qigong meditation was recorded in a jade pendant inscription (around 600 B.C.), which included 36 ancient Chinese words laying out the detailed process of Qigong exercise and qi movement within the body (see Figure 16.1):

> When you breathe deeply to a degree, internally refined qi will gather. When the refined qi is fully accumulated, it expands and descends downward (Dantian in the lower abdomen area). When the refined qi is reinforced to a certain level it begins to rise up (along the spinal cord) to the head, and then falls down (to the Dantian) again. The internal qi

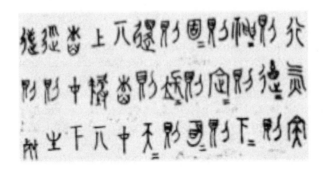

FIGURE 16.1. The script of a jade pendant (ca. 600 B.C.) described the process of Qigong exercises.

then circulates around the Ren-Du meridians during your daily practice. The universal qi becomes integrated. It comes in through the top of the head, with the earth qi, which enters the body through the feet. Thus you will be healthier and more alive while you follow it, and more prone to the effects of aging and death when you don't.

2. The period of *Qigong mixed with religion* (206 B.C.–500 A.D.). During the Han dynasty (206 B.C.), Buddhism meditation methods were imported from India, which brought Qigong practice and meditation into the religious Qigong era.

Not long after Buddhism had been introduced into China, Zhang Dao-Ling combined the traditional Daoist (Taoism) principles with Buddhism and created a religion called Dao Jiao. Many of the meditation methods were a combination of the principles and training methods from both sources. At that time Tibet had developed its own branch of Buddhism, with its own training system and methods of attaining Buddhahood. Later, these practices were integrated with Qigong cultivation and practice.

The development and cultivation of Qigong required a large time commitment and spiritual guidance outside of the secular society. Religious temples provided such a physical and spiritual environment. Meanwhile, Qigong practice might actually have helped religious practitioners to more effectively reach higher spiritual levels and deeper understanding of the religious scriptures through deep meditation. These integrative results made Qigong a popular practice among religions; however, Qigong in itself is not a religion.

At this stage, Qigong had shown its characteristics as an exercise of one's consciousness or intention. The founder of Zen (a Buddhist Qigong tradition), Bodhidharma (?–528 A.D.), spent 9 years in a deep meditation state, facing a rocky wall in a cave at the Shaolin Temple. As a Chinese saying stated, "Bodhidharma brought no word with him from the west but the skill to work with mind or consciousness." Bodhidharma was also considered a significant contributor to the creation and development of martial-art Qigong, which is the Qigong style he taught in the Shaolin Temple.

3. The period of *development with the appearance of martial-art Qigong* (500 A.D.–1950s). In the Liang dynasty (502–557 A.D.), people discovered that, in addition to improving health, Qigong training could also increase physical strength and be used for self-defense and fighting. The application of Qigong to martial arts increased the popularity of Qigong in society. Many Qigong forms were created for this purpose. In parallel, both religious and medical Qigong also developed rapidly during this period.

With modern conveniences of travel and communications, Chinese Qigong training because mixed with Qigong practices from India, Japan, and many other countries from 1911 on. However, until very recently, Qigong was still transmitted privately from generation to generation.

4. The period of *modern Qigong research and massive (large scale of promotion and practice) Qigong movement* (1950s–present). Qigong gradually emerged from traditional, secret transmission into a common practice by the public and a subject of scientific research when more and more Qigong practitioners left traditional private practices to openly display their healing abilities in public and to teach the public to practice Qigong. During the Cultural Revolution (1966–1976), Qigong was considered a "pseudoscience" or "idealism," and its practice was forbidden in China. In 1978 many scientists and practitioners became interested in reviving Qigong as one of the effective healing methods in health care. They tried to use advanced scientific measurements and technology to prove that Qigong was not purely "idealism" and did not depend on a placebo psychological

effect, but was, rather, an objective life phenomenon with measurable processes (Chen, 2004). Since then, thousands of scientific research studies have been conducted and published in China, and millions of people have started practicing Qigong for the purpose of health and healing rather than for spiritual purposes.

Different Traditions with Different Focuses

There have been numerous forms and schools of Qigong in Chinese history. Various methods can be used to classify these Qigong forms. Although Qigong was well known for its healing and health potential, most forms of Qigong were not created for the purpose of healing but for the cultivation of mind and spirituality. Currently, the Chinese government classifies all contemporary Qigong into two categories—preventive health Qigong and medical Qigong—ignoring its spiritual tradition.

Historically, Qigong can be divided into five major disciplines or traditions: Confucianist, Buddhist, Taoist, medical, and martial arts. Each discipline has its own set of goals, methods, and forms. Following are brief descriptions of these five major traditions in Chinese Qigong development (Liang & Wu, 1997).

Confucianist Qigong, developed by the followers of Confucius, is designed for the attainment of higher moral character and intelligence, focusing on education and moral cultivation. This form of meditation had relatively few followers historically, but it reflects one of the essences of Qigong—an exercise of consciousness. Typical forms in this tradition are "listening to breathing" (a meditation form with a focus on slow breathing and attention to listening to the breathing) and the "sitting and forgetting self" exercise (a meditation form similar to mindfulness [see Chapter 15, this volume] with an empty mind as the optimal goal).

Buddhist Qigong aims to liberate the mind by emphasizing the cultivation of virtue and enlightening wisdom, and it considers the human body to be just a "stinking bag" holding the honorable spirit (claiming 58,000 schools or forms in history, it is the most popular). With this philosophy, a pure Buddhist Qigong form is not concerned with much reason to building a healthy body; however, health and healing could be a side effect of developing a positive mind and relaxation state. The famous Buddhist Qigong traditions include Zen, Mi (Tibetan), and Tiantai.

Daoist (or Taoist) Qigong emphasizes the preservation of the physical body first, and then the higher levels of virtue and spiritual cultivation (3,600 schools have taught this form throughout history). Most Daoist Qigong consisted of training both the body (*qi*, or "*ming*" = life) and the spirit (*yi*, or "*xing*" = spirituality). Some encouraged body, or qi, cultivation before spiritual, or yi, cultivation, whereas others considered spiritual training more important than body training. Because Daoism put emphasis on the current life and explored the techniques of preserving long life, many Daoist Qigong masters lived extremely long lives. Biographies of Daoist Qigong masters throughout history show that most of them lived to be more than 90 years old in times in which the average life expectancy was around 40 (Zhang, Gu, Wang, Liu, & Song, 1994). The famous Daoist Qigong traditions include Taiji, Danding (including Nei Dan Qigong), Jianxian (Sward Qigong), Fulu (*fu* implies "symbol"), Xuanzeng, and others.

Medical Qigong refers to those Qigong forms created or practiced for healing of self or others. It emphasizes how to use human vital energy (qi) to help eliminate imbalances and disharmonies, which are considered the root causes of many illnesses and diseases, and how to prevent them. It was influenced greatly by Daoist philosophy but was developed independently, mostly by TCM practitioners. Historically, the most famous TCM doctors were also good Qigong practitioners. Medical Qigong teaches medical practitioners how to use the inner qi in a dynamic way for diagnosis, healing, and preventing diseases (discussed further later in the chapter). Today, medical Qigong is still a standard course in many schools of Chinese medicine. The typical medical Qigong forms include Five-Animal-Acts Qigong (by Hua Tuo), Six-Healing-Sounds Qigong (Liu et al., 2005), Brighten-Eye Qigong, and Taiji Five-Element Qigong (He, 2003).

Martial Arts Qigong tends to train the practitioner for self-defense, protecting and preparing the body to better endure sword cuts or sharp weapons or attacks by a powerful punch or kick. Such methods include Iron Shirt and Golden-Bell Qigong. It also trains the body to deliver powerful blows that are enhanced with qi, such as the Burning-Palm or Iron-Palm methods. Demonstrations of martial-art Qigong can be seen from time to time. However, many martial-art Qigong practitioners have died prematurely due to overexertion of their bodies or to an imbalance of inner qi (Zhang et al., 1994). For example, Bruce Lee, a well-known contemporary martial-art Qigong practitioner, he died in his mid-30s.

In short, all forms of Qigong are not the same. As Qigong gains popularity, it is very important for a beginner to know which Qigong form is most appropriate for him or her. The preceding classifications may also help beginners learn how to determine the authenticity of a Qigong form and thus gain some protection against fraudulent Qigong "masters" who are not educated and qualified in Qigong and therefore tend to provide incomplete or misleading instruction.

Most Qigong practice may involve a combination of such elements as relaxation, breathing work, guided imagery, slow movement, biofeedback, tranquil state, mindfulness meditation (see Chapter 15, this volume), and mind–body integration. Qigong practice is said to help relax and develop a balance between the body, mind, and spirit, and relaxation and balance are the basic ingredients of good health (Zhang et al., 1994; Liu et al., 2005).

Various forms of Qigong have reported some health benefits, but not all forms were designed for the purpose of health care or healing. Only medical Qigong makes treating illness or curing disease its major purpose.

THEORETICAL FOUNDATIONS

Basic Theory

According to TCM, good health is a result of a free-flowing, well-balanced qi (energy) system, whereas sickness or the experience of pain is the result of qi blockage or unbalanced energy in the body. Acupuncture and Qigong share the same qi flow and meridian theory. The meridian system charts the major channels of qi flow. The difference between acupuncture and Qigong is that acupuncture uses external force (needles or pressure stimulation) to help the qi flow and balance, whereas Qigong uses mostly internal force (qi cultivation and self-practice) to help smooth the qi flow and break the qi blockages.

In addition to the concept of qi, the concept of yi (mind or intention) also plays a key role in Qigong practice and Qigong healing. TCM believes that qi tends to follow the yi (*"qi shui yi xing"*). When a person is under stress or is disturbed by many random thoughts for a long time, his or her qi cannot flow smoothly or normally, and he or she will soon experience qi imbalance (emotional disturbance) or qi blockage (psychosomatic symptoms). Therefore, having the consciousness focus on one thing or on nothing (mindfulness) is the key to training in Qigong practice. This focus creates a state of empty mind without desire. Cultivation of the mind can be practiced at any time without Qigong or meditation.

Medical Qigong or Qigong Therapy

Medical Qigong refers to the Qigong forms or therapies used by medical practitioners who emphasize using vital energy (qi) to assist with diagnosis and to control and prevent illness and disease. Medical Qigong, or Qigong therapy, consists of both internal Qigong exercise (self-practice) and external qi healing (through the clinician's involvement). Although Qigong is a self-training method, the emission of qi (or external Qigong therapy) has always been part of the medical Qigong practice that attempts to help others regain their health, similar to the practice of *reiki* in Japan and of therapeutic touch in the United States. Therefore the difference between internal training and external Qigong therapy in the history and development of medical Qigong must be examined.

Internal Qigong training is the major component of medical Qigong and refers to the self-practice of Qigong forms. There are three major categories of these Qigong forms: movement (active) Qigong (*dong gong*), "standing pole" (*zhuang gong*) Qigong, and static forms or meditation (*jing gong*). Movement Qigong (mostly an introductory form) uses guided physical movements or gestures to help practitioners concentrate and induce the qi energy flow in the body. Earlier forms of taiji quan may be considered as typical movement Qigong. Static Qigong is mostly meditation, which may include relaxation, breathing manipulation, mindful meditation, guided imagery, incantation, seal palm symbols, and mindfulness state. The main purpose of static Qigong is the training of intentional power, or consciousness stability, when cultivating qi energy. It was said that the intention or consciousness, once well-trained, will lead qi flow in the body, direct it to where it is needed, and break through the blocked area. Blocked qi is considered to be the origin of many illnesses and diseases. The "standing pole" is a form between movement and static Qigong, which usually starts with a standing position. Then, as the qi is cultivated or moved, various spontaneous movements will follow. The magnitude or degree of the movement varies, and sometimes it may even be greater than during movement Qigong.

External Qigong therapy (EQT) refers to the process by which a Qigong practitioner directs or emits his qi to help break qi blockages in others and induce the sick qi out of the body so as to relieve pain or to balance the qi flow in the body and get rid of disease. EQT can be practiced through the use of either qi (emitting vital energy) or yi (the consciousness or intentional therapy) or a combination of the two techniques (the type most commonly used). Most schools of medical Qigong will teach both techniques. Many Qigong clinics in Chinese hospitals provide external qi therapy.

Although the physical nature of qi remains as yet unproven, there are intriguing reports that suggest the possibility of physical, biophysical, and/or biochemical alterations induced by external qi therapy or "qi emission" (Chen, 2004). For example, qi emissions by Qigong masters have been reported to be associated with significant structural changes in aqueous solutions, to alter the phase behavior of dipalmitoyl phosphatidyl choline (DPPC) liposomes, to enable the growth of Fab protein crystals (Yan et al., 1999), to inhibit tumor growth in mice (Chen, Li, Liu, & He, 1997), to change the conformation of such biomolecules as polyglutamic acid, polylysine, and metallothionein (Chu, He, Zhou, & Chen, 1998), and to reduce phosphorylation of a cell-free preparation (Muehsami, Markow, & Muehsami, 1994). Thus there is a small but growing body of scientific evidence that suggests the physical existence of qi, as well as the healing power of Qigong therapy (Agishi, 1998; Chen, 2004; Loh, 1999; Sancier, 1996; Sancier, 1999; Wirth, Cram, & Chang, 1997; Wu et al., 1999).

Qigong Meditation versus Other Meditations

The term *meditation* refers to a mental state or the continued thought or reflection or contemplation on sacred or solemn subjects. For many who are troubled by the stresses of modern life, it is an age-old method, particularly in the East, that people turn to for help in coping with anxiety and in finding a deeper meaning in life. Mindfulness meditation has become popular in the United States and has been integrated with cognitive therapy to help improve outcomes in the treatment of depression (Segal et al., 2002).

Meditation is one of the most important components in Qigong practice. In some sense, all meditations could be called *Qigong* in China, but internal practice of medical Qigong is more than meditation. In order to differentiate medical Qigong from other meditation forms, I discuss how medical Qigong is thought to work toward health and healing from a TCM perspective. Some of these explanations have not yet been scientifically verified.

1. In terms of practice, most meditations involve a single practice or focus, for example, concentration on one's breathing. Medical Qigong consists of three major components for stimulating a balanced qi flow and a tranquil state, as described earlier: movement Qigong, static Qigong (meditation), and "standing pole." Standing meditation, accompanied by spontaneous movement, is actually a powerful means of qi generation and qi balance by nature.

2. Qi plays an important role in medical Qigong practice but not necessarily in most other types of meditation. Qigong uses the qi-flow meridian theory. One of the healing mechanisms of Qigong, from a TCM perspective, is the belief that motivated qi (vital energy moving more powerfully after Qigong practice) strikes against areas of illness in the body and removes destructive blocks to allow healthy qi to flow. There is experiential evidence that Qigong practitioners may clearly feel pain or soreness during practice as a result of this qi-striking process.

3. Although most meditation requires the role of mind or intention, medical Qigong meditation puts the role of yi (mind and intention) above anything else in two distinct ways: (1) the induced state of "empty mind without desire" and emphasis on tranquility helps a practitioner to calm conflicting emotions and resolve mental disturbances, and (2) the resulting tranquil state strengthens a practitioner's power of intention. The qi meditation introduced here to treat stress engages these components through a guided imagery process.

4. In addition to the relaxation response common to other types of meditation, medical Qigong meditation generates healing results by rapidly uncovering the body's self-healing potential through modulated breathing, liberated tranquility, intentional qi induction, guided imagery, and an enhanced mind–body communication. The increased immune functions that are facilitated by these processes result in a strengthened self-repair and self-regeneration capability. Sancier (1996) concluded, after reviewing the literature on medical applications of Qigong, that "Qigong enables the body to heal itself" (p. 44).

ASSESSMENT OF EFFECTIVENESS

Although most Qigong forms were not designed for healing or for treating specific health conditions, Qigong practice is said to be very effective in ameliorating the effects of many stress-related conditions, such as hypertension, allergy, asthma, back or neck pain, premenstrual syndrome, insomnia, headache, depression, anxiety, and addiction. It is said that Qigong works by increasing the practitioners' self-healing capabilities, including immune functions, self-recovery capability, and self-regeneration capability (He, 2003; Liu et al., 2005; Sancier, 1996). The potential applications of Qigong in health and healing are too numerous to list, and to some extent, the potential of Qigong challenges our current understanding of life and health in general. Most practitioners credit their Qigong meditation with improving daily life in many ways, including:

- A more relaxed, harmonious state of mind and body.
- A noticeable reduction in prior ailments and a reduction in feelings of stress.
- An increased resistance to illness.
- A heightened sensitivity to the body's internal organs, with a developed ability to regulate their own health and vitality.

Not many clinical studies have been done in the United States to assess the effectiveness of Qigong. I searched the computerized database by keywords related to Qigong (*Qigong, chi kung; taiji, tai chi*[1]) and stress and found 15 cites on Medline and 13 on PsycINFO. Most of the scientific and clinical research on the effectiveness of Qigong has been done in China and Japan (which are not included in the English database), although increasing numbers of clinical studies are being carried out in the United States and around the world. The Qigong Institute in California has put together a Qigong Database, updated every other year, with many scientific assessments and Qigong studies from publications and conference proceedings around the world. The latest Qigong database (version 7.0) contains more than 3,500 entries (*www.qigonginstitute.org*). If we do a similar keyword search in this database, we find many more entries and studies related to Qigong and stress. For example, *stress* appears in 248 entries; *anxiety*, 134; *hypertension*,, 151; *headache*, 74; *insomnia*, 37; *pain*, 261; *psychosomatic symptoms*, 61; *respiration symptoms*, 132; and *cardiovascular*, 113.

Qigong Exercise Directly Reduces Stress

Research has suggested that 80% of the patients in a primary care setting show evidence of significant psychosocial distress (Sobel, 1995). Many common health problems are related to stress, such as headache, hypertension, obesity, lower back pain, asthma, allergy, insomnia, and more. Therefore, an effective strategy for managing stress will greatly reduce health problems and increase the quality of life. The relaxation and energetic response produced by Qigong exercise has been well documented in clinical studies of the health benefits of Qigong (Liu et al., 2005; Sandlund & Norlander, 2000; Wall, 2005).

Sandlund and Norlander (2000) reviewed more than 20 studies published from 1996 to 1999 on the effects of tai chi chuan (a slow-movement form of Qigong) on stress response and well-being and concluded that, although the slow-movement Tai chi may not achieve aerobic fitness, it could enhance flexibility and overall psychological well-being. Tai chi exercises led to an improvement of mood. The researchers concluded that all studies on the benefits of tai chi have revealed positive results and that tai chi was an effective way to reduce stress. Wang, Collet, and Lau (2004) reviewed general health outcomes of tai chi. Among the six studies they reviewed with psychological measures, five reported positive or significant effects of tai chi exercise on reducing stress and anxiety.

Some research applied advanced technology and measurements in direct assessment of the differences between Qigong and other relaxation techniques. He, Li, Xi, and Zhang (1999) applied a "stress meter" (a piece of equipment measuring body conductivity under 5 volts of direct current with a 128-pin sensor) to evaluate the degree of relaxation achieved through Qigong meditation training in comparison with other, non-Qigong techniques (relaxation meditations). After testing 73 participants during Qigong meditation and 56 participants during the non-Qigong techniques with 10 separate measures during the meditation state, the researchers reported that participants in the Qigong meditation group were able to reach deeper levels of relaxation than those in regular meditation (measured by skin conductance and other electronic sensors).

Some studies exploring Qigong effects focused on physiological changes or hormone levels that are related to stress. A randomized controlled study by Lee et al. (2001) examined the psychoneuroimmunological effects of external qi therapy and reported that 10 minutes of external qi therapy could significantly reduce participants' anxiety, negative mood, and cortisol levels and increase the cellular activities of neutrophil and natural killer cells in comparison with the participants in placebo control. Guo, Tang, and Liang (1996) applied the measures of change in urine catecholamine and cortisol levels under both physical and psychological stress conditions to examine the difference in stress reduction through Qigong practice and reported that the levels of catecholamine and cortisol in the Qigong group were significantly lower than those of the control group ($p < .05$) immediately after exposure to the stressor, but no difference was reported either at baseline or 1 hour after the stressor, suggesting that Qigong practice could suppress the reaction to mental and physical distress.

We also found laboratory studies of animals that were given external qi therapy for stress reduction. Zhang, Wang, Yan, Ge, and Zhou (1993) applied external qi therapy in cold-stressed mice. The mice were divided into three groups: the normal control group, the stress control group (mice underwent 5 minutes of 1°C cold-stress exposure per day for 8 days), and the Qigong group (in addition to cold stress, mice received emitted qi 30 minutes per day for 8 days). Then, the thymus, spleen, and brain were dissected, and T-cell and B-cell proliferation and the RDCC activities of K-cells were used to investigate the immune adjusting effect of the emitted qi on cold-stressed mice. They found that the T-cell and B-cell proliferation rate and the activities of K-cells of the stressed mice were significantly lower than those of the nonstressed controls; however, the T- and B-cell proliferation and the activities of K-cells in the Qigong group were significantly higher than those in the stress control group ($p < .01$). Although the immune organs (thymus and spleen) of the stressed mice were atrophied more significantly than those of the nonstressed mice ($p < .01$), the external-qi-treated group had no injuries to the thymus and spleen in comparison with the controls ($p < .01$). Itoh, Shen, Itoh, and Tamura (2000) in Japan explored the effects of external qi therapy on rats under stress based on urinary excretion measurements of catecholamine. In their study, rats received external qi treatment for 4 days. The researchers then conducted a stress load test (swimming) and measured the urinary excretion of catecholamines (adrenaline, noradrenaline, and dopamine). They reported that, for both control and Qigong groups, the quantity of adrenaline increased greatly after the stress load. The quantity of noradrenaline increased after the stress load for the control group but not for the Qigong group. In the Qigong group, the quantity of noradrenaline decreased significantly after stress load, which suggests that external qi might have some influence on the autonomic nervous system.

Qigong Therapy for Stress-Related Symptoms

Many studies focus on the effectiveness of Qigong therapy for stress-related symptoms. Following are examples of these studies and their conclusions.

Control of Hypertension

Mayer (1999) reviewed 30 representative studies, mostly in China, that explored the therapeutic effects of Qigong therapy for hypertension, including a 30-year longitudinal follow-up study, and concluded that Qigong is an effective way to control hypertension without any adverse side effects.

In Wang et al.'s (2004) recent review of tai chi, four studies (two with randomized control) were discussed in terms of the effects of tai chi on hypertension, and all of them reported that tai chi significantly decreased blood pressure among hypertension patients.

Recently, Lee, Kim, and Moon (2003) conducted a clinical study to evaluate the efficacy of Qigong as a nonpharmacological treatment for hypertension in Korea. Fifty-eight patients were randomly assigned into the Qigong group and a wait-list control group (n = 29 each). After 10 weeks of Qigong practice, the Qigong group reported significant reduction in systolic and diastolic blood pressure, rate pressure product, norepinephrine, epinephrine, cortisol, and stress level, in comparison with the control group. These results suggest that Qigong may reduce blood pressure and catecholamines by stabilizing the sympathetic nervous system. They considered Qigong to be an effective nonpharmacological modality to reduce blood pressure in essential hypertensive patients.

Improvement of Cardiovascular Conditions

Improvement of cardiovascular conditions through Qigong practice has been documented (Sancier, 1996). For example, Lu, Liu, and Zhuang (1996) compared the treatment outcomes for patients with heart disease in their clinical studies of Qigong therapy with music and found that the patients treated with Qigong and music reported significantly higher rates of complete freedom from symptoms and significant improvement (10% and 32%, respectively) than the conventional medication group (5% and 21%, respectively; $p < .01$).

Wang et al. (2004) reviewed 16 studies of tai chi with patients with cardiorespiratory conditions and reported that regular practice of tai chi will delay the decline of cardiorespiratory function in older adults and might be prescribed as a suitable exercise for them.

Reduction of Chronic Pain Syndrome and Arthritis Symptoms

Wu and colleagues studied patients who recieved qi emission and Qigong instruction by a Qigong master and patients who received the same set of instruction by a sham master (the "sham" group). After 10 weeks, 91% of the Qigong patients reported a transient drop in pain compared to only 36% of the control group. A long-term reduction in anxiety in patients suffering from treatment-resistant complex regional pain syndrome type I was found (Wu et al., 1999).

Chen and Liu (2004) reviewed more than 20 studies of Qigong therapy in the treatment of various forms of arthritis, including osteoarthritis, rheumatoid arthritis, scapulohumeral periarthritis, cervical spondylopathy, and arthromyodynia. Most participants in these studies did not respond to the conventional therapies for their chronic pains and functional problems. However, Qigong therapy (self-practice and/or external qi therapy) produced significant improvement or complete freedom from symptoms for a large proportion of these patients in many of the reviewed studies.

Reduction of Anxiety and Depression

Although there are few studies that focus on the mental benefits of Qigong, Pavek (1988) reported that Qigong therapy was very useful to patients suffering from anxiety, depression, blocked grief, and sleep disorders. Wang (1993) used the Symptom Checklist 90 (SCL-90) to examine the effect of Qigong exercise on mental health and found that the group with more Qigong practice reported significantly lower scores in most of the mental health indicators, including anxiety and depression. Shan, Yan, Sheng, and Hu (1989) used Qigong therapy to treat anxiety in psychiatric clinics and reported that five of the eight patients were anxiety-free after 1 month of Qigong practice, that two reported significant improvements, and that only one failed to respond.

Wu et al. (1999) examined the effect of Qigong therapy on late-stage complex regional pain syndrome, as well as on anxiety, for each of the participants in a randomized placebo-controlled trial and found that anxiety was reduced in both groups over time but that the reduction was significantly greater in the group practicing genuine Qigong than in the control group. The reduction of anxiety had a long-term effect, whereas the pain relief was only short term. The preexisting differences in hypnotic susceptibility cannot explain the significant and long-lasting improvement in anxiety in the Qigong group. Another group of scientists in Baltimore applied Qigong therapy and cognitive-behavioral therapy with fibromyalgia patients and reported significant reduction in pain, fatigue, and insomnia and improved function and mood state after an 8-week intervention (Singh, Berman, Hadhazy, & Creamer, 1998).

How Qigong Works for Health and Healing

The mechanism of how Qigong works to achieve health benefits is still the subject of scientific exploration. Various Qigong forms posit different explanations of how Qigong works in healing. Throughout its history, Qigong has been employed and developed as a method for curing illness and strengthening the mind and body. Qigong's main therapeutic properties may well lie in its regulation of the respiratory system, metabolism, activity of the cerebral cortex and central nervous system, and the cardiovascular system, as well as its effect in correcting abnormal reactions of the organs, its massaging effect on the organs of the abdominal cavity, and its effect on self-control of the physical functions of one's body. However, not enough research or data exist to document these effects. According to TCM and available scientific literature in Chinese, Qigong may work to benefit the practitioners through the following possible paths.

1. Motivated qi (vital energy flowing more strongly in the meridian after Qigong practice) strikes against locations of illness in the body. According to TCM, good health is a result of a free-flowing and well-balanced qi (energy) system, whereas sickness and the experience of pain are the results of qi blockage or unbalanced energy in certain areas

of the body. Qi imbalance is the precursor of any physical illness. One way to stay healthy and function well is to perform Qigong exercises in order to keep the qi flowing smoothly in the body so that each cell in the body gets a constant supply of vital energy. Once the supply of qi to the cells becomes blocked, blood flow to that area will change, and disease or pain may occur. One possible mechanism of Qigong therapy for pain relief and symptom reduction is motivating qi and energy within the body, breaking the qi blockage and balancing the energy system. Therefore, it is common for Qigong practitioners to report more serious symptoms or pain on a temporary basis due to qi's striking against sites of illness. These pains or symptoms go away completely with continued practice.

2. Cultivation of yi (consciousness and intention) and the emphasis on an "empty mind without desire" in Qigong practice may help the practitioners strengthen their consciousness and intention, release suppressed emotions, and resolve mental disturbances. It is said that Qigong training of the mind or intention helps the practitioner to release him- or herself from the socialized self, or consciousness (the source of all stress), and return to the original self without social pressure or natural consciousness. Many chronic diseases of unknown origin may well be related to mental disturbances, social pressures, or emotional twists. Qigong practice may lead to the release of these emotional disturbances, which may have been the sources of many chronic diseases. It is a common phenomenon for Qigong practitioners to tear, cry, or laugh during Qigong practice and then to feel complete relief after the practice.

In addition, the increased power of focused mind and energy level of intention could also work with the human body by reaching the locations of illness (similarly to the mechanism of guided imagery), changing the features of illness, and turning the abnormal into normal (He, 2003; Chen, 2004). Scientific evidence from parapsychological studies suggests such human consciousness or intention potential, even though we still do not know exactly how it works.

3. Quality Qigong practice may rapidly reveal or uncover the body's potential self-healing capability. This includes increasing the immune functions, the self-repair capability, and the self-regeneration capability (Chen & Yueng, 2002; He, 2003). For example, the relaxation and tranquility status achieved during Qigong practice may relieve stress, build up vital energy, and rapidly increase immune-system function (Lee et al., 2001). There is some scientific evidence to connect relaxation and guided imagery with increased immune function while connecting stress and depression with malfunction of the immune system. We have also observed that many patients have completely recovered from multiple complicated diseases or symptoms with Qigong therapy in a short period of time without any medications, and some middle-aged adults and seniors have experienced new growth of hair and teeth. In this sense, Qigong therapy has challenged the current medical practice of depending on the use of symptom-releasing pharmaceutical drugs.

SIDE EFFECTS AND CONTRAINDICATIONS

Many people think that Qigong practice has no side effects. However, strictly speaking, some side effects could occur from practicing Qigong exercise if the practitioner is not prepared. If one practices Qigong extensively on a daily basis without an appropriate understanding of the natural process of Qigong or without having the right instructor to assist him or her, one may run into some qi phenomena, or side effects. These effects more likely occur among those who learn Qigong from books or tapes without proper guidance or who had an unqualified instructor. However, if one understands what kind of effects may be experienced in intensive Qigong practice, there is no danger at all in practicing.

Generally speaking, three common types of responses occur during intensive Qigong practice that have been mislabeled as potential side effects or reported as "Qigong deviations" in the literature:

1. Appearance of new symptoms or increased severity of old symptoms. This is typical for medical Qigong practice when qi strikes against a location of illness or a blocked area. As stated previously, TCM practitioners believe that sickness or experience of pain is the result of qi blockage or unbalanced energy in the body. One mechanism of Qigong therapy for pain relief and symptom reduction is motivating qi and energy within the body, breaking the qi blockage and balancing the energy system. Therefore, it is common for beginning Qigong practitioners to report more serious symptoms or pain temporarily when qi is striking against sick locations. These pains or symptoms will go away completely with continuous practice (He, 2003; Liu et al., 2005). For example, a person with a history of arthritis of the knee might feel increased pain at the knee for a period of time after intensive Qigong practice. If he stops practicing at that moment, the pain will continue for a while; if he continues practicing Qigong, the qi strikes against the blockage (arthritis), and the pain will completely disappear forever.

2. Pain or soreness through the back and neck area. Some practitioners may even feel as though they have the pressure of a mountain on their heads. This occurs when strengthened qi starts flowing upward in the Du meridian (along the spinal cord) and strikes through the "Jiaji gateway" and the "Yuzeng gateway" in the lower back and at the back of the neck, the common qi striking points. Under close supervision and with proper understanding, the practitioner can easily correct this problem by continuing practice and getting over the blockage and can reach a higher level of cultivation. However, uninformed practitioners may consider that there is something wrong in their practice and stop the Qigong practice altogether at this stage. Many psychiatrists who do not practice Qigong might also consider this a psychosomatic symptom due to Qigong practice (Shan, Yan, Xu, et al., 1989).

3. Hallucinations and Qigong psychoses. It is quite common for the advanced Qigong practitioner to experience some hallucinations or illusions during Qigong practice, such as photism or phonism (Ng, 1999; Lee, 2000). However, as long as the practitioners do not believe what they see or hear or sustain these hallucinations, and as long as they continue their practice, these hallucinations will eventually go away. There is no danger of becoming disoriented so long as the practitioner knows in advance that this might happen. Unfortunately, most Qigong instructors have not had such experiences themselves and do not tell their students about this potential. Therefore, practicing with a misunderstanding of Qigong hallucinations or practicing with strong intentions or inappropriate purposes (such as to communicate with higher beings, to develop supernatural ability, or to reach self-completion, as some sham Qigong practitioners advocate), may lead to various forms of psychosis or even to schizophrenia or other types of abnormal behaviors (Shan, Yan, Xu, et al., 1989; Lee, 2000).

As discussed earlier, most of the so-called side effects of Qigong practice may simply arise from the natural pathways of qi cultivation, and they can be overcome by continuous practice. The key in dealing with these issues is for the practitioner to be informed in advance, to try not to believe in what appears during practice, and to continue practicing Qigong until the stage is over. However, the unfortunate end result for those who do not understand these phenomena would be discontinuing practice at the time it is most needed.

Qigong practice can be improved rapidly and successfully if the practitioner can avail him- or herself of the natural flow of qi and adhere to the notion of "a life of simplicity and empty mind without desires" during practice. It is crucial to understand the potential discomfort while qi is striking at the gateways and to increase practice when qi strikes against locations of illness with more symptoms. When confronted with Qigong hallucinations during practice, the person should simply ignore them all and continue to practice without interruptions. This way the practitioner will never deviate or lose control. The Qigong practice may become harmful to the practitioner or others if he or she practices with wants and desires, seeking a quick fix or immediate success, or practices under the misguided influence of a fraudulent Qigong master.

THE METHOD

A thousand different Qigong forms or methods exist, most of which contain the basic elements of relaxation, tranquility, and breathing works, and, therefore, they may have some therapeutic effect for stress management. It is difficult to introduce a specific method as representing Qigong without misleading the student. Although there are many different elements and components in different traditions of Qigong, there are also some common methods—three basic adjustments before Qigong meditation and the key components during Qigong practice, which can be found in most Qigong traditions. I describe these, then briefly introduce the taiji five-element medical Qigong forms as an example of medical Qigong practice.

The Three Adjustments: Basics of Qigong

1. Adjust your body position by finding a comfortable position to sit, lie down, or stand (as instructed by the specific form), and relax completely in the position you choose. Sometimes, if it is a meditation form, you can smile gently and keep your eyes and mouth lightly closed.
2. Adjust your breathing. Different breathing techniques may be used by different Qigong forms or traditions. In the Taoist Qigong that is taught at the World Institute for Self-Healing (*www.wishus.org*), the students are asked to pay special attention to the area around the abdomen (lower Dantian), to begin abdominal breathing, and to breathe softly, evenly, deeply, and slowly.
3. Adjust your mind or mental state by clearing your mind of all thoughts and letting your awareness stay at the lower Dantian area, relaxed and peaceful. In the optimal Qigong state, your mind will always be on either one thing (the instructed subject) or nothing (the mindfulness state).

It is said that advanced Qigong meditation is the integration of the three adjustments into oneness without any distinction.

Key Components of Qigong Exercise

The essential points during Qigong practice include: (1) relaxation (completely relaxing both physically and psychologically, without falling asleep); (2) tranquility (a mind state of quiet and concentration, ignoring surroundings, focusing on one thing or nothing); and (3) naturalness (following the natural way both physically and emotionally, without wants and intents).

Most Qigong forms also emphasize maintaining a state of empty mind without desire during practice (reports of this are mostly subjective and difficult to measure). Only those who can minimize desire and intention during practice can achieve the optimal status for both mind and body. Practicing Qigong with strong purpose or desire is considered a deviation from the tradition of cultivating qi essence. Researchers and practitioners have noticed many stages of achievement and development during Qigong practice and cultivation, and there are significant differences among various schools or traditions on the designated stages. For example, the complete Qigong cultivation process for the Daoist tradition may include the following stages: cultivating sperm or blood (for men or women, respectively) into qi, cultivating qi into spirit (*shen*), cultivating the spirit return to emptiness (*xu*), and cultivating emptiness up to Dao. However, medical Qigong, for the purpose of healing, focuses only on the first two stages of this process.

Taiji Five-Element Medical Qigong

As one of the medical Qigong systems from China, Taiji Five-Element Medical Qigong (TFMQ) is based on the Daoist philosophy of self-cultivation and the assumption that there are meridians of circulating qi energy throughout the entire body. TFMQ applies the five-element theory of TCM to systematically absorb the universal qi energy and to rapidly uncover and strengthen self-healing capabilities. It is simple and easy to learn, yet powerful and effective in helping to relieve symptoms, improve recovery, and gain general health resilience.

TFMQ is a complete healing system that uses one formula for various health conditions by working on improving the immune system, self-recovery, and self-regeneration capabilities. This Qigong works directly on the root source of many health problems instead of just the symptoms of the defined illnesses. TFMQ is suitable for people of any age group and any physical condition, as long as they are able to follow the instructions in the practice. The system includes three forms: one-step classic meditation, standing meditation for magnification, and meditation for purification.

Common Components for TFMQ Meditation

- Find a quiet place with a comfortable position without any interference for at least 30 minutes.
- Regulate your body by finding a comfortable position to sit, lie down, or stand, relax completely (in both physical and psychological sense), and lightly close your eyes.
- Regulate your breath by paying special attention to the area around your abdomen (lower Dantian), and apply abdominal breath softly, evenly, deeply, and slowly.
- Regulate your mental state by clearing your mind of all thoughts and letting your awareness stay at the lower Dantian area peacefully. Use one thought to replace other random thoughts, gradually reaching an empty-minded, or mindfulness, state.
- In order to achieve an empty-minded state without any desire, you need to forget about your diseases, about your troubles or worries, about the environment, and about yourself.
- Let everything go through complete relaxation without falling asleep (maintain your awareness); get into a tranquil state without being distracted by random thoughts or

the noises around you; follow the natural way both physically and emotionally when something comes up (such as a physical movement or emotional release), let it come and let it go; do not restrain anything.

- Always do the closing[2] after the meditation; make sure you close at the end of each practice completely before you do anything else. Should you fall asleep during practice, do a closing immediately after you wake up.

Major Procedures in One-Step Classic Meditation

- This is the core of TFMQ. It takes 50 minutes to complete the entire form.
- TFMQ can be practiced at any time, anywhere, and as often as you like. There are five major stages in this form of classic meditation.
- The first step is "light up the furnace." Set up a warm place for qi cultivation at your lower Dantian, where all qi goes to and comes from. Start with strong intention, coordinated with your breathing; you need to feel warmth in the lower Dantian at the end of this step so as to let the qi move around. (This is achieved through focused intention plus coordinated breathing, an important technique in Daoist Qigong meditation.)
- The second step is to gather energy from the sun and the moon. Consciousness or intention should be light and not too strong. Try to stay in a state of seemingly thinking but not thinking, seemingly sleeping but not sleeping.
- Keep all pores on the skin open. Keep attention on the two ends of the process, not the in-between process—that is, think of skin and pores while inhaling, and think of the lower Dantian while exhaling (keep attention on exhalation and inhalation).
- The third step is to gather five-color universal energy from five planets through five key senses, and send them to five major organs. These five elements and order are not random but specifically follow the five-element theory of traditional Chinese medicine in the attempt to make them orderly and healthy.
- The fourth step is to wash out sickness with sacred water, similarly to the process of meditation for detoxification, which needs relatively strong consciousness and clear visualization.
- Wash from outside to inside with a strong whirlpool and from head to feet, with five organs and five colors being reinforced. Visualize the location(s) of sickness changing from black to white or to the appropriate color (a five-element chart may be used as supplemental material).
- The fifth step is to reach an empty-mind state through a fading-out technique. This is a relatively higher level of Qigong cultivation, a transition from guided form to formless meditation. It may be difficult to achieve in the beginning. Some techniques can be used to help at this stage, such as letting the awareness stay at the lower Dantian if in a conscious state; or you can think about your childhood, happy images of yourself, and so forth.
- You may use this stage to communicate with your locations of sickness, a mind-healing technique. Visualize the area getting smaller or disappearing, or talk with it with good intentions.
- You can do this portion of the practice (empty mind) anytime and anywhere.
- Always close as instructed previously.

Example: Relaxation through Smiling Exercise

The following introduces a special Qigong form for relaxation. Note that instead of simply teaching the practitioner to relax physically, this Qigong exercise achieves the relaxation state by inducing internal smiling or psychological/spiritual relaxation, as the psychological relaxation is more important in the mind–body–spirit integration.

Here are the instructions for this internal smiling exercise:

This exercise is designed to help you quickly recover from fatigue, reduce stress, and increase your energy and efficacy. You can do this at anytime and anywhere.

You can do this exercise standing, sitting, or lying down. Whichever position you select, make sure you are comfortable and relaxed. Clear your mind of all thoughts.

Lightly close your eyes. Breathe naturally, paying special attention to the area around your abdomen. Let your breathing be soft, even, deep, and slow.

Now you are relaxed. As you breathe naturally and relax, focus your attention on the area between your two eyebrows. Visualize a small smiling face in between your two eyebrows, smiling, and smiling happily at you. The smiling face begins to grow bigger and bigger until it covers your entire head.

The smiling face continues to expand, and it covers your entire chest. Your entire chest becomes a smiling face. It continues to expand. . . . Your entire body becomes a smiling face. Your organs, your nervous system, all your cells and pores are smiling . . . Smiling . . . and smiling.

The smiling face continues to expand from your body outward to become a very large smiling face covering the entire room, and then to the surrounding environment. It continues to expand, smiling and expanding, smiling and expanding until it covers the earth. The entire earth and everything in it turns into a huge smiling face, smiling, smiling, and smiling!

The huge smiling face continues to expand, reaching the entire universe, and the entire universe becomes an endless smiling face.

Everything is smiling,

Everything becomes the smiling face,

There is no one, not you, or anyone else—just smiles.

There are no desires, no wants, no demands, just smiles.

There is no disease, no illness, no disasters; just smiles.

There is no heaven, no earth, just smiles, smiles, and smiles.

Continue to visualize and feel the smiling face for a few minutes, or for as long as you want.

Now, you can finish the exercise by letting the smiling face gradually become smaller and smaller and come back into your body, then reduce it to the size of an egg and send it to your lower Dantian. Visualize the small smiling face in your lower Dantian for a minute as you continue to breathe naturally.

You feel completely relaxed, content, and worry-free.

Briskly rub your palms together until they feel warm, and then use your palms to stroke your face downward a few times. Your smiling exercise is now completed.

CASE EXAMPLE

Following are a few cases of patients who benefited significantly from TFMQ.

Case 1

A 58-year-old Caucasian man in New Jersey had a series of chronic conditions, some of which could be directly related to psychological distress. These conditions include a high prostate specific antigen (PSA) mark (but not a confirmed cancer), atrial septal defect, asthma, allergies, hypertension, multiple injuries from an auto accident, and edema in both legs. He started the practice of TFMQ and Qigong therapy due to his concern about his elevated PSA mark (around 11) and the family history of cancer. The Qigong therapy was introduced to him through an intensive Qigong workshop, which involved the training and practice of gathering qi, magnifying qi energy and using it for self-healing with visualization and guided imagery, and supervised energetic fasting. The patient practiced Qigong for more than 4 hours a day during intensive training and about 1 to 2 hours daily thereafter. About 10 sessions of external qi healing were performed by a Qigong master for his pain relief and systematic adjustment. After the intensive workshop and Qigong therapy, plus 36 days of *Bigu* (energetic water fasting), the patient discontinued all medications (8 in total) and lost 35 pounds in 2 months. His blood pressure dropped from 220/110 with medication to 120/75 without medication in 2 weeks; his pulse rate dropped from 88 beats per minute (BPM) resting to 68 BPM in the mornings and 55 BPM in the evenings; the edema in his legs went away; symptoms of asthma and allergies disappeared; and his PSA level dropped from 11 to 4 (normal), all without any medications (Chen & Turner, 2004).

Although the patient's original motive for participating in Qigong practice was to lower his elevated PSA level, the outcome of the intensive Qigong training was really much better than he had expected—a complete recovery from multiple chronic symptoms. One of the unique characteristics of this case is that most of his previous physical conditions were not curable by known conventional medications or healing procedures, yet he achieved simultaneous recovery with Qigong therapy in a very short period and has stayed medication-free for more than 2 years. None of his doctors can offer an explanation as to the source of his simultaneous recovery from multiple symptoms in such a short time.

Case 2

A female patient from Japan in her mid-30s weighed 215 pounds and suffered from heart disease, diabetes, high cholesterol, arthritis, and major depression. She had lost her job, her boyfriend, and her self-confidence at the time when she was introduced to Qigong therapy in 1999. She came to China to learn to practice the TFMQ system with the Bigu technique (energetic fasting). After she had practiced Qigong therapy intensively for 40 days (more than 6 hours a day)—including 25 days of Bigu—not only had her weight dropped to 143 pounds, but also her depression and other chronic conditions had disappeared completely. Now she enjoys a renewed physical and emotional well-being, is back in the workforce, and is living a normal life.

Case 3

An Asian male in his 40s, a practitioner of Chinese medicine and acupuncture in southern California, had suffered from diabetes, headache, and back pain for quite some time. He had not practiced Qigong previously. Within 2 weeks after attending the TFMQ training class, he reported regaining the energy level that he had had about 15 years ago. Practicing only 1½ hours of Qigong and sleeping deeply for 4 hours a day, he said "the benefits for my health are unmistakable." As a doctor himself, he kept very detailed records of his health conditions during the Qigong class period, which involved intensive Qigong meditation with group qi adjustment (a healer placed and monitored the qi field in the classroom). Table 16.1 presents some observations of his personal conditions before and after Qigong training.

TABLE 16.1. Patient Self-Reported Improvement in 2 Weeks of Qigong Training

Conditions	Before Qigong class	After Qigong class
Blood sugar	293	110 (normal)
Weight	192 pounds	172 pounds
Blood pressure	135/95	118/78
Arthritis pain	Finger joints	Disappeared after 3 days
Sleep time	8–9 hours	5 hours
Other pains I	Liver, stomach, and colon for over 2 years	Recovered after 2 days
Other pains II	Headache, backache, and pain in right waist area	Recovered after 3 days
Other	Bleeding teeth and baldness	Stopped bleeding and numerous new hair growth after class

SUMMARY AND CONCLUSIONS

Qigong, an ancient Chinese energy healing practice that combines the elements of relaxation, breathing work, guided imagery, biofeedback (Chapters 9–11, this volume), mindfulness meditation (Chapter 15, this volume), mind manipulation, and mind–body integration, is a very effective option for stress management. As the case studies demonstrated, Qigong therapy works for more than just stress management and can be applied to a variety of health conditions to achieve simultaneous recovery. These results present a great challenge to current medicine and health care.

Qigong therapy might be an effective tool in stress management. What is more important is that a complete self-healing-based medical system to promote self-care and to find the healer within accompanies Qigong therapy. The TFMQ described in this chapter is simple and easy to learn yet powerful and effective for helping to relieve symptoms, improve recovery, and gain general health resilience. The factors that contribute to its efficacy in healing include a drug-free approach, to avoid the side effects of pharmaceuticals; use of innate self-healing power; the following of TCM philosophies; and a healthy lifestyle.

Although Qigong has a lot of common elements with other effective stress reduction methods, it encompasses more than other therapies in terms of its concept and the application of human vital energy (qi) and intention power (yi), which manage stress both physically and psychologically, and achieves a result that goes beyond reduction of stress. It is hoped that more scientists and health care professionals will become interested in research and applications of Qigong therapy.

ACKNOWLEDGMENTS

I would like to thank the Qigong Institute (*www.Qigonginstitute.org*) in California for supporting my Chinese literature review with a small research grant. I also appreciate the help of Mrs. Denise Dehnbostel, Ms. Joy Staller, and Dr. Yinong Chong in editing and commenting on an earlier version of this chapter.

NOTES

1. Taiji, or tai chi, is considered the movement form of Qigong, at least at the beginning of the tai chi exercises.
2. Here, *closing* refers to the procedure that ends a Qigong meditation or practice, usually for example, like rubbing palms together until feel warm; stroking the face from top down; combing the hair by running fingers through it; chomping teeth; and so forth. The procedure is intended to bring the practitioner from meditation back to a normal state.

REFERENCES

Agishi, T. (1998). Effects of the external Qigong on symptoms of arteriosclerotic obstruction in the lower extremities evaluated by modern medical technology. *Artificial Organs, 22*(8), 707–710.

Chen, K. (2004). An analytic review of studies on measuring effects of external qi in China. *Alternative Therapies in Health and Medicine, 10*(4), 38–50.

Chen, K., & Liu, T. J. (2004). Effects of Qigong therapy on arthritis: A review and report of a pilot trial. *Medical Paradigm, 1*(1), 36–48.

Chen, K., & Turner, F. D. (2004). A case study of simultaneous recovery from multiple physical symptoms with medical Qigong therapy. *Journal of Alternative and Complementary Medicine, 10*(1), 159–162.

Chen, K., & Yeung, R., (2002). Exploratory studies of Qigong therapy for cancer in China. *Integrative Cancer Therapies, 1*(4), 345–370.

Chen, X., Li, Y., Liu, G., & He, B. (1997). The inhibitory effects of Chinese Taijing Five-Element Qigong on transplanted hepatocarcinoma in mice. *Asian Medicine, 11*, 36–38.

Chu, D. Y., He, W. G., Zhou, Y. F., & Chen, B. C. (1998). The effect of Chinese Qigong on the conformation of biomolecule. *Chinese Journal of Somatic Science, 8*(4), 155–159.

Guo, Y. J., Tang, C. M., & Liang, F. (1996). Urine catecholamine and cortisol levels in Qigong practitioners under stress conditions. *Proceedings of the third National Academic Conference on Qigong Science, Beijing* (pp. 8, 90).

He, B. H. (2003). *Taiji five-element self-recovery system: Comprehensive Qigong therapy.* Hong Kong: Qingwen.

He, H. Z., Li, D. L., Xi, W. B., & Zhang, C. L. (1999). A "stress meter" assessment of the degree of relaxation in Qigong vs. non-Qigong meditation. *Frontier Perspectives, 8*(1), 37–42.

Itoh, T., Shen, Z., Itoh, Y., & Tamura, A. (2000). The effects of *wai qi* on rats under stress based on urinary excretion measurements of catecholamines . *Journal of the International Society of Life Information Science, 18*(2), 338–345.

Lee, M. S., Huh, H. J., Hong, S. S., Jang, H. S., Ryu, H., Lee, H. S., et al. (2001). Psychoneuroimmunological effects of Qi-therapy: Preliminary study on the changes of level of anxiety, mood, cortisol and melatonin and cellular function of neutrophil and natural killer cells. *Stress Health, 17*, 17–24.

Lee, M. S., Lee, M. S., Kim, H. J., & Moon, S. R. (2003). Qigong reduced blood pressure and catecholamine levels of patients with essential hypertension. *International Journal of Neuroscience, 113*, 1707–1717.

Lee, S. (2000, March 18). Chinese hypnosis can cause Qigong-induced mental disorders. *British Medical Journal, 320*(7237), 803.

Liang, S. Y., & Wu, W. C. (1997). *Qigong empowerment: A guide to medical, Taoist, Buddhist, and Wushu energy cultivation.* East Providence, RI: The Way of the Dragon.

Liu, T., Hua, W. G., et al. (2005). *Qigong study in Chinese medicine.* Beijing: China Publisher of Chinese Medicine.

Loh, S. H. (1999). Qigong therapy in the treatment of metastatic colon cancer. *Alternative Therapies in Health and Medicine, 5*(4), 111–112.

Lu, L. T., Liu, Y. K., & Zhuang, Y. B. (1996). The clinical study of coronary heart disease treated by Qigong with music. *Proceedings of the third World Conference on Medical Qigong, Beijing, China.*

Mayer, M. H. (1999). Qigong and hypertension: A critique of research. *Journal of Alternative and Complementary Medicine, 5*(4), 371–382.

Muehsami, D. J., Markow, M. S., & Muehsami, P. A. (1994). Effects of Qigong on cell-free myosin phosphorylation: Preliminary experiments. *Subtle Energies, 5*, 103–104.

Ng, B. Y. (1999). Qigong-induced mental disorders: A review. *Australian and New Zealand Journal of Psychiatry, 33*(2), 197–206.

Pavek, R. R. (1988). Effects of Qigong on psychosomatic and other emotionally rooted disorders. *Proceedings of the First World Conference of Academic Exchange on Medical Qigong*, Beijing, China, p. 150.

Sancier, K. M. (1996). Medical applications of Qigong. *Alternative Therapies in Health and Medicine, 2*(1), 40–45.

Sancier, K. M. (1999). Therapeutic benefits of Qigong exercises in combination with drugs. *Journal of Alternative and Complementary Medicine, 5*, 383–389.

Sandlund, E. S., & Norlander, T. (2000, April). The effects of Tai Chi Chuan relaxation and exercise on stress responses and well-being: An overview of research. *International Journal of Stress Management, 7*(2), 139–149.

Segal, Z. V., Williams, J. M. G., & Teasdale, J. D. (2002). Mindfulness-based cognitive therapy for depression: A new approach to preventing relapse. New York: Guilford Press.

Shan, H., Yan, H., Sheng, H., & Hu, S. (1989). A preliminary evaluation on Chinese Qigong treatment of anxiety. *Proceedsing of the Second International Conference on Qigong*, Xian, China, p.165.

Shan, H. H., Yan, H. Q., Xu, S. H., Zhang, M. D., Yu, Y. P., Zhao, J. C., et al. (1989, June). Clinical phenomenology of mental disorders caused by Qigong exercise. *Chinese Medicine Journal, 102*(6), 445–448.

Singh, B., Berman, B., Hadhazy, V., & Creamer, P. (1998). A pilot study of cognitive behavioral therapy in fibromyalgia. *Alternative Therapies in Health and Medicine, 24*(2), 67–70.

Sobel, D. S. (1995). Rethinking medicine: Improving health outcomes with cost-effective psychosocial interventions. *Psychosomatic Medicine, 57*(3), 234–244.

Wall, R. B. (2005, July–August). Tai Chi and mindfulness-based stress reduction in a Boston public middle school. *Journal of Pediatric Health Care, 19*(4), 230–237.

Wang, C. C., Collet, J. P., & Lau, J. (2004). The effect of Tai Chi on health outcomes in patients with chronic conditions. *Archive of Internal Medicine, 164*, 493–501.

Wang, J. (1993). Role of Qigong on mental health. *Proceedings of the Second World Conference of Academic Exchange on Medical Qigong*, Beijing, China.

Wirth, D. P., Cram, J. R., & Chang, R. J. (1997). Multisite electromyographic analysis of therapeutic touch and Qigong therapy. *Journal of Alternative and Complementary Medicine, 3*(2), 109–118.

Wu, W. H., Bandilla, E., Ciccone, D. S., Yang, J., Cheng, S. S., Carner, N., et al. (1999). Effects of Qigong on late-stage complex regional pain syndrome. *Alternative Therapies in Health and Medicine, 5*(1), 45–54.

Yan, X., Lin, H., Li, H., Traynor-Kaplan, A., Xia, Z. Q., Lu, F., et al. (1999). Structure and property changes in certain material influenced by the external Qi of Qigong. *Material Research Innovation, 2*, 349–359.

Yang, J. M. (1991). *Qigong for arthritis: The Chinese way of healing and prevention*. Jamaica Plain, MA: YMAA.

Zhang, L., Wang, L., Yan, Y. Z., Ge, D. Y., & Zhou, Y. (1993). Adjusting effect of emitted qi on the immune function of cold-stressed mice. *Proceedings of the 2nd World Conference of Academic Exchange of Medical Qigong*, 109.

Zhang, Z. H., Gu, P. D., Wang, S. L., Liu, Z. B., & Song, T. B. (Eds.). (1994). *The encyclopedia of Chinese Qigong*. Beijing, China: United.

CHAPTER 17

Yoga as a Therapeutic Intervention

SAT BIR S. KHALSA

HISTORY OF THE METHOD

In its earliest form, yoga was a practical discipline incorporating techniques whose goal was the development of a state of mental and physical health, well-being, inner harmony, and, ultimately, an experience involving "a union of the human individual with the universal and transcendent Existence" (Aurobindo, 1999, p. 6). It can, therefore, be considered a form of practical mysticism, the primary goal of which is the ultimate manifestation or achievement of the unitive experience that has been described with terms such as *cosmic, universal, transcendental* or *God consciousness, oneness,* or *bliss.* Although imbued with this clear philosophical underpinning, it has not been traditionally considered a religious practice. Yoga practices are believed to have originated in early civilizations on the Indian subcontinent, and they have been practiced historically in India and throughout East Asia and have evolved distinctly separately from Oriental religions.

Over the past century yoga has been introduced into and practiced in the West, where it has become increasingly popular (Saper, Eisenberg, Davis, Culpepper, & Phillips, 2004). In its modern, Western manifestation, yoga includes the practices of meditation, regulation of respiration, and physical exercises and postures in which the focus is more on isometric exercise and stretching than on aerobic fitness. However, there are now a wide variety of styles of yoga practice, some of which focus less on the philosophical, meditative, and even respiratory components and more (or entirely) on the physical exercises and postures.

Historically, the limited application of yoga techniques for specific disorders is recent relative to the ancient origins of yoga (Gharote, 1982). In fact, "the therapeutic aspect of yoga does not feature in any of the traditional systems of self-help . . . yoga therapy was not a developed branch of yogic discipline as such" (Gharote, 1987, p. 4). Because the primary goal of yoga practice is spiritual development, its beneficial medical consequences can more precisely be described as positive side effects (Goyeche, 1979).

The first systematic medical application of yoga started in India as early as 1918 at the Yoga Institute near Mumbai (Yogendra, 1970) and at the Kaivalyadhama Yoga Institute in Lonavala under Swami Kuvalyananda in the 1920s (Gharote, 1991; Willoughby, 2000). Subsequently, yoga therapy has proliferated in India with the establishment of yogic hospitals and clinics, notably the Vivekananda Yoga Research Institute near Bangalore (SVYASA), and with the widespread application of yoga treatments by other yoga therapy clinics and individual clinicians (Bhole & Karambelkar, 1972; Vinekar, 1976; Willoughby, 2000). It has also proliferated internationally, with the appearance of yoga therapy centers, the inclusion of yoga programs in alternative medicine centers and hospital cancer programs, and the emergence of "yoga therapists." For the latter there are yoga therapy training programs and a representative society, the International Association of Yoga Therapists (IAYT), based in the United States. Several dozen books are available specifically on the topic of yoga therapy in general and on yoga therapy for specific disorders (e.g., Gharote & Lockhart, 1987; Monro, Nagarathna, & Nagendra, 1990).

THEORETICAL FOUNDATIONS

A general feature of these practices is their capability of inducing a coordinated psychophysiological response that is the antithesis of the stress response. This "relaxation response" consists of a generalized reduction in both cognitive and somatic arousal, as observed in the modified activity of the hypothalamic–pituitary axis and the autonomic nervous system (Benson, 1975). Bagchi and Wenger (1957), in their early classic research study of yoga practitioners in India, wrote "physiologically Yogic meditation represents deep relaxation of the autonomic nervous system without drowsiness or sleep and a type of cerebral activity without highly accelerated electrophysiological manifestation but probably with more or less insensibility to some outside stimuli for a short or long time" (p. 146). A large number of subsequent research studies examining the effects of these techniques both in isolation and in combination have further confirmed these early results (Pratap, 1971; Funderburk, 1977; Delmonte, 1984; Arpita, 1990; Jevning, Wallace, & Beidebach, 1992; Murphy & Donovan, 1999). Studies have shown that both short-term and long-term practice of yoga techniques are associated with a number of physiological and psychological changes, including reductions of basal cortisol and catecholamine secretion, a decrease in sympathetic activity with a corresponding increase in parasympathetic activity, reductions in metabolic rate and oxygen consumption, salutary effects on cognitive activity and cerebral neurophysiology, and improved neuromuscular and respiratory function (Kamei et al., 2000; Malathi, Damodaran, Shah, Patil, & Maratha, 2000; Patki, Makwana, Karmarkar, & Wadikar, 2003; Ray, Mukhopadhyaya, et al., 2001; Ray, Singha, et al., 2001; Schell, Allolio, & Schonecke, 1994; Schmidt, Wijga, Von Zur, Brabant, & Wagner, 1997; Telles, Nagarathna, Nagendra, & Desiraju, 1993; Telles & Vani, 2002; Tran, Holly, Lashbrook, & Amsterdam, 2001; Udupa, Madanmohan, Bhavanani, Vijayalakshmi, & Krishnamurthy, 2003; Vempati & Telles, 2002; Watanabe, Fukuda, Hara, & Shirakawa, 2002; Yadav & Das, 2001).

Accordingly, it has been suggested that yoga practice appears to be especially effective in counteracting the negative impact of stress (Serber, 2000; Udupa, 1985). Studies comparing the effects of yoga with those of other exercise modalities have revealed that it has superior effects on some measures of stress tolerance and mood (Berger & Owen, 1992; Johnson, Walker, Heys, Whiting, & Eremin, 1997; Netz & Lidor, 2003; Szabo, Mesko, Caputo, & Gill, 1998). Research evaluating yoga as an intervention in healthy individuals and patients under stress has suggested that a yoga intervention is an effective countermeasure (Damodaran et al., 2002; Khasky & Smith, 1999; Malathi et al., 1998; Malathi & Damodaran, 1999; Moadel et al., 2003; Waelde, Thompson, & Gallagher-Thompson, 2004). Not surprisingly, the ability of yoga practice to positively affect psychophysiological functioning has also led to the implementation of these techniques as a therapeutic intervention in a number of disorders that have psychosomatic or stress-related components.

ASSESSMENT

Research on the psychophysiological effects of yoga practice began with Kuvalyananda's work in the 1920s, and there are a number of published reviews of this basic research literature (Arpita, 1990; Funderburk, 1977; Gharote, 1991; Pratap, 1971; Udupa, 1976). Research on therapeutic applications of yoga and meditation began more recently (Gharote, 1991), and although there are some reviews of this literature, these have focused on specific disorders (Raub, 2002; Taylor & Majmundar, 2000; Kaushal, Behera, & Grover, 1988; Telles & Naveen, 1997). A good deal of yoga therapy research has been published in specialty yoga journals, particularly the journal *Yoga Mimamsa*. These are not easily accessible and therefore not consistently reviewed or cited. Although meditation is an integral part of yoga practice, there is a extensive body of research literature that examines meditation alone (without incorporation of yogic breathing and/or specific yoga postures), and this literature has been reviewed previously (Baer, 2003; Jacobs, 2001; Murphy & Donovan, 1999; Perez-de-Albeniz & Holmes, 2000; Proulx, 2003). The most well-known meditation techniques that have been used clinically include transcendental meditation (TM), mindfulness meditation (or Vipassana, which is the basic technique in the mindfulness-based stress reduction program), and Herbert Benson's relaxation response technique (see Carrington, Chapter 14, this volume, on mantra meditation and Kristeller, Chapter 15, this volume, on mindfulness meditation).

My recent bibliometric analysis of yoga therapy research (which has not included studies of meditation alone) has revealed a total of 181 publications in 81 different journals published by researchers in 15 different countries from 1967 to early 2004 (Khalsa, 2004b). The first substantive published research in yoga therapy did not appear until the late 1960s and early 1970s. From that time, there was a consistent increase in frequency of publications up until the late 1980s, since which time the frequency has been stable, suggesting the possibility of saturation or a ceiling effect of productivity in this field. However, it is more likely that an ongoing sharp increase is occurring in the present and will continue in the near future. This may be due in part to the recent increased interest in yoga as an alternative medical intervention, particularly in the West (Barnes, Powell-Griner, McFann, & Nahin, 2004; Saper et al., 2004), and to increased funding by government agencies, such as the National Center for Complementary and Alternative Medicine in the United States.

A clear majority of the studies have been conducted in Indian institutions; followed by those in the United States, with fewer than half as many publications; and then by investigators in England, Europe, and elsewhere. This dominance of Indian investigators stands in contrast to the usual trend in scientific research, in which the United States, England, Europe, and Japan dominate productivity, but it is perhaps not surprising in this case given the Indian origin of yoga practice. However, many of the studies performed in India have been published in Indian journals, and the peer-review procedures of some of these journals are not as rigorous as those of Western journals. Furthermore, Indian investigators have generated proportionately fewer randomized controlled trials (RCTs) than their Western counterparts. With the dramatic increase in popularity of yoga in the West, it is possible that Western laboratories may begin increasing the frequency of research in this area to a pace faster than that in India. For example, for the time period

1973–1989, the number of Indian- and U.S.-published RCTs was 11 and 2, respectively. From 1990 to 2004, the number of Indian-based studies was 21, a twofold increase, whereas the number of U.S. studies was 16, an eightfold increase (Khalsa, 2004b).

A wide variety of yoga techniques contribute to the interventions used in this literature, ranging from individual physical postures or breathing techniques to complete yoga lifestyle interventions involving dietary and psychospiritual components. Application of the interventions is equally varied and ranges from individual practice to group sessions, from daily practice sessions to weekly sessions, and from short-duration to long-duration sessions.

An analysis of the experimental protocols described in the methodology sections of all of the publications in the bibliometric analysis revealed that just under half of the publications reported on studies that incorporated the RCT, a study design with wide recognition as the best evaluation of treatment effectiveness. Few of the yoga specialty journal publications incorporated RCTs. Therefore, although these publications may provide valuable preliminary data, they are not as rigorous as those published in nonyoga journal publications. The fact that almost half of the nonyoga journal publications have reported RCTs is encouraging, as these trials provide the most valuable and conclusive information. A sample-size analysis on these publications, however, suggests that the vast majority of these studies have been relatively small RCTs (Khalsa, 2004b).

The three types of disorders most evaluated in yoga studies have been psychiatric conditions, cardiovascular disorders, and respiratory disorders. These are followed in turn by diabetes, neurological conditions, musculoskeletal conditions, and a variety of other disorders. About one-third of the psychiatric conditions consisted of depressive disorders, and these were followed, in order of prevalence, by anxiety, addictive disorders, and a variety of other psychopathological conditions. Publications on cardiovascular conditions were almost evenly split between hypertension and heart disease. The predominant respiratory condition was asthma, with a smaller contribution of chronic obstructive pulmonary disease (COPD) and a few other respiratory conditions. Neurological conditions included mostly headache and epilepsy, whereas musculoskeletal disorders included a wide array of unrelated conditions. In order of prevalence, the discrete disorders that were studied the most were asthma, hypertension, heart disease, diabetes, depression or dysthymia, and anxiety. It is likely that a number of factors contributed to the choice of disorders evaluated for the effectiveness of yoga. One of these factors is the suitability of yoga in counteracting stress and reducing autonomic arousal, which are known to contribute to these disorders. Another factor is likely the sociopolitical drive to address disorders that have the highest mortality rates—heart disease, asthma, diabetes, and hypertension among them. It is therefore unlikely that an analysis of the existing research literature can provide much information as to which disorders can be most effectively treated with yoga. The appropriate study for that determination would be a meta-analysis that would evaluate relative effect sizes for yoga treatments across disorders (Khalsa, 2004b). A brief review of published research reporting on yoga treatments for asthma, hypertension and heart disease, and depression and anxiety follows.

Asthma

Of all the studies of yoga therapy, those on asthma are the most common, with more than 40 publications (Khalsa, 2004b). The involvement of a psychological or stress component in asthma provides a rationale for the use of yoga techniques, as does the use of yogic breathing techniques, which have been shown to improve respiratory function in normal participants (Goyeche, Abo, & Ikemi, 1982; Lehrer, Feldman, Giardino, Song, &

Schmaling, 2002; Raub, 2002). Interventions used in asthma research studies range from individual breathing practices to a full multicomponent yoga practice. Although at least a half-dozen uncontrolled studies have reported improvements in lung function parameters (Khalsa, 2004b; Lehrer et al., 2002; Raub, 2002; Goyeche et al., 1982), the results from RCTs have been mixed. A yogic breathing technique that involves maintaining the duration of the exhale to twice that of the inhale has been reported to have some benefit in an uncontrolled study (Singh, 1987), but in two RCTs with this technique, improvements in the main outcome measures were not statistically significant (Cooper et al., 2003; Singh, Wisniewski, Britton, & Tattersfield, 1990). In RCT studies with multicomponent yoga practice, two studies showed positive benefits in lung function and in other measures (Manocha, Marks, Kenchington, Peters, & Salome, 2002; Nagarathna & Nagendra, 1985), whereas two studies did not show statistically significant improvements in lung function, although improvement was observed in ancillary measures (Vedanthan et al., 1998; Fluge et al., 1994).

Hypertension and Heart Disease

As in the case of asthma, psychological factors and stress are potential contributing factors to the pathophysiology of hypertension and heart disease, providing a rationale for treatment with yoga (Patel, 1997), which has been shown to be effective in increasing cardiovascular health and reducing risk factors in healthy individuals (Raub, 2002). Accordingly, a number of uncontrolled studies have reported improvements in blood pressure and other measures in hypertensive patients (Khalsa, 2004b; Raub, 2002). Research using yoga-based treatments for hypertension is notable for the contribution of Chandra Patel and colleagues, who conducted an early series of studies that included RCTs. They showed the effectiveness of yoga-based stress management techniques in the treatment of patients with hypertension, including significant reductions in blood pressure and reduction in medication requirements (Patel, 1997). Of five other RCTs that evaluated blood pressure changes with yoga in hypertension (Aivazyan, 1990; Broota, Varma, & Singh, 1995; Latha & Kaliappan, 1991; Murugesan, Govindarajulu, & Bera, 2000; Van Montfrans, Karemaker, Wieling, & Dunning, 1990), four of these reported statistically significant reductions in blood pressure (Aivazyan, 1990; Broota et al., 1995; Latha & Kalrappan, 1991; Murugesan et al., 2000).

The majority of studies evaluating yoga-based treatments for heart disease have incorporated a variety of additional treatment modalities, such as dietary restrictions and counseling, into a treatment package that can be considered more of a "yoga lifestyle" intervention. Most notable are the studies by Dean Ornish and colleagues, who were the first to demonstrate that it was possible not only to arrest the progression of coronary artery disease but also to actually reverse it (Koertge et al., 2003; Ornish et al., 1998; Ornish, 1998). Other investigators have applied similar lifestyle programs, mostly in RCTs, and have reported improvements in a number of cardiovascular measures (Jatuporn et al., 2003; Mahajan, Reddy, & Sachdeva, 1999; Manchanda et al., 2000; Yogendra et al., 2004).

Depression and Anxiety

Of studies evaluating the effectiveness of yoga treatment for psychiatric or psychological conditions, those that evaluate patients with depression, dysthymia, or anxiety make up a strong majority (Khalsa, 2004b). Research on yoga's effectiveness in treating these disorders was among the earliest in studies of yoga therapy. In particular, the studies by Vahia and colleagues were among the first, beginning with a case series report in 1966 (Vahia, Vinekar, & Doongaji, 1966), followed by an uncontrolled study (Vahia, 1972) and then three reports with RCTs (Balkrishna, Sanghvi, Rana, Doongaji, & Vahia, 1977; Vahia, Doongaji, Jeste, Kapoor, et al., 1973; Vahia, Doongaji, Jeste, Ravindranath, et al., 1973). These studies, as did two other studies (Sethi, Trivedi, Srivastava, & Yadav, 1982; Platania-Solazzo et al., 1992), all employed a multicomponent yoga practice to study populations with a mix of disorders, most of whom had depression or anxiety, and reported significant improvements using qualitative clinical assessments and/or self-report questionnaires specific for anxiety and/or depression.

Despite the improvements in anxiety reported in the studies described above, very little research has evaluated yoga treatments specifically for anxiety disorder (Sahasi, Mohan, & Kacker, 1989), as almost all published studies have reported on treatments in patients with depression. Improvements in depression have been reported in a study of severely depressed students using a single yoga exercise (Khumar, Kaur, & Kaur, 1993) and in another short-term study of psychiatry outpatients diagnosed with depression using a limited set of exercises (Broota & Dhir, 1990). A series of reports has appeared that have evaluated a very specific yoga practice called Sudarshan Kriya yoga, which involves a series of breathing exercises in the treatment of depression and dysthymia (Janakiramaiah et al., 1998; Janakiramaiah et al., 2000; Murthy, Gangadhar, Janakiramaiah, & Subbakrishna, 1997; Murthy, Janakiramaiah, Gangadhar, & Subbakrishna, 1998; Rohini, Pandey, Janakiramaiah, Gangadhar, & Vedamurthachar, 2000). One of these was an RCT with hospitalized patients with severe depression that showed that this treatment was as effective as treatment with the antidepressant imipramine (Janakiramaiah et al., 2000). Most recently, a randomized case–control study in the United States has reported findings suggestive of a significant improvement in participants with mild depression who were treated with another popular style of yoga practice in which the emphasis was on exercises specifically believed to be useful for depression (Woolery, Myers, Stemlieb, & Zeltzer, 2004).

SIDE EFFECTS AND CONTRAINDICATIONS

Yoga practices are associated with minimal risk of negative side effects or adverse consequences. Although it has been suggested that meditation practice is contraindicated for some psychiatric conditions, such as psychosis, there is no reliable research evidence for or against this contention. A number of case reports of negative consequences associated with yoga practice have appeared. A major problem with evidence restricted to only case reports of psychological adverse events "triggered" by meditation is that one cannot rule out the possibility that such events were simply spontaneously generated in accordance with the natural history of the disorder and may have been triggered by other ongoing ordinary life circumstances. Furthermore, many of these negative case reports involve individuals who are practicing techniques on their own in an overintensive or contraindicated manner. It should go without saying that treatment of any medical or psychiatric condition with potentially serious consequences (e.g., psychosis, major depression, epilepsy, diabetes) should be treated under the careful and regular supervision of an appropriately qualified clinician, regardless of the presumed benign nature of a treatment. Under the supervision of a qualified and experienced yoga instructor, yoga therapy would usually be practiced in a less intensive format, which would likely minimize the risk of adverse events. In general, it is more likely that unexpected positive benefits might appear with yoga therapy, such as resolution of stress-related symptoms other than those that constitute the primary complaint.

THE METHOD

From the perspective of a patient who wishes to benefit therapeutically from yoga, a number of important issues arise with respect to identifying the appropriate practice (Riley, 2004). Referrals to specific yoga practices or yoga therapists by health care professionals is not commonplace. This leaves the patient in the position of evaluating potential practice options from information in the public domain, including the Internet, print advertisements and directory listings of yoga centers, and books and magazines.

The first issue a patient faces is the choice of the yoga style to practice. To some extent, this choice will be influenced by the availability of different styles in any particular region, the location of the class, and the cost and the timing of class offerings. There is no single standardized practice format, nor is this likely or necessarily desirable in the future. The current practice of yoga is characterized by a wide variety of styles, many of these from specific schools of practice that are tied to specific masters or traditional styles in India. On the one hand, some styles may include practice of only a few physical postures with virtually no attention to breathing, meditation, or philosophy and with the focus entirely on physical fitness. At the other extreme are styles that promote all elements of a yogic lifestyle, including not only postures, breathing, and meditation but also the use of mantras, diet, philosophy, and spirituality. In the West, yoga instruction is also offered in a wide variety of settings, ranging from dedicated yoga centers and ashrams to fitness centers, local recreation facilities, community centers, libraries, and so forth. Despite the lack of a universal standardization of yoga teaching and practice, individual schools or styles of yoga practice may adopt standards for how classes are taught and may specify strict requirements for certification as teachers within that style. However, it is probably safe to conclude that the emphasis that an individual yoga instructor exerts on how the yoga is taught and practiced is also highly variable; different teachers certified in the same style may provide a very different experience.

Depending on the nature of a patient's medical complaint, personality, and psychology, a style that is restricted to physical postures alone may not have as much therapeutic benefit as a style that incorporates multiple techniques (i.e., breathing exercises, meditation). The latter would have greater probability of providing benefits, particularly in disorders in which physiological and cognitive hyperarousal are strong contributors. Specific physiological benefits have been ascribed to different individual yoga exercises, and it is therefore possible that a patient may derive more benefit from practicing techniques specific for his or her disorder, if such techniques can be identified. However, there is some variability as to what the claimed benefits are for individual exercises among the different yoga styles. Instructors may or may not be in a position to provide such specific recommendations, and few research studies have provided any information about the relative efficacy of different individual exercises or programs for specific conditions. However, there are a growing number of instructors who consider themselves "yoga therapists," and there is a prolific growth in the number of books and Internet sources from which one might derive specific yoga practice recommendations for a specific disorder. On the other hand, it is likely that a comprehensive practice of yoga that includes postures, breathing, and meditation will be adequately effective for almost all disorders. In fact, such interventions have been used most commonly in clinical yoga treatment research trials.

Other important patient practice issues are compliance and frequency of practice. Generally, yoga classes offered in group settings involve class attendance from once to several times per week; it is uncertain whether a patient will derive significant benefits from a once-per-week practice session. It is more likely that multiple sessions per week, or even daily practice sessions, would be more effective in generating therapeutic benefits on a reasonable time scale. As with all techniques in behavioral and mind–body medicine, self-care practices require a commitment on the part of the patient to devote sufficient time and effort to the intervention. In the case of yoga and meditation, these are currently undergoing a popularity boom, and patients are likely to view undertaking these practices favorably (Saper et al., 2004). Furthermore, most individuals beginning a regular yoga practice experience relatively immediate positive benefits of improved relaxation and well-being, which in turn helps facilitate compliance with a regular regimen. In general, clinical studies employing yoga treatments have reported good compliance and patient satisfaction.

CASE EXAMPLE

The following case report was conducted in the context of a pilot study evaluating the effectiveness of a yoga treatment for insomnia (Khalsa, 2004a). The research protocol used was approved by Brigham and Women's Hospital, and informed consent was obtained. The participant was 54 years old with a 7-year history of sleep-onset insomnia, fibromyalgia, and posttraumatic stress disorder (PTSD). The participant also reported significant daytime fatigue and sleepiness, although a prior sleep study had ruled out the presence of other sleep disorders, including sleep apnea. The subject also reported lifelong bouts of recurring depression and had recently discontinued antidepressant medication. The participant had been recently diagnosed with insulin-dependent diabetes and also reported sexual dysfunction and shortness of breath. At the time of the study, the participant was taking Valium as needed for fibromyalgia and anxiety and daily neurontin for back pain, and was undergoing chiropractic treatment three times per week for fibromyalgia symptoms.

Throughout a 2-week pretreatment baseline evaluation, an 8-week treatment phase, and a 2-week follow-up at 6 months posttreatment, the participant maintained daily sleep diaries, which provided information on subjective sleep characteristics. In addition, sleep, mood, and other questionnaires were completed on a regular basis. The participant underwent a 1-hour treatment session, followed by a brief in-person follow-up meeting 1 week later, and then was contacted by telephone every 2 weeks to address any problems or concerns with the treatment. The treatment consisted of a daily 31-minute breathing meditation called Shabad Kriya, from the Kundalini yoga style (as taught by Yogi Bhajan). This meditation involved a segmented breathing pattern, in which the majority of each breath cycle involved breath retention, and also required meditation on a silently repeated mantra.

The participant's compliance with the treatment was regular, and time of practice gradually increased so that by the final 2 weeks of treatment the yoga practice was fairly consistent for the full duration. The participant also reported practicing the technique occasionally during the daytime, especially under stressful circumstances, and reported that it resulted in a lightening of fibromyalgia symptoms and decreased sensitivity of fibromyalgia trigger points. Accordingly, during the treatment phase, the participant reported reducing the number of chiropractic treatments for fibromyalgia to once per week. By the end of the treatment, the participant reported experiencing significantly reduced fibromyalgia symptoms and had stopped chiropractic treatments altogether. Furthermore, the participant also reported a reduction in insulin dose, reductions in PTSD symptoms and back pain, a restoration of sexual function, and an improvement in respiratory function.

Results from the sleep–wake logs and questionnaires are shown in Figure 17.1. Sleep-onset latency averaged 101 minutes during the 2-week pretreatment baseline pe-

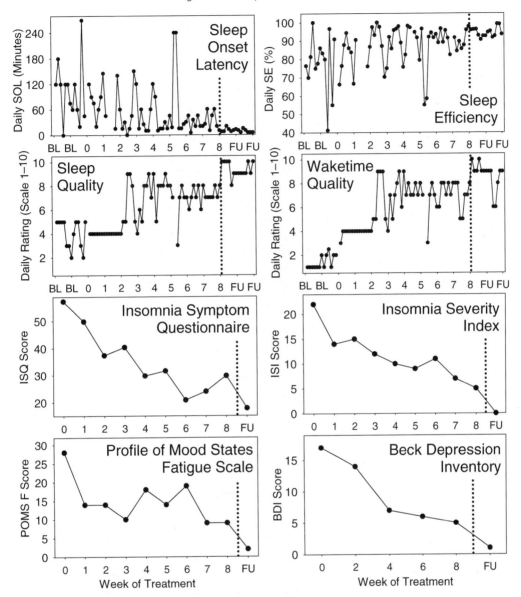

FIGURE 17.1. The top four panels show plots of raw data derived directly or calculated from daily sleep–wake diaries, with the value of the sleep characteristic on the vertical axis and time in weeks on the horizontal axis; each data point represents one night's sleep. A 2-week baseline (BL) precedes the intervention, which starts at week zero. Data for the 2-week follow-up interval (FU) at 6 months posttreatment are plotted after week 8, starting at the vertical dotted line. The bottom four panels show scores of self-report questionnaires, with zero indicating the pretreatment baseline score, followed by scores every 1 or 2 weeks and the 6-month posttreatment follow-up (FU) questionnaire.

riod, well above the commonly accepted cutoff point for clinically significant sleep-onset insomnia. The top left panel of the figure shows the high degree of irregularity in sleep-onset latency that is characteristic of chronic insomnia. However, shortly after initiating treatment, the irregularity, as well as the overall average of sleep-onset latency, was notably reduced, and further reduction continued throughout the 8-week treatment phase. In the last 2 weeks of treatment, sleep-onset latency averaged 30 minutes. Sleep-onset latency was further reduced to an average of 9 minutes during the 2-week follow-up 6 months later, well below any clinical criterion for insomnia. Similarly, sleep efficiency, a measure of the time asleep relative to the total time in bed, also showed a gradual increase and progressive reduction in variability, with average sleep efficiency during baseline of 78% increasing to 91% at end of treatment, and further to 95% at follow-up, well above the clinical benchmark for insomnia of 80–85%. The participant's daily ratings of sleep quality and feeling of restedness at wake time (wake time quality) on a scale from 1 to 10 also showed gradual improvement from average baseline ratings of 4.0 and 1.4, respectively, to end-treatment averages of 7.2 and 7.1, respectively, to follow-up values of 9.4 and 8.6, respectively. Accordingly, ratings on two insomnia questionnaires, the Insomnia Symptom Questionnaire and the Insomnia Severity Index, also showed gradual but substantial improvement throughout the treatment and during follow-up. Both of these questionnaires also incorporate self-evaluation of daytime impairments, such as drowsiness and fatigue, suggesting that the treatment was also effective in improving daytime functioning, an important consideration in insomnia. This result was further confirmed by the scores on the Profile of Mood States Fatigue Scale, shown in the bottom left panel, which indicate steady improvement throughout the treatment. Finally, the participant also showed a steady decline in depression, as shown by the Beck Depression Inventory scores in the bottom right panel.

SUMMARY AND CONCLUSIONS

Through its incorporation of multiple practices, including physical exercise, breath regulation, and meditation, yoga is perhaps the most comprehensive approach in mind–body medicine, and therefore it is an ideal stress management intervention. The appreciable body of research on its psychophysiological benefits in normal participants and in patients attests to the effectiveness of yoga in both the maintenance of wellness and the treatment of medical and psychiatric/psychological disorders, particularly those that are stress-related. Its strong popularity makes it an attractive practice for patients. However, due in part to the lack of integration of yoga therapy into the medical system, the choice of a specific yoga intervention is dependent on the patient's evaluation of potential instructors and styles of yoga practice. As a therapeutic intervention, yoga shares with the rest of behavioral medicine the requirement of compliance and regular practice in order to ensure effectiveness. Patients are likely to experience negligible negative side effects and may actually derive potential ancillary benefits in mood, quality of life, and relief of other stress-related symptomatology.

ACKNOWLEDGMENTS

I am deeply indebted to my spiritual teacher Yogi Bhajan, a master of Kundalini yoga, for his inspiration and guidance and for his service in promoting the practice of yoga in the West. Supported in part by a Mentored Research Career Development Award (No. 5K01AT000066) from the National Center for Complementary and Alternative Medicine of the National Institutes of Health.

REFERENCES

Aivazyan, T. A. (1990). Psychological relaxation therapy in essential hypertension: Efficacy and its predictors. *Yoga Mimamsa, 29*, 27–39.

Arpita. (1990). Physiological and psychological effects of hatha yoga: A review of the literature. *Journal of the International Association of Yoga Therapists, 1*, 1–28.

Aurobindo, S. (1999). *The synthesis of yoga* (5th ed.). Pondicherry, India: Sri Aurobindo Ahram.

Baer, R. A. (2003). Mindfulness training as a clinical intervention: A conceptual and empirical review. *Clinical Psychology: Science and Practice, 10*, 125–143.

Bagchi, B. K., & Wenger, M. A. (1957). Electro-physiological correlates of some Yogi exercises. *Electroencephalography and Clinical Neurophysiology* (Suppl. 7), 132–149.

Balkrishna, V., Sanghvi, L. D., Rana, K., Doongaji, D. R., & Vahia, N. S. (1977). The comparison of psychophysiological therapy with drug therapy. *Indian Journal of Psychiatry, 19*, 87–91.

Barnes, P. M., Powell-Griner, E., McFann, K., & Nahin, R. L. (2004). *Complementary and alternative medicine use among adults: United States, 2002* (NCHS Report No. 343). Hyattsville, MD: National Center for Health Statistics.

Benson, H. (1975). *The relaxation response*. New York: Morrow.

Berger, B. G., & Owen, D. R. (1992). Mood alteration with yoga and swimming: Aerobic exercise may not be necessary. *Perceptual and Motor Skills, 75*, 1331–1343.

Bhole, M. V., & Karambelkar, P. V. (1972). Yoga practices in relation to therapeutics. *Yoga Mimamsa, 14*, 27–34.

Broota, A., & Dhir, R. (1990). Efficacy of two relaxation techniques in depression. *Journal of Personality and Clinical Studies, 6*, 83–90.

Broota, A., Varma, R., & Singh, A. (1995). Role of relaxation in hypertension. *Journal of the Indian Academy of Applied Psychology, 21*, 29–36.

Cooper, S., Oborne, J., Newton, S., Harrison, V., Thompson, C. J., Lewis, S. et al. (2003). Effect of two breathing exercises (Buteyko and pranayama) in asthma: A randomised controlled trial. *Thorax, 58*, 674–679.

Damodaran, A., Malathi, A., Patil, N., Shah, N., Suryavansihi, & Marathe, S. (2002). Therapeutic potential of yoga practices in modifying cardiovascular risk profile in middle-aged men and women. *Journal of the Association of Physicians of India, 50*, 633–640.

Delmonte, M. M. (1984). Physiological concomitants of meditation practice. *International Journal of Psychosomatics, 31*, 23–36.

Fluge, T., Richter, J., Fabel, H., Zysno, E., Weller, E., & Wagner, T. O. (1994). Long-term effects of breathing exercises and yoga in patients with bronchial asthma. *Pneumologie, 48*, 484–490.

Funderburk, J. (1977). *Science studies yoga: A review of physiological data*. Glenview, IL: Himalayan International Institute.

Gharote, M. L. (1982). Yoga therapy: Its scope and limitations. *Journal of Research and Education in Indian Medicine, 1*, 37–42.

Gharote, M. L. (1987). The essence of yoga therapy. In M. L. Gharote & M. Lockhart (Eds.), *The art of survival: A guide to yoga therapy* (pp. 3–6). London: Unwin Hyman.

Gharote, M. L. (1991). Analytical survey of researches in yoga. *Yoga Mimamsa, 29*, 53–68.

Gharote, M. L., & Lockhart, M. (Eds.). (1987). *The art of survival: A guide to yoga therapy*. London: Unwin Hyman.

Goyeche, J. R. (1979). Yoga as therapy in psychosomatic medicine. *Psychotherapy and Psychosomatics, 31*, 373–381.

Goyeche, J. R., Abo, Y., & Ikemi, Y. (1982). Asthma: The yoga perspective. Part II: Yoga therapy in the treatment of asthma. *Journal of Asthma, 19*, 189–201.

Jacobs, G. D. (2001). Clinical applications of the relaxation response and mind–body interventions. *Journal of Alternative and Complementary Medicine, 7*(Suppl. 1), S93–101.

Janakiramaiah, N., Gangadhar, B. N., Naga Venkatesha Murthy, P., Harish, M. G., Subbakrishna, D. K.,

& Vedamurthachar, A. (2000). Antidepressant efficacy of Sudarshan Kriya yoga (SKY) in melancholia: A randomized comparison with electroconvulsive therapy (ECT) and imipramine. *Journal of Affective Disorders*, 57, 255–259.

Janakiramaiah, N., Gangadhar, B. N., Naga Venkatesha Murthy, P., Harish, M. G., Taranath Shetty, K., Subbakrishna, D. K., et al. (1998). Therapeutic efficacy of Sudarshan Kriya yoga (SKY) in dysthymic disorder. *NIMHANS Journal*, 16, 21–28.

Jatuporn, S., Sangwatanaroj, S., Saengsiri, A. O., Rattanapruks, S., Srimahachota, S., Uthayachalerm, W., et al. (2003). Short-term effects of an intensive lifestyle modification program on lipid peroxidation and antioxidant systems in patients with coronary artery disease. *Clinical Hemorheology and Microcirculation*, 29, 429–436.

Jevning, R., Wallace, R. K., & Beidebach, M. (1992). The physiology of meditation: A review: A wakeful hypometabolic integrated response. *Neuroscience and Biobehavioral Reviews*, 16, 415–424.

Johnson, V. C., Walker, L. G., Heys, S., Whiting, P. H., & Eremin, O. (1997). Can relaxation training and hypnotherapy modify the immune response to stress, and is hypnotizability relevant? *Alternative Therapies in Health and Medicine*, 3, 89–90.

Kamei, T., Toriumi, Y., Kimura, H., Ohno, S., Kumano, H., & Kimura, K. (2000). Decrease in serum cortisol during yoga exercise is correlated with alpha wave activation. *Perceptual and Motor Skills*, 90, 1027–1032.

Kaushal, R., Behera, D., & Grover, P. (1988). The theory and practice of yoga therapy for nasobronchial allergy. *Lung India*, 6, 108–116.

Khalsa, S. B. S. (2004a). Treatment of chronic insomnia with yoga: A preliminary study with sleep–wake diaries. *Applied Psychophysiology and Biofeedback*, 29(4), 269–278.

Khalsa, S. B. S. (2004b). Yoga as a therapeutic intervention: A bibliometric analysis of published research studies. *Indian Journal of Physiology and Pharmacology*, 48, 269–285.

Khasky, A. D., & Smith, J. C. (1999). Stress, relaxation states, and creativity. *Perceptual and Motor Skills*, 88, 409–416.

Khumar, S. S., Kaur, P., & Kaur, S. (1993). Effectiveness of Shavasana on depression among university students. *Indian Journal of Clinical Psychology*, 20, 82–87.

Koertge, J., Weidner, G., Elliott-Eller, M., Scherwitz, L., Merritt-Worden, T. A., Marlin, R., et al. (2003). Improvement in medical risk factors and quality of life in women and men with coronary artery disease in the Multicenter Lifestyle Demonstration Project. *American Journal of Cardiology*, 91, 1316–1322.

Latha & Kaliappan, K. V. (1991). Yoga, pranayama, thermal biofeedback techniques in the management of stress and high blood pressure. *Journal of Indian Psychology*, 9, 36–46.

Lehrer, P., Feldman, J., Giardino, N., Song, H. S., & Schmaling, K. (2002). Psychological aspects of asthma. *Journal of Consulting and Clinical Psychology*, 70, 691–711.

Mahajan, A. S., Reddy, K. S., & Sachdeva, U. (1999). Lipid profile of coronary risk subjects following yogic lifestyle intervention. *Indian Heart Journal*, 51, 37–40.

Malathi, A., & Damodaran, A. (1999). Stress due to exams in medical students: Role of yoga. *Indian Journal of Physiology and Pharmacology*, 43, 218–224.

Malathi, A., Damodaran, A., Shah, N., Krishnamurthy, G., Namjoshi, P., & Ghodke, S. (1998). Psychophysiological changes at the time of examination in medical students before and after the practice of yoga and relaxation. *Indian Journal of Psychiatry*, 40, 35–40.

Malathi, A., Damodaran, A., Shah, N., Patil, N., & Maratha, S. (2000). Effect of yogic practices on subjective well-being. *Indian Journal of Physiology and Pharmacology*, 44, 202–206.

Manchanda, S. C., Narang, R., Reddy, K. S., Sachdeva, U., Prabhakaran, D., Dharmanand, S., et al. (2000). Retardation of coronary atherosclerosis with yoga lifestyle intervention. *Journal of the Association of Physicians of India*, 48, 687–694.

Manocha, R., Marks, G. B., Kenchington, P., Peters, D., & Salome, C. M. (2002). Sahaja yoga in the management of moderate to severe asthma: A randomised controlled trial. *Thorax*, 57, 110–115.

Moadel, A. B., Shah, C., Patel, S., Wylie-Rosett, J., Siedlecki, H., Porcelli, T., et al. (2003). Randomized controlled trial of yoga for symptom management during breast cancer treatment [Abstract]. *Proceedings of the American Society of Clinical Oncology*, 22, 726.

Monro, R., Nagarathna, R., & Nagendra, H. R. (1990). *Yoga for common ailments*. New York: Fireside Simon & Schuster.

Murphy, M., & Donovan, S. (1999). *The physical and psychological effects of meditation: A review of contemporary research with a comprehensive bibliography, 1931–1996* (2nd ed.) Sausalito, CA: Institute of Noetic Sciences.

Murthy, P. J., Gangadhar, B. N., Janakiramaiah, N., & Subbakrishna, D. K. (1997). Normalization of P300 amplitude following treatment in dysthymia. *Biological Psychiatry, 42,* 740–743.

Murthy, P. J., Janakiramaiah, N., Gangadhar, B. N., & Subbakrishna, D. K. (1998). P300 amplitude and antidepressant response to Sudarshan Kriya yoga (SKY). *Journal of Affective Disorders, 50,* 45–48.

Murugesan, R., Govindarajulu, N., & Bera, T. K. (2000). Effect of selected yogic practices on the management of hypertension. *Indian Journal of Physiology and Pharmacology, 44,* 207–210.

Nagarathna, R., & Nagendra, H. R. (1985). Yoga for bronchial asthma: A controlled study. *British Medical Journal, 291,* 1077–1079.

Netz, Y., & Lidor, R. (2003). Mood alterations in mindful versus aerobic exercise modes. *Journal of Psychology, 137,* 405–419.

Ornish, D. (1998). Avoiding revascularization with lifestyle changes: The Multicenter Lifestyle Demonstration Project. *American Journal of Cardiology, 82,* 72T–76T.

Ornish, D., Scherwitz, L. W., Billings, J. H., Brown, S. E., Gould, K. L., Merritt, T. A., et al. (1998). Intensive lifestyle changes for reversal of coronary heart disease. *Journal of the American Medical Association, 280,* 2001–2007.

Patel, C. (1997). Stress management and hypertension. *Acta Physiologica Scandinavica, 161,* 155–157.

Patki, R. A., Makwana, J. J., Karmarkar, G., & Wadikar, S. S. (2003). Effect of regular yogic practice on autonomic functions. *Indian Practitioner, 56,* 9–11.

Perez-de-Albeniz, A., & Holmes, J. (2000). Meditation: Concepts, effects and uses in therapy. *International Journal of Psychotherapy, 5,* 49–58.

Platania-Solazzo, A., Field, T. M., Blank, J., Seligman, F., Kuhn, C., Schanberg, S., et al. (1992). Relaxation therapy reduces anxiety in child and adolescent psychiatric patients. *Acta Paedopsychiatrica, 55,* 115–120.

Pratap, V. (1971). Scientific studies on yoga: A review. *Yoga Mimamsa, 13,* 1–18.

Proulx, K. (2003). Integrating mindfulness-based stress reduction. *Holistic Nursing Practice, 17,* 201–208.

Raub, J. A. (2002). Psychophysiologic effects of hatha yoga on musculoskeletal and cardiopulmonary function: A literature review. *Journal of Alternative and Complementary Medicine, 8,* 797–812.

Ray, U. S., Mukhopadhyaya, S., Purkayastha, S. S., Asnani, V., Tomer, O. S., Prashad, R., et al. (2001). Effect of yogic exercises on physical and mental health of young fellowship course trainees. *Indian Journal of Physiology and Pharmacology, 45,* 37–53.

Ray, U. S., Sinha, B., Tomer, O. S., Pathak, A., Dasgupta, T., & Selvamurthy, W. (2001). Aerobic capacity and perceived exertion after practice of Hatha yogic exercises. *Indian Journal of Medical Research, 114,* 215–221.

Riley, D. (2004). Hatha yoga and the treatment of illness. *Alternative Therapies in Health and Medicine, 10,* 20–21.

Rohini, V., Pandey, R. S., Janakiramaiah, N., Gangadhar, B. N., & Vedamurthachar, A. (2000). A comparative study of full and partial Sudarshan Kriya yoga (SKY) in major depressive disorder. *NIMHANS Journal, 18,* 53–57.

Sahasi, G., Mohan, D., & Kacker, C. (1989). Effectiveness of yogic techniques in the management of anxiety. *Journal of Personality and Clinical Studies, 5,* 51–55.

Saper, R. B., Eisenberg, D. M., Davis, R. B., Culpepper, L., & Phillips, R. S. (2004). Prevalence and patterns of adult yoga use in the United States: Results of a national survey. *Alternative Therapies in Health and Medicine, 10,* 44–49.

Schell, F. J., Allolio, B., & Schonecke, O. W. (1994). Physiological and psychological effects of hatha yoga exercise in healthy women. *International Journal of Psychosomatics, 41,* 46–52.

Schmidt, T., Wijga, A., Von Zur, M., Brabant, G., & Wagner, T. O. (1997). Changes in cardiovascular risk factors and hormones during a comprehensive residential three-month kriya yoga training and vegetarian nutrition. *Acta Physiologica Scandinavica Supplementum, 640,* 158–162.

Serber, E. (2000). Stress management through yoga. *International Journal of Yoga Therapy, 10,* 11–16.

Sethi, B. B., Trivedi, J. K., Srivastava, A., & Yadav, S. (1982). Indigenous therapy in practice of psychiatry in India. *Indian Journal of Psychiatry, 24,* 230–236.

Singh, V. (1987). Effect of respiratory exercises on asthma: The Pink City lung exerciser. *Journal of Asthma, 24,* 355–359.

Singh, V., Wisniewski, A., Britton, J., & Tattersfield, A. (1990). Effect of yoga breathing exercises (*pranayama*) on airway reactivity in subjects with asthma. *Lancet, 335*, 1381–1383.

Szabo, A., Mesko, A., Caputo, A., & Gill, E. T. (1998). Examination of exercise-induced feeling states in four modes of exercise. *International Journal of Sport Psychology, 29*, 376–390.

Taylor, M. J., & Majmundar, M. (2000). Incorporating yoga therapeutics into orthopaedic physical therapy. *Orthopaedic Physical Therapy Clinics of North America, 9*, 341–360.

Telles, S., Nagarathna, R., Nagendra, H. R., & Desiraju, T. (1993). Physiological changes in sports teachers following 3 months of training in Yoga. *Indian Journal of Medical Sciences, 47*, 235–238.

Telles, S., & Naveen, K. V. (1997). Yoga for rehabilitation: An overview. *Indian Journal of Medical Sciences, 51*, 123–127.

Telles, S., & Vani, P. R. (2002). Increase in voluntary pulse rate reduction achieved following yoga training. *International Journal of Stress Management, 9*, 236–239.

Tran, M. D., Holly, R. G., Lashbrook, J., & Amsterdam, E. A. (2001). Effects of hatha yoga practice on the health-related aspects of physical fitness. *Preventive Cardiology, 4*, 165–170.

Udupa, K., Madanmohan, Bhavanani, A. B., Vijayalakshmi, P., & Krishnamurthy, N. (2003). Effect of pranayam training on cardiac function in normal young volunteers. *Indian Journal of Physiology and Pharmacology, 47*, 27–33.

Udupa, K. N. (1976). A manual of science and philosophy of yoga. *Journal of Research in Indian Medicine, Yoga and Homeopathy, 11*, 1–103.

Udupa, K. N. (1985). *Stress and its management by yoga.* Delhi, India: Motilal Banarsidass.

Vahia, N. S. (1972). A deconditioning therapy based upon concepts of Patanjali. *International Journal of Social Psychiatry, 18*, 61–66.

Vahia, N. S., Doongaji, D., Jeste, D., Kapoor, S., Ardhapurkar, I., & Ravindranath, S. (1973). Further experience with the therapy based upon concepts of Patanjali in the treatment of psychiatric disorders. *Indian Journal of Psychiatry, 15*, 32–37.

Vahia, N. S., Doongaji, D. R., Jeste, D. V., Ravindranath, S., Kapoor, S. N., & Ardhapurkar, I. (1973). Psychophysiologic therapy based on the concepts of Patanjali: A new approach to the treatment of neurotic and psychosomatic disorders. *American Journal of Psychotherapy, 27*, 557–565.

Vahia, N. S., Vinekar, S. L., & Doongaji, D. R. (1966). Some ancient Indian concepts in the treatment of psychiatric disorders. *British Journal of Psychiatry, 112*, 1089–1096.

Van Montfrans, G. A., Karemaker, J. M., Wieling, W., & Dunning, A. J. (1990). Relaxation therapy and continuous ambulatory blood pressure in mild hypertension: A controlled study. *British Medical Journal, 300*, 1368–1372.

Vedanthan, P. K., Kesavalu, L. N., Murthy, K. C., Duvall, K., Hall, M. J., Baker, S., et al. (1998). Clinical study of yoga techniques in university students with asthma: A controlled study. *Allergy and Asthma Proceedings, 19*, 3–9.

Vempati, R. P., & Telles, S. (2002). Yoga-based guided relaxation reduces sympathetic activity judged from baseline levels. *Psychological Reports, 90*, 487–494.

Vinekar, S. L. (1976). Scientific basis of yoga. *Yoga Mimamsa, 18*, 89–97.

Waelde, L. C., Thompson, L., & Gallagher-Thompson, D. (2004). A pilot study of a yoga and meditation intervention for dementia caregiver stress. *Journal of Clinical Psychology, 60*, 677–687.

Watanabe, E., Fukuda, S., Hara, H., & Shirakawa, T. (2002). Altered responses of saliva cortisol and mood status by long-period special yoga exercise mixed with meditation and guided imagery. *Journal of International Society of Life Information Science, 20*, 585–587.

Willoughby, D. (2000, August). Yoga therapy. *Yoga International*, 39–46.

Woolery, A., Myers, H., Stemlieb, B., & Zeltzer, L. (2004). A yoga intervention for young adults with elevated symptoms of depression. *Alternative Therapies in Health and Medicine, 10*, 60–63.

Yadav, R. K., & Das, S. (2001). Effect of yogic practice on pulmonary functions in young females. *Indian Journal of Physiology and Pharmacology, 45*, 493–496.

Yogendra, J. (1970). The study of clinical-cum-medical research and yoga. *Journal of the Yoga Institute, 16*, 3–10.

Yogendra, J., Yogendra, H. J., Ambardekar, S., Lele, R. D., Shetty, S., Dave, M., et al. (2004). Beneficial effects of yoga lifestyle on reversibility of ischaemic heart disease: Caring Heart Project of International Board of Yoga. *Journal of the Association of Physicians of India, 52*, 283–289.

Cognitive Methods

CHAPTER 18

Cognitive Approaches to Stress and Stress Management

JAMES L. PRETZER
AARON T. BECK

Imagine three individuals who each face a normatively stressful situation: being stuck in a traffic jam on the way to work.

Sue overslept, had to rush to get ready, just grabbed a cup of coffee for breakfast, and now finds herself trapped in bumper-to-bumper traffic. She is thinking "Oh my God! Now I'm going to be late for work! My boss will be furious. I'm already in trouble for getting in late last week. Why does this always happen to me?" Her heart is racing, her muscles are tense, and she can feel a migraine coming on.

Ann got up just in time, dressed hurriedly, and had time for a quick breakfast. She is now stuck in bumper-to-bumper traffic and finds herself thinking "Oh no! I'm going to be late!" Then she pauses and says to herself, "Actually, at this pace I'll only be a little late, it won't be a big deal. People will understand, they have to deal with this traffic, too." She feels somewhat tense and tries to relax as she drives on in to work.

Mary remembered that traffic often is bad in the morning. She got up in time to get ready without rushing, had her breakfast, and allowed a little extra time in case traffic was bad. Now she is stuck in the same traffic jam and is thinking "Boy, traffic is terrible today. It's a good thing I allowed extra time. Oh well, there's nothing to do but put up with it." She turns on the radio and relaxes as she drives slowly to work.

It appears that each of the preceding individuals responding to the same situation (being stuck in a traffic jam on the way to work), and yet each experiences very different levels of stress and distress. How are we to understand individual variation in response to stressful events? How are we to help those who encounter problems coping with stress?

COGNITIVE THERAPY'S PERSPECTIVE ON STRESS

The Role of Cognitive Processes in Stress

One aspect of cognitive therapy's approach to understanding the enormous individual variation in responses to stressors is the assertion that humans respond to their internal representations of situations, not to the objective situation itself. As Lazarus (1966) emphasized, humans are constantly and automatically appraising the situations they encounter, and these appraisals play a central role in our response to those situations. Aaron Beck's analysis of individual variations in response to stress (Beck, 1983, 1984; Pretzer, Beck, & Newman, 1989) has resulted in a series of propositions (see Table 18.1) that provide a conceptual framework for understanding individual variation in response to stressors and for effectively using the wide range of stress management techniques that are available to us.

TABLE 18.1. Propositions Regarding the Role of Cognition in Stress

1. The individual's construction of a situation is an active, continuing process that includes successive appraisals of the external situation, as well as of the risks, costs, and likely gains of possible responses. When the individual's vital interests appear to be at stake, this appraisal process provides a highly selective conceptualization of the situation and possible responses.

2. The cognitive structuring of a situation is responsible for mobilizing the organism to action. If the mobilization is not adequately discharged, it forms the precursor to a stress reaction.

3. Overt behavior stems directly from the mobilization of impulses, drives, or wishes (behavioral inclinations). The emotional experience is parallel to the behavioral inclination and is not a determinant of overt action.

4. Depending on the content of the cognitive constellation, the behavioral inclination may be a desire to flee, attack, approach, or avoid; the corresponding affect would be anxiety, anger, affection, or sadness, respectively. The responses can be regarded as organized into structures, with primacy assigned to the controlling cognitive constellation, which activates and controls the behavioral inclination and the affective response.

5. The stressors lead to a disruption of the normal activity of the cognitive organization. In addition to erosion of the ability to concentrate, recall, and reason and to control impulses, there is a relative increase in primitive (primary-process) content.

6. Specific primitive cognitive constellations are "chained" to specific stimuli. This pairing constitutes the specific sensitivity of a given individual and prepares the way for inappropriate or excessive reactions. Because people vary widely in their specific sensitivities, an event that is a stressor for one person may be a benign situation for another.

7. Differences in personality organization account for some of the wide variations in individual sensitivities to stressors. Thus the autonomous and sociotropic personality types differ in the kinds of stressors to which they are sensitive. The occurrence of a stress reaction is thus contingent to a large degree on specific vulnerabilities related to personality.

8. Each of the stress syndromes (such as hostility, anxiety, and depression) consists of hyperactive schemas with an idiosyncratic content specific to that syndrome. Each syndrome comprises a specific controlling cognitive constellation and the resultant behavioral inclinations and affect.

9. The principal stressor may be internal, with no apparent referent in the outside world. The assumption that the only road to fulfillment is through total success is intrinsic in achievement-oriented persons prone to stress reactions.

10. Stressful interactions with other people occur in a mutually reinforcing cycle of maladaptive cognitive reactions. Specific mechanisms, such as the egocentric cognitive mode, framing, and polarization, lead to increased mobilization and, consequently, to stress.

11. An individual experiences an inclination to respond physically, although the stimulus may be psychosocial or symbolic and although ultimate overt behavior is verbal. The mobilization for "fight or flight" involves the same cognitive–motoric systems, regardless of whether the level of meaning of a threat or challenge is physical or psychosocial.

The individual's construction of a particular situation may be likened to taking a snapshot. In taking a photograph, the individual scans the relevant environment and then focuses on specific aspects of the situation. The photograph reduces a three-dimensional situation to two dimensions and consequently sacrifices a great deal of information; it also may introduce a certain amount of distortion. Similarly, in perceiving a particular event, the cognitive set influences the "picture" obtained by an individual. Whether the mental image or conception is broad or narrow, clear or blurred, accurate or distorted depends on the characteristics of the existing cognitive set. The individual's cognitive set automatically determines which aspects are to be magnified, which minimized, and which excluded.

It is probable that a person takes a series of "pictures" before reaching a final conceptualization. The first "shot" of an event provides a very basic appraisal of the situation—whether it is likely to be pleasant, neutral, or noxious and whether it directly affects the individual's vital interests. This first "shot" provides feedback that either reinforces or modifies the preexisting cognitive set. If the initial appraisal is that the situation affects the individual's vital interests, he or she shows a "critical response." One type of critical response is the "emergency response." This response is activated when the individual perceives a threat to his or her survival, domain, individuality, functioning, status, or attachments—that is, attack, depreciation, encroachment, thwarting, abandonment, rejection, or deprivation. Another type of critical response occurs when the individual perceives an event as increasing or facilitating self-enhancement—the attainment of personal goals, exhibitionism, or receiving admiration.

An essential feature of the critical response is that it is egocentric. The situation is conceptualized in terms of "How does it affect me?" The immediate interests of the individual are central in the conceptualization, and the details are selected and molded (or distorted) to focus solely on self-interest. The critical response tends to be simplistic and to focus on situations that were of central importance in more primitive times—physical danger, predation, social bonding, and so forth. Generally, the critical response tends to be overly inclusive. Events that actually are not related to issues of personal identity, survival, or self-enhancement may be perceived as though they are relevant to these issues.

For our present purpose, let us assume that the individual's first impression of a situation is that it is noxious. This appraisal activates a particular *mode* (assembly of *schemas*[1]), which is used to refine the classification of the stimulus situation. The initial impression of a situation fits into the category of "primary appraisal" (Lazarus, 1966). If the primary appraisal is that the situation is noxious, successive "reappraisals" are made to provide immediate answers to a series of questions:

1. Is the noxious stimulus a threat to the individual or his or her interests?
2. Is the threat concrete and immediate or abstract, symbolic, and remote?
3. What is the content and magnitude of the threat?
   a. Does it involve possible physical damage to the individual?
   b. Is the threat of a psychosocial nature—for example, disparagement or devaluation?
   c. Does the threat involve violation of some rules that the individual relies on to protect his or her integrity or interest?

At the same time that the nature of the threat is being evaluated, the individual is assessing his or her resources for dealing with it. This assessment, labeled "secondary appraisal" by Lazarus (1966), aims to provide concrete information regarding the individual's coping mechanisms and ability to absorb the impact of any assault. The final picture or construction of the noxious situation is based on an equation that takes into account the amount and the probabilities of damage inherent in the threat as opposed to the individual's capacity to deal with it (the "risk–resources equation"). These assessments are not cool, deliberate computations but to a large degree are automatic. The equation is based on highly subjective evaluations that are prone to considerable error; two individuals with similar coping capacities might respond in a vastly different manner to the same threatening situation.

If the risk is judged to be high in relation to the coping resources available, the individual is mobilized to reduce the degree of threat through avoidance or escape ("flight reaction"), preparing for defense, or self-inhibition ("freezing"). If the individual judges the threat to be low in relation to available coping mechanisms, he or she is mobilized to eliminate or deflect the threat ("fight reaction").

Another type of critical response, as noted earlier, occurs when the stimulus situation is perceived as potentially self-enhancing. For example, a person is challenged or invited to compete for a prize. The person then makes rapid evaluations of the desirability of the goal, his or her capacity for reaching it, and the costs to him or her in terms of expenditure of time, energy, and sacrifice of other goals. These factors may be reduced to a cost–benefit ratio analogous to the risk–resources ratio. The final construction of the stimulus situation determines whether or not the person accepts the challenge or invitation and, consequently, whether or not the person becomes mobilized to attain the goal.

The processes involved in the critical response are automatic, involuntary, and typically not within awareness. Because of the exclusionary and categorical nature of thinking at this primitive level, critical responses are typically based on a one-sided, exaggerated view of the stimulus situation. As pointed out by Bowlby (1981), current studies of human perception show that before a person is aware of seeing or hearing a stimulus, the sensory inflow coming through the eyes or ears has already passed through many stages of selection, interpretation, and appraisal. This processing is done at extraordinary speeds, almost all of it is outside awareness, and it is quite selective. Many potentially relevant aspects of the stimulus situation are excluded in the course of this initial processing. The criteria applied to sensory inflow that determine what information is to be accepted and what is to be excluded reflect what appears to be in the person's best interests at any one time. Thus, when a person is hungry, information regarding food is given priority, whereas other information that might ordinarily be useful is excluded. However, some aspects of the situation take precedence over others. Bowlby (1981) writes that, should the individual perceive danger, priorities would immediately change so that input concerned with issues of danger and safety would take precedence and input concerned with food would temporarily be excluded. He asserts that this change regarding which inputs are accepted and which are excluded is effected by systems that are central to cognitive organizations.

Of course, not all stimuli are interpreted as noxious, and not all psychophysiological reactions are "fight" or "flight." Depending on the kind of appraisal, a host of different reactions may be stimulated by a given situation. These reactions may range from a wish to engage in some recreational activity to a desire to undertake a dangerous mission. They have a common theme, however: The individual is mobilized to engage in some kind of action. For a variety of reasons, he or she may not yield to the desire, wish, or drive; nonetheless, the mobilization has a powerful effect. Recent writings have emphasized the emotional response to a stressful stimulus but have largely neglected the importance of the motivated response.

If a person is activated to perform a particular behavior, the directing force may be labeled a *behavioral inclination*. The behavioral inclinations, or action tendencies, constitute one type of motivation. Another class of motivations is concerned with "receiving" rather than "doing" and includes wishes for love, praise, or approval, as well as the appetitive wishes. The intensity of the behavioral inclination is reflected in the degree of arousal. If the behavioral inclination is not translated into action, then the individual remains in a state of arousal for a period of time, even though the instigating stimulus is no longer present. The mobilization of the individual for action is the key to understanding stress reactions. If the arousal is intense and is not dissipated by action, then the individual is likely to experience some degree of stress.

At the same time that an individual is aroused to action, he or she may experience an affective response. For example, people who believe they are in a dangerous situation generally experience subjective anxiety, as well as a desire to escape; if they judge that other people are mistreating them, they are likely to experience anger, as well as a desire to attack. Similarly, people may experience feelings of excitement as they prepare to engage in a competitive sport. In each case, the behavioral inclination represents the catalyst to action. The affective response occurs independently of the behavior (although these two phenomena are often fused in technical as well as popular concepts). Both the behavioral inclination and the affective response stem from the individual's conceptualizations of the situation and are related to each other only insofar as they are both related to the cognitive structuring of the situation. It should be noted that a behavioral inclination may be aroused with minimal or no evidence of an emotional response. Persons exposed to a sudden dangerous situation (e.g., an impending automobile collision) may react to avert the danger without experiencing subjective anxiety.

The popular concept of emotions, which is also reflected to some degree in psychoanalytic theory, revolves around the notion that these phenomena are like a fluid in a reservoir. When the internal hydraulic system reaches a certain level, it builds up a pressure for overt expression. According to the same metaphor, the suppression of certain emotions such as anger can lead to a wide variety of ills, ranging from headache to hypertension. By the same token, it has been stated that the free and open expression of emotions such as anger or sadness can relieve the psychosomatic disorders.

The question naturally arises: How do we know that people are suppressing or expressing their emotions? Let us take the example of angry people, who may stamp their feet, yell, shout epithets, or physically attack persons whom they regard as adversaries. They may state that they have been unjustly injured and that they are going to "get even" with the other persons. According to the conventional notions, we would label the observed behavior as "anger" or as an "angry reaction." Further reflection, however, forces us to raise questions about this notion. Are we actually seeing in the observed behavior a manifestation of some endopsychic process other than emotion? When we see an individual shake a fist and express condemning words, it seems more logical to infer that we are seeing the direct expression of a motivation (behavioral inclination) rather than the expression of an emotion. (As a matter of fact, an individual can play-act this scenario without feeling angry at all.)

If we question individuals who are behaving in this way, they may explain that they are "blowing off steam" or "expressing angry feelings." Similarly, people who have tightened their muscles in an attempt to prevent themselves from engaging in antagonistic behavior are likely to explain this behavior as "bottling up my feelings." (Again, note the use of a fluid metaphor to refer to feelings.) If we ask such persons "What would you like to do?" they may respond with a description of a series of actions, such as "I would like to punch him in the nose. . . . I would like to humiliate him, I'd like to make him feel the way I feel." If we inquire about such individuals' feelings, they may describe them in terms of "anger swelling up inside me." They believe that if they could release (and thus reduce) the anger, they would feel better. Suppose that such an individual does scold the offender and that the offender then apologizes. The individual feels better and is no longer angry. This sequence of events thus appears to be consistent with the person's notions regarding the release of anger: He or she felt angry, expressed the anger, is no longer angry, and feels better. Thus the person "demonstrates" to his or her own satisfaction that the problem lay in "suppressing my anger."

Does this experience really confirm the validity of the conventional notions regarding the expression of emotions? Let us examine the earlier phase of the process, when an individual feels "anger bursting out all over." When we analyze the situation, we might question whether the person is transforming the anger into overt behavior or whether he or she is simply carrying out an inclination to act against the adversary. The second formulation—that what we are observing are the effects of an impulse to scold, berate, or attack the other person—seems more plausible, because it does not require the notion of some "transmutation" of an emotion into behavior and because it fits in general with our idea that goal-directed physical activity is preceded by a wish, drive, or impulse (behavioral inclination). According to this formulation, the behavioral inclination and not the emotional response is involved in the mobilization for action.

The way in which the cognitive organization processes the information determines the behavioral inclinations and affect. Thus we can conceive of a chain of events proceeding from the environmental event to the cognitive processing system (the controlling cognitive constellation) to the action-arousing system (the behavioral inclination) to the motoric system and finally to the observable actions. Concomitantly, the controlling cognitive constellation may activate the affect-arousing system.

The role of the cognitive organization in processing information has been described previously (Beck, 1967, 1976). Briefly, the organization is composed of systems of structural components—namely, *cognitive schemas*. When an external event occurs, specific cognitive schemas are activated and are used to classify, interpret, evaluate, and assign a meaning to the event. In normal functioning, the schemas that are activated are relevant to the nature of the event. A series of adjustments occurs so that the appropriate schemas are "fitted" to the external stimulus. The final interpretation of an event represents an interaction between that event and the schemas.

The thematic content of the cognitive schemas determines the nature of the affective response and of the behavioral inclinations. Thus, if the content is relevant to danger, then a wish to flee and the feeling of anxiety are experienced. The theme of personal encroachment stimulates anger and the wish to attack. The perception of receiving desired interpersonal "supplies" (such as love) may stimulate feelings of affection and the desire to approach the other person. Perceived disapproval, on the other hand, produces sadness and often the desire to avoid the other person.

Whether an impulse will be expressed in overt behavior is dependent on the controlling cognitive constellation. For example: an individual, confronted by a stranger who approaches with an aggressive stance and makes aggressive threats in a raised voice, construes the situation as presenting the threat of an unjustified attack and consequently becomes mobilized to attack or to flee depending on his or her appraisal of his or her ability to handle the threat. The impulse to attack or to flee will be transformed into actual behavior unless the individual decides that this action is unwise and that the impulse to do so should be inhibited.

Translating this example into structural terms, we propose that the activation of the cognitive constellation leads directly to the activation of the motor apparatus, which "prepares for action." The feedback to the cognitive schemas may trigger a new signal—namely, to control or inhibit action. The result of this interaction is that the organism is mobilized for action but is prevented by internal controls from carrying it out. It should be noted that the controlling signal does not deactivate the mobilization, which persists. This formulation suggests the need for postulating a system of controls whose functions range from blanket inhibition to sensitive modulation of the impulses. (In a later section, we discuss how modifications in the cognitive constellation can facilitate *demobilization*.)

It should be noted that although affect may be stimulated, it has no role in the mobilization for action. Moreover, although the individual may inhibit the inclination to attack or flee, he or she nonetheless experiences anger or fear. Similarly, if the individual carries out the hostile inclinations, he or she also experiences anger. Furthermore, he or she will continue to experience both the inclination and the affect (anger) until there is some modification in the controlling cognitive constellation.

Under ordinary conditions, the activation of the cognitive–behavioral–affective configuration does not cause any particular problems. In fact, the configuration can be viewed as the mechanism for producing the wide range of normal emotions and normal behavior. Under certain circumstances, however, the primitive, egocentric cognitive system is activated (Beck, 1967, pp. 281–290). This activation is likely to occur when the individual perceives that vital interests are at stake. Specific idiosyncratic cognitive schemas become hyperactive if the resultant behavioral and affective mobilization is sufficiently intense or prolonged; distress, conceptual distortions, cognitive dysfunctions, and, frequently, disturbance of physiological functions (such as appetite and sleep) are produced.

In stress reactions, deviations in the thinking process play a major role. The stress-prone individual is primed to make extreme, one-sided, absolute, and global judgments. Because the appraisals tend to be extreme and one-sided, the behavioral inclinations also tend to be extreme. For example, a hostility-prone employer may be primed to react to a relatively minor error by an employee as though it were criminal negligence and, consequently, will be inclined to attack the employee verbally or physically. A person who is susceptible to fear reactions may interpret an unfamiliar noise as the firing of a revolver or the rumble of an earthquake and will have an overpowering urge to escape. A depression-prone individual may interpret a humorous comment as a rejection and will want to withdraw. In the primitive mode of thinking, the complexity, variability, and diversity of human experiences are reduced to a few crude categories. In contrast, mature cognition (*secondary-process thinking*) integrates stimuli into many dimensions or qualities, is quantitative rather than categorical, and is relativistic rather than absolutistic.

It is interesting to note that the characteristics of the primitive cognitive organization are also reflected in the systems relevant to behavioral inclinations, control, and affect. Thus the content of the impulses tends to be more extreme, and the mechanisms of control also show a dichotomous character. Just as the individual's capacity to fine-tune cognitive responses is impaired, so his or her modulation of behavioral inclinations deteriorates into a "choice" between total inhibition and no control at all. For example, a hostile person may manifest an inclination to respond to an insult with a violent counterattack, as well as reduced control over this impulse. A depressed person has strong regressive desires, such as staying in bed and avoiding constructive action; he or she also has attenuated control over these inclinations. A fearful person has exaggerated impulses to escape from "noxious" stimuli; he or she experiences overcontrol (inhibition) of assertiveness and undercontrol of the wish to escape.

Another feature of cognitive stress or strain is the relative diminution of what has been described in the psychoanalytic literature as "secondary-process thinking" (Beck, Rush, Shaw, & Emery, 1979, p. 15). Thus stressed individuals lose, to varying degrees, their capacity to observe their automatic thoughts (cognitions) objectively, to subject them to reality testing, and to adjust them to reality. Furthermore, the idiosyncratic cognitions are often so intense that such individuals have difficulty in "turning them off" and shifting their focus to other topics.

Why does one person tend to react to life experiences with chronic hostility, another with depression, and a third with severe or chronic anxiety? People differ not only in their types of responses to stressors but also in the kinds of stressors to which they overreact. Thus they are likely to demonstrate individualized hypersensitivities to specific stressors and to experience specific patterns of responses. The differences in the types of susceptibility and response patterns may be attributed to differences in cognitive organization and, in many cases, to differences in personality as well.

The construct of *specific sensitivity*, first described by Saul (1947) as "specific emotional vulnerability," refers to the individual's predilection to overreact to certain highly specific situations (specific stressors). This theoretical formulation postulates that the individual has a number of sensitive areas and that, when a given situation impinges on one of these areas, he or she is likely to respond cognitively in the kind of relatively crude, categorical form characteristic of primary-process cognition. The idiosyncratic cognitive response sets in motion the motivational systems that may lead to stress.

To illustrate the concept of specific sensitivity, let us take a commonplace example. A young man was bitten by a dog as a child. From that time on, he has responded with anxiety to the sight of any dog, to the sound of a dog barking, or even to the picture of a dog. Any stimulus relevant to a dog elicits the thought "It will bite my leg off" and generally an image of the leg being severed at the calf. He then experiences anxiety and a wish to flee. Thus the young man reacts to an innocuous stimulus as though it were dangerous. The specific stressor in this case is any dog, and the specific cognitive response is automatic, stereotyped, and undifferentiated. Even though he "knows" at one level (the mature cognitive system) that there is no danger, the primitive cognitive system is prepotent for as long as the stimulus is present. Because the reaction disappears after the stimulus is removed, this case can be considered a specific phobia and not regarded as a stress reaction (unless the exposure to the stressor is prolonged or intense enough to produce a residual dysfunction).

In order to illustrate how a specific sensitivity predisposes an individual to a stress reaction, let us consider the case of a middle-aged man with intense chronic anxiety. The episode of anxiety started shortly after his brother died of a heart attack, when he himself began to have pains in his chest. From that point on, he has been acutely aware of changes in his breathing or heart rate and any perceptible sensations in his chest—all of which make him believe he is having a heart attack and lead to chest pain (because of splinting of the intercostal muscles), anxiety, and a desire to rush to the hospital. He has a similar reaction when he hears of anybody dying of a heart attack. This case qualifies as a stress reaction, because the psychophysiological effects last after exposure to a stimulus and are represented in continued dysfunctional thinking ("I am in danger of dying"), impaired concentration, chronic feelings of discomfort, and increased heart rate.

This anecdote illustrates how a person responds selectively (fear reaction) to an initial stressor (his brother's death) with hypersensitivity to any stimuli suggestive of coronary disease. The hypersensitivity can be understood in terms of the predominance of a cognitive constellation relevant to the danger of "instant death." This constellation remains prepotent, so that most internal stimuli are scanned for signs of an impending heart attack. Moreover, even external stimuli relevant to the concept of heart attack (such as news of a friend's having a coronary episode) are capable of activating or intensifying his fear.

A wide variety of sensitivities and response patterns may exist. People with a sensitivity to the same stressor may have notably different response patterns; others may have the same type of response, but to dissimilar stimuli. For example, two students studying together may react strongly when they hear a loud noise, such as the backfiring of a car—one with hostility, the other with fear. The first regards the noise as an encroachment; the other perceives it as a danger (namely, gunfire). Other people may show the same type of response (e.g., fear of bodily harm or death) to quite different stimuli, such as the sight of blood or a barking dog. It is therefore expedient to categorize stress reactions in terms of the cognitive response rather than the specific stimulus.

In the course of development, individuals gradually form a number of concepts (schemas) about themselves and their world. As these concepts are structuralized, they become embedded in a cluster of related memories, meanings, assumptions, expectations, and rules, which the individuals utilize to process incoming data and to mobilize themselves into action. The related schemas (Beck, 1964) may be so broad and pervasive across situations that they may constitute a major dimension of personality type. On the other hand, the schemas may be relatively narrow and applicable only to a highly specific set of stimuli. If a schema has been formed under stressful conditions, it may assume the characteristic structures of the primitive cognitive system (primary-process thinking): rigid, global, categorical, and absolutistic.

To illustrate a primitive concept, let us return to the example of the young man who was bitten by the dog. According to the proposed theory, the severity of the trauma was responsible for the formation not only of an extremely negative memory of the dog but also of an extreme, unidimensional, undifferentiated construction of the category "dog." The primitive concept has a content such as "Dogs are dangerous." When this schema is activated, dogs are appraised according to only one dimension: not whether they are large or small, frisky or passive, shaggy or smooth-coated, but only as dangerous. Since the schema is categorical and absolute, the specific appraisal excludes the notion "safe." Hence, the cognitive response to the sight of any dog is uniform: "This dog is dangerous." This response occurs even when the dog is objectively harmless, geographically remote, or safely chained. Associated with the concept are a number of assumptions and expectations, such as "If it comes closer, it will bite me" and "I won't be able to ward off the attack." Furthermore, several rules (imperatives)—such as "You must get to a safe place," "Get ready to be attacked," and "Freeze!"—are derived from the concept. Of course, when the primitive schema is not invoked, the individual is capable of responding realistically to the category "dog" (mature cognitive system).

It is important to recognize that when a concept or schema is highly structuralized and hypervalent, the power of mature thinking to subject the construction to reality testing, to make discriminations, and to correct the distortion is greatly diminished. Nonetheless, it is possible in psychotherapy to counterbalance the primitive concept by helping the patient to strengthen and to apply realistic, flexible, multidimensional concepts (secondary-process thinking). As becomes clear later, the task of psychotherapy is much more difficult when the individual has a large assembly of broad primitive concepts organized around a single major theme relevant to a large proportion of his or her experience, such as interpersonal relations.

It may not be difficult to understand how a person can react excessively to a highly specific type of stimulus. However, it is puzzling to observe that certain individuals over-react in a relatively uniform way to a wide variety of apparently dissimilar situations. As we get to know such persons better, we find that most of the situations fit into a pattern. Thus one individual may react with fear and inhibition when making requests, making a phone call, asking for directions, associating with strangers, or traveling alone—in other words, whenever there is any conceivable risk of rejection or isolation. Another person may react with hostility in situations that demand conformity to social norms or to institutional requirements. These observations suggest that such people are governed by certain broad expectations and conceptions that they carry with them into every situation. The situations are found to have a common thread—namely, a similar individualized meaning to the person.

In some cases, the individualized meanings seem to pervade every interaction. In structural terms, it appears that a few schemas whose contents are relevant to this individualized meaning are activated by the diverse situations. For example, we can return to the anecdote of the student who becomes hostile when he hears a loud noise while he is studying. In reviewing his reaction to a multitude of varied life situations, we find that he is extremely sensitive to any characteristic of a situation that represents an incursion on his "life space" or an impediment to his goals. He becomes hostile if interrupted while talking, studying, or daydreaming. He is intolerant of being crowded by other people in restaurants, elevators, or conference rooms. He prefers to sit near the exit in theaters or other public places. He reacts strongly against formal rules, orders, and restrictions. He insists on "leaving his options open" and may, for example, break off a love relationship rather than accept a limitation on his freedom of action.

For this individual, a host of related concepts are applied to all interpersonal, as well as impersonal, relationships. These are organized into a value system whose themes are fulfillment through action, expression of individuality, and preservation of autonomy. (In contrast, the sociotropic person is oriented to receiving, togetherness, and dependency.) Thus even minimal encroachment on this system elicits such cognitions as "She is pushing me around," "She is trying to trap me," or "I am boxed in." These extreme ideas occur in interactions as diverse as someone's expressing an interest in his work, asking him to participate in a group project, asking him personal questions, or expressing love and affection. Whereas these situations might elicit gratitude, cooperativeness, friendliness, or affection in other people, they stir up hostility in this individual.

Some individuals of this type may show exorbitant reactions even when the noxious situation is impersonal or physical (e.g., crawling through a narrow tunnel). For example, a man who had received many decorations for bravery in World War II experienced a crippling (and demoralizing) anxiety attack when he attempted to crawl through a large cylinder in an amusement park. The possibility of being immobilized in the cylinder threatened his notion of his autonomy, on which his concept of his identity was based. He could not tell even his best friend about his emotional reaction, because he was afraid of being ridiculed. It is of interest to note that this paratrooper's heroic exploits had centered around escaping from closed-in environments: He had shown extraordinary daring in jumping out of aircraft behind enemy lines and in breaking out of prison camps.

A characteristic of all the syndromes is that once the cognitive constellation becomes overactive, it tends to select and process stimuli that are congruent with it—a process described by Mahoney (1982) as "feedforward." As a result of extracting only congruent stimuli, the cognitive constellation continues to be hyperactive or becomes more active. Thus individuals who are fixated on ideas of personal danger are likely to scan their environment for signs of potential harm and to misread innocuous events as dangerous. Consequently, the notion of imminent harm becomes progressively greater. Similarly, the tendency of depressed patients to direct their attention to negative events and to misinterpret or blot out positive events intensifies their negative constructions of their experience. The same vicious cycle may be observed in acute hostile reactions: As hostile individuals misinterpret successive events as challenges or affronts, they are more likely to interpret subsequent neutral occurrences in the same way.

The principal stressor may be internal rather than external. A stereotypical example of this sort of "self-stressing" would be the hard-driving businessperson or scientist. Such persons typically set high goals and drive themselves and others in order to achieve them. This leads to a constant state of tension. Although there may be no objective evidence of pressure from the outside, such patients' occupations present problems for them because of the way they perceive their work. Because they regard each specific task as a major confrontation, they are continually driving, nagging, and pressing themselves. Their self-imposed psychological stress is accompanied by overloading of one or more of their psychophysiological systems.

The excessive momentum behind the work drive may be these persons' chronic concern that they will not reach their goals or that they or their subordinates will make costly errors. These "worried achievers" react to each new task with strong doubts. They exaggerate the importance or the difficulty of a task (a faulty cognitive appraisal) and underestimate their capacity to deal with it (also a faulty cognitive appraisal). Not only do they magnify the obstacles to completing a task, but they also exaggerate the consequences of failure. They may, for example, visualize a chain of events leading to bankruptcy whenever the outcome of a particular financial venture is uncertain. These individuals are predisposed to excessive tension, because they exaggerate not only the dire consequences of falling short of their goals but also the probability of these consequences occurring.

These "irritable achievers" are also in a continuous state of tension because of what they conceive of as unnecessary obstacles in the paths toward their goals. They may experience hostility toward their coworkers or subordinates whenever their systems fail to operate at maximum efficiency. Alternatively, they may reproach themselves savagely if they perceive that they have been inefficient or negligent. A system may be so important that the end becomes more important than the means.

Stress does not occur in a vacuum. When we look at the interpersonal relations of stressed individuals, we realize that their behavior evokes responses from other people, which are fed back to them and stimulate further responses in them. Ordinarily, interpersonal responses are modulated in such a way as to minimize the amount of friction among people and also the degree of disturbance within individuals. Thus people operate as though they have a kind of "thermostat" that regulates their behavior. When these adjustments in behavior do not occur in an adaptive way, the stage is set for stress in individuals and/or in the persons with whom they are interacting (see Lazarus, 1981).

A more comprehensive reciprocal, or interactional, model demands the inclusion of cognitive structuring. Thus an individual structures a particular situation with another person in a specific way. The individual's structuring of the situation will lead to a particular behavior. His or her behavior is interpreted in a specific way by the other person, who then manifests a behavioral response to this interpretation. Thus we get a continuous cycling of cognition–behavior–cognition–behavior. For example, Bob thinks that it would be nice to do something with Harry and suggests that they go to a ball game. Harry reacts to the overt behavior (the suggestion) with an idiosyncratic interpretation—"He is making an unwarranted demand"—and starts to criticize Bob for "being demanding." Bob responds to this critical behavior with his own interpretation: "He is treating me unfairly. I can't let him get away with this." He then verbally counterattacks.

Harry responds cognitively with the notion "This guy is useless to me; I might as well write him off," and tells Bob, "Look, we just can't get along. Why don't we call the whole thing off?" Bob's cognitions then run something like this: "Harry is being unreasonable. He regards me as a pushover. I can't let him get away with it, or other people will think they can push me around." Bob then becomes overmobilized for further attack. At this point, what he says will be insufficient to restore his mobilization to a baseline level. Consequently, the state of overmobilization persists for a period of time. This kind of overmobilization is the immediate factor in producing stress. If sustained and repeated over a long enough period, the individual's reactions may move from heightened activity in the neuroendocrine system to specific physiological dysfunctions.

As pointed out previously, when people consider their vital interests to be at stake, they are likely to shift into the egocentric mode. The egocentric mode organizes present, past, and future situations or events predominantly in terms of how they affect the individuals' own vital interests. Because such individuals are focused on the meanings of the events to them, the meanings of other persons are not part of their phenomenal field. Even when they attempt to view situations from the standpoints of other persons, they will, as long as they are in the egocentric mode, come up with interpretations that are heavily laden with the meanings the events have for them.

In interpersonal relations, clashes are likely to occur when each individual is operating solely within the egocentric mode. Even though an individual may have no desire to hurt (and, indeed, may even want to help), his or her egocentricity places a burden on the other person and ultimately on himself or herself. A clash is inevitable when both individuals view things according to their highly personalized formulations. Each person's constructions of his or her own behavior and of the other person's behavior will inevitably lead to a conflict of interest.

The stressful nature of interactions is well illustrated in the form of the widely recognized frictions that develop in marital relationships. The stressful interactions derived from one couple's conflict serve as a model to exemplify the mutually reinforcing nature of stressors. The couple demonstrated completely different cognitive sets in the following situation: The wife asked the husband to stay home with her on a particular night because she felt sick. He refused, because he had already committed himself to spending the evening with a business colleague. They then slipped into such a screaming match that each started to think seriously about getting a divorce.

On exploration, it became apparent that each partner not only was viewing the disagreement in egocentric terms but also was "catastrophizing." The wife's thoughts were these: "If he won't do this small favor for me, how can I count on him when I have a major problem? It shows I can't count on him for anything." The husband's interpretation was this: "She is completely unreasonable. She won't give me any freedom. She looks for any excuse to keep me home. If I have to give in, I can't survive."

This anecdote illustrates several characteristics of the egocentric mode. First, neither person was aware of the meaning conveyed by his or her behavior to the spouse. Second, each believed that his or her interpretation of the event was so valid that its reasonableness should be apparent to anybody. The wife, for example, was convinced that her husband's noncompliance with minor requests proved that she would not be able to rely on him for help when she needed it. The husband believed that compliance with the "small request" would place him in a straitjacket. Because the egocentric mode precludes the possibility of integrating crucial interpersonal feedback (in this case, understanding the spouse's perspective), each individual tended to attempt maladaptively to force the spouse to accept his or her frame of reference. The result was that each partner became frozen in his or her own perspective.

It is interesting that the egocentric mode tends to highlight certain dominant personality patterns. In the preceding example, the husband, who had a strong autonomous bent, needed to maintain a certain freedom of action in his relationships. His specific vulnerability was "being tied down." The wife, on the other hand, had a strong sociotropic/dependent pattern and, consequently, was especially sensitive to being left alone. Continued abrasion of the sensitive areas could lead to stress in either or both partners.

When people view other people with whom they are in conflict, they tend to make an appraisal not only of the others' behavior but also of the other persons themselves. Generally, the type of actions that people consider to be most typical of these others or most salient in terms of their interaction with them are transformed into images or concepts of the other individuals. For example, somebody who is regarded as acting deviously will emerge in an image as a "sneak" or "cheat." In the preceding example, the husband pictured his wife as a demanding, needy, rigid person; the wife visualized the husband as a self-centered, insensitive, undependable person.

Framing consists of focusing on some characteristic that one attributes to another person and portraying this individual in such a way that this attribute dominates the picture of that person. The term *frame* is applied to the specific image or concept of an individual with whom one is in conflict. In creating a frame, one not only reduces a highly complex individual to a few (usually negative) character traits but also manufactures additional elements to flesh out the image (which inevitably is a distortion or caricature of the other person). It is possible to have more than one frame of another person: A wife may see her husband at one time as kind and generous and at other times as selfish and rejecting. The wife in this instance becomes sensitized to certain types of behavior, which she correlates with the negative attributes. When a particular instigating event occurs, the frame that is anchored to that type of stimulus is aroused. For example, whenever the husband places a priority on his interests, the wife is likely to visualize him as a bully.

As the spouses in the "framing" example discussed their opposing wishes, they became increasingly angry at each other. Moreover, as their discussion progressed, they took more extreme, inflexible, opposing positions. We see two interacting phenomena here: "external polarization" (moving further apart in their expressed opinions) and "internal polarization" (thinking more negatively of each other). Their view of each other became more and more negative until it was finally hardened into a specific frame. The view was expressed also in a vague image, which might be verbalized as follows:

HUSBAND: She is weak, demanding, incapable of helping herself. She is mush, a weakling.

WIFE: He is insensitive, ruthless, rejecting, inconsiderate.

The negative constructions by the husband led him to withdraw more. This behavior in turn was processed cognitively by the wife as rejection and abandonment and led her to become more dependent, clinging, scolding—and ultimately depressed. He viewed her depressed behavior as manipulation to induce guilt and force him to comply. Thus he wanted even more to be free of her. Over time, each person developed extreme, unrealistic evaluations of the other person, selectively focused on data consistent with the "frame" each had imposed on the other, overlooked favorable data through inattention or forgetting, misinterpreted the other's behavior, and attributed unworthy motives to explain the other's behavior.

To describe the phenomena of the interaction, the model must be expanded still further. Cognitive structuring does not lead directly to overt behavior. Interposed between the cognitive process and behavior is the motivational component labeled *behavioral inclination*. In this case, the behavioral inclination emerged from the cognitive constellation in the form of a wish to scold, demand, complain, withdraw, or punish. The overt behavior (speech) of one spouse was consequently tinged with phrases, inflections, and tones that connoted disapproval and devaluation of the other spouse.

An individual may show the same type of response, regardless of whether the noxious stimulus is physical or abstract (psychosocial): The person responds in much the same way to a psychosocial challenge, threat, or injury as he or she does to an actual physical confrontation or attack (see Wolff, 1950). To illustrate, let us examine one of these "real-life dramas." A man was shoved in a ticket line by somebody wanting to move the line along. As he felt the pressure on his back, he became mobilized to counterattack: His voluntary muscles became tense, and he experienced an increase in heart rate and blood pressure as he braced himself to push back the offender. A few weeks later, one of his coworkers was pressing him to speed up his work. The individual experienced the same type of physical pressure across his back as when he was shoved in line. Moreover, he felt the same wish and bracing of his muscles to push away his coworker.

The crucial observation is that our protagonist became mobilized to counteract the challenge in the same fashion (voluntary nervous system, autonomic nervous system) when he was psychosocially pressured to do something he did not want to do as when he was subjected to physical pressure from an adversary. Although it may be conceded that there might be some adaptational benefit in preparing to defend oneself against physical encroachments (such as being shoved), there seems little benefit from this total kind of physical mobilization when an adequate response would be a verbal statement employing only the muscles of articulation: "Leave me alone," "Get off my back," "I don't want to do it." Why do people who are confronted with minor psychosocial challenges respond with a mobilization of the fight-or-flight apparatus when their conscious desire is simply to utter a few words? Certainly, the total mobilization is at best superfluous and at worst self-destructive. It seems that even though humans are generally well trained to respond overtly in an appropriate, "civilized" way to minor challenges, they are nonetheless the victims of an inherited primitive response system. Although they may have a well-functioning system of controls to keep the primitive responses in check, they nonetheless have to contend continually with being mobilized for aggressive action far in excess of the demands of the real situations.

If our protagonist were to be "attacked" verbally, say, by somebody insulting him, he might experience an urge to strike the offender just as though he had been attacked physically. These examples indicate that there is an equivalence between the abstract verbal stimulus and the concrete physical stimulus. The initial response to both psychosocial and physical transgressions is identical: Each elicits an impulse to counterattack physically. Whether the transgression is concrete or symbolic in nature, a basic physical response occurs.

It is easy to confirm the observation that individuals who have hostile reactions generally experience tightening of their shoulder, arm, back, or leg muscles, even though they may not be aware of the behavioral inclination to use these muscles against an adversary. With introspection, individuals who are retaliating verbally may recognize a concomitant impulse to strike their adversaries. In the disorders that are characterized by chronic muscular tension, it is important to determine whether individuals are experiencing this kind of behavioral inclination to defend themselves or to counterattack.

The reactions of the fear syndrome are analogous to those of the hostility syndrome. The noxious stimulus may be a threat of psychological injury (e.g., betrayal) or of physical injury (e.g., being stabbed in the back). Such persons may respond both verbally (e.g., by shouting "How can you do this to me?") and physically (by an impulse to protect themselves or to flee). The typical reactions of the voluntary and involuntary (autonomic) nervous systems occur, and such individuals become mobilized for self-protection or flight, regardless of whether the fear is of an abstract (e.g., psychosocial) injury or a concrete (physical) injury.

The similarities in response to either a psychosocial or a physical stimulus suggest the presence of a generalized meaning that encompasses both types of stimulus. In the hostile reaction, the generalized meaning occurs in the form of an idea such as "That person is transgressing against me." In the fear reaction, the meaning assumes a general form such as "I am in danger of having a damaging experience." An encroachment on or danger to the physical integrity of an individual would appear logically to be more serious than a transgression or threat to an individual's psychological status. This notion is exemplified in the old saw "Sticks and stones may break my bones, but words will never hurt me." Despite the common-sense utility of such a saying, the meaning of a verbal assault is so close to that of a physical assault that the same cognitive and motor systems are activated in response to each stimulus.

This formulation suggests that in our "civilized" society, the symbolic meanings of countless social interactions are continuously arousing us to flight, defend, or flee. It seems plausible that because we rarely allow this arousal to be transformed into physical action, our voluntary and autonomic nervous systems are continually overloaded. Beyond a certain point, this overloading leads to a stress reaction.

A Cognitive Model of Stress

The cognitive model of stress is summarized graphically in Figure 18.1. Humans constantly and automatically appraise the situations they encounter in terms of the demands those situations place on them and in terms of their capacity to cope with those demands. These appraisals elicit both behavioral inclinations and emotional responses. Once elicited, these behavioral inclinations and emotional responses become part of the situation with which the individual must cope. One must cope both with the external situation and with the emotions and impulses that occur in response to the situation. Those behavioral inclinations that are acted on and any emotions that are expressed may have effects on the situation with which the individual is faced, may elicit or discourage social support, and may expand or decrease the individual's coping skills and resources. Thus the cognitive model sees stress as the result of a dynamic interaction between the individual and his or her environment in which cognition plays an important role. Note, however, that the actual demands of the situation, the individual's coping skills and resources, social support, behavior, and emotion also play important roles in the model.

If humans perceived and interpreted the situations they encounter accurately, problematic levels would arise only when objectively stressful situations persisted and the individual was unable to either escape the situation or overcome it. Unfortunately, humans are quite capable of misperceiving and misinterpreting both the situations they face and

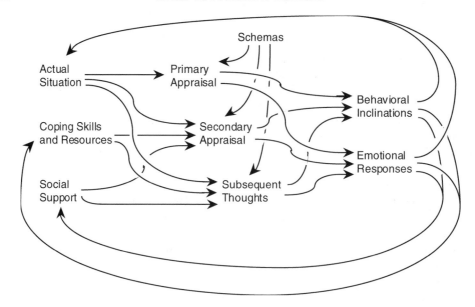

FIGURE 18.1. Cognitive model of stress.

their capacities for coping with those situations. Thus problematic levels of stress can arise for a variety of reasons:

1. The demands of the situation may exceed the individual's capacity for coping with the situation.
2. The individual may overestimate the demands of the situation and/or underestimate his or her capacity for coping with the situation and thus perceive the demands of the situation as exceeding his or her ability to cope when this is not the case.
3. The individual may exaggerate the consequences of being unable to cope with the situation.
4. The individual may attempt to cope with the situation in ways that prove to be ineffective or dysfunctional.
5. Fears, inhibitions, beliefs, expectations, and so forth may block the individual from using necessary coping skills.
6. The individual may not have an adequate support system.
7. Fears, inhibitions, beliefs, expectations, and so forth may block the individual from making use of his or her support system.

This perspective on stress provides a basis for a strategic approach to stress management. Rather than applying a single stress management technique to all individuals who consult us or choosing haphazardly from among the myriad of stress management techniques that are available, we can assess which of the preceding factors contribute to the individual's problems with stress and then choose interventions targeted to those specific difficulties. Thus we would use very different interventions with an individual who is grossly overestimating the demands of the situation than we would use with an individual who is perceiving the situation realistically but who lacks the skills needed to cope with it effectively.

COGNITIVE THERAPY AND STRESS MANAGEMENT

To understand the cognitive approach to treatment of stress reactions, let us take a commonplace example and see how this problem would be approached.

> Mr. A was a hard-driving businessman who presented for treatment with hypertension, headaches, and a sleep disturbance. Every day he left his house at 7 A.M. in order to avoid the heavy traffic. However, by the time he arrived at his office half an hour later, his face was red, he was perspiring, his pulse was racing, and he had a headache. What happened in the interim?
>
> Although Mr. A initially stated that he was simply driving his car to work, a more detailed assessment made it clear that he approached his drive to work as a competitive situation. Practically every second of his trip, he was engaged in confrontations and challenges with other drivers. The competitive struggle led him to cut in and out of lanes and to attempt to get the jump on the other drivers at stop signals. He believed that the other drivers were similarly trying to beat him, and he was impelled to counterattack if one of them did get an advantage.
>
> Aside from his competitive reactions, Mr. A had a personal goal of making the best possible time on his drive. He reacted to any loss of momentum as though he were blocked by a major barrier. He mentally or verbally attacked any slow driver who impeded forward progress. He regarded it as a personal defeat if he did not beat out a yellow light before it turned red.
>
> Far from simply traveling to work, Mr. A was engaged in a personal survival course. His maneuvering was not a game but rather a series of fierce encounters. He was mobilized for aggressive physical action, as manifested by his muscular tension, increased blood pressure, and increased heart rate. The drive provided little opportunity to transform the mobilization into action other than the minimal exertion involved in driving his car, and by the time he reached the office his muscles were taut and he was coiled, prepared to strike. Once he arrived at the office, there was no opportunity to engage in the kind of physical action that would facilitate "demobilization." Moreover, because his cognitive set revolved around the notion of "attack," he tended to interpret further encounters in terms of this construct and to remain in a state of mobilization.

Adopting a Strategic Approach to Stress Management

How can the cognitive approach be applied to alleviating Mr. A's symptoms? The first step in the management of stress reactions is the application of the principles outlined in the first part of this chapter to understanding this individual. An individualized understanding of this particular case provides a basis for selecting the interventions that are most likely to prove useful in alleviating Mr. A's difficulties. Although cognitive and behavioral interventions play a major role in cognitive therapy's approach to stress management, it is important to note that none of these interventions is mandatory. Cognitive therapy's understanding of stress provides a conceptual framework within which a wide range of interventions can be utilized. We advocate a strategic approach to treatment in which the therapist develops an understanding of the individual's problems and then selects interventions appropriate for that individual (Beck, 1995, pp. 13–24; Persons, 1989). As a result, the goals of therapy, the interventions used, and the duration of treatment can vary considerably from case to case.

It is traditional to think of stress as an isolated response to stressful events and to think of stress management as a narrowly focused intervention that addresses only the individual's response to those events. Very short-term, narrowly focused interventions are often appropriate, especially if the individual has a history of doing well until faced with an objectively stressful situation. However, a somewhat broader intervention approach is likely to be appropriate when the individual has a history of repeated difficulties in coping with stress, a history of psychosocial difficulties when not dealing with stressful situations, or idiosyncratic beliefs and assumptions that play a significant role in his or her problems with stress. When broader issues are addressed, the individual should be less vulnerable to similar problems in the future.

In Mr. A's case, treatment consisted of much more than simply focusing on his stress during his commute to work each morning. In part the reason was that more narrowly focused stress management interventions had not proven to be very effective. Mr. A had been referred for psychotherapy for hypertension and chronic muscle tension after relaxation techniques and biofeedback applied by a very experienced therapist had been only mildly effective. Treatment began with an initial evaluation intended to provide a basis for an initial conceptualization which would aid in selecting an intervention approach.

In the initial interview, Mr. A was extremely restless and unable to sit still. He asked whether he could move around and then paced the floor for the first part of the interview. He said that although he was successful in business and had a happy marriage and a good relationship with his children, he got little enjoyment out of life. He complained that he was unable to relax at home and that he and his wife had to take frequent vacations in order for him to have periods of rest and relaxation. He also complained of being chronically depressed. The initial evaluation provided information about a number of factors relevant to understanding of Mr. A's problems.

Stressors

It goes without saying that the occurrence of stressful life events plays a major role in understanding an individual's problems with stress. The situations in which Mr. A experiences stress were fairly "ordinary" events to which he reacted quite strongly. In addition to the stress he experienced on his drive to work, he also reacted strongly to the initiation of any new contract, project, or account, as well as to any action by one of his employees that impeded his progress in any way. Taking on a new project added substantially to the feeling of pressure that he chronically experienced. Furthermore, he interpreted anything less than optimum efficiency on the part of one of his employees as "negligence" and would feel hostile toward that employee. Because he considered it unwise to scold his employees, he carried a constant load of hostility.

Mr. A also was hypersensitive to a variety of events that would only minimally disturb other people. If asked to do anything, he would feel "put upon," as though the additional tasks made his burden unbearable. Any limitation of his freedom of action made him feel "locked in" or "trapped," whether the limitation was physical or psychological. He was sensitive to any perceived interference in his goal-directed activity. These included interruptions, being in crowds, finding that a door was locked or was difficult to open, being told that a rule prohibited a certain course of action, or being asked to finish a project before he felt ready.

The Importance of Meanings

Apparently minor events can have a substantial emotional impact if the individual invests them with additional meaning. Mr. A reacted intensely to an assortment of trivial matters. For example, he demanded that his staff always have sharp pencils available to him and reacted to any lapses in this routine with the same degree of seriousness with which he would react to problems obtaining financing for one of his business ventures.

On exploration, it was discovered that his overreaction to not having sharp pencils available was based on his conviction that his success depended on flawless operation of his "system." As he saw it, any imperfection in the workings of his business organization meant that there was a breakdown in the system and therefore meant that his success was jeopardized. His line of reasoning was something like: "If I can't count on my staff for something simple like pens and pencils, how can I count on them for something really important?" Any event that weakened his confidence in the efficient operation of his employees led to a complete loss of confidence in his system and a fear that disaster was imminent.

Not surprisingly, his sense of having been let down by his staff led to anger at the offenders and a wish to punish them. However, he feared that angry outbursts or excessive punishment would impair the efficiency of his system. As a result, he suppressed these reactions and experienced chronic frustration and aggravation.

Dysfunctional Thoughts

As discussed previously, humans constantly and automatically appraise and reappraise the situations they encounter. The results are automatic thoughts such as "That was too damn close! That bastard did it on purpose" in response to being cut off in traffic. The individual may or may not be aware of these automatic thoughts, and the thoughts may or may not be realistic. However, these thoughts can have a major impact on emotion and behavior. We tend to react as though these unexamined thoughts are literally true, whether they are or not. Thus when the thoughts are exaggerated or unrealistic they can play a major role in the individual's problems.

Cognitive Distortions

Humans are subject to a variety of thinking errors, such as viewing situations in black-and-white terms, jumping to conclusions, or anticipating catastrophic consequences. These "cognitive distortions" (see Freeman, Pretzer, Fleming, & Simon, 2004, pp. 5–6) can have a significant impact on the individual's interpretation of events. Stress-prone individuals often interpret impersonal events egocentrically ("Why does this have to happen to *me*?"), exaggerate the frequency of noxious events ("He *always* does that!"), and exaggerate the severity of noxious events ("He *never* shows me *any* respect!").

Mr. A had a strong tendency to view situations in black-and-white terms. For example, he viewed employees as either "careful" or "negligent," without any gradations in between the two extremes. He constantly interpreted impersonal situations as though they were directed at him personally, as when a driver who had been weaving through traffic cut in front of him, and his reaction was "He did that to show me up!" He also reacted to small events as though they were likely to have catastrophic consequences. These cognitive errors resulted in mundane events being much more stressful than was necessary.

Core Beliefs

Core beliefs are the individual's most central ideas about the self. These beliefs develop in childhood as the child interacts with significant others in a variety of situations. Once core beliefs are acquired, they can be quite persistent and can have important impacts in many areas. Although Mr. A was seen as quite successful by most, he was haunted by persistent feelings of inadequacy. During his childhood he had experienced many interactions in which his older siblings pointed out his inadequacies, treated him with contempt, and ridiculed him. As a result, he had developed a persistent view of himself as inadequate and a persistent expectation that he would be ridiculed unless he proved his competence by succeeding at whatever tasks he undertook.

Interpersonal Strategies

Individuals also develop beliefs about what they need to do in interpersonal interactions in order to obtain the results they desire. These beliefs are based on experiences acquired in interactions with significant others, on the examples the child grows up with, and on the lessons the child is taught, both implicitly and explicitly. For example, a parent who reacts strongly to anything he or she perceives as disrespect implicitly communicates that respect is very important. The same parent may also explicitly teach the child certain strategies for obtaining respect, such as "You have to *make* people respect you. Show them that you *can* do it."

Mr. A believed that financial success was *the* way of gaining the respect of his peers. Thus making money was a source of gratification for him because it enhanced his social image, not just because of the financial rewards. His financial success provided him with a sense that he was safe from ridicule as long as he was successful. However, whenever there seemed to be a risk of the loss of financial security, he began to experience anxiety and to visualize the contempt that he expected his business associates to have for him if he were to fail.

Mr. A's sense of confidence depended on the tangible evidence of success. When he did well on a business deal, he would think, "I am successful. I am really bright." If he did not do well, he would think, "I am stupid." Apparently, he had not built up any solid core of self-esteem that would persist independent of fluctuations in his cash flow. Instead, he conducted his life as though he really were stupid and inadequate and could be acceptable only if he could prove he was competent by succeeding. Unfortunately, he defined *competence* only in terms of the outcome of his most recent venture, and he needed a steady stream of successes to prove that he was competent. He took great pride in the material satisfactions that his family had, but he always had a nagging sense that he would "lose everything" if his business went under. His dichotomous thinking was evident in his considering his business (and himself) as either a success or a failure. There was nothing in between.

Lifestyle

It may seem that whether one experiences many stressful life events or not is simply a matter of luck. However, often individuals make choices that have a significant impact on the likelihood of stressful life events. Decisions such as whether one accepts a job offer that entails a long commute through an urban setting, obtains a large mortgage rather than buying a more modest home, or encourages one's spouse to become a full-time homemaker can have a lasting impact on the frequency and severity of stressful life events. In his overall approach to life, Mr. A placed a very high value on financial success and success in his business. He set high standards for success and was driven to achieve his objectives at all costs. He was intolerant of any obstacles, delays, or detours.

Throughout his life, he was constantly pressing toward a goal and was continually monitoring his progress toward the goal, just as he did when driving to work. He attached great significance to each goal, regarded each activity as a do-or-die matter, and was chronically overmobilized. When unexpected problems or minor mistakes were encountered, he reacted as though a major disaster were imminent. He was impelled to constantly work toward his objectives even on evenings and weekends or when there was nothing to be done.

Developing an Individualized Conceptualization

By conducting an initial evaluation and collecting detailed information about thoughts, feelings, and actions in problem situations, the therapist can obtain the information needed to develop a working understanding of the individual and the problems he or she is encountering. However, it often is not easy for a therapist to organize all the information he or she has obtained in order to make use of it. Several cognitive therapists (Beck, 1995; Persons, 1989) have developed conceptualization forms designed to help therapists make sense of the information they obtain over the course of therapy. Figure 18.2 shows how Judith Beck's cognitive conceptualization diagram (Beck, 1995) would be used to organize the information presented about Mr. A thus far.

The cognitive therapists' goal is to use an understanding of the individual and his or her problems to guide intervention. The therapist's understanding of the patient is initially based on information gathered during the initial evaluation, but it is constantly updated and refined as additional information is collected over the course of therapy. The information summarized in Figure 18.2 was obtained over the course of the initial evaluation and several treatment sessions.

Collaborative Empiricism

The preceding conceptualization is intended to facilitate a strategic approach to intervention in which the therapist thinks in terms of what needs to be accomplished and the available options for achieving those ends. However, there are many possible ways of going about this. The idea of *collaborative empiricism* is central to the practice of cognitive therapy (see Table 18.2 for a summary of the general principles of cognitive therapy). In the initial evaluation, the cognitive therapist works *with* his or her patient to collect detailed information regarding the specific thoughts, feelings, and actions that occur in problem situations. These observations provide a basis for developing an individualized understanding of the patient that facilitates strategic intervention. Collaborative empiricism continues to play an important role as the focus of therapy shifts from assessment to intervention. Many of the specific techniques used to modify dysfunctional thoughts, beliefs, and strategies emphasize firsthand observation and "behavioral experiments" to test the validity of dysfunctional automatic thoughts or dysfunctional beliefs and to develop more adaptive alternatives. Rather than relying on the therapist's expertise, theoretical deductions, or logic, cognitive therapy assumes that empirical observation is the most reliable means for developing valid conceptualizations and effective interventions.

Persons unfamiliar with cognitive therapy sometimes assume that cognitive therapists focus solely on modifying the individual's cognitions and ignore behavior and emotions. It is important to remember that a broad range of behavioral interventions and emotion-focused interventions are also a part of cognitive therapy.

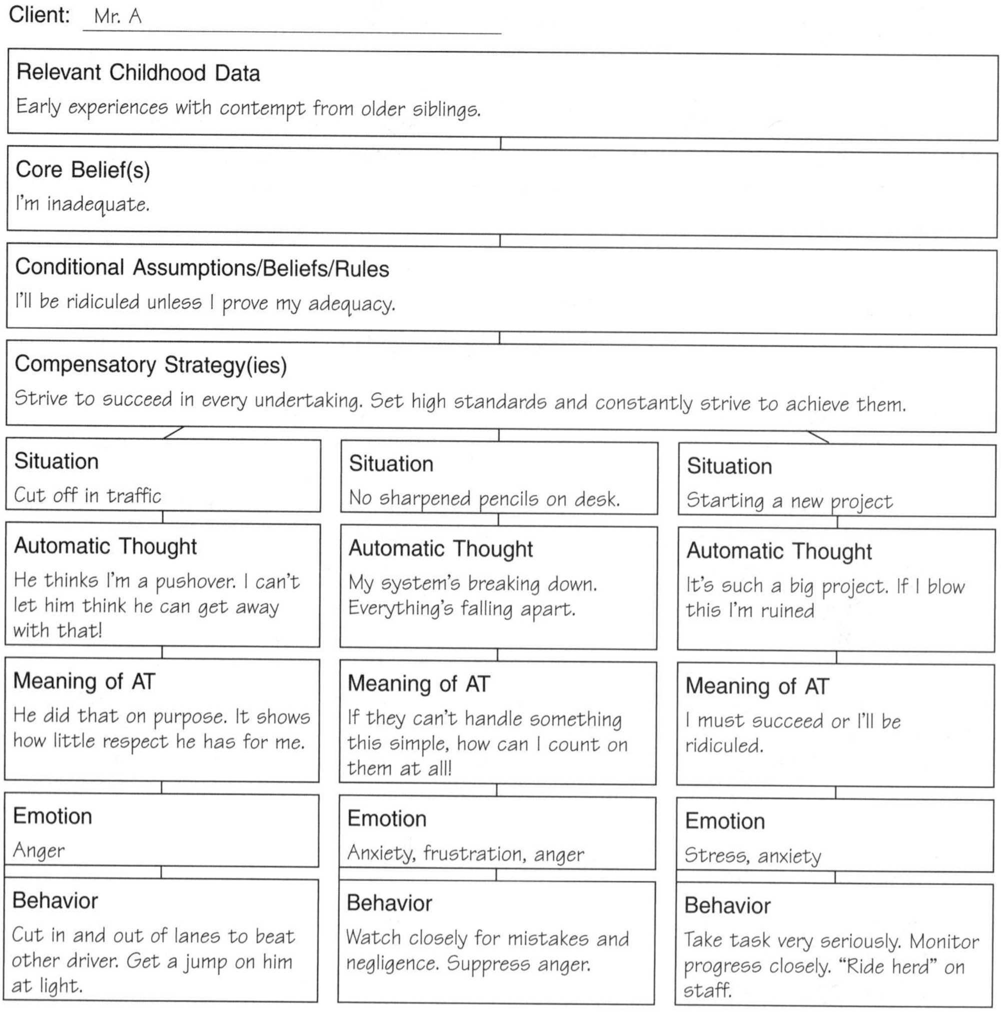

Client: Mr. A
_____

| Relevant Childhood Data |
| Early experiences with contempt from older siblings. |

| Core Belief(s) |
| I'm inadequate. |

| Conditional Assumptions/Beliefs/Rules |
| I'll be ridiculed unless I prove my adequacy. |

| Compensatory Strategy(ies) |
| Strive to succeed in every undertaking. Set high standards and constantly strive to achieve them. |

Situation	Situation	Situation
Cut off in traffic	No sharpened pencils on desk.	Starting a new project
Automatic Thought	**Automatic Thought**	**Automatic Thought**
He thinks I'm a pushover. I can't let him think he can get away with that!	My system's breaking down. Everything's falling apart.	It's such a big project. If I blow this I'm ruined
Meaning of AT	**Meaning of AT**	**Meaning of AT**
He did that on purpose. It shows how little respect he has for me.	If they can't handle something this simple, how can I count on them at all!	I must succeed or I'll be ridiculed.
Emotion	**Emotion**	**Emotion**
Anger	Anxiety, frustration, anger	Stress, anxiety
Behavior	**Behavior**	**Behavior**
Cut in and out of lanes to beat other driver. Get a jump on him at light.	Watch closely for mistakes and negligence. Suppress anger.	Take task very seriously. Monitor progress closely. "Ride herd" on staff.

FIGURE 18.2. Cognitive conceptualization diagram.

TABLE 18.2. General Principles of Cognitive Therapy

- Therapist and patient work collaboratively toward clear goals.
- The therapist takes an active, directive role.
- Interventions are based on an individualized conceptualization.
- The focus is on specific problem situations and on specific thoughts, feelings, and actions.
- Therapist and patient focus on modifying thoughts, coping with emotions, and/or changing behavior as needed.
- The patient continues the work of therapy between sessions.
- Interventions later in therapy focus on identifying and modifying predisposing factors, including schemas and core beliefs.
- At the close of treatment therapist and patient work explicitly on relapse prevention.

Using Specific Intervention Techniques

In cognitive therapy's approach to stress management, the therapist's overall aim is to modify any cognitive processes that contribute to the client's stress, to increase his or her ability to cope adaptively with stressful situations, and to do what can be done to reduce stressors and increase social supports. A variety of cognitive, behavioral, interpersonal, and other interventions can be used to achieve these aims. In Mr. A's case, a number of cognitive and behavioral interventions were used.

"Taking a Break"

Often, cognitive processes that contribute to the individual's stress (such as Mr. A's perception of his drive to work as a competitive situation in which he must beat other drivers) become hypervalent. Mr. A's stress and frustration from his drive to work on Monday increased the likelihood that he would approach his workday and his drive to work on Tuesday with an aggressive, competitive mindset and thus tended to be self-perpetuating. When this is the case, one promising initial intervention is to temporarily reduce the individual's exposure to the situations that serve as stressors. For example, if Mr. A could take time off from work, stop driving himself to work, or drive to work at a time when there was very little traffic, this would be likely to reduce the activation of his competitive, aggressive schemas. When it is not practical for the individual to reduce exposure to stressors, relaxation techniques, biofeedback, or meditation techniques can be used to decrease arousal and decrease the activity of stress-related cognitions. As the overactivity of this cognitive constellation is reduced, there is not only a reduced mobilization of the neuromuscular endocrine system but also a relative increase in the adaptive functions (particularly objectivity and perspective).

Although a simple reduction in the overactivity of stress-related cognitions usually is not sufficient to resolve the individual's stress-related problems, it makes it easier for the therapist to help the individual to reflect on his or her reactions, to recognize overreactions, to test some of his or her conclusions, and to adopt a broader view regarding his or her problems. Specific cognitive techniques can be used to identify and address the cognitions that contribute to the individual's stress.

Identifying Dysfunctional Cognitions

It is important to recognize that although we might label Mr. A's symptoms as manifestations of a "stress reaction," the environmental stressors he faces are ordinary situations that many people face regularly without experiencing the level of stress that Mr. A encounters. If we were to think simply in terms of external factors, we might have difficulty explaining why Mr. A experienced his trip as more stressful than the other drivers did. In order to achieve an understanding of his problem, we would need to examine the internal factors: his thoughts, impulses, and feelings. However, this often is easier said than done. Mr. A may be focused on the behavior of other drivers, not on his own cognitive processes. In fact, he may well assert that there are no thoughts going through his head as he drives and that the problem is just all the people who drive like idiots.

The easiest way to identify the relevant cognitions is to have the patient choose one specific situation that provides a good example of a time when stress becomes a problem. Then the therapist can elicit a detailed description of the events that led up to the situation, the chain of events as the stress developed, and the individual's emotional reactions.

It usually is then possible to obtain useful reports of cognitions by asking about the individual's immediate, spontaneous reactions at key points in the chain of events:[2]

> THERAPIST: So let me recap. It's last Monday. You've had to rush to get out of the house on time and now you're pulling onto the freeway. A guy in a beat-up old car cuts you off rather than leaving room for you to merge. Immediately you feel yourself tense up and your heart starts pounding. What do you remember running through your head right then?
>
> MR. A: I was thinking that I couldn't let him get away with treating me like that.
>
> THERAPIST: Usually it works best if we come as close as we can to an exact quote of what ran through your head because sometimes the wording makes a big difference. Do you remember just how that was worded?
>
> MR. A: Let me think. . . . It was "That bastard did it on purpose. He must think I'm a pushover. I can't let him get away with this shit."

Mr. A gradually became aware of his thoughts and impulses while driving. Each time he was able to identify these cognitions, he increased his objectivity toward them. Some of the categories were these:

1. Projections (mind reading): "They think I am a pushover."
2. Exaggeration: "I'll never get to work at this rate. . . . This bottleneck is awful."
3. Imperatives: "I must get to work as fast as I can," "I can't let him think he can get away with edging me out," "I must show him," "I must not allow myself to be jammed in."
4. Negative attributions: "They are deliberately trying to cut me off."
5. Punitive wishes: "I will show him how stupid he is by cutting in front of him."

Understanding the Meanings

Once a sampling of the patient's thoughts in problem situations has been identified, it usually becomes apparent that he or she is attaching additional meanings to the situations encountered. Initially, Mr. A was not fully conscious of how he was driven to fight off the other drivers, nor did he see the connection between his combativeness on the road and his symptoms. By identifying the specific thoughts that occurred while Mr. A was driving and pointing out their connection to his physical and emotional reactions, his therapist was able to prepare him to make additional observations during subsequent drives so that they could develop a more detailed understanding of his cognitions while driving. Over the course of several drives to work, he was able to recognize that he has a pervasive tendency to react as though his commute was a matter of challenge, confrontation, and competition, to react to any difficulty as though it were a major barrier, and to react as though any delay in getting to work would have disastrous consequences. He also recognized that his thoughts led to the overmobilization manifested in his stress symptoms: increased heart rate, increased blood pressure, and headache. He also came to see that these cognitive patterns carried over into his workday. Throughout his working day, he reacted to each encounter as though he were engaged in hand-to-hand combat.

One of the most important characteristics that Mr. A detected (with his therapist's help) was his own egocentrism. He viewed all events as though he were the central character in a drama; the behavior of all the other characters had meaning only insofar as he related it to his own "vital interests." He personalized events that were essentially imper-sonal and perceived confrontations and challenges when others were conducting their own lives oblivious to him.

Modifying Dysfunctional Cognitions

Cognitive therapy is well known for emphasizing the identification of dysfunctional cognitions and for using a variety of interventions to modify those cognitions or minimize their impact. These interventions can be quite useful when dysfunctional cognitions play a role in the individual's problems with stress.

A useful first step in addressing dysfunctional cognitions is to frame the cognitions as ideas that may or may not be true and to collaboratively engage the patient in looking critically at his or her own thoughts. It is essential that patients attain distance from their reactions so that they can look at their experiences as phenomena instead of being totally absorbed by them. Then they may be able to recognize that their thoughts and conclu-sions are inferences, not facts—that their beliefs are derived from an internal process and are not pure images of external reality. They may consequently realize that, because their cognitive processes are fallible, they may have been accepting misinterpretations, distor-tions, and exaggerations as "truth." Furthermore, they can observe that the laws and rules that they apply to themselves and others are not immutable, natural laws (such as the laws of gravity and thermodynamics) but are often arbitrary and self-defeating.

With increasing objectivity, patients can recognize that the meanings and significance of events are "man-made" and do not occur independently in nature. Although they do not voluntarily attach irrelevant and self-defeating meanings to events, it is possible to undo the assignment of meaning—to strip away the excess baggage from events. It is worth emphasizing that simply taking a history and asking the "right" questions can in-crease a patient's objectivity (and perspective). As a therapist probes for meanings, a pa-tient may spontaneously begin to question the validity of his or her conclusions and to see the symptoms in a new light.

The therapist can then work to expand the frames of reference by which the patient judges events, him- or herself, and others. Individuals may then be able to obtain a more realistic conception of the magnitude, seriousness, and duration of the stressors they face. This can be done by considering how others view the situation, the relative importance of the situation when compared with the individual's true priorities, and the magnitude of the likely consequences.

For example, with increasing perspective Mr. A could come to see that beating other drivers and getting to work fast was relatively unimportant—not a life-and-death strug-gle; and he could further realize that the encounter with other drivers was time-limited and not a part of a continuous war. The conceptualizations involved in a broader per-spective are far more complex and involve many more kinds of shading than those de-rived from the narrow egocentric frame of reference.

A crucial element in facilitating demobilization of the neuroendocrine system is changing the cognitive set. Each time Mr. A went out to his car, a specific cognitive set was induced—that is, his view of his world shifted from a relatively peaceful, harmonious outlook during breakfast to an expectation of confrontation and competition. A cogni-tive set is the final product of the network of associated attitudes, expectations, memo-ries, and meanings that are activated by a given situation. This set may be induced by spe-cific situations (e.g., Mr. A's trip to work), or it may be relatively stable across all situations, as when a person is depressed. In the earlier portion of this chapter, we applied the term *controlling cognitive constellation* to designate the basic cognitive structures (schemas) that are reflected in the cognitive set. Although the structures operate outside of awareness, the individual has access to the content represented in the set. A change in the cognitive set may be achieved by changing the nature of the environmental stimuli, by transferring attention to a different set of stimuli, or by subjecting the content of the set to logical and empirical analysis.

The cognitive set induced by specific stimuli may also be conceptualized as consisting of a composite of primary and secondary appraisals. Thus therapeutic work may be directed toward modifying the conception of threat or challenge (primary appraisal) or toward the evaluation of coping resources (secondary appraisal). The validity of the primary and secondary appraisals is tested by subjecting them to a series of questions: What is the evidence of a threat? How serious is it? What coping resources are available? The individual can also reduce exaggerated threats through coping self-statements (Ellis, 1962; Goldfried, 1977; Meichenbaum, 1977; Novaco, 1975; Turk, Meichenbaum, & Genest, 1983).

An alternative to the idea of taking a break, discussed previously, would be for Mr. A to mentally take a break from the situation by shifting his attention away from the other drivers and from thinking about competition, occupying his mind with nonstressful stimuli. Thus he might focus on listening to an audiotape or to the radio or observe features of his environment to which he had formerly been oblivious. The diversion would vitiate the power of the cognitive set and would thus reduce the frequency and intensity of Mr. A's hostile inferences regarding confrontations and challenges.

Cognitive restructuring and reality testing often are an important part of cognitive therapy. The techniques of cognitive modification are aimed at improving a patient's way of processing information and, consequently, his or her grasp of reality. Take, for example, Mr. A's notion that other drivers were trying to beat him out or to obstruct his progress. A series of questions could be raised: (1) What is the evidence for this conclusion? (2) Is there evidence that contradicts this conclusion? (3) Are there alternative explanations for their presumed hostile behavior? Such a joint inquiry between therapist and patient has been labeled *collaborative empiricism* elsewhere (Hollon & Beck, 1979). The technique consists of framing the individual's conclusion as a hypothesis, which is then jointly investigated. By assuming an investigative role, the therapist encourages the patient to view his or her ideas as conclusions or inferences to be examined, rather than as beliefs to be defended. The approach has the benefit of increasing the patient's objectivity and reality testing.

For example, after Mr. A had been asked to look for evidence either consistent with or contradictory to his notion that the other drivers were trying to beat him out (or obstruct him), he reported the following incident: "There was a truck ahead of me. I thought it was deliberately trying to block me, so I gunned my engine to pass it. Then I saw that the driver was busy talking to his buddy and didn't even notice me." Through looking for evidence, he came to realize that, far from engaging in a battle with him, the drivers of other vehicles often were not even aware of him. Such an observation not only can correct a misconception but can also help shake the egocentric perspective.

It can be particularly important to identify and address the dysfunctional interpersonal strategies that play a role in the individual's problems. Imagine an individual who operates on the basis of an interpersonal strategy such as "The way to get a kid to be good is to punish them when they are bad." He or she will be likely to respond to any perceived transgressions by punishing the child. If the punishment results in "good" behavior on the part of the child (i.e., no further transgressions), it appears that the strategy worked. If the punishment is followed by further transgressions, the individual is likely to conclude that he or she needs to "try harder" and thus is likely to proceed with more frequent punishment and more intense punishment rather than recognizing that punishment is proving to be ineffective with this child and considering other strategies.

In Mr. A's case, because he attributed responsibility for success or failure to both himself and his staff, he was constantly prepared to identify and punish the offending party when something went wrong. Typically, he would investigate any "foul-up" and would feel a strong urge to "come down hard" on the offending party, whether it was himself or an employee. However, he also was aware that he could not continually badger his staff without this having a negative impact on morale and productivity. As a result, he often had hostile reactions to his staff that he did not express while being harshly critical of any mistakes on his own part.

Mr. A's punitive attitude had to do with several related issues. As he saw it, his vital interests were at stake; thus any offense by the staff struck at the heart of these interests. This caused pain and raised a desire to retaliate because of the pain that they had caused him. The punishment was also intended to "teach them a lesson" in order to prevent a recurrence of the offense. He also believed that he needed to punish members of the staff periodically in order to "tighten the reins" and keep his organization running efficiently.

It is notable that much of his hostility was engendered simply as a result of the rules being broken rather than of any real damage having been done. Because Mr. A saw his "system" as being crucial to his success, he was continually vigilant to make sure that the rules were followed closely. Thus he would check his secretary's work to make sure that there were no mistakes in punctuation, and he would monitor the arrival and departure times of the employees to make sure that they were not cheating. Because of this vigilance, he did indeed perceive a fair number of minor infractions. Unfortunately, he responded to each as though it was a major transgression that would lead to immediate disaster.

Once the interpersonal strategies behind his vigilant, punitive approach to his staff and to himself was understood, it was possible to help Mr. A consider the benefits and drawbacks of this approach and to help him to consider alternative approaches to succeeding in business. He eventually adopted an approach that included distinguishing between major and minor transgressions, using rewards for good behavior and punishment for bad behavior, decreasing his vigilance for small infractions, and accepting that a good but imperfect performance did not mean that the individual was either incompetent or malicious. As he tested this alternative approach in practice, he found that it was much less stressful and worked at least as well as his original approach.

Behavioral Interventions

Despite the name *cognitive therapy*, cognitive techniques are by no means the only interventions used. Behavioral interventions play a prominent role as well and are used both to change behavior and to facilitate cognitive change. Although verbal interventions conducted in the therapist's office are often quite useful in identifying and modifying dysfunctional cognitions, words alone often have only a limited impact. One of the most effective methods for modifying dysfunctional automatic thoughts, beliefs, and interpersonal strategies is to frame the cognition in question as a testable hypothesis and then to help the patient find ways to test the hypothesis in real-life situations through "behavioral experiments."

Sometimes this process is quite simple and straightforward. For example, the individual who believes "It won't do any good to speak up, they won't take me seriously" can be coached through "speaking up" in a variety of real-life situations and observing the actual results. If it turns out that the patient is taken seriously at least some of the time, the belief is likely to change. If it turns out that the patient is not taken seriously when he or she speaks up, therapist and patient can consider whether work on assertion skills is needed or whether there are more promising ways to deal with situations in which the patient is not taken seriously. However, there are many situations in which some thought and effort is needed to figure out how to reframe a problematic cognition as a testable hypothesis. See Bennett-Levy et al. (2004) for detailed discussion of the use of behavioral experiments with a wide range of problems.

Relaxation techniques are often used as a part of stress management. However, previous attempts to use these techniques with Mr. A had been unsuccessful, in part due to his conviction that constant vigilance was necessary. Once this issue had been addressed, training Mr. A in a relaxation technique such as progressive relaxation training (Jacobson, 1938), in meditation, or in using biofeedback to learn to relax might serve several purposes. First, these interventions may result directly in a damping down of his physiological arousal and alleviate some of his physical symptoms. In addition, relaxation practice during the day might lower Mr. A's overall level of arousal and decrease his reactivity to potential stressors.

Beyond this, relaxation techniques would probably help to modify Mr. A's cognitive set in several ways. Certainly, a focus on relaxing his muscles might divert Mr. A from his overvigilant attention to the other drivers. In addition, the instruction to "relax" implies powerful meanings, such as "Things are not as serious as I make them out to be" or "It is OK to sit back and take it easy." Because the motive force behind Mr. A's tension was the drive to action, the assignment to relax would activate competing cognitive structures relevant to inaction and passivity.

Although the individual's misinterpretations of mundane situations, the additional meanings he or she attaches to the situation, and a hypervalent cognitive set often play important roles in stress, they rarely constitute the full story. Usually, another part of the problem is that the individual lacks the skills needed to cope effectively with the situation or fails to make effective use of the skills he or she possesses. If the therapist helps the patient to adopt a problem-solving orientation, to clearly identify his or her goals, to consider a range of options for achieving those goals, to select promising options, and then to put those options into practice, it often is possible to substantially improve the patient's ability to cope with stressful situations.

With some patients, the primary problem is that they have not mastered the skills needed to cope with problem situations. In this case, they are likely to need help in mastering those skills and learning to apply them effectively in practice. Other patients have the needed skills but fail to use them because of fears, inhibitions, and unrealistic expectations that block them from using the skills they have. When this is the case, the therapist can work to identify the cognitions that interfere with effective coping and to address them.

Often, interpersonal conflict plays an important role in stress-related problems. Appropriate assertion often proves to be an effective method for dealing with interpersonal problems and to be a good alternative to aggression. A nonassertive individual may have the skills necessary for appropriate assertion but be inhibited by fears and expectations such as "If I speak up for myself, no one will take me seriously," or "If I speak up for myself, they'll get mad at me." When this is the case, interventions that address these cognitions often are sufficient to enable the individual to deal with problem situations more effectively. However, many individuals are not skilled in dealing with interpersonal conflict effectively and assertively. In this case, it may be necessary to work to improve the individual's skills through instruction, coaching, and practice (see Rakos, 1991).

Lifestyle Changes

When aspects of the individual's lifestyle contribute to chronic or recurrent stress, it can be quite valuable to help him or her recognize this and make appropriate changes. Something as simple as waking up at the last minute so that one has to rush to get ready each morning can make a significant difference in one's level of stress.

It might seem as though "simple" steps such as getting adequate sleep, nutrition, and exercise, taking time for fun and relaxation, or spending part of one's time engaged in rewarding activities rather than unpleasant responsibilities would be easy for the patient to do. However, unspoken beliefs such as "I shouldn't waste time" can complicate this process. Often, it is important to identify and modify the cognitions that block the individual from making the necessary changes.

Relapse Prevention

If the therapist simply helps the patient make the necessary cognitive, behavioral, and lifestyle changes and then terminates treatment at that point, a significant portion of patients will gradually revert back to their dysfunctional patterns following treatment. Cognitive therapy ends with the therapist and patient working explicitly on relapse prevention. The therapist and patient identify high-risk situations and make sure that the patient is equipped to cope with them effectively. They also work together to identify early "warning signs" of reversion to dysfunctional patterns and plan ways for the patient to respond to them. See Wilson (1992) for a detailed discussion of relapse prevention with a wide range of problems.

Ideally, the patient leaves treatment with a written relapse prevention plan to refer to if he or she encounters difficulties in the future (see Figure 18.3 for one possible format for a relapse prevention plan). Usually, termination includes the therapist and patient discussing whether occasional "booster sessions" would be useful in maintaining changes, as well as a discussion of when the patient should recontact the therapist.

CONCLUSIONS

The cognitive approach to the treatment of stress reactions focuses on reducing the hyperactivity of the individual's controlling schemas, modifying dysfunctional cognitions, and improving the individual's ability to cope effectively. The patient is encouraged to examine the internal factors—thoughts, impulses, and feelings—that contribute to the stress response. The patient also identifies the meanings he or she has assigned to events that are connected to both behavioral activation and affect. Cognitive techniques such as identifying automatic thoughts, recognizing and correcting cognitive distortions, and identifying broad beliefs and assumptions that underlie cognition are used to clarify the problems.

Through a process of collaborative empiricism, the cognitive therapist and the patient frame the patient's conclusions as hypotheses, which are investigated and tested by

Relapse Prevention Plan	
High-Risk Situation(s) What situations have been hard to handle in the past? What situations are hard to handle currently? What situations are likely to be hard to handle in the future?	Plan How do I want to deal with it?
Early Warning Signs What feelings, thoughts, or actions would be early noticeable signs that I'm having difficulty?	Plan What would be good for me to do if I see these signs?
If this doesn't work, then what?	

FIGURE 18.3. One possible format for a relapse prevention plan

increasing both objectivity and perspective. The process of logically evaluating dysfunctional cognitions and testing them in real-life situations leads to shifts in thinking, with the ultimate goal being structural change. Structural change may come about through the analysis of specific stressors and of vulnerabilities, rules, and imperatives that have governed the person's responses. Structural change, then, extends beyond modifying habitual cognitive errors to the underlying organization of rules, formulas, assumptions, and imperatives that misclassify events as threatening. Cognitive interventions may also facilitate behavior change, especially when fears, expectations, and beliefs interfere with effective coping.

Behavioral interventions are used not only to help the individual cope more effectively but also to facilitate cognitive change. In particular, behavioral experiments provide a powerful way to modify many dysfunctional cognitions. Behavioral interventions are also used to improve coping skills and to accomplish broader lifestyle changes when necessary. Practical steps such as "taking a break" from dealing with stressful situations, obtaining necessary information, and making better use of available social support can also play an important role in stress management.

A large body of research provides evidence that cognitive therapy is effective with mental health problems ranging from depression to schizophrenia. In addition, many of the interventions discussed in this chapter have been tested empirically in relation to stress management. However, the precise approach to stress management discussed in this chapter has not yet been subjected to controlled outcome studies. Therefore, we do not yet have empirical evidence to document the effectiveness of the approach to stress management presented in this chapter. Given our clinical experience and cognitive therapy's strong empirical base, we are look forward to empirical tests of this treatment approach.

NOTES

1. *Schemas* are cognitive structures for screening, coding, and evaluating experiences. Their content consists of unconditional core beliefs (e.g., "I'm no good"; "Others can't be trusted"; "Effort does not pay off") that are derived from previous experience. Schemas typically operate outside of the individual's awareness and often are not clearly verbalized.
2. For a detailed discussion of methods for identifying dysfunctional cognitions, see Beck (1995, Ch. 6).

REFERENCES

Beck, A. T. (1964). Thinking and depression: 2. Theory and therapy. *Archives of General Psychiatry, 10,* 561–571.

Beck, A. T. (1967). *Depression: Clinical, experimental, and theoretical.* New York: Hoeber.

Beck, A. T. (1976). *Cognitive therapy and the emotional disorders.* New York: International Universities Press.

Beck, A. T. (1983). Cognitive approaches to stress reactions. In P. Lehrer & R. L. Woolfolk (Eds.), *Clinical guide to stress management.* New York: Guilford Press.

Beck, A. T. (1984). Cognitive approaches to stress. In R. Woolfolk & P. Lehrer (Eds.), *Principles and practice of stress management.* New York: Guilford Press.

Beck, A. T., Rush, A. J., Shaw, B. F., & Emery, G. (1979). *Cognitive therapy of depression.* New York: Guilford Press.

Beck, J. (1995). *Cognitive therapy: Basics and beyond.* New York: Guilford Press.

Bennett-Levy, J., Butler, G., Fennell, M., Hackman, A., Mueller, M., & Westbrook, D (Eds.). (2004). *Oxford guide to behavioural experiments in cognitive therapy.* New York: Oxford University Press.

Bowlby, J. (1981, April). *Cognitive processes in the genesis of psychopathology.* Invited address to the biennial meeting of the Society for Research in Child Development, Boston.

Ellis, A. (1962). *Reason and emotion in psychotherapy.* New York: Lyle Stuart.

Freeman, A., Pretzer, J., Fleming, B., & Simon, K. (2004). *Clinical applications of cognitive therapy* (2nd ed.). New York: Kluwer Academic/Plenum.

Goldfried, M. R. (1977). The use of relaxation and cognitive relabeling as coping skills. In R. B. Stuart (Ed.), *Behavioral self-management: Strategies and outcomes.* New York: Brunner/Mazel.

Hollon, S. D., & Beck, A. T. (1979). Cognitive therapy of depression. In S. D. Hollon & P.C. Kendall (Eds.), *Cognitive-behavioral interventions: Theory, research, and procedures.* New York: Academic Press.

Jacobson, E. (1938). *Progressive relaxation* (2nd ed.). Chicago: University of Chicago Press.

Lazarus, R. S. (1966). *Psychological stress and the coping process.* New York: McGraw-Hill.

Lazarus, R. S. (1981). The stress and coping paradigm. In C. Eisdorfer, D. Cohen, A. Kleinman, & P. Maxim (Eds.), *Conceptual models for psychotherapy.* New York: Spectrum.

Mahoney, M. (1982). Psychotherapy and human change processes. In J. H. Harvey & M. P. Parke (Eds.), *Psychotherapy research and behavior change.* Washington, DC: American Psychological Association.

Meichenbaum, D. H. (1977). *Cognitive behavior modification: An integrative approach.* New York: Plenum Press.

Novaco, R. (1975). *Anger control: The development and evaluation of an experimental treatment.* Lexington, MA: Heath.

Persons, J. (1989). *Cognitive therapy in practice: A case formulation approach.* New York: Norton.

Pretzer, J., Beck, A. T., & Newman, C. F. (1989). Stress and stress management: A cognitive view. *Journal of Cognitive Psychotherapy: An International Quarterly, 3,* 163–179.

Rakos, R. (1991). *Assertive behavior: Theory, research, and training.* New York: Routledge.

Saul, L. J. (1947). *Emotional maturity.* Philadelphia: Lippincott.

Turk, D. C., Meichenbaum, D., & Genest, M. (1983). *Pain and behavioral medicine: A cognitive-behavioral perspective.* New York: Guilford Press.

Wilson, P. H. (Ed.). (1992). *Principles and practice of relapse prevention.* New York: Guilford Press.

Wolff, H. G. (1950). Life stress and bodily disease: A formulation. In *Life stress and bodily disease: Proceedings of the Association for Research in Nervous and Mental Disease, December 2 and 3, 1949, New York.* Baltimore: Williams & Wilkins.

CHAPTER 19

Stress Inoculation Training
A Preventative and Treatment Approach

DONALD MEICHENBAUM

Clinicians who seek to provide help to stressed individuals, either on a treatment or on a preventative basis, are confronted with a major challenge. As Elliott and Eisdorfer (1982) observed, stressful events come in diverse forms that include exposure to:

1. *Acute time-limited stressors*, including such events as preparing for specific medical procedures (e.g., surgery, dental examination) or for invasive medical examinations (e.g., biopsies, cardiac catherization) or having to confront specific evaluations (e.g., a PhD defense)
2. *A sequence of stressful events* that may follow from the exposure to traumatic events, such as a terrorist attack, a rape, a natural disaster that results in a major loss of resources, or exposure to stressors that require *transitional adjustments* due to major losses (e.g., death of a loved one, becoming unemployed), each of which gives rise to a series of related challenges
3. *Chronic intermittent stressors* that entail repeated exposures to stressors such as repetitive evaluations and ongoing competitive performances (e.g., musical or athletic competitions), recurrent medical tests or treatments, or episodic physical disorders such as recurrent headaches, as well as the exposure to intermittent stress that accompanies certain occupational roles, such as military combat
4. *Chronic continual stressors* such as debilitating medical or psychiatric illnesses, physical disabilities resulting from exposure to traumatic events (e.g., burns, spinal cord injuries, traumatic brain injuries), or exposure to prolonged distress, including marital or familial discord, urban violence, poverty, and racism, as well as exposure to persistent occupational dangers and stressors in professions such as police work, nursing, and teaching

These varied stressful events may range from those that are time-limited and require situational adjustments to those chronic stressful events that are persistent and that require long-term adaptation. Stressors may also differ between those that are potentially controllable (i.e., can be lessened, avoided, or eliminated by engaging in certain behaviors) and those judged to be uncontrollable (i.e., an incurable illness, exposure to ongoing threats of violence, caring for a spouse with severe dementia) and whether they are predictable or unpredictable; of short duration (i.e., an examination) or chronic (i.e., living in a racist society, being exposed to poverty, having a stressful job); intermittent or recurrent; current or distant in the past. Distant stressors are traumatic experiences that occurred in the distant past yet that have the potential to continually affect one's well-being and even modify the individual's immune system because of the long-lasting emotional, cognitive, and behavioral sequelae (Segerstrom & Miller, 2004).

In some instances, individuals are exposed to multiple features of such stressful events. As an example, I was asked to consult in the possible application of cognitive-behavioral stress inoculation techniques for a highly distressed population. In July 2002 the Canadian government established a treatment team to address the clinical needs of a native Inuit people in the newest Canadian province of Nunavit. The Inuit people had been dislocated, being forced to shift from a nomadic existence to confined resettlements with accompanying economic deprivations (substandard living conditions, overcrowding, poverty) and disruptions to traditional roles and relationships. On top of having to cope with all of these chronic stressors, a subset of young male Inuit youths experienced a prolonged period of victimization. Over a period of 6 years in the early 1980s, in three native Inuit communities, a self-confessed male pedophile schoolteacher, who was appointed by the government, sexually abused 85 male Inuit youths. The aftermath of this exposure to multiple stressors has been a high rate of depression, substance abuse, and domestic violence. Most telling is the high suicide rate among the Inuit, who are twice as likely to commit suicide as other native populations and four times as likely to engage in self-destructive behaviors. They also have the highest completion rate of suicide attempts (some 38% of attempters; Brody, 2000; Meichenbaum, 2005).

What clinical tools exist to help individuals and communities cope with the diversity of such stressors (acute, sequential, and chronic)? What empirically based stress management procedures exist that can be used in a culturally sensitive fashion to aid individuals in their adaptation processes? How can clinicians help individuals prepare for and prevent maladaptive responses to stressors and help them build on the strengths and resilience that they bring to such challenging situations?

For the past 30 years, I have been involved in the development of stress prevention and reduction procedures to address these challenging questions, under the label of *stress inoculation training* (SIT; Meichenbaum, 1975, 1976, 1977, 1985, 1993, 1996, 2001; Meichenbaum & Deffenbacher, 1988; Meichenbaum & Fitzpatrick, 1993; Meichenbaum & Fong, 1993; Meichenbaum & Jaremko, 1993; Meichenbaum & Novaco, 1978; Meichenbaum & Turk, 1976, 1987; Turk, Meichenbaum & Genest, 1983).

In this chapter, I bring together these clinical experiences and research from this 30-year journey, highlighting the work of other clinical researchers who have adapted SIT or who have developed related cognitive-behavioral stress management interventions. In lieu of the multiple ongoing stressors that society now confronts, including possible terrorist attacks, wars, AIDS, increasing poverty, and urban and family violence, the need for effective empirically based interventions is all the more pressing. This need is more evident to me since I retired from the University of Waterloo in Ontario, Canada, and became the research director of the Melissa Institute for Violence Prevention and Treatment of Victims of Violence in Miami, Florida (see *www.melissainstitute.org*).

The discussion of stress reduction interventions begins with a consideration of the concept of inoculation that gave rise to the SIT treatment approach. I then consider the theoretical underpinnings of SIT and provide a detailed description of the clinical procedural steps involved in conducting SIT. Illustrative applications of how SIT has been applied on both a treatment and a preventative basis are offered. For a detailed summary of the empirical status and meta-analytical review of SIT, the interested reader is directed to reviews by Maag and Kotlash (1994), who examined SIT with children and adolescents; by Saunders, Driskell, Johnston, and Salas (1966), who reviewed patients with anxiety; by Meichenbaum (1993), who provided a 20-year update of some 200 SIT case studies, demonstration projects, and clinical research outcome studies; and by Meichenbaum (1996, 2001), who offered a review of SIT with adults with posttraumatic stress disorder (PTSD) and adults with anger-control problems and aggressive behaviors.

The primary focus of this chapter is on the "clinical wisdom" that has been garnered over 30 years of applying SIT on both a treatment and a preventive basis.

THE CONCEPT OF INOCULATION

A central concept underlying SIT is that of *inoculation*, which has been used both in medicine and in social–psychological research on attitude change. In 1796 Edward Jenner noted that inoculation of humans with cowpox conferred immunity against the more deadly smallpox virus. In medicine, vaccinations often involve exposure to weaker forms of a disease so as to ward off more severe reactions. In such cases, the earlier exposure is generally to a more moderate form of the stress or disease to be guarded against. Such exposure produces antibodies and physically prepares the body for future attacks.

Consistent with the concept of inoculation, Aldwin and Levenson (2004) highlight an area of biology called *hormesis* that studies the *positive* results that derive from exposure to small amounts of toxins that in larger amounts might prove lethal. A series of studies on animals indicated that small and brief exposure to stressors can contribute to the development of repair mechanisms that protect against the impact of subsequent, more intense stressors (Calabrese & Baldwin, 2002). In a comparable fashion SIT, which is designed to intervene with humans at the psychosocial level, provides individuals with experience with minor stressors that fosters psychological preparedness and promotes resilience.

Similarly, in the area of attitude change, McGuire (1964) has observed that prior exposure to attitudinal information can protect or "inoculate" individuals from subsequent, more intense efforts at persuasion. Such prior exposure to persuasive efforts mobilizes counterattitudinal strategies that can be used in subsequent conversion efforts. In both medical and attitudinal inoculations, a person's resistance is enhanced by exposure to a stimulus strong enough to arouse defenses and coping processes without being so powerful that it overwhelms the individual. SIT is based on the notion that exposing clients to milder forms of stress can bolster both coping mechanisms and the individual's (group's, community's) confidence in using his or her coping repertoire. SIT is designed to bolster individual's preparedness and develop a sense of mastery.

THEORETICAL UNDERPINNINGS

SIT adopts a transactional view of stress and coping as espoused by Lazarus and Folkman (1984). Their model proposed that stress occurs whenever the perceived demands of a situation tax or exceed the perceived resources of the system (individual, family, group, or community) to meet those demands, especially when the system's well-being is judged or perceived as being at stake. This relational process-oriented view of stress emphasizes the critical role of cognitive–affective appraisal processes and coping activities. According to the transactional perspective, stress is neither a characteristic of the environment alone nor a characteristic of the person alone. Instead, stress is defined as a particular type of transactional, bidirectional, dynamic relationship between the person and the environment in which the individual or group perceives the adaptive demands as taxing or exceeding their perceived available coping resources to meet those demands. Like beauty, stress is in large part "in the eye of the beholder."

Another related literature that has influenced the development of SIT is that deriving for a *constructive narrative perspective* (CNP). The CNP views individuals, groups, and communities as *storytelling entities* who construct narratives about themselves, others, the world, and the future. The nature and content of the "stories" that individuals tell themselves and others play a critical role in influencing the coping processes. A growing literature on the roles that cognitions and emotions play in the maintenance of stress reactions, especially in the case of persistent PTSD, has highlighted the potential usefulness of a CNP (Brewin & Holmes, 2003; Ehlers & Clark, 2000; Harvey, 2000; Howard, 1991; Janoff-Bulman, 1990; McAdams, Reynolds, Lewis, Patten, & Bowman, 2001; Neimeyer, 2001; Smucker, Grunet, & Weis, 2003). At both the personal and cultural levels, the narratives are organized around identifiable episodes, including intelligible plots and characters, and they convey goals and themes. In the case of traumatic stressful events, the narratives often highlight the perceived "defining moments" of the life stories. Meichenbaum (2005) has summarized the features of clients' narratives and behaviors that contribute to persistent stress reactions. These elements are enumerated in Table 19.1.

How distressed individuals and communities try to make sense of and transform their emotional pain can influence their coping processes. The more individuals and communities engage in the cognitions and behaviors enumerated in Table 19.1, the greater the likelihood that they will have persistent stressful reactions. SIT can be viewed as an engaging way to help clients become aware of the impact of their narratives and maladaptive stress-engendering behaviors (e.g., avoidance, rumination and brooding, catastrophizing, safety-seeking behaviors, absence of self-disclosure, and failure to access and employ social supports). SIT helps distressed individuals become aware of how they can engage in behaviors that maintain and exacerbate their distress. SIT helps clients construct a more adaptive narrative, find "meaning," and engage in more adaptive direct-action problem solving and palliative, emotional-regulation, accepting, and coping skills. SIT trainers are *not only* in the business of teaching coping skills and enhancing the clients' confidence and sense of efficacy in applying these coping skills; the SIT trainer is also in the business of helping clients construct new life stories that move them from perceiving themselves as "victims" to becoming "survivors," if not indeed "thrivers." How does SIT help clients achieve these challenging and laudable goals?

WHAT IS SIT?

SIT is a flexible, individually tailored, multifaceted form of cognitive-behavioral therapy. Given the wide array of stressors that individuals, families, and communities experience, SIT provides a set of general principles and clinical guidelines for treating distressed individuals, rather than a specific treatment formula or a set of "canned" interventions. SIT is *not* a panacea, and it is often used as a supplemental tool to other forms of interventions,

TABLE 19.1. Summary of Behaviors and Cognitions That Lead to Persistent PTSD and Prolonged Stress Responses: A Constructive Narrative Perspective

A. *Self-focused cognitions* that have a "victim" theme
   1. Seeing oneself as being continually *vulnerable*.
   2. Seeing oneself as being *mentally defeated*.
   3. Dwelling on negative *implications*.
   4. Being preoccupied with *others'* views.
   5. Imagining and ruminating about *what might have happened* ("near-miss experience").

B. *Beliefs*
   1. Changes are *permanent*.
   2. The world is *un*safe, *un*predictable, *un*trustworthy.
   3. The *future* will be negative.
   4. Life has *lost its meaning*.

C. *Blame*
   1. Blaming *others*, with accompanying anger.
   2. Blaming *oneself*, with accompanying guilt, shame, and humiliation.

D. *Comparisons*
   1. Oneself with others.
   2. Before with now.
   3. Now with what might have been.

E. *Actions taken*
   1. Being continually *hypervigilant*.
   2. Being *avoidant—cognitive level* (suppressing unwanted thoughts, dissociating, engaging in "undoing" behaviors).
   3. Being *avoidant—behavioral level* (avoiding reminders, using substances, withdrawing, abandoning normal routines, engaging in avoidant safety behaviors).
   4. *Ruminating* and engaging in *contrafactual* thinking ("Only if").
   5. *Delaying* change behaviors.
   6. Failing to *resolve* and *share* trauma story (keeping secrets).
   7. Putting oneself at risk for *revictimization*.

F. Actions *not taken*
   1. *Believing* that anything *positive* could result from trauma experience.
   2. Retrieving and accepting data of *positive self-identity*.
   3. *Seeking social supports*.
   4. Protecting oneself from *negative, unsupportive stress-engendering environments*.
   5. Using *faith* and *religion* as a means of coping.

such as prolonged exposure with traumatized patients or environmental and community supports with individuals confronting chronic stressors, as described later.

SIT consists of three interlocking and overlapping phases:

1. A conceptual educational phase.
2. A skills acquisition and skills consolidation phase.
3. An application and follow-through phase.

The ways that these SIT phases are implemented will vary depending on both (1) the nature of the stressors (e.g., acute time-limited stressors, such as a medical procedure, vs. prolonged ongoing repetitive stressors, such as working in a highly stressed occupation or living in a high-risk violent environment) and (2) the resources and coping abilities of the clients.

The treatment goals of SIT are to bolster the clients' coping repertoire (intra- and interpersonal skills), as well as their confidence in being able to apply their coping skills in a flexible fashion that meets their appraised demands of the stressful situations. Some stressors lend themselves to change and can be altered or avoided, whereas other stressors are *not* changeable (e.g., irreversible loss, incurable illness). Thus some stressful situations do *not* lend themselves to direct-action problem-solving coping efforts, because resolutions are not always attainable. In such instances, an emotionally palliative and accepting set of coping responses are most appropriate (e.g., mindfulness training, reframing, attention diversion, adaptive engaging in spiritual rituals, adaptive affective expression, and humor). SIT demonstrates that there is no one "correct" way to cope with the diversity of stressors. What coping efforts may work in one situation or at one time may not be applicable at other times or in other situations.

In the *initial conceptual education phase of SIT*, a collaborative working relationship and therapeutic alliance are established between the clients and the trainer. This relationship provides the basis, or the "glue," that allows and encourages clients to confront stressors and implement the variety of coping skills, both within the training sessions and *in vivo*, that constitute the needed "inoculation" exposure trials. Norcross (2004) has underscored the critical importance of therapy relationship factors that contribute to the change processes. Besides working on the formulation and maintenance of a therapeutic alliance, the second objective of this initial phase of SIT is to enhance the clients' understanding and awareness of the nature and impact of their stress and coping resources. A variety of clinical techniques are used to nurture this educational process. This informational exchange is *not* a didactic lecture by the trainer/therapist but rather a by-product of a discovery-oriented inductive Socratic exchange (i.e., the SIT trainer uses "curious" questions to promote the clients' processing). Moreover, this educational process is ongoing throughout the course of SIT training. Although at the outset of SIT, the focus may be on possible warning signs or triggers and on the chain analyses of clients' accounts, later on in SIT training the education process may focus on relapse prevention and self-attributional processes (i.e., how to ensure that clients take "personal credit" for changes they have brought about).

A variety of clinical techniques, including Socratic discovery-based interviewing; psychological testing with constructive feedback about deficits, styles of responding, and "strengths" or signs of resilience; self-monitoring activities; bibliotherapy; and exposure to modeling films are used to foster the clients' increased awareness and sense of personal control and mastery. Table 19.2 provides an enumeration of the informational content that is covered over the course of various phases of SIT.

In a collaborative fashion, a more facilitative reconceptualization of the clients' stressful experiences and reactions is formulated. Rather than conceiving their stressors as being overwhelming, uncontrollable, unpredictable, debilitating, and hopeless, the SIT trainer helps clients develop a sense of "learned resourcefulness."

The *second phase* of SIT, which follows naturally from the reconceptualization process, focuses on helping clients *acquire coping skills*, and on *consolidation of those coping skills* that they already possess, and on removing any intra- and interpersonal and systemic barriers that may exist. The intra- and interpersonal coping skills are taught and practiced in the clinical or training setting and then gradually practiced *in vivo*. A major focus of this skills-training phase is the emphasis placed on following guidelines to achieve generalization and maintenance of the treatment effects. Therapists cannot merely "train and hope" for generalization. SIT trainers need to explicitly build the technology of generalization training into the treatment protocol, as is later noted.

TABLE 19.2. Ongoing Educational Components of SIT

SIT helps clients . . .

1. Appreciate that the stress they experience is *not* abnormal and *not* a sign that they are "going crazy" or "losing their minds." Rather, their distressing reactions may be a "normal" reaction to a difficult and challenging stressful situation.

2. Appreciate that many of their reactions may be the "wisdom of the body," or "hature's way" of coping with overwhelming stressors. For example, intrusive ideation may be a way of trying to make sense of what has happened; denial may be a way to "dose oneself" in order to handle so much stress at a given time. (In fact, each of the symptoms of PTSD could be reframed as a coping efforts; see Meichenbaum, 1996).

3. View their current coping efforts as a reflection of being "stuck," namely using (or overusing) a coping pattern such as dissociation that at one time was adaptive (e.g., when being repeatedly raped in an incestuous situation) or being hypervigilant (i.e., continually being on "sentry duty" even when it is no longer required). The problem is that clients are "stuck" (not "crazy," or "inadequate," or "weak") using coping efforts that at one time were adaptive but are now being overemployed.

4. Recognize how they may inadvertently and perhaps even unknowingly employ intrapersonal coping efforts (avoidance, suppression, rumination and brooding, contrafactual thinking, and safety behaviors) that make the stressful situation worse; educate clients about the transactional nature of stress.

5. Appreciate that their stress reactions are made up of different components (biopsychological perspective, physiological arousal, plus cognitive appraisals) and that these reactions go through different phases (namely, the phase of preparing for a stressor, the phase of confronting the stressor, the phase of being truly tested or overwhelmed, and the phase of reflecting on how they handled or did not handle the stressor). In this way, their stress reactions are differentiated into several phases that are made up of different components. Patients are educated about how each phase can trigger appropriate coping efforts.

6. Notice the "cycle" by which internal and external triggering events (12 o'clock on an imaginary clock) elicit primary and secondary emotions (3 o'clock) and accompanying thoughts (automatic thoughts, thinking processes and schemas or beliefs; 6 o'clock), which, in turn, lead to specific behaviors and resultant consequences (9 o'clock). Clients can be asked to self-monitor if, indeed, they engage in such "vicious" (stress-engendering) cycles. Moreover, if they do, clients can be asked, "What is the impact, what is the toll, what is the price of engaging in such a cyclical pattern? Moreover, what can be done to break the cycle?" The various coping efforts follow naturally from such probes.

7. Appreciate the distinction between the changeable and unchangeable aspects of stressful situations and to match either problem-focused or emotion-focused coping efforts to meet the perceived demands of the stress-engendering situation.

8. Break down or disaggregate global stressors into specific short-term, intermediate, and long-term coping goals. Such goal-directed thinking nurtures a sense of hopefulness.

9. Debunk any myths held by the client or significant others concerning their presenting problems (e.g., myths concerning rape, sexual abuse) and challenge so-called stage models of reactions to stress. Also address any myths concerning stress and coping, such as: (1) people need to go through uniform emotional stages of reactions in response to stress; (2) there is a "right" way to cope; (3) distressed people cannot experience positive emotions in the aftermath of traumatic stress; and (4) people should *not* expect to *experience* stressful reactions well after stressful life events occur.

The *final application and follow-through phase* of SIT includes opportunities for clients to *apply the variety of coping skills* on a graduated basis across increasingly demanding levels of stressors (that is, following the "inoculation" concept). Such techniques as imagery and behavioral rehearsal, modeling, role playing, and graded *in vivo* exposure are employed. A central feature of this application phase is the use of relapse prevention procedures (Marlatt & Gordon, 1988; Witkiewitz & Marlatt, 2004). The SIT trainer explores with clients the variety of possible high-risk stressful situations that they may reexperience (e.g., reminders, anniversary effects, dysphoric emotions, interpersonal conflicts and criticisms, and social pressures). Then the clients rehearse and practice in a collaborative fashion with the trainer (and with other clients in a group setting or with significant others) the various intra- and interpersonal coping techniques that might be employed. As part of the relapse prevention intervention, clients are taught how to view any lapses, should they occur, as "learning opportunities" rather than as occasions to "catastrophize" and relapse. The follow-through features of SIT are designed to extend training into the future by including booster training sessions, active case management, engagement of significant others, and environmental manipulations.

Consistent with a transactional model of stress that SIT embraces, and consistent with the recognition that the stress clients experience may be endemic, societal, institutional and unavoidable, *SIT often goes beyond the clients* to involve significant others. For example, in preparing patients for stressful medical examinations, the SIT trainer can focus on teaching coping skills to distressed medical patients but can also attempt to work with hospital staff in order to reduce the nature and level of hospital and medical stress (see Kendall, 1983, for a description of work with catheterized patients and Wernick, Jaremko, & Taylor, 1981, and Wernick, 1983, for work with burn patients.) In competitive sports, an SIT trainer can help athletes develop their coping skills in order to handle the stress of competition (Long, 1980; Mace & Carroll, 1986; Mace, Eastman, & Carroll, 1986, 1987), but as Smith (1980) observes, a trainer can also attempt to influence the behaviors of the athlete's coaches and parents, thus reducing a major source of competitive stress. Similarly, in work with victims of rape or terrorist attacks, the unfortunate "secondary victimization" of the distressed individuals from community agents (doctors, police, judges, teachers, administrators, health care providers, parents, and peers) can exacerbate the stress responses (see Ayalon, 1983; Veronen & Kilpatrick, 1983). It would be short-sighted to delimit SIT interventions to just the targeted victims or distressed clients and not to attempt to influence the stress-engendering behaviors and attitudes of significant others and community members. SIT has adopted the dual-track strategy of working directly with stressed clients, as well as with significant others and community agents who may inadvertently, and perhaps even unknowingly, exacerbate stress. SIT trainers search for and enlist "allies" to support the ongoing coping efforts of clients.

HOW IS SIT CONDUCTED?

One of the strengths of SIT is its flexibility. SIT has been carried out with individuals, couples, families, and small and large groups. The length of the SIT intervention has varied, from as short as 20 minutes in preparing patients for surgery (Langer, Janis, & Wolfer, 1975) to 40 one-hour weekly and biweekly sessions administered to psychiatric patients with recurrent mental disorders and to individuals with chronic medical problems (Turk et al., 1983). In most instances in the clinical domain, SIT consists of some 8–15 sessions, plus booster and follow-up sessions conducted over a 3- to 12-month period.

Obviously, the manners in which the three phases of SIT (conceptualization, skills acquisition and consolidation, application and follow-through) are conducted will vary, depending on the nature of the clients and the length of SIT training. The content of the conceptualization phase, the specific skills that will be emphasized and trained, and the nature of the application phase (inoculation trials) will each be specifically geared to the targeted population. There is, however, sufficient congruence across SIT application that a procedural flowchart of the SIT treatment procedure can be outlined, as shown in Table 19.3. More detailed clinical presentations of SIT are offered by Meichenbaum (1996, 2001).

ILLUSTRATIVE APPLICATIONS OF SIT

SIT has been employed in both a treatment and a preventative manner with a wide variety of medical and psychiatric populations and with a variety of diverse professional groups who experience high rates of job-related stress. Elsewhere (Meichenbaum, 1993; Wertkin, 1985), these diverse applications have been reviewed, and more recent reviews are also available (Maag & Kotlash, 1994; Saunders et al., 1996). On a treatment basis, SIT and closely aligned cognitive-behavioral stress management procedures (Antoni et al., 2001; Antoni, 2003; Cruess et al., 2000), anxiety management approaches (Suinn, 1999), coping skills training (Folkman et al., 1991), and cognitive–affective stress management training (Smith & Rohsenow, 1987) have been employed with a wide variety of clients. These clinical applications have been used with:

1. *Medical patients* who have various acute and chronic pain disorders, patients with breast cancer and those with essential hypertension, burn patients, ulcer patients, and patients with rheumatoid arthritis; on a *preventive basis*, SIT has been employed with medical and dental patients who are preparing for surgery or invasive medical examinations, with type A individuals, and with the caretakers of both child and adult patients who are medically ill.
2. *Psychiatric patients* with PTSD as a result of sexual assault; adults and adolescent patients with severe problems of anxiety (e.g., panic attacks) and those with anger-control problems and aggressive behaviors, such as in the case of abusive parents; aggressive individuals who are developmentally delayed, and chronically distressed outpatients with mental illnesses.
3. Individuals with *performance anxiety*, such as public-speaking and dating anxiety or debilitating anxiety in athletic competitions; and with individuals with *circumscribed fears* (animal phobias, fear of flying).
4. *Professional groups*, such as probation officers, nurses, teachers, military personnel, psychiatric staff members, and disaster and safety workers.
5. *Individuals* who have to deal with *stress of life transitions*, including coping with unemployment, or who are transitioning into new settings, such as high school or reentering college, overseas placement, and joining the military.

In short, since its origin in 1976, SIT has been employed on both a treatment and a preventative basis with a wide variety of diverse clinical populations and with highly

TABLE 19.3. A Flowchart of SIT

Phase 1: Conceptualization

- In a collaborative fashion, identify the determinants of the presenting problem or the individual's stress concerns by means of (1) interviews with the client and significant others; (2) the client's use of an imagery-based reconstruction and assessment of a prototypical stressful incident; (3) psychological and environmental assessments; and (4) behavioral observations. (As Folkman et al., 1991, suggest, have the client address "who, what, where," and "when" questions: "Who is involved?" "What kind of situations cause stress?" "When is this kind of situation likely to occur?" "When did it occur last?" Also see interviews in Meichenbaum, 1996, 2001)
- Permit the client to tell his or her "story" (solicit narrative accounts of stress and coping and collaboratively identify the client's coping strengths and resources). Help the client to transform his or her description from global terms into behaviorally specific terms.
- Have the client disaggregate global stressors into specific stressful situations. Then help him or her break stressful situations and reactions into specific behaviorally prescriptive problems. Have the client consider his or her present coping efforts and evaluate which are maladaptive and which are adaptive.
- Have the client appreciate the differences between changeable and unchangeable aspects of stress situations.
- Have the client establish short-term, intermediate, and long-term behaviorally specifiable goals.
- Have the client engage in self-monitoring of the commonalities of stressful situations and the role of stress-engendering appraisals, internal dialogue, feelings, and behaviors. Help the client appreciate the transactional nature of his or her stress. (Use the clock metaphor of a "vicious cycle" in Table 19.2). Train the client to analyze problems (e.g., to conduct both situational and developmental analyses and to seek disconfirmatory data—"check things out").
- Ascertain the degree to which coping difficulties arise from coping-skills deficits or are the result of "performance failures" (namely, maladaptive beliefs, feelings of low self-efficacy, negative ideation, secondary gains).
- Collaboratively formulate with the client and significant others a reconceptualization of the client's distress. Socratically educate the client and significant others about the nature and impact of stress and the resilience and courage individuals manifest in the face of stressful life events. Using the client's own "data," offer a reconceptualization that stress consists of different components (physiological, cognitive, affective, and behavioral) and that stress reactions go through different "phases," as described in Table 19.2. The specific reconceptualization offered will vary with the target population; the plausibility of the reconceptualization is more important than its scientific validity. In the course of this process, facilitate the discovery of a sense of meaning, nurture the client's hope, and highlight the client's strengths and feelings of resourcefulness.
- Debunk any client myths, as noted in Table 19.2.

Phase 2: Skills acquisition and consolidation

A. *Skills training* (tailor to the needs of the specific population and to the length of training)
- Ascertain the client's preferred mode of coping. Explore with the client how these coping efforts can be employed in the present situation. Examine what intrapersonal or interpersonal factors are blocking such coping efforts.
- Train problem-focused instrumental coping skills that are directed at the modification, avoidance, and minimization of the impact of stressors (e.g., anxiety management, cognitive restructuring, self-instructional training, communication, assertion, problem solving, anger control, applied cue-controlled relaxation training, parenting, study skills, using social supports). Select each skill package according to the needs of the specific client or group of clients. Help the client to break complex, stressful problems into more manageable subproblems that can be solved one at a time.
- Help the client engage in problem solving by identifying possibilities for change, considering and ranking alternative solutions and practicing coping behavioral activities in the clinic and *in vivo*.
- Train emotionally focused palliative coping skills, especially when the client has to deal with unchangeable and uncontrollable stressors (e.g., perspective taking; selective attention-diversion procedures, as in the case of chronic pain patients; adaptive modes of affective expression such as humor, relaxation, reframing the situation, acceptance skills, and spiritual rituals).

(continued)

TABLE 19.3. *(continued)*

- Train clients how to use social supports effectively (i.e., how to choose, obtain, and maintain support). As Folkman et al. (1991) observe, help clients identify what kind of support is needed (informational, emotional, tangible), from whom to seek such support, and how to maintain support resources.
- Aim to help the client develop an extensive repertoire of coping responses in order to facilitate flexible responding. Nurture gradual mastery.

B. Skills rehearsal and consolidation
  - Promote the smooth integration and execution of coping responses by means of behavioral and imagery rehearsal.
  - Use coping modeling (either live or videotape models). Engage in collaborative discussion, rehearsal, and feedback of coping skills.
  - Use self-instructional training to help the client develop internal mediators to self-regulate coping responses.
  - Solicit the client's verbal commitment to employ specific efforts.
  - Discuss possible barriers and obstacles to using coping behaviors and ways to anticipate and address such barriers.
  - Follow treatment guidelines to enhance the likelihood transfer or generalization of coping skills (see Meichenbaum, 1996, 2001).

Phase 3: Application and follow-through

A. *Encouraging application of coping skills in the form of stress inoculation trials*
  - Prepare the client for application by using coping imagery, together with techniques in which early stress cues act as signals for coping.
  - Expose the client in the session to graded stressors via imagery and behavioral exposure to stressful and arousing scenes.
  - Use graded exposure and other response induction aids to foster *in vivo* responding.
  - Employ relapse prevention procedures: Identify high-risk situations, anticipate possible stressful reactions, and rehearse coping responses.
  - Use counterattitudinal procedures to increase the likelihood of treatment adherence (i.e., ask and challenge the client to indicate where, how, and why he or she will use coping efforts).
  - Bolster self-efficacy by reviewing both the client's successful and unsuccessful coping efforts. Ensure that the client makes self-attributions ("takes credit") for success or mastery experiences (provide attribution retraining).

B. *Maintenance and generalization*
  - Gradually phase out treatment and include booster and follow-up sessions.
  - Involve significant others in training (e.g., parents, spouse, coaches, hospital staff, police, administrators), as well as peer and self-help groups.
  - Have the client coach someone with a similar problem (i.e., put client in a "helper" or consultative role).
  - Help the client to restructure environmental stressors and develop appropriate escape routes. Ensure that the client does not view the desire for escape or avoidance as a sign of failure but rather as a sign of taking personal control.
  - Help the client to develop coping strategies for recovering from failure and setbacks, so that lapses do not become relapses.
  - Work with clients to avoid revictimization.

stressed occupational groups. The following description provides examples of some of these diverse applications.

Patients with Medical Problems

The SIT interventions with medical patients have a heavy educational component in which patients and often their caretakers receive procedural and sensory information and are then afforded opportunities to practice coping skills. SIT highlights ways in which patients can use their own preferred idiosyncratic coping strategies. The coping training may include the use of coping-modeling films, both imaginal and behavioral rehearsal, and *in vivo* graded exposure. Such behavioral practice is accompanied by corrective feedback; personal attribution training, in which patients "take credit" for the changes they have been able to bring about; and relapse prevention strategies should lapses occur. The manner in which SIT is conducted needs to be individually tailored to the age of the patient and to the patient's preferred mode of coping. Finally, the research on the application of SIT to medical patients has underscored the need to ensure that the length of SIT treatment should be performance-based rather than time-based (an arbitrarily set number of sessions). Instead of all medical patients receiving treatment of a prescribed length, the length of treatment or the number of multiple practice and "inoculation" trials should be tailored to some behavioral criteria of mastery and accompanying expressed self-efficacy, especially for patients with intense and chronic medical problems. The following three examples illustrate the varied applications of SIT to medical problems.

1. Langer et al. (1975) provided 20 minutes' worth of coping skills training to medical patients prior to their surgeries. The conceptualization phase of SIT highlighted the manner in which stress can be affected by selective attentional and cognitive processes, how to focus on the benefits that can accrue from the surgery, and immediate coping efforts (relaxation, self-guided rethinking efforts, imaginal rehearsal). The SIT group, relative to both the informational and assessment control groups, evidenced significantly less preoperative anxiety and fewer postoperative requests for pain relievers and sedatives. The SIT-treated patients also stayed in the hospital for a shorter period of time. Siegal and Peterson (1980) have used a similar multifaceted coping skills package of relaxation training, calming self-talk, and guided imagery to help young dental patients reduce stress.

2. Jay and Elliott (1990) developed an SIT videotape film for parents of 3- to 12-year-old children with pediatric leukemia who have to undergo bone marrow aspirations and lumbar punctures. One hour prior to each child's medical procedure, the parents were shown a brief film of a model parent who employed coping self-statements, relaxation efforts, and coping imagery rehearsal. The parents were then given an opportunity to practice these coping skills. Relative to parents who received a child-focused intervention, the SIT-treated parents evidenced significantly less anxiety and enhanced coping skills. Videotaped SIT-modeling films have been used in a variety of clinical settings, including anger control, with rape victims preparing for forensic examination, and parenting (see Meichenbaum, 1996, 2001).

3. Finally, cognitive-behavioral stress management (CBSM), which overlaps with many of the features of SIT, has been used most impressively with female early-stage breast cancer patients. Like SIT, this 10-week group CBSM comprises (1) an educational component that debunks myths about breast cancer, enhances patients' awareness of stress and of ways to reduce it, and nurtures hope; (2) a skills acquisition and practice

phase in which patients learn ways to use intra- and interpersonal coping skills that range from emotional expression of concerns and feelings and acceptance skills to relaxation, problem-solving benefit finding, and ways to preserve and augment the patients' social support networks; and (3) an application phase in which patients are given opportunities and encouraged to practice the learned coping skills. Moreover, the patients are encouraged to take credit for the changes they are able to bring about in order to further promote a positive self-image. The CBSM not only resulted in improved behavioral adjustment and posttraumatic growth, but CBSM also continued to improve immune functioning (i.e., greater lymphocyte proliferative responses at a 3-month follow-up) relative to a control group (Cruess et al., 2000).

Psychiatric Patients

SIT has been employed with a variety of psychiatric groups on both an inpatient and an outpatient basis. In most studies, SIT has been compared or combined with other multifaceted psychoeducational and pharmacological interventions; for example, Holcomb (1986) has examined the relative efficacy of eight 1-hour SIT sessions with and without psychotropic medications in the treatment of psychiatric inpatients. In terms of anxiety, depression, and overall subjective distress, Holcomb reported that SIT with and without medication was superior to pharmacological interventions alone; impressively, this relative improvement was evident at a 3-year follow-up, as indicated by fewer patient readmissions for psychiatric problems.

SIT and related cognitive-behavioral interventions have been applied to psychiatric patients who have specific disorders such as panic attacks, PTSD, and anger-control problems and aggression. In many instances, these patients have overlapping comorbid disorders.

In the anxiety domain, the panic-control treatment procedures of Barlow (1988), Clark and Salkovskis (1989), and Rapee (1987) have extended the SIT treatment model to patients with anxiety disorders. During the initial conceptualization phase, the patients are offered an explanatory and conceptual model, based on their symptoms, that highlights the interactive role that hypervigilance about bodily cues, their "catastrophic" misinterpretations of their physiological arousal, and their hyperventilation play in eliciting and exacerbating their anxiety reactions. Such a reconceptualization of panic attacks readily leads to the second phase of treatment, which is the acquisition and practice of a variety of coping responses that include (1) relaxation skills in order to control physical tenseness and hyperventilation, (2) cognitive coping skills in order to control "catastrophic" misrepresentation, and (3) cognitive restructuring procedures in order to alter the patients' appraisal attributions, expectations, and avoidance behaviors.

Following the SIT model, the final application and follow-through phase provides the patients with "inoculation" trials by means of imaginal and behavioral rehearsal, both in the clinic and *in vivo*. The behavioral coping trials include opportunities to cope with self-induced hyperventilation and the symptoms of panic attacks, coping imagery to anxiety-producing scenes, and, finally, graduated exposure to panic-inducing situations. Relapse prevention and self-attribution treatment components are included in this last phase of treatment. Michelson and Marchione (1991) have documented the relative efficacy of this three-phase cognitive-behavioral intervention.

Another anxiety disorder that has been treated by means of SIT is PTSD. For instance, Veronen and Kilpatrick (1982) used SIT to successfully treat rape victims. The SIT intervention consisted of a psychoeducational component concerning the nature and impact of rape and the acquisition and practice of coping skills aimed at management of assault-related anxiety and postassault problems. The coping skills that were taught included cue-controlled relaxation, thought stopping, cognitive restructuring, guided self-dialogue, covert modeling, and role playing. Homework assignments consisted of patients practicing the various coping skills *in vivo*. Foa and her colleagues have also found that SIT can reduce PTSD symptoms that result from sexual assaults. These reductions were maintained at follow-up assessments conducted up to 1 year posttreatment (Foa, Rothbaum, Riggs, & Murdock, 1991; Foa et al., 1999). In two well-controlled studies, SIT demonstrated more improvement in PTSD symptoms than supportive counseling and wait-list conditions (Foa et al., 1991; Foa et al., 1999). In a study comparing SIT, prolonged exposure (PE), and PE/SIT, SIT demonstrated significant reduction in PTSD and related symptoms. There was a trend, however, for clients who received PE to obtain higher levels of overall functioning, as evident in a composite reduction of PTSD, anxiety, and depressive symptoms (Foa et al., 1999).

In evaluating the relative efficacy of PE and SIT in these studies, it is important to keep in mind that, in the original SIT treatment protocol, clients were confronted with anxiety-engendering situations, either imaginally or by means of role playing and graded *in vivo* exposure. In the Foa et al. comparative studies, this exposure–rehearsal component that fosters inoculation was eliminated because of the possible overlap with the exposure comparison condition. Thus the SIT was delimited to only the initial two phases of psychoeducational and coping skills training. The critical exposure and accompanying self-attribution and relapse prevention components that constitute the final phase were omitted from the SIT comparison group.

The results of these studies (Foa et al., 1991; Foa et al., 1999) underscore the additional therapeutic benefits that accrue from including the third, experiential practice, component of SIT. Educating clients and teaching coping skills are necessary but insufficient components to lead to sustained improvement. Similar conclusions have been drawn by other clinical researchers who have used variations of cognitive therapy to treat clients with PTSD (Marks, Lovell, Noshirvani, Livanou, & Thrasher, 1998; Resick & Schnicke, 1992; Tarrier et al., 1999). The results of these studies have also highlighted the fact that various forms of cognitive-behavioral therapies, such as SIT, prolonged exposure, and cognitive restructuring, have broad effects in reducing associated negative emotional states such as anger, depression, and anxiety, as well as PTSD symptomatology. For example, Cahill, Rauch, Hembree, and Foa (2003) report that SIT, but not PE, produced a greater decrease in anger in female assault victims than did the combination treatment of PE/SIT. Thus those interventions that included SIT seem particularly well suited for treating clients with issues of anger control.

Cahill et al. (2003) caution that several clinical studies, both theirs and others', have also demonstrated that combining treatments (e.g., SIT with PE and cognitive restructuring) did *not* result in better outcomes and sometimes resulted in slightly worse outcomes than those obtained by individual treatments (Foa et al. 1999; Marks et al., 1998; Paunovic & Ost, 2001). Such attempts to combine various interventions within a time-limited treatment protocol may dilute the effectiveness of the respective interventions.

Anger is an often overlooked emotional disorder in the psychiatric community, although it overlaps with some 19 different psychiatric conditions. Anger is often experienced among various survivors of sexual assault, motor vehicle accidents, torture, and combat and among refugees. A number of clinical researchers, including Jerry Deffenbacher, Eva Feindler, Arthur Hains, and Ray Novaco and their colleagues, have applied SIT with adolescents and adults who have problems with anger control and aggressive behaviors (see Deffenbacher & McKay, 2000; Feindler & Ecton, 1986; Hains, 1992; Novaco, 1975). Novaco has also applied SIT to several occupational groups for whom anger control is an important part of their job (namely, law enforcement officers, probation officers, and Marine drill instructors; Novaco, 1977a, 1977b, 1980; Novaco, Cook, & Sarason, 1983).

The potential usefulness of SIT and related cognitive-behavioral interventions with adolescents and adults who have anger-control problems and who manifest aggressive behaviors was highlighted by DiGuiseppe and Tafrate (2001). They conducted a meta-analytic review and concluded that the cognitive-behavioral treatments "seem to work equally well for all age groups and all types of populations and are equally effective for men and women. The average effect sizes across all outcome measures ranged from .67 to .99 with a mean of .70" (p. 263).

The results of this meta-analysis revealed that the cognitive-behavioral SIT was "moderately successful" (p. 263). Patients in the SIT group were better off than 76% of the control group of untreated patients and that 83% of the treated patients improved in comparison to their pretest scores. This level of improvement was maintained at a follow-up period that ranged from 2 to 64 weeks. These findings are similar to conclusions drawn by Beck and Fernandez (1998), who conducted a similar meta-analysis of 50 SIT and cognitive-behavioral interventions that involved 1,640 participants across the full age range. In both meta-analytic reviews, they found that those treatment programs that used standardized manuals and treatment fidelity checks were found to be most effective.

An example of SIT with individuals with anger-control problems was offered by Chemtob, Novaco, Hamada, and Gross (1997), who targeted the treatment of anger among a group of veterans who experienced both PTSD and elevated levels of anger. They added SIT to routine Veterans Administration clinical care and found that, relative to a control group that continued to receive only routine care, adding SIT was effective in significantly reducing state anger, increasing anger control and coping skills, decreasing general anxiety, and decreasing PTSD symptoms of reexperiencing. The SIT treatment of anger not only decreased the targeted level of anger but also decreased PTSD symptoms, highlighting the robustness of SIT. See Meichenbaum (2001) for a detailed description of how to apply SIT on both a treatment and preventative basis with individuals who have problems controlling their anger and their accompanying aggressive behaviors.

Individuals with Evaluative Anxiety and Those Requiring Transitional Adjustment

From its origin, SIT has been employed with individuals who experience debilitating anxiety in evaluative situations. This may take the form of treating individuals with anxiety in such areas as testing, speech, math, computer use, dating, writing, and performance in an athletic competition (see Hembree, 1988, and Meichenbaum, 1993, for reviews of these studies). In most of these treatment studies, SIT was combined with population-specific skills training, such as public-speaking training, writing, and study skills. In each domain, SIT has been adapted to and "packaged" in ways that would make SIT most appealing. For instance, Smith (1980) has characterized the stress management features of SIT as a form of "mental toughness training" for athletes and their coaches. SIT was designed to help athletes "control their emotional responses that might interfere with performance and is also designed to help athletes focus their attention on the task at hand" (Smith, 1980, p. 157). The rationale of "mental toughness training" is more likely to be acceptable than the rationale of "reducing stress," as if stress is something to be avoided.

Many athletes and coaches believe that athletes need to experience stress in order to achieve peak performance. Under the aegis of "mental toughness training," Smith (1980) has developed a cognitive-behavioral group-training program that is offered in six twice-weekly, 1-hour sessions. The initial educational/conceptualization phase orients the participants to the nature of stress and emotions, the role mental processes play, and various ways to develop an "integrated coping response." The skills-acquisition phase focuses on cue-controlled relaxation, imagining stressful situations, and cognitive rehearsing of "antistress" coping self-statements. The goal of training is *not* to eliminate emotional arousal but rather to give athletes greater control over their emotional responses. The athletes are given an opportunity to rehearse their coping skills under conditions of trainer-induced high arousal and strong affect, which are stimulated by the trainer's offering of highly charged imagery scenes. In this inoculation fashion, the athletes are taught to focus their attention on intense feelings and then to practice reframing, accepting, and/or turning them off again in order to reduce and prevent high arousal levels from getting out of hand. The trainer also attends to the excessively high performance standards and distorted fear of the consequences of possible failure that distressed athletes, their coaches, and their parents may hold. In addition, the trainer, in collaboration with a coach and an athlete, can set up *in vivo* practice trials and can implement a training program to improve relevant sports skills. In short, SIT with athletes is packaged as an educational program in self-control, not as a form of psychotherapy.

Another anxiety-producing situation in which SIT has been employed successfully is that accompanying the transitional adjustment to unemployment. A randomized field experiment conducted by Caplan, Vinokur, Price, and van Ryan (1989) provides encouraging data. As part of a comprehensive intensive intervention, eight 3-hour sessions were conducted with the unemployed over a 2-week period. Following the educational phase on the impact of the stress of being laid off and the acquisition and practice of job-seeking and problem-solving skills, the participants were given inoculation trials concerning how to cope with possible rejection and setbacks. This comprehensive cognitive-behavioral intervention contributed to higher rates of reemployment, higher motivation, and greater job satisfaction in the SIT treatment group relative to a matched attention-control group.

Meichenbaum (1993) reviewed the literature on the potential usefulness of SIT in helping individuals adjust to entry into the military, senior students reentering a university, and individuals taking up overseas assignments.

CONCLUSIONS

The past 30 years have witnessed a broad application of SIT to a variety of stressed populations, in both a treatment and a preventative manner. In each instance, the clinical application of SIT has been individually tailored to the specific target population and circumstances. It is the flexibility of the SIT format that has contributed to its robust effectiveness. It should also be apparent that SIT is a complex, multifaceted cognitive-behavioral intervention that comprises key elements of nurturing a therapeutic working alliance with clients; psychoeducational features that include inductive Socratic discovery-oriented inquiry, collaborative goal setting that nurtures hope, and direct-action problem-solving and acceptance-based-coping skills training that incorporates training generalization guidelines; relapse prevention; and self-attributional training procedures. In those instances in which clients have been victimized, SIT can be readily supplemented with symptom-specific interventions (e.g., cognitive-behavioral coping techniques to address physiological arousal, dissociation, emotional dysregulation, and physical pain) and "memory work" such as imaginal and *in vivo* exposure-based techniques. From an SIT perspective, the treatment goal is *not* merely to have clients relive and retell their abuse histories but rather to have them consider the nature of the "stories" they tell both themselves and others as a result of such trauma exposure. SIT is designed to help clients consider the conclusions that they draw about themselves, the world, and the future as a result of such trauma experiences. SIT is designed to help clients construct a more adaptive narrative and to change their views of themselves from "victims" to "survivors" to "thrivers." The SIT concludes with a consideration of how to help clients find meaning or to transform their emotional pain into healing processes and activities and to learn how to reclaim their lives. Finally, SIT focuses on ways to ensure that such victimized individuals are *not* revictimized.

In short, SIT is more than a mere collection and application of a variety of coping techniques. The coping-skills features of SIT are critical, but without the other contextual features of SIT, especially the "inoculation" trials and application opportunities, the skills-training components are unlikely to prove effective or sufficient. SIT is not a chapter heading for a collection of cognitive-behavioral coping techniques but rather a client-sensitive, highly collaborative intervention that is as much concerned about working with clients as it is about working with significant others and agencies who may inadvertently and unknowingly engender and help maintain even more stress. As noted, the SIT model embraces both the transactional model of stress and coping and the mandate for clinicians and trainers to be involved in assessing both the clients and their environments. Such an SIT treatment plan will go a long way toward helping individuals and communities cope more effectively in the stressful post–September 11 environment in which we live.

REFERENCES

Aldwin, C. M., & Levenson, M. R. (2004). Posttraumatic growth: A developmental perspective. *Psychological Inquiry, 15*, 19–22.

Antoni, M. H. (2003). *Stress management intervention for women with breast cancer.* Washington, DC: American Psychological Association.

Antoni, M. H., Lehman, J. M., Kilburn, K. M., Boyers, A. E., Yont, S. E., & Culver, J. L. (2001). Cognitive-behavioral stress management intervention decreases the prevalence of depression and enhances the sense of benefit among women under treatment for early-stage breast cancer. *Health Psychology, 20*, 20–32.

Ayalon, O. (1983). Coping with terrorism: The Israeli case. In D. Meichenbaum & M. Jaremko (Eds.), *Stress prevention and management: A cognitive behavioral approach.* New York: Plenum Press.

Barlow, D. (1988). *Anxiety and its disorders: The nature and treatment of anxiety and panic.* New York: Guilford Press.

Beck, R., & Fernandez, E. (1998). Cognitive-behavioral self-regulation of the frequency, duration and intensity of anger. *Journal of Psychopathology and Behavioral Assessment, 20*, 217–229.

Brewin, C. R., & Holmes, E. A. (2003). Psychological theories of posttraumatic stress disorder. *Clinical Psychological Review, 23*, 339–376.

Brody, H. (2000). *The other side of Eden.* New York: North Point Press.

Cahill, S. P., Rauch, S. A., Hembree, E. A., & Foa, E. B. (2003). Effect of cognitive-behavioral treatment for PTSD on anger. *Journal of Cognitive Psychotherapy, 17*, 113–131.

Calabrese, E. J., & Baldwin, L. A. (2002). Hormesis: A dose–response revolution. *Annual Review of Pharmacology and Toxicology, 43*, 175–197.

Caplan, R. D., Vinokur, A. D., Price, R. H., & van Ryan, M. (1989). Job seeking, reemployment, and mental health: A randomized field trial in coping with job loss. *Journal of Applied Psychology, 74,* 10–20.

Chemtob, C. M., Novaco, R. W., Hamada, R. S., & Gross, D. M. (1997). Cognitive-behavioral treatment for severe anger in posttraumatic disorder. *Journal of Consulting and Clinical Psychology, 65,* 184–189.

Clark, D. M., & Salkovskis, P. M. (1989). *Panic disorder treatment manual.* Oxford, UK: Pergamon Press.

Cruess, D. G., Antoni, M. H., McGregor, B. A. S., Kilbourn, K. M., Boyers, A. E., et al. (2000). Cognitive behavioral stress management reduces serum cortisol by enhancing benefit finding among women being treated for early-stage breast cancer. *Psychosomatic Medicine, 62,* 304–308.

Deffenbacher, J. L., & McKay, M. (2000). *Overcoming situations and general anger.* Oakland, CA: New Harbinger.

DiGuiseppe, R., & Tafrate, R. C. (2001). *Anger treatment for adults: A meta-analytic review.* Unpublished manuscript, St. John's University, Jamaica, New York.

Ehlers, A., & Clark, D. M. (2000). A cognitive model of posttraumatic stress disorder. *Behaviour Research and Therapy, 38,* 319–345.

Elliott, G. R., & Eisdorfer, C. (1982). *Stress and human health.* New York: Springer.

Feindler, E. L., & Ecton, R. B. (1986). *Adolescent anger control: Cognitive-behavioral techniques.* Elmsford, NY: Pergamon Press.

Foa, E. B., Dancu, C., Hembree, E. A., Jaycox, L. H., Meadows, E. A., & Street, G. D. (1999). A comparison of exposure therapy, stress inoculation training and their combination for reducing posttraumatic stress disorder in female assault victims. *Journal of Consulting and Clinical Psychology, 67,* 194–200.

Foa, E. B., Rothbaum, B. O., Riggs, D. S., & Murdock, T. B. (1991). Treatment of posttraumatic stress disorder in rape victims: A comparison between cognitive-behavioral procedures and counseling. *Journal of Consulting and Clinical Psychology, 59,* 715–723.

Folkman, S., Chesney, M., McKusik, L., Ironson, G., Johnson, D. G., & Coates, T. J. (1991). Translating coping theory into an intervention. In J. Eckenrode (Ed.), *The social context of coping.* New York: Plenum Press.

Hains, A. A. (1992). A stress inoculation training program for adolescents in a high school setting: A multiple baseline approach. *Journal of Adolescence, 15,* 163–175.

Harvey, J. H. (2000). *Embracing the memory.* Needham Heights, MA: Allyn & Bacon.

Hembree, R. (1988). Correlates, causes, effects of test anxiety. *Review of Educational Research, 58,* 47–77.

Holcomb, W. R. (1986). Stress inoculation therapy with anxiety and stress disorders of acute psychiatric patients. *Journal of Clinical Psychology, 42,* 864–872.

Howard, G. S. (1991). Cultural tales: A narrative approach to thinking, cross-cultural psychology and psychotherapy. *American Psychologist, 46,* 187–197.

Janoff-Bulman, R. (1990). Understanding people in terms of their assumptive worlds. In D. J. Ozer, J. M. Healy, & A. J. Stewart (Eds.), *Perspectives in personality: Self and emotion.* Greenwich, CT: JAI Press

Jay, S. M., & Elliott, C. H. (1990). A stress inoculation program for parents whose children are undergoing painful medical procedures. *Journal of Consulting and Clinical Psychology, 58,* 799–804.

Kendall, P. C. (1983). Stressful medical procedures: Cognitive-behavioral strategies for stress management and prevention. In D. Meichenbaum & M. Jaremko (Eds.), *Stress prevention and management: A cognitive behavioral approach.* New York: Plenum Press.

Langer, T., Janis, I., & Wolfer, J. (1975). Reduction of psychological stress in surgical patients. *Journal of Experimental Social Psychology, 11,* 155–165.

Lazarus, R. S., & Folkman, S. (1984). *Stress, appraisal, and coping.* New York: Springer-Verlag.

Long, B. C. (1980). Stress management for the athlete: A cognitive-behavioral model. In C. H. Nadeau, W. R. Halliwell, K. M. Newell, & G. C. Roberts (Eds.), *Psychology of motor behavior and sport.* Champaign, IL: Human Kinetics.

Maag, J., & Kotlash, J. (1994). Review of stress inoculation training with children and adolescents: Issues and recommendations. *Behavior Modification, 18,* 443–469.

Mace, R. D., & Carroll, D. (1986). Stress inoculation training to control anxiety in sports: Three case studies in squash. *British Journal of Sports Medicine, 20,* 115–117.

Mace, R. D., Eastman, C., & Carroll, D. (1986). Stress inoculation training: A case study in gymnastics. *British Journal of Sports Medicine, 20,* 139–141.

Mace, R. D., Eastman, C., & Carroll, D. (1987). The effects of stress inoculation training in gymnastics on the pommeled horse: A case study. *Behavioral Psychotherapy, 15,* 272–229.

Marks, I., Lovell, K., Noshirvani, H., Livanou, M., & Thrasher, S. (1998). Treatment of post-traumatic stress disorder by exposure and/or cognitive restructuring: A controlled study. *Archives of General Psychiatry, 55,* 317–325.

Marlatt, G. A., & Gordon, J. R. (Eds.). (1988). *Relapse prevention: Maintenance strategies in the treatment of addictive behaviors.* New York: Guilford Press.

McAdams, D. P., Reynolds, J., Lewis, M., Patten, A. V., & Bowman, P. J. (2001). When bad things turn good and good things turn bad: Sequences of redemption and contamination in life narratives and their relation to psychological adaptation in midlife adults and in students. *Personality and Social Psychology Bulletin, 27,* 474–485.

McGuire, W. (1964). Inducing resistance to persuasion: Some contemporary approaches. In L. Berkowitz (Ed.), *Advances in social psychology* (Vol. 1). New York: Academic Press.

Meichenbaum, D. (1975). Self-instructional methods. In F. H. Kanfer & A. P. Goldstein (Eds.), *Helping people change* (pp. 357–391). New York: Pergamon Press.

Meichenbaum, D. (1976). A self-instructional approach to stress management: A proposal for stress inoculation training. In C. Spielberger & I. Sarason (Eds.), *Stress and anxiety in modern life.* New York: Winston.

Meichenbaum, D. (1977). *Cognitive behavior modification: An integrative approach.* New York: Plenum Press.

Meichenbaum, D. (1985). *Stress inoculation training.* Elmsford, NY: Pergamon Press.

Meichenbaum, D. (1993). Stress inoculation training: A 20-year update. In P. M. Lehrer & R. L. Woolfolk (Eds.), *Principles and practice of stress management* (pp. 373–406). New York: Guilford Press.

Meichenbaum, D. (1996). *Treating adults with post-traumatic stress disorder.* Waterloo, Ontario, Canada: Institute Press.

Meichenbaum, D. (2001). *Treating individuals with anger-control problems and aggressive behaviors.* Waterloo, Ontario, Canada: Institute Press.

Meichenbaum, D. (2005). Trauma and suicide: A constructive narrative perspective. In T. E. Ellis (Ed.), *Cognition and suicide: Theory, research and practice.* Washington, DC: American Psychological Association.

Meichenbaum, D., & Deffenbacher, J. L. (1988). Stress inoculation training. *Counseling Psychologist, 16,* 69–90.

Meichenbaum, D., & Fitzpatrick, D. (1993). A narrative constructivist perspective of stress and coping: Stress inoculation applications. In L. Goldberger & S. Breznitz (Eds.), *Handbook of stress* (2nd ed.). New York: Free Press.

Meichenbaum, D., & Fong, G. (1993). How individuals control their own minds: A constructive narrative perspective. In D. M. Wegner & J. W. Pennebaker (Eds.), *Handbook of mental control.* New York: Prentice Hall.

Meichenbaum, D., & Jaremko, M. E. (Eds.). (1993). *Stress reduction and prevention.* New York: Plenum Press.

Meichenbaum, D., & Novaco, R. (1978). Stress inoculation: A preventative approach. In C. Spielberger & I. Sarason (Eds.), *Stress and anxiety* (Vol. 5). Washington, DC: Hemisphere.

Meichenbaum, D., & Turk, D. C. (1976). The cognitive behavioral management of anxiety, anger and pain. In P. Davidson (Ed.), *The behavioral management of anxiety, depression and pain.* New York: Brunner/Mazel.

Meichenbaum, D., & Turk, D. C. (1987). *Facilitating treatment adherence: A practitioner's guidebook.* New York: Plenum Press.

Michelson, L. K., & Marchione, K. (1991). Behavioral, cognitive and pharmacological treatment of panic disorder with agoraphobia: Critique and synthesis. *Journal of Consulting and Clinical Psychology, 59,* 100–114.

Neimeyer, R. A. (2001). *Meaning reconstruction and the experience of loss.* Washington, DC: American Psychological Association.

Norcross, J. (2004). Empirically supported therapy relationships. *Clinical Psychologist, 57,* 19–24.

Novaco, R. (1975). *Anger control: The development and evaluation of an experimental treatment.* Lexington, MA: Heath.

Novaco, R. (1977a). Stress inoculation: A cognitive therapy for anger and its application to a case of depression. *Journal of Consulting and Clinical Psychology, 45,* 600–608.

Novaco, R. (1977b). A stress inoculation approach to anger management in the training of law enforcement officers. *American Journal of Community Psychology, 5,* 327–346.

Novaco, R. (1980). Training of probation officers for anger problems. *Journal of Consulting Psychology, 27,* 385–390.

Novaco, R., Cook, T., & Sarason, I. (1983). Military recruit training: An arena for stress-coping skills. In D. Meichenbaum & M. Jaremko (Eds.), *Stress prevention and management: A cognitive-behavioral approach.* New York: Plenum Press.

Paunovic, N., & Ost, L. G. (2001). Cognitive-behavioral therapy vs. exposure therapy in treatment of PTSD in refugees. *Behaviour Research and Therapy, 39,* 1183–1197.

Rapee, R. (1987). The psychological treatment of panic attacks: Theoretical conceptualization and review of evidence. *Clinical Psychology Review, 7,* 427–438.

Resick, P. A., & Schnicke, M. K. (1992). Cognitive processing therapy for sexual assault victims. *Journal of Consulting and Clinical Psychology, 60,* 748–756.

Saunders, T., Driskell, J. E., Johnston, J. H., & Salas, E. (1996). The effect of stress inoculation training on anxiety and performance. *Journal of Occupational Psychology, 1,* 170–186.

Segerstrom, S. C., & Miller, G. E. (2004). Psychological stress and the human immune system: A meta-analytic study of 30 years of inquiry. *Psychological Bulletin, 130,* 601–630.

Siegal, L. J., & Peterson, L. (1980). Stress reduction in young dental patients through coping skills and sensory information. *Journal of Consulting and Clinical Psychology, 48,* 785–787.

Smith, R. E. (1980). A cognitive–affective approach to stress management training for athletes. In C. H. Nadeau, W. R. Halliwell, K. M. Newell, & G. C. Roberts (Eds.), *Psychology of motor behavior and sport.* Champaign, IL: Human Kinetics.

Smith, R. E., & Rohsenow, D. J. (1987). *Cognitive–affective stress management training: A treatment and resource manual.* San Rafael, CA: Select Press.

Smucker, M. P., Grunet, B. K., & Weis, J. M. (2003). Posttraumatic stress disorder: A new algorithm treatment model. In R. L. Leahy (Ed.), *Roadblocks in cognitive-behavioral therapy* (pp. 175–194). New York: Guilford Press.

Suinn, R. M. (1990). *Anxiety management training.* New York: Plenum Press.

Tarrier, N., Pilgrim, H., Sommerfield, C., Faragher, B., Reynolds, M., Graham, E., et al. (1999). A randomized trial of cognitive therapy and imagined exposure in the treatment of chronic posttraumatic stress disorder. *Journal of Consulting and Clinical Psychology, 29,* 12–18.

Turk, D. C., Meichenbaum, D., & Genest, M. (1983). *Pain and behavioral medicine: A cognitive-behavioral perspective.* New York: Guilford Press.

Veronen, L. J., & Kilpatrick, D. G. (1982, November). *Stress inoculation training for victims of rape: Efficacy and differential findings.* Symposium conducted at the annual convention of the Association for the Advancement of Behavior Therapy, Los Angeles.

Veronen, L. J., & Kilpatrick, D. G. (1983). Stress management for rape victims. In D. Meichenbaum & M. Jaremko (Eds.), *Stress prevention and management: A cognitive behavioral approach.* New York: Plenum Press.

Wernick, R. L. (1983). Stress inoculation in the management of clinical pain: Applications to burn patients. In D. Meichenbaum & M. Jaremko (Eds.). *Stress reduction and prevention: A cognitive behavioral approach* (pp. 191–218). New York: Plenum Press.

Wernick, R. L., Jaremko, M., & Taylor, P. (1981). Pain management in severely burned adults: A test of stress inoculation. *Journal of Behavioral Medicine, 4,* 103–109.

Wertkin, R. A. (1985). Stress inoculation training: Principles and applications. *Social Casework, 12,* 611–616.

Witkiewitz, K., & Marlatt, G. A. (2004). Relapse prevention for alcohol and drug problems: That was Zen, this is Tao. *American Psychologist, 59,* 224–235.

Other Methods

CHAPTER 20

Music Therapy
Applications to Stress Management

CHERYL DILEO
JOKE BRADT

HISTORY OF THE METHOD

Music is ubiquitous in the vast majority of cultures. It is integral to daily life; it is pervasive in all areas of human functioning. Aside from its aesthetic and entertainment values, repeated and consistent descriptions testify to its use for nonaesthetic or nonentertainment goals. Out of the interest in examining its uses to promote human health and well-being has grown the discipline of music therapy. Its use to facilitate relaxation has been one of its most important therapeutic aspects (Scartelli, 1989).

The use of music to treat health problems is firmly rooted in history. The close association between music and medicine can be traced to ancient cultures, in which music was closely allied with medical practice (Boxberger, 1962). The oldest account of medical practices, the Kahum Papyrus, details the use of incantations for healing purposes (Light, Love, Benson, & Morch, 1954, cited in Standley, 1986).

Although the use of music to treat various psychological and physiological problems extends throughout antiquity, the Middle Ages, and the Renaissance, its modern history began at the end of the 19th century. This period marked the advent of empirical studies on physiological and psychological responses to music. These studies pointed to the effects of music on neurosis (Corning, 1899); insomnia and fevers (Davison, 1899); and blood pressure, circulation, cardiac contraction, and respiration (Dogiel, 1880, cited in Eagle, 1972). Davison (1899) further postulated that it was important to match the music to the psychological state of the patient (Pratt & Jones, 1987). Other early researchers concluded that physiological functions responded reflexively to music (Hyde, 1927) and that the individual's appreciation for the music was the important determinant of physiological response (Vincent & Thompson, 1929). These ideas, among others, have established a foundation for using music to affect health.

Music therapy as a formalized discipline began during and immediately following World War II, when its effects on convalescing and "shell-shocked" patients were noted. To advance scientific knowledge in this discipline and to provide standards and support

TABLE 20.1. Examples of Clinical Conditions for Which Music Therapy Is Used

- Developmental disabilities (Gfeller, 1999; Jellison, 2000)
- Physical disabilities (Thaut, 1999)
- Medical conditions (Dileo, 1999a; Dileo & Bradt, 2005; Standley, 2000)
- Behavior disturbances (Montello & Coons, 1998; Rickson & Watkins, 2003)
- Offenders (Thaut, 1989)
- Stress (Dileo & Bradt, 2005; Pelletier, 2004)

- Sensory impairments (Codding, 2000; Robb, 2003)
- Autism (Gold & Wigram, 2003; Thaut, 1992)
- Gerontology and Alzheimer's disease (Clair, 1996; Koger, Chapin, & Brotons, 1999)
- Psychiatric conditions(Silverman, 2003; Unkefer & Thaut, 2002; Maratos & Gold, 2003; Gold, Bentley, & Wigram, 2003)
- Terminal illness (Dileo & Loewy, 2005; Hilliard, 2003)

for its practitioners, the National Association for Music Therapy was formed in 1950, the American Association for Music Therapy was founded in 1971, and the American Music Therapy Association (a merger of these two groups) was founded in 1998.

Music therapy as a discipline embraces a wide range of clinical applications, and examples of these are presented in Table 20.1. Medical applications of music therapy have burgeoned during the past 20 years, and examples of these are presented in Table 20.2.

THEORETICAL FOUNDATIONS

Defining Music Therapy

Because music therapy is such a broad discipline, with many possible clinical applications, a working definition must be adopted that provides a foundation for its therapeutic potential in stress management. Thus "music therapy is a systematic process of intervention wherein the therapist helps the client to promote health, using music experiences and the relationships that develop through them as dynamic forces of change" (Bruscia, 1998, p. 20). Necessary components of music therapy based on this definition are: a client with a defined health need, a trained music therapist, a relationship between client and therapist, a goal-oriented music process, music materials, and an evaluation of therapeutic effectiveness.

TABLE 20.2. Medical Specialties within Which Music Therapy Is Used

- Neonatology (Caine, 1991; Standley, 2002)
- Obstetrics and gynecology (Davis, 1992; Liebman & MacLaren, 1991)
- Intensive care (Chlan, 1998; Wong, Lopez-Nahas, & Molassiotis, 2001)
- Physical Rehabilitation (Nayak, Wheeler, Shiflett, & Agostinelli, 2000; Stanley & Ramsey, 1998)
- Surgery (MacDonald et al., 2003; Robb, Nichols, Rutan, Bishop, & Parker, 1995)
- Dentistry (Aitken, Wilson, Coury, & Moursi, 2002; Goff, Pratt, & Madrigal, 1997)

- Pediatrics (Malone, 1996; Robb, 2001)
- Cardiology (Hamel, 2001; White, 1992, 1999)
- Oncology (Burns, 2001; Burns, Harbuz, Hucklebridge, & Bunt, 2001)
- Alzheimer's disease (Koger, Chapin, & Brotons, 1999; Kumar et al., 1999)
- Hospice (Dileo & Loewy, 2005; Hilliard, 2003)

Types of Music Experiences

The full range of possible experiences within music is used in music therapy. These include (1) listening to live, improvised, or prerecorded music, or listening to and also "feeling" low-frequency music vibrations, (2) performing music or learning/practicing on an instrument, (3) improvising music spontaneously using voice and/or instruments, (4) composing music (music and/or lyrics), and (5) music combined with other arts modalities (e.g., art, dance, drama).

Classification of Approaches

The presence of both music experiences and a relationship between the client and the therapist differentiates *music therapy* from other uses of music (e.g., self-help methods). Whereas both are always present in music therapy, each may assume a greater, lesser, or equal degree of importance in stress management treatment depending on the needs of the client (Maranto, 1991, 1992). In addition, music therapy can be used as the primary mode of intervention to effect health changes in the individual, or it can be equal or subordinate to other methods of stress management intervention, such as autogenic training, meditation, or medication.

Music therapy may also be offered to the client at various levels of practice depending on his or her needs and the level of and specialized training of the therapist (e.g., bachelor's level, graduate training, or specialized training in a particular method). At the more basic levels of music therapy practice, music therapy activities may be used as a distraction from stress and anxiety; music may be used in combination with other, traditional approaches to stress management; and music may be used in an attempt to palliate the client's symptoms of stress. In addition, music may be used within a psychoeducational approach to stress management. At more advanced levels of music therapy practice, the therapist addresses the full range of the client's issues besides those that cause anxiety and utilizes methods that will enhance insight into these issues and support change. In addition to implementing a greater range and sophistication of music-based stress management methods, the therapist uses music to facilitate self-exploration and awareness and a new way of being for the client. Furthermore, specialized methods of music therapy, such as the Bonny Method of Guided Imagery and Music, Analytical Music Therapy, or Creative Music Therapy, may be used as primary modes of intervention.

In addition to this brief classification of music therapy practice, it is important to further differentiate music therapy from other types of practices involving music (see Table 20.3), such as music medicine and music for self-help.

Music medicine (Dileo, 1999b) refers to the use of music by medical or health care professionals to affect changes in various domains (physical, psychological, etc.). In this practice, taped music is used to elicit desired clinical effects or to enhance other types of treatment. Specifically, music *alone* is used as the intervention. Some research studies support the effectiveness of these procedures and, indeed, music listening is known to yield therapeutic benefits.

In addition, there appears to be widespread use of music for *self-help purposes*, and many music tapes and CDs that claim to assist an individual in achieving relaxation are available in the marketplace. Although there is little literature on the effectiveness of these mass-market products, it is possible that some individuals may derive benefits. As we describe later in this chapter, there is little support for a "one-size-fits-all" approach to music for stress reduction.

TABLE 20.3. Music Therapy Compared with Other Music Practices in Stress Reduction

	Music therapy	Music medicine	Music for self-help
Trained music therapist	Yes	No	No
Trained professional	Yes	Yes	No
Type of music experience	Listening, performing, creating/improvising, composing	Listening	Listening
Type of music stimulus	Mostly live and/or improvised; some prerecorded	Prerecorded	Prerecorded
Relationship with therapist	Yes, through music	No, not through music	No
Assessment used	Yes	Not typically	No
Goal-oriented process	Yes	Not typically	No
Individualized treatment	Yes	Not typically	No
Evaluation of treatment	Yes	Not typically	Only personal evaluation

Responses to and Effects of Music and Music Therapy

Research indicates that both music and music therapy elicit physiological, psychological, cognitive, social, and spiritual responses (Dileo & Bradt, 2005), and these effects can clearly support a rationale for the use of music and music therapy in stress management (see Table 20.4). It is important to emphasize that both music and music therapy affect all of these domains in the person, and it is likely that these effects are interrelated. Thus it is not always possible to discuss "physiological" responses separately from responses in other human domains.

A number of individual factors also influence responses to music, as identified in the literature. These include, but are not limited to: age, gender, cognitive function, severity of stress, training in music, familiarity with and preference for the music, culture, and personal associations with the music (see Pelletier, 2004; Standley, 1986, 2000). Because of these individual factors, it becomes obvious that specific pieces of music cannot be universally prescribed for stress reduction. With that said, however, there are pieces of music that have been tested in more than one study with similarly positive outcomes (see Pelletier, 2004). In music therapy clinical practice, the music and music experiences selected for stress reduction are the result of an individualized assessment process that involves the client.

Thus, when one examines the effects of music on various human domains, inconsistencies in the research findings may become apparent (Hanser, 1985). Because of the aforementioned variables and the complexity of the musical stimuli, it is not always possible to predict the direction of human responses to music (Bartlett, 1996). Musical stimuli are not often standardized across different studies; for example, researchers' interpretations of what constitutes "sedative" versus "stimulative" music may indeed differ (Bartlett, 1996). Also, because music is not a static phenomenon, many pieces of music include periods of both tension and resolution of tension. The experience of music is a moment-to-moment phenomenon, and, as such, responses to music also may vary in the moment (Edwards, Eagle, Pennebaker, & Tunks, 1990); these changes are not sensitive to pre–post measurement tools. In addition, the volume, quality, instrumentation, arrangement, and so forth of the music may be mitigating factors in the musical experience. Elements of music, as well as the music gestalt, may evoke differential responses. Last, live music stimuli may evoke different responses than does prerecorded music (Bailey, 1983).

Furthermore, when one considers the complexity of individual differences in response to music, one may not assume that responses among participants are similar and predictable (Thaut, 1989). One must take into account individuals' attention to the music (Dainow, 1977), their current emotional and physical status, their processing differences (Lacey, 1956), and their cognitive and emotional interpretations of the music, as well as nonmusical associations that often accompany specific pieces or genres of music. Music also evokes various types of imagery in many individuals. Thus the individual's unique imagery will influence his or her responses to the music.

ASSESSMENT

Applications of Music and Music Therapy to Stress Management

A number of uses of music in stress management have been described in the literature. Studies have dealt with the influence of music on anxiety, as well as with the uses of music to manage stress in a number of anxiety-provoking situations, ranging from university and occupational settings to clinical settings to medical settings.

Dileo and Bradt (2005) completed a meta-analysis of all the research literature concerning the use of music therapy in medical treatment. Eleven categories of medical specialization were identified in this analysis: neonatology, pediatrics, obstetrics and gynecology, cardiac and intensive care, rehabilitation, surgery, oncology and terminal illness, general medicine, gerontology, fetal responses, and dentistry. In this analysis, 183 studies were included, and music's effects on 40 categories of dependent variables were assessed. The anxiety associated with medical conditions and procedures was a dependent variable in a number of the studies reviewed. The results of this analysis that are relevant to stress reduction are presented in Table 20.4. In the following data, r scores of 0.10 are considered small effect sizes, scores of 0.25 are considerate moderate effect sizes, and scores of 0.40 and above are considered large effect sizes. In addition, the effect size scores represent the effectiveness of music or music therapy treatment in comparison to a no-treatment control condition.

Larger overall effect sizes for music interventions that employ patient-preferred as opposed to nonpreferred music were also found in this analysis. In addition, the overall effect size for music therapy as a treatment intervention was much larger (0.40) than that for music medicine interventions (0.24).

Pelletier (2004) conducted a meta-analytic review of 22 research studies involving the effects of music-assisted relaxation (recorded music combined with relaxation strategies) on participants who were experiencing stress and anxiety. In this review, she compared music interventions with no-music interventions and found a large overall mean effect size for the music conditions ($d = +0.6711$). No significant differences were found among types of dependent measures (i.e., physiological, behavioral, self-report). However, the homogeneity Q value was significant ($p = 0.00$), and a quality analysis was performed. The results of this revealed enhanced effects of music-assisted relaxation: with individuals under 18, with musicians (as opposed to nonmusicians), with individual as

TABLE 20.4. Effect Sizes of Music/Music Therapy Conditions versus No-Treatment Conditions on Selected Variables for Patients in Medical Treatment

Variable	k	r_u	N	95% CI
Overall heart rate	44	0.28*	1,883	+.17 to +.40
Overall respiration rate	22	0.32*	738	+.18 to +.44
Diastolic blood pressure	25	0.27*	2,028	+.09 to +.42
Systolic blood pressure	25	0.28*	1,194	+.10 to +.45
Cortisol	7	0.05	218	−.09 to +.19
Skin temperature	4	0.27	342	−.31 to +.70
Secretory IgA	4	0.35*	136	+.05 to +.58
Use of sedatives	6	0.31*	405	+.15 to +.45
Anxiety—non-STAI	19	0.28*	831	+.15 to +.40
Anxiety—STAI scores	40	0.30*	1,921	+.21 to +.39
Mood	11	0.44*	358	+.23 to +.60

Note. k, the number of independent samples; N, the total number of participants in these samples (music group and nonmusic group); r_u, the unbiased effect size estimate; 95% CI, 95% confidence interval for r_u; IgA, immunoglobulin A; STAI, Stait–Trait Anxiety Inventory.
* significant at $p < .05$.

opposed to group treatment, with multiple treatment sessions, with musical stimuli that had been previously tested and shown effective, and with the addition of verbal suggestion or low-frequency stimulation to the music protocol.

Dileo and Bradt (2005) also completed a meta-analysis of the research literature on music therapy and stress in nonmedical populations. Forty-one studies comparing a music or music therapy experimental condition with a no-music control condition were included (these studies are included in the reference section of this chapter, marked by *). In Table 20.5, correlational effect sizes are presented for the study level mean and for a variety of stress-related variables. Overall, self-report measures resulted in a higher effect size than did physiological measures.

In addition, studies using classical music resulted in lower study level effect sizes and a lower effect size for anxiety than studies using nonclassical music (e.g., new age, easy listening; Table 20.6). Unfortunately, many studies described in general terms only the music selected for the experimental condition. Although these results suggest that greater stress reduction is achieved with the use of nonclassical music, great care should be taken when interpreting these results. Most studies ($N = 34$) did not take into account participants' musical preferences. As pointed out previously, musical preference is of great importance when selecting music for use in stress management. It could well be that the classical music studies resulted in lower effect sizes because of a mismatch between the music used and participants' musical preference. The results suggest that classical music is not superior to other musical styles in terms of its effects on outcomes of stress reduction.

Although not included in the meta-analyses described here, several research studies highlight the effects of music on heart rate variability and stress reduction either through passive listening (Umemura & Honda, 1998; White, 1999; Yanagihashi, Ohira, Kimura, & Fujiwara, 1997) or through active involvement, such as singing (Grape, Sandgren, Hansson, Ericson, & Theorell, 2003) or chanting (Bernardi et al., 2001). The potential for both types of experiences within music to enhance heart rate variability is seen as very encouraging, and the mechanisms for such effects warrant further investigation. It is pos-

TABLE 20.5. Effect Sizes for Music/Music Therapy Condition versus No-Treatment Condition in a Nonmedical Population

Outcome	k	N	r_u	95% CI	p	Q
Study level mean	41	2,588	0.21	+.15 to +.26	.00**	67.99*
Study level mean (outliers removed)	39	2,510	0.21	+.15 to +.26	.00**	57.60*
Anxiety	21	1,351	0.33	+.21 to +.44	.00**	74.03*
Relaxation	9	642	0.23	+.13 to +.33	.00**	9.75
Tension	4	403	0.35	+.07 to +.63	.01**	11.96*
Mood	4	140	0.32	+.10 to +.54	.00**	4.39
Heart rate/Pulse rate	10	694	0.23	+.08 to +.38	.00**	26.40*
IgA	3	137	0.37	+.20 to +.55	.00**	1.19
Cortisol	3	115	0.04	–.15 to +.23	.69	1.67
Beta-endorphin	3	59	0.03	–.24 to +.31	.81	0.52
Finger temperature	3	169	0.00	–.15 to +.15	1.00	0.00

* $p < .05$, indicating that the sample is not homogeneous.
** $p < .01$.

sible that music experiences such as singing or wind instrument playing may structure and facilitate one's breathing at his or her individual resonant frequency rate, especially when the musical phrases of slow, sedative music (e.g., 9–12 seconds in length) mirror the resonant frequency of the cardiovascular system, in which resonance properties can be activated by respiration (Paul Lehrer, personal communication, January 2005). Further, it is possible that the moment-to-moment variation in music entrains with heart rate, enhancing its variability during music listening.

In addition, biofeedback equipment (e.g., RESPeRATE®; *www.resperate.com/MD*) that employs personalized musical tones to facilitate slow respiration (< 10 breaths per minute) and prolonged exhalation has been found to significantly lower blood pressure (Elliott, Black, Alter, & Gavish, 2004; Elliott, Izzo, et al., 2004; Grossman, Grossman, Schein, Zimlichman, & Gavish, 2001; Meles et al., 2004; Parati, Izzo, & Gavish, 2003; Rosenthal, Alter, Peleg, & Gavish, 2001; Schein et al., 2001; Viskoper et al., 2003). This device analyzes the person's breathing rate and pattern and creates a melody comprising

TABLE 20.6. Effect Sizes for Classical Music versus Nonclassical Music Treatment Conditions

Outcome	Classical	k	N	r_u	95% CI	p	Q
Study level mean	Yes	25	1,797	0.18	+.11 to +.24	.00**	0.06
Study level mean	No	14	713	0.27	+.17 to +.37	.00**	18.60
Anxiety	Yes	10	865	0.31	+.15 to +.47	.00**	39.42*
Anxiety	No	11	408	0.36	+.18 to +.55	.00**	33.80*

* $p < .05$, indicating that the sample is not homogeneous.
** $p < .01$.

two different tones: one for inhalation and another for exhalation. The patient is instructed to synchronize his or her respiration to these tones, and the exhalation tone is gradually extended and the breathing rate slowed to less than 10 breaths per minute.

Adverse Effects

Perhaps one of the main advantages of using music in stress reduction is its relative lack of negative side effects, particularly when it is implemented by a trained music therapist. In the vast majority of the literature, the only negative effect of music reported (if, indeed, it can be considered a negative effect) was the lack of the desired response. Thus the adverse reactions mentioned next have been observed in our clinical practice. Adverse reactions may happen more frequently when music is used by professionals who have not had sufficient training in these methods; that is, when music is used casually as a supplement to other techniques and without a full music therapy assessment process. Music can be a very powerful tool in therapy because of its ability to access physiological, psychological, and cognitive reactions simultaneously; thus it cannot be used in a cavalier manner. Moreover, because music can access feelings and responses directly and immediately, caution should be exercised in its use without consultation with trained music therapy professionals.

In this section, we list possible adverse reactions as determined in clinical work and suggest remedial measures in the event that these adverse responses occur.

Displeasure with the Music

Arbitrary selections of music by an untrained clinician can elicit responses that are counterproductive to treatment. This may be considered the most common reason for any adverse reactions. It cannot be assumed that one particular piece or genre of music is universally effective with patients; rather, music can be selected for therapeutic use only following an individualized assessment process with direct input from the client. It has been observed that clinicians may select music based on their own personal preferences (as opposed to the client's), and clinicians should be aware that the client may not respond to the music selected in the same manner as the clinician.

A variety of psychological and physiological reactions have been observed to occur when inappropriate music is used, including irritation, anger, frustration, and increases in psychological and physiological measures of tension. For example, we have observed escalations in the client's anxiety; a request to end the session; direct verbalizations about the nature of the music; fidgeting; and lack of compliance with the procedures used. The severity of these reactions can be minimized and remediated by a careful observation of the patient's physiological and behavioral reactions while experiencing the music. If adverse effects are noted, a change in music or discontinuation of the music is warranted immediately. Also, a discussion with the client about these reactions should take place; the clinician should obtain more feedback from the client on the nature of his or her reactions, so that they can be avoided in the future. Throughout this process, it is important that the integrity of the therapeutic relationship be preserved and that the patient–therapist trust inherent in this relationship be maintained. This can be accomplished only by an open relationship with the client in which the client's feedback on the music and methodology is acknowledged and respected.

Cathartic Reactions

Even when a careful assessment of the client has been completed, it is possible that very strong feelings, associations, memories, and imagery may be elicited by the music. It is even possible that music that has been used successfully for stress reduction at one time may cause stress reactions at another time. The reason for this is that relaxed states minimize the client's defenses and allow psychological issues to be more readily evoked by music. A relaxed state makes a client more vulnerable to imagery and feelings; this vulnerability is intensified when imagery-evoking music is used (Quittner & Glueckauf, 1983). It may be impossible for the inexperienced or untrained therapist to know how evocative a particular piece of music may be for a given individual or what memories (negative, traumatic, etc.) the music may summon. We have observed that these reactions may include intense affect, vivid memories, and physiological reactions. When the goal of treatment is the resolution of psychotherapeutic issues in the client, the uncovering of these reactions may be an important component of the process and may facilitate therapy. However, if stress reduction is the goal of therapy, these reactions may be considered counterproductive in the short term. Furthermore, they must be handled with therapeutic skill and cannot be dismissed by an ethical therapist.

Once these reactions occur, they usually will not be averted by simply changing the music. However, they can be minimized by gently stopping the music and guiding the person back to an alert state. If these reactions are considered part of the goals of therapy, and if the therapist is competent in dealing with these issues, the therapy may be continued. Again, it must be emphasized that these reactions can be minimized by careful selection of the music by a trained music therapist. In addition, therapeutic skill is necessary to deal with these reactions when they occur, to give the client the needed support, and to refer the client to appropriate resources (if the therapist is not trained in doing this) for further work on issues that have come to the surface.

It is important to note at this point that music selected for psychotherapeutic work and music selected for stress reduction may be vastly different both in nature and quality.

Combining Techniques

Music is often used in combination with many methods of stress reduction, such as hypnosis, biofeedback, progressive muscle relaxation, meditation, and directed visualization (e.g., Clark, McCorkle, & Williams, 1981; Guzzetta, 1989; Liebman & MacLaren, 1991; Logan & Roberts, 1984; Robb et al., 1995). In her meta-analysis of the stress literature, Pelletier (2004) found significant differences among the following approaches combined with music, in descending order of effect size: verbal suggestion, vibroacoustic stimulation, and progressive muscle relaxation.

When combining music and stress reduction approaches that involve a great deal of verbal direction or other auditory stimuli (e.g., clicks in biofeedback), the clinician should be careful not to create a sensory overload for the client that might actually enhance the client's tension. It is important to understand the individual client's experience of and ability to integrate these different auditory stimuli and not create an experience in which the client must cognitively switch back and forth between the stimuli. For most clients, the combining of verbal instruction with music does not create a sensory overload (as suggested by Robb, 2000), especially when the verbal instructions and the nature of the music are consistent with each other and can form a gestalt.

In combining music with another stress reduction technique, several factors must be addressed:

1. Can music enhance the technique, or can music alone be used to facilitate the desired response?
2. If music is used in combination with the technique, what is the perceptual role of the music? That is, is it designed to be in the foreground or the background, and does this role change?
3. Is the music appropriate for the technique? For example, if verbal instructions are used, does the music match these instructions in content or does it divert the person from the instructions?
4. Would it be more appropriate to sequence the music following the technique or to provide music simultaneously?
5. Is the timing of verbal directions planned in advance to coincide with the music? Are there gaps in the music (e.g., in between music selections)?

Contraindications

Music therapy–based stress reduction approaches are contraindicated for clients with various psychiatric diagnoses for whom relaxed or altered states of consciousness may further exacerbate the illness. These include psychotic individuals, those with borderline personality disorder, and people with autism. Furthermore, music therapy listening approaches are not suitable for clients who have hearing difficulties, although these clients may benefit from low-frequency music stimulation. Clients with musicogenic epilepsy, a rare condition in which music stimuli may cause seizures, are also not suitable for music therapy approaches. Last, clients suffering from brain injury, brain dysfunction, and/or severe auditory processing difficulties may require music that is highly structured and without a wide range of overtones, for example, synthesized music, to benefit from its use in stress reduction.

METHODS

As mentioned previously, the full range of experiences available within music is utilized in music therapy. These include (1) listening experiences, (2) performing/learning/practicing experiences, (3) improvisational experiences, (4) music composition, and (5) combined arts experiences.

Listening Experiences

In listening experiences, the client assumes a relatively passive role when listening to music with or without verbal instructions or when receiving music and low-frequency sounds through the body. Client responses include following directions for relaxing or creating images suggested by the therapist and/or stimulated by the music. The following categories of listening experiences may be used in music therapy for stress reduction.

Music listening experiences are perhaps the most frequently used in stress reduction, and a variety of methods exist. Indeed, music alone, that is, without verbal directions or suggestions for imagery, may be used to facilitate stress reduction (e.g., Hamel, 2001). The music used may be (1) prerecorded with or without low-frequency tones (e.g.,

Wigram & Dileo, 1997) (2) improvised by the therapist, (3) composed by the therapist, or (4) cocreated by client and therapist.

The therapist may select prerecorded music for the client based on its sedative qualities, along with a consideration of its familiarity to and preference by the client. This is done through an assessment process involving input from the client, as well as a pretesting of the musical selections themselves with the client. Sedative music may be found within a variety of musical styles: classical, jazz, popular, new age, country, and so forth, according to the preference of the client. Qualities of sedative music may include: simplicity in structure, melody, and harmonies; repetition; absence of lyrics; slow tempos; relative lack of harmonic tension; and instrumentation that involves strings, woodwinds, and piano, as opposed to brass and percussion. Nature sounds, such as waves, bird sounds, and so forth, may be included in the music. The therapist must ascertain that the music used does not stimulate memories, associations, or images for the client that are inconsistent with the goal of relaxation.

Prerecorded music may also contain low-frequency sounds. This approach (known as *vibroacoustic* or *vibrotactile* therapy) requires specialized equipment, such as a bed or chair in which the client can recline and hear the music while the low-frequency tones provide direct stimulation to the body. Depending on the frequencies used (either superimposed on the music or provided through other means), various areas of the body are "vibrated." Frequencies can also be varied to produce "waves" of vibration throughout the body. There are a number of clinical applications for these methodologies besides relaxation (Wigram & Dileo, 1997).

The therapist may also improvise music for the client according to the client's preferred musical style and/or musical instruments (including voice; see Turry, 1997). This may be done spontaneously and freely by the therapist or in accordance with a physiological parameter of the client (*iso music*; Saperston, 1995). For example, the therapist may match the pulse of the improvised music to the client's respiration rate. Once matched and sustained for a short period of time, the therapist will gradually decrease the pulse of the music to encourage a slowing down of the breath. The therapist may also improvise music based on a physiological parameter that is being monitored (e.g., heart rate). Again, the music will be created first to match the physiological response, and once this is done, the therapist will change the music in the direction of the desired outcome, with the physiological response following suit (Saperston, 1995).

The therapist may also precompose music especially for a client according to his or her preferences. This music may include cues or instructions or messages for relaxation, either musically or through lyrics (see Saperston, 1999).

Last, the therapist may improvise music under the direction of the client in a process called *music therapy entrainment* (Dileo, 1997; Dileo & Bradt, 1999; Rider, 1997a, 1997b, 2000). In entrainment, the specially trained music therapist creates music that matches the client's description of his or her anxiety, as well as music that the client describes as "healing" or "relaxing." After this is done, the client closes his or her eyes and listens to the therapist begin improvising the music that matches the anxiety, gradually moving to the "healing" music. The therapist also "resonates" with the client's experience through the music. Following the music, the experience is processed verbally with the client, and a tape recording of the music may be provided to the client for use outside the session (see the case examples later in the chapter).

Prerecorded, improvised, vibroacoustic, and/or precomposed music may be combined with other, traditional stress reduction approaches, such as biofeedback, progressive muscle relaxation, autogenic training, systematic desensitization, and imagery work.

When combined with biofeedback, music may be used as a cue and facilitator for a relaxed state or as a contingency for the achievement of the desired criterion for relaxation. In either case, to be effective, the music should be sedative in quality (as described earlier) and also in accordance with the client's preferences (see Scartelli, 1989).

When combining music with progressive muscle relaxation (PMR) and autogenic training, the music may initially provide the eliciting stimulus for the client's entering into a relaxed state and/or the means for sustaining such. We suggest that, when using these combined methods, it is important to match the verbal instructions with the music; for example, when the verbal instructions in PMR involve tensing a particular muscle or muscle group, the music should reflect this tension. Similarly, there should be a release of tension in the music as the client releases the tension in the muscle. To facilitate this intimate connection between music and verbal instruction, the music therapist will often improvise music in the moment, selecting instruments for the improvisation that closely match the desired clinical outcome. In this manner, the music and the verbal stimuli provide a seamless gestalt to deepen and enhance the client's experience of relaxation. Appropriate music is provided following the verbal input to sustain the client's relaxation.

As another example, when combining music and autogenic training, the music therapist might use the verbal self-suggestions as lyrics in an original song composed for the client. With repeated application of the song as a prompt for relaxation, the client may further internalize this song to be used as a prompt for dealing with anxiety in daily life (see Saperston, 1999).

When music is combined with systematic desensitization, precomposed, vibroacoustic, and/or improvised music may be used to provide a cue for relaxation and may sustain the body in a relaxed state as anxiety-provoking situations are described by the therapist and imagined by the client (Reitman, 1999).

Precomposed and/or improvised music may also be used in facilitating imagery experiences that lead to relaxation. Research suggests that music enhances imagery vividness (McKinney, 1990; McKinney & Tims, 1995; Peach, 1984; Quittner & Glueckauf, 1983), the accessibility of images (Quittner & Glueckauf, 1983), and their quality and length (McKinney & Tims, 1995; Quittner & Glueckauf, 1983). When used for this purpose, music may support imagery directed by the therapist or the client's spontaneous imagery as elicited by the music. In the latter case, an initial imagery focus is provided for the client (e.g., escape to a favorite, relaxing place; an imaginal journey; visualizations of the self coping with a stressful situation), and music is used to amplify, deepen, support, and provide a structure for the imagery.

At an advanced level of practice and with specialized institute training, the music therapist may utilize the Bonny Method of Guided Imagery and Music. As a psychotherapeutic method, it is not designed specifically for relaxation goals and thus may not have anxiety-reducing effects (Pelletier, 2004). However, potential outcomes of this approach, for example, may lead to the resolution of issues related to the client's stress and to the enhancement of emotional expression (Burns, 2001). This approach is structured to include the components that follow.

1. An initial conversation takes place between the client and therapist to determine the focus for the session (usually lasting about 2 hours). During this conversation, the client discusses events that have happened since the last session, further insights about images or additional images that have occurred, and how in general he or she is feeling. If this is the first session for the client, the practitioner will complete a thorough clinical assessment and describe the method in detail to the client. Based on this preliminary discus-

sion, the practitioner selects an imagery induction, imagery focus, and music for exploring the issue or theme that has been identified for that session.

2. A relaxation induction is provided by the therapist to facilitate the client's entrance into an altered state of consciousness. The relaxation induction chosen will vary, depending on the client's preferences, ease of entering into an altered state, and focus for the session. The induction will thus vary in length and detail depending on these factors. For example, the therapist may use a form of PMR or an imagery-based induction.

3. The therapist suggests an initial imagery focus as a starting place for the client's imagery. This focus is related to the issue the client will explore in the session. For example, the therapist might suggest that the client imagine him- or herself in a favorite or safe place, with others in his or her life, or in a place in nature. The range of these starting images varies widely.

4. A specially designed music program from the classical genre is selected according to the client's needs. These programs are available for professionals trained in this method and contain classical pieces that have been chosen, sequenced, and tested to evoke rich imagery that may enhance personal exploration. The musical programs are designed around specific clinical themes, for example, creativity, grieving, emotional expression, and so forth (see Bruscia, 2002, for additional information on the development of these music programs).

5. As the music plays, the client reports his or her imaginal experiences verbally to the therapist as they occur, and a dialogue between the therapist and client ensues, as the therapist provides support and suggestions for deepening and fully experiencing the imagery. The therapist enters into the client's imagery as fully as possible and accompanies him or her in the process. The therapist records a verbatim transcript of the client's imagery during the session.

6. At the end of the music and imagery experience, the therapist processes the experiences with the client either verbally or through other creative means, such as mandala work or clay. The therapist does not interpret the client's imagery but supports him or her in doing this and in making connections between the imagery and the client's life and needs. (For a comprehensive description of this method, see Bruscia & Grocke, 2002.)

Performing/Practicing/Learning Experiences

The act of performing, practicing, or learning precomposed music using voice and/or instruments may also serve as an approach to stress reduction. We have observed that these activities may serve as a diversion from stress and may enhance the client's mood, boost self-esteem, provide opportunities for self-nurturance, and allow for "centering" experiences, after which coping mechanisms may be more effective. These experiences also encourage the individual to refocus his or her attention on a creative experience that may enhance empowerment and control and promote normalization even in difficult circumstances (see Chetta, 1981).

This approach is suitable for both trained and untrained musicians. For clients who have not had musical training, music therapists often utilize specialized music instruction methods designed to minimize the learning curve in playing an instrument. At the same time, most individuals are able to use their voices for singing favorite songs on or off pitch and without judgment by the therapist regarding vocal quality. Emphasis is always on the process of performing rather than on the musical product.

Clients who are confined to stressful circumstances, for example, a hospital, may use learning or practicing an instrument as an effective means of coping with boredom and stress. For example, one of us (C. D.) has used music therapy with heart failure inpatients waiting for a transplant. The stresses of these circumstances defy description, as these patients are literally "in between" life and death; a heart transplant is their only hope for survival, and there are not enough hearts available for all. As they may be hospitalized for extended periods of time, some patients may choose to learn to play an instrument or to maintain their skills on an instrument during their hospital stay. Not only were these music experiences helpful in structuring their time and in reducing the stress they were experiencing, but playing instruments also represented to them hope for the future and an investment in their lives beyond their current circumstances. Thus the process of learning the instrument addressed multiple needs and contributed to an improved quality of life even in the most difficult of situations (Dileo & Zanders, 2005).

Besides the psychological benefits that may contribute to stress reduction, direct physical benefits may result from the act of singing, musically chanting, and/or toning (Bernardi et al., 2001; Rider, Mickey, Weldin, & Hawkinson, 1990). In toning, the client experiments with different pitches and observes how these pitches vibrate within the body. Based on these sensations, he or she will select a pitch to sustain using repeated long breaths. No words are used—only the vowel sounds that best support the production of the tones. The client is encouraged to continue toning until a state of relaxation is achieved, and this often occurs quite rapidly, that is, in a matter of minutes. Chanting may involve a similar process, although words are selected to accompany tone. Chanting may be designed by the therapist to progress from faster to slower tempos, thus entraining with the client's physical process of moving from a state of arousal to a state of relaxation.

Thus toning, chanting, and singing provide a means for structuring the breath in a pleasurable manner by facilitating deep and sustained breathing. In addition, toning and chanting create a sensation of internal vibration, the location of which can be controlled by the client according to need. Furthermore, when words are used in singing or chanting, they may enhance the meaning of the experience, as lyrics can also provide messages of significance to the client. These experiences may be easily combined with other stress reduction approaches that center on the breath.

Improvisational Experiences

Music improvisation involves creating music spontaneously in the moment, using voice and/or instruments (most often percussion). Music improvisation allows for the immediate expression of feelings nonverbally, and a wide range of music therapy methods exist that employ improvisation as a primary method (Bruscia, 1987; Wigram, 2004). Music improvisation, whether as a solo, in a dyad with the therapist or another person, or within a group, facilitates self-awareness and encourages exploration of personal and life options and new ways of being. In addition, it allows one to explore new identities while also receiving feedback from others on aspects of the self previously undiscovered (Bruscia, 1987).

Whereas the expression of feelings regarding stress is perhaps one of the most immediate outcomes of music improvisation experiences, use of these methods can have a number of psychological benefits for the client that go beyond the moment. Music therapy improvisation is often an important means of client assessment; that is, examining elements of a client's music may provide important insight into his or her coping mechanisms and ways of relating to self and others (Bruscia, 1987). In addition, it may serve as an important supplement to traditional methods of assessment.

Compositional Experiences

Songwriting is the most common type of compositional method used in music therapy. In songwriting, either new lyrics are created for existing music or completely original lyrics and music are composed. Clients without musical training are often assisted in the process by the therapist, who provides appropriate structure for the experience as well as assistance with musical aspects of the piece (O'Callaghan, 2001). Songwriting is used in a wide range of clinical situations and for a variety of therapeutic purposes.

As a method of stress reduction, songwriting assists the client in expressing feelings in a creative and contained manner and in having these feelings acknowledged and validated in musical form. As original musical lyrics may often reveal aspects of an individual's belief system, this approach may be quite useful in assessment, especially within a cognitive framework. Furthermore, specially composed song lyrics may provide an alternate means of countering a client's irrational belief systems, and, when internalized by the client, they can be a cue for more rational thinking as automatic thoughts occur. The melody and rhythm that accompanies the lyrics may further enhance their meaning for the client (O'Callaghan, 2005).

Physical Environment and Equipment

Equipment and settings vary, depending on the music therapy relaxation method used. For the most part, however, the following are needed:

1. A small, comfortable room with minimal visual and auditory distractions. This is essential, because auditory distractions in particular will interfere with the music procedures. Lighting in the room should be controllable via shades and lamps. The furnishings of the room should be conducive to relaxation.
2. A comfortable bed, cot, mat, or reclining chair for the client. Several of these should be available to accommodate different clients' preferences and physical conditions.
3. An appropriate audio system with clear, nondistorted delivery and high-quality headphones. The system should include capabilities for both audiocassettes and compact discs.
4. A wide selection of pretested tapes and discs from various musical genres (classical, jazz, new age, popular, country-western, etc.), which can be selected according to clients' preferences. It is important that the therapist be familiar enough with these tapes and discs to make selections on the basis of their sedative and entrainment qualities, their potential for eliciting or not eliciting imagery, and the preferences of different clients.
5. Appropriate equipment for physiological monitoring, including biofeedback equipment. Software designed to permit music or vibrational feedback instead of auditory or visual feedback is optimal.
6. Musical instruments (piano, rhythm instruments, etc.) to be used for live music, improvisation, and entrainment.
7. Vibroacoustic equipment.

The Therapist–Client Relationship in Music Therapy

As the definition of music therapy and the classification model presented earlier in this chapter indicate, a supportive therapist–client relationship, characterized by empathy, trust, and safety, is an essential component of music therapy interventions. The client–therapist relationship in music therapy, particularly in its application in medicine, may differ from other clinical relationships for several reasons:

1. In music therapy, the personal qualities of the therapist and the relationship developed with the client through the music may each and in combination effect change (Maranto, 1991, 1992). The ability of the music therapist to be "present" and "resonate" with the client's experience both in and outside of the music is vital, as these are considered essential factors in healing.
2. The therapist, because of the medium used, is able to focus on "healthy" or creative parts of the individual rather than on aspects of the illness.
3. Clients associate music therapy with pleasure and relaxation rather than discomfort and stress.
4. Because music is pervasive in everyday life, it may be less threatening to clients than other forms of therapy.
5. The use of music as a therapy may be less stigmatizing to the client than other methods of intervention.

As stated previously, the presence of a trained therapist differentiates music therapy from other uses of music. Curricula for training music therapists have been in existence for almost 50 years. These studies, accomplished either at the graduate or the undergraduate level, provide students with training in music, music therapy, behavioral sciences, social sciences, and physiology. Students learn how to use music therapy techniques with a wide variety of clinical conditions. Following an internship of 900–1,040 hours, students are eligible to sit for the national board certification examination, administered by the Certification Board for Music Therapy, Inc. Graduate work in music therapy is strongly encouraged if individuals are to use more in-depth methods of music therapy, including applications in medicine. Approximately 70 universities offer undergraduate training and certification coursework; 17 offer master's degrees; and 7 offer PhD studies in related areas with an emphasis in music therapy. One program offers the DA degree in music therapy, and one has a full PhD program in music therapy.

Methods for Enhancing Compliance

Music therapy has the ability to be transferred into the client's own environment. Relevant music therapy sessions may be tape-recorded for the client for follow-up use. Music may be portable, via a Walkman, iPod, or similar devices, and thus may be used in a variety of nonclinical settings (e.g., in the car, at home, at work, or wherever there is a perceived need). Again, there is no stigma attached to listening to music.

Typically, following music therapy sessions and the learning of skills therein, clients are given detailed instructions on how to transfer skills to their own situations and use them most efficiently for their own needs. Because music is a pleasurable experience, resistance is not generally an issue.

Change is maintained through the music therapist's continued monitoring of the client and the evaluation of self-report data. Ways of incorporating music in the day-to-day environment that are compatible with the client's own routine and lifestyle are explored and implemented. Indeed, the inclusion of music as a stress management device can be virtually effortless when it is done creatively and in conjunction with the client's own preferences. Clients can use music in a cue-controlled manner or in a preventative way to deter stress. The accessible aspects of music allow clients to feel in control of their treatment and perhaps more motivated to continue its use in stress reduction.

CASE EXAMPLES

Music and Imagery with the Terminally Ill

Joe was a 75-year-old man with inoperable cancer of the lung and diaphragm. He lived at home with his wife; prior to his diagnosis, he had enjoyed a very active lifestyle that included dancing several times a week and part-time employment. He was referred to the therapist by his surgeon because of his interest in music to improve the quality of his life and to reduce his anxiety concerning his illness. Joe was a very quiet, gentle person who was unable to share his feelings about his illness with his family for fear of creating a burden for them.

Joe was seen in his home for sessions that lasted for 2 hours each. Sessions were held every 2–3 weeks; he received no other interventions besides medical treatment. Joe was very interested in assuming an active role with regard to his illness, and he read the latest books and articles on the topic of mind–body relationships. Still, he was worried about the progression of the disease, about not being able to continue his former level of activity, and about becoming a burden to the family that he continued to care for. An assessment by the therapist indicated that "big-band" music was his favorite, yet he liked many styles of music and was willing to experiment with new types.

During the first session, a version of progressive relaxation that involved tensing and releasing various muscle groups was used; an imagery focus of going to a favorite comfortable place was given; and sedative new-age music was used. The music played for 15 minutes, after which Joe was guided back to an alert state, and he and the therapist discussed the feelings and imagery that had occurred during the music. Because biofeedback equipment was unavailable throughout therapy, the achievement of relaxation was gauged from observation of physiological signs such as respiration rate, muscle tension, and movement; also, information was gleaned from the patient's self-report. After the music and imagery of the first session, the patient reported that it was the most relaxed he had been in months. His imagery had been very comforting to him, and he couldn't believe that he could feel that peaceful again. Tears of gratitude came to his eyes as the session was concluded.

At subsequent sessions, similar techniques were used. However, different imagery was suggested to reflect Joe's needs in different sessions, as determined via initial discussions; music was chosen in a similar manner. For example, at one session Joe reported having difficulty breathing because of his tumor and the humid weather. The imagery chosen was that of being on a beach; music was chosen that could entrain slow, relaxed breathing. Guided imagery was used throughout the music selection—imagery of "breathing in" the music and letting it open his airways, as well as imagery of letting the music enter the body through the breath, allowing it to travel to different parts of the body, and letting any tension found be removed from the body via exhalation. The results of this session were extraordinary. The effects of the music and imagery procedures lasted several days. During the course of treatment, relaxation inductions were also varied, but consistently less and less time was needed until relaxation was achieved. The procedures never failed to elicit a deep state of relaxation in the patient.

Following the music sessions, the therapist spent considerable time processing the images with Joe, along with the feelings that emerged. It seemed that the music was able to relax him sufficiently to allow him to address his fears and concerns about the illness, as well as to release emotions that had been pent up for many years. The music-facilitated relaxation also permitted the patient to attempt a review of difficult situations in his life and to come to resolutions on various issues. Joe commented on several occasions that because of music therapy, he was able to gain control again over his life.

The therapist provided tapes, and Joe used them daily, particularly when he felt tension mounting. However, he reported that this was not as effective as having sessions with the therapist.

Although the cancer ultimately took Joe's life, he remained fairly active until his demise, and his family reported that music therapy was the only thing that appeared to help him deal with his illness. He knew that music therapy was a safe place to "let go" of tension and to face and resolve his fears concerning his illness.

Music Therapy Entrainment for Stress Management

Maria, a 25-year-old professional, self-referred to the therapist with feelings of no longer being able to manage all the varied responsibilities in her life, including a promising and demanding job, two small children, a husband with an equally demanding job, and a mother who had just been diagnosed with cancer. She was experiencing headaches, rapid heartbeat, exhaustion, and an inability to concentrate. She reported feeling pressured throughout her waking hours and had difficulty sleeping. A physical examination had revealed no physical problems, and her physician had recommended medication, but she wanted to explore complementary approaches to her stress. She turned to music therapy as a possible treatment because she had heard of it through a friend whose handicapped son had benefited greatly from it. She was also a lifelong music lover, although she had never been trained musically.

During the initial intake and assessment by the music therapist, Maria reported having tried listening to calm music but was unable to relate to it; her mind raced, and she was unable to focus. Also, she didn't have much time in her day to devote to relaxation practices; she needed a method that would match what she was experiencing. She also needed a method that she could use during the day for a rapid stress reduction. The therapist described the entrainment process to her, and she thought that this might work well for her.

As the first step in the process, the music therapist asked Maria to try to describe her main stress symptoms (rapid heartbeat, headaches, and inability to concentrate) in detail and in musical terms (pitch, rhythm, timbre, etc.). The therapist asked specific questions about each symptom, and Maria had no difficulty in describing her symptoms as follows: (1) a rapid, even pulse on a low, single-pitched tone bar; (2) her headache as a sharp, arrhythmic, and sporadic strike on a cymbal; and (3) her inability to concentrate as a hand moving in circles over the head of a large hand drum producing a fuzzy, unfocused, multipitched sound. After the timbres, rhythms, and pitches of her symptoms were identified, Maria was asked to describe how these sounds fit together to best depict her experience of stress, for example, the underlying persistent rapid rhythm of her heartbeat, the intrusive, unpredictable pangs of pain with her headache, and the regular, periodic, though not continual sound of her lack of concentration. The therapist experimented with these sounds and, with feedback from Maria, was able to accurately match her stress symptoms musically.

In a similar manner, Maria was then asked to describe which musical sounds could heal her symptoms of stress. The therapist experimented with different sounds, and Maria selected the sound of the rain stick. On experimenting with these sounds, she felt that a noninstrumental, personal sound was needed. The therapist suggested vocal sounds and provided soft pitches for her in a lullaby-like, three-quarter meter. As the therapist demonstrated it for her, Maria immediately agreed that this was the exact nurturing music she needed. Again, the therapist reviewed with Maria how she felt these two sounds (rainstick and voice) should be integrated in the healing music.

In the next stage of the process, the therapist directed Maria in some simple breathing exercises, as she felt that Maria was becoming tense. The therapist told Maria about what would happen next Maria would lie back, close her eyes and listen, and the therapist would begin playing the "stress" music and gradually change to the "healing" music. She would be in charge of the points at which the "stress" music would begin and end and also when the "healing" music would begin and end. She would use predetermined hand signals to the therapist to indicate this. She would also use a different hand signal to tell the therapist if the music should be louder or softer. The therapist also told Maria that she would audiotape the music.

Maria felt very comfortable with her degree of control over the music and was able to lie back, close her eyes, and signal that the "stress" music should begin. The therapist placed the instruments close to Maria's body, and as she played the music improvisation, she used her own images, feelings, and cognitions, along with the music, to closely resonate with Maria's experience of stress. Maria listened intently to the music, signaling to the therapist to increase and lower its volume at different points.

After approximately 2 minutes of having the "stress" music played, Maria signaled that the "healing" music should begin. The therapist made a gentle and gradual transition between the two types of music, fading out the "stress" music and letting the "healing" music begin softly. The therapist noticed a dramatic decrease in Maria's breathing and muscle tension as she began to sing in lullaby-like musical phrases. Maria's face muscles lost their tension, and her breathing became shallow and regular; at times, she thought that Maria had drifted off to sleep. Again, the therapist used both the music and her own feelings, images, and thoughts to "be" with Maria in this experience. After about 10 minutes of the "healing" music, Maria signaled to the therapist to end the improvisation.

After the music stopped, the therapist gave Maria as much time as she needed to return to an alert state, after which time she processed the session verbally with her. Maria was amazed at how deeply she had relaxed. When asked how this had happened for her, she reported feeling that she was not alone during this experience and that she had felt the therapist's intimate presence and empathy, both musically and personally. This had been a very poignant experience for her, and she indicated that it was very rare for her to feel this level of support and emotional attunement with anyone. She was profoundly grateful for this, as she felt understood and validated. She also reported that when hearing the "stress" music, what had started as symptoms inside of her became externalized in the music. She was able to feel separate from them and look at them in a more objective manner. In doing this, she felt a level of control and empowerment over these reactions. The opposite happened with the "healing" music: What began as sounds external to her became internalized, and she could feel the voice and sounds of the rain stick as her own self-nurturing music. After further discussion, Maria revealed that she was very optimistic about the possibilities of entrainment in helping her overcome her stress. The therapist provided her with the tape of the music, and she was encouraged to use the tape during the day when her stress became problematic.

During subsequent sessions, Maria told the therapist that she used the tape regularly as she needed it. She was surprised to find that the headache, rapid heartbeat, and lack of focus had diminished significantly and were no longer as bothersome to her. She was also able to hear the healing music inside of herself without using the tape, and she did this frequently during the day as she found herself becoming anxious. As the symptoms of stress changed in quality, the therapist provided and audiotaped "stress" music that more closely matched her symptoms, although the "healing" music remained relatively the same. After four music therapy sessions over an 8-week period, Maria's stress seemed to be at a manageable level for her, and she was happier and more in charge of her life. Music therapy was terminated with the agreement that she would return in the future if her stress again became problematic.

COMMENTS AND REFLECTIONS

Music therapy is and will continue to be an important therapeutic modality for treating stress associated with a variety of conditions. We believe that the value of this therapeutic modality lies in its ability to address the *whole* person concurrently and simultaneously— that is, on physical, affective, cognitive, social, and spiritual levels. In addition, the range and flexibility of music therapy experiences, whether used as primary treatment or in combination with other stress management approaches, is extremely adaptable to use with an array of clients' needs. Music may provide a useful accompaniment to stress management approaches used by other professionals. Music is a noninvasive technique with few side effects and contraindications, with a relative ease of administration, with no stigma attached, and with evidence-based outcomes.

It is predicted that the need for music therapy as a primary or supportive therapy in stress reduction will continue to grow, as individuals seek treatment that is consistent with their need to manage their own health.

Ongoing music therapy research, particularly that concerning the immune system's responsiveness to music and the entrainment possibilities of music, will certainly open many new frontiers to music therapy practitioners. In addition, exciting new possibilities exist for further exploration of music's ability to enhance heart rate variability.

SUMMARY AND CONCLUSIONS

Music is a method of treatment that humankind has relied on for many centuries. Although music is a complex stimulus, and although responses to music are equally complex, research has supported the effectiveness of music therapy as a treatment modality for many clinical issues. Because music is a personal and unique experience for each individual, an individual's relationship to music is an important factor in designing music therapy treatment. It is unlikely that music programs designed "for the masses" will be ever be effective for all. Of all the reasons for the existence of music in virtually every culture, most salient is its ability to elicit and maintain human health, well-being, and quality of life.

REFERENCES

Note. * Indicates studies included in Dileo and Bradt (2005).

Aitken, J. C., Wilson, S., Coury, D., & Moursi, A. M. (2002). The effect of music distraction on pain, anxiety and behavior in pediatric dental patients. *Pediatric Dentistry, 24* (2), 114–118.

Baer, B. (1981). *An exploration of creative expression and relaxation as stress-resolving experiences: Some implications for chronically ill and severely disabled populations.* Unpublished doctoral dissertation, Ohio State University.*

Bailey, L. M. (1983). The effects of live music versus tape-recorded music on hospitalized cancer patients. *Music Therapy, 3,* 17–28.

Barger, D. A. (1979). The effect of music and verbal suggestion on heart rate and self-reports. *Journal of Music Therapy, 16*(4), 158–171.*

Bartlett, D. L. (1996). Physiological responses to music and sound stimuli. In D. Hodges (Ed.), *Handbook of music psychology* (pp. 343–386). San Antonio, TX: IMR Press.

Bernardi, L., Sleight, P., Bandinelli, G., Cencetti, S., Fattorini, L., Wdowczyc-Szulc, J., et al. (2001). Effect of rosary prayer and yoga mantras on autonomic cardiovascular rhythms: Comparative study. *British Medical Journal, 323,* 1446–1449.

Blanchard, B. (1979). The effect of music on pulse rate, blood pressure, and final exam scores of university students. *Journal of Sports Medicine, 19,* 305–307.*

Blood, D., & Ferriss, S. (1993). Effects of background music on anxiety, satisfaction with communication, and productivity. *Psychological Reports, 72,* 171–177.*

Boxberger, R. (1962). Historical bases for the use of music in therapy. In E. H. Schneider (Ed.), *Music therapy 1961: Eleventh book of proceedings of the National Association for Music Therapy* (pp. 125–166). Lawrence, KS: National Association for Music Therapy.

Brennan, F., & Charnetski, C. J. (2000). Stress and immune system function in a newspaper's newsroom. *Psychological Reports, 87,* 218–222.*

Bruscia, K. E. (1987). *Improvisational models of music therapy.* Springfield, IL: Thomas.

Bruscia, K. E. (1998). *Defining music therapy* (2nd ed.). Gilsum, NH: Barcelona.

Bruscia, K. E. (2002). Developments in music programming for the Bonny method. In K. E. Bruscia & D. E. Grocke (Eds.), *Guided imagery and music: The Bonny method and beyond* (pp. 307–316). Gilsum, NH: Barcelona.

Bruscia, K. E., & Grocke, D. E. (Eds.). (2002). *Guided imagery and music: The Bonny method and beyond.* Gilsum, NH: Barcelona.

Burns, D. S. (2001). The effect of the Bonny Method of Guided Imagery and Music on the mood and life quality of cancer patients. *Journal of Music Therapy, 38,* 51–65.

Burns S. J., Harbuz, M. S., Hucklebridge, F., & Bunt, L. (2001). A pilot study into the therapeutic effects of music therapy at a cancer help center. *Alternative Therapies in Health and Medicine, 7*(1), 48–56

Caine, J. (1991). The effects of music on the selected stress behaviors, weight, caloric and formula intake and length of hospital stay of premature and low birth weight neonates in a newborn intensive care unit. *Journal of Music Therapy, 28,* 180–192.

Chetta, H. D. (1981). The effect of music and desensitization on preoperative anxiety in children. *Journal of Music Therapy, 18,* 74–87.

Chlan, L. (1998, May–June). Effectiveness of a music therapy intervention on relaxation and anxiety for patients receiving ventilatory assistance. *Heart and Lung, 27*(3), 169–176.

Clair, A. A. (1996). *Therapeutic uses of music with older adults.* Baltimore: Health Professions Press.

Clark, M. E., McCorkle, R. R., & Williams, S. R. (1981). Music therapy-assisted labor and delivery. *Journal of Music Therapy, 18,* 88–100.

Codding, P. A. (2000). Music therapy literature and clinical applications for blind and severely visually impaired persons 1940–2000. In D. S. Smith (Ed.), *Effectiveness of music therapy procedures: Documentation of research and clinical practice* (pp. 159–198). Silver Spring, MD: American Music Therapy Association.

Corning, T. L. (1899). The uses of musical vibrations before and during sleep. *Medical Record, 55,* 79–86.

Dainow, E. (1977). Physical effects and motor responses to music. *Journal of Research in Music Education*, 25, 211–221.

Davis, C. A. (1992). The effects of music and basic relaxation instruction on pain and anxiety of women undergoing in-office gynecological procedures. *Journal of Music Therapy*, 29, 202–216.

Davis, W. B., & Thaut, M. H. (1989). The influence of preferred relaxing music on measures of state anxiety, relaxation, and physiological responses. *Journal of Music Therapy*, 26(4), 168–187.*

Davison, J. T. H. (1899, October). Music in medicine. *Lancet*, 1159–, 1162.

Dileo, C. (1997). Reflections on medical music therapy: Biopsychosocial aspects of the treatment process. In J. Loewy (Ed.), *Music therapy and pediatric pain* (pp. 125–144). Cherry Hill, NJ: Jeffrey Books.

Dileo, C. (Ed.). (1999a). *Music therapy and medicine: Theoretical and clinical applications*. Silver Spring, MD: American Music Therapy Association.

Dileo, C. (1999b). Introduction to *Music Therapy and Medicine:* Definitions, theoretical orientations and levels of practice. In C. Dileo (Ed.), *Music therapy and medicine: Theoretical and clinical applications* (pp. 1–10). Silver Spring, MD: American Music Therapy Association.

Dileo, C., & Bradt, J. (1999). Entrainment, resonance and pain-related suffering. In C. Dileo (Ed.), *Music therapy and medicine: Theoretical and clinical applications* (pp. 181–188). Silver Spring, MD: American Music Therapy Association.

Dileo, C., & Bradt, J. (2005). *Music therapy and medicine: A meta-analysis and agenda for future research*. Cherry Hill, NJ: Jeffrey Books.

Dileo, C., & Loewy, J. (Eds.). (2005). *Music therapy at the end of life*. Cherry Hill, NJ: Jeffrey Books.

Dileo, C., & Zanders, M. (2005). In-between: Music therapy with inpatients awaiting a heart transplant. In C. Dileo & J. Loewy (Eds.), *Music therapy at the end of life* (pp. 65–76). Cherry Hill, NJ: Jeffrey Books.

Eagle, C. T., Jr. (1972). *A review of human physiological systems and their response to musical stimuli*. Paper presented at the Southeastern Conference of the National Association for Music Therapy, Tallahassee, FL.

Edwards, M. C., Eagle, C. T., Jr., Pennebaker, J., & Tunks, T. (1990). Relationships among elements of music and physiological responses of listeners. In C. Dileo-Maranto (Ed.), *Applications of music in medicine* (pp. 41–57). Washington, DC: National Association for Music Therapy.

Elliott, W., Black, H. R., Alter, A., & Gavish, B. (2004). Blood pressure reduction with device-guided breathing: Pooled data from 7 controlled studies. *Journal of Hypertension*, 22(2), S116.

Elliott, W., Izzo, J., Jr., White, W. B., Rosing, D., Snyder, C. S., & Alter, A., (2004). Graded blood pressure reduction in hypertensive outpatients associated with use of a device to assist with slow breathing. *Journal of Clinical Hypertension*, 6(10), 553–559.

Field, T., Quintino, O., Henteleff, T., Wells-Keife, L., & Delvecchio Feinberg, G. (1997). Job stress reduction therapies. *Alternative Therapies in Health and Medicine*, 3(4), 54–56.*

Fisher, S., & Greenberg, R. (1972). Sedative effects upon women of exciting and calm music. *Perceptual and Motor Skills*, 34, 987–990.*

Fudin, N. A., Tarakanov, O. P., & Klassina, S. Y. (1996). Music as a means of improvement of students' functional state before an exam. *Human Physiology*, 22(3), 349–356.*

Gerra, G., Zaimovic, A., Franchini, D., Palladino, M., Guicastro, G., Reali, N., et al. (1998). Neuroendocrine responses of healthy volunteers to "technomusic": Relationships with personality traits and emotional state. *International Journal of Psychophysiology*, 28, 99–111.*

Gfeller, K. E. (1999). Music therapy in the schools. In W. B. Davis, K. E. Gfeller, & M. H. Thaut (Eds.), *An introduction to music therapy: Theory and practice* (pp. 259–272). Dubuque, IA: McGraw-Hill.

Goff, L. C., Pratt, R. R., & Madrigal, J. L. (1997). Music listening and S-IgA levels in patients undergoing a dental procedure. *International Journal of Arts Medicine*, 5(2), 22–26.

Gold, C., Bentley, K., & Wigram, T. (2003). Music therapy for schizophrenia or schizophrenia-like illnesses [Protocol for a Cochrane Review]. *Cochrane Database of Systematic Review*, 4. Chichester, UK: Wiley.

Gold, C., & Wigram, T. (2003). Music therapy for autistic spectrum disorder. In *Cochrane Database of Systematic Reviews*, 4. Chichester, UK: Wiley.

Grape, C., Sandgren, M., Hansson, L. O., Ericson, M., & Theorell, T. (2003). Does singing promote well-being? An empirical study of professional and amateur singers during a singing lesson. *Integrative Physiological and Behavioral Science*, 38(1), 65–74.

Grossman, E., Grossman, A., Schein, M. H., Zimlichman, R., & Gavish, B. (2001). Breathing control lowers blood pressure. *Journal of Human Hypertension*, 15(4), 263–269.

Guzzetta, C. E. (1989). Effects of relaxation and music therapy on patients in a coronary care unit with presumptive myocardial infarction. *Heart and Lung, 18,* 609–616.

Hamel, W. J. (2001). The effects of music intervention on anxiety in the patient waiting for cardiac catheterization. *Intensive and Critical Care Nursing, 17,* 279–285.

Hammer, S. E. (1996). The effects of guided imagery through music on state and trait anxiety. *Journal of Music Therapy, 33*(1), 47–70.*

Hanser, S. B. (1985). Music therapy and stress reduction research. *Journal of Music Therapy, 22,* 194–206.

Hilliard, R. E. (2003). The effects of music therapy on the quality and length of life of people diagnosed with terminal cancer. *Journal of Music Therapy, 40,* 133–137.

Hirokawa, E., & Ohira, H. (2003). The effects of music listening after a stressful task on immune functions, neuroendocrine responses, and emotional states in college students. *Journal of Music Therapy, 40*(3), 189–211.*

Hyde, I. M. (1927). Effects of music upon electrocardiograms and blood pressure. *Journal of Experimental Psychology, 7,* 213–224.

Jellison, J. A. (1975). The effects of music on automatic stress responses and verbal reports. In C. K. Madsen, R. D. Greer, & C. H. Madsen, Jr. (Eds.), *Research in music behavior: Modifying music behavior in the classroom* (pp. 206–219). New York: Teachers College Press, Columbia University.*

Jellison, J. A. (2000). A content analysis of music research with disabled children and youth (1974–1999): Applications in special education. In D. S. Smith (Ed.), *Effectiveness of music therapy procedures: Documentation of research and clinical practice* (pp. 199–264). Silver Spring, MD: American Music Therapy Association.

Keller, S., & Seraganian, P. (1984). Physical fitness level and autonomic reactivity to psychosocial stress. *Journal of Psychomatic Research, 28*(4), 279–287.*

Kibler, V., & Rider, M. (1983). Effects of progressive music relaxation and music on stress as measured by finger temperature response. *Journal of Clinical Psychology, 39*(2), 213–215.*

Knight, W. E., & Rickaed, N. (2001). Relaxing music prevents stress-induced increases in subjective anxiety, systolic blood pressure, and heart rate in healthy males and females. *Journal of Music Therapy, 38*(4), 254–272.*

Koger, S. M., Chapin, K., & Brotons, M. (1999). Is music therapy an effective intervention for dementia? A meta-analytic review of the literature. *Journal of Music Therapy, 36,* 2–15.

Kumar, A. M., Tims, F., Cruess, D. G., Mintzer, M. J., Ironson, G., Loewenstein, D., et al. (1999). Music therapy increases serum melatonin levels in patients with Alzheimer's disease. *Alternative Therapies in Health and Medicine, 5*(6),49–57.

Lacey, J. I. (1956). The evaluation of autonomic responses: Toward a general solution. *Annals of the New York Academy of Sciences, 67,* 123–164.

Lata, S., & Dwivedi, K. (2001). The effect of music on anxiety. *Psycho-Lingua, 31*(2), 143–146.*

Liebman, S. S., & MacLaren, A. (1991). The effects of music and relaxation on third trimester anxiety in adolescent pregnancy. *Journal of Music Therapy, 28,* 89–100.

Light, G. A., Love, D. M., Benson, D., & Morch, E. T. (1954). Music in surgery. *Current Researches in Anesthesia and Analgesia, 33,* 258–264.

Logan, T. G., & Roberts, A. R. (1984). The effects of different types of music on tension level. *Journal of Music Therapy, 21,* 177–183.

MacDonald, R., Mitchell, L., Dillon, T., Serpell, M. G., Davies, J. B., & Ashley, E. A. (2003). An empirical investigation of the anxiolytic and pain reducing effects of music. *Psychology of Music, 31*(2), 187–203.

Malone, A. (1996). The effects of live music on the distress of pediatric patients receiving intravenous starts, venipunctures, injections, and heel sticks. *Journal of Music Therapy, 23,* 19–33.

Maranto, C. D. (1991). A classification model for music and medicine. In C. D. Maranto (Ed.), *Applications of music in medicine* (pp. 1–6). Washington, DC: National Association for Music Therapy.

Maranto, C. D. (1992). A comprehensive definition of music therapy with an integrative model for music medicine. In R. Spintge & R. Droh (Eds.), *MusicMedicine* (pp. 19–29). St. Louis, MO: MMB Music.

Maratos, A., & Gold, C. (2003). Music therapy for depression [Protocol]. In *Cochrane Database of Systematic Reviews, 4.* Chichester, UK: Wiley.

McKinney, C. H. (1990). The effect of music on imagery. *Journal of Music Therapy, 27,* 34–46.

McKinney, C. H., Antoni, M. H., Kumar, A., & Kumar, M. (1995). The effects of guided imagery and music on depression and beta-endorphin levels in healthy adults: A pilot study. *Journal of the Association for Music and Imagery, 4, 67–78.* *

McKinney, C. H., Antoni, M. H., Kumar, M., Tims, F. C., & McCabe, P. M. (1997). Effects of guided imagery and music (GIM) therapy on mood and cortisol in healthy adults. *Health Psychology, 16,* 390–400.*

McKinney, C. H., & Tims, F. (1995). Differential effects of selected classical music on the imagery of high versus low imagers: Two studies. *Journal of Music Therapy, 32,* 22–45.

McKinney, C. H., Tims, F. C., Kumar, A. M., & Kumar, M. (1997). The effect of selected classical music and spontaneous imagery on plasma ß-endorphin. *Journal of Behavioral Medicine, 20*(1), 85–99.*

Meles, E., Giannattasio, C., Failla, M., Gentile, G., Capra, A., & Mancia, G. (2004). Nonpharmacologic treatment of hypertension by respiratory exercise in the home setting. *American Journal of Hypertension, 17,* 370–374.

Metera, A., Metera, A., & Warwas, I. (1975). Influence of music on the minute oxygen consumption and basal metabolic rate. *Anaesthesia, Resuscitation, and Intensive Therapy, 3* (3), 259–264.*

Montello, L. M., & Coons, E. E. (1998). Effects of active versus passive group music therapy on preadolescents with emotional, learning and behavioral disorders. *Journal of Music Therapy, 26,* 155–166.

Mornhinweg, G. (1992). Effects of music preference and selection on stress reduction. *Journal of Holistic Nursing, 10*(2), 101–109.*

Nayak, S., Wheeler, B., Shiflett, S. C., & Agostinelli, S. (2000). Effect of music therapy on mood and social interaction among individuals with acute traumatic brain injury and stroke. *Rehabilitation Psychology, 45*(3), 274–283.

Nieman, B. K., Pratt, R. A., & Maughan, M. L. (1993). Biofeedback training, selected coping strategies and music relaxation interventions to reduce debilitative musical performance anxiety. *Internaional Journal of Arts Medicine, II*(2), 7–15.*

O'Callaghan, C. C. (2001). Bringing music to life: A study of music therapy and palliative care experiences in a cancer hospital. *Journal of Palliative Care, 17*(3), 155–160.

O'Callaghan, C. C. (2005). Song-writing in threatened lives. In C. Dileo & J. Loewy (Eds.), *Music therapy at the end of life* (pp. 117–128). Cherry Hill, NJ: Jeffrey Books.

Parati, G., Izzo, J. L., Jr., & Gavish, B. (2003). Respiration and Blood Pressure. In J. L. Izzo & H. R. Black (Eds.), *Hypertension primer* (3rd ed., pp. 117–120). Baltimore: Lippincott, Williams & Wilkins.

Peach, S. (1984). Some applications for the clinical use of guided imagery and music. *Journal of Music Therapy, 21,* 27–34.

Pelletier, C. L. (2004). The effect of music on decreasing arousal due to stress: A meta-analysis. *Journal of Music Therapy, 41*(3), 192–214.

Peretti, P. (1975). Changes in galvanic skin response as affected by musical selection, sex, and academic discipline. *Journal of Psychology, 89,* 183–187.*

Peretti, P., & Zweifel, J. (1983). Affect of music preference on anxiety as determined by physiological skin responses. *Acta Psychiatrica Belgica, 83,* 437–442.*

Pratt, R. R., & Jones, R. W. (1987). Music and medicine: A partnership in history. In R. Spintge & R. Droh (Eds.), *Music in medicine* (pp. 377–388). Berlin, Germany: Springer-Verlag.

Quittner, A., & Glueckauf, R. (1983). The facilitative effects of music on visual imagery: A multiple measures approach. *Journal of Mental Imagery, 7,* 105–119.

Reitman, A. D. (1999). Performing arts medicine: Music therapy to treat anxiety in musicians. In C. Dileo (Ed.), *Music therapy and medicine: Theoretical and clinical applications* (pp. 53–68) Silver Spring, MD: American Music Therapy Association.

Rickson, D. J., & Watkins, W. G. (2003). Music therapy to promote prosocial behaviors in aggressive adolescent boys: A pilot study. *Journal of Music Therapy, 40*(4), 283–301.

Rider, M. (1997a). Entrainment music, healing imagery, and the rhythmic language of health and disease. In J. V. Loewy (Ed.), *Music therapy and pediatric pain* (pp. 81–88). Cherry Hill, NJ: Jeffrey Books.

Rider, M. (1997b). *The rhythmic language of health and disease.* St. Louis, MO: MMB Music.

Rider, M. (2000). Homeodynamic mechanisms of improvisational music therapy. In C. Dileo (Ed.), *Music therapy and medicine: Theoretical and clinical applications* (pp. 107–114). Silver Spring, MD: American Music Therapy.

Rider, M., Floyd, J., & Kirkpatrick, J. (1985). The effect of music, imagery, and relaxation on adrenal corticosteriods and the reentrainment of circadian rhythms. *Journal of Music Therapy, 22*(1), 46–58.*

Rider, M., Mickey, C., Weldin, C., & Hawkinson, R. (1990). The effects of toning, listening and singing on psychophysiological responses. In C. Dileo-Maranto (Ed.), *Applications of music in medicine* (pp. 73–84). Washington, DC: National Association for Music Therapy.

Robb, S. L. (2000). Music-assisted progressive muscle relaxation, progressive muscle relaxation, and silence: A comparison of relaxation techniques. *Journal of Music Therapy, 37*(1), 2–21.*

Robb, S. L. (2001). The effect of therapeutic music interventions on the behavior of hospitalized children in isolation: Developing a contextual support model of music therapy. *Journal of Music Therapy, 37*, 118–146.

Robb, S. L. (2003). Music interventions and group participation skills of preschoolers with visual impairments: Raising questions about music, arousal and attention. *Journal of Music Therapy, 40*(4), 266–282.

Robb, S. L., Nichols, R. J., Rutan, R. L., Bishop, B. L., & Parker, J. C. (1995). The effect of music assisted relaxation on preoperative anxiety. *Journal of Music Therapy, 32*(1), 2–21.

Rohner, S., & Miller, R. (1980). Degrees of familiar and affective music and their affects on state anxiety. *Journal of Music Therapy, 17*(1), 2–15.*

Rosenthal, T., Alter, A., Peleg, E., & Gavish, B. (2001). Device-guided breathing exercises reduce blood pressure and ambulatory and home measurement. *Americal Journal of Hypertension, 14*(1), 74–76.

Routhieaux, R. L., & Tansik, D. A. (1997). The benefits of music in hospital waiting rooms. *Health Care Supervisor, 16*(2), 31–40.*

Russell, L. (1992). Comparisons of cognitive, music and imagery techniques on anxiety reduction with university students. *Journal of College Student Development, 33*, 516–523.*

Saperston, B. (1995). The effects of consistent tempi and physiological interactive tempi on heart rate and EMG responses. In T. Wigram, B. Saperston, & R. West (Eds.), *The art and science of music therapy: A handbook* (pp. 58–82). London: Routledge.

Saperston, B. (1999). Music-based individualized relaxation training in medical settings. In C. Dileo (Ed.), *Music therapy and medicine: Theoretical and clinical applications* (pp. 41–52). Silver Spring, MD: American Music Therapy Association.

Scartelli, J. P. (1989). *Music and self-management methods: A physiological model.* St. Louis, MO: MMB Music.

Schein, M. H., Gavish, B., Herz, M., Rosner-Kahana, D., Naveh, P., Knishkowy, B., et al. (2001). Treating hypertension with a device that slows and regularises breathing: A randomised, double-blind controlled study. *Journal of Human Hypertension, 15*(4), 271–278.

Scheufele, P. M. (1999). Effects of progressive relaxation and classical music on measurements of attention, relaxation, and stress responses. *Journal of Behavioral Medicine, 23*(2), 207–228.*

Silverman, M. J. (2003).The influence of music on the symptoms of psychosis: A meta-analysis. *Journal of Music Therapy, 40*, 27–40.

Smith, C., & Morris, L. (1977). Differential effects of stimulative and sedative music on anxiety, concentration, and performance. *Psychological Reports, 41*, 1047–1053.*

Standley, J. M. (1986). Music research in medical/dental treatment: Meta-analysis and clinical implications. *Journal of Music Therapy, 23*(2), 50–55.

Standley, J. M. (2000). Music research in medical/dental treatment. In D. S. Smith (Ed.), *Effectiveness of music therapy procedures: Documentation of research and clinical practice* (pp. 1–64). Silver Spring, MD: American Music Therapy Association.

Standley, J. M. (2002). A meta-analysis of the efficacy of music therapy for premature infants. *Journal of Pediatric Nursing, 17*(2), 107–113.

Stanley, P., & Ramsey, D. (1998). The effects of electronic music-making as a therapeutic activity for improving upper extremity active range of motion. *Occupational Therapy International, 5*(3), 223–237.

Stanton, H. E. (1975). Music and test anxiety. *British Journal of Educational Psychology, 45*, 80–82.*

Staum, M. J., & Brotons, M. (2000). The effect of music amplitude on the relaxation response. *Journal of Music Therapy, 37*(1), 22–39.*

Stratton, V. (1992). Influence of music and socializing on perceived stress while waiting. *Perceptual and Motor Skills, 75*, 334.*

Stratton, V., & Zalanowski, A. (1984). The relationship between music, degree of liking, and self-reported relaxation. *Journal of Music Therapy, 21*(4), 184–192.*

Strauser, J. M. (1997). The effects of music versus silence on measures of state anxiety, perceived relaxation, and physiological responses of patients receiving chiropractic interventions. *Journal of Music Therapy, 34*(2), 88–105.*

Summer, S., Hoffman, J., Neff, J. A., Hanson, S., & Pierce, K. (1990). The effect of 60 beats per minute music on test taking anxiety among nursing students. *Journal of Nursing Education, 29,* 66–70.*

Thaut, M. H. (1989). The influence of music therapy interventions on self-rated changes in relaxation, affect and thought in psychiatric prisoner-patients. *Journal of Music Therapy, 26,* 155–166.

Thaut, M. H. (1992). Music therapy with autistic children. In W. B. Davis, K. E. Gfeller, & M. H. Thaut (Eds.), *An introduction to music therapy: Theory and practice* (pp. 180–196). Dubuque, IA: Brown.

Thaut, M. H. (1999). Music therapy in neurological rehabilitation. In W. B. Davis, K. E. Gfeller, & M. H. Thaut (Eds.), *An introduction to music therapy: Theory and practice* (pp. 259–272). Dubuque, IA: McGraw-Hill.

Thaut, M. H., & Davis, W. B. (1993). The influence of subject-selected versus experimenter-chosen music on affect, anxiety, and relaxation. *Journal of Music Therapy, 30*(4), 210–223.*

Tsao, C. (1989). Health communication: The relationship of the immune system to relaxation, music, imagery and emotional affect. (Doctoral dissertation, Temple University, 1989). *Dissertation Abstracts International, 50*(11A), 3537.*

Turry, A. (1997). The use of clinical improvisation to alleviate procedural distress in young children. In J. V. Loewy (Ed.), *Music therapy and pediatric pain* (pp. 89–96). Cherry Hill, NJ: Jeffrey Books.

Umemura, M., & Honda, K. (1998). Influence of music on heart rate variability and comfort: A consideration through comparison of music and noise. *Journal of Human Ergology, 27*(1–2), 30–38.

Unkefer, R. F., & Thaut, M. H. (2002). *Music therapy in the treatment of adults with mental disorders* (2nd ed.). St Louis, MO: MMB Music.

VanderArk, S., & Ely, D. (1994). University biology and music majors' emotional ratings of musical stimuli and their physiological correlates of heart rate, finger temperature and blood pressure. *Perceptual and Motor Skills, 79,* 1391–1397.*

Vincent, S., & Thompson, J. H. (1929). The effects of music upon the human blood pressure. *Lancet, 1,* 534–537.

Viskoper, R., Shapira, I., Priluck, R., Mindlin, R., Chornia, L., Laszt, A., et al. (2003). Non-pharmacological treatment of resistant hypertensives by device-guided slow breathing exercises. *American Journal of Hypertension, 16,* 484–487.

Walworth, D. D. (2003). The effect of preferred music genre selection versus preferred song selection on experimentally induced anxiety levels. *Journal of Music Therapy, 40*(1), 2–14.*

White, J. M. (1992). Music therapy: An intervention to reduce anxiety in the myocardial infarction patient. *Clinical Nurse Specialist, 6*(2), 58–63.

White, J. M. (1999). Effects of relaxing music on cardiac autonomic balance and anxiety after acute myocardial infarction. *American Journal of Critical Care, 8*(4), 220–230.

Wigram, T. (2004). *Improvisation: Methods and techniques for music therapy clinicians, educators and students.* London: Kingsley.

Wigram, T., & Dileo, C. (Eds.). (1997). *Music, vibration and health.* Cherry Hill, NJ: Jeffrey Books.

Wong, H. L. C., Lopez-Nahas, V., & Molassiotis, A. (2001). Effect of music therapy on anxiety in ventilator-dependent patients. *Heart and Lung, 30*(5), 376–387.

Yanagihashi, R., Ohira, M., Kimura, T., & Fujiwara, T. (1997). Physiological and psychological assessment of sound. *International Journal of Biometeorology, 40*(3), 157–161.

CHAPTER 21

Eye Movement Desensitization and Reprocessing and Stress

Research, Theory, and Practical Suggestions

LEE HYER
BONNIE KUSHNER

HISTORY OF THE METHOD

Eye-movement desensitization and reprocessing (EMDR) is now more than 15 years old. It was introduced by Francine Shapiro (1989) as a new treatment for traumatic memories. EMDR has been promulgated as a treatment for several disorders, including anxiety disorders, and especially posttraumatic stress disorder (PTSD) and other stress reactions (Shapiro, 1995). It has been applied with success to a variety of traumas and disorders, most notably combat trauma (e.g., Carlson, Chemtob, Rusnak, & Hedlund, 1996). In addition, it has been found to be effective for panic disorder (e.g., Feske & Goldstein, 1997), claustrophobia (Lohr, Tolin, & Kleinknecht, 1996), spider phobia (e.g., Muris & Merckelbach, 1997), and blood and injection phobias (Kleinknecht, 1993); for somatoform disorders, including chronic pain (Brown, McGoldrick, & Buchanan, 1997; Grant, 1999; Ray & Zbik, 2001; Wilson, Tinker, Becker, Hofmann, & Cole, 2000); dissociative disorders (e.g., Fine, 1994; Lazrove & Fine, 1996; Marquis & Puk, 1994; Rouanzoin, 1994; Young, 1994), and grief reactions (e.g., Solomon, 1994, 1995, 1998). It has been found effective with crime victims and police officers (e.g., Baker & McBride, 1991), with children suffering trauma from assault or natural disasters (e.g., Chemtob, Nakashima, Hamada, & Carlson, 2002; Cocco & Sharpe, 1993; Datta & Wallace, 1994, 1996; Greenwald, 1994, 1998, 1999), with sexual assault victims (Hyer, 1995; Parnell, 1994, 1999), with victims of accidents and patients having surgery (Blore, 1997; Hassard, 1993; McCann, 1992; Puk, 1992; Solomon & Kaufman, 1994), with victims of sexual dysfunction who are now able to maintain healthy sexual relationships (Levin, 1993; Wernik, 1993), with victims of chemical dependency and pathological gamblers (Henry, 1996; Shapiro & Forrest, 1997). It has also been shown to enhance performance (Crabbe, 1996; Foster & Lendl, 1995, 1996).

This chapter addresses several things. First, we consider the key features of EMDR, its theoretical foundations, and later its integration with other therapies. We consider the merits of the key (and controversial) components of EMDR and discuss the integration of EMDR in psychotherapy. We then consider the efficacy of EMDR in PTSD and examine meta-analyses and studies that evaluate this therapeutic program. We rate the salient studies of EMDR and PTSD. Then we discuss EMDR and its limitations and contraindications. Finally, we present the EMDR protocol and three cases that demonstrate the use of EMDR.

THEORETICAL FOUNDATIONS

EMDR is best formulated as a psychotherapy method with several component parts. It was developed as a treatment for PTSD. Over time, EMDR has been applied to many problems unrelated to trauma. In fact, EMDR addresses problems, not DSM diagnoses. Anything that the person finds problematic can serve as a target. From this position, adaptive information processing, the theory proposed by Shapiro (1995), has evolved. This theory argues that physiologically new information is processed to an adaptive state. Adaptive processing occurs because associations are forged with previously stored data, resulting in learning, in relief of emotional stress, and in growth. Memory networks in the cortex develop to contain these data, allowing links to occur and, by so doing, assisting a free flow of information. Trauma disrupts this process and is stored just as it is input, with all its distorted parts and perceptions. Given stasis, intrusions of the unprocessed sensory, affective, and cognitive elements result, causing dysfunctional reactions or symptoms. Eye movements or other dual-attention tasks, the theory holds, enhance information processing.

Shapiro (2001) applies the metaphor of trauma to all therapy problems as "little t" and "big T." "Big T" consists of trauma as it would be defined in the Diagnostic and Statistical Manual (DSM) for PTSD. "Little t" is just as pernicious. It consists of the barely noticeable and seemingly negligible occurrences that represent the slights of development that result in a position (on that issue) and a response (coping). Even a minor slight results in a lasting effect and a reaction that is persistent. If one is humiliated, for example, a whole series of internal and external movements occur to handle the humiliation. A person reacts to present stimuli with emotional–cognitive–physiological reactions that are stored in memory. The past is then repeated in the present through these filters. Over time, the person develops a personality style to handle situations. In the parlance of EMDR, in the case of little t's or big T's, memories are not metabolized, and new, related data are not fully processed, resulting in stress reactions. In this way, the past wraps around the present, and the present is perceived through the lens of the past. Data then are stored dysfunctionally. Van der Kolk (2002) believes that data are stored as sensations: "Trauma is not primarily imprinted on people's consciousness but in their sensate experience" (p. 78).

Consistent with many psychological therapies, then, EMDR assumes that most problems arise from faulty learning. In EMDR, however, the concept of learning is defined very broadly. Learning is viewed as a process that is not only cognitive but also sensory, affective, and physiological. This more holistic view of learning distinguishes EMDR somewhat from many other therapies. EMDR then targets data from the person—sensations, emotions, cognitions, behaviors.

TABLE 21.1. Candidates for Theoretical Foundations of EMDR

- Exposure—dosed exposure
- Placebo (expectation)
- Demand characteristics
- Distraction
- Neurobiological balance (pacemaker mechanism of rhythmic repetition)
- Rapid eye movement (sleep)
- Relaxation response
- Orienting response that disrupts the trauma associative network
- Mastery
- Counterconditioning
- Assimilation, as negative cognitions are assimilated and accommodated
- State-specific learning with corrective information
- Adaptive information processing

This, then, represents the theory of EMDR. At present, however, a lack of clarity about the influence of the operative mechanisms of EMDR remains. Dismantling studies are suspect. We do not yet know, for example, how thoughts, feelings, and behaviors are linked so that we can identify dysfunctional thoughts and common cognitive errors and help clients to generate more rational responses and to better appraise the world, themselves, and their trauma. This is no different from traditional cognitive-behavioral therapy (CBT) in which, for example, changes occur in the client even before they occur in the client's cognitive processes. Logically, in EMDR, a discrimination between remembering and reencountering occurs, as well as a differentiation of traumatic events from similar but safe ones. We can speculate that an association of trauma with mastery ("I can do this") also results. As a by-product, we also speculate that trauma memories are renarrated and become better organized.

Table 21.1 lists other constructs that have been offered as explanations for the processes of EMDR in trauma. Many apply to therapy in general, and all appear to have merit. Most are overlapping.

Speculation on EMDR Theory

Exposure is central to the theory of and intervention for PTSD. Too many data exist to eschew exposure as a curative component. There are, however, other characteristics that define EMDR. First and foremost, EMDR highlights cognition. EMDR addresses cognitions, both positive and negative, in a clear and transparent way. EMDR fosters living consciously. To think clearly is to liberate a process of thinking clearly. Consciousness then can operate at higher and lower levels of clarity and intensity. In any situation, the question is not whether one brings consciousness to it or not but whether one brings to it the level of consciousness required to be effective. As in most disorders, avoidance is the enemy—passivity, surrender, excessive need for help, loss of control, surrender, giving in to emotions. Branden (1997) says, "Like a light that can be turned brighter or dimmer, consciousness exists on a continuum" (p. 22).

EMDR also addresses affect and sensations. The client is asked to experience the moment and process the data. Often the client is directed to attend to the experience of the body and affect. In some ways such interventions are treasured above other experiences. Ideally, the person is activated at moderate levels of arousal, as the therapy is directed by the client. EMDR addresses all these with a "good enough" understanding of the person. Again, EMDR moves information. Van der Kolk (2002) says: "Because PTSD creates a kind of frozen sensory world, the therapeutic challenge is to open patient's minds to new possibilities so that they can encounter new experiences with openness and flexibility rather than interpreting the present as a continuous reliving of the past" (p. 64).

In therapy, EMDR keeps to the present. "Stay with that" is the mantra. It optimizes being present and experiencing sensations and emotions in the context of safety and ritualistic structure. It does so as a self-directed assimilation. Shapiro (1995) notes that it allows "the work of letting the person I am take over from the person I was." EMDR loosens up the free associative process, giving people rapid access to memories. Eventually other memories or ideas are connected. Hyer and Brandsma (1997) labeled this as *desensitization with free association*. These authors argued that EMDR is effective because it embodies sound principles of psychotherapy. According to Hyer and Brandsma (1997) and Fensterheim (1996), EMDR is a complex multicomponent, multistage process, blending many elements of other effective therapies into a comprehensive treatment protocol. Shapiro (1995, 1999) maintains that EMDR, with its brief exposures to associated material, external–internal focus, and structured therapeutic protocol, is a distinctly different form of therapy.

Table 21.2 lists EMDR treatment components and the integrative elements noted by Hyer and Brandsma (1997).

The fact that similar results may occur with exposure or other cognitive restructuring treatments does not mean that EMDR is a similar treatment. Based on Striker and Gold's (1996) criteria for psychotherapy integrative models, EMDR is a theoretical integration model that offers different perspectives at the levels of theory and practice. EMDR, then, is compatible with other techniques and can be used as a supplement. In her edited book, Shapiro (2002) provides a forum for varied therapists to provide input on the interaction of EMDR with their therapies. Lazarus and Lazarus (2002), for example, note that EMDR is an elegant BASIC-ID, a multimodal therapy that addresses Behavior, Affect, Sensations, Imagery, Cognition, Interpersonal actions, and Drugs. Wachtel (2002) also interacts with the client in a psychodynamic way and periodically interrupts with the question "Would you like to try EMDR for. . . . " Young and colleagues (Young, Zangwill, & Behary, 2002) also apply schema-focused therapy with EMDR.

Table 21.3 summarizes several treatment strategies to be followed by eye movements and perhaps other EMDR components.

TABLE 21.2. EMDR Treatment Components and Integrative Elements

EMDR components	EMDR components of psychotherapy
• Structure of method • Subjective units of distress • Exposure to feared stimuli • Negative and positive cognitions • Provision of new and corrective information • Relaxation • Instruction in self-control coping • Homework logs between sessions • Mindfulness emphasis • Minimal relationship	• Associative networks are unique to each person. • Growth motives control processing; unexpected sensations, associations, thoughts, images ascend. • Movement rules. • Nondirective therapy. • Power of treatment expectations. • Clean language. • Data chunked and alternatively experienced and processed. • Positive and negative cognitions. • Affect/sensation is respected most. • Therapist is blank screen.

TABLE 21.3. Integrative Methods with EMDR

1. Interpretation: "It sounds like . . . " and saccades
2. Interpretation: "What else comes to mind?" and saccades
3. Functional analysis and saccades
4. Socratic questions and saccades
5. Schemas and saccades
6. BASIC-ID and saccades
7. Accessing emotions and saccades
8. Relaxation method and saccades
9. Resources and saccades
10. Schema and saccades

Finally, we note that in the past 5 years, perhaps as a result of the empirically supported treatment (EST) debate, a synthesis is forming of the common factors approach, case-based methods, and the EST movement. On the case-based side, the emphasis has been on a nomothetically influenced, yet individual, case formulation of a patient. The disciplined inquiry (Peterson, 1991) has been supplemented by the pragmatic case study method (Fishman, 1999), as well as by evidence-based practice (Messer, 2004). Persons's (Persons, Davidson, & Tomkins, 2000) model of case formulation is a representation of this thinking. Under such a model, the case is assessed, formulated, and altered as a result of progress. Modules of treatment are applied as the case warrants, presumably as a result of empirically supported efficacy. On the EST side is the recommendation for the flexible manual (Wilson, 2005) and the process-influenced practice of the use of manuals (Schulte, 1996). This format obviates a stereotypic and routinized application of a manual.

EMDR represents a model of therapy for such a fusion. On the one side, it is manualized and is empirically supported. It has a set of procedures that allow for a structure in therapy that is reasonably specific. On the other side, EMDR is flexible. It allows the client to direct the process and progress of therapy. The therapist can apply more open interventions (e.g., cognitive interweave) or elect to use distinct protocols (see Shapiro, 1995). In addition, EMDR has been applied as a supplement to other therapies. In this context, then, EMDR is integrative, as it provides a theoretical structure and technology for use with related therapies.

Theory and PTSD

Based on reviews and data from Van Etten and Taylor (1998), Foa and Kozak (1997), Foa and Meadows (1997), and Marks (2000), as well as others, prolonged exposure (PE) and cognitive restructuring (CR) are the two curative components in the treatment of PTSD. In fact, they are equal in efficacy, and their combination is not supported. Only the combination of imaginal exposure and *in vivo* exposure is superior to either alone, and combining imaginal exposure with CR is preferable (Taylor et al., 2003). In practice, however, for most therapists the combination of PE and CR is one of emphasis, and optimal integration can be case based.

In truth, there have been successes in combining treatments for PTSD. Cloitre, Koenen, Cohen, and Han (2002) applied the skills training in affective and interpersonal regulation (STAIR) method that targets affect regulation, interpersonal skills, and PTSD symptoms. This treatment was found to be efficacious. The patient labels feelings, manages emotions, tolerates distress, and identifies trauma-based cognitions as a forerunner to exposure. This allows for an exposure in which appropriate coping can occur and in which the experience is more tolerable. Cognitive processing therapy (CPT; Resick & Schnicke, 1992), too, applies psychoeducational methods liberally before and during trauma exposure. Exposure is also "milder." The educational session describes the PTSD process and asks victims to write about the trauma. "Stuck points" are identified, and these problematic beliefs are targeted as the connection between events, thoughts, and feelings surfaces. In effect, the account of the trauma takes precedence over the exposure. Themes of safety, trust, control, esteem, and intimacy are identified and arguments practiced (Resick & Schnicke, 1992). This, too, is done carefully with trauma exposure. Interestingly, the application of CR and PE was found to have an especially great impact in cases of guilt (Resick & Schnicke, 1992) or of alienation and defeat (Ehlers et al., 1998).

Bryant and colleagues (Bryant, Harvey, Dang, Sackville, & Basten, 1998; Bryant, Moulds, Gutherie, Dang, & Nixon, 2003) also teach clients cognitive restructuring before imaginal exposure. Clients learn about dysfunctional unrealistic and catastrophic thoughts. In another study, Chard (2000) has clients read and process trauma accounts in individual sessions and only then participate in more in-depth CBT. This study, as well as the other studies reviewed on CR training, have yielded positive outcomes.

PTSD studies, then, suggest that both CR and PE are effective by themselves and that, if exposure is considered, it is most helpful to apply CR in careful doses at the beginning as a way to prepare for the coming exposure. This can be done in various ways. From the EMDR perspective, this process unfolds naturally. According to the theory, stored perceptions of the etiological event, which are defined as affect, are considered to be the core of the problem. This is state-dependent learning. The physiological storage of earlier life experiences is key to understanding behavior, personality, and experiences. As noted, data are stored in memories. In EMDR the process is one of information allocation: Data are moved and other information is accessed. Eventually there is an adaptive resolution: What is useful is learned and "placed," and what is useless is discarded. Internal "brain" connections are made. Van der Kolk (2002) notes, "EMDR activates a wide variety of unexpected sensations, feelings, images, and thoughts that are ordinarily not accessed in conjunction with other memories" (p. 162).

One additional aspect is added in the treatment of PTSD—relaxation. In EMDR, relaxation training is part of the protocol. It is probable that participants who are given relaxation training actually engage in more exposure due to their greater ability to handle stress. In fact, relaxation may work in the treatment of PTSD because it allows the patient to access action tendencies that are different from the usual trauma-related ones.

Data on the added value of relaxation as a treatment for PTSD, however, are lacking. Little information is available on the breadth or speed of its effects or on the incidence of symptom worsening. Marks, Lovell, Noshirvani, Livanou, and Thrasher (1998), for example, found that relaxation training was moderately effective in reducing the global severity of PTSD symptoms. Although these investigators found that relaxation tended to be less effective than exposure therapy, the effects of relaxation are noteworthy, because PTSD often remains unchanged in the absence of treatment (Taylor et al., 2003; van Etten & Taylor, 1998). Relaxation, then, might exert its effects by reducing hyperarousal symptoms. Once hyperarousal is reduced, the patient may be less distressed by trauma-related stimuli and, therefore, less avoidant. Thus relaxation training might encourage therapeutic exposure, even in the absence of formal exposure exercises.

One method of relaxation, autogenic training (AT), is related to EMDR. AT is similar to EMDR because it combines relaxing imagery, cognitive processing, and anxiety-provoking scenes directed by the client. In AT, sensations of the autonomic nervous system are activated cognitively by mantras related to areas of the body (arms, legs, solar plexus, heart rate, forehead). AT addresses both cognition and somatic elements. In fact, AT has been shown to have greater effects than progressive muscle relaxation (PMR) or electromyographic (EMG) biofeedback on autonomic measures and disorders associated with autonomic dysfunction. These effects have involved heart rate, blood pressure, and plasma norepinephrine (see Lehrer & Woolfolk, 1999). There is also evidence that AT may produce more vivid images and emotions than progressive relaxation (Borgeat, Stravynski, & Chalout, 1983). It also reduces cognitive problems, as in self-reported anxiety (see Lehrer & Woolfolk, 1999).

It may be, then, that relaxation as a component of EMDR has a robust effect on trauma or stress as it mixes well with self-regulation and cognitive elements, as well as reduced hyperarousal. Other processes involved in relaxation may include primary-process thinking, heightened suggestibility, rhythmical and monotonous stimulation, increased alpha and theta activity, and generally lower physiological activity. EMDR also fosters other mechanisms of relaxation, such as selective attention, reduced exteroceptive and proprioceptive sensory input, a receptive attitude, and relaxed posture.

ASSESSMENT/EFFICACY

Overall

A broad base of published case reports and controlled research support EMDR as an empirically validated treatment for trauma. The Department of Defense/Department of Veterans Affairs Practice Guidelines (2004) have placed EMDR in its highest category, recommended for all trauma populations. The American Psychiatric Association (2004) recommended EMDR for its empirical support and demonstrated effectiveness. In addition, current treatment guidelines of the International Society for Traumatic Stress Studies have designated EMDR as an effective treatment for PTSD (Chemtob, Tolin, van der Kolk & Pitman, 2000; Foa, Keane, & Friedman, 2000) as have the Northern Ireland Department of Health (CREST, 2001), the Israeli National Council for Mental Health (Belich, Kotler, Kutz, & Shaley, 2002), Swedish (Sjöblom et al., 2003), Dutch (Dutch National Steering Committee Guidelines for Mental Health Care, 2003), French (INSERM, 2004), and British (National Institute for Clinical Excellence, 2005). Most recently, Chambless et al. (1998) outlined criteria for empirically supported therapies. According to a task force of the Clinical Division of the American Psychological Association, the only methods empirically supported for the treatment of any PTSD population were EMDR, exposure therapy, and stress inoculation therapy (Chambless, et al., 1997). The American Psychiatric Association's *Practice Guideline on Acute Stress Disorder and Posttraumatic Stress Disorder* (2004) also has placed EMDR in the category of highest level of effectiveness.

EMDR has been compared with several types of controls, including waiting list and nonspecific treatment, as well as such accepted treatment methods as exposure (imaginal and *in vivo*). Like any evaluated treatment, it has been used with various populations using varied measures and with therapists trained at different levels, and it has been applied over different time periods. Its components have also been dismantled. In general, the results have been favorable and effect sizes acceptable. This applies even to those studies in which exposure has been the control treatment. Additionally, there have been several nonrandomized trials (Silver, Brooks, & Obenchain, 1995; Solomon & Kaufman, 1994; Sprang, 2001), which we do not review.

Meta-Analysis

Several meta-analyses have been done (Bradley, Greene, Russ, Dutra, & Westen, 2005; Davidson & Parker, 2001; Corsini, Lombardo, & DeGennaro, 2001; Van Etten & Taylor, 1998). Van Etten and Taylor (1998) assessed 61 treatment outcome trials from 39 studies of chronic PTSD. They examined the comparative efficacy of treatments using pharmacotherapies, psychological therapies (behavior therapy, EMDR, relaxation training, hypnotherapy, and dynamic therapy), and control conditions (pill-placebo, wait-list controls, supportive psychotherapies, and nonsaccade EMDR control). Results indicate that behavior therapy, selective serotonin reuptake inhibitors (SSRIs), and EMDR were the most effective treatments for PTSD. Salient findings were that EMDR needed fewer sessions than behavior therapy (3.7 vs. 10.1 weeks), with the best effect sizes.

Davidson and Parker (2001) evaluated 34 studies that examined EMDR with a variety of populations and measures. Many of the same studies were included. Process (validity of cognition [VoC] and subjective units of distress [SUDs]) and outcome measures were examined separately. When outcomes of EMDR treatment are compared with those of no treatment, and when outcomes are compared with pretreatment status, clients are better off with EMDR treatment than without. The median effect size, against a comparison of no treatment is robust ($r = .44$, $d = 0.98$), and this result is reproduced across studies, measures, and complaints. In addition, EMDR seems to be effective compared with nonspecific therapies. This median effect also is strong ($r = .40$, $d = 0.87$). When EMDR is assessed relative to other exposure-based treatments, the result is less optimistic. When outcome measures are considered, EMDR falls into an effect-size category with other treatments that have proven effective, such as exposure treatments for anxiety and cognitive-behavioral therapy for mood. The differences between EMDR and other effective exposure treatments are small ($r = .19$, $d = 0.39$ against exposure treatment not *in vivo* and $r = -.19$, $d = -0.39$ against *in vivo* exposure or cognitive-behavioral therapy).

Studies

We review the most relevant controlled studies investigating EMDR treatment of PTSD. Most of these studies involve civilian populations. Traumas include rape, physical violence, childhood abuse, natural disaster, accidents, and others. In general, there is a reduction in PTSD diagnosis of 60–90% in three to eight sessions. In the randomized studies, EMDR was roughly equivalent to cognitive-behavioral therapy (CBT), but EMDR took less treatment time and was well maintained at follow-up. Four controlled studies involve combat-related trauma. All addressed one or two memories or involved 1 to 12 sessions.

Boudewyns and Hyer (1996) built on an earlier study (Boudewyns, Stwertka, Hyer, Albrecht, & Sperr, 1993) and sought to evaluate the addition of EMDR and an EMDR analogue with eyes closed (EC) to standard group therapy. They randomly assigned 61 combat veterans with chronic PTSD to one of three conditions, EMDR, EC, or standard group therapy, the first two being add-ons to standard group therapy. Every participant received group therapy, with the EMDR and EC conditions also receiving five to seven treatment sessions of either EMDR or EC. Targets were one or two trauma memories. Participants in the EC and EMDR conditions showed superior improvement on mood and physiological (EMG and skin conductance) measures compared with group-therapy controls. Participants in all three conditions improved significantly on a structured interview measuring PTSD symptoms. There were no group differences. Limitations of the study include nontreatment of the majority of traumatic memories and concurrent group treatment received by participants. Treatment fidelity was assessed as a variable, based on reviews of videotapes of randomly selected sessions. A blind, trained independent interviewer conducted pre- and posttests. In sum, results indicate that the procedures of EMDR and an analogue of EMDR were effective in a treatment milieu of combat veterans.

In perhaps the best designed study on combat veterans, Carlson, Chemtob, Rusnak, Hedlund, and Muraoka (1998) randomly assigned 35 Vietnam War combat veterans with PTSD to a wait-list control or to 12 treatment sessions of biofeedback relaxation or EMDR. At posttreatment, the EMDR group had significantly lower scores on instruments measuring PTSD and depression than the wait-list group. At 3-month follow-up, the EMDR group had significantly lower scores than the biofeedback relaxation group on measures of PTSD and self-reported symptoms. Surprisingly, both treatment groups, as well as the wait-list control group, showed significant improvement on physiological measures, with no differences between groups and with the decrease in physiological arousal maintained at 3-month follow-up. The strengths of this study include provision of a full course of treatment to combat veterans and comparison with another treatment, relaxation. This study controlled for therapist allegiance, as the participants who did not receive EMDR received the therapist's preferred treatment. Only one posttreatment assessment was conducted by a trained independent rater blinded to conditions at 9-month follow-up. It was completed for 9 of the 10 EMDR participants, and confirmed the maintenance of treatment effects, with 78% of the EMDR participants no longer meeting diagnostic criteria for PTSD.

Lee and Gavriel (1998) randomly assigned 22 civilian participants with PTSD to stress inoculation training with prolonged exposure (SITPE) or to EMDR. After serving as their own controls during a wait-list period, participants were provided with seven 60-minute treatment sessions. Measures were collected at pre- and posttreatment and at 3-month follow-up. Both EMDR and SITPE were found to be effective, with significant improvement on PTSD and depression measures. At follow-up 83% of the EMDR and 75% of the SITPE participants no longer met PTSD criteria. The only difference found between groups was on the Intrusion subscales of the PTSD measures, with the EMDR group showing significantly greater improvement. The trained interviewer was not blind or independent. Fidelity checks were satisfactory for both treatments. Strengths of this study include its comparison with an empirically validated treatment, SITPE. This study indicates that EMDR and SITPE may be fairly equivalent in treatment effectiveness. Interestingly, EMDR required an average of only 3 hours of homework; SITPE required 28 hours.

Marcus, Marquis, and Sakai (1997) compared EMDR with "standard Kaiser care" (SKC) at Kaiser Permanente in an outpatient health maintenance organization (HMO). SKC consisted of individual therapy (cognitive, psychodynamic, or behavioral). Sixty-seven individuals with PTSD (with both single and multiple traumas) were randomly assigned to either EMDR or SKC treatment and received an unlimited number of 50-minute treatment sessions. EMDR participants attained symptom reduction with significantly greater rapidity and had significantly fewer treatment sessions than SKC participants. EMDR produced significantly lower scores than SKC, after 3 sessions and at posttreatment, on measures of PTSD symptoms, depression, and anxiety. After three sessions, 50% of the EMDR participants no longer met criteria for PTSD, compared with 20% of the SKC group. At posttreatment, 77% of the EMDR group (including 100% of the single-trauma victims) no longer met criteria for PTSD compared with 50% of the

SKC group. The following complications were noted: independent interviewer (with unspecified training) not blind to treatment condition due to participant response; excessive treatment comparisons made without statistical corrections; the unknown quality of the comparison condition; and a confusing number of medication-related supervision appointments. Strengths of this study include its high external validity: This study indicates that EMDR may be superior to the wide variety of treatments used in an HMO setting. A follow-up study revealed similar results (Marcus, Marquis, & Sakai, 2004).

Rogers et al. (1999) provided a single session of EMDR or exposure therapy treatment. Twelve combat veterans with PTSD were randomly assigned to one of the treatment conditions. The session focused on the most distressing identified combat memory and used measures designed to be sensitive to change on that one treated memory. Both groups significantly improved on a trauma measure as it was applied to that particular memory. A posttest measure in which participants monitored the severity of intrusive recollections for the one memory showed a significant decrease for the EMDR group compared with the exposure group. Pre- and postassessments were done by an independent blind assessor. This study had many weaknesses: There was only one session (especially problematic for the exposure group); treatment fidelity was not reported; outcome measures consisted of self-reports; and process measures were applied.

Rothbaum (1997) treated 18 adult female rape victims with PTSD. They were randomly assigned either to four 90-minute sessions of EMDR or to a wait-list control group. The self-report scores of the EMDR participants on PTSD and depression scales were significantly lower than those of wait-list controls. At posttreatment, 90% of the participants in the EMDR group no longer met full criteria for PTSD compared with 12% of the wait-list group. Results were evaluated by a trained, blind independent assessor using structured interviews and self-report measures. Rothbaum was the only therapist for participants in the initial EMDR condition, but other therapists were added for the delayed treatment condition, which followed the same pattern of recovery, mitigating against the confound of therapist effects. Other weaknesses included the small sample size, the fact that participants received concurrent treatment, and that a wait-list control was used.

Scheck, Schaeffer, and Gillette (1998) compared EMDR with an active-listening (AL) control in a group of 60 traumatized young women who were engaging in high-risk behavior, such as sexual promiscuity, running away, or substance abuse. Using a structured interview, 77% were diagnosed with PTSD. The women received two 90-minute treatment sessions and were given a homework assignment of journal writing. The effects of EMDR were significantly greater than those of AL on all measures except self-concept. Treatment gains were maintained at 3-month follow-up for both groups. Posttreatment measures were collected by a trained, independent, blind assessor, but they did not include a structured diagnostic interview. Limitations of this study include the reduced dose of EMDR, the mixed sample (some did not have PTSD), the lack of posttreatment assessment of PTSD diagnosis, the weakness of the control condition, and the lack of treatment integrity ratings. Strengths of this study include use of a blind independent assessor and reliable measures. These results indicate that EMDR is superior to a condition that controls for some of the nonspecific effects of treatment, such as attention, therapeutic rapport, and active listening.

Vaughan et al. (1994) assigned 36 civilian participants, 78% of whom were diagnosed with PTSD, to either EMDR, imaginal exposure (image habituation training; IHT), applied muscle relaxation (AMR) training or a wait list. Those participants without PTSD failed to meet only criterion C of the DSM-IV, which requires three avoidance symptoms. Three to five treatment sessions were administered, with daily homework assigned to the IHT and AMR groups only. The IHT group listened daily for 60 minutes to an audiotaped description of their trauma and recorded their thoughts and feelings. All treatments led to significant decreases in depression and PTSD symptoms for participants in the treatment groups as compared with those on the waiting list. A comparison between treatment groups found a significantly greater reduction at posttreatment for the EMDR group on PTSD intrusive symptoms. At follow-up, 70% of participants in all treatment groups no longer met PTSD diagnostic criteria. Limitations of this study include the lack of treatment fidelity ratings, a limited number of treatment sessions, and different amounts of treatment received by the groups, with additional daily homework time in the AMR and IHT groups. Strengths include blind independent assessments and reliable measures, as well as a comparison of EMDR with an exposure treatment.

Wilson, Becker, and Tinker (1995) randomly assigned a sample of 80 traumatized individuals to wait-list or EMDR conditions. Only half the participants met criteria for PTSD. Participants received three 90-minute sessions of EMDR. At posttreatment and 3-month follow-up, significant differences were found between EMDR and wait-list groups on measures of PTSD symptoms, depression, and anxiety. When treatment was provided to the wait-list group, treatment effects were replicated, with significant effects for all measures. A linear regression analysis indicated that treatment gains did not vary as a function of pretreatment symptom severity or PTSD diagnosis. Treatment fidelity was assessed, and a trained, blind independent assessor administered all self-report measures. In a 15-month follow-up study (Wilson, Becker & Tinker, 1997), 32 of the original 37 participants with PTSD were interviewed by an independent assessor. There was an 84% reduction in PTSD diagnosis compared with pretreatment. The original study is limited by the lack of a structured interview to assess posttreatment diagnosis and by the wait-list design. Because this design does not control for influences during the 15-month period, it is not possible to conclude that the maintenance of posttreatment outcome resulted solely from EMDR treatment effects.

Devilly, Spence, and Rapee (1998) assigned 51 combat veterans with PTSD in nonrandom blocks to one of three conditions: standard psychiatric support (SPS) at other settings, two sessions of EMDR, or two sessions of an EMDR variant (REDDR) in which participants concentrated on a stationary flashing light. Most participants were also receiving other concurrent mental health treatment. At posttreatment all groups showed significant improvement on measures of PTSD, depression, anxiety, and problem coping. There were no differences between the three groups. Measures of reliable change, a more stringent measure indicating change, showed that 67% of the EMDR group, 42% of the REDDR group, and 10% of the SPS group were reliably improved. Forty-six percent of the veterans did not mail back their follow-up measures, and the authors note a diminishing of treatment effect over time. Unfortunately, this study lacked random assignment, because participants were assigned in nonrandom blocks. There was also only one therapist. Additionally, a trained assessor was not blinded to conditions, and treatment delivery did not follow standard protocols. Other limitations include use of different assessment procedures at pre- and posttest, concurrent mental health treatment, and an insufficient number of sessions for multiply traumatized veterans.

Devilly and Spence (1999) compared a CBT variant developed by Devilly, trauma treatment protocol (TTP), with EMDR. TTP is a treatment package combining elements of CBT, stress inoculation training, and prolonged exposure. Twenty-three civilian participants with PTSD were assigned in nonrandom blocks to eight sessions of either EMDR or TTP. After the initial session, 31% of EMDR participants dropped out of treatment before receiving any EMDR. Both EMDR and TTP were significantly effective on all measures. TTP was significantly more effective than EMDR on combined PTSD measures and on a scale of global function. At 3-month follow-up, scores on a self-report PTSD measure indicated that 58% of the TTP participants no longer met PTSD criteria on a self-report measure compared with only 18% of the EMDR group. Limitations of this study include the large dropout rate, the number of statistical analyses done (allowing type I error), change in assessment procedures at posttest, lack of an independent blind assessor, and partial randomization. One therapist provided treatment to every participant in the TTP condition and to most EMDR participants. Furthermore, indications are that there were deficiencies in treatment delivery of EMDR.

In an early study, Jensen (1994) randomly assigned 25 Vietnam War combat veterans suffering from PTSD to a wait-list condition or to two sessions of EMDR. Most of the veterans were receiving concurrent treatment. No difference was found between groups at posttreatment. Instead of improving, the condition of the veterans actually deteriorated. To assess outcome, the researchers used a diagnostic instrument that was insufficient to measure the small amount of change that may have been achieved in two sessions. Other limitations include poor treatment fidelity, lack of a trained, blind, independent assessor, an insufficient number of sessions, and concurrent treatment. The wait-list condition was confounded by participants' being informed that no treatment would be provided and encouraged to seek treatment elsewhere.

Taylor et al. (2003) examined the efficacy, speed, and incidence of symptom worsening of three treatments for PTSD: prolonged exposure, relaxation training, and EMDR. Participants all received eight 90-minute sessions of individual therapy. Sixty people with PTSD (45 of whom completed treatment) received treatment. All three treatments were effective. The percentages of patients who no longer met criteria for PTSD at both posttreatment and follow-up were: 80% for the exposure group, 53% for the EMDR group, and 33% for the relaxation group. Exposure was significantly superior to relaxation. EMDR and exposure were no different. Exposure did produce greater reductions in avoidance and reexperiencing symptoms than did EMDR or relaxation. In a follow-up study (Taylor, 2004), treatment credibility was related to better treatment outcomes. Strengths include defined target symptoms, reliable and valid measures, blind evaluators, adequately trained assessors, manualized treatments, random assignment to treatment, and evaluation of treatment adherence. Limitations included a sample that had severe, chronic PTSD.

In a later study, Lee, Gavriel, Drummond, Richards, and Greenwald (2002) evaluated the effectiveness of SITPE versus EMDR. Participants ($N = 24$: mean age = 35.3 years) who had diagnoses of PTSD were randomly assigned to one of the treatment conditions. Participants also served as their own wait-list controls. Outcome measures included self-report and observer-rated measures of PTSD and self-report measures of depression. On global PTSD measures, there were no significant differences between the treatments at the end of therapy. However, on the subscale measures of the degree of intrusion symptoms, EMDR did significantly better than SITPE. At follow-up EMDR was found to lead to greater gains on all measures. Participants in the EMDR condition showed greater gains at 3-month follow-up. As before, the trained interviewer was not blind or independent. Strengths of this study include the comparison with an empirically validated treatment, SITPE. Again, EMDR required an average of only 3 hours of homework; SITPE required 28 hours.

Ironson, Freund, Strauss, and Williams (2002) conducted a pilot study that compared the efficacy of EMDR and PE for PTSD. Data were analyzed for 22 patients from a university-based clinic serving the outside community (predominantly rape and crime victims) who completed at least one active session of treatment after three preparatory sessions. Results showed that both approaches produced a significant reduction in PTSD and depression symptoms, which was maintained at 3-month follow-up. Successful treatment was faster with EMDR, as a larger number of people (7 of 10) showed a 70% reduction in PTSD symptoms after three active sessions, compared with 2 of 12 with PE. EMDR had a lower dropout rate than PE (0 of 10 vs. 3 of 10). However, all patients who remained in treatment with PE showed a reduction in PTSD scores. Weaknesses of this study included pretreatment preparation, no diagnostic evaluation, use of only self-report measures, no blind reviewers, application of few sessions, use of graduate students as therapists, and use of process measures.

Summary

Other reviews exist. They argue for PTSD but do so for other reasons than objectively evaluating studies (e.g., Shapiro & Maxfield, 2002; Maxfield, Lake, & Hyer, 2004). One review (Rubin, 2003) noted that although EMDR is effective with adults with single trauma, it is less effective when the focus is not children, combat PTSD, and multiple-trauma PTSD. Other earlier reviews (e.g., Herbert et al., 2000 [au, not in refs]; Lohr, Tolin, & Lilienfeld, 1998) believe that EMDR is basically exposure and that the use of eye movements is unnecessary and even gimmicky. EMDR is effective as a treatment for PTSD. In general, on outcome measures EMDR is effective when posttest measures are compared with pretest measures within participants and when EMDR is compared with wait-list/no-treatment or nonspecific treatment controls, regardless of the training of the therapists. Several studies compared EMDR with treatments whose efficacy for PTSD was unknown or not established. These include biofeedback relaxation (Carlson et al., 1998), applied muscle relaxation training (Taylor et al., 2003; Vaughan et al., 1994), active listening (Scheck et al., 1998), and standard care in an HMO (Marcus et al., 1997). Because these treatments provide nonspecific therapeutic effects, such as attention, therapeutic alliance, expectations, and placebo effects, these studies can be said to control for such effects. Such treatments may also contain some active ingredients whose role cannot be specified. These studies found EMDR to be significantly more effective than the other comparison treatments. EMDR was also superior to wait-list conditions (Rothbaum, 1997; Wilson et al., 1995, 1997).

Other studies also exist that find for the efficacy of EMDR; female survivors (Edmond, Rubin, & Wambach, 1999; Edmond, Sloan, & McCarty, 2004; Jaberghaderi, Greenwald, Rubin, Dolatabadim, & Zand, 2004; Rothbaum, Astin, & Marsteller, 2005; Scheck, Schaeffer, & Gillette, 1998), adults (Power, McGoldrick, Brown, et al., 2002, children (Soberman, Greenwald, & Rule, 2002), as well as medications (e.g., van der Kolk, Burbridge, & Suzuki, 1997). The best test of a treatment is a comparison with another treatment known to be effective. EMDR is not shown to be more effective than exposure therapies. Five of the covered studies compared EMDR with behavioral and CBT therapies. Three of these studies (Lee & Gavriel, 1998; Rogers et al., 1999; Vaughan et al., 1994) indicated that EMDR and CBT were equivalent, although EMDR may have been more effective with intrusive symptoms and also more efficient, requiring no homework and less time. This is in contrast to the findings of Taylor et al. (2003) and one of the three less rigorous studies (Devilly & Spence, 1999), both of which found CBT superior to EMDR.

Table 21.4 provides a brief view of EMDR and outcomes. EMDR fares well in the treatment of PTSD, being marginally superior to exposure and equal in effectiveness to CBT.

TABLE 21.4. EMDR Outcomes

- Waiting-list controls: EMDR effective.
- Placebo: EMDR effective.
- Extant non-CBT treatments: EMDR effective.
- Exposure: EMDR and exposure effective.
- CBT: Both EMDR and CBT effective.
- Maintenance effects: EMDR effective.
- Necessity of eye movements: Mild or little effect, but some element of dual attention seems important.

Maxfield and Hyer

We can see that the efficacy of EMDR varies across studies. The results attained in treatment outcome studies are intrinsically related to the methods employed to evaluate outcome. Research design, type of measures, sample selection and size, treatment delivery, and assessment are elements that may influence treatment outcome (Kazdin, 1994). Many methodological concerns permeated the research we have reviewed here. They include nonblind raters, too few sessions, poor treatment integrity, samples given multiple therapies, and insensitive measures.

Maxfield and Hyer (2002) sought to determine whether differences in outcome were related to methodological differences. They reviewed the research to identify methodological strengths, weaknesses, and empirical findings. They assessed the relationships between effect size and methodology ratings using the Gold Standard (GS) Scale (modified criteria from Foa & Meadows, 1997). Results indicated a significant relationship between scores on the GS Scale and effect size and between effect size and treatment fidelity. Unfortunately, the GS Scale did not assess everything important. Additional methodological components not detected by the GS Scale were identified and assessed. The researchers hypothesized that concurrent treatment confounds, lack of interviews, absence of multimodal measures, and inadequate course of treatment length would be associated with lower effect sizes. To determine whether these factors influenced outcome, three more methodological standards were devised and added to the GS Scale, creating the Expanded GS Scale.

The Expanded GS Scale consists of the original seven standards plus three additional standards. To evaluate methodology in treatment outcome studies, Foa and Meadows (1997) developed a set of seven GSs. These include the following: (1) *Clearly defined target symptoms*, so that appropriate measures can be employed to assess improvement, with specifications of inclusion and exclusion criteria; (2) *reliable and valid measures*, with good psychometric properties; (3) *use of blind evaluators*, other than the treatment provider, to collect assessment measures; (4) *assessor training*, with demonstrated interrater reliability; (5) *manualized, replicable, specific treatment programs*, to ensure consistent and replicable treatment delivery; (6) *unbiased assignment to treatment*, either random assignment to conditions or stratified sampling, with treatment delivered by at least two therapists; (7) *treatment adherence*, evaluated by treatment fidelity ratings. Additional items were designed to measure each of the preceding possible methodological shortcomings: GS 8, *no confounded conditions*; GS 9, *use of multimodal measures*; GS 10, *adequate course of treatment*. Based on the observation that multiple-trauma survivors require more extensive treatment, GS 10 was operationalized to evaluate the adequacy of treatment length, differentiating between combat veterans (multitrauma) and civilian participants. GS 10 differentiates by actual number of sessions. Differences between raters were resolved by consensus and/or by assigning the lower rating (Table 21.5).

Fifteen controlled studies noted previously in this chapter were reviewed. Where information in the studies was incomplete or unclear, the researchers were contacted to ensure accuracy. The methodological rigor of each study was assessed by three raters who had applied Foa and Meadow's (1997) GS to pre- and posttreatment methods. Pre–post effect sizes and comparison effect sizes were calculated. Pre–post effect sizes (ESs) were calculated for the primary PTSD measure used in each study using Cohen's d statistic (the difference of the pretreatment mean minus posttreatment mean, divided by the pooled standard deviation). Comparison ESs were also calculated (the difference of posttreatment means, divided by the pooled standard deviation).

Each of these GSs was measured on a 3-point Likert scale, and the scores are given in Table 21.6. Also, the group that had the higher ES was checked on reliable measures. In fact, the Expanded GS Scale scores ranged from 4.0 to 8.5, with a mean of 6.9 and a SD of 1.41. The addition of these three methodological items appeared to provide better differentiation among the studies and to result in a more comprehensive evaluation of methodological strength. The studies that were above the mean GS had an average ES of 1.63; the studies below the mean had an average ES of 0.66.

There was a significant relationship between outcome and methodology for the EMDR condition, $R = .81$, $F(1,10) = 19.52$, $p = .001$, and for the control conditions, $R = .63$, $F(1,10) = 6.7$, $p = .03$. To explore the relationship between ES and the additional GS items, regressions were conducted between ES and GS 8, 9, and 10. One-tailed tests were used for these secondary analyses. ES had significant correlations with GS 8 (no confounded conditions), $R = .56$, and with GS 10 (adequate course of treatment), $R = .56$. The correlation between ES and number of sessions was not significant ($R = .28$). The correlation for GS 9 (use of multimodal measures) was nonsignificant, even when GS 3 (use of blind independent assessor) was controlled for. The results suggest that when the aggregate evidence for EMDR's efficacy is considered, greater weight should be given to studies with more rigorous methodology; such studies found EMDR to be an efficacious treatment for PTSD.

These findings indicate a strong relationship between methodology and outcome. As methodology becomes more rigorous, the treatment effect becomes larger. The relationship between methodology and outcome is apparent when the studies are grouped according to methodological strength. The more rigorous methodological studies achieved large ESs and indicated that EMDR was efficacious, and more efficacious than control conditions.

Critical Issues

We now consider problems related to EMDR research. First, the EMDR protocol applies process measures as part of the treatment. Several studies have tested EMDR using process measures, ratings of subjective units of distress (SUDs) elicited by the fear-provoking images and validity of cognition (VoC) ratings of the new cognitions to be associated with the images. This was true of Shapiro's original study (Shapiro, 1989). These are measures used to determine when phases of treatment end. Ideally, EMDR treatment generally continues until both SUD and VoC reach a criterion value (Shapiro, 1995). These measures are integral to the treatment. In the meta-analysis by Davidson and Parker

TABLE 21.5. Gold Standard (GS) Scale

GS 1 Clearly defined target symptoms.
    0: no clear diagnosis, symptoms not clearly defined.
    .5: not all participants with PTSD, clear defined symptoms.
    1: all participants with PTSD

GS 2 Reliable and valid measures.
    0: did not use reliable and valid measures.
    .5: measures used were inadequate to measure change.
    1: reliable, valid, and adequate measures.

GS 3 Use of blind independent assessor.
    0: assessor was therapist.
    .5: assessor was not blind.
    1: assessor was blind and independent.

GS 4 Assessor training.
    0: no training in administration of instruments used in the study.
    .5: training in administration of instruments used in the study.
    1: training with performance supervision, or reliability checks.

GS 5 Manualized, replicable, specific treatment.
    0: treatment was not replicable or specific.
    1: treatment followed EMDR training manual (Shapiro, 1995).

GS 6 Unbiased assignment to treatment.
    0: assignment not randomized.
    .5: only one therapist *or* other semirandomized designs.
    1: unbiased assignment to treatment.

GS 7 Treatment adherence.
    0: treatment fidelity poor.
    .5: treatment fidelity unknown, or variable.
    1: treatment fidelity checked and adequate.

GS 8 No confounded conditions.
    0: most participants receiving concurrent psychotherapy.
    0.5: a few participants receiving concurrent psychotherapy, or
       unspecified and no exclusion for concurrent treatment.
    1: no subjects receiving concurrent psychotherapy.

GS 9 Use of multimodal measures.
    0: self-report measures only.
    .5: self-report plus interview or physiological or behavioral measures.
    1: self-report plus two or more other types of measures.

GS 10 Adequate course of treatment: Length of treatment for civilian
      participant studies.
    0: 1–2 sessions.
    .5: 3–4 sessions.
    1: 5+ sessions

    Length of treatment for combat veteran participant studies.
    0: 1–6 sessions.
    .5: 7–10 sessions.
    1: 11+ sessions.

Note. Data from Foa and Meadows (1997).

TABLE 21.6. Gold Standards and Effect Size

Study	Total 10	EMDR	Control
Boudewyns & Hyer (1996)	7.5	×	
Carlson et al. ()	8.5	×	
Devilly et al. (1998)	4.0	×	
Devilly & Spence (1999)	6.5		×
Jensen (1994)	4.5		×
Lee & Gavriel (1998)	8.0	×	
Marcus et al. (1997)	8.0	×	
Rogers et al. (1999)	6.5	×	
Rothbaum (1997)	8.0	×	
Scheck et al. (1998)	6.5	×	
Vaughan et al. (1994)	7.5	×	
Wilson et al. ()	7.5	×	
Taylor et al. (2003)	8.0		×
Ironson et al. (2002)	7.0	×	
Lee et al. (2002)	7.5	×	

(2001), within-subject comparisons on process measures (SUD and VoC) do show a robust ES ($r = .81$, $d = 2.71$, based on 12 comparisons). The ESs for better outcome measures are, however, much more modest. Several (e.g., Lohr, Tolin, & Kleinknecht, 1996; Lohr et al., 1998) have raised the criticism that progress through the stages of EMDR is conditional on changes in reported SUD and VoC measures. Critics (Acierno, Hersen, Van Hasselt, Tremont, & Mueser, 1994; Herbert & Mueser, 1992) advocated standardized measures of treatment outcome, and most recent studies have included a variety of these.

Second, recent descriptions of EMDR suggest that more than a single session is needed (Feske, 1998). The treatment manual (Shapiro, 1995) indicates that EMDR is "not one-session therapy" (p. 117), often requiring at least 12 sessions (p. 325). It is now reasonably established that EMDR requires a full protocol (discussed later in the chapter), including adequate time within session to allow the dose of assimilation and exposure, as well as the unique features of the method, to take hold.

Third, the relationship of EMDR and exposure is still in doubt. The effects of EMDR may be due largely to imaginal exposure during sessions. Interestingly, done well, exposure (in EMDR) may facilitate more time on task and result in more naturally occurring in vivo exposure. The key question is how EMDR fares with exposure therapy in the strict sense. As noted earlier, the results have been mixed; some research suggests that exposure-based treatment is more effective than EMDR (Devilly & Spence, 1999; Taylor et al., 2003), whereas other studies suggest that EMDR is somewhat more effective (Ironson et al., 2002; Lee et al., 2002; Vaughan et al., 1994).

Table 21.7 highlights differences between EMDR and classic exposure. Two features, at least, are apparent. First, EMDR is not classic exposure. In fact, the chunking of trauma data that occurs in EMDR may be an improved method of accessing trauma material, allowing for discomfort at acceptable levels. Second, the use of the eye movements, while not necessary by themselves, seems to facilitate the process of unearthing trauma material and to create a curative milieu for change.

TABLE 21.7. Differences between EMDR and Classic Exposure

EMDR	Exposure
1. EMDR uses frequent brief episodes of exposure.	1. Exposure should be continual and uninterrupted.
2. EMDR is structured but uses free association.	2. Exposure is structured.
3. EMDR often does not foster high anxiety.	3. Exposure fosters high levels of anxiety for long periods.
4. EMDR shows a rapid reduction of SUDs.	4. Exposure is gradual.

Third, the near-zero ESs indicate that eye movement is unnecessary. As noted earlier, eye movements were originally described as "the crucial component of the . . . procedure" (Shapiro, 1989, p. 220). Although some reviews have been far less critical of the procedure (Feske, 1998), most reviews (e.g., Lohr, Tolin, & Kleinknecht, 1995; Lohr et al., 1998) found little evidence that eye movements, or even other methods of lateral stimulation, are necessary. Evidence suggests that the "eye movements integral to the treatment, and to its name, are unnecessary" (Davidson & Parker, 2001, p. 305). In the main, dismantling studies that examined the use of alternating movements other than with the eyes were not shown to be different from EMDR. Some studies have shown that alternatives to eye movements, such as bilateral finger tapping, are equally as effective as eye movements. More recently, therapist finger movements are seen as part of a group of external alternating stimuli to which a client's attention is directed (Shapiro, 1996, p. 209). Rather than being seen as disconfirming EMDR, then, the alternatives used in these studies have been incorporated by Shapiro as valid alternative techniques of EMDR (Shapiro, 1994).

Unfortunately, when eye movements are used in evaluations of treatment efficacy, faulty designs may result, as the control condition may still contain the possible effective mechanism, which could be focused attention, distraction, stimulation of an orienting response, bilateral activation, or rhythmic activity (Shapiro, 1995). Studies that attempt to control for eye movements (Boudewyns & Hyer, 1996; Pitman et al., 1996; Renfrey & Spates, 1994; Wilson, Silver, Covi, & Foster, 1996) control for only one aspect (eye movements) of a complex process. Of course, a further concern is the lack of a convincing rationale for expecting eye movements and hand tapping to reduce PTSD (Foa & Rothbaum, 1998). On balance, then, there is little evidence that eye movements or other alternating stimuli are necessary.

That said, eye movements do appear to have some effect. Exactly what this effect is remains an empirical question. Eye movements decrease hyperarousal, enhance semantic recall, and decrease vividness of memory images (Wilson et al., 1996). This task elicits an "orienting response," causing multilayered simultaneous activations with focal attentions and working memory (Lipke, 2000). Eye movements seem to facilitate access to more data and often result in faster resolution, as well as relaxation. In addition, the bilateral stimulation possibly integrates the two hemispheres and allows the right (intuitive) and left (speech encoding) areas (Nicosia, 1995) to communicate better. The prefrontal cortex provides further integration. A "compelled relaxation response" has been documented (Wilson et al., 1996). This response includes slowed heart rate, a decreased galvanic skin response (GSR), respiration that matches the rhythm of the saccades, and initial increase and then decrease in blood pressure in the sets of saccades. Data also suggest that eye movements decrease the vividness of imagery (van der Hout, Muris, Salemink, & Kindt, 2001) and result in the differential processing of data at the level of the brain.

In positron emission tomography (PET) scans it appears that the "lower" areas of the brain are now not inhibited by the orbitofrontal cortex. Levin, Lazrove, and van der Kolk (1999) performed scans on patients who had had three sessions of EMDR. After the session, scans showed that the anterior cyngulate gyrus evidenced increased activation, as did the prefrontal cortex. Based on scan data, there appears to be a state-dependent inhibition of the orbitofrontal region (hippocampus, cingulate, thalamus, and dorsolateral prefrontal cortex) and activation of the limbic system and right hemisphere in trauma imagery. After EMDR processing, the PET data show that the prefrontal lobe is activated and the trauma is better narrativized. Practically, then, it appears that cognitive and emotional information are processed in different areas of the brain. It has been supposed (Shapiro, 1995) that EMDR facilitates the movement of information.

CONTRAINDICATIONS

As with most psychotherapies, there are few contraindications, if this term is construed as meaning causing harm. In general, problems with EMDR have developed because it has extended its internal validity markers and because the technique addresses many types of psychiatric problems with varied populations. This psychotherapy is not intended for psychiatric problems that involve direct brain disorders (e.g., traumatic brain injury, dementia), severe depression, disorders in which psychosis exists (notably schizophrenia, bipolar disorder, and depression with psychosis), intractable disorders such as obsessive–compulsive disorder (OCD), or structurally deficient Axis II disorders (e.g., paranoid, schizotypal, and borderline personality disorders). Debate about its merits regarding the somatoform and dissociative disorders continues. There exists little validation on both sides. Additionally, EMDR has not been evaluated to any degree with older adults or children.

Problems occur due to the just discussed problem diagnostic areas, to patient factors (resistance), to faulty belief systems that prevent the full experience of the procedure, and to EMDR protocols that are not applied well. One diagnosis less responsive to EMDR is depression. Patients repeat negative cognitions and cannot process and move information easily. Unless the therapist can adapt the technique for these patients (e.g., cognitive interweaving and more active involvement), the patient will not show change. Patient resistance, another category of problem, can occur for many reasons. Shapiro (1995) outlines several of these, including secondary gain, more central targets, and patient inability to embrace the process of the eye movements. EMDR has developed untested protocols for resistance. Faulty beliefs were also noted as problematic. Often there are secondary gain issues or a lack of belief in the procedure. Often, too, the patient goes through the motions but is not "present."

The issue of therapist competence is also important. Competence is especially troublesome, as many of the studies reviewed did not meet this criterion, both in terms of training and of therapy monitoring. As a rule, EMDR is appealing because it appears simple. When the patient is not able to show change, however, the therapist is instructed to intervene more. Although Shapiro (1995) provides suggestions for this process, it is less precise and is not empirically supported; we provide further suggestions on Table 21.9.

The therapist, then, is faced with two principal tasks in therapy: to promote basic patient behaviors that allow therapy to thrive (e.g., seeking treatment, cooperating with the technique, self-disclosing, exploring and testing out new patterns, and reducing obvious resistance) and to successfully apply a protocol (Schulte, 1996). When the basic patient behaviors are lacking, therapist flexibility is important. The therapist must know when to switch from the method-based to process-based modalities (Schulte, 1996). Although EMDR is not protected from this task to any degree more than any other therapy, it has one advantage: Immediate feedback is received from the patient, and changes can be made quickly. This allows moment-to-moment processing of the therapy tasks. The therapist, then, is always receiving data on the progress of the therapy. When there is little or no movement, the task requires that the therapist become more active. It is at these moments that the therapy becomes more complex and that problems can result.

METHOD/PROTOCOL

The protocol of EMDR involves eight phases of treatment (see Table 21.8). A complete procedural description of EMDR is given in Shapiro's (1995) treatment manual. EMDR is a complex eight-phase therapy that is transferable to other therapies. EMDR is hypothesized to facilitate the accessing and processing of traumatic memories and to bring these to an adaptive resolution, indicated by desensitization of emotional distress, reformulation of associated cognitions, and relief of accompanying physiological arousal. During EMDR the client focuses on emotionally disturbing material in sequential doses while simultaneously focusing on an external stimulus. This stimulus is bilateral. Therapist-directed eye movements are the most commonly used external stimulus, but a variety of other stimuli, including hand tapping and aural stimulation, are often used (Shapiro, 1991, 1993, 1994, 1995, 1999). This dual (external–internal) focus is combined with frequent brief periods of focusing on new associations as they arise.

All eight phases can be completed within one session, but the number of sessions can vary from one to many.

TABLE 21.8. Phases of EMDR Treatment

1. *Client history*: The therapist obtains information about the client's current level of functioning and current symptoms and assesses the client's stability, negative belief systems, and support systems. With this information, targets are established for treatment.

2. *Preparation of the client*: Tasks in this phase include rapport building, establishing methods for helping the client handle incomplete sessions, and helping the client build ego strength. Often relaxation is taught.

3. *Assessment*: This involves helping the client decide on the scenes to target and exploring the client's negative beliefs, as well as positive cognitions. Measures taken at this stage include the VoC (validity of cognition) and SUDs (subjective units of distress).

4. *Desensitization*: Series of bilateral stimulations are used to reduce the negative effects of the targeted memories.

5. *Installation*: Positive beliefs are installed using bilateral stimulation. Negative thoughts are replaced with positive ones.

6. *Double check*: Call up the original scene and see whether any residual unresolved feelings remain.

7. *Closure*: Help the client reestablish equilibrium and stability.

8. *Reevaluation*: Done at the beginning of the next session to see whether the treatment effects are being maintained.

If problems result, several procedures are available to alleviate them. Use of guided imagery, grounding techniques, positive statements, breathing, and the like, with the eye movements, are especially helpful. Just adding a positive statement ("It's over") can be of value. Working through traumatic memories, including those to which the client has clear access, should not occur until the client's self-structure is relatively stable and he or she can tolerate strong affect. The client's ability to tolerate exposure to new, painful material can be gauged through assessments of his or her ability to engage in introspection, to manage and limit self-loathing and self-deprecation, and to engage in self-soothing and calming activities, especially. Self-capacities are enhanced as a client learns concrete coping skills, including thought-stopping and stress-inoculation techniques, as well as "dosing" exposure to emotional discomfort or stressful events and transforming events by developing positive imagery.

In many ways EMDR is designed to be flexible in the therapy room. The two more recent edited books by Shapiro (Shapiro & Maxfield, 2002; Shapiro, Kaslow, & Maxfield, 2007) confirm what many therapists know and do: EMDR is used differently by different therapists from different therapeutic orientations (DiGiorgio, Arnkoff, Glass, Lyhus, & Walter, 2004). Table 21.9 presents one way to think about EMDR. It outlines the basic therapeutic interventions and honors the least restrictive principle. When more assistance is required, the needed input is specified. Above all, the EMDR ideals of staying out of the client's way, providing choice, facilitating movement, identifying blockages, and applying the technology of the method are important. In addition to specifying interventions that proceed from least to most intrusive, Table 21.9 also considers resources and assimilative techniques. Resources are intended to be supportive and to guide behavior. The assimilative techniques are intended to amplify the Socratic methods in EMDR and can be used at any time in the desensitization processing.

It is interesting that EMDR also has a procedure for acute trauma. As trauma has not had time to consolidate, the therapeutic reaction requires a fast-line method to unearth all its parts. Table 21.10 provides this sequence.

CASES EXAMPLES

Ellie

Ellie is a female in her late 30s who came specifically for EMDR. She had recently had an abortion and since then had been depressed. She thought that with time, she would feel better, but instead she began to feel worse. When she found herself withdrawing emotionally from her family and friends, she finally realized that she needed help. She was hoping to find tools that she could use that would help her recover. She found EMDR.

In the first session, Ellie told her story (client history). She and her husband wanted a second child (they had one 3-year-old son). Eventually she became pregnant, and after some tests she was told that the child had a rare disorder called "Edward's syndrome" and that she would be wise to abort the baby. (The child might not survive the pregnancy and most likely would not live long after birth.) The doctor recommended that she do this, and her husband and parents agreed. Ellie was in a state of shock and reluctantly agreed. But inside she was not ready to do it. Even on the way to the hospital, she told her mother that she didn't want to go through with it, but she was told she had no choice. She gave in. Since then she had had many regrets and doubts, and she was upset that she had aborted her child. She told me (B. K.) that even though she was early on in her pregnancy, she had found out that it was a girl, and she had begun to develop a relationship with the child.

TABLE 21.9. Potential EMDR Responses

1. Narrative attunement

Empathic exploration: Do *not* be an active therapist, but have the client listen and trust the process.
- "Stay with that."
- "Attend to that."
- "Focus on that."
- "Bring that up."

Help—Do what is natural:
- Alter mode (e.g., feelings for thoughts).
- Get SUDs rating.
- Four helpers:
  a. When positive or negative features of processing arise, go with negative.
  b. If choice of feelings, images, or content, choose feelings.
  c. Body sensations, however, are the true test of movement.
  d. When there is a change, say: "Pay attention to tension that *remains*."

2. Doing therapy

Help 1—Support:
- Empower—"This is no worse than the original trauma and you survived that."
- Reframe—"Something positive is happening."
- Choice—"In the past you had no choice; now you have one."

Help 2—Light resistance (no change):
- "When else in the past were you like this?"
- "What prevents you from ... ?"
- "What would you need to have happen to move this along?"
- "I can't give up this memory because ... "

Help 3—Heavy resistance:
- *Query for the potential resistance*: "Imagine yourself" (opposite of resistance components).
- Secondary gain:
  "Who would you be without the problem?"
  "How would you like to be living?"
  "What would you need?"
  "What is preventing this?"
  "What would happen if ... ?"
- Early learning:
  "Where did you learn this?"
  "Access early memory/event of this learning."

Help 4—Be a therapist:
- "What would unblock this?"
- "What might symbolize this cycle?"
- "Focus on body or feeling."
- Partialize events in the loop.
- Frame-by-frame iteration of process.
- "Concentrate on blocking out this scene."
- "What would allow you to feel ... ?"

Help 5—Be real, active:
- Cognitive interweave
- Guided imagery
- Relaxation

3. Support–resources

Future orientation:
- See yourself in the future with this issue.
- Install the positive cognition.

(continued)

TABLE 21.9. *(continued)*

Resource building:
- *Now* resources:
  How would the client prefer to be acting?
  What are goals for the future?
  What is called for now in the day-to-day functions of living?RWhat metaphors, images, symbols, stories are available to represent the resource?
  Who is the key mentor/model for the person?
- *Then* resources:
  Embryonic resources for change?
  What are the missing resources for each personality?
  What metaphors, images, symbols, stories are available to represent the resource?
  What about generic issues of safety, trust, self-esteem, independence, intimacy, and power?

4. Assimilation queries
   - "What evidence do you have to support this thought?"
   - "Is there any alternative way of looking at the situation or yourself?"
   - "Is there any alternative explanation?"
   - "How do you think I, your therapist, would view this situation? How would [valued person] think of it?"
   - "Are you 'shoulding or musting' on yourself or the world?"
   - "What's the worst possible outcome?"
   - "How long will this unpleasant situation last?"
   - "On the grand scale of injustice or badness, how unjust or bad is it?"
   - "Are you confusing a remote possibility with a high-probability outcome?"
   - "Are you overestimating the amount of control or responsibility you have for the situation?"
   - "Are you discounting or discrediting positive aspects of the situation or your ability to cope with it?"
   - "What does this problem say about who you are?"

In the session, Ellie was in tears explaining what happened. After I told her how EMDR works and what to expect, we agreed to use both bilateral sound and bilateral tactile stimulation (client preparation). Assessment took place via the standard protocol—target, VoC, SUDs, and so forth—and then desensitization was initiated. She noticed the sensations in her body, the sadness, the target, and the negative belief and then simply noticed what was happening. She stayed with the processing until she wanted to talk about what was happening.

Ellie is an exceptionally bright, articulate, and sensitive woman. She responded to the processing and wanted to do very long sets. She cried often. She also wanted to tell

TABLE 21.10. EMDR: Acute Sequence

1. Obtain a narrative history of the event.

2. Target the most disturbing aspect of the memory (if necessary).

3. Target the remainder of the narrative in chronological order.

4. Have client visualize the entire sequence of the event with eyes closed and reprocess it as disturbance arises. Repeat until the entire event can be visualized from start to finish without distress.

5. Have client visualize the event from start to finish with eyes open, and install positive cognition.

6. Conclude with body scan.

7. Process present stimuli, if necessary.

me how she was feeling and what she was thinking about. She remembered the doctor commenting that something was wrong with the baby during the first ultrasound. Her heart sank. Bilateral stimulation was continued, as she was able to process several difficult pieces of trauma. She processed many incidents during that first session, and she cried deeply for most of the processing. Toward the end of the 2-hour session, she indicated that she felt improved (SUD = 3). Installation was also positive. She commented that she felt relief for the first time in months (closure). We prepared for the week and the next session.

During the next several sessions, Ellie processed many incidents that had upset her— her doctor seeming to be pleased that he had found a problem without seeming to care about her; her husband believing that there was no choice and accepting this readily; her parents accepting the decision and not discussing other options with her. She realized that the worst thing about this experience was that nobody had given her the time to make the decision for herself. She had no control. She told me that finally she was beginning to understand why she had been so depressed. She hadn't understood her reactions, because she was prochoice. She hadn't realized that she had not been allowed to make the decision for herself.

After each session, Ellie was feeling better and better. The last important piece that she processed was her fear that her baby would not have been able to understand her actions. With EMDR processing, she accepted the situation and her role in it. She realized that it was the lack of control that was at the root of her depression. Her feelings of "no control" were discussed in the present, as well as in the past. She then processed events from throughout her life in which she had felt no control. At one point she indicated that she thought she had been born with a preset role—that of taking care of everybody else and not being in control of her own life.

Her depression lifted, and she began to be her "old self" again. She noticed that she was different with her family and friends. She felt much more in control of her life. During a recent conversation, she remarked that her son seemed to be very much happier, and she wondered whether the reason was that she was so much happier.

In EMDR, it is also important to address the future. Ellie processed ideas about what she was going to do to honor her daughter's memory. She was to celebrate the birthdate. She and her husband were going to plant a lilac tree in the backyard and spend the day remembering the baby and feeling her presence in their hearts.

Ellie's EMDR sessions continued, at first weekly and then in alternate weeks, for 6 months. She accepted the loss of her baby and felt noticeably better. This carried over into all other areas of her life. She indicated that before beginning EMDR she had hoped that therapy might be like "going into a happy hour and being given a glass of wine at half price." She then said that it had turned out that therapy was like "being given a very large case of the best wine."

Lesley

Client History

Lesley is a teller in a bank who had been held up in a robbery. A brief history was taken regarding the current symptoms and functioning. Her target was a robbery in which she was given a note by a customer that instructed her to give him a sum of money or she would die. During her training she had been told that if something like that happened, she was to follow instructions. Nevertheless, the incident shook her, and she found that at first she feared going to work, then she began to fear using public transportation, and shortly after that she became afraid to leave her house unless somebody accompanied her. She feared that the holdup man would find her and kill her. This was evident when she came to the first therapy session with a friend.

Preparation/Rationale and Demonstration of Procedure

Lesley was given the standard introduction (Shapiro, 1995). She was also introduced to the desensitization procedure. She referred eye movements of all the modalities. A pointer was used with a light at one end. She followed the light with her eyes while I (B. K.) moved the pointer back and forth in series. She was not taught a relaxation method at this point, as she preferred to be given the desensitization immediately.

Assessment

THERAPIST: When you think about the holdup and everything related to it, what do you think about it now? [negative cognition]

LESLEY: I keep thinking that I almost died.

THERAPIST: What picture represents the worst part of that for you now?

LESLEY: When he passed me the note—and I read it, that was the worst part.

THERAPIST: Do you have a negative belief about yourself now that relates to that picture?

LESLEY: Yes, I'm in danger.

THERAPIST: When you think about that picture, what would you like to believe about yourself now? [validity of cognition]

LESLEY: I'd like to believe that I can be safe.

THERAPIST: When you think of the picture of him passing you the note and you reading it, how true do the words "I can be safe" feel to you now on a scale of 1 to 7, where 1 feels completely false and 7 feels completely true?

LESLEY: 1.

THERAPIST: When you think about you receiving the note and reading it, what emotion or emotions do you feel now? [emotions]

LESLEY: Fear. I feel scared.

THERAPIST: On a scale of 0 to 10, where 0 is neutral or no disturbance and 10 is the highest disturbance that you can imagine, how disturbing does the incident feel to you right now? [SUDs]

LESLEY: Very disturbing—9.

THERAPIST: Where do you feel that in your body? [location of body sensations]

LESLEY: In my heart, in my stomach.

Desensitization

Think of the picture of you being handed the note and reading it, the negative words "I'm in danger," and notice where in your body you are feeling that, and now, follow the light with your eyes.

During the desensitization phase in her therapy sessions, Lesley recalled many aspects of what happened—her uncertainty about giving the robber the money, her fears about being killed even if she followed his instructions, and, most of all, her fears about him coming after her. As we worked on these, she gradually came to realize that he probably feared her more than she feared him. Even after he was caught, at first she was still frightened, but gradually and steadily her fears lessened and eventually disappeared. The SUD was finally at 0.

Installation

The link of the positive cognition "I can feel safe" with the original picture (being handed the note and reading it) is called installation.

> THERAPIST: Do the words "I can feel safe" feel right to you, or is there another positive statement that would feel more accurate?
>
> LESLEY: I think that's okay.
>
> THERAPIST: Think about the original picture and the words "I can feel safe" and follow the light. (*Eye movements are done.*) Now, on a scale of 1 to 7, how true do the words "I can feel safe" feel to you now?
>
> LESLEY: It's almost true—probably 6½.

Check

> Now keep in mind the original memory and the words "I can feel safe" and mentally scan your body, from the top of your head to your feet, and see if you notice any tension or tightness or anything that doesn't feel right to you. [body scan]

> Sets of eye movements were done until she felt fine.

Closure

Lesley was rewarded and validated. She was also informed that the processing might continue and that it would be okay to telephone the therapist if necessary. She was also provided with basic relapse rubrics and encouraged not to become risk-averse.

Rachel

Rachel is a woman in her 40s who came because she was suffering from multiple chemical sensitivity (MCS). She had numerous allergy symptoms and experienced sensitivities to a variety of substances—pesticides, scented shampoos, nail polish, hair dye, synthetic materials, and so forth. A greater problem was that she needed to have some dental work done and was upset because she was having bad reactions to all of the dental substances that were available. She had been in therapy before with little success; her symptoms worsened.

During an initial telephone conversation, we discussed the possibility that the problems she was dealing with might be the result of memories from unresolved past traumas that were stored in her body and experienced as symptoms. If this were the case, then EMDR might be appropriate. During the history-taking phase, it became clear that Rachel had experienced many traumas in her life. To provide safety and reassurance for her, I (B. K.) encouraged her to contact me if she wanted to discuss anything about her sessions that was puzzling or uncomfortable.

Many clients with MCS don't believe that their symptoms might be emotionally based. With these clients, much of the beginning part of therapy consists of encouraging them to be willing to look at possible emotional causes. Rachel, on the other hand, was willing to accept the belief that emotional problems caused her symptoms.

When we began the desensitization phase of the EMDR protocol, we used both auditory and tactile stimulation simultaneously. She responded well. With problems such as Rachel's, it is often the case that long sets of bilateral stimulation are appropriate. In general, when working with people who are suffering from specific physical symptoms (people with syndromes such as fibromyalgia or chronic fatigue syndrome), we target body sensations, emotions, and thoughts. Like many clients with MCS, Rachel felt comfortable processing her feelings and thoughts and often processed for 5 to 10 minutes at a time.

Rachel remembered many traumas, and these memories brought out a great deal of sadness in her. The more sadness she felt, the more her symptoms lessened in intensity. One of her main symptoms, when she came into contact with a substance to which she was "sensitive," was difficulty breathing. During the sessions, her breathing returned to normal.

During each session she seemed different—calmer, more relaxed, her voice lowered. She began trying new things, such as scented shampoo and conditioner for her hair. One time she brought in a substance in a box that her dentist had given to her. She wanted to put it in her mouth and process the sensations. Often she couldn't breathe when she took the substance out of the box. In the session, she opened the box and immediately developed difficulty breathing. Bilateral stimulations proved effective. Almost immediately the symptoms remitted.

Sessions were held weekly and, later, biweekly. She continued to make progress. On one occasion she arrived at the session with "streaks in her hair." She had just left the hairdresser. She was more confident and now "knew" that her symptoms represented unresolved feelings that could be controlled.

At follow-up, she reported that she had had substantial dental work without incident. She said, "I had expected to live a life with no teeth and gray hair and look at me now." She was now aware of how interrelated her emotions and symptoms were and of how symptoms resulted from her associations and feelings. She was aware now that MCS symptoms were emotionally driven.

CONCLUSION

EMDR should no longer be considered controversial. Probably misnamed, EMDR encompasses more than eye movements, and it is here to stay. It is empirically supported for PTSD and has some applicability for most anxiety disorders, as well as general stress reactions. Like CBT, EMDR functions with a brief case formulation, cognitive assessment, and understanding of the core problems and applies modules that directly address affect, behaviors, imagery, and sensations. Like CBT, EMDR requires a case formulation that is a deliberate and conjoint effort to identify the etiological, precipitant, and maintaining problems of the person. It is a formulation of the necessary components to address psychological problems and to provide practical interventions. The patient is informed totally about therapy. Each becomes a participant observer and active collaborator in his or her own care. Like CBT, EMDR is also integrative and dynamic. EMDR places symptoms in the context of the person's life and the cyclic patterns, both internally and externally driven. Like CBT, EMDR fosters an emphasis on the patient as participant observer. Like CBT, EMDR allows the therapist to assess whether "treatment receipt" (is the client getting what is called for?) and "treatment enactment" (is the patient doing what is requested?) are in process.

Many of the studies we have reviewed are written well. The EMDR literature is now mature enough that less sophisticated studies can be left unpublished. The current literature, however, still suffers from excessive variance in findings from study to study, and this may be reduced by improved methodological rigor. The noncombat PTSD population is an especially fruitful area for application and study. As always, the scientific literature needs carefully designed, executed, and analyzed research that pays attention to issues of effect size, power, measurement, and reproducibility, as well as to issues of clinical significance. Although it makes sense to report SUD and VoC scores for completeness, the use of valid outcomes is essential for the assessment of effectiveness. The progress on dismantling studies should continue, especially as regards the other components of this treatment method (e.g., positive and negative cognition, SUDs, instillation, etc.).

In the two most controversial areas of EMDR, exposure and use of eye movements, the jury is still in deliberation. As discussed earlier, EMDR is different from exposure. Strikingly, EMDR does what is a central element of exposure for PTSD problems: Fear memory is activated, new information is added, repeated exposure results in habituation within and across sessions, and changes occur in threat appraisals. Whether eye movements are necessary, only time and study will tell. As this therapy has grown and recursively accepted feedback from the professional literature, statements about its efficacy have been more tempered. In time, any inappropriate extension of the method to disorders and populations for which efficacy has not been demonstrated will disappear. Hopefully, the generalizability (along with the internal validity discussed earlier) of EMDR will be a major focus in the next decade.

The premise of therapy across different types of PTSD is to help people integrate their traumatic experiences in such a way that their old models of the world are not shattered and replaced by perverse traumatic models, yet they also do not ignore or deny the impact of their traumatic experiences. EMDR seems to walk this tightrope well for the trauma victim, providing methods to negotiate the perils of denial and devastation. Statistician John Tukey is reputed to have said, "All models are wrong; some are useful." At this moment in time and at this place in the progress of psychotherapy, EMDR can be considered useful.

REFERENCES

American Psychiatric Association. (2004). *Practice guideline for the treatment of patients with acute stress disorder and posttraumatic stress disorder.* Arlington, VA: Author.

American Psychiatric Association. (2004). *Practice guidelines.*

Baker, N., & McBride, B. (1991, August). *Clinical applications of EMDR in a law enforcement environment: Observations of the psychological service unit of the L.A. County Sheriff's Department.* Paper presented at the annual meeting of the American Psychological Association, Police Psychology (Division 18, Police & Public Safety Subsection) miniconvention, San Francisco, CA.

Belich, A., Kotler, M., Kutz, E., & Shaley, A. (2002). *A position paper of the (Israeli) National Council for Mental Health: Guidelines for the assessment and professional intervention with terror victims in the hospital and in the community.* Jerusalem, Israel: Israeli National Council for Mental Health.

Blore, D. C. (1997). Reflections on "a day when the whole world seemed to be darkened." *Changes: An International Journal of Psychology and Psychiatry, 15,* 89–95.

Borgeat, F., Stravynski, A., & Chalout, L. (1983). A controlled comparison of thermal biofeedback and relaxation training in the treatment of essential hypertension: II. Effects on cardiovascular reactivity. *Health Psychology, 7,* 13–33.

Boudewyns, P. A., & Hyer, L. A. (1996). Eye movement desensitization and reprocessing (EMDR) as treatment for post-traumatic stress disorder (PTSD). *Clinical Psychology and Psychotherapy, 3*(3), 185–195.

Boudewyns, P. A., Stwertka, S. A., Hyer, L. A., Albrecht, J. W., & Sperr, E. V. (1993). Eye movement desensitization and reprocessing: A pilot study. *Behavior Therapist, 16,* 30–33.

Bradley, R., Greene, J., Russ, E., Dutra, L., & Westen, D. (2005). A multidimensional meta-analysis of psychotherapy for PTSD. *American Journal of Psychiatry, 162,* 214–227.

Branden, N. (1997). *The art of living consciously: The power of awareness to transform everyday life.* New York: Simon & Schuster.

Brown, K. W., McGoldrick, T., & Buchanan, R. (1997). Body dysmorphic disorder: Seven cases treated with eye movement desensitization and reprocessing. *Behavioural and Cognitive Psychotherapy, 25,* 203–207.

Bryant, R., Harvey, A., Dang, S., Sackville, T., & Basten, C. (1998). Treatment of acute stress disorder: A comparison of cognitive behavioral therapy and supportive counseling. *Journal of Consulting and Clinical Psychology, 66,* 862–866.

Bryant, R., Moulds, M., Gutherie, R., Dang, S., & Nixon, R. (2003). Imaginal exposure alone and imaginal exposure with cognitive restructuring in treatment of posttraumatic stress disorder. *Journal of Community and Clinical Psychology, 71,* 206–212.

Carlson, J. G., Chemtob, C. M., Rusnak, K., & Hedlund, N. L. (1996). Eye movement desensitization and reprocessing treatment for combat PTSD. *Psychotherapy, 33,* 104–113.

Carlson, J. G., Chemtob, C. M., Rusnak, K., Hedlund, N. L., & Muraoka, M. Y. (1998). Eye movement desensitization and reprocessing for combat-related posttraumatic stress disorder. *Journal of Traumatic Stress, 11,* 3–24.

Chard, K. (2000). *Cognitive processing therapy for sexual abuse: An economic study.* Unpublished Manuscript, University of Kentucky.

Chambless, D. L., Baker, M. J., Baucom, D. H., Beutler, L. E., Calhoun, K. S., Crits-Christoph, P., et al. (1998). Update on empirically validated therapies. *Clinical Psychologist, 51,* 3–16.

Chemtob, C. M., Nakashima, J., Hamada, R. S., & Carlson, J. G. (2002). Brief treatment for elementary school children with disaster-related posttraumatic stress disorder: A field study. *Journal of Clinical Psychology, 58,* 99–112.

Chemtob, C. M., Tolin, D. F., van der Kolk, B. A., & Pitman, R. K. (2000). Eye movement desensitization and reprocessing. In E. B. Foa, T. M. Keane, & M. J. Friedman (Eds.), *Effective treatments for PTSD: Practice guidelines from the International Society of Traumatic Stress Studies* (pp. 139–155, 333–335). New York: Guilford Press.

Cloitre, M., Koenen, K., Cohen, L., & Han, H. (2002). Skills training in affective and interpersonal regulation followed by exposure: A phase-based treatment related to childhood abuse. *Journal of Consulting and Clinical Psychology, 70,* 1067–1075.

Cocco, N., & Sharpe, L. (1993). An auditory variant of eye movement desensitization in a case of childhood posttraumatic stress disorder. *Journal of Behavior Therapy and Experimental Psychiatry, 24,* 373–377.

Crabbe, B. (1996, November). Can eye-movement therapy improve your riding? *Dressage Today,* 28–33.

Datta, P. C., & Wallace, J. (1994, May). *Treatment of sexual traumas of sex offenders using eye movement desensitization and reprocessing.* Paper presented at the Annual Symposium in Forensic Psychology, San Francisco.

Datta, P. C., & Wallace, J. (1996, November). Enhancement of victim empathy along with reduction of anxiety and increase of positive cognition of sex offenders after treatment with EMDR. Paper presented at the annual convention of the Association for the Advancement of Behavior Therapy, EMDR Special Interest Group, New York.

Davidson, P. R., & Parker, K. C. H. (2001). Eye movement desensitization and reprocessing: A meta-analysis. *Journal of Consulting and Clinical Psychology, 69,* 305–316.

Department of Veterans Affairs and Department of Defense. (2004). *VA/DoD clinical practice guideline for the management of post-traumatic stress*. Washington, DC: Author.

Devilly, G. J., & Spence, S. H. (1999). The relative efficacy and treatment distress of EMDR and a cognitive-behavioral trauma treatment protocol in the amelioration of posttraumatic stress disorder. *Journal of Anxiety Disorders, 13*(1–2), 131–157.

Devilly, G. J., Spence, S. H., & Rapee, R. M. (1998). Statistical and reliable change with eye movement desensitization and reprocessing: Treating trauma with a veteran population. *Behavior Therapy, 29*, 435–455.

DiGiorgio, K., Arnkoff, D., Glass, C., Lyhus, K., & Walter, R. (2004). EMDR and theoretical orientation: A qualitative study of how therapists integrate eye movement desensitization and reprocessing into their approach to psychotherapy. *Journal of Psychotherapy Integration, 14*, 227–253.

Dutch National Steering Committee Guidelines for Mental Health Care. (2003). *Multidisciplinary guidelines on anxiety disorders*. Utrecht, the Netherlands: Quality Institute Heath Care CBO/Trimbos Institute.

Edmond, T., Rubin, A., & Wambach, K. (1999). The effectiveness of EMDR with adult female survivors of childhood sexual abuse. *Social Work Research, 23*, 103–116.

Edmond, T., Sloan, L., & McCarty, D. (2004). Sexual abuse survivors' perceptions of the effectiveness of EMDR and eclectic therapy: A mixed-methods study. *Research on Social Work Practice, 14*, 259–272.

Ehlers, A., Clark, D. M., Dunmore, E., Jaycox, L., Meadows, E., & Foa, E. (1998). Predicting response to exposure treatment in PTSD: The role of mental defeat and alienation. *Journal of Traumatic Stress, 11*, 457–471.

Fensterheim, H. (1996). Eye movement desensitization and reprocessing with complex personality pathology: An integrative therapy. *Journal of Psychotherapy Integration, 6*, 27–38.

Feske, U. (1998). Eye movement desensitization and reprocessing treatment for posttraumatic stress disorder. *Clinical Psychology: Science and Practice, 5*, 171–181.

Feske, U., & Goldstein, A. (1997). Eye movement desensitization and reprocessing treatment for panic disorder: A controlled outcome and partial dismantling study. *Journal of Consulting and Clinical Psychology, 36*, 1026–1035.

Fine, C. G. (1994, June). *Eye movement desensitization and reprocessing (EMDR) for dissociative disorders*. Paper presented at the Eastern Regional Conference on Abuse and Multiple Personality, Alexandria, VA.

Fishman, D. (1999). *The case for pragmatic psychology*. New York: New York University Press.

Foa, E., Keane, T., & Friedman, M. (Eds.). (2000). *Effective treatments for PTSD: Practice guidelines from the International Society of Traumatic Stress Studies*. New York: Guilford Press.

Foa, E. B., & Kozak, M. J. (1997). Beyond the efficacy ceiling? Cognitive behavior therapy in search of theory. *Behavior Therapy, 28*, 601–611.

Foa, E. B., & Meadows, E. A. (1997). Psychosocial treatments for posttraumatic stress disorder: A critical review. *Annual Review of Psychology, 48*, 449–480.

Foa, E. B., & Rothbaum, B. O. (1998). *Treating the trauma of rape: Cognitive behavioral therapy for PTSD*. New York: Guilford Press.

Foster, S., & Lendl, J. (1995). Eye movement desensitization and reprocessing: Initial applications for enhancing performance in athletes. *Journal of Applied Sport Psychology, 7*(Suppl.), 63.

Foster, S., & Lendl, J. (1996). Eye movement desensitization and reprocessing: Four case studies of a new tool for executive coaching and restoring employee performance after setbacks. *Consulting Psychology Journal, 48*, 155–161.

Grant, M. (1999). *Pain control with EMDR*. New Hope, PA: EMDR Humanitarian Assistance Program.

Greenwald, R. (1994). Applying eye movement desensitization and reprocessing to the treatment of traumatized children: Five case studies. *Anxiety Disorders Practice Journal, 1*, 83–97.

Greenwald, R. (1998). Eye movement desensitization and reprocessing (EMDR): New hope for children suffering from trauma and loss. *Clinical Child Psychology and Psychiatry, 3*, 279–287.

Greenwald, R. (1999). *Eye movement desensitization and reprocessing (EMDR) in child and adolescent psychotherapy*. New York: Aronson.

Hassard, A. (1993). Eye movement desensitization of body image. *Behavioural Psychotherapy, 21*, 157–160.

Henry, S. L. (1996). Pathological gambling: Etiological considerations and treatment efficacy of eye movement desensitization/reprocessing. *Journal of Gambling Studies, 12* 395–405.

Herbert, J. D., & Mueser, K. T. (1992). Eye movement desensitization: A critique of the evidence. *Journal of Behavior Therapy and Experimental Psychiatry, 23,* 169–174.

Hyer, L. (1995). Use of EMDR in a "dementing" PTSD survivor. *Clinical Gerontologist, 16,* 70–73.

Hyer, L., & Brandsma, J. M. (1997). EMDR minus eye movements equals good psychotherapy. *Journal of Traumatic Stress, 10,* 515–522.

INSERM. (2004). *Psychotherapy: An evaluation of three approaches.* Paris: French National Institute of Health and Medical Research.

Ironson, G. I., Freund, B., Strauss, J. L., & Williams, J. (2002). A comparison of two treatments for traumatic stress: A community based study of EMDR and prolonged exposure. *Journal of Clinical Psychology, 58,* 113–128.

Jaberghaderi, N., Greenwald, R., Rubin, A., Dolatabadim S., & Zand, S. O. (2004). A comparison of CBT and EMDR for sexually abused Iranian girls. *Clinical Psychology and Psychotherapy, 11,* 358–368.

Jensen, J. A. (1994). An investigation of eye movement desensitization and reprocessing (EMDR) as a treatment for posttraumatic stress disorder (PTSD) symptoms of Vietnam combat veterans. *Behavior Therapy, 25,* 311–325.

Kazdin, A. E. (1994). Methodology, design, and evaluation in psychotherapy research. In A. E. Bergin & S. L. Garfield (Eds.), *Handbook of psychotherapy and behavior change* (4th ed., pp. 19–71). New York: Wiley.

Kleinknecht, R. A. (1993). Rapid treatment of blood and injection phobias with eye movement desensitization. *Journal of Behavior Therapy and Experimental Psychiatry, 24,* 211–217.

Lazarus, C. N., & Lazarus, A. A. (2002). EMDR: An elegantly concentrated multimodal procedure. In F. Shapiro (Ed.), *EMDR as an integrative psychotherapy approach: Experts of diverse orientations explore the paradigm prism* (pp. 209–224). Washington, DC: American Psychological Association Books.

Lazrove, S., & Fine, C. G. (1996). The use of EMDR in patients with dissociative identity disorder. *Dissociation, 9,* 289–299.

Lee, C., & Gavriel, H. (1998). Treatment of post-traumatic stress disorder: A comparison of stress inoculation training with prolonged exposure and eye movement desensitization and reprocessing. *Proceedings of the World Congress of Behavioral and Cognitive Therapies, Acapulco.*

Lee, C., Gavriel, H., Drummond, P., Richards, J., & Greenwald, R. (2002). Treatment of posttraumatic stress disorder: A comparison of stress inoculation training with prolonged exposure and eye movement desensitization and reprocessing. *Journal of Clinical Psychology, 58,* 1071–1089.

Lehrer, P. M., & Woolfolk, R. (Eds.). (1993). *Principles and practice of stress management* (2nd ed.). New York: Guilford Press.

Levin, C. (1993, July–August). The enigma of EMDR. *Family Therapy Networker,* 75–83.

Levin, P., Lazrove, S., & van der Kolk, B. A. (1999). What psychological testing and neuroimaging tell us about the treatment of posttraumatic stress disorder (PTSD) by eye movement desensitization and reprocessing (EMDR). *Journal of Anxiety Disorders, 13,* 159–172.

Lipke, H. (2000). *EMDR and psychotherapy integration: Theoretical and clinical suggestions with focus on traumatic stress.* New York: CRC Press.

Lohr, J. M., Tolin, D. F., & Kleinknecht, R. A. (1995). An intensive investigation of eye movement desensitization of medical phobias. *Journal of Behavior Therapy and Experimental Psychiatry, 26,* 141–151.

Lohr, J. M., Tolin, D. F., & Kleinknecht, R. A. (1996). An intensive investigation of eye movement desensitization of claustrophobia. *Journal of Anxiety Disorders, 10,* 73–88.

Lohr, J. M., Tolin, D. F., & Lilienfeld, S. O. (1998). Efficacy of eye movement desensitization and reprocessing: Implications for behavior therapy. *Behavior Therapy, 29,* 123–156.

Marcus, S., Marquis, P., & Sakai, C. (2004). Three- and 6-month follow-up of EMDR treatment of PTSD in an HMO setting. *International Journal of Stress Management, 11,* 195–208.

Marcus, S. V., Marquis, P., & Sakai, C. (1997). Controlled study of treatment of PTSD using EMDR in an HMO setting. *Psychotherapy, 34,* 307–315.

Marks, I. M. (2000). Forty years of psychosocial treatment. *Behavioural and Cognitive Psychotherapy*, 28, 323–334.

Marks, I., Lovell, K., Noshirvani, H., Livanou, M., & Thrasher, S. (1998). Exposure and cognitive restructuring alone and combined in PTSD: A controlled study. *Archives of General Psychiatry*, 55, 317–325.

Marquis, J. N., & Puk, G. (1994, November). *Dissociative identity disorder: A common sense and cognitive-behavioral view.* Paper presented at the annual meeting of the Association for Advancement of Behavior Therapy, San Diego.

Maxfield, L., & Hyer, L. A. (2002). The relationship between efficacy and methodology in studies investigating EMDR treatment of PTSD. *Journal of Clinical Psychology*, 58, 23–41.

Maxfield, L., Lake, K., & Hyer, L. (2004). Some answers to unanswered questions about the empirical support for EMDR in the treatment of PTSD. *Traumatology*, 10, 73–89.

McCann, D. L. (1992). Post-traumatic stress disorder due to devastating burns overcome by a single session of eye movement desensitization. *Journal of Behavior Therapy and Experimental Psychiatry*, 23, 319–323.

Messer, S. (2004). Evidence-based practice: Beyond empirically supported treatments. *Professional Psychology: Research and Practice*, 33, 580–588.

Muris, P., & Merckelbach, H. (1997). Treating spider phobics with eye movement desensitization and reprocessing: A controlled study. *Behavioral and Cognitive Psychotherapy*, 25, 39–50.

National Institute for Clinical Excellence. (2005). *Posttraumatic stress disorder (PTSD): The management of adults and children in primary and secondary care.* London: NICE Guidelines.

Nicosia, G. J. (1995, March). Eye movement desensitization and reprocessing is not hypnosis. *Dissociation*, 8(1), 69.

Northern Ireland Department of Health. (2001). *Treatment choice in psychological therapies and counselling: Evidence based clinical practice guideline.* London: Author. Retrieved March 15, 2002, from *www.doh.gov.uk/mentalhealth/treatmentguideline/*

Parnell, L. (1994, August). *Treatment of sexual abuse survivors with EMDR: Two case reports.* Paper presented at the annual meeting of the American Psychological Association, Los Angeles.

Parnell, L. (1999). *EMDR in the treatment of adults abused as children.* New York: Norton.

Persons, J., Davidson, J., & Tomkins, M. (2000). *Essential components of cognitive behavioral therapy for depression.* Washington, DC: American Psychological Association.

Peterson, D. (1991). Connection and disconnection of research and practice in the education of professional psychologists. *American Psychologist*, 46, 422–429.

Pitman, R. K., Orr, S. P., Altman, B., Longpre, R. E., Poiré, R. E., & Macklin, M. L. (1996). Emotional processing during eye movement desensitization and reprocessing therapy of Vietnam veterans with chronic posttraumatic stress disorder. *Comprehensive Psychiatry*, 37, 419–429.

Power, K. G., McGoldrick, T., Brown, K., et al. [au, need up to 6 names] (2002). A controlled comparison of eye movement desensitization and reprocessing versus exposure plus cognitive restructuring, versus waiting list in the treatment of post-traumatic stress disorder. *Journal of Clinical Psychology and Psychotherapy*, 9, 299–318.

Puk, G. (1992, May). *The use of eye movement desensitization and reprocessing in motor vehicle accident trauma.* Paper presented at the annual meeting of the American College of Forensic Psychology, San Francisco.

Ray, A. L., & Zbik, A. (2001). Cognitive behavioral therapies and beyond. In C. D. Tollison, J. R. Satterthwaite, & J. W. Tollison (Eds.), *Practical pain management* (3rd ed., pp. 189–208). Philadelphia: Lippincott.

Renfrey, G., & Spates, C. R. (1994). Eye movement desensitization: A partial dismantling study. *Journal of Behavior Therapy and Experimental Psychiatry*, 25, 231–239.

Resick, P., & Schnicke, M. (1992). Cognitive processing therapy for sexual assault victims. *Journal of Consulting and Clinical Psychology*, 60, 748–756.

Rogers, S., Silver, S., Goss, J., Obenchain, J., Willis, A., & Whitney, R. (1999). A single session, controlled group study of flooding and eye movement desensitization and reprocessing in treating posttraumatic stress disorder among Vietnam War veterans: Preliminary data. *Journal of Anxiety Disorders*, 13(1–2), 119–130.

Rothbaum, B. O. (1997). A controlled study of eye movement desensitization and reprocessing in the treatment of posttraumatic stress disordered sexual assault victims. *Bulletin of the Menninger Clinic, 61,* 317–334.

Rothbaum, B. O., Astin, M. C., & Marsteller, F. (2005). Prolonged exposure versus eye movement desensitization (EMDR) for PTSD rape victims. *Journal of Traumatic Stress, 18,* 607–616.

Rouanzoin, C. (1994, March). *EMDR: Dissociative disorders and MPD.* Paper presented at the annual meeting of the Anxiety Disorders Association of America, Santa Monica, CA.

Rubin, A. (2003). Unanswered questions about the empirical support for EMDR in the treatment of PTSD: A review of research. *Traumatology, 9,* 4–30.

Scheck, M. M., Schaeffer, J. A., & Gillette, C. S. (1998). Brief psychological intervention with traumatized young women: The efficacy of eye movement desensitization and reprocessing. *Journal of Traumatic Stress, 11,* 25–44.

Schulte, D. (1996). Tailor-made and standardized therapy: Complementary tasks in behavior therapy: A contrarian view. *Journal of Behavior Therapy and Experimental Psychiatry, 27,* 119–126.

Shapiro, F. (1989). Efficacy of the eye movement desensitization procedure in the treatment of traumatic memories. *Journal of Traumatic Stress, 2,* 199–223.

Shapiro, F. (1991). Eye movement desensitization and reprocessing procedure: From EMD to EMDR—A new treatment model for anxiety and related traumata. *Behavior Therapist, 14,* 133–135.

Shapiro, F. (1993). Eye movement desensitization and reprocessing (EMDR) in 1992. *Journal of Traumatic Stress, 6,* 417–421.

Shapiro, F. (1994). Alternative stimuli in the use of EMD(R). *Journal of Behavior Therapy & Experimental Psychiatry, 25,* 89.

Shapiro, F. (1995). *Eye movement desensitization and reprocessing: Basic principles, protocols and procedures.* New York: Guilford Press.

Shapiro, F. (1996). Eye movement desensitization and reprocessing (EMDR): Evaluation of controlled PTSD research. *Journal of Behavior Therapy and Experimental Psychiatry, 27,* 209–218.

Shapiro, F. (1999). Eye movement desensitization and reprocessing (EMDR) and the anxiety disorders: Clinical and research implications of an integrated psychotherapy treatment. *Journal of Anxiety Disorders, 13,* 35–67.

Shapiro, F. (2001). *Eye movement desensitization and reprocessing: Basic principles, protocols and procedures* (2nd ed.). New York: Guilford Press.

Shapiro, F. (Ed.). (2002). *EMDR as an integrative psychotherapy approach: Experts of diverse orientations explore the paradigm prism.* Washington, DC: American Psychological Association Books.

Shapiro, F., & Forrest, M. (1997). *EMDR: The breakthrough therapy for overcoming anxiety, stress and trauma.* New York: Basic Books.

Shapiro, F., Kaslow, F., & Maxfield, L. (2007). *Handbook of EMDR and family processes.* Hoboken, NJ: Wiley.

Silver, S. M., Brooks, A., & Obenchain, J. (1995). Eye movement desensitization and reprocessing treatment of Vietnam war veterans with PTSD: Comparative effects with biofeedback and relaxation training. *Journal of Traumatic Stress, 8,* 337–342.

Sjöblom, P. O., Andréewitch, S., Bejerot, S., Mörtberg, E., Brinck, U., Ruck, C., et al. (2003). *Regional treatment recommendation for anxiety disorders.* Stockholm: Medical Program Committee/Stockholm City Council, Sweden.

Soberman, G. B., Greenwald, R., & Rule, D. L. (2002). A controlled study of eye movement desensitization and reprocessing (EMDR) for boys with conduct problems. *Journal of Aggression, Maltreatment, and Trauma, 6,* 217–236.

Solomon, R. M. (1994, June). *Eye movement desensitization and reprocessing and treatment of grief.* Paper presented at International Conference on Grief and Bereavement in Contemporary Society, Stockholm, Sweden.

Solomon, R. M. (1995, February). *Critical incident trauma: Lessons learned at Waco, Texas.* Paper presented at the Law Enforcement Psychology Conference, San Mateo, CA.

Solomon, R. M. (1998). Utilization of EMDR in crisis intervention. *Crisis Intervention, 4,* 239–246.

Solomon, R. M., & Kaufman, T. (1994, March). *Eye movement desensitization and reprocessing: An effective addition to critical incident treatment protocols.* Paper presented at the annual meeting of the Anxiety Disorders Association of America, Santa Monica, CA.

Sprang, G. (2001). The use of eye movement desensitization and reprocessing (EMDR) in the treatment of traumatic stress and complicated mourning: Psychological and behavioral outcomes. *Research on Social Work Practice, 11*, 300–320.

Taylor, S., et al. (2004). Efficacy and outcome predictors for three PTSD treatments: Exposure therapy, EMDR, and relaxation therapy. In S. Taylor (Ed.), *Advances in the treatment of posttraumatic stress disorder: Cognitive-behavioral perspectives* (pp. 13–38). New York: Springer.

Taylor, S., Thordarson, D. S., Maxfield, L., Fedoroff, I. C., Lovell, K., & Ogrodniczuk, J. (2003). Comparative efficacy, speed, and adverse effects of three PTSD treatments: Exposure therapy, EMDR, and relaxation training. *Journal of Consulting and Clinical Psychology, 71*, 330–338.

van den Hout, M., Muris, P., Salemink, E., & Kindt, M. (2001). Autobiographical memories become less vivid and emotional after eye movements. *British Journal of Clinical Psychology, 40*, 121–130.

van der Kolk, B., et al. (in press). A randomized clinical trial of EMDR, fluoxetine and pill placebo in the treatment of PTSD: Treatment effects and long-term maintenance. *Journal of Clinical Psychiatry.*

van der Kolk, B. A. (2002). Beyond the talking cure: Somatic experience and subcortical imprints in the treatment of trauma. In F. Shapiro (Ed.), *EMDR as an integrative psychotherapy approach: Experts of diverse orientations explore the paradigm prism* (pp. 57–84). Washington, DC: American Psychological Association Books.

van der Kolk, B. A., Burbridge, B. A., & Suzuki, J. (1997). The psychobiology of traumatic memory: Clinical implications of neuroimaging studies. In R. Yehuda & A. C. McFarland (Eds.), *Annals of the New York Academy of Sciences: Vol. 821. Psychobiology of posttraumatic stress disorder.* New York: New York Academy of Sciences.

Van Etten, M. L., & Taylor, S. (1998). Comparative efficacy of treatments for posttraumatic stress disorder: A meta-analysis. *Clinical Psychology and Psychotherapy, 5*, 126–144.

Vaughan, K., Armstrong, M. S., Gold, R., O'Connor, N., Jenneke, W., & Tarrier, N. (1994). A trial of eye movement desensitization compared to image habituation training and applied muscle relaxation in post-traumatic stress disorder. *Journal of Behavior Therapy and Experimental Psychiatry, 25*(4), 283–291.

Wachtel, P. L. (2002). EMDR and psychoanalysis. In F. Shapiro (Ed.), *EMDR as an integrative psychotherapy approach: Experts of diverse orientations explore the paradigm prism* (pp. 123–150). Washington, DC: American Psychological Association Books.

Wernik, U. (1993). The role of the traumatic component in the etiology of sexual dysfunctions and its treatment with eye movement desensitization procedure. *Journal of Sex Education and Therapy, 19*, 212–222.

Wilson, S. A., Becker, L. A., & Tinker, R. H. (1995). Eye movement desensitization and reprocessing (EMDR) treatment for psychologically traumatized individuals. *Journal of Consulting and Clinical Psychology, 63*(6), 928–937.

Wilson, S. A., Becker, L. A., & Tinker, R. H. (1997). Fifteen-month follow-up of eye movement desensitization and reprocessing (EMDR) treatment for psychological trauma. *Journal of Consulting and Clinical Psychology, 65*(6), 1047–1056.

Wilson, S. A., Tinker, R., Becker, L. A., Hofmann, A., & Cole, J. W. (2000, September). *EMDR treatment of phantom limb pain with brain imaging (MEG).* Paper presented at the annual meeting of the EMDR International Association, Toronto, Ontario, Canada.

Wilson, T. (2005, March 16). *Value of manualized therapies.* Paper presented at the Veterans Administration Medical Center, Lyons, NJ

Wilson, D. L., Silver, S. M., Covi, W. C., & Foster, S. (1996). Eye movement desensitization and reprocessing: Effectiveness and autonomic correlates. *Journal of Behavior Therapy and Experimental Psychiatry, 27*, 219–229.

Young, J. E., Zangwill, W. M., & Behary, W. E. (2002). Combining EMDR and schema- focused therapy: The whole may be greater than the sum of the parts. In F. Shapiro (Ed.), *EMDR as an integrative psychotherapy approach: Experts of diverse orientations explore the paradigm prism* (pp. 181–208). Washington, DC: American Psychological Association Books.

Young, W. (1994). EMDR treatment of phobic symptoms in multiple personality. *Dissociation, 7*, 129–133.

CHAPTER 22

Pharmacological Approach to the Management of Stress and Anxiety Disorders

LASZLO A. PAPP

Although stress is part of human existence, the severity of a given stress does not usually predict the kind and degree of the subsequent reaction. Such reactions range from benign, transitional anxiety to severe, debilitating anxiety disorders. Although the pharmacological approach has been traditionally reserved for the management of anxiety disorders, the availability of efficacious and safe medications makes this approach a compelling alternative in the treatment of many stress reactions. At the same time, it should be emphasized that an equally efficacious nonpharmacological treatment is almost always preferable to medications. This chapter, an update of the original written by Laszlo Papp and Jack Gorman for the previous editions of this book, outlines the current principles of the pharmacological management of anxiety. Major changes include a significant expansion within the three traditional categories of antianxiety medications. Antidepressant anxiolytics, specifically the selective serotonin reuptake inhibitors (SSRIs), are now considered first-line agents for most anxiety disorders. In addition to the SSRIs, the traditional tricyclic antidepressants (TCAs), and monoamine oxidase inhibitors (MAOIs), this category now includes a number of newer "atypical" or "third-generation" antidepressants with proven anxiolytic properties. The information on the second group, benzodiazepines (BZDs), has been substantially revised and updated. Reflecting the rapid development of the field, the third category under "other antianxiety medications" has been expanded as well to include neuroleptics and a relatively new, but increasingly significant, class, the anticonvulsants. New sections have been added to describe the general principles of pharmacotherapy, to address controversies in the use of anxiolytic antidepressants, and to provide preliminary data on pharmacotherapy for specific phobias. The anxiety disorder categories discussed have been made consistent with the most recent (4th, text revised) edition of the *Diagnostic and Statistical Manual of Mental Disorders* (DSM-IV-TR; American Psychiatric Association, 2000). Although significant recent advances in anxiety disorders research outside of pharmacology are presented, only if clinically relevant.

MEDICATIONS AND ANXIETY

"Normal" anxiety serves many useful purposes. Anxiety ensures that we prepare for a job interview, seek the doctor's advice when feeling sick, and pay our taxes on time. In these situations, anxiety motivates us to take necessary actions and prevent potential dangers; once the problem is resolved, the anxiety lifts. Eliminating this type of "normal" anxiety by the use of prescription medications, alcohol, or other licit and illicit drugs is counterproductive and can be quite dangerous.

In some instances, however, anxiety can become excessive. A critical comment from one's superior may be blown out of proportion. Undue rumination about being fired from one's job may then spread to social and family functioning and may cause temporary disruption in sleep. After a few weeks and some reassurance, normal functioning is usually restored. This type of "excessive" anxiety serves no useful purpose when it lasts beyond the duration of the stressor. Although treatment is usually recommended, medications are rarely required.

Unlike "normal" and "excessive" anxiety, anxiety disorders in general (with the exception of posttraumatic stress disorder, or PTSD) do not directly result from, although they are frequently complicated by, real-life stresses. For instance, early childhood trauma is increasingly recognized to play a significant role in anxiety disorders (Safren, Gershuny, Marzol, Otto, & Pollack, 2002). Anxiety disorders have been found to be the most common psychiatric illnesses in the United States, with a lifetime prevalence rate of 28.8% (Kessler, Berglund, Demler, Jin, & Walters, 2005). Untreated, they can become lifelong disabilities that seriously interfere with everyday functioning. Nevertheless, these patients rarely receive adequate psychiatric evaluation and treatment. Some will decline help because of the stigma attached to psychiatric treatment, some will be disappointed by their physicians' approach and their lack of empathy, and others will resort to self-medication with alcohol or some other licit or illicit substance (Papp, 2004).

Anxiety disorders are highly treatable, and many of the treatments involve the judicious use of medications. The strategy of "pharmacological dissection" (Klein, 1964) of the formerly homogeneous category of "anxiety neurosis" into distinct and meaningful diagnostic groups has contributed to an unprecedented growth in the field of anxiety research. The establishment of separate anxiety disorder categories has given renewed impetus to the development of anxiety-disorder-specific medications. Basic science, including neuroimaging, neuroreceptor physiology, and genetics, involving both animals and human subjects, has begun to reveal the theoretical bases and underlying neurobiology of the differential and specific efficacy of anxiolytic agents. At the same time, symptom clusters that frequently cut across DSM diagnostic categories are increasingly recognized as legitimate targets of pharmacological interventions. The efficacy of some of these medications in several, distinct diagnostic categories suggests shared etiology and pathophysiology.

Pharmacological advances continue to generate both overenthusiasm about and unjustified skepticism toward the use of psychotropic medications in general. Fortunately, the artificial dichotomy and the subsequent hostility between the so-called biological and psychological approaches that has damaged the image of the profession and confused patients is rapidly fading; a growing number of clinicians and researchers recognize that this division is unjustified and unproductive (Alexopoulos, 2004). Rather than insisting on "purity," these "pragmatists" successfully advocate an eclectic approach based on scientific evidence. This chapter provides guidelines for the use of medications by the "pragmatic" practitioner.

HISTORICAL BACKGROUND

The oldest antistress drug is alcohol; to date, it remains the most frequently used nonspecific tranquilizer. The introduction of paraldehyde in 1882 and bromides in the early 20th century, followed shortly by the first use of barbiturates in 1903, heralded the beginning of modern anxiolysis. Although at present the use of these drugs should be strictly limited by the availability of safer and more effective anxiolytics, paraldehyde and some of the barbiturates retain certain specialized utilities.

Intramuscular or oral paraldehyde is an old-fashioned treatment for alcohol withdrawal. Phenobarbital is still used in the emergency treatment of seizures, as well as in cases of congenital hyperbilirubinemia (elevated blood bilirubin concentration). It is also used to decrease oxygen utilization during anesthesia and to reduce cerebral edema (swelling) following head trauma. Barbiturates may exert their sedative effects by decreasing presynaptic neurotransmitter release, by enhancing the postsynaptic effects of the inhibitory neurotransmitter gamma-aminobutyric acid (GABA), or by blocking calcium entry into neurons. Barbiturates are respiratory depressants and are contraindicated in patients with respiratory insufficiency, including sleep apnea. Abrupt discontinuation of these drugs may result in severe, potentially life-threatening withdrawal reactions. Barbiturates are clearly addicting and lethal in overdose.

In the 1930s, in response to the deficiencies of barbiturates, a series of non-barbiturate, non-BZD hypnotics were developed. Unfortunately, these drugs turned out to be just as problematic as the barbiturates, and most of them have retained only historic significance. Glutethimide (Doriden) overdose, for instance, can result in convulsions and fluctuating coma, as the drug is episodically released from tissue stores. Methaqualone (Quaalude) and methyprylone (Noludar) are both highly addicting and can be fatal in overdose. Meprobamate (Miltown) and tybamate (Benvil, Solacen) are modestly effective anxiolytics but possess a very low therapeutic index (therapeutic–toxic ratio).

The synthesis in 1957 of the first BZD, chlordiazepoxide (Librium), introduced a new era in the safe pharmacological management of anxiety. The demonstration of the specific anxiolytic effects of antidepressants, starting with imipramine and the MAOIs in the 1960s, followed by fluoxetine and other SSRIs in the 1980s and the continued steady flow of other "atypical" neurotransmitter-specific agents and anticonvulsants in the 1990s, provides many safe options in the pharmacological management of anxiety today. Novel pharmacological targets in anxiolysis under development include the glutaminergic system, substance P, neuroactive peptides, and the hypothalamic–pituitary–adrenal (HPA) system, among others. Advances in the emerging field of pharmacogenetics/pharmacogenomics have begun to yield clinically relevant results; genetic variations between and within populations could clearly influence response rates, metabolism, and side effects of most anxiolytics (Phillips & Van Bebber, 2005).

Although the current pharmacological management of anxiety disorders ranks among the most successful therapies in medicine, response rates still vary widely, from over 70% for panic disorder to only under 30% for chronic posttraumatic stress disorder. Increased efficacy and tolerability of newer medications have led to the recognition that treatment to full remission, as opposed to "improvement," confers significantly better long-term outcome. Consequently, the goal of modern anxiolytic therapies has been updated from partial symptom relief to restoring premorbid functioning.

GENERAL PRINCIPLES

One of the most important principles of pharmacotherapy is to use the lowest effective dose for the shortest possible period of time. This principle easily accommodates a range of needs, from the as-needed use of small doses of benzodiazepines for the occasional airplane ride for patients whose anxiety is limited to apprehension about flying to the lifelong need for high doses of antidepressants for severe obsessive–compulsive disorder. In other words, pharmacotherapy, just like most therapeutic interventions, requires careful consideration of the specific needs of the patient. Although this may sound like a commonsense truism, unnecessarily rigid prescribing schedules are not uncommon. The only recourse for patients is being well informed. The best predictor of a successful outcome is continued open discussion between physician and the informed patient. The following brief summary could form the basis of pharmacotherapy for all anxiety disorders.

The comprehensive psychiatric interview should assess onset, course, symptomatology, and comorbidity. Comorbid conditions (e.g., depression, bipolar disorder, substance use, personality disorders) will usually complicate the management of anxiety disorders and predict poorer outcome. Making the correct diagnosis is the basis of any therapy. The initial interview should elicit the history of prior treatments (doses, length of treatment periods, response, and side effects for each medication), prejudices, attitudes, and reservations about taking medications in general. The most common misperception is that psychiatric medications inevitably lead to addiction; many patients, as well as some clinicians, use the terms *dependence* and *addiction* interchangeably. Most prescription medications, both psychiatric and nonpsychiatric, will result in dependence. Patients with chronic conditions, such as diabetes, hypertension, recurrent depression, and anxiety, "depend" on their medications in order to function normally; stopping them abruptly could result in withdrawal symptoms and the return of their original symptoms. Addiction connotes pathological use, the goal of which is to reach a "high," which usually requires increasing doses of illicit and licit drugs and leads to significantly impaired functioning. In addiction, the risks of drug use clearly outweigh the potential benefits. Proper use of prescription medications almost never leads to addiction. A treatment history of family members may help with diagnosis and could predict the medication response of the patient.

Most patients will have had a comprehensive physical exam prior to the psychiatric evaluation, including blood tests for chemistry, hematology, and thyroid function, a urinalysis, and an electrocardiogram (EKG). Signs of neurological abnormalities should prompt a neurological exam and the appropriate brain imaging studies. Sleep abnormalities may warrant a referral for somnography in a sleep laboratory.

If the decision to use medications is made, the physician may rely on treatment algorithms, or decision trees, ideally based on scientific evidence. But many times, the choice can be based only on anecdotal information and published consensus statements. One guiding principle of these algorithms is that, in the absence of conclusive evidence for differential efficacy, the choice is usually determined by side-effect profiles. Clearly, longer maintenance treatments lower relapse rates, but the optimal duration of medication maintenance is generally unknown. Most anxiety disorders are chronic conditions, requiring continued, frequently lifelong but possibly intermittent, treatments.

Abrupt discontinuation of most medications, including anxiolytics/antidepressants, after long-term, continuous use results in withdrawal symptoms. Although medically dangerous withdrawal symptoms are rare and associated with only a few anxiolytics (discussed later), sudden discontinuation of most could result in significant discomfort. As a general rule, anxiolytics should be tapered gradually, unless continued exposure to the drug might be unsafe (e.g., nonelective surgery or other emergencies). Patients should be warned not to run out of their medications. Setting aside a week's worth in a separate container should remind them that they have only a few days to get their refill on time. This simple tool will spare them from making the frantic last-minute calls to doctors, insurance companies, and pharmacies.

Slow, gradual tapering of medication may be attempted after 1 year in symptom-free patients. The benefits of taper should be balanced against the potential complication of drug resistance. Retreatment with the same agent may not produce benefits, and a former drug responder needs several trials before an efficacious drug is found again. Another potential complication of long-term pharmacotherapy of anxiety, drug "burnout," refers to patients who, after a few months of response, develop drug resistance. Dose adjustment up or down might help, but frequently it is necessary to augment or replace the original agent.

Failure to respond should trigger reassessment of the diagnosis of comorbid conditions and target symptoms, review of side effects, and checking compliance, and potential drug interactions. The most frequent reason for medication nonresponse remains undermedication. Noncompliance is frequently related to anticipated or actual side effects. Thus side-effect profiles have been increasingly considered a major factor in choosing a drug. A less efficacious drug with a more favorable side-effect profile may be preferred.

Patients should be well informed, but an overinclusive presentation of side effects may be unnecessary and alarming, particularly because most side effects are benign and do not represent clinically significant limitations. A generic approach to the most commonly reported side effects of antianxiety medications should begin with the fact that lower than therapeutic starting doses are generally better tolerated; gradual, slow increase gives the patient with anxiety the best chance to accommodate to adverse reactions. Complaints of dry mouth respond to increased fluid intake, sugarless gum or candy, and possibly to bethanecol. Excessive perspiration may diminish with time; if it persists, a low-dose, strongly anticholinergic antidepressant (e.g., amitriptyline) or terazosin could be added. Constipation is alleviated with a high-bulk diet with plenty of fluid, stool softeners, or milk of magnesia. Avoiding sudden positional or postural changes and wearing support hose should minimize orthostatic/positional hypotension. More severe cases require increased fluid and salt intake, salt tablets, mineralocorticoids, or amphetamines, unless specifically contraindicated. Urinary hesitancy should prompt dose reduction and/or bethanecol. Anticholinergic side effects (dry mouth, constipation, positional hypotension, etc.) are best handled by switching to a less anticholinergic drug. Anticholinergic drugs are contraindicated in cases of prostate hypertrophy or closed-angle glaucoma. Sexual dysfunction is a common side effect, mostly of serotonergic drugs. Dose reduction is rarely helpful. Delayed or lack of orgasm (anorgasmia) may respond to bethanecol, cyproheptadine, sildenafil, or yohimbine. Diminished libido may improve with bupropion or buspirone. Unfortunately, the combined efficacy of the antidotes to sexual dysfunction is disappointing, and the anxiolytic medication may have to be discontinued.

Insomnia may improve over time, but switching the dose to the morning may help as well. Severe insomnia usually responds to hypnotics (zolpidem [Ambien], zaleplon [Sonata], eszopiclone [Lunesta], ramelteon [Rozerem], benzodiazepines or trazodone

[Desyrel]). Sedating drugs are given at bedtime. Most antidepressants cause photo-sensitivity. Antidepressant-induced hypomania may respond to dose reduction, but, especially if the patient has a history of bipolarity, mood stabilizers may be indicated. Weight gain is one of the most troublesome and limiting side effects of antidepressant antianxiety drugs. Tricyclic antidepressants with strong anticholinergic profile and MAOIs are probably the worst offenders, followed by the serotonergic class. Atypical antidepressants such as bupropion, trazodone, and nefazadone are less likely to cause weight gain, but due to their weak anxiolytic effects, they are mostly used to counter side effects and/or to augment other anxiolytics. If diet and exercise fail, certain diet pills, appetite suppressants, or bupropion can be tried, but frequently only dose reduction or a switch to a different agent will be successful.

Many of the anxiolytic antidepressants can induce hyponatremia (Kinzie, 1987) in the context of the syndrome called "inappropriate antidiuretic hormone secretion" (SIADH). Most of the SSRIs, TCAs, neuroleptics, and several others (reboxetine, bupropion) have been implicated in the syndrome, manifesting clinically as weakness, lethargy, confusion, nausea, and headache that could progress to convulsions, coma, and death if not treated. The management of the condition includes fluid restriction and intravenous administration of hypertonic saline.

Duration and frequency of contact between the patient and the medicating doctor vary depending on many factors (logistics, severity of illness, patient's response to the medication, availability and utilization of ancillary mental health and medical services), but general guidelines apply. The initial evaluation should last for at least 1 hour. If the patient begins to take medication, a follow-up visit, lasting from 20 to 30 minutes, should occur within a week or two after the first visit. Another follow-up visit is usually indicated approximately 1 month after the initial evaluation, and if the condition of the patient is stable, monthly visits are usually sufficient to monitor progress. Face-to-face contact could be less frequent in certain situations, but a visit every 3 months is usually the outside limit. The prescribing physician should make arrangements for 24-hour coverage and should be available to answer questions on the phone.

BENZODIAZEPINES

Despite the wide availability of alternatives, BZDs remain the most popular anxiolytics. Other therapeutic indications for BZDs include insomnia, seizures, muscle spasms, and the induction of anesthesia. All BZDs possess similar anxiolytic, sedative, and anticonvulsant properties; pharmacokinetic differences explain their various indications. Because of their safety, efficacy, and high therapeutic index, BZDs have almost entirely replaced barbiturates and most nonbarbiturate, non-BZD sedatives. From the time they became available in the mid-1960s, BZD use in the United States increased steadily until 1985. Since then, the number of BZD prescriptions filled annually in retail pharmacies has leveled off. The most commonly prescribed BZD was chlordiazepoxide in 1965, surpassed by diazepam by 1970 and alprazolam by 1987 (Nelson, 1987). According to a recent survey, approximately 1 out of every 10 American adults had taken BZDs during the previous year, whereas 1 out of every 4 psychiatric patients used BZDs during the same time period. Nevertheless, only a small fraction of those found to be in need of pharmacological treatment for an anxiety disorder received any medication (Salzman, Goldenberg, Bruce, & Keller, 2001). Contrary to public perception, scientific data conclusively show that BZDs are safe, that they are not overused, and that tolerance to their therapeutic effects is extremely rare (American Psychiatric Association Task Force, 1990). When used properly, doses of BZDs remain constant over several years of continued use, and dose escalation is quite rare (Soumerai et al., 2003). A case can be made that, given the high prevalence of severe anxiety disorders, BZDs, along with other anxiolytics, are, in fact, underprescribed.

Pharmacology of BZDs

BZDs bind to the BZD–GABA receptor complex and enhance the postsynaptic inhibitory effects of GABA. This process is mediated by the opening of postsynaptic chloride channels (Tallman, Paul, Skolnick, & Gallagher, 1980; Pritchett et al., 1989). Because of their high lipid solubility, all BZDs readily cross the blood–brain barrier. Many of the compounds discussed later, in the section on anticonvulsants, also have putative effects on GABA, but, possibly due to higher selectivity and alternative mechanisms of action on the GABA receptor complex, their therapeutic and side-effect profiles are different.

The so-called long-acting BZDs (e.g., chlordiazepoxide or diazepam) produce active metabolites that require the hepatic mixed-oxidase system for degradation. The elimination half-life (time needed for the plasma concentration to fall by 50%) of these BZDs tends to be more than 24 hours, sometimes several days. By contrast, short-acting BZDs (e.g., lorazepam or oxazepam) have no active metabolites, do not require the mixed-oxidase system, and therefore have half-lives that are shorter than 24 hours. The active metabolites of alprazolam and triazolam do not lengthen their half-lives. Due to shared metabolic pathways that primarily involve the cytochrome P450 isoenzymes, clinically significant changes in drug concentrations may occur when BZDs are combined with other anxiolytics (e.g., SSRIs). Currently available BZDs, used as anxiolytics in the United States, are listed in Table 22.1.

Principles of BZD Use

A number of factors should be taken into account when BZDs are used for anxiety.

1. All BZDs are equally sedating. Tolerance to this sedative–hypnotic effect usually develops within a few weeks of continued use. Tolerance to their anxiolytic effects, however, is extremely rare. Evidence consistently shows that once a therapeutic dose of a BZD is reached, it is rarely necessary to raise the dose again in order to maintain the same level

TABLE 22.1 Benzodiazepine Anxiolytics

Generic name	Trade name	Usual daily dose (mg)
Long-acting		
Chlordiazepoxide	Librium	15–100
Clonazepam	Klonopin, wafer Klonopin	0.5–6
Clorazepate	Tranxene	7.5–60
Diazepam	Valium	2–60
Short-acting		
Alprazolam	Xanax/XR/Niravam	0.5–6
Lorazepam	Ativan	1–6
Oxazepam	Serax	30–120

of therapeutic benefit (Rickels, Schweizer, Csanalosi, Case, & Chung, 1988). In fact, patients with panic disorder have been shown to reduce their BZD dose over time (Sheehan, 1987). Because of their increased vulnerability to sedation and cognitive side effects, older patients should take significantly lower doses of BZDs. Other occasionally observed side effects that necessitate dose reduction include ataxia or incoordination, dysarthria (slurred speech), vertigo, impaired memory, and dizziness. Hence it is critical that patients on BZDs be regularly monitored by a physician.

2. Some patients, frequently those with histories of organic brain disease or significant character pathology, become "disinhibited" (lacking appropriate inhibitions, disregarding social conventions) on BZDs. These patients should be placed on a significantly reduced BZD dose and followed carefully.

3. BZD abuse by patients with prior histories of alcohol or other substance abuse is common (Ciraulo, Sands, & Shader, 1988). Only as a last resort should BZDs be prescribed for these patients.

4. Like most drugs, if BZDs are taken for a long period of time, they may produce physiological dependence, as evidenced by discontinuance syndrome when stopped abruptly (Roy-Byrne, Dager, Cowley, Vitaliano, & Dunner, 1989). The symptoms of this discontinuance syndrome commonly include insomnia, anxiety, agitation, muscle twitching, tremor, diarrhea, photophobia, headache, and nausea. They may represent a transient and more intense return of the original anxiety symptoms (rebound), the return of the pattern of the original anxiety (recurrence or relapse), and/or the development of new symptoms that were not part of the original anxiety (withdrawal). The most severe, but fortunately the least frequent, discontinuance symptom is withdrawal seizure. The severity of the discontinuance syndrome is proportional to the dose and duration of use and the rate of taper. Therefore, as a rule, BZDs should be used at the lowest efficacious dose and for the shortest time needed for improvement. In tapering, the dose should be reduced by no more than 10% every 3 days.

5. Some studies suggest that benzodiazepines can induce or exacerbate depression, although causality has not been established. If depression develops during the course of BZD treatment, lowering the dose, discontinuing the drug, and/or adding an antidepressant may be indicated.

6. Although reported fetal abnormalities (cleft palate, lip deformities) associated with BZD use have not been confirmed, the consensus is that BZDs should be avoided during the first trimester and preferably during the entire pregnancy. BZDs belong to pregnancy class D. They are not contraindicated in pregnancy but should be used with caution, following careful risk–benefit analysis.

BZD Treatment Recommendations

The presence of anxiety does not necessarily indicate the need for anxiolytics. As noted earlier, mild anxiety may actually improve performance. Even moderate anxiety that interferes with performance may still be best managed with psychotherapy. If it is determined that drug treatment is necessary for an acute anxiety episode, rapid relief is usually achieved by a single oral dose of diazepam or alprazolam. Because of its high lipid solubility, diazepam works within 15 minutes. Placed under the tongue, alprazolam also dissolves rapidly, with a comparable speed of onset of action. Clonazepam in a wafer form and an orally dissolving formulation of alprazolam also speed absorption and serve as alternatives for patients fearful of swallowing pills. On the other hand, if the intramuscular route is preferred, lorazepam is a better choice. Contrary to earlier claims of better efficacy for the "high-potency" alprazolam compared with the "low-potency" diazepam in patients with panic disorder, current evidence strongly suggests that all BZDs are equally efficacious (Charney & Woods, 1989). Nevertheless, for reasons other than lack of efficacy (cost, marketing, tradition), not all BZDs are used for anxiolysis.

For short-term use (less than 1 week), short-half-life BZDs have the advantage of having no "hangover effect" and of causing less sedation than long-half-life BZDs. Those with rapid, simple metabolism are preferred in the elderly and in patients with impaired liver function. For longer term use, long- and short-half-life BZDs are equally useful. Studies provide mixed results as to whether the discontinuance syndrome is any less troublesome with long-acting than with short-acting BZDs.

The length of BZD treatment is highly individual. Some patients continue their medications at stable doses for several years without any evidence of loss in efficacy. Short-term anxiolytic treatment should probably continue for at least 2 to 4 weeks beyond complete symptom remission. At that point the dose could be reduced and, if possible, discontinued. If the original symptoms return, the medication should be reinstituted; at a later date, tapering could be attempted again. Rebound anxiety and/or withdrawal symptoms should not be confused with the return of the original symptoms; they are best managed by slower tapering. Cognitive-behavioral strategies have been shown to facilitate successful BZD taper (Gorenstein et al., 2005). Because learning and retention may be affected directly, and because the as-needed use of benzodiazepines may serve as an avoidance strategy, some psychotherapists advocate anxiolytics other than benzodiazepines if used in combination with cognitive-behavioral therapy (CBT) (Westra, Stewart, & Conrad, 2002). Recommendations for the use of BZDs in the treatment of specific anxiety disorders are given later in the chapter.

ANTIDEPRESSANTS

The success of imipramine in controlling panic attacks in patients with panic disorder provided the first evidence that antidepressants may alleviate anxiety independently of their antidepressant effect (Klein & Fink, 1962). This historic observation in the late 1950s also marked the beginning of attempts to differentiate among the anxiety disorders on the basis of their response to medications. The introduction of fluoxetine in the 1980s, followed by a series of similarly acting agents, began a new era of anxiolysis with a focus on serotonergic neurotransmission. Because of their broad spectrum of efficacy and favorable side-effect profile, this new class of antidepressants, the SSRIs, provided an important alternative to patients intolerant of the side effects of older agents and for those suffering from comorbid conditions such as depression. By 1990, fluoxetine became the number-one-selling antidepressant, and a few years later the SSRIs became the first-line treatment choice for most anxiety disorders. Over the past several years, "third-generation" antidepressants, including the serotonin–norepinephrine reuptake inhibitors (SNRIs) such as venlafaxine and duloxetine, have been added as broad-spectrum anxiolytic alternatives.

The efficacy of antidepressants is most likely related to their ability to alter neurotransmission in the synapse. They can block the reuptake of neurotransmitters back into the presynaptic nerve ending, antagonize certain receptors (directly or indirectly, partially or fully), or inhibit specific neurotransmitter-degrading enzymes. Patients with anxiety disorders show diminished physiological flexibility (Hoehn-Saric et al., 2004). The normalization of heart rate variability in anxiety disorders by antidepressants implies relevant cardiovascular etiopathology (Yeregani et al., 1995). Similarly, correcting respiratory abnormalities in these patients with antidepressants may be an important aspect of their utility; most antidepressants directly affect the central regulation of respiration (Papp, Klein, & Gorman, 1993).

An alternative theory focuses on the neuroprotective effects of antidepressants; they may be beneficial by countering neurodegenerative processes associated with aging, trauma, and other insults to the central nervous system. The anxiolytic effects of disrupting the integration of pathological, aversive memories using fluoxetine in an animal model suggests still another potential mechanism (Degroot & Nomikos, 2005). The potentiating effect of D-cycloserine in exposure therapy (Ressler et al., 2004) also supports the significance of memory and learning theory in anxiolysis. The exact mechanism of anxiolysis remains the subject of intensive research (Snyder & Peroutka, 1984).

Most antidepressants have long elimination half-lives and a number of active metabolites. Therefore, most of them can be taken once a day. Other than for monitoring compliance, antidepressant blood levels have limited use in clinical practice. The exception is nortriptyline: A blood level of nortriptyline between 50 and 150ng has been found to be associated with good results and should be maintained. In the case of other antidepressants, however, blood levels fluctuate widely and do not predict or correspond with clinical status (American Psychiatric Association Task Force, 1985).

The currently available antidepressants with anxiolytic properties are listed in Table 22.2. They include TCAs, MAOIs (including reversible MAOIs, or RIMAs), SSRIs, SNRIs, and "other" or "atypical" antidepressants.

Tricyclic Antidepressants

Following the seminal studies with imipramine, a series of TCAs (this traditional category include a few heterocyclic compounds as well) were tested in patients with panic disorder and other anxiety disorders. Most controlled studies found these drugs to be superior to placebo in most anxiety disorders (Liebowitz et al., 1988). The advantages of TCAs over BZDs (once-a-day administration, fewer and less troublesome withdrawal symptoms, less sedation, less dependence, broader efficacy), in spite of some disadvantages (later onset of action, anticholinergic side effects, initial agitation, metabolic effects, and sexual effects), make them a good treatment alternative for patients with anxiety disorders.

Most side effects of the TCAs, though they can be quite bothersome, do not represent clinically significant limitations. Orthostatic hypotension is problematic only in the elderly, who are more susceptible to falls and subsequent injuries. In most cases the inconvenience of positional drops in blood pressure can be minimized by avoiding sudden postural changes, increasing salt intake, or using constrictive support hose. For patients with severe orthostatic hypotension, nortriptyline can still be successfully utilized.

Most TCAs prolong the PR and QRS intervals on the EKG, but in an otherwise healthy patient, these EKG changes are not clinically significant. Anticholinergic side effects are the most frequent causes of premature termination or intolerance of TCAs. Significant weight gain, urinary hesitancy or block, severe constipation, sexual dysfunction, and cognitive impairment may be managed by lowering the dose or by adding bethanecol, stool softeners, or (in the case of anorgasmia) yohimbine, ginkgo, or the antihistamine cyproheptadine. Most TCAs cause photosensitivity.

If medications with anticholinergic side effects are contraindicated (i.e., because of prostate hypertrophy or closed-angle glaucoma), the least anticholinergic TCA, desipramine, or an antidepressant with no anticholinergic side effects (e.g., SSRIs, bupropion) should be used. The only TCA found beneficial in the treatment of patients with obsessive–compulsive disorder (OCD) is clomipramine, most likely due to its powerful serotonergic properties.

TABLE 22.2. Antidepressant Anxiolytics

Generic name	Trade name	Usual daily dose (mg)
Tricyclic antidepressants		
Amitriptyline	Elavil, Endep	150–300
Clomipramine	Anafranil	50–250
Desipramine	Norpramin, Pertofrane	150–300
Doxepin	Sinequan, Adapin	150–300
Imipramine	Tofranil (PM) Jamimine	75–300
Nortriptyline	Aventyl, Pamelor	50–150
Protriptyline	Vivactil	20–60
Trimipramine	Surmontil	100–300
Monoamine oxidase inhibitors		
Isocarboxazide	Marplan	20–50
Pargyline	Eutonyl	75–150
Phenelzine	Nardil	45–90
Selegiline/deprenyl	Eldepryl/Emsam	30–60/6–12
Tranylcypromine	Parnate	30–60
Moclobemide (RIMA)	Manerix	75–150
Brofaromine (RIMA)		100–250
Atypical antidepressants		
Bupropion	Wellbutrin (SR/XL)/Zyban	200–450
Trazodone	Desyrel	50–400
Nefazodone	Serzone	100–400
Mirtazepine	Remeron (Sol Tab)	15–60
Reboxetine	Edronax/Vestra	4–8
Selective serotonin reuptake inhibitors		
Fluoxetine	Prozac/Sarafem	5–80
Sertraline	Zoloft	50–200
Paroxetine	Paxil/Pexeva	10–60
Fluvoxamine	Luvox	50–200
Citalopram	Celexa	10–40
Escitalopram	Lexapro	5–20
Selective serotonin–norepinephrine reuptake inhibitors		
Venlafaxine	Effexor/XR	75–250
Duloxetine	Cymbalta	40–120

Monoamine Oxidase Inhibitors

Close to the time of the identification of imipramine as an antipanic drug in the United States, investigators in England showed that "hysterical" patients with phobic symptoms responded favorably to MAOIs. Patients in this diagnostic category share a number of features with patients with agoraphobia and panic disorder. Subsequent comparative trials in patients with phobias have shown that the MAOI phenelzine is marginally more effective than imipramine and that both drugs are significantly more effective than placebo (Sheehan, Bach, Ballenger, & Jacobsen, 1980). The more recently introduced antidepressants (SSRIs, SNRIs, atypicals) have not been compared directly with MAOIs in clinical trials.

The reluctance to prescribe MAOIs and the relative absence of clinical trials with this class stem from the fact that, unless patients adhere to a special tyramine-free diet, MAOIs can induce hypertensive crisis. Following in the footsteps of their British colleagues, American psychiatrists increasingly acknowledge the unique benefits of MAOIs and realize that the diet is easy to follow and that hypertensive reactions are exceedingly rare (Tollefson, 1983). The introduction of reversible inhibitors of MAO-A (RIMAs, not currently available in the United States) gave new impetus to increased utilization. Due to their selective and reversible inhibition of the MAO-A, this subclass of MAOIs (moclobemide, brofaromine) poses only minimal risk of tyramine-induced hypertensive crisis. Preliminary data indicate that RIMAs may be comparable in efficacy to the traditional MAOIs and may possess an improved risk–benefit ratio. A transdermal delivery system for selegiline, recently marketed in the United States under the trade name Emsam, further reduces the risk of hypertensive crisis. Diet restriction is not required at the lowest (6 mg) dose, but given the limited experience, caution is still warranted.

Orthostatic hypotension is a more common and more serious side effect of MAOI than of TCA treatment; its management includes the techniques recommended for the TCAs. Severe postural hypotension usually responds well to the addition of fludrocortisone (0.1 mg two to three times a day) for 2 weeks. Weight gain, sexual dysfunction, peripheral edema, and hypomania, in addition to weak anticholinergic symptoms, may require adjusting the dose or switching to a different class of antidepressant (after at least 2 weeks off the MAOI, while also remaining on the diet). Agitation and insomnia are more likely with tranylcypromine. As a precaution, patients are advised to carry a wallet card and/or wear a bracelet to alert caregivers of the potential drug interactions (e.g., all sympathomimetics, most decongestants, meperidine, etc.). Some clinicians recommend that patients on MAOIs carry the antihypertensive nifedipine (with some advantage over the more traditional chlorpromazine) to be used in case of severe headache, usually the sign of a hypertensive crisis. Cases of nifedipine-induced sudden drop in blood pressure makes this recommendation controversial. Following taper and discontinuation of MAOIs, diet restrictions should continue for at least 2 weeks.

Selective Serotonin Reuptake Inhibitors

Fluoxetine (Prozac), the first SSRI introduced in the United States, proved to be a real advance over the previous generations of antidepressants. By 1990, after only 2 years on the market, fluoxetine was the best-selling antidepressant in the country. Over the next decade, five more SSRIs have been marketed in the United States (paroxetine [Paxil], sertraline [Zoloft], fluvoxamine [Luvox], citalopram [Celexa], escitalopram [Lexapro]). Contrary to various claims, none of them presents a clear and substantive advance over fluoxetine. Also contrary to their marketed, disorder-specific indications, they all possess comparable efficacy for most anxiety disorders. Whereas the pharmacological profiles of the SSRIs are quite similar, their side effects differ, due to varying affinity to the subtypes of the 5-HT receptors. They also differ in their ability to inhibit the isoenzymes of the hepatic P450 system, and therefore they can induce differential drug–drug interactions. Selecting one over the other is usually based on these side effects and drug–drug interactions. These drugs are serotonin-specific, with only minimal effects on noradrenergic and dopaminergic neurotransmission. Their advantages over the more traditional antidepressants are numerous.

SSRIs, in general, are well tolerated (no anticholinergic and only minimal cardiovascular side effects) and easily administered. Moreover, they are not lethal in overdose. The disadvantages include delayed onset of action and the fact that most patients with panic attacks cannot tolerate the usual starting dose of the more activating fluoxetine and sertraline due to increased initial anxiety. Benzodiazepines have been used successfully in combination with these activating SSRIs during the first few weeks and then tapered gradually when the SSRI becomes effective (Goddard et al., 2001). Also, because of the initial agitation and insomnia, these activating drugs are usually taken in the morning, whereas the more sedating paroxetine is given at bedtime.

As became obvious over the years, up to 50% of patients also complain of delayed orgasm and decreased libido while on SSRIs. Less than half of the patients who experience sexual side effects will get partial relief from the usual antidotes (lower doses, addition of bupropion, sildenafil, yohimbine, cyproheptadine, ginkgo, etc.). Another postmarketing surprise was the significant weight gain many patients experienced on SSRIs. Paroxetine and fluoxetine seem to be the worst offenders, but weight monitoring is advised with all SSRIs. Increased appetite, food cravings, and slowed metabolism are all implicated. Because the countermeasures (addition of bupropion, topiramate, appetite suppressants, or thyroid hormones) are rarely effective, poorly tolerated, and frequently contraindicated, weight gain is one of the most common reasons for stopping SSRIs. Fluoxetine's long half-life of several days allows administration less than once a day and, in select patients, even once a week. Careful monitoring of electrolytes in elderly patients may identify SSRI-induced hyponatremia due to inappropriate antidiuretic hormone secretion. Treatment with SSRIs may be associated with reduced bone density (Richards et al., 2007).

If clinically justified, SSRIs are not contraindicated during pregnancy (Kulin et al, 1998); they do appear in breast milk, but the effects on the newborn seem temporary and relatively benign (Misri, Kim, Riggs, & Kostras, 2000). Because of recent reports of increased risks of cardiovascular malformations and premature births in babies born to mothers exposed to paroxetine during pregnancy, paroxetine's pregnancy category has been changed from C to D, indicating elevated risk. Drugs in category D are not contraindicated in pregnancy, but they should be used with caution and avoided if safer alternatives are available. For now, all other SSRIs remain in pregnancy category C.

Compared with other patients with anxiety disorders, those with OCD usually require substantially higher doses and longer duration of exposure before they respond to the SSRIs. Abrupt discontinuation of SSRIs in an emergency is not contraindicated medically; withdrawal symptoms (flu-like syndrome, insomnia, agitation) are not dangerous, are transient, and are generally less problematic than those of BZDs. Nevertheless, gradual tapering is still recommended to minimize the occasionally quite severe discomfort.

Serotonin–Norepinephrine Reuptake Inhibitors

The first SNRI, venlafaxine (Effexor), was introduced in the late 1990s. The efficacy of venlafaxine has been demonstrated in several large clinical trials, first in the treatment of depression and then in several anxiety disorders, including generalized anxiety, panic, social anxiety, and posttraumatic stress disorders. Although venlafaxine resembles tricyclic antidepressants in its dual action on serotonergic and noradrenergic reuptake, it is relatively devoid of anticholinergic and cardiovascular side effects. Dose-dependent reuptake inhibition (5-HT at lower doses, norepinephrine at higher doses) may explain the sequence of side effects during titration (Frazer, 2001). The reported elevation in blood pressure is less likely on low doses (Thase, 1998), and the initial nausea usually responds to more gradual dose increase. Large randomized trials found that the extended-release form of venlafaxine was also effective for generalized anxiety disorder (GAD; Gelenberg et al., 2000) and that 90% of those maintained on the drug were able to control GAD for 6 months (Montgomery et al., 2002). As a dual-mechanism agent, venlafaxine may be particularly advantageous in patients with comorbid anxiety disorder and depression (Silverstone & Salinas, 2001). Compared with the dose required in depression, a substantially lower level (mean dose under 100mgs) may benefit patients with panic disorder, with the added advantage of significantly fewer side effects (Papp et al., 1998). Unfortunately, withdrawal from venlafaxine can be problematic due to clinically significant withdrawal symptoms, including nausea, lethargy, gastrointestinal upset, and a "flu-like" syndrome that could last for several weeks. Gradual, prolonged taper is the only antidote.

A second medication in this class was introduced in 2004 in the United States. Duloxetine (Cymbalta) has been approved for the treatment of depression, GAD, and neuropathic pain, and preliminary data also suggest efficacy in other anxiety disorders in doses comparable to those used in patients with depression. At the usual dose of 60–120 mgs/day, the most frequently observed side effects were nausea, dry mouth, constipation, sedation, and increased sweating. Sexual side effects and weight gain may be less common than seen with SSRIs, but this claim has not been confirmed in controlled trials.

"Atypical" Antidepressants

Medications in this class are not easily categorized by their mechanisms of action. They tend to affect several neurotransmitter systems as agonists and/or antagonists (partial or full), autoreceptor modulators, and/or reuptake inhibitors. In general, they are less efficacious as anxiolytics when used alone, but they can potentiate the benefits and/or counter some of the side effects of other anxiolytics.

The selective alpha$_2$ and 5-HT$_{2/3}$ antagonist mirtazapine (Remeron) has shown promising anxiolytic effects in open trials. Its common side effects of sedation and weight gain could benefit older patients with insomnia and loss of appetite as well as when used in combination with activating antidepressants.

Trazodone (Desyrel) is a relatively weak anxiolytic but can be beneficial for anxious patients with prominent insomnia or those who develop sleep problems on SSRIs. Trazodone is well tolerated but has been reported to exacerbate preexisting ventricular irritability (Pohl, Bridges, Rainey, Boudoulas, & Yeragani, 1986), and can induce priapism (sustained, painful erection) and orthostatic hypotension (Ellison, Milofsky, & Ely, 1990).

The 5-HT$_2$ antagonist nefazodone (Serzone) has been tested extensively and has demonstrated clear benefits in patients with PTSD, panic disorder (PD) and GAD. Reports of possible nefazodone-induced liver damage caused the manufacturer to stop marketing the brand name product in the United States, and most practitioners stopped prescribing it altogether. Unless the association with liver damage is refuted, nefazodone is not likely to survive.

Bupropion (Wellbutrin, Zyban) is a powerful antidepressant but failed as an anxiolytic. Due to its significant activating properties, most patients with anxiety disorders are unable to tolerate it even when given in combination with other antidepressants (usually to counter sexual and metabolic side effects). As potential exceptions, the mood symptoms of patients with PTSD may respond favorably to bupropion (Canive, Clark, Calais, Qualls, & Tuason, 1998), and some patients with social anxiety disorder may also benefit (Emmanuel et al., 2000).

The selective norepinephrine reuptake inhibitor reboxetine (not yet available in the United States) is a likely anxiolytic that has shown significant benefits in patients with PD (Dannon et al., 2002; Versiani et al., 2002).

Antidepressant Treatment Recommendations

Antidepressants are not recommended for the treatment of episodic anxiety or excessive anxiety; they should be reserved for managing anxiety disorders. Disorder-specific recommendations are given later in the chapter. In the absence of conclusive evidence for differential efficacy, the choice among them depends on side effects, history of prior response to drugs (either of the patient or of their first-degree relatives), comorbid medical (endocrine, cardiac, gastrointestinal, neurological, etc.) and psychiatric conditions (depression, mania, other anxiety disorders), drug–drug interactions (for patients on multiple-drug regimens), and patient preference. The exception to this rule is to favor primarily serotonergic drugs (SSRIs, clomipramine) in patients with OCD.

In order to minimize initial agitation, the starting dose of the antidepressant may have to be a small fraction of the usual antidepressant dose. The dose of antidepressant needed for symptom control varies widely from individual to individual. The general rule here is to raise the dose either until symptoms remit completely or until bothersome side effects prevent further increase. The eventual effective anxiolytic dose is comparable to the antidepressant dose for the majority of patients with anxiety disorders (with the possible exception of venlafaxine). Patients with OCD, and possibly with GAD, tend to require higher doses and longer duration of initial drug exposure before they respond to treatment. Slow titration, usually recommended for the elderly and those with known drug sensitivity, will also extend the length of initial drug exposure needed.

In general, although exceptions do exist, most anxiety disorders run a chronic, fluctuating course. The pharmacological approach should match this course, with periodic attempts to taper and discontinue the drug following a prolonged—typically more than 1 year—symptom-free period. Relapse should warrant the consideration of even longer medication maintenance; life-long maintenance is indicated after multiple relapses and/or failed attempts to discontinue medications. Antidepressants may trigger hypomania in vulnerable patients. Bipolar comorbidity may be particularly prevalent in patients with Pd (MacKinnon et al., 2002). Careful history and close monitoring are the best strategies for minimizing this problem. Patients with positive histories for either drug-induced or spontaneous manic or hypomanic episodes should not be started on antidepressants without a mood stabilizer. These patients may preferentially respond to an anticonvulsant with anxiolytic properties (see the section on anticonvulsants later in the chapter).

Serotonin syndrome is a rare but potential risk for patients receiving two or more serotonergic agents. An SSRI added to another serotonergic antidepressant (clomipramine) or metoclopramide (an antiemetic) or to any of the several serotonergic diet pills (sibutramine [Meridia]) could trigger the syndrome, which consists of confusion, agitation, diaphoresis, fever, and tachycardia (Fisher & Davis, 2002). Drug–drug interactions are increasingly recognized as important factors in selecting the appropriate agent. Inhibition or induction of the numerous hepatic P450 isoenzymes could result in significant alteration of plasma levels. Fluoxetine, paroxetine, and fluvoxamine are most likely to affect the metabolism of several classes of medications (e.g., TCAs, neuroleptics, beta blockers, macrolide antibiotics, benzodiazepines, antihistamines, calcium channel blockers, antiarrhythmics), whereas sertraline and escitalopram are relatively free of this problem.

Suicide Risk and Antidepressants

The association between increased suicidal ideation and treatment with antidepressants has been considered ever since the introduction of the first antidepressants. It is possible that the initial agitation associated with most antidepressants (including SSRIs) is responsible for this clinically significant phenomenon (Papp & Gorman, 1990).

More recently, the controversy has focused on SSRIs (Fava & Rosenbaum, 1991) and specifically on their use in depressed children and adolescents. Based on questionable evidence the SSRIs, with the exception of fluoxetine, have been suspended for the treatment of depression in youths in the United Kingdom, and similar restrictions are under review by the Food and Drug Administration (FDA) in the United States. For now, a "black box" warning has been added to the product label of all antidepressants stating the increased risk of suicide. The increased media and public attention have generated much-needed scrutiny and careful review of the data. Unfortunately, at present, factors other than medical or scientific ones are driving the debate, to the detriment of patients. Many patients and concerned parents of younger patients, frightened by sensationalized and unsubstantiated reports, have stopped effective medication regimens or switched to medications that are not implicated (even though some of these alternative medications are more dangerous and less effective).

As the available data are being analyzed and a definitive statement is being prepared, the following guidelines seem reasonable: depressed patients, treated or untreated, are at increased risk for suicide; suicidal risk is also increased in patients with primary anxiety disorders, especially if comorbid depression or certain personality disorders are also present; most antidepressants, including SSRIs, SNRIs, TCAs, and MAOIs, could cause initial activation and agitation and therefore require careful monitoring, particularly during the first few weeks following treatment initiation; adolescents and children, possibly regardless of the initial and/or primary diagnosis, might be at elevated risk compared with adults when exposed to all antidepressants.

OTHER ANTIANXIETY MEDICATIONS

Neuroleptics

As a general rule, neuroleptics or antipsychotics (also incorrectly referred to as "major tranquilizers") should not be used in the treatment of anxiety or anxiety disorders, mainly because of the possibility of inducing movement disorders such as tardive dyskinesia. Tardive dyskinesia (TD), characterized by involuntary muscle movements, is a cumulative, frequently irreversible side effect of neuroleptics following long-term use. As possible exceptions to this rule, neuroleptics may be necessary to treat agitation in the elderly and to manage anxiety in patients with organic brain disease. These patients may become delirious on usual doses of antianxiety medications such as BZDs, but they may benefit greatly from low doses of preferably atypical neuroleptics. Short-term treatment with neuroleptics reduces the risk in these patients of developing TD. The reported association in demented older patients between increased cardiovascular and cerebrovascular mortality and atypical antipsychotics (Herrmann, Mamdani, & Lanctor, 2004) should also be considered in deciding the most appropriate approach in this patient population.

In select situations, neuroleptics may be indicated as "last resort" antianxiety agents. For example, in managing patients with borderline personality disorder or severe, refractory PTSD, patients with histories of drug dependence, or patients for whom all other alternatives have failed, periodic short-term use of neuroleptics may be justified (Klein, Gittelman, Quitkin, & Rifkin, 1980). Extrapyramidal side effects must be monitored during any length of neuroleptic treatment.

In spite of their improved side-effect profile, including significantly lower risk of TD, second-generation or atypical antipsychotics (clozapine [Clozaril], olanzapine [Zyprexa], risperidone [Risperdal], quetiapine [Seroquel], ziprasidone [Geodon], aripiprazole [Abilify]) should also be used only as last-resort options. The likely association between this new class of antipsychotics and increased rates of diabetes, obesity, and dyslipidemia (Consensus Development Conference on Antipsychotic Drugs and Obesity and Diabetes, 2004) suggests that the risks of using antipsychotics in patients with anxiety disorders remain substantial (Gao, Muzina, Gajwani, & Calabrese, 2006). Due to the fixed ratio and differential half-lives of two agents, combination preparations containing an antidepressant and an antipsychotic (e.g., Triavil, Symbyax) are even more problematic and should be avoided.

Beta-Adrenergic Receptor Antagonists (Beta Blockers)

Beta blockers are probably the most frequently used medications in the treatment of hypertension, angina, and migraine headache. Their mechanism of action is to reduce adrenergic stimulation by antagonizing beta-adrenergic receptors located in the cardiovascular system (Frishman, 1981).

Autonomic symptoms (e.g., rapid heartbeat, tremor, tingling, perspiration, blushing, and chest constriction) are frequent concomitants of anxiety. These symptoms may be induced by increased adrenaline secretion during anxiety. Patients with anxiety may have a tendency to misinterpret these symptoms as dangerous, and they are also often hyperaware of normal adrenergic functioning. For instance, innocuous palpitations may be perceived as evidence of an impending heart attack. Catastrophic thinking, in turn, may augment the original symptom. Beta-adrenergic receptor antagonist drugs may derive their benefits from blocking these symptoms. A number of beta blockers have been found effective in the treatment of both generalized anxiety and situationally provoked anxiety, such as social phobia and performance anxiety (Kathol, Noyes, & Slymen, 1980; Gorman, Liebowitz, Fyer, Campeas, & Klein, 1985).

It is somewhat controversial at present as to whether these drugs exert their beneficial effects only through the reduction of peripheral autonomic symptoms or whether they work through central mechanisms as well (Gottschalk, Stone, & Gleser, 1974; Gorman et al., 1983). In support of peripheral action are treatment studies that divide patients with anxiety into predominantly psychic versus somatic groups. Somatic anxiety seems to respond both to BZDs and to beta blockers more than to placebo, but only BZDs, not beta blockers, seem superior to placebo in treating psychic anxiety. Also, practolol and atenolol, two selective peripheral beta blockers, seem to be effective antianxiety agents. Because neither of these beta blockers enters the brain to any significant degree, this finding is consistent with peripheral efficacy for beta blockers.

Beta blockers are contraindicated in patients with a history of asthma or serious allergies that produce wheezing. Relative contraindications include hypotension, bradycardia, congestive heart failure, and diabetes mellitus. Given these potentially severe complications, beta blockers should be administered only by a physician.

All beta blockers are rapidly absorbed from the gastrointestinal tract. Depending on their lipid solubility, they may cross the blood–brain barrier. For instance, the highly lipid-soluble propranolol may exert considerable central effects, such as sedation. The weakly lipid-soluble atenolol does not cross the blood–brain barrier and has many fewer central effects. Some of the beta blockers are local anesthetics, and some are intrinsically sympathomimetic (i.e., they also stimulate some beta-adrenergic receptors).

Selective beta blockers (atenolol, metoprolol) antagonize only beta-adrenergic receptors, located primarily in the myocardium. Nonselective beta blockers (propranolol, pindolol) antagonize both $beta_1$ and $beta_2$ adrenergic receptors. Because $beta_2$-adrenergic receptors are located in the vascular and bronchial smooth muscles, nonselective beta blockers can cause airway constriction. In general, beta blockers are safe and relatively easy to administer; their side effects are generally mild and may include nightmares, depression, tingling sensations in the hands and feet, and, occasionally, sexual dysfunction, fatigue, and sedation. Beta blockers are not habit forming. Although there are no significant withdrawal symptoms, tapering is recommended on discontinuation in order to avoid rebound blood pressure changes.

Anticonvulsants

All medications in this class reduce seizures, but they do not have the same mechanism of action, and not all possess anxiolytic activity. Furthermore, their anxiolytic properties may be related to diverse putative mechanisms, including antagonism on sodium (lamotrigine, carbamazepine, phenytoin, topiramate) or calcium channels (gabapentin, pregabalin), inhibition of glutamate (topiramate) and/or to modulating of the GABA complex (tiagabine, barbiturates, valproic acid); for some, the mechanism of action is "complex" or not known (levetiracetam, valproic acid). None of these anticonvulsants are currently indicated for the treatment of anxiety disorders. Although anecdotal information is promising for many, only those drugs with substantial clinical data suggestive of anxiolytic potential are discussed under the recommendations for specific anxiety disorders. BZDs are also considered anticonvulsants, but they are discussed as a separate group.

In general, anticonvulsants tend to be less efficacious anxiolytics than the first-line agents (SSRIs, MAOIs, TCAs, BZDs) but better tolerated due to more favorable side effects. They are less likely to be associated with weight gain (with the possible exception of carbamazepine), sexual dysfunction, and the initial agitation and insomnia typical of most antidepressants. Unlike the BZDs, they are not habit forming, and their taper and discontinuation are usually uneventful. Given the current state of clinical and research information on this class of anxiolytics, they are reserved for refractory cases, for patients intolerant of the aforementioned side effects, as augmenting agents added to other anxiolytics, and as alternatives to BZDs for those with comorbid substance use disorder.

Buspirone

For a while, the 5-HT1$_A$ agonist azapirone, buspirone (BuSpar), was promoted as the best alternative to benzodiazepines. Buspirone is pharmacologically unrelated to BZDs or any other marketed anxiolytics. However, earlier controlled studies suggesting comparable efficacy with benzodiazepines (Enkelmann, 1991; Rickels & Schweizer, 1987; Rickels, Schweizer, Csanalosi, Case, & Chung, 1988) have not been confirmed, and clinical experience with buspirone has been disappointing, especially in patients previously exposed to benzodiazepines (De Martinis, Rynn, Rickles, & Mandos, 2000). Although buspirone is safe and well tolerated and is less likely to induce drowsiness, dependence, and psychomotor impairment than to benzodiazepines, the initial side effects of nausea, dizziness, and gastrointestinal irritation may be problematic, especially in the elderly. The onset of action for buspirone is delayed for an average of 4 to 5 weeks. Effect sizes are relatively low, and dropout rates are high in buspirone trials for GAD (Gould, Otto, Pollack, & Yap, 1997). Because buspirone is not effective for panic disorder (Pohl, Balon, Yeragani, & Gershon, 1989) or depression, it is not recommended for anxious patients with these comorbid conditions.

Antihistamines

Although also promoted as anxiolytics, antihistamines such as diphenhydramine and hydroxazine induce excessive daytime sedation, irritability, cognitive impairment, and ataxia. They can be lethal in overdose and tolerance to their sedating properties develops quickly. Therefore, these drugs are of limited use as long-term anxiolytics.

D-Cycloserine

The antituberculotic NMDA partial agonist D-cycloserine, an intriguing parallel to the antidepressant and anxiolytic properties of other antituberculotic agents, has been found to facilitate extinction of conditioned fear, possibly by direct modulation of the fear circuits (Walker, Ressler, Lu, & Davis, 2002; Davis, 2002). In a double-blind, randomized, placebo-controlled study, single-dose administration of D-cycloserine combined with exposure therapy improved the symptoms of acrophobia significantly more than combined placebo and exposure therapy (Ressler et al., 2004). The mechanism of action is thought to be related to D-cycloserine's effect as a cognitive enhancer of associative learning. If confirmed, D-cycloserine's acute efficacy, compared with the delayed effects of most other anxiolytics, is also of heuristic interest, possibly leading to novel theories of the psychopathology of anxiety.

COMBINED PSYCHOTHERAPY AND PHARMACOTHERAPY

Combining psychotherapy, usually cognitive-behavioral treatment (CBT), and pharmacotherapy involving antidepressants and other anxiolytics is common practice in the treatment of anxiety disorders. Studies have just begun to evaluate the value of this approach empirically, and the results have been mixed. Westra and Stewart (1998) reviewed studies on combined treatment for anxiety disorders and concluded that most studies do not show a clear advantage of combined therapy over CBT alone and that high-potency benzodiazepines may actually detract from CBT's efficacy. Sample studies exemplifying this pattern have investigated fluvoxamine (Sharp, Power, Simpson, & Swanson, 1996) and imipramine (Barlow et al., 2000) combined with CBT for panic disorder and clomipramine (Kozak, Liebowitz, & Foa, 2000) and fluvoxamine (van Balkom et al., 1998) combined with CBT for obsessive compulsive disorder.

Other studies have found clear advantages of combined therapy, generally in those populations in which CBT produces more limited benefits. Patients with CBT-resistant OCD respond significantly more to combined fluvoxamine and CBT than to fluvoxamine alone (Neziroglu, Yaryura-Tobias, Walz, & McKay, 2000; Hohagen et al., 1998). The combination of clomipramine and CBT had clear advantages over monotherapy among patients with OCD with more widespread symptoms. The benefits of added CBT may manifest after patients taper their medications. Those in combined treatments seem to better maintain treatment gains with a lower rate of relapse at follow-up, compared with those receiving medication alone (Barlow, Gorman, Shear, & Woods, 2000).

While confirming the benefits of combined treatment, these studies also imply that for the majority of patients one of the treatments is probably superfluous; 60–65% of patients receiving combined treatment would achieve responder status with either CBT or medication alone (Gorenstein & Papp, 2007). A clinical approach that starts with a single treatment and then adds a second on evidence of inadequate response seems more cost-effective and less burdensome, and, due to improved patient compliance, it should be at least as efficacious as combined treatment.

DISORDER-SPECIFIC TREATMENT RECOMMENDATIONS

Generalized Anxiety Disorder

Patients with GAD suffer from "unrealistic or excessive anxiety and worry" for at least 6 months. They experience motor tension, autonomic hyperactivity, and hypervigilance. The usual course of GAD includes periods of quiescence and exacerbation (Papp & Kleber, 2001). Functional impairment is comparable to that seen in depression (Kessler, DuPont, Berglund, & Wittchen, 1999). Comorbid depression is a common complication and adds substantially to morbidity and disability (Wittchen, Zhao, Kessler, & Eaton, 1994).

BZDs are the traditional pharmacological choice in the treatment of GAD. They have been clearly established as efficacious in relieving the symptoms of GAD (Rickels, Case, Downing, & Winoku, 1983, 1987). Data do not support the advantage of any one BZD over others, and correlation has not been established between clinical response and dose or plasma level. A daily equivalent of 15–25 mg of diazepam is usually sufficient to relieve the symptoms in up to 70% of patients with GAD (Greenblatt, Shader, & Abernathy, 1983). Most of the somatic and some of the psychic anxiety symptoms respond within the first week of treatment. Tolerance to the sedative effects of BZDs develops quickly, but the antianxiety effect of a given dose is well maintained over time.

However, BZDs are no longer considered the first-line choice because of the problems associated with the physiological and psychological dependence that develop after long-term use, and relapse rates on discontinuation of BZDs are high. Even more important is the lack of benefits of BZDs in the majority of patients with GAD who also suffer from comorbid depression. Therefore, antidepressants (SSRIs, SNRIs, TCAs) have replaced BZDs as first-, second-, and frequently even third-line options for GAD treatment (Hoehn-Saric, McLeod, & Zimmerli, 1988; Davidson, Bose, & Wang, 2005). The choice among the many efficacious antidepressants is usually made based on side effects and individual patient characteristics. Only for those unable to tolerate the side effects of or who fail to respond to at least two antidepressants (preferably with different mechanisms of action) should BZDs be considered. Doses and response patterns of antidepressants are similar to those observed in depression and in most other anxiety disorders. Increased initial physiological symptoms and anxiety may be related to side effects rather than to the hypersensitivity syndrome described in PD.

Isolated but prominent GAD symptoms, such as palpitation, tremor, and sweating, may respond to beta blockers within 1 week of treatments, but the full GAD picture usually requires the use of antidepressants. Although controlled studies are unavailable, clinical experience and studies in PD (Goddard et al., 2001) suggest the benefits of combination treatments for GAD. For instance, the combination of BZDs or beta blockers with antidepressants could result in rapid response. When the antidepressant becomes effective, the BZD or beta blocker can be tapered and then discontinued. If all other options are contraindicated or fail, buspirone can be tried. In spite of the relatively high doses (> 60 mgs) usually needed, response rates to buspirone remain low (Olajide & Lader, 1987), particularly in patients with prior BZD exposure (Schweizer, Rickels, & Lucki, 1986).

Because GAD is a chronic, frequently lifelong condition, treatment should probably be continued indefinitely, though it could be tried intermittently. The option of intermittent, relatively short-term (6 months) treatment could be limited to symptomatic periods

(Rickels & Schweizer, 1998). The treatment of elderly patients with GAD presents specific challenges. Given their sensitivity to side effects and frequent comorbid conditions requiring multiple-drug regimens, the preferred treatment for the elderly is CBT alone. Unfortunately, CBT for GAD is about 50% less effective for the elderly than it is for younger adults, and the dropout rate among the elderly is almost twice as high (Stanley, Beck, & Zebb, 1996; Stanley et al., 1993; Wetherell, Gatz, & Craske, 2003). Therefore, the combination of CBT and pharmacotherapy is probably the best treatment strategy in this patient population (Gorenstein et al., 2005).

Longer treatments seem to confer the benefits of improved functioning, fewer residual symptoms, and lower relapse rates, but it is unknown whether the type of treatment—pharmacological, psychological, or the combination of the two—matters in conferring the long-term benefits. Because of significant comorbidity, the efficacy of antidepressants in GAD may not be independent of their anxiolytic and antidepressant properties. Patients with predominantly somatic symptoms and/or early-onset GAD may require ongoing pharmacotherapy, whereas the excessive worry and late-onset GAD are better controlled by regularly practiced CBT techniques. Because it is not known what is required for the optimal maintenance treatment of patients with GAD who responded to either CBT or medication, the most prudent approach is to schedule follow-up appointments at increasing intervals.

Panic Disorder with or without Agoraphobia

The hallmark of PD is the panic attack. These sudden, unexpected, episodic bursts of anxiety are characterized by autonomic symptoms (e.g., sweating, hyperventilation, palpitation, light-headedness) and fear of impending doom. They last from 5 to 30 minutes. Frequent complications include anticipatory anxiety, which is the almost constant fear of panic attacks; agoraphobia, or phobic avoidance of situations associated with panic attacks; and secondary demoralization, occasionally leading to severe depression.

Medication treatment is targeted at the panic attacks, but treatment outcome should be assessed across the full symptom spectrum, including quality of life (Shear et al. 1997). Once the attacks are blocked, the anticipatory anxiety, agoraphobia, and depression usually remit, as well. Antidepressants and BZDs are the medications most often used to treat panic attacks. The traditional antipanic drug, the TCA imipramine (Zitrin, Klein, Woerner, & Ross, 1983), has been largely replaced by the SSRIs due to their ease of administration and more favorable side-effect profile. In addition to most TCAs, SSRIs, SNRIs, the MAOIs, including phenelzine and tranylcypromine, most BZDs, and several "other" or "atypical" antidepressants, such as nefazodone, bupropion, and reboxetine, have been shown to possess antipanic properties. A large meta-analysis of effect sizes showed no significant difference in efficacy among the most frequently prescribed antipanic agents (Otto, Tuby, Gould, McCleon, & Pollack, 2001).

Regardless of the agent chosen, approximately 60–70% of the patients are expected to respond to monopharmacotherapy; an additional 10–15% will respond to a combination or to sequential pharmacotherapy. Concomitant psychotherapy (CBT, interpersonal therapy [IPT]) could boost the overall response rate to 80–90%. The goal of treatment is full remission, which could take several months to achieve after the initial response. Full remission, the elimination of phobic avoidance and anticipatory anxiety, in addition to the absence of full- and limited-symptom panic attacks, confers superior long-term outcome and diminished relapse rates.

SSRIs are currently considered first-line antipanic medications. Relatively low starting doses will minimize initial agitation and triggering of severe panic attacks during the first few days of treatment. Starting patients on a benzodiazepine at the same time might be necessary, either only as needed or as a standing order. Severe insomnia is an indication for a more sedating SSRI such as paroxetine, but insomnia will also respond to as-needed hypnotics.

If the first-line drug fails following an adequate trial (at least 4–5 weeks on a therapeutic dose), the current algorithm suggests a choice between a second SSRI, a TCA, or venlafaxine. MAOIs are reserved as fifth choice (while carefully observing the rules of transitioning to an MAOI and maintaining the diet restrictions), preceded by BZDs and anticonvulsants (valproic acid, gabapentin, levetiracetam, tiagabine, etc.) as third or fourth choice.

If speedy recovery is the main goal and/or antidepressants are inappropriate, BZDs are the best choice. The initial sedation usually lifts after the first 10 days, but the anxiolytic effect remains unaltered. Although the high-potency BZDs (alprazolam and clonazepam) are well-established antipanic medications for short- and long-term treatments, contrary to previous claims, all BZDs, including low-potency BZDs such as diazepam, seem equally efficacious if used at comparable doses. Once the appropriate dose has been established, dose adjustment is rarely needed. Patients with PD with no histories of substance use disorder do not abuse BZDs. Withdrawal from BZDs is more problematic than withdrawal from antidepressants, but it can be managed by slow taper and the use of cognitive-behavioral strategies (Gorenstein et al., 2005). In addition to controlling the initial agitation or insomnia, BZDs are also useful add-ons to SSRIs to speed up the response, which can be delayed for up to 5 weeks on most antidepressants. Although augmentation strategies for partial response to antidepressants have not been investigated systematically, anecdotal evidence supports the benefit of added BZDs.

Only preliminary data support the utility of the anticonvulsants tiagabine, gabapentin, pregabalin, and levetiracetam in the management of panic disorder. Valproic acid (at plasma levels between 60 and 120ng/ml) has shown clear antipanic effects (Lum, Fontaine, Elie, & Ontiveros, 1990; Keck, Taylor, Tugrul, McElroy, & Bennett, 1993). A controlled trial showed efficacy for gabapentin in patients with moderately severe PD (Pande et al., 2000). The antipanic effects of levetiracetam may be comparable to those of more established agents (Papp, 2006). The advantages of anticonvulsants are easy administration, favorable side-effects profile, early onset of action, and an early hypnotic effect that benefits patients with PD and insomnia (Papp & Ray, 2003; Papp, 2004). Unlike BZDs, these drugs are not contraindicated in substance use disorders and can be discontinued without unpleasant withdrawal symptoms, but they seem to share the disadvantage of BZDs of not addressing comorbid depression. Anticonvulsants should be used as first-line agents or add-ons for patients with PD and clear bipolar comorbidity (Rotondo et al., 2002). Partial response to anticonvulsants can be augmented with antidepressants, and the addition of anticonvulsants can complement the antipanic effects of antidepressants.

Effective antipanic medications should be continued for a minimum of 6–9 panic-free months, although recent reports support the benefits of even longer maintenance. Relapse rates seem significantly lower after 2 years of treatment (Mavissakalian & Perel, 1992). Patients with PD who have had several prior episodes may need to be treated indefinitely. Once a patient is panic-free, exposure to fearful situations should be encouraged. Panic disorder is a cyclical illness, with sometimes many months or years of complete remission. A treatment approach that helped once is likely to be successful again.

Focused, time-limited CBT is a good alternative in situations in which medications are contraindicated or resisted by patients. Even if formal antipanic psychotherapy is not employed, such techniques as breathing retraining, relaxation exercise, and exposure will prolong remission in the drug-free state. Combining pharmacotherapy and CBT may confer longer term benefits, particularly following medication taper (Barlow et al., 2000). Even a less-than-optimal CBT added to pharmacotherapy can significantly enhance overall outcome in primary care (Roy-Byrne et al., 2005). A comprehensive, and still mostly valid, set of treatment recommendations, based on thorough review of the literature, was published by the American Psychiatric Association's Committee on Practice Guidelines in 1998. A revision and update of the *Guideline for Panic Disorder* is scheduled for publication in 2008.

Social Phobia or Social Anxiety Disorder

Patients with social phobia (social anxiety disorder [SAD] in DSM-IV) experience significant anxiety, usually coupled with alarming autonomic symptoms (palpitation, sweating, shortness of breath, chest pain, etc.), in one or more social situations. Their fear of embarrassing or humiliating themselves in these situations usually leads to significant avoidance. Limited social phobia involves one or two situations (e.g., public speaking). Patients with generalized social phobia are anxious in and tend to avoid many different social situations. Social phobia appears to be a chronic condition, beginning in late adolescence and often resulting in lifelong disability. Substance abuse and secondary depression are frequent complications. Nevertheless, research on social phobia was largely neglected by American psychiatry until the publication of DSM-III in 1980.

Over the past two decades the disorder has been increasingly recognized as more common and more disabling, but also more treatable, than originally believed. The results of many large-scale medication trials indicate the efficacy of several classes of antidepressants, starting with the MAOI phenelzine (Liebowitz et al., 1990), the SNRI venlafaxine (Liebowitz, Gelenberg, & Munjack, 2005), and most of the SSRIs (Stein, Ipser, & Balkom, 2004). Several of them (paroxetine, venlafaxine, sertraline) have received regulatory approval for the treatment of social phobia. Evidence also supports the benefits of these drugs in maintenance and relapse prevention trials; they reduce comorbid depression and functional disability.

As a result, in parallel to the recommendations for many other anxiety disorders, SSRIs have become first-line agents, replacing the more traditional choices, such as beta blockers (Hartley, Ungapen, & Davie, 1983) and BZDs. The selective, reversible MAOIs (RIMAs) with significantly improved side-effect profiles and no diet restrictions provide attractive and powerful alternatives for treatment-resistant generalized SAD (Versiani et al., 1992; Fahlen, Nilsson, Borg, Humble, & Pauli, 1997). Given the relative nonresponse to TCAs coupled with the results of neuroimaging studies (Schneier et al., 2000), the pathophysiology of SAD is likely to involve serotonergic as well as dopaminergic neurotransmission.

BZDs and beta blockers retain their utility as the as-needed medications for limited social and performance anxiety (public speaking, musical performances) but fail in the treatment of generalized social anxiety (Turner et al., 1994). Clonazepam may be beneficial for generalized social anxiety (Davidson, Tupler, & Potts, 1994) as well. The high rate of alcohol problems in this population is a major limitation to the use of BZDs. Only if self-medication is clearly established as the cause of alcoholism should BZDs be tried under close monitoring. Because the anticonvulsants gabapentin and pregabalin have also been found efficacious in social anxiety (Pande et al., 1999), these medications should be considered as alternatives for patients with preexisting and/or comorbid substance use disorders.

The beneficial effects of beta blockers, if any, for performance anxiety are obvious after the first week of treatment; approximately 50% of these patients will benefit substantially. Because of their relative safety, rapid onset of action, and ease of administration, an initial trial with beta blockers is a reasonable first choice for the relief of simple performance anxiety (possibly a mild version of limited social phobia). In cases of predictable and relatively infrequent performance anxiety, propranolol (10–40 mgs) may be taken approximately 1 hour before the stressful event. The medication will control such symptoms as trembling, sweating, blushing, or palpitation for about 3–6 hours. If the performance anxiety is less predictable and more frequent, a longer acting drug (e.g., atenolol, 25–100 mgs, taken at night) will usually provide symptom control for the subsequent 24-hour period. Patients should be advised to test the medications prior to the actual performance and to titrate the dose for optimal benefits and minimal side effects. As an example, many musicians use beta blockers regularly, but they fail to appreciate that although their anxiety is reduced, important aspects of their performance (rhythmic and dynamic intensity) may be compromised (James & Savage, 1984). Although casual self-medication with beta blockers, mostly for performance anxiety, is common, due to potential side effects and drug–drug interactions, unsupervised use should be strongly discouraged (Lehrer, Rosen, Kostis, & Greenfield, 1987).

Generalized social anxiety disorder usually requires the use of antidepressants (Liebowitz et al., 2005). The acute response may be delayed for up to 10–12 weeks, and continued treatment at full dose is usually needed to maintain gains. The choice and dosing of the SSRI, as first-line agent, as well as the duration of treatment, follow the recommendations given above for PD. Refractory cases with prominent sympathetic overdrive (blushing, sweating) may respond to surgical sympathectomy (Pohjavaara, Telaranta, & Vaisanen, 2003) or to repeated botulinum toxin injections. Response rates of over 90% have been reported following bilateral sympathetic block. The success rates from botulinum injections are lower and less predictable. Mild but subjectively significant and disabling perspiration may respond to topical agents, to terazosin, or to strongly anticholinergic medications.

As is the case for most anxiety disorders, the benefits of targeted psychotherapies (CBT, social skills training) are substantial and can be comparable to that of medications (Turner, Beidel, & Jacob, 1994; Heimberg et al., 1998).

Obsessive–Compulsive Disorder

Patients with OCD experience repetitive, usually senseless thoughts or impulses (obsessions), occasionally accompanied by repetitive and also senseless behaviors (compulsions) such as washing, counting, or checking. OCD is a highly disabling disorder with poor prognosis. With a usual onset before age 18, a lifetime prevalence of approximately 2%, and the need for long-term treatment, it is one of the most costly medical conditions to manage. Spontaneous remissions are rare, and without appropriate treatment most patients with OCD will remain symptomatic and impaired. Because of its distinct features, OCD may be reclassified under a new DSM category tentatively named "impulse control disorders."

The treatment of OCD is difficult. Although cognitive-behavioral treatments seem just as effective as medications (Kobak, Greist, Jefferson, Katzelnick, & Henk, 1998), most patients will resort to taking medications and add psychotherapy only if it is readily available. The most effective medications are the SSRIs and clomipramine, suggesting that reuptake inhibition of serotonin is the underlying mechanism of beneficial drug effect in OCD.

Clomipramine, a TCA with powerful serotonergic-reuptake-blocking properties, was the first successful anti-OCD drug (Pato, Zohar-Kadouch, Zohar, & Murphy, 1988).

Although it has only been available in the United States only since 1990, the drug has been tested extensively around the world. With the exception of a slightly higher dose-related risk of seizure, the side effects are identical to those described for TCA. Clomipramine will substantially reduce the duration and/or the amount of obsessions and compulsions and alleviate the anxiety experienced in about 50% of patients with OCD.

The preferred pharmacological alternatives to clomipramine are the SSRIs (Turner, Jacob, & Beidel, 1985). Most clinicians consider the SSRIs as first-line drugs for OCD because of their fewer and more favorable side effects. The effective doses of most anti-OCD medications tend to be higher and the needed duration of treatment longer than for those customary in depression. In spite of progress in management, full remission is rare, and continued maintenance treatment does not always protect from relapse. Refractory cases may benefit from combining SSRIs, preferably fluvoxamine, with clomipramine, and, especially in the presence of psychotic features, with atypical antipsychotics (McDougle, Epperson, Pelton, Waslynk, & Price, 2000, Koran, Ringold, & Elliott, 2000). Comorbid tic disorder may respond to pimozide or haloperidol (McDougle et al., 1994), and comorbid attention-deficit disorder will benefit from psychostimulants when added to the SSRI. Other augmenting strategies (with lithium, fenfluramine, buspiron, gabapentin, etc.) have been less successful. The significant benefits of once-a-week oral morphine added to standard pharmacotherapy may imply the relevance of mu-receptors and glutamate in the pathophysiology of treatment-refractory OCD (Koran et al., 2005). Intravenous clomipramine (Fallon et al., 1992) and psychosurgery, most commonly capsulotomy or cingulotomy (Baer et al., 1995), are usually reserved as last resorts. If effective, medications usually have to be taken permanently. Drug discontinuation likely results in rapid relapse. Behavioral psychotherapy is strongly recommended to supplement the medication treatment of OCD. Combination treatment is considered the most successful approach by the Expert Consensus Panel for Obsessive–Compulsive Disorder (1997).

Posttraumatic Stress Disorder

PTSD is diagnosed when the patient persistently reexperiences a traumatic event that is usually life-threatening, although the perceived severity of the trauma may be more relevant diagnostically and clinically. Features of the illness include flashbacks to the trauma, nightmares, "psychic numbness," and affective symptoms, in addition to anxiety and symptoms of increased arousal. A large percentage of patients with acute PTSD will develop a chronic illness. With a lifetime prevalence rate of 12% and a women-to-men ratio of 2 to 1, PTSD is one of the most common, as well as the most treatment-resistant, conditions. The rate of suicidal behavior, 19%, is the highest among the anxiety disorders and is comparable to that in depression (Ballenger et al., 2000). Possibly due to complex pathophysiology that involves several neurotransmitter systems, the HPA axis, and cognitive functions involving memory, only about a third of the patients will respond to pharmacotherapy.

In general, pharmacological treatment should focus on the presenting symptoms (depression, anxiety, insomnia, irritability, etc.), but optimally it should address the full spectrum of PTSD symptomatology. Combat-related PTSD may differ significantly from PTSD in civilian populations. Differences in the nature of the trauma, gender distribution, comorbid conditions, and course of illness translate to differential response to treatments. Supported by several large-scale, well-controlled trials, SSRIs, with the possible exception of fluoxetine (Hertzberg, Feldman, Beckham, Kudler, & Davidson, 2000), are now considered the first-line agents of choice for PTSD. With priority among them determined by the prominent symptoms of the disorder and the side effects of the agent (severe insomnia responds well to paroxetine, clear lethargy may benefit from sertraline, weight gain is most likely from paroxetine, etc.), SSRIs are most likely to cover the broad range of PTSD symptoms (Marshall, Beebe, Oldhan, & Zanielli, 2001; Rapaport, Endicott, & Clary, 2002). The Expert Consensus Guidelines (1999) recommend psychotherapy for mild PTSD and the combination of medication and psychotherapy for severe or chronic PTSD. Treatment should continue for at least 12 months, and severe cases should be treated for 24 months, with continued "booster" sessions as needed. Over half of "nonresponders" to 12 weeks of pharmacotherapy were converted to "responders" with continued treatment (Londborg et al., 2001), confirming the need for longer-term initial trials for PTSD.

Other antidepressant anxiolytics with demonstrated, but more narrow, benefits for PTSD include phenelzine, and, to a lesser degree, the TCAs amitriptyline and imipramine (Kosten, Frank, Dan, McDougle, & Giller, 1991). Civilian PTSD and the mood symptoms of veterans with chronic PTSD may respond to bupropion, suggestive of noradrenergic dysfunction (Canive et al., 1998; Dong & Blier, 2001). Mirtazepine (Davidson et al., 2003) and venlafaxine (Smajkic et al., 2001) were also found effective in single controlled pilot trials. Nefazodone has shown benefits for chronic PTSD in veterans as well as in civilians and children (Davis, Nugent, Murray, Kramer, & Petty, 2000; Hidalgo et al., 1999; Domon & Anderson, 2000), but due to recently reported potential liver damage, nefazodone is not likely to gain acceptance. Doses, onset of benefits, duration of treatment, and side effects, including the initial agitation for patients with significant anxiety, are similar to those described earlier.

Of the anticonvulsants, lamotrigine, topiramate, tiagabine, carbamazepine, levetiracetam, and gabapentin have been reported to be beneficial in PTSD; clear reductions in nightmares, flashbacks, irritability, and insomnia were found, compared with relatively more modest or no effects on depression (Yehuda, 1999). Lamotrigine seemed particularly useful for the symptoms of avoidance and reexperiencing (Hertzberg et al., 1999). As in other anxiety disorders, anticonvulsants do not seem to address the full core pathology of PTSD, but they are useful augmenting agents with relatively few side effects or drug–drug interactions (Berlant & van Kammen, 2002; Kinrys, Wygent, Pardo, & Melo, 2006).

Unless contraindicated (current or past history of substance use, BZD dependence, etc.), BZDs can be used to manage prominent irritability, muscle tension, insomnia, startle response, and other symptoms of hyperarousal (Gelpin, Bonne, Peri, Tszandes, & Shaler, 1996). BZDs given to patients immediately following a trauma do not appear to prevent or temper the symptoms of PTSD. Given their relatively narrow range of benefits, BZDs are not recommended as monotherapy for PTSD.

There is some evidence that beta blockers (Yudofsky, Williams, & Gorman, 1981) and the alpha$_2$-adrenergic agonist clonidine (Bond, 1986) may control explosive behavior, hyperalertness, intrusive thoughts, and nightmares. Although controversial, beta blockers might also have a protective effect against PTSD if given preventively (Pitman et al., 2002). If these results are replicated, they would also point toward noradrenergic dysfunction as a possible etiology in PTSD. Buspirone may be added to alleviate hyperarousal as well. Severe treatment-resistant PTSD, with or without psychotic symptoms, may require the judicious use of preferably atypical antipsychotics added to antidepressants (Stein et al., 2004). The addition of triiodothyronine (Cytomel) to SSRIs might be a good augmenting strategy for prominent and treatment-resistant depression (Agid, Shalev, & Lerer, 2001) and the alpha antagonist prazosin could be added for patients with severe nightmares (Raskind et al., 2000). Psychotherapy or, at the very least, counseling is probably needed to supplement pharmacotherapy, although this has not been studied in a controlled design. The most comprehensive treatment recommendations for PTSD have recently been published in the American Psychiatric Association *Practice Guideline* series (2004).

Specific Phobias

Although specific phobias are quite common, most patients with the condition are not dysfunctional and therefore do not seek treatment. When treatment is required, the recommendation is usually exposure. Medications are used only to facilitate psychotherapy. Mostly anecdotal evidence and only a handful of controlled studies support the benefits of medications in specific phobias. It appears that single or as-needed use of BZDs and beta blockers is most common, and only the most severe cases require regular prolonged pharmacotherapy. Paroxetine (Benjamin, Ben-Zion, Karbofsky, & Dannon, 2000), but not imipramine (Zitrin et al., 1983), seemed beneficial in controlled trials in mixed phobic populations. Patients with blood–injury phobias may benefit from prolonged treatment with clonazepam (Davidson et al., 1994). Acute administration of the glucocorticoid cortisol reduced phobic fear in spider phobia in an intriguing controlled trial (Soravia et al., 2006). As discussed earlier, D-cycloserine may also facilitate exposure therapy for acrophobia (Ressler et al., 2004). If the theory (Goisman et al., 1998) proposing that specific phobia may be a prodrome of a more severe anxiety and/or mood disorder is confirmed, early intervention in this population should gain significantly more support.

CONCLUSION

Significant progress has been made in the pharmacological management of anxiety disorders since the first edition of this book. A series of new compounds have been introduced and found to be effective in large controlled clinical trials. Led by the SSRIs, these newer medications have largely replaced or curtailed the utility of most traditional anxiolytics. Although the efficacy of newer and older compounds seems comparable, the side-effect profiles of the more recent anxiolytics are clearly more favorable. Given that most anxiety disorders are chronic conditions requiring long-term treatment, the tolerability of side effects has become one of the most important factors in making the most appropriate choice. The wider availability of specific, effective, and well-tolerated antianxiety medications has significantly increased the number of patients with anxiety disorders who seek and receive psychiatric treatment. Although the goal of treatment is to achieve full remission, for most anxiety disorders, just like for most other medical conditions, cure is not yet possible. However, as a result of these new developments, patients with anxiety disorders have become less disabled, and many can return to full function.

Because the currently recommended antianxiety medications are increasingly safe and not known to produce permanent side effects even after long-term use, medication treatment has become a viable alternative to a less effective nonpharmacological treatment. Given the comparable efficacy of pharmacotherapy and specific, time-limited, targeted psychotherapies, an unbiased, open approach that also respects and considers patient preference is strongly recommended. Whenever available, integrated treatment approaches are most likely to provide maximum benefits to patients. If formal psychotherapy is not available, simple, easily learned psychological techniques (stress management, problem solving, cognitive-behavioral strategies, etc.) should effectively supplement pharmacotherapy, reduce symptoms, and shorten the length of needed pharmacotherapy and could facilitate the tapering of ineffective medications or the discontinuation of medications in asymptomatic patients.

REFERENCES

Agid, O., Shalev, A. Y., & Lerer, B. (2001). Triiodothyronine augmentation of selective serotonin reuptake inhibitors in posttraumatic stress disorder. *Journal of Clinical Psychiatry, 6,* 169–173.

Alexopoulos, G. S. (2004). On the "infallibility" of psychopathology and its implications for action. *American Journal of Psychiatry, 161*(12), 2151–2154.

American Psychiatric Association. (2000). *Diagnostic and statistical manual of mental disorders* (4th ed., text rev.). Washington, DC: Author.

American Psychiatric Association Task Force. (1985). Tricyclic antidepressants: Blood level measurements and clinical outcome. *American Journal of Psychiatry, 142,* 155–165.

American Psychiatric Association Task Force. (1990). *Benzodiazepine dependence, toxicity, and abuse.* Washington, DC: American Psychiatric Association Press.

American Psychiatric Association. (1998). Practice guidelines for the treatment of patients with panic disorder. *American Journal of Psychiatry, 155,* 1–34.

American Psychiatric Association. (2004). Practice guidelines for the treatment of patients with acute stress disorder and posttraumatic stress disorder. Washington, DC: American Psychiatric Association Press.

Baer, L., Rauch, S. L., Ballentine, H. T., Martuga, R., Cosgrove, R., Cassem, E., et al. (1995). Cingulotomy for untreatable obsessive–compulsive disorder. *Archives of General Psychiatry, 52,* 384–392.

Ballenger, J. C. (1999). Clinical guidelines for establishing remission in patients with depression and anxiety. *Journal of Clinical Psychiatry, 60*(Suppl. 22), 29–34.

Ballenger, J. C., Davidson, J. R., Lecrubier, Y., Nutt, D. J., Marshall, R. D., Neweroff, C. B., et al. (2000). Consensus statement on posttraumatic stress disorder from the International Consensus Group on Depression and Anxiety. *Journal of Clinical Psychiatry, 61*(Suppl. 5), 60–66.

Barlow, D. H., Gorman, J. M., Shear, M. K., & Woods, S. W. (2000). Cognitive-behavioral therapy, imipramine, or their combination for panic disorder: A randomized controlled trial. *Journal of the American Medical Association, 283,* 2529–2536.

Benjamin, J., Ben-Zion, I. Z., Karbofsky, E., & Dannon, T. (2000). Double-blind placebo-controlled pilot study of paroxetine for specific phobia. *Psychopharmacology, 149,* 194–196.

Berlant, J., & van Kammen, D. P. (2002). Open-label topiramate as primary or adjunctive therapy in chronic civilian posttraumatic stress disorder: A preliminary report. *Journal of Clinical Psychiatry, 63,* 15–20.

Bond, W. S. (1986). Psychiatric indications for clonidine: The neuropharmacologic and clinical basis. *Journal of Clinical Psychopharmacology, 6,* 81–90.

Canive, J. M., Clark, R. D., Calais, L. A., Qualls, C., & Tuason, V. B. (1998). Bupropion treatment in veterans with posttraumatic stress disorder; an open study. *Journal of Clinical Psychopharmacology, 18*(5), 379–383.

Charney, D. S., & Woods, S. W. (1989). Benzodiazepine treatment of panic disorder: A comparison of alprazolam and lorazepam. *Journal of Clinical Psychiatry, 50*(11), 418–423.

Ciraulo, D. A., Sands, B. F., & Shader, R. I. (1988). Critical review of liability for benzodiazepine abuse among alcoholics. *American Journal of Psychiatry, 145,* 1501–1506.

Consensus Development Conference on Antipsychotic Drugs and Obesity and Diabetes. (2004). *Journal of Clinical Psychiatry, 65*(2), 267–272.

Dannon, P. N., Iancu, I., & Gzunhaus, L. (2002). The efficacy of reboxetine in treatment-refractory patients with panic disorder: An open-label study. *Human Psychopharmacology, 17*(7), 329–333.

Davidson J., Bose, A., & Wang, Q. (2005). Safety and efficacy of escitalopram in the long term treatment of generalized anxiety disorder. *Journal of Clinical Psychiatry*, 66, 1441–1446.

Davidson, J. R. T., Tupler, L. A., & Potts, N. L. S. (1994). Treatment of social phobia with benzodiazepines. *Journal of Clinical Psychiatry*, 55(Suppl. 6), 28–32.

Davidson, J. R. T., Weisler R. H., Butterfield, M. I., Casat, C. D., Connor, K. M., & Barnett, S. (2003). Mirtazepine vs. placebo in posttraumatic stress disorder: A pilot trial. *Biological Psychiatry*, 53, 261–264.

Davis, L. L., Nugent, A. L., Murray, K., Kramer, G. L., & Petty, F. (2000). Nefazodone treatment for chronic posttraumatic stress disorder: An open trial. *Journal of Clinical Psychopharmacology*, 20(2), 159–164.

Davis, M. (2002). Role of NMDA receptors and MAP kinase in the amygdale in extinction of fear: Clinical implications for exposure therapy. *European Journal of Neuroscience*, 16(3), 395–398.

Degroot, A., & Nomikos G. G. (2005). Fluoxetine disrupts the integration of anxiety and aversive memories. *Neuropsychopharmacology*, 30(2), 391–400.

DeMartinis, N., Rynn, M., Rickels, K., & Mandos, L. (2000). Prior benzodiazepine use and buspirone response in the treatment of generalized anxiety disorder. *Journal of Clinical Psychiatry*, 62(8), 657–658.

Domon, S. E., & Anderson, M. S. (2000). Nefazodone for PTSD. *Journal of American Academy of Child and Adolescent Psychiatry*, 39(8), 942–943.

Dong, J., & Blier, P. (2001). Modifications of norepinephrine and serotonin, but not dopamine, neuron firing by sustained bupropion treatment. *Psychopharmacology*, 155(1), 52–57.

Ellison, J. M., Milofsky, J. E., & Ely, E. (1990). Fluoxetine-induced bradycardia and syncope in two patients. *Journal of Clinical Psychiatry*, 51, 385–386.

Emmanuel, N. P., Brawman-Mintzer, O., Morton, W. A., Book, S. W., Johnson, M. R., & Lorberbaum, J. P. (2000). Bupropion-SR in the treatment of social phobia. *Depression and Anxiety*, 12(2), 111–113.

Enkelmann, R. (1991). Alprazolam versus buspirone in the treatment of outpatients with generalized anxiety disorder. *Psychopharmacology*, 105(3), 428–432.

Expert Consensus Guideline Series. (1999). Treatment of posttraumatic stress disorder. *Journal of Clinical Psychiatry*, 60(Suppl. 16), 3–76.

Expert Consensus Panel for Obsessive–Compulsive Disorder. (1997). Treatment of obsessive–compulsive disorder. *Journal of Clinical Psychiatry*, 58(Suppl. 4), 2–72.

Fahlen, T., Nilsson, H. L., Borg, K., Humble, L., & Pauli, U. (1997). Social phobia: The clinical efficacy and tolerability of the monoamine oxidase-A and serotonin uptake inhibitor brofaromine: A double-blind placebo-controlled study. *Journal of Clinical Psychopharmacology*, 171, 255–260.

Fallon, B. A., Campeas, R., Schneier, F. R., Hollander, E., Feerick, J., & Hatterer, J. (1992). Open trial of intravenous clomipramine in five treatment-refractory patients with obsessive–compulsive disorder. *Journal of Neuropsychiatry and Clinical Neuroscience*, 4, 70–75.

Fava, M., & Rosenbaum, J. F. (1991). Suicidality and fluoxetine: Is there a relationship? *Journal of Clinical Psychiatry*, 52(3), 108–111.

Fisher, A. A., & Davis, M. W. (2002). Serotonin syndrome caused by selective serotonin reuptake inhibitors–metoclopramide interaction. *Annals of Pharmacotherapy*, 36(1), 67–71.

Frazer, A. (2001). Serotonergic and noradrenergic reuptake inhibitors: Prediction of clinical effects from in vitro potencies. *Journal of Clinical Psychiatry*, 62(Suppl. 12), 16–23.

Frishman, W. H. (1981). Beta-adrenoceptor antagonists: New drugs and new indications. *New England Journal of Medicine*, 305, 500.

Gao, K., Muzina, D., Gajwani, P., & Calabrese, J. R. (2006). Efficacy of typical and atypical antipsychotics for primary and comorbid anxiety symptoms or disorders: A review. *Journal of Clinical Psychiatry*, 67, 1327–1340.

Gelenberg, A. J., Lydiard, R. B., Rudolph, R. L., Aguiar, L., Haskins, J. T., & Salinas, E. (2000). Efficacy of venlafaxine extended-release capsules in nondepressed outpatients with generalized anxiety disorder: A 6-month randomized controlled trial. *Journal of the American Medical Association*, 283(23), 3082–3088.

Gelpin, E., Bonne, O., Peri, T., Tszandes, D., & Shalev, A. Y. (1996). Treatment of recent trauma survivors with benzodiazepines: A prospective study. *Journal of Clinical Psychiatry*, 57, 390–394.

Goddard, A. W., Brouette, T., Almai, A., Jetty, P., Woods, S. W., & Charney, D. (2001). Early coadministration of clonazepam with sertraline for panic disorder. *Archives of General Psychiatry*, *58*, 681–686.

Goisman, R. M., Allsworth, J., Rogers, M. P., Warshaw, M. G., Goldenberg, I., & Vasile, R. G. (1998). Simple phobia as a comorbid anxiety disorder. *Depression and Anxiety*, *7*, 105–112.

Gorenstein, E. E., Kleber, M. S., de Jesus, M., Mohlman, J., Gorman, J. M., & Papp, L. A. (2005). Cognitive-behavioral therapy for management of anxiety and medication taper in older adults. *American Journal of Geriatric Psychiatry*, *13*, 901–909.

Gorenstein, E. E., & Papp, L. A. (2007). Cognitive-behavioral therapy for anxiety in the elderly. *Current Psychiatry Reports*, *9*(1), 20–25.

Gorman, J. M., Levy, G. F., Liebowitz, M. R., McGrath, P., Appleby, I. L., Dillon, D. J., et al. (1983). Effect of acute beta-adrenergic blockade on lactate-induced panic. *Archives of General Psychiatry*, *40*, 1079.

Gorman, J. M., Liebowitz, M. R., Fyer, A. J., Campeas, R., & Klein, D. F. (1985). Treatment of social phobia with atenolol. *Journal of Clinical Psychopharmacology*, *5*, 298.

Gottschalk, L. A., Stone, W. N., & Gleser, C. G. (1974). Peripheral versus central mechanisms accounting for antianxiety effects of propranolol. *Psychosomatic Medicine*, *36*, 47.

Gould, R. A., Otto, M. N., Pollack, M. H., & Yap, L. (1997). Cognitive-behavioral and pharmacological treatment of generalized anxiety disorder: A preliminary meta-analysis. *Behavior Therapy*, *28*, 285–305.

Greenblatt, D. J., Shader, R. I., & Abernethy, D. R. (1983). Drug therapy: Current status of benzodiazepines. *New England Journal of Medicine*, *309*(7), 410–416.

Hartley, L. R., Ungapen, S., & Davie, T. (1983). The effect of beta adrenergic blocking drugs on speaker's performance and memory. *British Journal of Psychiatry*, *142*, 512.

Heimberg, R. G., Liebowitz, M. R., Hope, D. A., Schneier, F. R., Holt, C. S., & Welkowitz, L. A. (1998). Cognitive-behavioral group therapy vs. phenelzine therapy for social phobia. *Archives of General Psychiatry*, *55*, 1133–1141.

Herrmann, N., Mamdani, M., & Lanctot, K. L. (2004). Atypical antipsychotics and risk of cerebro-vascular accidents. *American Journal of Psychiatry*, *161*(6), 1113–1115.

Hertzberg, M. A., Butterfield, M. I., Feldman, M. E., Beckham, J. C., Sutherland, S. M., & Connor, K. M. (1999). A preliminary study of lamotrigine for the treatment of posttraumatic stress disorder. *Biological Psychiatry*, *45*(9), 1226–1229.

Hertzberg, M. A., Feldman, M. E., Beckham, S. C., Kudler, H. S., & Davidson, J. R. (2000). Lack of efficacy for fluoxetine in PTSD: A placebo-controlled trial in combat veterans. *Annals of Clinical Psychiatry*, *14*(2), 101–105.

Hidalgo, R. M., Hertzberg, M. A., Mellman, T., Petty, F., Tucker, T., & Weisler, R. (1999). Nefazodone in post-traumatic stress disorder: Results from six-open-label trials. *International Clinical Psychopharmacology*, *14*(2), 61–68.

Hoehn-Saric, R., McLeod, D. R., Funderburk, F., & Kowalski, P. (2004). Somatic symptoms and physiologic responses in generalized anxiety disorder and panic disorder: An ambulatory monitor study. *Archives of General Psychiatry*, *61*(9), 913–921.

Hoehn-Saric, R., McLeod, D. R., & Zimmerli, W. D. (1988) Differential effects of alprazolam and imipramine in generalized anxiety disorder: Somatic versus psychic symptoms. *Journal of Clinical Psychiatry*, *49*, 293–301.

Hohagen, F., Winkelmann, G., Rasche-Raeuchle, H., Hand, I., Koenig, A., Muenchau, et al. (1998). Combination of behaviour therapy with fluoxamine in comparison with behaviour therapy and placebo: Results of a multicentre study. *British Journal of Psychiatry*, *173*, 71–78.

James, I. M., & Savage, I. (1984). Beneficial effects of nadolol on anxiety-induced disturbances of musical performance in musicians; A comparison with diazepam and placebo. *American Heart Journal*, *108*, 1150–1155.

Kathol, R. G., Noyes, R., Jr., & Slymen, D. J. (1980). Propranolol in chronic anxiety disorders: A controlled study. *Archives of General Psychiatry*, *37*, 1361.

Keck, P. E., Taylor, V. E., Tugrul, K. C., McElroy, S. L., & Bennett, J. A. (1993). Valproate treatment of panic disorder and lactate-induced panic attacks. *Biological Psychiatry*, *35*, 775–780.

Kessler, R. C., Berglund, P., Demler, O., Jin, R., & Walters, E. E. (2005). Lifetime prevalence and age-of-onset distributions of DSM-IV disorders in the National Comorbidity Survey Replication. *Archives of General Psychiatry*, *62*(6), 593–602.

Kessler, R. C., DuPont, R. L., Berglund, P., & Wittchen, H. (1999). Impairment in pure and comorbid generalized anxiety disorder and major depression at 12 months in two national surveys. *American Journal of Psychiatry, 156*(12), 1915–1923.

Kinrys, G., Wygent, L. E., Pardo, T. B., & Melo, M. (2006). Levetiracetam for treatment-refractory post-traumatic stress disorder. *Journal of Clinical Psychiatry, 67,* 211–214.

Kinzie, B. J. (1987). Management of the syndrome of inappropriate secretion of antidiuretic hormone. *Clinical Pharmacy, 61*(8), 625–633.*

Klein, D. F. (1964). Delineation of two drug-responsive anxiety syndromes. *Psychopharmacology Bulletin, 5,* 397.

Klein, D. F., & Fink, M. (1962). Psychiatric reaction patterns to imipramine. *American Journal of Psychiatry, 119,* 432–438.

Klein, D. F., Gittelman, R., Quitkin, F. M., & Rifkin, A. (1980). *Diagnosis and treatment of psychiatric disorders: Adults and children* (2nd ed.). Baltimore: Williams & Wilkins.

Kobak, K. A., Greist, J. H., Jefferson, J. W., Katzelnick, D. J., & Henk, H. J. (1998). Behavioral versus pharmacological treatments for obsessive–compulsive disorder: A meta-analysis. *Psychopharmacology, 136,* 205–216.

Koran, L. M., Aboujaoude, E., Bullock, K. D., Franz, B., Gamel, N., & Elliott, M. (2005). Double-blind treatment with oral morphine in treatment-resistant obsessive–compulsive disorder. *Journal of Clinical Psychiatry, 66*(3), 353–359.

Koran, L. M., Ringold, A. L., & Elliott, M. A. (2000). Olanzapine augmentation for treatment-resistant obsessive–compulsive disorder. *Journal of Clinical Psychiatry, 61,* 514–517.

Kosten, T. R., Frank, J. B., Dan, E., McDougle, C. J., & Giller, E. L. (1991). Pharmacotherapy for post-traumatic stress disorder using phenelzine or imipramine. *Journal of Nervous and Mental Disease, 179,* 366–370.

Kozak, M. J., Liebowitz, M. R., & Foa, E. B. (2000). Cognitive behavior therapy and pharmacotherapy for obsessive-compulsive disorder: The NIMH-sponsored collaborative study. In W. K. Goodman & M. V. Rudorfer (Eds.), *Obsessive–compulsive disorder: Contemporary issues in treatment. Personality and clinical psychology series* (pp. 501–530). Mahwah, NJ: Erlbaum.

Kulin, N. A., Pastuszak, A., Sage, S. R., Schick-Boschetto, B., Spivey, G., Feldkamp, M. et al. (1998). Pregnancy outcome following maternal use of the new selective serotonin reuptake inhibitors: A prospective controlled multicenter study. *Journal of the American Medical Association, 279*(8), 609–610.

Lehrer, P. M., Rosen, R. C., Kostis, J. B., & Greenfield, D. (1987). Treating stage fright in musicians: The use of beta-blockers. *New Jersey Medicine, 84*(1), 27–33.

Liebowitz, M. R., Fyer, A. J., Gorman, J. M., Campeas, R. B., Sandberg, D. P., Hollander, E., et al. (1988). Tricyclic therapy of the DSM-III anxiety disorders: A review with implications for further research. *Journal of Psychiatric Research, 22*(Suppl. 1), 7–31.

Liebowitz, M. R., Gelenberg, A. J., & Munjack, D. (2005). Venlafaxine extended release vs. placebo and paroxetine in social anxiety disorder. *Archives of General Psychiatry, 62*(2), 190–198.

Liebowitz, M. R., Schneier, F., Campeas, R., Gorman, J., Flyer, A., Hollander, E., et al. (1990). Phenelzine and atenolol in social phobia. *Psychopharmacology Bulletin, 26*(1), 123–125.

Londborg, P. D., Hegel, M. T., Goldstein, S., Goldstein, D., Himmelhoch, J. M., & Maddock, R. (2001). Sertraline treatment of posttraumatic stress disorder: Results of 24 weeks of open-label continuation treatment. *Journal of Clinical Psychiatry, 62,* 325–331.

Lum, M., Fontaine, R., Elie, R., & Ontiveros, A. (1990). Divalproex sodium's antipanic effect in panic disorder: A placebo-controlled study. *Biological Psychiatry, 27,* 164A.

MacKinnon, D. F., Zandi, P. P., Cooper, J., Potash, J. B., Simpson, S. G., Gershon, E., et al. (2002). Comorbid bipolar disorder and panic disorder in families with a high prevalence of bipolar disorder. *American Journal of Psychiatry, 159*(1), 30–35.

Marshall, R. D., Beebe, K. L., Oldham, M., & Zanielli, R. (2001). Efficacy and safety of paroxetine treatment for chronic PTSD: A fixed-dose, placebo-controlled study. *American Journal of Psychiatry, 158*(12), 1982–1988.

Mavissakalian, M., & Perel, J. M. (1992). Protective effects of imipramine maintenance treatment in panic disorder with agoraphobia. *American Journal of Psychiatry, 149,* 1053–1057.

McDougle, C. J., Epperson, C. N., Pelton, G. H., Waslynk, S., & Price L. H. (2000). A double-blind, placebo controlled study of risperidone addition in serotonin reuptake inhibitor–refractory obsessive–compulsive disorder. *Archives of General Psychiatry, 57,* 794–801.

McDougle, C. J., Goodman, W. K., Keckman, J. F., Lee, N. C., Heninger, G. R., & Price, L. H. (1994). Haloperidol addition in fluvoxamine-refractory obsessive–compulsive disorder: A double-blind, placebo-controlled study in patients with and without tics. *Archives of General Psychiatry, 51*, 302–308.

Misri, S., Kim, J., Riggs, K. W., & Kostaras, X. (2000). Paroxetine levels in postpartum depressed women, breast milk, and infant serum. *Journal of Clinical Psychiatry, 61*(11), 828–832.

Montgomery, S. A., Mahe, V., Haudiquet, V., & Hackett, D. (2002). Effectiveness of venlafaxine, extended release formulation, in the short-term and long-term treatment of generalized anxiety disorder: Results of a survival analysis. *Journal of Clinical Psychopharmacology, 22*(6), 561–567.

Nelson, R. C. (1987). *Estimates of benzodiazepine use, doses, and duration of use: Data on seizures and other reported withdrawal.* Washington DC: U.S. Food and Drug Administration.

Neziroglu, F., Yaryura-Tobias, J. A., Walz, J., & McKay, D. (2000). The effect of fluvoxamine and behavior therapy on children and adolescents with obsessive–compulsive disorder. *Journal of Child and Adolescent Psychopharmacology, 10, 295–306.*

Olajide, D., & Lader, M. (1987). A comparison of buspirone, diazepam and placebo in patients with chronic anxiety states. *Journal of Clinical Psychopharmacology, 7*, 148–152.

Otto, M. W., Tuby, K. S., Gould, R. A., Mclean, R. Y., & Pollack, M. H. (2001). An effect-size analysis of the relative efficacy and tolerability of serotonin selective reuptake inhibitors for panic disorder. *American Journal of Psychiatry, 158*(12), 1989–1992.

Pande, A. C., Davidson, J. R. T., Jefferson, J. W., Janney, C. A., Katzelnick, A. J., & Weisler, R. H. (1999). Treatment of social phobia with gabapentin: A placebo-controlled study. *Journal of Clinical Psychopharmacology, 19*, 341–348.

Pande, A. C., Pollack, M. H., Crockatt, J., Greiner, M., Chuinard, G., & Lydiard, R. T. S. (2000). Placebo-controlled study of gabapentin treatment of panic disorder. *Journal of Clinical Psychopharmacology, 20*, 467–471.

Papp, L. A. (2004). Generalized anxiety disorder: Evaluation and treatment. In R. L. Spitzer, M. B. First, M., Gibbon, & J. B. W. Williams (Eds.), *Treatment companion to the DSM-IV-TR casebook.* Washington, DC: American Psychiatric Association Press.

Papp, L. A. (2006). Safety and efficacy of levetiracetam: Results of an open label, fixed–flexible dose study for patients with panic disorder. *Journal of Clinical Psychiatry, 67*(10), 1573–1576.

Papp, L. A., Gorenstein, E. E., & Kleber, M. (1998). *Treatment of late-life anxiety disorders.* Paper presented at the annual meeting of the American Psychiatric Association, Toronto, Canada.

Papp, L. A., & Gorman, J. M. (1990). Suicidal preoccupation during fluoxetine treatment. *American Journal of Psychiatry, 147*, 1380.

Papp, L. A., & Kleber, M. (2001). Diagnosis and epidemiology of generalized anxiety disorder. In D. J. Stein & E. Hollander (Eds.), *Textbook of anxiety disorders.* Washington, DC: American Psychiatric Association Press.

Papp, L. A., Klein, D. F., & Gorman, J. M. (1993). Carbon dioxide hypersensitivity, hyperventilation, and panic disorder. *American Journal of Psychiatry, 150*, 1149–1157.

Papp, L. A., & Ray, S. (2003, May). *The SGRI tiagabine for the treatment of generalized anxiety disorder.* Paper presented at the annual meeting of the American Psychiatric Association. San Francisco.

Papp, L. A., Sinha, S. S., Martinez, J. M., Coplan, J. D., Amchin, J., & Gorman, J. M. (1998). Low-dose venlafaxine treatment in panic disorder. *Psychopharmacology Bulletin, 34*(2), 207–209.

Pato, M. T., Zohar-Kadouch, R., Zohar, J., & Murphy, D. L. (1988). Return of symptoms after discontinuation of clomipramine in patients with obsessive–compulsive disorder. *American Journal of Psychiatry, 145*(12), 1531–1525.

Phillips, K. A., & Van Bebber, S. L. (2005). Measuring the value of pharmacogenomics. *Nature Reviews Drug Discovery, 4*(6), 500–509.

Pitman, R. K., Sanders, K. M., Zusman, R. M., Healy, A. R., Cheema, F., & Lasko, N. B. (2002). Pilot study of secondary prevention of posttraumatic stress disorder with propanolol. *Biological Psychiatry, 51*(2), 189–192.

Pohjavaara, P., Telaranta, T., & Vaisanen, E. (2003). The role of the sympathetic nervous system in anxiety: Is it possible to relieve anxiety with endoscopic sympathetic block? *Norwegian Journal of Psychiatry, 57*(1), 55–60.

Pohl, R., Balon R., Yeragani, V. K., & Gershon, S. (1989). Serotonergic anxiolytics in the treatment of panic disorder: A controlled study with buspirone. *Psychopathology, 22*(Suppl. 1), 60–67.

Pohl, R., Bridges, M., Rainey, J. M., Jr., Boudoulas, H., & Yeragani, V. K. (1986). Effects of trazodone and desipramine on cardiac rate and rhythm in a patient with preexisting cardiovascular disease. *Journal of Clinical Psychopharmacology, 6*, 380–381.

Pritchett, D. B., Sontheimer, H., Shivers, B., Ymer, S., Kettenmann, H., & Schofield, P. R. (1989). Importance of a novel GABA$_A$ receptor subunit for benzodiazepine pharmacology. *Nature, 338*, 582–590.

Rapaport, M. H., Endicott, J., & Clary, C. M. (2002). Posttraumatic stress disorder and quality of life: Results across 64 weeks of sertraline treatment. *Journal of Clinical Psychiatry, 63*(1), 59–65.

Raskind, M. A., Dobie, D. J., Kanter, E. D., Petrie, E. C., Thompson, C. E., & Perskind, E. R. (2000). The ?$_1$-adrenergic antagonist prazosin ameliorates combat trauma nightmares in veterans with posttraumatic stress disorder: A report of 4 cases. *Journal of Clinical Psychiatry, 61*, 129–133.

Ressler, K. J., Rothbaum, B. O., Tannenbaum, L., Anderson, P., Graap, K., Zimand, E., et al. (2004). Cognitive enhancers as adjuncts to psychotherapy. *Archives of General Psychiatry, 61*, 1136–1144.

Rickels, K., Case, W. G., Downing, R. W., & Winokur, A. (1983). Long-term diazepam therapy and clinical outcome. *Journal of the American Medical Association, 50*, 767–771.

Rickels, K., & Schweizer, E. (1987). Current pharmacotherapy of anxiety and panic. In H. Y. Meltzer (Ed.), *Psychopharmacology: The third generation of progress.* New York: Raven Press.

Rickels, K., Schweizer, E., Csanalosi, I., Case, W. G., & Chung, H. (1988). Long-term treatment of anxiety and risk of withdrawal. *Archives of General Psychiatry, 45*(5), 444–450.

Rotondo, A., Mazzanti, C., Dell'Osso, L., Rucci, P., Sullivan, P., & Bouanani, S. (2002). Catechol o-methyltransferase, serotonin transporter, and tryptophan hydroxylase gene polymorphisms in bipolar disorder patients with and without comorbid panic disorder. *American Journal of Psychiatry, 159*(1), 23–29.

Roy-Byrne, P. P., Craske, M. G., Stein, M. B., Sullivan, G., Bystritsky, A., Katon, W., et al. (2005). A randomized effectiveness trial of cognitive-behavioral therapy and medication for primary care panic disorder. *Archives of General Psychiatry, 62*, 290–298.

Roy-Byrne, P. P., Dager, S. R., Cowley, D. S., Vitaliano, P., & Dunner, D. L. (1989). Relapse and rebound following discontinuation of benzodiazapine treatment of panic attacks: Alprazolam versus diazepam. *American Journal of Psychiatry, 146*, 860–864.

Safren, S. A., Gershuny, B. S., Marzol, P., Otto, M. W., & Pollack, M. H. (2002). History of childhood abuse in panic disorder, social phobia and generalized anxiety disorder. *Journal of Nervous and Mental Disease, 190*, 453–456.

Salzman, C., Goldenberg, I., Bruce, S. E., & Keller, M. B. (2001). Pharmacologic treatment of anxiety disorders in 1989 versus 1996: Results from the Harvard/Brown Anxiety Disorders Research Program. *Journal of Clinical Psychiatry, 62*, 149–152.

Schneier, F. R., Liebowitz, M. R., Abi-Dargham, A., Zea-Ponce, Y., Lin, S. H., & Laruelle, M. (2000). Low dopamine (D2) receptor binding potential in social phobia. *American Journal of Psychiatry, 157*, 457–459.

Schweizer, E., Rickels, K., & Lucki, O. (1986). Resistance to the anti-anxiety effect of buspirone in patients with a history of benzodiazepine use. *New England Journal of Medicine, 314*, 719–720.

Shaomei, L., et al. (2001). Combination of clomipramine with exposure therapy in treatment of obsessive-compulsive disorder [English abstract]. *Chinese Mental Health Journal, 15*, 239–240.

Sharp, D. M., Power, K. G., Simpson, R. J., & Swanson, V. (1996). Fluvoxamine, placebo, and cognitive behavior therapy used alone and in combination in the treatment of panic disorder and agoraphobia. *Journal of Anxiety Disorders, 10*, 219–242.

Shear, M. K., Brown, T. A., Barlow, D. H., Money, R., Gorman, J. M., & Papp, L. A. (1997). Multicenter collaborative Panic Disorder Severity Scale, *American Journal of Psychiatry, 154*, 1571–1575.

Sheehan, D. (1987). Benzodiazepines in panic disorder and agoraphobia. *Journal of Affective Disorders, 13*, 169–181.

Sheehan, D., Bach, M. B., Ballenger, J., & Jacobsen, G. (1980). Treatment of endogenous anxiety with phobic, hysterical, and hypochondriacal symptoms. *Archives of General Psychiatry, 37*, 51–59.

Silverstone, P. H., & Salinas, E. (2001). Efficacy of venlafaxine extended release in patients with major depressive disorder and comorbid generalized anxiety disorder. *Journal of Clinical Psychiatry, 62*(7), 523–529.

Smajkic, A., Weine, S., Duric-Bijedic, Z., Boskaile, E., Lewis, J., & Pavkovic, T. (2001). Sertraline, paroxetine, and venlafaxine in refugee posttraumatic stress disorder with depression symptoms. *Journal of Trauma and Stress, 14*, 445–452.

Snyder, S. H., & Peroutka, S. J. (1984). Antidepressants and neurotransmitter receptors. In R. M. Post & J. C. Ballenger (Eds.), *Neurobiology of mood disorders.* Baltimore: Williams & Wilkins.

Soravia, L. M., Heinrichs, M., Aerni, A., Maroni, C., Schelling, G., Ehlert, U., et al. (2006). Glucocorticoids reduce phobic fear in humans. *Proceedings of the National Academy of Sciences of the USA, 103*(14), 5585–5590.

Soumerai, S. B., Simoni-Wastila, L., Singer, C., Mah, C., Gao, X., Salzman, C., et al. (2003). Lack of relationship between long-term use of benzodiazepines and escalation to high dosages. *[journal title?]* , *54*(7), 1006–1011.

Stanley, M. A., Beck, J. G., Novy, D. M., Averill, P. M., Swann, A. C., Diefenbach, G. J., et al. (2003). Cognitive-behavioral treatment of late-life generalized anxiety disorder. *Journal of Consulting and Clinical Psychology, 71*, 309–319.

Stanley, M. A., Beck, J. G., & Zebb, B. J. (1996). Psychometric properties of four anxiety measures in older adults. *Behaviour Research and Therapy, 34*, 827–838.

Stein, D. J., Ipser, J., & Balkom, A. (2004). Pharmacotherapy for social phobia. *Cochrane Database of Systematic Reviews, 4*. Chichester, UK: Wiley.

Tallman, J. F., Paul, S. M., Skolnick, P., & Gallagher, D. W. (1980). Receptors for the age of anxiety: Pharmacology of the benzodiazepines. *Science, 201*, 274–281.

Thase, M. E. (1998). Effects of venlafaxine on blood pressure: A meta-analysis of original data from 3,744 depressed patients. *Journal of Clinical Psychiatry, 59*(10), 502–508.

Tollefson, G. D. (1983). Monoamine oxidase inhibitors: A review. *Journal of Clinical Psychiatry, 44*, 280.

Turner, S. M., Beidel, D. C., & Jacob, R. (1994). Social phobia: A comparison of behavior therapy and atenolol. *Journal of Consulting and Clinical Psychology, 62*, 350–358.

Turner, S. M., Jacob, R. G., & Beidel, D. C. (1985). Fluoxetine treatment of obsessive–compulsive disorder. *Journal of Clinical Psychopharmacology, 5*, 201–212.

van Balkom, A. J. L. M., de Haan, E., van Oppen, P., Spinhoven, P., Hoogduin, K. A. L., & van Dyck, R. (1998). Cognitive and behavioral therapies alone versus in combination with fluvoxamine in the treatment of obsessive–compulsive disorder. *Journal of Nervous and Mental Disease, 186*, 492–499.

Versiani, M., Cassano, G., Perugi, G., Benedetti, A., Mastalli, L., & Nardi, A. (2002). Reboxetine, a selective norepinephrine reuptake inhibitor, is an effective and well-tolerated treatment for panic disorder. *Journal of Clinical Psychiatry, 63*(1), 31–37.

Versiani, M., Nardi, A. E., Mundim, F. D., Alves, A., Liebowitz, M. R., & Amtein, R. (1992). Pharmacotherapy of social phobia: A controlled study with moclobemide and phenelzine. *British Journal of Psychiatry, 161*, 353–360.

Walker, D. L., Ressler, K. J., Lu, K. T., & Davis, M. (2002). Facilitation of conditioned fear extinction by systemic administration of intra-amygdala infusions of D-cycloserine as assessed with fear-potentiated startle in rats. *Journal of Neuroscience, 22*(6), 2343–2351.

Westra, H. A., & Stewart, S. H. (1998). Cognitive-behavioral therapy and pharmacotherapy: Complementary or contradictory approaches to the treatment of anxiety? *Clinical Psychology Review, 18*, 307–340.

Wetherell, J. L., Gatz, M., & Craske, M. G. (2003). Treatment of generalized anxiety disorder in older adults. *Journal of Consulting and Clinical Psychology, 71*, 31–40.

Wittchen, H. U., Zhao, S., Kessler, R. C., & Eaton, W. W. (1994). DSM-III-R generalized anxiety disorder in the National Comorbidity Survey. *Archives of General Psychiatry, 51*(5), 355–364.

Yehuda, R. (1999). Managing anger and aggression in patients with posttraumatic stress disorder. *Journal of Clinical Psychiatry, 60*(Suppl. 15), 33–37.

Yeragani, V. K., Pohl, R., Stinivasan, K., Balou, R., Romesti, C., & Berchou, R. (1995). Effects of isoproterenol infusions on heart rate variability in patients with panic disorder. *Psychiatry Research, 56*(3), 289–293.

Yudofsky, S., Williams, D., & Gorman, J. (1981). Propranolol in the treatment of rage and violent behavior in patients with chronic brain syndromes. *American Journal of Psychiatry, 138*, 218–220.

Zitrin, C. M., Klein, D. F., Woerner, M. G., & Ross, D. C. (1983). Treatment of phobias: I. Comparison of imipramine hydrochloride and placebo. *Archives of General Psychiatry, 40*, 125–138.

PART III

INTEGRATION

CHAPTER 23

Sport Psychophysiology and Peak Performance Applications of Stress Management

PAUL DAVIS
WESLEY E. SIME
JAMES ROBERTSON

THEORETICAL FOUNDATIONS

The elite sport environment, with its culture of extreme ego orientation, is inherently threatening for many athletes. Whether threats emanate internally or externally, few elite athletes have totally escaped the grasp of performance-debilitating stress during their entire careers. Although it seems that some athletes cope easily with the multitude of possible stressors associated with the quest for elite athletic performance, unaided by specific psychological preparation, many other talented athletes struggle—often failing to achieve their expected performance potential. It is this gap between potential and performance that has driven much of the field of sport psychophysiology from both research and applied perspectives. Researchers have sought to identify the key causal variables of stress that lead to decrements in performance (Hanin, 2000; Janelle, 2002), and applied practitioners have developed a myriad of techniques in the hopes of mitigating or eliminating the often disastrous effects of stress (Elchami, 2003).

History of Stress Management in Sport

Sport psychophysiology was formally introduced little more than two decades ago, when a group of applied sport psychologists convened to write the first bold position paper on the critical role of stress and coping in sport performance titled "Stress Management for Sport" (Zaichowsky & Sime, 1982). Since then, others have continued to validate the physiological effects of psychological stress states in a variety of sports (Carlstedt, 2001; Hatfield & Landers, 1983; Janelle, 1999; Sime, 1985; Vickers, 1996). Recent research efforts have benefited from technological advances in equipment that enable the precise quantification of a variety of physiological indices. The application of this technology to performance enhancement protocols within sport psychology practice is becoming more widely accepted in spite of the ambivalence, technophobia, and dualist perspectives that exist among many athletes, coaches, and a large number of research or applied sport psychologists (Davis & Sime, 2005).

While the field of sport psychophysiology has steadily developed over the past two decades, some have questioned both current research approaches and applied practice, focusing on: (1) the validity of generalizing laboratory experiments to the competitive environment, (2) the reluctance to integrate neuroscience with sport psychology, and (3) the minimal attention devoted to the full range of emotional experience of individual athletes (Carlstedt, 2001; Cerin, 2003; Hanin, 2000; Holmes & Collins, 2001; Keil, Holmes, Bennett, Davids, & Smith, 2000).

This chapter has multiple purposes. We aim to provide an integrative definition of stress and explain how and why it originates, as well as the debilitating effect it has on sport performance. We also hope to provoke discussion of the evolving field of sport psychophysiology by providing both theory and applied examples that will inform the reader of the possibilities offered by an array of effective biofeedback protocols to reduce distress while enhancing athletic performance. Last, we wish to further highlight the role of emotions in sport (Cerin, 2003; Hanin, 2000; Skinner & Brewer, 2004)—both negative and positive—and to illustrate how positive psychology's "broaden and build theory" (Fredrickson, 1998; Fredrickson, 2000) and "undoing hypothesis" (Levenson & Fredrickson, 1998; Fredrickson, Mancuso, Branigan, & Tugade, 2000) provide valuable insight into the development of coping strategies and stress reduction within sport contexts. The question of whether the accumulated evidence meets criteria to state definitively that stress management applications are effective in sport psychology and performance enhancement venues is evaluated in accordance with the guidelines set forth by the Association for Applied Psychophysiology and Biofeedback (LaVaque et al., 2002). The following evaluative categories are employed in this review: level 1 = efficacious and specific, level 2 = efficacious, level 3 = possibly efficacious, and level 4 = further research needed to establish efficacy.

Evolving Role of Stress in Sport Contexts

Although stress is a prevailing theme throughout the general sport psychology literature, there remains disagreement among researchers and practitioners regarding its definition (Janelle, 1999). In past decades, the constructs of arousal (physiological and psychological activation associated with various levels of practice and competition) and anxiety (a state of arousal delineated into cognitive and somatic components) have been used as synonyms for stress (Janelle, 2002) and have been the focus of numerous studies illustrating their deleterious effects on performance (Gould & Udry, 1994; Martens, Burton, Vealey, Bump, & Smith, 1990; Weinberg & Gould, 2003). The terms *distress* and *eustress* have been used to differentiate between negative and positive forms of stress (Lazarus, 1999).

The very earliest measures of these constructs were neither sophisticated nor technologically advanced. Practitioners simply made observations of athletes who appeared tense, nervous, or scared and subsequently performed poorly, contrasting their behavior with the confidence and poise exhibited by more successful athletes. Anxiety, manifested in the form of "fidgeting" behavior, higher eye-blink rate, and other pragmatic behavioral observations, was considered a primary predictor of poor performance under stress (Kojima et al., 2002). Most early discussion regarding mind–body integration in sport was limited to purely cognitive information and retrospective self-reports derived from elite, world-class performers (Sime, 1982). Athletes were advised to recognize the symptoms of emotional arousal as warning signals that their bodily systems were getting "too charged up" and were provided with basic stress management and arousal reduction strategies such as deep breathing or thought stopping to help insulate them from distracting cognitive intrusions or emotional activation.

The prevailing conventional wisdom among sport psychologicsts as a result of this early research on stress sports is that precompetition anxiety levels are inversely related to performance outcomes (Hanton, Thomas, & Maynard, 2004). Yet recently some researchers have questioned this premise. Several meta-analyses have uncovered scant evidence of causal relationships between cognitive or somatic anxiety and performance. Instead, the data suggest that self-confidence displays a stronger and more consistent relationship to performance outcomes than either type of anxiety (Woodman & Hardy, 2003; Craft, Magyar, Becker, & Feltz, 2003; Thomas, Maynard, & Hanton, 2004). Others have argued that the subjective emotional experiences of athletes are so broad and varied that relying on the singular emotion of anxiety to inform the athlete–stress relationship is incomplete or inaccurate, as other threat-related negative emotions may be more important to the discussion (Cerin, 2003; Hanin, 2000; Jones, 2003). Also, as Hanin (2000) suggests, it is clear that athletic competition and performance is a multi-stage endeavor incorporating preparation (preperformance), execution (performance), and evaluation (postperformance). Accordingly, focusing solely on preperformance anxiety levels ignores a significant segment of the performance process and the information that could be derived from it.

Modern Definition of Stress in Sport

The cognitive–motivational–relational theory (CMRT) of emotion, wherein stress is a unitary phenomenon entwined with emotion, coping, and appraisal (Lazarus, 1999), forms the backbone of our definition of stress in sport. In this model, emotion is defined as a psychophysiological reaction to environmental or social variables, consisting of internal subjective experience, impulses for action, and physiological change driven by individual cognitive appraisal of motivational and relational variables that are mediating factors arousing, sustaining, modifying, or extinguishing the stress response. Emotion is considered the superior (controlling) element of the theory, since without it there is no need for coping (Lazarus, 1999). Coping plays a vital secondary role in the stress process, as perceived availability of coping resources affects how an individual appraises a situation, determining whether and what emotion is displayed, how one responds to the psychophysiological symptoms of the aroused negative emotion, and whether stress occurs (Lazarus, 1999). Understanding this process and how it leads to a wide range of individual differences in the manifestations of stress is critical to understanding our conceptualization of competitive stress and how to devise interventions to minimize it.

When present stimuli are consciously or unconsciously associated with past losses or potential harm (Johnson, 2003), a threat appraisal is generated, negative emotion aroused, and the coping process activated (Lazarus, 1999). When adequate coping resources are available, the perceived threat and negative emotion is minimized, and the individual is typically able to adapt. If the individual does not possess adequate coping resources, then stress and maladaptive behavior are the likely results. It would appear, then, that coping—how each athlete manages and regulates his or her emotional state aroused by the cognitive framing evoked by their own unique, subjective experience—is critical to defining stress, and thus understanding its effect on athletic performance (Lazarus, 2000). We shall define competitive stress as a situation occurring when psychological demands are perceived (consciously or subconsciously) by an athlete to exceed his or her available coping resources (Hanin, 2000; Janelle, 2002; Lazarus, 2000).

Emotion research from general psychology suggests that the primary function of negative emotion is to mobilize the mind and body in preparation to avoid or approach threatening stimuli (Lazarus, 1999; Levenson, 1992). Certainly, negative emotions such as fear or anxiety may function as approach motivators within the sport arena, prompting the athlete to get "psyched up" for the "battle" of competition. Indeed, for many athletes, experiencing uncertainty, nervousness, or fear before and/or during competition is viewed as natural and potentially helpful to performance. When the coping resources of an athlete are overwhelmed by the intensity or duration of negative emotion(s), stress occurs, triggering avoidance behaviors that are debilitating for athletic performance (Hanin, 2000; Janelle, Singer, & Williams, 1999; Murray & Janelle, 2003; Robazza, Bortoli, & Nougier, 2000).

While Lazarus (1999) suggests that the experience of positive emotion may also lead to stress, we disagree with this position, based upon the "psychophysiological reaction" that determines emotional valence. Although slight differences exist in the levels of autonomic arousal between various negative emotions, all produce increased cardiovascular measures, hormonal activation, skin response, and attentional changes designed to prepare the body for a specific overt action associated with each emotion (Levenson, 1992). Positive emotions, on the other hand, do not bear distinctive autonomic markers, and by themselves, in fact, their manifestation is rather benign (Fredrickson, 1998; Levenson & Fredrickson, 1998). Thus the psychological component of threat appraisal *and* the physiological arousal of negative emotion must occur together in order for an individual to experience stress.

Hanin's (2000) Individual Zones of Optimal Functioning (IZOF) model argues that in addition to the emotion of anxiety, other negative emotions such as anger, fear, guilt, shame, embarrassment, envy, and contempt often occur during the athletic performance cycle, leading to stress and performance decrements (Carlstedt, 2001). The goal of the IZOF model is to understand and shape each athlete's optimal emotional range during the performance cycle, since substantial individual differences exist among athletes that affect (1) the appraisal of experienced stimuli, (2) the emotion(s) those experiences elicit, and (3) how those emotions are regulated (Hanin, 2000). Multiple possible stimuli may cause threatening appraisals, negative emotions, and stress at any point during the performance cycle. If neglected, this stress may persist, further disrupting the preparation, execution, and evaluation of future performances and creating a downward spiral of chronic negative emotion and underachievement by the athlete (when the gap between potential and performance is persistently large). Often, chronically stressed athletes succumb to "burnout" and prematurely withdraw from sport participation.

Psychophysiological Effects of Stress on Athletes

The specific psychophysiological effects of stress and negative emotion may include increased heart rate, blood pressure, and electrodermal response; disruption in respiratory sinus arrhythmia; decreased skin temperature (less peripheral blood flow); the release of potent damaging hormones; and reduced brain functioning, especially related to attention (Bundy, Lane, Murray, & Fisher, 2002; Janelle, 2002; Levenson, 1992; McGrady, Chapter 2, this volume; Salvador, Suay, González-Bono, & Serrano, 2003). The resulting sweaty and/or cold hands are serious, debilitating factors in sports where an athlete's grip (e.g., golf, auto racing, gymnastics) or ball handling (e.g., basketball, football, baseball) is critical, as dexterity is compromised due to the reduced blood flow to extremities associated with increased sympathetic arousal. Negative emotions may cause attention to become either narrowed (resulting in hyperfocus on stimuli central to the task) or inefficient (consuming the resources available for the high working memory tasks required for highly skilled athletic movements) (Janelle et al., 1999). In addition, when emotion intensity increases to extreme levels, attentional narrowing may lead to distraction—the visual search wanders to threatening or irrelevant cues—and deterioration of performance and a greater risk of injury (Janelle et al., 1999; Rogers, Alderman, & Landers, 2003).

SENSORY INTEGRATION/DISTURBANCE AND SPORT PERFORMANCE

During optimal human functioning, numerous bodily systems are integrated seamlessly, however, as illustrated in several non-sporting contexts (Damasio, 1994; Meegan, Aslin, & Jacobs, 2000). Lacey and Lacey (1979) demonstrated how decreases in blood pressure and heart rate are associated with sensory reception and sensorimotor integration. More recent investigation on the complicated interaction between sensory functioning and human physiology has revealed that when vision is fixated upon a small target, heart rate decelerates dramatically (Richards & Cronise, 2000). Exploration of these interesting interrelationships continues below.

Rhythm, Timing, and Sensory Integration

The work of Carlstedt (2001, 2004) links these cardiovascular and sensory concepts to enhanced athletic performance. To execute performance efficiently at the highest levels of sport, athletes must integrate the visual, attentional, temporal, motor, limbic (emotion), and proprioception systems. At the elite level of sport, it would seem that many, if not most, physical errors have as their underlying cause a variety of sensory processing and integration disruptions that occur as a result of stress.

If an athlete has an attentional system deficit and improper sensorimotor integration, then timing and rhythm will be disrupted, thus making it more difficult to produce efficient movement (Libkuman, Otani, & Steger, 2002). Even millisecond delays in the sensory balancing and motor coordination process within the vestibular, visual, and proprioceptive subsystems result in imbalances that are evidenced by movement errors on the field of play. Within the sensory balancing and motor coordination process, it appears that breakdowns may first occur in the mental process of creating an accurate performance "blueprint," which leads to errors in the physical execution of that mental model. The specific intention of making a definitive sport movement (e.g., jumping, throwing) is best organized and executed in sequential fashion and at a preconscious level (Singer, 2002). However, sometimes an athlete's muscular effort does not respond precisely according to this blueprint because of systemic disruptions caused by stress. This creates inefficient timing and synchronicity between the motor planning and execution stages, ultimately leading to reductions in task performance (Hatfield & Hillman, 2001).

However, when dealing with stressful conditions, athletes may need to reallocate and/or shift resources from the visual to the motor system and back as they search for awareness of the target and body position. Stress may adversely affect the temporal system as well, leading the athlete to consciously process motor movements while taxing delicate sensory integration functions and disrupting the subtle, finite muscle contractions necessary for optimal performance (Hatfield & Hillman, 2001). This is what athletes are talking about when they say, "I didn't have any rhythm today."

"Quiet-Eye" Influence on Performance

Recent studies of the visual gaze patterns of athletes in selected sports have revealed that the experience of a phenomenon dubbed "quiet eye" is associated with improved performance (Martell & Vickers, 2004; Rodrigues, Vickers, & Williams, 2002; Vickers, 1992, 1996; Vickers & Adolphe, 1997; Williams, Vickers, & Rodrigues, 2002). Quiet-eye behavior is associated with smoother gaze patterns and less frequent (but longer) final visual fixations (defined as the final ocular connection to a target before motor movement is initiated). This pattern of visual attention appears necessary for organization and sequencing of motor execution, and it has been associated with higher alpha and beta power in the left hemisphere and a decrease of alpha and beta in the right hemisphere of expert marksmen (Deeny, Hillman, Janelle, & Hatfield, 2003; Janelle et al., 2000). In laboratory settings, negative emotions have been shown to disrupt optimal quiet-eye periods and to degrade performance (Rodrigues, Vickers, & Williams, 2002). Thus it appears that visual fixation and attention are critically linked elements of athletic performance subject to the debilitating consequences of negative emotion and threat appraisal (Janelle et al., 1999; Rogers et al., 2003).

Tempo of Movement

Temporal disruption during elite performance is also a result of stress, whether measured by reaction time (Williams & Andersen, 1997), by quiet-eye duration (Williams, Singer, & Frehlich, 2002), or by other means involving tempo. Recently, Novosel and Garrity (2004) have uncovered a relationship between temporal dimensions, motor performance, and stress. In video analysis of the golf swings of numerous male and female world-class professional golfers during actual competition, it was found that rhythm and tempo interact in the form of a defined ratio with which to swing a golf club—that is, a 3:1 ratio of video camera frames as measured from takeaway to the top of the backswing (3 units of time), followed by the downward swing to contact with the golf ball (1 unit of time). Although Novosel and Garrity (2004) assert this ratio to be the ideal and claim it to be associated with optimal brain functioning and lack of stress, there has been little first-level (efficacious and specific) scientific corroboration of this phenomenon. However, similar discovery of the salient value of this 3:1 ratio has been made in preliminary investigations by one of us (P. D.) among elite baseball and tennis performers, as well.

The sum total of evidence cited here in regard to tempo of movement, quiet eye, and the overall rhythm, timing, and sensory integration provides a solid rationale for the more sophisticated application of stress management principles in sport performance. This linkage merits the distinction of being possibly efficacious (LaVaque et al., 2002) as it relates to the interventions that are presented in the preceding subsections.

Sources of Athlete Stress

The threats associated with athletic competition are not limited to the obvious physical harm that may occur in rugged, violent sports (such as American football, rugby, boxing, or martial arts) but also encompass psychological strain, especially for those athletes whose personal identities are associated with successful sport performance. Although the actual competition itself, along with subsequent evaluation, is a potent source of stress, there are many other peripheral sources. These include issues affected by coaching leadership, team dynamics, and intra- or interpersonal issues relating to the athlete's relationships outside sport (Fletcher & Hanton, 2003; Giacobbi et al., 2004; Humphrey, Yow, & Bowden, 2000).

During the execution phase of performance, game errors, tough luck, a bad call by an official, or an exceptional performance by an opponent are common sources of stress (Anshel & Wells, 2000). Intrapersonal issues such as clinical depression, substance abuse, gambling, or eating disorders often filter from an athlete's personal life into his or her athletic performance. Negative emotions arising from interpersonal crises such as divorce, death of a loved one, sexual identity, sibling rivalry, or poor parental relationship may create stress that deleteriously affects performance. Unfortunately, many athletes hide these personal issues from coaches, teammates, and counseling or sport psychology professionals until they are free-falling helplessly. These problems illustrate the pervasive nature of stress and how chronic negative emotions may be difficult to eradicate unless the source of the stress is correctly identified.

The athlete–coach relationship may be a particularly acute source of athlete stress (Baker, Cote, & Hawes, 2000; Fletcher & Hanton, 2003; Kenow & Williams, 1999; Ryska & Yin, 2000). Often a coach is the most important figure in an athlete's life, and the coach–athlete relationship plays a critical role in the quality of performance. The personality and/or leadership effectiveness of an athlete's coach may be a source of conflict that elicits threatening appraisals by an athlete, causing negative emotion and stress to occur. Many coaches, unaware of the appraisal, coping, and emotion process, unwittingly undermine an athlete's performance by using excessive or inappropriate threatening behaviors in the misguided belief that they will motivate the athlete. As we have mentioned previously, negative emotions can provide motivation, but only if the athlete possesses the resources to cope with them.

A variety of other issues within elite sport environments may be stress-provoking. Organizational policies or role ambiguity within the team setting often lead to athlete uncertainty, anxiety, and stress (Beauchamp, Bray, Eys, & Carron, 2003). The grueling amounts of travel required to compete at the elite level (Waterhouse, Reilly, & Edwards, 2004), and issues such as team selection, financial support, and quality of facilities all may create threat appraisals that lead to stress (Fletcher & Hanton, 2003).

TRADITIONAL SPORT PSYCHOLOGY APPROACH TO STRESS AND PERFORMANCE

Sport psychologists have typically and traditionally presumed athletes' elevated heart rate, shallow respiration, and inability to focus their attentional processes to be classic symptoms of anxiety. Commonly used techniques to treat these symptoms (but without the benefit of simultaneous psychophysiological monitoring) are progressive relaxation, hypnosis, cognitive restructuring, mental rehearsal, imagery, self-monitoring, or a combination of interventions such as noted in visuomotor behavioral rehearsal (Elchami, 2003). The vast majority of these techniques aim to relieve the psychophysiological symptoms of stress at the most basic level rather than striving to empower the performer to develop understanding and self-awareness of his or her idiosyncratic stress process (Kirschenbaum, O'Connor, & Owens, 1999).

The development of mental rehearsal skills via imagery has long been a staple of traditional sport psychology interventions (Cumming & Hall, 2002). Imagery interventions often are used to reduce state anxiety by familiarizing the athlete with the required sport task through mental simulation of exact competitive situations culminating in a successful performance. It is believed that by visually imagining or getting the feel (kinesthetically) of successful sport-specific motor performance, athletes may reduce precompetition anxiety and develop greater self-confidence or self-efficacy in their sporting ability (Beauchamp, Bray, & Albinson, 2002; Taylor & Shaw, 2002; Jones, Bray, Mace, MacRae, & Stockbridge, 2002). Typical protocols include using a guided verbal script with the aim of enabling "game-like" visual vividness and concentration. In addition, scripts often suggest that an athlete attempt to experience the sensation of muscle contractions representative (kinesthetically) of those used during the specific sport movement.

Some researchers and practitioners question the validity of using verbal imagery scripts, however, contending that this process uses ventral processing pathways instead of the dorsal pathways that are more closely associated with the perception–action coupling of actual motor performance (Keil et al., 2000; Milner & Goodale, 1995). They instead suggest incorporating visuomotor imagery methods that integrate nonconscious visual and kinesthetic attentional processes that could lead to a reorganization in the dorsal pathway and to improved performance. Thus the challenge to sport psychologists is to design realistic methods of imagery that entrain mental rehearsal through the dorsal stream.

Davis and Sime (2006) provide an example of an innovative imagery protocol that combines the neuroscientific evidence of Keil et al. (2000) with neurofeedback. At present, though, it seems that very little sophisticated psychophysiology training exists without fairly assertive and innovative approaches by professionals (Carlstedt, 2001), which brings into question the weak level of efficacy (LaVaque et al., 2002) of the field at the present time. This may be due to (1) technophobia or lack of training for the applied practitioners, (2) unwillingness of coaches to relinquish control of their athletes, or (3) simply the lack of awareness by athletes and coaches as to the benefits of instrumented biofeedback training.

APPLIED PSYCHOPHYSIOLOGY IN A SPORT SETTING

Most traditional sport psychologists would agree that biofeedback is possibly efficacious (LaVaque et al., 2002) as an important tool in assisting athletes to manage cognitions and emotions associated with competition, to control activation levels, and ultimately to establish psychophysiological readiness of the body for optimum performance (Karteroliotis & Gill, 1987; Radeke & Stein, 1994; Silva & Stevens, 2002). Several biofeedback protocols have been used successfully to achieve a certain degree of arousal control and stress management within applied sport psychology (Blumenstein, Bar-Eli, & Tenenbaum, 1997; Carlstedt, 2001; Petruzzello, Landers, & Salazar; 1991; Strack, 2004). Elaborate integrative schemes of this nature are likely to aid in gaining a comprehensive understanding of the ideal individual levels of sympathetic and parasympathetic balance that fit for various open (externally paced, e.g., basketball) versus closed (internally paced, e.g., golf) sport events (Hanin, 2000).

Although many general conclusions have been made regarding the impact on performance of these psychophysiological parameters, it has been difficult to ascertain the true extent to which biofeedback training, over time, actually enhances performance (Carlstedt, 2001). Although a modest number of level-1 (efficacious and specific) scientific investigations on biofeedback in sport exist, problems arise because no two individuals appraise negative (or positive) competitive stimuli in the same way. This confounding variable results in a plethora of unique stress profiles, making it difficult to interpret individual biofeedback results. Few studies have been done to determine whether there are common standards or levels of heart rate (HR), electroencephalographic (EEG), or electromyographic (EMG) activity that are ideal for optimal performance to occur. The issue of conducting corroborating biofeedback research is complicated by several facts. First, because biofeedback is often used in combination with a comprehensive intervention package that includes professional consultation and/or other adjunctive techniques, such as imagery and relaxation training, it is difficult to ascribe specific amounts of performance variance solely to it. Second, because of the idiographic differences in emotional activation and stress, traditional large-sample social science research from which group means are derived may actually be counterproductive in these efforts (Hanin, 2000; Lazarus, 2003). Finally, the issue of ecological validity presents a theoretical problem. This issue centers on two contentions: (1) that many protocols neglect recent knowledge derived from the field of neuroscience (Keil et al., 2000), and (2) that traditional biofeedback monitoring requires the athlete to wear an array of sensors and wires that are somewhat obtrusive to athletic movement (Carlstedt, 2001). In other words, it is not possible in laboratory settings to capture the same psychophysiological data that would occur within the actual sport environment. Recent advances in technology that include wireless remote monitoring with unobtrusive sensing devices may correct this problem in the near future.

We encourage the use of sophisticated biofeedback and computer technology to allow sport psychophysiologists to create protocols that closely mimic performance conditions (Davis & Sime, 2006). Future generations of wireless biofeedback devices may allow practitioners not only to capture psychophysiological data such as HR, EMG, and EEG unobtrusively during actual competitive events but also to instantaneously reflect physiological and emotional states back to the athlete. In this way, we may shed further light on the practice of competitive stress management and sport psychophysiology techniques and methodologies in realistic settings, as opposed to the laboratory or clinic, wherein it is difficult to simulate actual performance demands.

Specific Protocols for Training in a Variety of Sport Settings

Biofeedback training using EMG biofeedback has been proven effective in reducing both anxiety and voluntary muscle tension, which often accompany one another, at rest and prior to competition (Blais & Vallerand, 1986). Any amount of residual muscle tension slows reaction time and the kinetic chain (the process whereby energy travels from spinal cord to feet or hands) that facilitates the fluid, yet whip-like, powerful (ballistic) actions observed in the execution of many sport motor movements carried to maximum (e.g., kicking for distance). Because excessive muscle tension is associated with slower reaction time, we believe that functional relaxation training is a relatively simple method of improving a critical aspect of performance in many sports (Fontani, Maffei, Cameli, & Finici, 1999).

Arena and Schwartz (2003) demonstrated that to make EMG particularly relevant to sport, it is desirable to use a modified FpN placement, with one sensor over the masseter muscle and the other in the posterior cervical region. This placement is ideal for validating the importance of relaxed facial and neck muscles just prior to motor performance (especially fine-motor tasks such as putting a ball in golf), because the residual tension created by teeth clenching often masks the critical perception necessary for success in these delicate movements. This method was used successfully in a professional consultation with the esteemed golfer Payne Stewart shortly before he won the U.S. Open Championship in 1999 and subsequently died in a plane crash (Sime, 2003). Similarly, thought-stopping techniques, along with muscle relaxation and biofeedback, have been used to reduce anxiety, gun vibration, heart rate, and catecholamine levels while increasing self-confidence and subsequent performance well above baseline levels in the demanding, stressful, individual sport of rifle shooting (Prapavessis, 2000).

Gaining control over autonomic functions during movement, as is needed in sport competition, is far more difficult to achieve than muscle control. For example, increases in peripheral blood flow are not easy to create on demand. Thermal biofeedback, however, has been shown to be effective in facilitating high performance in cold-weather sports such as hockey and curling (Kappes & Chapman, 1984). Because many football, baseball, and soccer games are often played outdoors under adverse weather conditions, and because hand temperature drops under stress, this thermal biofeedback approach has considerable utility. By contrast, electrodermal response (EDR) and temperature biofeedback have been used successfully, together with HR biofeedback, to achieve congruence among cognition, emotions, and stress reactions while facilitating optimal performance in the dance routines with elite rhythmic gymnastics (Schmidt & Peper, 1993). In this Olympic sport consultation, biofeedback was paired with mental rehearsal to enhance concentration and coordination between partners to achieve high levels of performance.

At the other temperature extreme, exaggerated fatigue and suppressed arousal have been observed during prolonged exercise in sweltering environments, wherein the ability to maintain a moderate core temperature in spite of extreme external heat and during heavy exercise was a critical factor in performance (Nielsen, Hydig, Bidstrup, Gonzalez-Alonso, & Christofferson, 2001). Learning how to cool core temperature is much more difficult than learning how to warm the periphery (hands and feet), however, because of the vasoregulatory microcirculation in distal parts of the body.

Heart Rate Variability (Respiratory Sinus Arrhythmia)

Respiratory sinus arrhythmia (RSA) is a relatively new concept in biofeedback (Lehrer, Smetankin, & Potapova, 2000; Gevirtz, Chapter 9, this volume), and it is even more unique to the competitive sport environment. RSA, the fluctuation in HR (rise and fall) cycling with each phase of inhalation and exhalation, is a relevant measure of composure and healthy, dynamic cardiovascular status. The degree of HR fluctuation can be disrupted by emotional reactions and enhanced by various behavioral interventions aimed at relaxation and composure. With finger or ear sensors or an electrocardiograph (EKG, for greater accuracy), it is possible to monitor beat-to-beat cardiac contractions via computer software, obtaining continuous measures and/or average per minute, providing an indication of the size of the RSA. In essence, a very regular up–down, smooth, sine-wave-like pattern indicates balanced autonomic nervous system functioning, referred to by some as *physiological entrainment* (McCraty, Atkinson, Tiller, Rein, & Watkins, 1995). By contrast, when HR oscillations are restricted and irregular in pattern, the composure needed for the performance of many complex motor skills is compromised (Hymes & Nuernberger, 1991; Kleiger, Miller, Bigger, & Moss, 1987). Heart rate variability (HRV) is quite simply an indicator of greater autonomic nervous system balance and is ultimately related to outstanding physical and mental performance.

RSA biofeedback training has been shown to be effective in reducing the effects of stress in a variety of sports. Twenty minutes of daily training significantly increased reaction times while also speeding recovery in relaxation of the quadriceps femoris muscle of elite wrestlers (Vaschillo, Disochin, & Rishe, personal communication, March 2001; Lehrer, Vaschillo, & Vaschillo, 2000). This rudimentary measure of coping with competitive stress (i.e., reaction time together with recovery time) was originated by Russian sport scientists and is also considered a valid measure of highly coordinated muscle effort and efficiency in energy conservation for endurance sports such as cross-country skiing and canoeing (Hedelin, Bjerle, & Henriksson-Larson, 2001). The parasympathetic activity produced by this training was found to be essential to achieving the supra conditioning levels necessary for these endurance athletes to excel. RSA biofeedback, together with instructions to strive for slow and deep respiration patterns, resulted in a quick return to more balanced central nervous functioning and cessation of sympathetic dominance among elite athletes under pressure of competition (Lehrer et al., 2000; Vaschillo et al., personal communication, 2001). In addition, when parasympathetic tone was higher (following RSA training), athletes had more open airways and greater airflow and oxygen intake during heavy exercise.

RSA training and cardiovascular efficiency are clearly essential training components for world-class endurance competitors (Langdeau, Turcotte, Desagne, Jobin, & Boulet, 2000; Strano et al., 1998). However, even archers and rifle shooters, who appear to have little need to be aerobically fit, still train with aerobic exercise because of the vagally mediated parasympathetic effect it induces, slowing heart rate and enhancing the emotional control needed within competition (Spalding, Jeffers, Torges, & Hatfield, 2000). Marksmen with the lowest resting HRs (bradycardia at rest) show greatly enhanced parasympathetic dominance, which leads to greater composure under stressful conditions. The ease with which RSA and cardiovascular training can be incorporated into "field training" of a variety of sports makes it a very appropriate physiological intervention (McCarty et al., 1995).

EEG Biofeedback and Attentional Control in Sport

Perhaps the most important recent development in the use of biofeedback in sport performance is the process of using selective brain-wave measures (neurofeedback) to shape and improve attention. In general, attention is defined as the process of facilitating selection of stimuli from the environment to the exclusion of other stimuli, resulting in an appropriate response to relevant stimuli only (Pfurtscheller, Stancak, & Neuper, 1996). A critical task necessary to achieving optimal performance in both open and closed sport events is the attainment of maximal concentration and attention to the most relevant details within the environment (Janelle, 2002; Radlo, Steinberg, Singer, & Barba, 2002; Singer, 2000; Singer, 2002). Considerable research on the relationships between attention, concentration, and elite sport performance has shown that the degree of attentional focus on specific task aspects is related to very specific EEG changes (Crews & Landers, 1993; Deeny et al., 2003; Gannon, Denot-Ledunois, Vardon, Perruchet, 1992; Loze, Collins, & Holmes, 2001; Smith et al., 2003). Therefore, EEG biofeedback appears to be an extremely valuable tool capable of shaping the ability of the athlete to appropriately shift visual attention from narrow to broad or from internal to external focus as might be needed in a difficult competitive situation.

One approach showed biofeedback to be successful in training attention to achieve enhanced alertness and task engagement by utilizing a complex array of peripheral biofeedback modalities (HR and skin conductance) together with neurofeedback specifically focusing on the parietal lobes to reinforce the occurrence of an optimal level of cortical attention (Freman, Mikulka, Scerbo, Prinzo, & Clouatre, 2000). This automated feedback system using a derived EEG (featuring Beta/Alpha + Theta from parietal and temporal regions) has been shown to be particularly effective for shooting sports, wherein vision and cortical activation are important variables. When visual attention was suppressed during the preshot routine, competitors were more likely to achieve an automatic flow of shots on target (Loze et al., 2001). Increased occipital lobe alpha during best shots and decreased readings during worst shots suggests that when shooters trust their full range of sensory data they are more accurate. In addition, high beta-wave activity from the occipital region has been associated with excessive cognitive activity (overanalysis and self-doubt) during the preshot period and decrements in shooting performance (Hillman, Apparies, Janelle, & Hatfield, 2000).

Another approach to optimizing performance is analyzing and shaping cognitive behavior on a moment-to-moment basis using neurofeedback (with the capability to actually separate levels of concentration and alertness while providing background audio tones as additional feedback prompts) in real time during performance of a competitive task (Sime, Allen, & Fazzano, 2001). This application is appropriate when the athlete is performing the event vicariously, using imagery in conjunction with video of the actual sport task (Davis & Sime, 2006). Some of the outcomes of this training include improving mental stamina in maintaining high levels of concentration and achieving momentary peaks in alertness and arousal as needed during critical moments, followed by periodic "micro breaks" to recharge the brain before taking on the next challenging activity (Sime et al., 2001). This sequence of alternating between high and low levels of concentration and alertness is the hallmark of elite performance, allowing athletes to focus when necessary while "spacing off" briefly when the opportunity permits for the purpose of recovery and renewal of complex cognitive processes (Davis & Sime, 2006).

The use of biofeedback in conjunction with imagery and video facilitates more rapid awareness of cognitive and emotional intrusions that might intrude on the experience of high-quality positive mental imagery (Davis & Sime, 2006). It also allows for "real-time" imagery without the use of verbal scripts, perhaps developing the ventral processing pathways that Keil et al. (2000) describe. Furthermore, EEG software provides the accurate feedback that is essential in the development of sensory integration for detecting and facilitating the ideal amount of effort needed for a given task performance. Although this research is very encouraging, it lacks first-level scientific investigation to support the outcomes at present (LaVaque et al., 2002).

POSITIVE PSYCHOLOGY: A NEW FRAMEWORK FOR STRESS COPING WITHIN SPORT

Positive psychology aims to illuminate positive subjective experiences, positive individual traits, and the institutions that enable positive experiences and positive traits (Peterson & Seligman, 2004). Because coping with stress during performance is informed and influenced by individual traits and personal resources (Lazarus, 2000), this burgeoning field provides a framework for understanding the stress process and how to create individualized stress-management interventions. The study of positive emotions and their effects is central to positive psychology, and several recently postulated theories regarding positive emotions may provide insight into how their use as coping resources may minimize the damaging effects of stress on athletic performance.

Broaden-and-Build Theory

Fredrickson's (1998) broaden-and-build theory has two distinct but complementary tenets. The first proposes that positive emotions have the ability to *broaden* the momentarily narrowed focus of attention brought forth by negative emotions that are commonly experienced during stress. By broadening attention, positive emotions increase global cognitive processing and the range of possible actions that individuals may pursue, as opposed to the hyperfocus or distraction that occurs when stressed (Fredrickson & Branigan, 2005). The second tenet theorizes that positive emotions *build* enduring physical, psychological, and social resources that may be drawn on by an individual within future contexts. These resources, such as confidence, hope, optimism, and resiliency (positive psychological capital; Luthans & Youssef, 2004), are posited to enable individuals to find positive meaning amid adversity (Tugade & Fredrickson, 2004). Each of these four constructs has positive relationships with optimal sport performance, suggesting that they are coping resources used to buffer athlete stress (Craft et al., 2003; Curry, Snyder, Cook, Ruby, & Rehm, 1997; Gaudreau & Blondin, 2004; Grove & Heard, 1997; Hanton, Evans, & Neil, 2003; Mummery, Schofield, & Perry, 2004; Woodman & Hardy, 2003).

Undoing Hypothesis

Fredrickson et al.'s (2000) undoing hypothesis suggests that one purpose of positive emotions might be to undo the damaging psychophysiological effects associated with negative emotions. The function of undoing is not to catapult the body into a benign state, however, but rather to move it back toward functional levels of autonomic arousal and cognition through faster recovery to baseline cardiovascular levels (Fredrickson et al., 2000; Levenson & Fredrickson, 1998; Tugade & Fredrickson, 2004). The undoing effect is unrelated to parasympathetic responsiveness in recovery from a stressful experience, and it appears to be limited to situations in which positive emotions may quickly follow negative ones. Furthermore, it does not appear to develop in response to events wherein positive emotions are experienced alone without negative emotions preceding, a fact that has important implications for coaching and leading behaviors in sport (Brown, 2004).

Positive Emotions and Coping with Stress in Sport

To perform optimally, emotional regulation and modulation of stress must occur continuously throughout the entire performance cycle. Preparation and evaluation phases, although appearing to be benign resting periods, are often critical moments of competition (Carlstedt, 2004), full of self-talk statements and cognitive appraisals that determine an athlete's emotional state (Conroy & Metzler, 2004). The broaden-and-build theory and the undoing hypothesis provide valuable insight into the cyclical stress–performance relationship and offer means by which sport psychologists can help athletes and their coaches mitigate the causes and effects of stress within the performance arena.

Precompetition threat appraisals arouse negative emotions and often lead to performance decrements, whereas positive emotions associated with precompetition challenge appraisals are positively correlated with perceived functionality of emotional states and optimal performance (Cerin, 2003). This implies that interventions that incorporate positive emotions may enable athletes to more effectively cope with stress, either by broadening their momentary thought processes or by undoing the associated physiological effects. The example of New England Patriots wide receiver Deion Branch perhaps illustrates how the undoing effect of positive emotions may work (Reilly, 2005). During the stressful hours prior to the NFL Super Bowl in 2005 (a game estimated to be watched live by several hundred million people), Branch telephoned 13 of his former coaches, from youth league to college, to express his gratitude for their support in helping him achieve professional success. Branch went on to perform exceptionally well, being named "Most Valuable Player" of the game, leading us to suggest that Branch had very effectively coped with the perceived stress of a threatening situation by using the positive emotion of gratitude. Branch's experience in the Super Bowl contrasts with those of numerous teammates and adversaries who performed somewhat below their past efforts in competition, suggesting that they fell victim to the insidious effects of competitive stress.

Another example, from the 2005 National Collegiate Athletic Association (NCAA) Division I basketball championships, illustrates how coaches may be able to undo the negative emotions and stress that athletes experience during the execution phase of competition by directing positive emotions toward their athletes. During a brief respite before two crucial free throw attempts at the end of a close game, coach John Beilein of the West Virginia Mountaineers instructed center Kevin Pitsnogle to "relax" by imagining the love he had for his wife and parents. Pitsnogle proceeded to knock down both shots and afterward remarked of the calming effect that Coach Beilein's suggestion had had on him (Jenkins, 2005). The capacity of coaches to engage in this type of behavior may vary greatly; however, it may be a mediating variable that differentiates coaching effectiveness (Davis, 2004). Obviously, these data (on the Super Bowl and the NCAA tournament) will be encouraging only on discovery of future confirmatory experimental studies designed to control for selection bias, expectation, and so forth.

The stressful symptoms that athletes experience during the postperformance stage of the performance cycle should not be overlooked, as the lingering psychological effects may lead to delays in beginning the preparation phase for the next contest, perhaps causing future poor performance. Arathoon and Malouff (2004) demonstrated that positive reappraisal increases positive affect following a competition loss, mitigating the consequences of negative emotions commonly experienced by athletes.

Upward Spiral of Positive Emotions

When the individual members of an organization experience the cumulative effects of positive emotions, the result is an "upward spiral" that creates a positive organizational climate through enhanced well-being and productivity of organization members (Frederickson, 2003). This process would appear to be valuable within team-sport contexts, reducing stress and providing the means to quickly recover from setbacks and ultimately affecting both short- and long-term performance (Ashkanasy & Daus, 2002; Wrisberg & Fisher, 2005; Smith, 2003).

The sum total of evidence cited here for the effects positive emotions on stress for and coping, provides a highly theoretical rationale for a more sophisticated role of positive emotion interventions in stress management and sport performance. However, these theories need much more research to establish efficacy (LaVaque et al., 2002) for interventions based upon these principles.

CASE EXAMPLE

As we discussed earlier in this chapter, coaches can play a critical role in the perception of stress by athletes. To investigate this phenomenon further, a qualitative instrumental case study was undertaken. Bounded by the 2002 and 2005 competitive Division I collegiate baseball seasons, the case study examined the effects of behavior on individual and team performance during a new head coach's first two seasons compared with the last two seasons of the prior head coach.

Data Collection

The study used extensive 90-minute interviews with the new head coach, the pitching coach, the university athletic director, the team's radio announcer, and three athletes who had been key members of the team during the period (2002–2005) binding the case. The interviews with the players were conducted in a focus-group format, whereas the other participants were interviewed individually. The team's win–loss record and other peripheral team statistics were analyzed in an attempt to triangulate interview data and as a means of corroborating the effects of the coach's leadership.

Data Analysis

Data analysis was performed using multiple methods. First, the data were analyzed typologically using categories derived from positive psychological capital theory (Luthans & Youssef, 2004). Next, data were aggregated into central recurring themes. Finally, detailed analyses of the team and individual statistical performance from the four seasons that make up the case were performed.

Findings

Positive Psychological Capital

One supposed effect of positive emotions posited by the broaden-and-build theory is the development of positive psychological capital—confidence, hope, optimism, and resilience (Fredrickson, 1998; Tugade & Fredrickson, 2004). Luthans and Avolio (2003) suggest that positive psychological capital is state-like and open to development and plays a central role in organizational outcomes. Specifically, Avolio, Gardner, Walumbwa, Luthans, and May (2004) suggest that among followers within an organization, these constructs are most influential when they are modeled positively by a leader. This positive modeling has the power to transform followers, increasing psychological well-being and producing enhanced performance and sustainable competitive advantages for the organization.

The highly negative psychological state of the baseball program during the 2003 season (the last year under the old head coach) was revealed in this description by the new head coach (who had been an assistant coach under the previous head coach):

> There was a hopeless feeling in the dugout during games . . . Even in the locker before games
> . . . a sense that *something* would go wrong. Somehow we'd find a way to lose, whether it was
> a bad hop, a great play by the opponent, or an inopportune call by an umpire against us. We
> played with very little confidence, and had no resiliency . . . other teams (coaches) knew that if
> they came out and jumped on us early, we'd fold.

As he began his tenure, the new head coach sought to specifically change this negative atmosphere. As he stated, "My sole purpose that fall was to change the mindset of the team, to establish that mental toughness within the program [confidence, optimism, resilience]."

The pitching coach observed and reported that the new head coach possessed confidence, hope, and optimism and began to model it immediately:

> He was confident in his ability to coach . . . he was confident that he knew the game and in his ability to teach the game, and because of that confidence he had a plan [hope]. He said, this is how we're going to do it . . . these are the key things we are going to focus on. This is what we will do and the other things will fall into place [optimism].

The positive modeling of these capacities by the new head coach was clearly evident in the comments of the players in focus-group discussion.

> We knew we could beat anyone we played. I remember coach was kind of mad after one loss. We had an eight-game winning streak broken and we just looked at each other like, big deal, we'll win tomorrow and start a new streak. And we did.

One player recalled driving to the ballpark in 2005 on the night of a big game against their highly ranked in-state rival. He looked at the teammate he was riding with (another focus group member) and asked, "Do you know how much fun it's going to be going out after we win tonight?" The player reported candidly that he had had no doubt that they would win that game. Game outcomes such as this and the team's overall statistics clearly demonstrate that the positive psychological capital influencing this team's confidence was greatly influenced by the head coach, whose leadership style was uniquely effective.

Challenge versus Threat Appraisals

A recurring theme of the interviews in this study was *challenge*. Everyone interviewed stated that the new head coach had consistently and effectively challenged team members, individually and collectively. The assistant coach stated, "he calls guys out and challenges them, like . . . you can do better than that, I've got confidence in you. I know you're better than what you showed."

The new head coach and players described several specific instances during the 2004–2005 seasons when the new head coach clearly challenged the team. The head coach described one of these instances: "I told them I was embarrassed by their performance, and they should be embarrassed too. We played as if we were afraid, and I told them that was not acceptable. I challenged them to come out the next night and play with passion and intensity."

A question that must be answered is why strong and/or autocratic messages from a leader are perceived as a challenge rather than as a threat. The team's radio announcer provided a valuable insight into this effect, stating that players knew that the head coach sincerely cared about them and wanted them to have success; thus his message was accepted as a challenge. The key, perhaps, lies in the frequency of the use of "other-directed" positive emotions by the leader (Davis, 2004; Michie & Gooty, 2005). Fredrickson and Losada (2005) suggest that the optimal ratio of positive to negative emotions is between 3:1 and 12:1 for enhanced organizational performance. This positivity ratio implies that negative emotions are important tools to be used by sport coaches to motivate their athletes. Yet in order for negative emotions to be effective (without producing stress), coaches must also express at least three times as many positive emotions in order to build positive psychological capital that athletes will use as a coping resource.

Statistical Analysis

The lack of psychological capital was evident in the team's peripheral statistics during the 2002 and 2003 seasons. The team's record in close games (decided by one or two runs) was 23 and 27. And they posted a woeful 10 and 24 record when they fell behind after the first inning, with only 17 come-from-behind wins during the two seasons.

Under the leadership of the new head coach, the team's performance improved dramatically during the 2004 and 2005 seasons, indicative of an improved psychological state. Besides their improved overall record (83–41 vs. 50–61), they were 29 and 16 in close games and had 34 come-from-behind wins. After trailing fewer times after the first inning (perhaps indicating greater confidence, hope, and optimism), they had a winning record of 13 and 12 when they did fall behind, thus exhibiting greater resilience in producing comeback victories.

The results of this case study illustrate how the behavior of coaches may affect the performance of athletes. Although no specific measures of stress were captured as part of this study, one can conclude that the improved performance of the team coincided with a reduction in stress perhaps because of the positive psychological capital that was developed and used as coping resources by the athletes on the team. Specifically, these coping resources enabled the athletes to experience more challenge and fewer threat appraisals, in which, as we have demonstrated, is critical to reducing negative emotions and stress in elite athletic environments.

SUMMARY AND CONCLUSIONS

Sport psychophysiology is a relatively new field that brings together an understanding of the psychophysiology of emotion with the psychology of sports performance. With the implementation of advanced technology, it is possible to monitor common physiological measures of stress in applied psychophysiology settings. Because of this, comprehensive and integrative stress management techniques are becoming more widely understood and incorporated within athletic domains. Applied practitioners with an understanding of psychophysiology and technology are finding increasing opportunities to synthesize their knowledge with standard sport psychology interventions into formal and extensive protocols within a variety of athletic settings (Carlstedt, 2004; Davis & Sime, 2006).

These techniques are especially important in light of recent news stories highlighting numerous problems with elite athletes in various sports who have chosen to seek competitive advantages by using illegal, unethical, and potentially harmful chemical drugs such as steriods (Canseco, 2005; Romanowski, Schefter, & Towle, 2005). In all of these highly publicized circumstances, it appears that comprehensive psychophysiological stress management practices were woefully neglected, perhaps due to lack of understanding or skepticism on the part of the athletes and/or their coaches and trainers. Because of these developments, sport psychophysiologists face great challenges but also tremendous opportunities. By developing collaborative relationships with coaches and sports medicine professionals and demonstrating the efficacy of various stress management techniques designed to develop the optimal neuromuscular and sensory integration necessary for optimal performance, well-trained sport psychophysiologists may become valuable assets in assisting athletes in striving for ethical strategies designed to gain competitive advantage.

It also appears that negative and positive emotions have distinct, yet complementary, roles. Thus sport psychologists must understand how and why multiple and varied emotions, both positive and negative, occur throughout the entirety of the performance cycle. Negative emotions are useful as motivators, yet when athletes lack the resources to properly regulate the adverse emotional process, they are prone to debilitating stress reactions. However, when the demands of a situation are within the capacity of their resources, athletes are likely to use the negative emotions induced by a potential harm or threat constructively and to appraise the situation as a challenge (Cerin, 2003; Skinner & Brewer, 2004). Building psychological resources is imperative to improve the coping ability of athletes, which will minimize stress. Positive psychology provides a theoretical foundation for understanding the role of positive emotions in the stress process and how psychological and social resources that improve coping may be developed within both individual and team-sport athletes. Concepts borrowed from positive organizational behavior provide an exciting new platform for both intraindividual and organizational-level sport psychology research and consultation.

This chapter has proposed two seemingly disparate approaches to understanding and applying stress management in sport—instrumented biofeedback and positive psychology. Perhaps the most exciting possibility for sport psychology and stress management practitioners lies in the marriage of these two approaches, especially when practiced in conjunction with Hanin's (2000) IZOF model. By using sophisticated yet simple and unobtrusive technologies such as wireless psychophysiology monitoring, for example (see *www.thoughttechnology.com*), or "smart fabrics" that enable unobtrusive body torso monitoring during live competition (see *www.sensatex.com*; *www.vivometrics.com*), it may be possible to determine which specific negative emotions are evoked within an athlete during the performance cycle and which positive emotions provide the quickest relief from stress (e.g., gratitude, for Deion Branch; love, for Kevin Pitsnogle; see the earlier discussion of highly publicized sport celebrities). Sport psychologists who are prepared to capitalize on these concepts will be able to provide a valuable service to athletes and coaches alike at the highest levels of sport.

Of course, this methodology is theoretical and in need of empirical validation through the use of both quantitative and qualitative research methodology. We expect that future results will document the individual differences that so many sport psychologists, coaches, and athletes themselves have experienced and observed repeatedly. Perhaps when these data linking psychophysiological indices with measurable outcomes of athletic performance are available, sport psychophysiology practitioners and stress management consultants will collaborate for the productive benefit of performers in many highly competitive and challenging sport and nonsport venues.

REFERENCES

Anshel, M., & Wells, B. (2000). Sources of acute stress and coping styles in competitive sport. *Anxiety, Stress, and Coping, 13*, 1–26.

Arathoon, S. M., & Malouff, J. M. (2004). The effectiveness of a brief cognitive intervention to help athletes cope with competition loss. *Journal of Sport Behavior, 27*, 213–230.

Arena, J., & Schwartz, M. (2003). Psychophysiological assessment and biofeedback baselines. In M. S. Schwartz & Associates (Eds.). *Biofeedback: A practitioners guide* (3rd ed., pp. 128–158). New York: Guilford Press.

Ashkanasy, N. M., & Daus, C. S. (2002). Emotion in the workplace: The new challenge for managers. *Academy of Management Executive, 16*, 76–86.

Avolio, B. J., Gardner, W. L., Walumbwa, F. O., Luthans, F., & May, D. R. (2004). Unlocking the mask: A look at the process by which authentic leaders impact follower attitudes and behaviors. *Leadership Quarterly, 15*, 801–823.

Baker, J., Cote, J., & Hawes, R. (2000). The relationship between coaching behaviors and sport anxiety in athletes. *Journal of Science and Medicine in Sport, 3*, 110–119.

Beauchamp, M. R., Bray, S. R., & Albinson, J. G. (2002). Pre-competition imagery, self-efficacy and performance in collegiate golfers. *Journal of Sports Sciences, 20*, 697–705.

Beauchamp, M. R., Bray, S. R., Eys, M. A., & Carron, A. V. (2003). The effect of role ambiguity on competitive state anxiety. *Journal of Sport and Exercise Psychology, 25*, 77–93.

Bittman, B., Berk, L., Shannon, M., Sharaf, M., Westengard, J., Guegler, K. J., & et al. (2005). Recreational music-making modulates the human stress response: A preliminary individualized gene expression strategy. *Medical Science Monitor, 11*, 31–40.

Blais, M. R., & Vallerand, R. J. (1986). Multimodal effects of electromyographic biofeedback: Looking at children's ability to control pre-competitive anxiety. *Journal of Sports Psychology, 8*, 283–303.

Blumenstein, B., Bar-Eli, N., & Tenenbaum, G. (1997). A five-step approach to mental training incorporating biofeedback. *Sport Psychologist, 11*, 440–453.

Brown, N. (2004, October). *The paradoxical power of negative emotions for positive psychology.* Paper presented at the International Positive Psychology Summit, Washington, DC.

Bundy, A. C., Lane, S. J., Murray, E. A., & Fisher, A. G. (2002). *Sensory integration: Theory and practice* (2nd ed.). Philadelphia: Davis.

Canseco, J. (2005). *Juiced: Wild times, rampant 'roids, smash hits, and how baseball got big.* New York: Regan.

Carlstedt, R. A. (2001). Ambulatory psychophysiology and ecological validity in studies of sports performance: Issues and implications for intervention protocols in biofeedback. *Biofeedback, 29*, 18–22.

Carlstedt, R. A. (2004). *Critical moments during competition: A mind–body model of sport performance when it counts the most.* New York: Psychology Press.

Cerin, E. (2003). Anxiety versus fundamental emotions as predictors of perceived functionality of precompetitive emotional states, threat, and challenge in individual sports. *Journal of Applied Sport Psychology, 15*, 223–238.

Conroy, D. E., & Metzler, J. N. (2004). Patterns of self-talk associated with different forms of competitive anxiety. *Journal of Sport and Exercise Psychology, 26*, 69–90.

Craft, L. L., Magyar, M., Becker, B. J., & Feltz, D. L. (2003). The relationship between the Competitive State Anxiety Inventory-2 and sport performance: A meta-analysis. *Journal of Sport and Exercise Psychology, 25*, 44–66.

Crews, D., & Landers, D. (1993). Electroencephalographic measures of attentional patterns prior to the golf putt. *Journal of American College of Sports Medicine, 25*, 116–126.

Cumming, J., & Hall, C. (2002). Deliberate imagery practice: The development of imagery skills in competitive athletes. *Journal of Sports Sciences, 20*, 137–145.

Curry, L. A., Snyder, C. R., Cook, D. L., Ruby, B. C., & Rehm, M. (1997). Role of hope in academic and sport achievement. *Journal of Personality and Social Psychology, 73*, 1257–1267.

Damasio, A. (1994). *Descartes' error: Emotion, reason, and the human brain.* New York: Gossett/Putnam.

Davis, P. A. (2004). *An investigation of the character strengths of exceptional high school coaches.* Unpublished master's thesis, University of Nebraska, Lincoln.

Davis, P. A., & Sime, W. E. (2005). Toward a psychophysiology of performance: Sport psychology principles dealing with anxiety. *International Journal of Stress Management, 12*(4), 363–378.

Deeny, S. P., Hillman, C. H., Janelle, C. M., & Hatfield, B. D. (2003). Cortico-cortical communication and superior performance in skilled marksmen: An EEG coherence analysis. *Journal of Sport and Exercise Psychology, 25*, 188–205.

Elchami, M. S. (2003). Emotions and athletic performance: An integrative critical analysis. *Dissertation Abstracts International, 64*, 2385. (UMI No. AAC3088914)

Fletcher, D., & Hanton, S. (2003). Sources of organizational stress in elite sports performers. *Sports Psychologist, 17*, 175–195.

Fontani, G., Maffei, D., Cameli, S., & Finici, P. (1999). Reactivity and event-related potentials during attentional tests in athletes. *European Journal of Applied Physiological and Occupational Physiology, 18*(5), 301–312.

Fredrickson, B. L. (1998). What good are positive emotions? *Review of General Psychology, 2*, 300–319.

Fredrickson, B. L. (2000). Extracting meaning from past affective experiences: The importance of peaks, ends, and specific emotions. *Cognition and Emotion, 14*, 577–606.

Fredrickson, B. L. (2003). Positive emotions and upward spirals in organizations. In K. Cameron, J. Dutton, & R. Quinn (Eds.), *Positive organizational scholarship* (pp. 163–175). San Francisco: Berrett-Koehler.

Fredrickson, B. L., & Branigan, C. (2005). Positive emotions broaden the scope of attention and thought–action repertoires. *Cognition and Emotion, 19*, 313–333.

Fredrickson, B. L., & Losada, M. (2005). Positive affect and the complex dynamics of human flourishing. *American Psychologist, 60*(7), 678–686.

Fredrickson, B. L., Mancuso, R. A., Branigan, C., & Tugade, M. M. (2000). The undoing effect of positive emotions. *Motivation and Emotion, 24*, 237–258.

Freman, F., Mikulka, P., Scerbo, M., Prinzo, L., & Clouatre, K. (2000). Evaluation of a psychophysiological controlled adaptive automation system, using performance on a tracking task. *Applied Psychophysiology and Biofeedback Journal, 25*, 102–115.

Gannon, T., Denot-Ledunois, F., Vardon, G., & Perruchet, T. (1992). An analysis of temporal electroencephalographic patterning prior to initiation of the arm curl. *Journal of Sport and Exercise Physiology, 14*, 87–100.

Gaudreau, P., & Blondin, J. (2004). Differential associations of dispositional optimism and pessimism with coping, goal attainment, and emotional adjustment during sport competition. *International Journal of Stress Management, 11*, 245–269.

Giacobbi, P. R., Lynn, T. K., Wetherington, J. M., Jenkins, J., Bodendorf, M., & Langley, B. (2004). Stress and coping during the transition to university for first-year female athletes. *Sport Psychologist, 18*, 1–21.

Gould, D., & Udry, E. (1994). Psychological skills for enhancing performance: Arousal regulation strategies. *Medicine and Science in Sport and Exercise, 26*, 478–485.

Grove, R. J., & Heard, N. P. (1997). Optimism and sport confidence as correlates of slump related coping among athletes. *Sport Psychologist, 11*, 400–410.

Hanin, Y. (2000). Individual zones of optimal functioning (IZOF) model: Emotion–performance relationships in sport. In Y. Hanin (Ed.), *Emotions in sport* (pp. 65–89). Champaign, IL: Human Kinetics.

Hanton, S., Evans, L., & Neil, R. (2003). Hardiness and the competitive trait anxiety response. *Anxiety, Stress, and Coping, 16*, 167–184.

Hanton, S., Thomas, O., & Maynard, I. (2004). Competitive anxiety responses in the week leading up to competition: The role of intensity, direction and frequency dimensions. *Psychology of Sport and Exercise, 5*, 169–182.

Hatfield, B., & Landers, D. (1983). Psychophysiology: A new direction of sports psychology. *Journal of Sports Psychology, 5*, 243–249.

Hatfield, B. D., & Hillman, C. H. (2001). The psychophysiology of sport: A mechanistic understanding of the psychology of superior performance. In R. N. Singer, H. A. Hausenblas, & C. M. Janelle (Eds.), *Handbook of sport psychology* (2nd ed., pp. 362–388). New York: Wiley.

Hedelin, R., Bjerle, P., & Henriksson-Larson, K. (2001). Heart rate variability in athletes: Relationship with central and peripheral performance. *Medicine and Science in Sports and Exercise, 33*(8), 1394–1398.

Hillman, C., Apparies, R., Janelle, C., & Hatfield, B. (2000). An electrocortical comparison of executed and rejected shots in skilled marksmen. *Biological Psychology, 52*(1), 71–83.

Holmes, P. S., & Collins, D. J. (2001). The PETTLEP approach to motor imagery: A functional equivalence model for sport psychologists. *Journal of Applied Sport Psychology, 13*, 60–83.

Humphrey, J. H., Yow, D. A., & Bowden, W. W. (2000). *Stress in college athletics: Causes, consequences, coping.* Binghamton, NY: Haworth Half-Court Press.

Hymes, A., & Nuernberger, P. (1991). Breathing patterns found in heart attack victims. *Journal of International Association of Yoga Therapists, 2*(25), 25–27.

Janelle, C. M. (1999). Ironic mental processes in sport: Implications for sport psychologists. *Sport Psychologist, 13*, 201–220.

Janelle, C. M. (2002). Anxiety, arousal and visual attention: A mechanistic account of performance variability. *Journal of Sports Sciences, 20*, 237–251.

Janelle, C. M., Hillman, C. H., Apparies, R. J., Murray, N. P., Melli, L., Fallon, E. A., et al. (2000). Expertise differences in cortical activation and gaze behavior during rifle shooting. *Journal of Sport and Exercise Psychology, 22*, 167–182.

Janelle, C. M., Singer, R. N., & Williams, A. M. (1999). External distraction and attentional narrowing: Visual search evidence. *Journal of Sport and Exercise Psychology, 21*, 70–91.

Jenkins, L. (2005, March 25). Mountaineers' climb isn't over. *Omaha World Herald*. Retrieved April 7, 2005, from *www.omaha.com*.

Johnson, S. (2003, March). Emotions and the brain: Fear. *Discover, 24*, 33–39.

Jones, M. V. (2003). Controlling emotions in sport. *Sport Psychologist, 17*, 471–486.

Jones, M. V., Bray, S. R., Mace, R. D., MacRae, A. W., & Stockbridge, C. (2002). The impact of motivational imagery on the emotional state and self-efficacy levels of novice climbers. *Journal of Sport Behavior, 25*, 57–74.

Kappes, B., & Chapman, S. (1984). The effects of indoor versus outdoor thermal biofeedback training in cold weather sports. *Journal of Sports Psychology, 6*, 305–311.

Karteroliotis, C., & Gill, D. (1987). Temporal changes in psychological and physiological components of state anxiety. *Journal of Sports Psychology, 9*, 261–274.

Keil, D., Holmes, P., Bennett, S., Davids, K., & Smith, N. (2000). Theory and practice in sport psychology and motor behaviour needs to be constrained by integrative modeling of brain and behaviour. *Journal of Sports Sciences, 18*, 433–443.

Kenow, L., & Williams, J. M. (1999). Coach–athlete compatibility and athlete's perception of coaching behaviors. *Journal of Sport Behavior, 22*, 251–260.

Kirschenbaum, D., O'Connor, E., & Owens, D. (1999). Positive illusions in golf: Empirical and conceptual analysis. *Journal of Applied Sports Psychology, 11*, 1–27.

Kleiger, R., Miller, P., Bigger, J., & Moss. A. (1987). The Multicenter Post-Infarction Research Group: Decreased heart rate variability and its association with increased mortality after acute myocardial infarction. *American Journal of Cardiology, 59*, 256–262.

Kojima, M., Shioiri, T., Hosoki, T., Sakai, M., Bando, T., & Someya, T. (2002) Blink rate variability in patients with panic disorder: New trial using audiovisual stimulation. *Psychiatry and Clinical Neurosciences, 56*(5), 545–549.

Lacey, J. I., & Lacey, B. C. (1979). Somatopsychic effects of interoception. In E. Meyer III & J. V. Brady (Eds.), *Research in the psychology of human behavior* (pp. 59–73). Baltimore: Johns Hopkins University Press.

Langdeau, J., Turcotte, H., Desagne, P., Jobin, J., & Boulet, L. (2000). Influence of sympatho-vagal balance on airway responsiveness in athletes. *European Journal of Applied Physiology, 83*(4–5), 370–375.

LaVaque, T., Hammond, D. C., Trudeau, D., Monastra, V., Perry, J., Lehrer, P., et al. (2002). Template for developing guidelines for the evaluation of the clinical efficacy of psychophysiological interventions. *Applied Psychophysiology and Biofeedback, 27*(4), 273–281.

Lazarus, R. S. (1999). *Stress and emotion: A new synthesis*. New York: Springer.

Lazarus, R. S. (2000). How emotions influence performance in competitive sports. *Sports Psychologist, 14*, 229–252.

Lazarus, R. S. (2003). Does the positive psychology movement have legs? *Psychological Inquiry, 14*, 93–109.

Lehrer, P. M., Smetankin, A., & Potapova, T. (2000). Respiratory sinus arrhythmia biofeedback therapy for asthma: A report of 20 unmedicated pediatric cases using the Smetankin method. *Applied Psychophysiology and Biofeedback, 25*, 193–200.

Lehrer, P. M., Vaschillo, E., & Vaschillo, B. (2000). Resonant frequency biofeedback training to increase cardiac variability: Rationale and manual for training. *Applied Psychophyisology and Biofeedback, 25*, 177–191.

Levenson, R. W. (1992). Autonomic nervous system differences among emotions. *Psychological Science, 3*, 23–27.

Levenson, R. W., & Fredrickson, B. L. (1998). Positive emotions speed recovery from the cardiovascular sequelae of negative emotions. *Cognition and Emotion, 12*, 191–220.

Libkuman, T., Otani, H., & Steger, N. (2002). Training in timing improves accuracy in golf. *Journal of General Psychology, 129*, 77–96.

Loze, G. M., Collins, D., & Holmes, P. S. (2001). Pre-shot EEG alpha-power reactivity during expert air-pistol shooting: A comparison of best and worst shots. *Journal of Sports Sciences, 19*, 727–733.

Luthans, F., & Avolio, B. (2003). Authentic leadership: A positive development approach. In K. S. Cameron, J. E. Dutton, & R. E. Quinn (Eds.), *Positive organizational scholarship* (pp. 241–258). San Francisco: Berrett-Koehler.

Luthans, F., & Youssef, C. M. (2004). Human, social, and now positive psychological capital management: Investing in people for competitive advantage. *Organizational Dynamics, 33*, 143–160.

Martell, S. G., & Vickers, J. N. (2004). Gaze characteristics of elite and near-elite athletes in ice hockey defensive tactics. *Human Movement Science, 22,* 689–712.

Martens, R., Burton, D., Vealey, R. S., Bump, L. A., & Smith, D. E. (1990). Development and validation of the Competitive State Anxiety Inventory-2. In R. Martens, R. S. Vealey, & D. Burton (Eds.), *Competitive anxiety in sport* (pp. 117–190). Champaign, IL: Human Kinetics.

McCraty, R., Atkinson, M., Tiller, W., Rein, G., & Watkins, A. (1995). The effects of emotions on short-term power spectrum analysis of heart variability. *American Journal of Cardiology, 76*(14), 1089–1093.

Meegan, D.V., Aslin, R. N., & Jacobs, R. A. (2000). Motor timing learned without motor training. *Nature Neuroscience, 3,* 860–862.

Michie, S., & Gooty, J. (2005). Values, emotions and authenticity: Will the real leader please stand up? *Leadership Quarterly, 16,* 441–457.

Milner, D. A., & Goodale, M. A. (1995). *The visual brain in action.* Oxford, UK: Oxford University Press.

Mummery, W. K., Schofield, G., & Perry, C. (2004). Bouncing back: The role of coping style, social support and self-concept in resilience of sport performance. *Athletic Insight: The Online Journal of Sport Psychology, 6.* Retrieved April 2005 from *www.athleticinsight.com.*

Murray, N. P., & Janelle, C. M. (2003). Anxiety and performance: A visual search examination of the processing efficiency theory. *Journal of Sport and Exercise Psychology, 25,* 171–188.

Nielsen, B., Hydig, T., Bidstrup, F., Gonzalez-Alonso, J., & Christofferson, G. (2001). Brain activity and fatigue during prolonged exercise in the heat. *Pfulgers Archives, 442*(1), 41–48.

Novosel, J., & Garrity, J. (2004). *Tour tempo: Golf's last secret finally revealed.* New York: Doubleday.

Peterson, C., & Seligman, M. E. P. (2004). *Character strengths and virtues: A handbook and classification.* New York: Oxford University Press.

Petruzzello, S., Landers, D., & Salazar, W. (1991). Biofeedback and sport/exercise performance: Applications and limitations. *Behavior Therapy, 22,* 379–392.

Pfurtscheller, G., Stancak, A., & Neuper, C. (1996). Event-related synchronization (ERS) in the alpha band—an electrophysiological correlate of cortical idling: A review. *International Journal of Psychophysiology, 24*(1–2), 39–46.

Prapavessis, H. (2000). The POMS and sports performance: A review. *Journal of Applied Sports Psychology, 12,* 34–48.

Radeke, T., & Stein, G. (1994). Felt arousal, thoughts/feelings, and ski performance. *Sports Psychologist, 8,* 360–375.

Radlo, S. J., Steinberg, G. M., Singer, R. N., & Barba, D. A. (2002). The influence of an attentional focus strategy on alpha brain wave activity, heart rate, and dart-throwing performance. *International Journal of Sport Psychology, 33,* 205–217.

Reilly, R. (2005, February 8). Making the right calls. *Sports Illustrated, 102,* 84.

Richards, J. E., & Cronise, K. (2000). Extended visual fixation in the early pre-school years: Look duration, heart rate changes, and attentional inertia. *Child Development, 71,* 602–620.

Robazza, C., Bortoli, L., & Nougier, V. (2000). Performance emotions in an elite archer: A case study. *Journal of Sport Behavior, 23,* 144–163.

Rodrigues, S. T., Vickers, J. N., & Williams, A. M. (2002). Head, eye and arm coordination in table tennis. *Journal of Sports Sciences, 20,* 187–200.

Rogers, T. J., Alderman, B. L., & Landers, D. M. (2003). Effects of life-event stress and hardiness on peripheral vision in a real-life stress situation. *Behavioral Medicine, 29,* 21–26.

Romanowski, B., Schefter, A., & Towle, P. (2005). *Romo: My life on the edge—living dreams and slaying dragons.* New York: Morrow.

Ryska, T. A., & Yin, Z. (2000). Testing the buffering hypothesis: Perceptions of coach support and pre-competitive anxiety among male and female high school athletes. *Current Psychology, 18,* 381–394.

Salvador, A., Suay, F., González-Bono, E., & Serrano, M. A. (2003). Anticipatory cortisol, testosterone and psychological responses to judo competition in young men. *Psychoneuroendocrinology, 28,* 364–376.

Schmidt, A., & Peper, E. (1993). Training strategies for concentration. In J. Williams (Ed.), *Applied sport psychology: Personal growth to peak performance.* Mountain View, CA: Mayfield.

Silva, J., & Stevens, D. (Eds.). (2002). *Psychological foundations of sport.* Boston: Allyn & Bacon.

Sime, W. E. (1982). Competitive stress management in perspective. In L. D. Zaichowsky & W. E. Sime

(Eds.), *Competitive stress management for sport* (pp. 120–129). Reston, VA: American Alliance for Health, Physical Education, Recreation and Dance.

Sime, W. E. (1985). Physiological perception: The key to peak performance in athletic competition. In J. Sandweiss & S. Wolf (Eds.), *Biofeedback and sport science* (pp. 33–62). New York: Plenum Press.

Sime, W. E. (2003). Sport applications of biofeedback. In M. Schwartz & F. Andrasik (Eds.), *Biofeedback: A practitioner's guide* (pp. 560–588). New York: Guilford Press.

Sime, W. E., Allen, T. W., & Fazzano, C. (2001). Optimal functioning in sport psychology: Helping athletes find their zone of excellence. *Biofeedback, 28*(5), 23–25.

Singer, R. N. (2000). Performance and human factors: Considerations about cognition and attention for self-paced and externally paced events. *Ergonomics, 43,* 1661–1680.

Singer, R. N. (2002). Preperformance state, routines, and automaticity: What does it take to realize expertise in self-paced events? *Journal of Sport and Exercise Psychology, 24,* 359–375.

Skinner, N., & Brewer, N. (2004). Adaptive approaches to competition: Challenge appraisals and positive emotion. *Journal of Sport and Exercise Psychology, 26,* 283–306.

Smith, A. M., Adler, C. H., Crews, D., Wharen, R. E., Laskowski, E. R., Barnes, K., et al. (2003). The "yips" in golf: A continuum between a focal dystonia and choking. *Sports Medicine, 33,* 13–31.

Smith, R. (2003, October). *Positive coaching and parenting in youth sports: Basic research and intervention.* Paper presented at the International Positive Psychology Summit, Washington, DC.

Spalding, T., Jeffers, L., Torges, S., & Hatfield, B. (2000). Vagal and cardiac reactivity to psychological stressors in trained and untrained men. *Medicine and Science in Sports and Exercise, 32*(3), 581–591.

Strack, B. (2003). Effect of heart variability biofeedback on batting performance in baseball. *Dissertation Abstracts International,* 3083450.

Strano, S., Lino, S., Calcagnini, G., Divirgilio, V., Ciardo, R., Cerutti, S., et al. (1998). Respiratory sinus arrhythmia and cardiovascular neuroregulation of athletes. *Medicine and Science in Sports and Exercise, 30*(2), 215–219.

Taylor, J. A., & Shaw, D. F. (2002). The effects of outcome imagery on golf-putting performance. *Journal of Sports Sciences, 20,* 607–613.

Thomas, O., Maynard, I., & Hanton, S. (2004). Temporal aspects of competitive anxiety and self-confidence as a function of anxiety perceptions. *Sport Psychologist, 18,* 172–188.

Tugade, M. M., & Fredrickson, B. L. (2004). Resilient individuals use positive emotions to bounce back from negative emotional experiences. *Journal of Personality and Social Psychology, 86,* 320–333.

Vickers, J. N. (1992). Gaze control in putting. *Perception, 21,* 117–132.

Vickers, J. N. (1996). Control of visual attention during the basketball free throw. *American Journal of Sports Medicine, 24,* S93–S97.

Vickers, J. N., & Adolphe, R. M. (1997). Gaze behavior during a ball tracking and aiming skill. *International Journal of Sports Vision, 4,* 18–27.

Waterhouse, J., Reilly, T., & Edwards, B. (2004). The stress of travel. *Journal of Sports Sciences, 22,* 946–967.

Weinberg, R. S., & Gould, D. (2003). *Foundations of sport and exercise psychology.* Champaign, IL: Human Kinetics.

Williams, A. M., Singer, R. N., & Frehlich, S. G. (2002). Quiet eye duration, expertise, and task complexity in a near and far aiming task. *Journal of Motor Behavior, 34,* 197–207.

Williams, A. M., Vickers, J., & Rodrigues, S. (2002). The effects of anxiety on visual search, movement kinematics, and performance in table tennis: A test of Eysenck and Calvo's processing efficiency theory. *Journal of Sport and Exercise Psychology, 24,* 438–455.

Williams, J. M., & Andersen, M. B. (1997). Psychosocial influences on central and peripheral vision and reaction time during demanding tasks. *Behavioral Medicine, 22,* 160–167.

Woodman, T., & Hardy, L. (2003). The relative impact of cognitive anxiety and self-confidence upon sport performance: A meta-analysis. *Journal of Sports Sciences, 21,* 443–458.

Wrisberg, C. A., & Fisher, L. E. (2005). Staying connected to teammates during rehabilitation. *Athletic Therapy Today, 10,* 62–63.

Zaichowsky, L., & Sime, W. (1982). *Stress management for sport.* Reston, VA: American Alliance for Health, Physical Education, Recreation and Dance.

CHAPTER 24

Differential Effects of Stress Management Therapies on Emotional and Behavioral Disorders

JONATHAN M. FELDMAN
ERIKA J. EISENBERG
EDUARDO GAMBINI-SUÁREZ
JACK H. NASSAU

This chapter reviews the literature on stress management techniques that have been used to treat emotional and behavioral disorders in adults and children. We evaluate each treatment to determine whether it meets criteria for an empirically supported therapy in accordance with the guidelines set forth by Chambless and Hollon (1998). The following categories are employed in this review: *efficacious and specific, efficacious, possibly efficacious*, and *further research needed to establish efficacy.*

STUDIES OF ADULTS

Anxiety Disorders

We review evidence of treatment efficacy of nonpharmacological therapies for four anxiety disorders: panic disorder (PD), posttraumatic stress disorder (PTSD), generalized anxiety disorder (GAD), and social anxiety disorder (SAD).

Panic Disorder

Since the last version of this chapter (Lehrer, Carr, Sargunaraj, & Woolfolk, 1993), stress management therapies for PD have received a substantial amount of attention. Three specific treatments have been researched: cognitive-behavioral therapy (CBT), applied relaxation, and eye movement desensitization and reprocessing (EMDR). CBT for PD consists of cognitive restructuring, breathing retraining and muscle relaxation, and exposure to bodily sensations (i.e., interoceptive exposure) and situations that are associated with panic attacks (Craske, Barlow, & Meadows, 2000). Applied relaxation (Öst, 1987) has been administered separately from other elements of CBT to determine its efficacy in the treatment of PD. Applied relaxation consists of progressive muscle relaxation (PMR) and differential and rapid relaxation. The goal of treatment is to apply these skills, once properly learned, in feared situations. Additionally, EMDR has been recently applied to the treatment of PD. EMDR consists of the patient describing an anxiety-provoking event (e.g., panic attack) while following a therapist's fingers from side to side with his or her eyes. The goal is to desensitize the patient to this fearful memory and to associate adaptive cognitions with this event and eye movements (Feske & Goldstein, 1997). Table 24.1 summarizes the efficacy of each of the interventions reviewed here for the treatment of PD.

CBT has been established as the first-line psychological treatment for PD. CBT for PD has been shown to be superior to applied relaxation (Arntz & van Den Hout, 1996; Clark et al., 1994; Craske, Brown, & Barlow, 1991), nondirective supportive therapy (Beck, Sokol, Clark, Berchick, & Wright, 1992; Craske, Maidenberg, & Bystritsky, 1995), and pill placebo (Klosko, Barlow, Tassinari, & Cemy, 1990). These positive findings have been maintained at follow-up periods ranging from 6 months (e.g., Arntz &

TABLE 24.1. Evaluation of Treatment Efficacy for Anxiety Disorders

Anxiety disorder	Intervention	Treatment efficacy
Panic disorder/ agoraphobia	CBT	Efficacious and specific
	Applied relaxation	Possibly efficacious
	EMDR	Further research needed to determine efficacy
	Respiratory biofeedback	Further research needed to determine efficacy
	Mindfulness meditation	Further research needed to determine efficacy
	Internet-based CBT and applied relaxation	Further research needed to determine efficacy
Posttraumatic stress disorder	CR/SIT	Efficacious
	Exposure	Efficacious
	CR/SIT + exposure	Efficacious
	EMDR	Possibly efficacious
	Relaxation	Further research needed to determine efficacy
Generalized anxiety disorder	CBT	Efficacious and specific
	Applied relaxation	Efficacious and specific
	CT	Efficacious and specific
	Biofeedback	Further research needed to determine efficacy
	Meditation	Further research needed to determine efficacy
Social anxiety disorder	Exposure + CT (CBT)	Efficacious
	Exposure	Efficacious
	CT	Efficacious
	Social skills training	Efficacious
	Applied relaxation	Possibly efficacious
	CBGT	Efficacious and specific
	IPT	Further research needed to determine efficacy

van Den Hout, 1996) to 24 months (e.g., Craske et al., 1991). The primary outcome measure for these studies has typically been the percentage of patients who are panic-free. A meta-analysis showed that the mean effect size was 0.68 for CBT versus control conditions (Gould, Otto, & Pollack, 1995). This meta-analysis showed that the mean percentage of panic-free patients who received CBT was 74.3% in comparison with only 27.1% for patients in control groups. However, reducing the length of CBT may reduce its efficacy. Craske et al. (1995) carried out four sessions of CBT and found that 53% of participants reported being panic-free, which is lower than the percentages typically found in the full-length CBT protocol of 12–16 sessions. Nevertheless, this finding was significant in comparison with those from a nondirective supportive therapy group, and it demonstrates the efficacy of brief CBT. At the present time, though, the standard 12- to 16-session protocol of CBT appears to yield the largest effect sizes and, therefore, is the recommended version. However, shorter CBT treatments may be useful for patients hesitant or not willing to engage in 4 months of therapy.

The hypothesized mechanism of change for cognitive restructuring, relaxation, and exposure is that each component will have treatment-specific effects on cognitive, physiological, and behavioral avoidance measures, respectively. Clark et al. (1994) provided evidence that misinterpretation of bodily sensations at the end of cognitive therapy (CT) was associated with worse outcome (e.g., relapse) at follow-up. This finding is consistent with cognitive theories of PD, which hypothesize that catastrophic misinterpretation of innocuous bodily sensations plays a key role in the development of PD (Clark, 1989). Michelson et al. (1990) showed that PMR and situational exposure administered separately were each more effective in reducing physiological arousal among PD patients with agoraphobia than paradoxical intention, a cognitively oriented therapy. On the other hand, Beck, Stanley, Baldwin, Deagle, and Averill (1994) failed to find evidence of treatment specificity for cognitive restructuring (CR) and relaxation therapy (RT) on cognitive and physiological measures, respectively.

The field has attempted to dismantle the components of CBT to determine which interventions are efficacious when administered separately from the entire protocol. However, a methodological issue inherent in this research is the difficulty in separating each treatment modality in order to conclude treatment specificity. For example, participants in CT-only conditions may engage in self-directed exposure, particularly as their self-efficacy increases during the course of CT. Beck et al. (1994) found that when CR and RT were administered separately, both were efficacious in reducing agoraphobic fears and panic-related symptoms without explicit use of exposure-based therapy. This finding raises questions about the necessity of exposure in treating agoraphobia symptoms. However, self-directed exposure needs to be carefully monitored in future studies before this conclusion can be reached. Bouchard et al. (1996) showed that separate administration of either CR or exposure led to improvements in panic and agoraphobia symptoms according to a similar time course. Furthermore, substantial evidence from other studies shows that exposure may be an important aspect of PD treatment. A meta-analysis showed that effect sizes for various interventions for PD were significantly reduced when exposure was included in the *comparison group* (Clum, Clum, & Surls, 1993). A separate meta-analysis showed that the combination of interoceptive exposure and CR produced a mean effect size of 0.88 (Gould et al., 1995). Situational exposure appears to be particularly important for agoraphobia. Ratings for *in vivo* anxiety levels during situational exposures were associated with global functioning at posttreatment and at 3-month follow-up among patients with PD and agoraphobia (Murphy, Michelson, Marchione, Marchione, & Testa, 1998). Therefore, the evidence to date suggests that both interoceptive and situational exposure (for agoraphobia) should be included as part of the treatment for PD.

The efficacy of relaxation as a separate treatment modality in PD has produced mixed evidence. Öst and colleagues (Öst & Westling, 1995; Öst, Westling, & Hellström, 1993) have not found differences on panic-related measures between applied relaxation, CT, and exposure. Participants receiving each of these treatments display clinically significant improvements in PD (e.g., high end-state functioning), which are maintained at 1-year follow-up. However, Clark et al. (1994) found that the combination of CR and interoceptive exposure was more efficacious than applied relaxation for treatment of PD (with or without agoraphobia), as reflected on multiple measures of anxiety and panic at 6- and 15-month follow-up. These findings by Clark et al. (1994) were replicated in patients with PD without agoraphobia by independent investigators (Arntz & van Den Hout, 1996) who were not involved in the development of Clark's (1989) CT or Öst's (1987) applied relaxation. Additionally, Beck et al. (1994) compared CR without any exposure with RT using the techniques of Bernstein and Borkovec (1973). A greater percentage of patients in both interventions were treatment responders, as measured by global PD severity, frequency of panic attacks, agoraphobia symptoms, and fear of body sensations, as compared with a minimal-contact control group. However, the effect size for each intervention group was lower than that typically found when using the combined CBT package. Given that two meta-analyses (Clum et al., 1993; Gould et al., 1995) have shown that CBT produces the most consistent and largest effect sizes, the multicomponent CBT package remains the first-line psychological treatment for PD.

Although numerous studies have demonstrated the efficacy of CBT over other treatments (as discussed), one study has provided data that question the specificity of CBT. Shear, Pilkonis, Cloitre, and Leon (1994) compared CBT with nondirective supportive therapy focusing on life stress. Both treatments consisted of 15 sessions. All participants received three initial sessions of psychoeducation concerning panic and its innocuous physiological sensations. No differences were found between the two groups with respect to the percentage of patients who reported being panic-free at posttreatment and at 6-month follow-up (75% for CBT; 68% for supportive therapy). Although the nondirective supportive therapy was intended to be noncognitive, discussions concerning misconceptions about panic attacks were permitted throughout the course of treatment as part of the psychoeducation component. Therefore, this part of the protocol may have been more similar to CT than intended and may have contributed to reductions in panic (Arntz & van Den Hout, 1996). Given that there is substantially more evidence from randomized controlled trials (RCTs) showing that CBT is superior to other forms of psychological treatment, we conclude that CBT is an efficacious and specific treatment for PD.

Psychological treatments other than traditional CBT have also been proposed as stress management therapies for PD. EMDR was more effective than a wait-list control and than EMDR without the eye movement component for some panic symptoms, although these differences were not maintained at 3-month follow-up (Feske & Goldstein, 1997). A separate study found no differences between EMDR and an attention-placebo control (PMR and associative therapy) on panic symptoms (Goldstein, de Beurs, Chambless, & Wilson, 2000). Furthermore, the effect size was small for both interventions. Therefore, further research would be needed to establish the efficacy of EMDR for PD. Additionally, respiratory biofeedback has been recently applied to the treatment of PD to increase partial pressure of end-tidal carbon dioxide (PCO_2) and normalize dysfunctional breathing patterns. Case studies have shown promising results in reducing panic symptoms and suggest the need for controlled studies (Meuret, Wilhelm, & Roth,

2001, 2004). Kabat-Zinn et al. (1992) administered a group mindfulness meditation program and showed that a small number of patients with PD (n = 10) showed reductions in self-reported and interview-rated anxiety and depression. Finally, it has recently been shown that CBT and applied relaxation may be effectively administered via the Internet, with only minimal therapist contact (Carlbring, Ekselius, & Andersson, 2003). However, control groups are needed to determine the efficacy of these promising interventions.

Posttraumatic Stress Disorder

Psychological therapies for PTSD include stress inoculation training (SIT), exposure therapy, relaxation, and EMDR. The theoretical rationale for CBT is based on Mowrer's (1939) two-factor theory of classical and operant conditioning. Experience of a traumatic event leads to a conditioned fear response to stimuli associated with the original trauma. Avoidance of these stimuli is then maintained over time via negative reinforcement. Habituation occurs by exposing patients to trauma-related but innocuous stimuli. CR teaches patients to identify and modify maladaptive thoughts and expectations associated with harmless, feared stimuli. SIT is a form of CBT, and it consists of CR, breathing retraining, tensing and relaxing muscle groups, and guided self-dialogue (Meichenbaum, 1975, 1985; also see Meichenbaum's discussion of SIT in Chapter 19, this volume). Exposure therapy is a behavioral therapy (BT) that uses either imagery or *in vivo*–based exposure to feared but harmless stimuli. Relaxation training is another form of BT that targets hyperarousal, which may also facilitate exposure to feared stimuli. The theoretical rationale for the use of eye movements in EMDR for the treatment of PTSD is less well developed. Table 24.1 provides a summary of treatment efficacy for each intervention.

The work of Foa et al. (1999) and of Marks, Lovell, Noshirvani, Livanou, and Thrasher (1998) has shown that the combination of cognitive techniques and exposure do not appear to offer an advantage to the administration of either treatment alone. RCTs have tested the efficacy of SIT, exposure therapy, and the combination of SIT and exposure in the treatment of PTSD. Foa and colleagues (1999; Foa, Rothbaum, Riggs, & Murdock, 1991) have examined female assault victims and shown that all three interventions were superior to wait-list control on reductions in the severity of PTSD. At 12-month follow-up, only 32–35% of participants in the three intervention conditions met criteria for PTSD. However, all participants in the control group still met criteria for PTSD at follow-up (Foa et al., 1999). Marks et al. (1998) examined PTSD among outpatients with a diverse range of traumas and found that exposure, CR, and their combination were each superior to relaxation across clinician and self-rated measures of PTSD. Few significant differences emerged between exposure, CR, and the combination group. The effect sizes on the primary outcome measures of PTSD ranged from 1.0 to 2.5, and improvement was still present at 6-month follow-up.

EMDR may also be an efficacious treatment for PTSD, although methodological flaws have limited many studies of EMDR. A meta-analysis of psychological treatments of PTSD found that BT (which included exposure therapy as well as CBT) and EMDR produced the largest effect sizes when compared with control groups (Van Etten & Taylor, 1998). Relaxation and hypnosis were less efficacious than EMDR and BT, although only one study of each was included in the meta-analysis. BT was more efficacious than EMDR on observer-rated PTSD symptoms at posttreatment, but this difference disappeared at follow-up (mean effect size = 1.93 for BT and 2.27 for EMDR). However, methodological flaws (e.g., failure to use structured PTSD interviews, failure to assess treatment integrity) in many of the studies employing EMDR limit the conclusions from this meta-analysis. Additionally, studies have failed to show a difference between EMDR that includes the saccadic eye movements and EMDR with fixed eyes (Pitman et al., 1996). Long-term maintenance of treatment gains at 5-year follow-up has also not been supported (Macklin et al., 2000).

Recent studies have directly compared EMDR with BT and produced conflicting findings. Taylor et al. (2003) carried out the most rigorous comparison to date of exposure, EMDR, and relaxation training. Exposure therapy produced greater statistically and clinically significant reductions than EMDR and relaxation on reexperiencing of PTSD symptoms (e.g., flashbacks) and avoidance symptoms at posttreatment and follow-up. Additionally, exposure was associated with more rapid reductions in avoidance symptoms. No differences were found between EMDR and relaxation on PTSD symptoms. Two prior studies compared EMDR to BT, but conclusions are limited by failure to use blind, independent evaluators of PTSD symptoms. Devilly and Spence (1999) found that the combination of SIT and exposure was superior to EMDR in reducing PTSD symptoms at both posttreatment and 3-month follow-up. On the other hand, Lee, Gavriel, Drummond, Richards, and Greenwald (2002) found that more participants in the EMDR group achieved clinically significant reductions (i.e., reductions of ≥ 2 standard deviations [*SD*] in PTSD symptoms) than the SIT–exposure group at 3-month follow-up.

In summary, these findings demonstrate that either CT (SIT) or BT (exposure) is the first-line psychological treatment for PTSD. Although there is some evidence to support the efficacy of EMDR, methodological limitations and lack of a developed, theoretical rationale for treatment of PTSD have hampered this body of research. It has been suggested that EMDR may simply work via the use of imaginal exposure during the protocol and *in vivo* exposure on the part of the patient (Taylor et al., 2003). Further research would be needed to test this theory.

Generalized Anxiety Disorder

CBT for GAD has been the primary psychological treatment studied in RCTs. CBT for GAD consists of self-monitoring of worry, relaxation, and cognitive restructuring. The patient then uses imagery-based or *in vivo* exposure to anxiety-provoking stimuli (e.g., thoughts, situations) to practice using these coping skills.

Borkovec and Ruscio (2001) conducted a meta-analysis of 11 studies that used CBT for treatment of GAD. There is strong support from CBT studies for the maintenance of treatment gains at 2-year follow-up (Borkovec, Newman, Pincus, & Lytle, 2002). The meta-analysis showed that for CBT the mean within-group effect sizes on the State–Trait Anxiety Inventory (STAI; Spielberger, Gorsuch, & Lushene, 1970) trait subscale and the Hamilton Anxiety Rating Scale (HARS; Hamilton, 1959) were 2.48 and 2.44 at posttherapy and follow-up, respectively (Borkovec & Ruscio, 2001). A similar pattern of results was also found for CBT on reductions in depressive symptoms. Between-group comparisons showed that CBT was superior to wait-list control groups, with a large effect size on measures of anxiety. CBT was also more effective than placebo (e.g., nondirective psychotherapy) or alternative therapy (e.g., psychodynamic) and yielded a large effect size on anxiety measures at posttherapy (0.71 for STAI trait subscale and 0.86 for HARS). Although CBT was still more effective at follow-up, the effect size was reduced (0.30 for STAI trait subscale and 0.41 for HARS). Finally, CBT was superior to BT and CT alone at posttherapy with small to moderate effect sizes, which increased to moderate effect sizes at follow-up (0.54 for STAI trait subscale and 0.59 for HARS).

More recent evidence from RCTs has shown that CBT and its individual components appear to produce similar results, without a clear advantage for any one of these interventions. Borkovec and colleagues (2002) recently conducted the most rigorous study to date comparing CBT, applied relaxation combined with self-control desensitization, and CT (CR and self-monitoring). No differences were found between these treatments on measures of anxiety and depression. All three interventions produced large effect sizes at posttherapy (2.38–2.95), and treatment gains were maintained at 24-month follow-up (2.31–2.67). Although this study did not include a nonspecific or no-treatment control condition, these effect sizes were all larger than effect sizes reported for nonspecific treatment groups in previous studies (Borkovec & Ruscio, 2001). Borkovec and Costello (1993) directly compared CBT, applied relaxation, and nondirective psychotherapy. Both CBT and applied relaxation were superior to nondirective therapy in reducing anxiety at posttreatment and at 12-month follow-up. No differences were found between CBT and applied relaxation at posttreatment. However, a greater percentage of patients who received CBT (58%) achieved high end-state functioning than did participants who received applied relaxation (33%). Öst and Breitholtz (2000) found no differences between applied relaxation and CT at posttreatment or at 12-month follow-up. Clinically significant improvements were found in 67% of patients receiving applied relaxation and 56% of those receiving CT at follow-up. Arntz (2003) also found no differences between applied relaxation and CT at 6-month follow-up and very similar rates of clinically significant changes.

These findings collectively support the efficacy and specificity of CBT and its individual components, as indicated by superior performance compared with nondirective therapy. However, these treatments do not produce the same level of clinically significant improvements for GAD as compared with CBT for other anxiety disorders, such as PD (Arntz, 2003; Borkovec & Costello, 1993; Öst & Breitholtz, 2000). Borkovec, Newman, and Castonguay (2003) have recommended incorporating elements of interpersonal therapy (IPT) with traditional CBT, and this area of research is currently being explored. The finding that interpersonal difficulties were a predictor of poorer treatment responses to CBT provides support for the role of IPT in the treatment of GAD (Borkovec et al., 2002).

Biofeedback and meditation have also been used in the treatment of GAD, although there is limited research on these interventions. Rice, Blanchard, and Purcell (1993) compared frontal EMG biofeedback, biofeedback to increase EEG alpha activity, biofeedback to decrease EEG alpha activity, and meditation, which was conceptualized as an attention-placebo condition. Contrary to the authors' hypotheses, no differences were found between any of the groups on self-reported anxiety, as assessed by the STAI trait subscale. However, all participants displayed within-group decreases in anxiety at posttreatment and 6-week follow-up. Conclusions from this study are limited by the short follow-up period and the small sample size, as only 38 participants had DSM-III diagnoses of GAD. Nevertheless, these results for biofeedback and meditation are promising and await further research from RCTs to determine their efficacy for the treatment of GAD.

Recent psychophysiological studies of patients with GAD also suggest that certain types of biofeedback, such as heart rate variability (HRV) biofeedback, may be useful treatment interventions. Hoehn-Saric, McLeod, Funderburk, and Kowalski (2004) used ambulatory monitoring to examine physiological measures throughout the day among patients with GAD and PD and controls without a psychiatric diagnosis. Patients with GAD and PD displayed reduced interbeat interval and skin conductance variability compared with controls. Furthermore, comparisons between subjective and objective measurement of anxiety revealed that controls were more accurate in detecting changes in these physiological measures. Interventions such as HRV biofeedback may be useful for restoring normal cardiac rhythms and autonomically mediated homeostatic regulation (see Chapter 10, this volume). This research on psychophysiological interventions awaits formal evaluation of its efficacy for GAD.

Social Anxiety Disorder

CBT is the only empirically supported psychological treatment for SAD at the present time (Chambless & Ollendick, 2001). CBT for SAD consists of relaxation training, social skills training, exposure to fearful social situations, and CR (Hambrick, Weeks, Harb, & Heimberg, 2003). The goal of CBT is for the patient to use these skills to achieve competent social performance in previously feared social situations.

Several meta-analyses have examined the efficacy of CBT and its individual components (Chambless & Hope, 1996; Federoff & Taylor, 2001; Feske & Chambless, 1995; Gould, Buckminster, Pollack, Otto, & Yap, 1997; Taylor, 1996). These meta-analyses have shown that exposure alone and exposure in combination with CT are the first-line psychological treatments for SAD. Taylor (1996) examined 42 studies and found that social skills training, exposure alone, CT (i.e., CR without exposure), and the combination of exposure and CT were each superior to wait-list control in reducing social anxiety. However, only exposure and CT had a larger effect size versus pill-placebo or attention-placebo conditions, thereby providing some evidence of specificity. Gould et al. (1997) included 27 CBT studies of SAD in a meta-analysis and found large effect sizes for exposure alone (0.90) and exposure plus CT (0.80) but medium effect sizes for social skills training (0.60) and CT (0.60). Federoff and Taylor (2001) also found large effect sizes for pre- to posttreatment changes when using exposure alone (1.08) and exposure plus CT (0.84), moderate to large effects for CT (0.72) and social skills training (0.64), and a medium effect size for applied relaxation (0.51). However, large variability among the seven exposure studies resulted in the 95% confidence interval overlapping with zero, and thus there was no significant treatment effect for exposure. The two studies included in the meta-analysis that examined applied relaxation were conducted by the same team of investigators (Jerremalm, Jansson, & Öst, 1986; Öst, Jerremalm, & Johansson, 1981). Exposure plus CT was the only treatment superior to attention placebo. Feske and Chambless (1995) conducted a meta-analysis of 24 studies and found that, among controlled studies, exposure had a large effect size (1.06) and exposure plus CT produced a small to medium effect size (0.38). However, exposure studies were compared only with wait-list controls, whereas the comparison groups for exposure plus CT sometimes included placebo and psychoeducational groups. Furthermore, the authors did not include several studies of exposure plus CT that showed positive findings (Hambrick et al., 2003).

These meta-analyses have also shown the durability of CBT, as treatment gains have been maintained at follow-up periods ranging from 2 to 6 months. In fact, Taylor (1996) showed that effect sizes increased significantly when examining within-group effects at follow-up (mean = 3 months) versus posttreatment. All other meta-analyses reviewed to this point also showed that the follow-up effect sizes for CBT modalities were at least as large as posttreatment effect sizes (Chambless & Hope, 1996; Federoff & Taylor, 2001; Feske & Chambless, 1995; Gould et al., 1997).

Group administration of CBT (CBGT) has been shown to be an efficacious and specific treatment for SAD, with long-term durability of treatment gains. Heimberg, Juster,

Hope, and Mattia (1995) have developed CBGT, which incorporates CR and exposure to fearful social situations. CBGT is typically administered to groups of six patients across a 12-session protocol. CBGT has been shown to be superior to wait-list controls (Hope, Heimberg, & Bruch, 1995), to pill placebo, and to psychoeducational support groups (Heimberg et al., 1998). Treatment gains from CBGT have been maintained at 5-year follow-up (Heimberg, Saltzman, Holt, & Blendell, 1993). Hofmann (2004) compared CBGT with group exposure therapy and found that both interventions were more efficacious than a wait-list control. However, CBGT was superior to group exposure at 6-month follow-up, and this difference appeared to be mediated by reduced social costs. Patients who complete CBGT also report increases in quality of life that are maintained at 6-month follow-up, although these scores still remain below those of normative populations (Eng, Coles, Heimberg, & Safren, 2001). The components of quality of life that appear to show the greatest improvements are achievement and social functioning (Eng, Coles, Heimberg, & Safren, 2005).

Even less attention has been devoted to alternative treatments in the SAD literature compared with other anxiety disorders. Lipsitz and Marshall (2001) have discussed the need for such alternative treatments, particularly for nonresponders to CBT approaches. Lipsitz, Markowitz, Cherry, and Fyer (1999) conducted an uncontrolled pilot study of IPT with nine patients with SAD. Seven of the patients were considered treatment responders based on clinician and self-ratings of social anxiety symptoms. These preliminary findings are promising for developing other efficacious psychological treatments for SAD.

Combining Pharmacological and Nonpharmacological Treatments for Anxiety Disorders

There has been considerable interest in the idea of combining pharmacological treatment with CBT, although surprisingly few well-controlled studies have been conducted. Proponents of combined treatment have argued that medication may allow the patient to engage in greater amounts of exposure due to reductions in anxiety caused by the medications. Therefore, the addition of pharmacological treatment with behavioral techniques may have a synergistic effect. Alternatively, critics argue that combined treatment may lead to worse long-term outcome. Pharmacological treatment may attenuate the physiological response during exposure to anxiety-provoking situations and thus prevent the patient from altering maladaptive beliefs. Additionally, the patient may attribute gains in psychotherapy to the medications, which can undermine self-efficacy. Therefore, the patient may be more likely to relapse after treatment is terminated (Foa, Franklin, & Moser, 2002).

Barlow, Gorman, Shear, and Woods (2000) conducted the largest multisite RCT to date, comparing combined treatment with monotherapies for PD. This study compared five groups: CBT (n = 77), imipramine (a tricyclic antidepressant; n = 83), pill placebo (n = 24), CBT plus imipramine (combined treatment; n = 65), and CBT plus pill placebo (n = 63). Patients received 11 CBT sessions (50 minutes) and/or 11 medication management sessions (30 minutes) across 12 weeks. Patients who were considered treatment responders entered the maintenance phase, which consisted of monthly CBT and/or medication management sessions across 6 months. Treatment was then discontinued, and a follow-up assessment was conducted 6 months later. Primary outcome measures included the Panic Disorder Severity Scale (PDSS; Shear et al., 1997) and the Clinical Global Impression Scale (CGI; Guy, 1976). At posttreatment, the combined group was superior to the CBT-alone group on the PDSS. At the end of the maintenance phase, the combined-treatment group was superior to the CBT-alone, CBT-plus-pill placebo, and imipramine-alone groups. However, participants in the combined-treatment group had the highest relapse rates at 12-month follow-up. CBT alone (85% treatment responder rate) and CBT plus pill placebo (83%) were superior to combined treatment (50%) at follow-up. Therefore, the combination of medication and CBT did not appear to offer long-term benefits. CBT was not able to protect against relapse rates following discontinuation of medication. Additionally, imipramine may have impeded the durability of CBT. Direct comparisons between imipramine and CBT alone showed that each treatment offered unique advantages. Imipramine produced a better quality of response on the PDSS among treatment responders at posttreatment. However, CBT was associated with lower relapse rates and greater durability of treatment gains.

A meta-analysis of treatments for PTSD showed that both CBT and selective serotonin reuptake inhibitors (SSRIs) have large effect sizes compared with control conditions (Van Etten & Taylor, 1998). The SSRIs appeared to be particularly effective for treating intrusive PTSD symptoms and comorbid depressive symptoms. However, the dropout rate for SSRIs (mean = 36%) was more than double the dropout rate for CBT (mean = 15%). The authors hypothesized that patients with PTSD may be hypersensitive to physiological side effects of SSRIs. Unfortunately, follow-up data from SSRI trials were not available for inclusion in this meta-analysis. Research on the combination of pharmacological and nonpharmacological treatments for PTSD has lagged behind that on other anxiety disorders.

The efficacy of CBT plus diazepam (a benzodiazepine) in the treatment of GAD was assessed by Power, Simpson, Swanson, and Wallace (1990). This study randomly assigned 101 participants to one of five groups: CBT, diazepam, pill placebo, CBT plus diazepam, and CBT plus pill placebo. Treatment was conducted for 10 weeks, and follow-up assessment was conducted at 6 months for both self-report and clinician-rated measurement of GAD symptoms. All treatments that included CBT were superior to diazepam at posttreatment and at 6-month follow-up. These findings also showed that the combination of CBT plus medication offered no additional benefit over CBT alone.

The combination of CBT and SSRIs for treatment of SAD has been examined in two RCTs. Davidson et al. (2004) conducted a multisite study comparing CBT, fluoxetine (an SSRI), pill placebo, CBT plus fluoxetine, and CBT plus pill placebo. Treatment was conducted for 14 weeks and administered to 295 participants. Clinician ratings using the CGI and Brief Social Phobia Scale (Davidson et al., 1997) served as the primary outcome measures. All active treatments were superior to pill placebo, and no differences were found between the active treatments at posttreatment. These results provide additional evidence showing that the combination of CBT plus pharmacotherapy offers no advantage over monotherapies at posttreatment. Blomhoff et al. (2001) randomized 375 participants with SAD to sertraline (SSRI) only (*n* = 95), to sertraline plus exposure (*n* = 95), to pill placebo plus exposure (*n* = 93), and to pill placebo only (*n* = 92). This study did not include a treatment arm to examine exposure alone. Participants received 24 weeks of sertraline or pill placebo and exposure or general medical care during the first 12 weeks of treatment. Exposure therapy consisted of eight sessions (15–20 minutes). This naturalistic study was carried out in primary care settings in Norway and Sweden, and general practitioners provided treatment. Both clinician and self-ratings were used as outcome measures. Sertraline alone and sertraline plus exposure were superior to the pill placebo–only condition. However, assessments conducted 28 weeks after discontinuation of treatment revealed a different pattern (Haug et al., 2003). Patients who received sertraline alone or sertraline plus exposure experienced exacerbation of symptoms across multiple measures. Patients in the exposure plus placebo condition displayed additional treatment gains at follow-up.

The literature has shown that combining pharmacological treatment with CBT for anxiety disorders does not offer additional benefits to either monotherapy alone. Although the combination treatment appears to offer short-term benefits at posttreatment, follow-up studies have shown that relapse rates increase when CBT is combined with medication. Additional research is needed to evaluate the efficacy of SSRIs in combination with CBT. The SSRIs are considered the first-line pharmacological agents for treatment of anxiety disorders. However, in the reviewed literature, only studies of SAD included SSRIs. Nevertheless, there is no support at the present time for long-term benefits of treatments that combine CBT and pharmacotherapy.

Anger

Anger is a widely prevalent emotional problem that has been linked to both physical and mental disease. Anger has been associated with increased risk for stroke (Williams, Nieto, Sanford, Couper, & Tyroler, 2002), myocardial infarction (Chang, Ford, Meoni, Wang, & Klag, 2002), hypertension and cardiovascular mortality (Harburg, Julius, Kaciroti, Gleiberman, & Schork, 2003). Additionally, anger has been linked to depression (Koh, Kim, & Park, 2002; Pasquini, Picardi, Biondi, Gaetano, & Morosini, 2004), substance abuse (Tivis, Parsons, & Nixon, 1998), and physical aggression (Tafrate, Kassinove, & Dundin, 2002). Treatment strategies have focused on anger as the primary problem and also an anger comorbid with other psychological disorders, typically depression and anxiety. These treatment approaches have been applied in a wide variety of environments and populations (e.g., in correctional settings, with students and drivers).

The treatment of anger has included CBT, CT, relaxation, skills training, and multicomponent interventions. The cognitive-behavioral approach originally developed by Novaco (1975) is still the basis for many anger management interventions. This treatment is based on Meichenbaum's SIT (1975, 1985; see also Chapter 19, this volume). The first stage of SIT focuses on CT. The client is asked to identify anger-triggering situations and to reframe the situations through adaptive self-statements. The second stage involves tensing and relaxing muscle groups, followed in later sessions by exposure to anger-provoking situations. Imagery or role plays are also utilized to practice these skills. Exercise is another technique that has been used for anger management. Aerobic exercise (e.g., swimming, walking, running, bicycling; see Chapter 13, this volume) and anaerobic exercise (e.g., weightlifting) may both affect the physiology of anger, although the specific mechanism has not yet been determined. Regular physical exercise has been associated with psychological benefits, such as reduced depression (Byrne & Byrne, 1993; Klein et al., 1985), anxiety (Cameron & Hudson, 1986), and anger (Buchman, Sallis, Criqui, Dimsdale, & Kaplan, 1991). Exercise may alter the style of anger expression and serve as an effective coping response to feelings of anger.

Several outcome measures have been used to assess the various dimensions of anger. The emotional state of anger (i.e., state anger) is typically measured by the intensity and duration of anger episodes. Trait anger refers to an individual's disposition to have angry feelings in response to situations. Anger suppression refers to holding in anger, whereas anger expression refers to the release of anger. The construct of anger has been typically assessed by self-report measures. The Novaco Anger Scale (NAS; Novaco, 1991) measures the experience of anger across three domains: cognition, arousal, and behavior. The

State–Trait Anger Scale (STAS; Spielberger, 1988) also measures the tendency to experience anger. The Spielberger State–Trait Anger Expression Inventory (STAXI; Spielberger, 1996) assesses the experience and expression of anger and also differentiates between expression and suppression of anger. Finally, the Driving Anger Scale (DAS; Deffenbacher, Oetting, & Lynch, 1994) measures anger that is experienced specifically in driving situations (i.e., "road rage"), such as being stuck in traffic or being cut off by another driver. The Profile of Mood States (POMS; McNair, Lorr, & Droppleman, 1992) also has an anger subscale.

CBT is an efficacious treatment for anger disorders. Beck and Fernandez (1998) conducted a meta-analysis of 50 studies that compared CBT with control groups (40 studies) or utilized a within-groups design with no control group (10 studies). These studies included participants of varying ages and with diverse conditions (e.g., abusive parents or spouses, juvenile offenders, inmates in detention facilities, aggressive schoolchildren). This meta-analysis showed that CBT yielded a medium to large effect size (weighted mean = 0.70) for the treatment of anger.

A recent meta-analysis of controlled studies (Del Vecchio & O'Leary, 2004) compared CBT, CT, and RT for various dimensions of anger. This meta-analysis showed that these three treatments for anger produced effect sizes ranging from medium to large (CBT = 0.68, CT = 0.82, RT = 0.90). However, it is important to consider the differential effects of each intervention for the specific dimensions of anger. CBT appears to be the most efficacious treatment for the expression of anger ($d = 0.61$), as compared with CT ($d = 0.38$) and relaxation ($d = 0.51$). CT appears to be the treatment of choice for anger suppression ($d = 0.64$), as compared with CBT ($d = 0.45$) and RT ($d = 0.16$). All three treatments had large effect sizes for the treatment of driving anger (CBT = 1.07, CT = 2.11, RT = 1.59), although only one study of CT was included in this analysis. RT appears to be the most efficacious approach ($d = 1.21$) for state anger, although CBT ($d = 0.91$) also displayed a large effect size. Trait anger responded similarly to all three approaches (CBT = 0.74, CT = 0.80, RT = 0.65). Finally, participants with difficulty controlling their anger appeared to respond best to CBT ($d = 0.60$). These findings suggest that clinicians should consider the specific dimension of anger when considering treatment options.

Table 24.2 provides a summary of evidence for treatment efficacy and recommendations for anger management. The treatment efficacy of CBT is supported across more dimensions of anger than are its individual components (CT, relaxation). Nevertheless, first-line treatments for anger suppression and state anger are CT and relaxation, respectively.

TABLE 24.2. Evaluation of Treatment Efficacy for Anger

Intervention	Treatment efficacy	Dimensions of anger
CBT	Efficacious	Driving anger, trait anger, anger expression, anger control, state anger
CT	Efficacious	Driving anger, trait anger, anger suppression
Relaxation	Efficacious	Driving anger, trait anger, state anger
Exercise	Further research needed to determine efficacy	

Note. Recommendations concerning dimensions of anger are based on the meta-analysis conducted by Del Vecchio and O'Leary (2004).

The study population also may be an important consideration in determining treatment responses to anger management interventions. Studies of anger have focused on caregivers, military personnel, angry drivers, and individuals diagnosed with medical conditions. Coon, Thompson, Steffen, Sorocco, and Gallagher-Thompson (2003) carried out an RCT comparing anger management (Novaco's approach), depression management (based on social learning and CBT principles), and a wait-list control group among female caregivers of relatives with dementia. Both treatment groups reported reductions in symptoms of anger, hostility, and depression, which were mediated by increases in self-efficacy in managing behavior problems and controlling upsetting thoughts. However, effect sizes for both interventions were relatively small. A separate, although uncontrolled, study showed that female caregivers of relatives with dementia who received pyscho-education, problem-solving therapy, and a combination of autogenic training and PMR reported pre–post decreases on anger and hostility (Mizuno, Hosaka, Ogihara, Higano, & Mano, 1999).

Conclusions regarding the efficacy of CBT anger management for military populations are limited by the uncontrolled nature of these studies. Military personnel who participated in a four-session CBT anger management protocol reported pre- to post-treatment decreases on the STAXI (Linkh & Sonnek, 2003). However, the high attrition rate (49%) is a major limitation of this study. Another uncontrolled multicomponent CBT study (Devilly, 2002) also showed decreases in anger, as measured by the Novaco Anger Inventory—Short Form (NAI; derived from the NAS).

Aggressive drivers may be good candidates for multicomponent CBT interventions. Galovski, Blanchard, Malta, and Freidenberg (2003) implemented a CBT protocol that included PMR for anger-provoking driving situations. Aggressive drivers displayed pre–post intervention decreases in heart rate and in systolic and diastolic blood pressure while listening to aggressive driving audio vignettes. This research should be replicated in controlled studies, but it offers promising findings due to the inclusion of physiological measures.

CT is also an efficacious treatment for anger. Deffenbacher, Dahlen, Lynch, Morris, and Gowensmith (2000) applied Beck's CT (Beck, Rush, Shaw, & Emery, 1979; Beck & Emery, 1985) to a sample of college students. The CT intervention yielded a large effect size for reduction in symptoms on 11 dimensions of anger in comparison with a no-treatment control group. These significant effects were maintained at 15-month follow-up. The reductions in anger among the CT group were considered to be clinically significant, as established by moderate to large effect sizes and an index of clinically significant change. However, a separate study showed that reductions in anger via cognitive techniques do not appear to be specific (Dua & Swinden, 1992). This RCT showed that participants trained to reduce their negative thoughts and individuals trained in meditation demonstrated greater reductions on self-report and physiological measures of anger than a no-treatment control group. In addition, a placebo group trained in guided imagery of anger-provoking situations also showed greater reductions on anger-related measures than the control group. The improvements in the placebo group may be attributed to imaginal exposure to an anger-producing situation and expectations of change. Therefore, CT appears to be efficacious, but not specific, for anger management.

Relaxation has also been established as an efficacious treatment for certain types of anger management. Deffenbacher, Filetti, Lynch, Dahlen, and Oetting (2002) compared relaxation coping skills (RCS), cognitive relaxation coping skills (CRCS), and a no-treatment control group among a group of high-anger drivers. RCS incorporated progressive relaxation, slow breathing, relaxation without tensing muscles, cue-controlled relaxation, and guided imagery relaxation. The CRCS intervention consisted of CR and cognitive coping skills training, in addition to relaxation. At posttreatment, individuals in both treatment conditions (RCS and CRCS) reported lower levels of trait anger and driving anger than the control group. Effect sizes were large, and results were maintained at 4-week follow-up. Additionally, the CRCS group reported engaging in less risky driving behavior. These findings provide evidence that relaxation is an efficacious treatment for driving anger, although adding a cognitive component may yield additional benefits.

Individualized stress management programs have applied traditional stress management techniques and adapted these protocols to address anger among people diagnosed with medical conditions. Inouye, Flannelly, and Flannelly (2001) conducted an RCT comparing stress management with a wait-list control among individuals with HIV/AIDS. The intervention included self-management techniques (biofeedback-assisted relaxation, guided imagery, abdominal breathing, PMR, and autogenic training), cognitive coping strategies (CR, anger and depression management) and psychoeducation on HIV/AIDS. Participants in the intervention reported greater reduction on the anger–hostility scale of the POMS than the control group. An RCT of patients with hypertension showed that participants receiving 10 hours of individualized stress management therapy had greater reductions in blood pressure than a wait-list control group (Linden, Lenz, & Con, 2001). These significant results were maintained at 6-month follow-up. Additionally, reductions in systolic blood pressure were associated with changes in anger coping style. Therefore, individualized stress management programs appear to be efficacious when tailored to specific medical populations. More research is needed to test the specificity of these interventions by including active placebo groups.

Exercise may be another application of stress management that reduces anger levels. A population-based study of Finnish participants showed that self-report of regular exercise, defined as two to three times per week, was associated with reports of less anger and depression (Hassmen, Koivula, & Uutela, 2000). Exercise may have an immediate effect on anger, as a single exercise class that involved either running, karate, or weight lifting was found to reduce anger among college students in comparison with a lecture class (McGowan, Pierce, & Jordan, 1991). Additionally, an uncontrolled study found that traditional judo training was associated with reductions in aggressiveness across training sessions (Lamarre & Nosanchuck, 1999). However, an outdoor walking exercise program for elderly Korean women failed to change anger levels, as assessed by the POMS (Shin, 1999). Nevertheless, the authors noted that the lack of significant findings might be explained by overall low levels of anger consistent with cultural values of Korean elders, who tend not to express their feelings of anger. Finally, an uncontrolled study of cardiac patients incorporated exercise, yoga, meditation, prayer, and spirituality (Kennedy, Abbott, & Rosenberg, 2002). Participants reported decreases in anger levels from pre- to postintervention. However, methodological flaws (e.g., no control group, no follow-up period, subjective report of outcomes) substantially limit conclusions concerning this intervention. Additional research is required to determine whether exercise interventions are efficacious as a form of anger management.

Future studies of treatments for anger should rely less on self-report measures to assess changes in anger. Observational studies in real-life situations or virtual reality environments, along with physiological measures (e.g., heart rate, blood pressure, adrenaline), will provide a more complete understanding of anger. The use of collateral informants (e.g., spouse) has also been underutilized in studies of anger. These additional assessment tools would provide valuable information on the assessment of anger, particularly among individuals who tend to underreport anger. Furthermore, the lack of a precise definition of anger and its exclusion from DSM-IV as a specific diagnosis has hampered the effort to distinguish between its emotional, behavioral, and physiological components. Finally, the ecological validity of anger needs to be established by studying cultural components of anger and differences that exist both within and across various ethnic groups.

Depression

IPT and CBT are the two types of psychotherapy that have been identified as efficacious treatments for major depression. IPT emphasizes the connection between identified problems (depression) and current relationship issues. IPT is not focused on the etiology of depression (Bolton et al., 2003), and it acknowledges the biopsychosocial aspects of depression (Gillies, 2001). IPT pinpoints interpersonal interactions as the mechanism for improving symptoms of depression. Therefore, treatment is focused on grief, interpersonal conflicts, role transitions, and interpersonal deficits (Imber et al., 1990; Bolton et al., 2003). CBT for depression focuses on the cognitive aspects of treatment, which include eliciting and testing automatic thoughts and identifying schemas in order to help both the patient and the therapist understand the patient's reality. Behavioral techniques, such as scheduling activities that include mastery and pleasure exercises, cognitive rehearsal, self-reliance training, and role playing, are utilized in order to help modify automatic thoughts (Young, Weinberger, & Beck, 2001).

Research has indicated that, although each of these psychological treatments is efficacious, these treatments do not appear to be specific (Elkin et al., 1989). The National Institute of Mental Health (NIMH) Treatment of Depression Collaborative Research Program (TDCRP) conducted a large multisite study that compared three types of treatment for depression: CBT, IPT, and imipramine plus clinical management. Outpatients with depression ($N = 239$) were randomly assigned to one of these three groups or to a control group, which consisted of placebo pill plus clinical management. No differences in treatment effects were found between CBT and IPT, as assessed by the two primary outcome measures used in the study: HRSD (Hamilton Rating Scale for Depression) and the BDI (Beck Depression Inventory). The effects of both CBT and IPT were significantly better than those of placebo; however, they were not as strong as the effects of imipramine plus clinical management at postassessment (Elkin et al., 1989; Chambless & Ollendick, 2001; Imber et al., 1990). After controlling for variables that were predictive of treatment outcome, no differences were found between CBT and IPT at posttest. However, participants in the CBT and IPT groups rated their life adjustment as being more positive than those in the imipramine and placebo groups at 18-month follow-up (Blatt, Zuroff, Bondi, & Sanisolow, 2000; Chambless & Ollendick, 2001).

Secondary analysis of data from the large-scale multisite NIMH study showed that patient characteristics may predict treatment response (Sotsky et al., 1991). Treating people with a modality that is more consistent with their strengths than their weaknesses may predict better responses. For example, low social dysfunction predicted better response to IPT. The authors also found that low cognitive dysfunction predicted superior responses to CBT and imipramine than to placebo.

The NIMH collaborative research program also assessed whether the reduction in depressive symptoms could be accounted for by mode-specific techniques of the interventions or whether there were common underlying mechanisms shared by all three treatments. The authors selected instruments for outcome measures that were designed to show whether each treatment modality had a differential and specific effect on outcome.

For example, the Social Adjustment Scale (SAS) was administered to determine whether participants in the IPT condition would display improvements in social adjustment (Imber et al., 1990). The investigators found that patients in CBT displayed the greatest improvements on the Need for Social Approval factor of the Dysfunctional Attitude Scale (DAS). This was the only measure that had a predicted differential effect. However, the authors concluded that a more comprehensive measure of social and interpersonal functioning was needed to assess whether IPT showed a differential treatment effect (Imber et al., 1990; Chambless & Ollendick, 2001). This study demonstrates the lack of specificity for psychotherapy treatments for depression. Therefore, factors that are common to psychotherapy may be more responsible for improvements in depressive symptoms than those that are specific to individual types of psychotherapy (Chambless & Ollendick, 2001; Imber et al., 1990).

In the last edition of this book, Lehrer et al. (1993) noted that IPT had recently emerged as a new treatment option for depression. Over the past decade, additional studies of IPT have been conducted, and IPT is now considered able to produce results that are comparable with those of CBT for treatment of depression. IPT is viewed as one of the most efficacious treatments available (Elkin et al., 1989; Chambless & Ollendick, 2001; Imber et al., 1990). IPT has been shown to produce significant reductions in depressive symptoms as compared with placebo plus clinical management (Chambless & Ollendick, 2001; Imber et al., 1990). Group administration of IPT has also been shown to be efficacious. One RCT study ($N = 224$) showed that IPT group therapy is efficacious when compared with a control group that did not receive any treatment (Bolton et al., 2003). Men and women in Uganda who met criteria for depression (on an adapted Hopkins Symptom Checklist) were assigned either to an intervention group, which consisted of sixteen 90-minute group IPT sessions for depression, or to a control group. The control group was not assessed to determine whether participants were involved in alternative treatments to relieve their depressive symptoms; thus this group cannot be considered a no-treatment group. After the intervention was completed, 6.5% and 54.7% of the participants in the intervention and control groups, respectively, met criteria for major depression as compared with 86% and 94%, respectively, before the intervention.

A meta-analysis of 48 studies assessed the efficacy of group therapy for depression. The analysis included 47 studies that utilized a CBT group. Eight of the 47 studies also included either a psychodynamic or IPT group. Group therapy may be particularly well suited for depressed patients because interpersonal functioning and social support have consistently predicted relapse of depression (McDermut, Miller, & Brown, 2001). Group therapy is also more cost effective than individual therapy. The authors found that group therapy was associated with greater improvement in depressive symptoms. The average effect size for pretreatment and posttreatment means on well-established self-report or interviewer-based measures of depression was 1.03 ($SD = .81$). This implies that patients treated with group therapy demonstrated greater reductions in depressive symptoms than 85% of the untreated patients. This meta-analysis was not able to determine that group therapy is more effective than individual treatment; however, it did show that CBT group therapy may be efficacious (McDermut et al., 2001).

Epidemiological studies have shown that exercise (see Chapter 13, this volume) is related to mental health and, in particular, to depressive symptoms (Babyak et al., 2000; Farmer et al., 1988; Stephens, 1988; Lobstein, Mosbacher, & Ismail, 1983). Studies have shown that when people increase their levels of exercise, they have the same reduced risk for depression as those who had exercised all along (Babyak et al., 2000; Camacho, Roberts, Lazarus, Kaplan, & Cohen, 1991). However, the risk for depression appears to increase among people who had previously been active but who stopped exercising. This implies that there are no build-up effects of exercise and that the effects are short term. These findings suggest that exercise may be a possible form of treatment for depression. However, a recent review of the literature on exercise and depression (Hausenblas, Dannecker, & Focht, 2001) concluded that although research has indicated an association between exercise and depression, it is not possible to identify a causal relationship due to a lack of methodologically stringent studies.

A recent meta-analysis of 14 studies examined the efficacy of exercise as a treatment for depression (Lawlor & Hopker, 2001). Ten of the studies that compared exercise with no treatment showed that exercise reduced symptoms of depression. Only RCTs were included in this analysis; however, all of the studies had methodological weaknesses, such as inadequate concealment of randomization, lack of intent-to-treat designs, no follow-up, or inadequate blinding. Furthermore, nine of them included populations that did not meet criteria for major depression. Therefore, these findings are difficult to generalize to a clinically depressed population, in which motivation for treatment tends to be low (Lawlor & Hopker, 2001).

Blumenthal and colleagues (1999) provided evidence that exercise may be efficacious in the treatment of depression. This study examined adults between the ages of 50 and 77 who met DSM-IV criteria for major depressive disorder (MDD). The participants were randomly assigned to receive either a group aerobics class three times a week, antidepressant medication (sertraline hydrochloride), or a combination of the two. A significant within-group reduction in depressive symptoms occurred after the 16-week intervention in all groups. There were no significant differences in reduction of depressive symptoms across the three treatment groups, and 60–69% of all participants no longer met criteria for MDD. The authors did note a significantly faster response in the medication group. However, at 10-month follow-up, participants in the exercise group had significantly lower relapse rates than those in the medication group. Also, regardless of which group the participants were assigned to, continued exercise on one's own during the follow-up period was associated with reduced probability of depression diagnosis at the end of the follow-up period (Babyak et al., 2000).

Anecdotal evidence supports the positive effect of yoga (see Khalsa, Chapter 17, this volume) on mood. However, few controlled research studies have examined the efficacy of yoga (Lawlor & Hopker, 2001; Manber, Allen, & Morris, 2002). One RCT studied the short-term effect of yoga (Iyengar) on mood among mildly depressed young adults (Woolery, Myers, Sternlieb, & Zeltzer, 2004). The participants were assigned either to 10 yoga classes or to a wait-list control group. The yoga intervention group reported significantly greater decreases in symptoms of depression on the BDI than the control group. However, methodological limitations of the study included lack of follow-up, the sole use of self-report, and the lack of placebo or alternate treatment. Additionally, it is not clear which aspects of yoga may be associated with improvements in mood. The findings may be attributed to breathing and relaxation, to physical movement, to group support and consistency or, as the authors point out, to an increase in sense of mastery. All of these limitations should be addressed in future research.

Janakiramaiah et al. (2000) examined the effects of yoga, electroconvulsive therapy (ECT), and imipramine on melancholic depression among 45 psychiatric patients who had an HRSD score of 17 or greater. No differences in remission rates of depression were found between patients taking imipramine (73%) and those practicing yoga (67%). Both of these rates were lower than that of the patients receiving ECT (93%). This study indicates that yoga has similar effects to those of imipramine, which is accepted as an efficacious treatment. Although these results are promising, further research is needed to show that yoga would be efficacious with outpatients suffering from other types of depression.

The cognitive behavioral analysis system of psychotherapy (CBASP) is an intervention designed specifically for patients with depression. It is a contingency program that utilizes negative reinforcement and is intended to highlight the connection between a patient's actions and the consequences of his or her behavior with the intention of facilitating adaptive behavioral changes. The treatment is composed of three techniques: situational analysis (SA), interpersonal discrimination exercise (IDE), and behavioral skills training/rehearsal (BST/R; McCullough, 2003). Keller et al. (2000) randomized 681 participants who met criteria for MDD into one of three treatment conditions: nefazodone, CBASP, or a combination group. Unfortunately, there was no placebo group. The investigators showed that response to treatment, which included both remission and satisfactory treatment response, as measured by the HRSD, did not differ significantly between nefazodone (55%) and CBASP (52%). However, the response rate when the two treatment modalities were combined was significantly higher (85%). These findings imply that CBASP may be efficacious because it is as efficacious as nefazodone (Feiger et al., 1999) when used independently. Although this was a large-scale multisite study, future research will need to include RCTs conducted by other teams of investigators in order to determine whether CBASP is an efficacious treatment for depression.

Behavioral activation (BA) therapy focuses on encouraging the patient with depression to increase overt behaviors that are commonly associated with positive environmental contingencies, which will in turn improve the client's thoughts, affect, and quality of life (Hopko, Lejuez, Ruggeiro, & Eifert, 2003). One RCT (Jacobson, Dobson, Truax, Addis, & Koerner, 1996) was designed to test the efficacy of CBT for depression and to compare and contrast its components. Three types of treatments were compared: BA, BA plus skills used to modify automatic thoughts, and full cognitive therapy treatment (CT). No significant differences were found among the three types of treatment, as measured by the BDI and HRSD at posttest. The mean improvement rate was 62% for the entire sample. Because BA was found to be as efficacious as BA plus cognitive skills, which is essentially CBT, BA may be an efficacious treatment for depression. There is also preliminary evidence supporting the efficacy of BA in a group format (Porter, Spates, & Smitham, 2004). However, replication by additional investigators is needed to supplement these promising findings for individual and group BA.

Two types of psychological treatments (IPT and CBT) have been shown to be efficacious in the treatment of depression (see Table 24.3). Neither of these treatments has been shown to have specificity, and, therefore, there is no clear first choice treatment for patients presenting with depressive symptoms. The TDCRP indicated that people tend to do better with treatments that specifically utilize their strengths rather than focusing on their weaknesses. For example, low cognitive dysfunction appears to be associated with better responses to CBT. Group therapy using IPT and CBT has been shown to be efficacious compared with no treatment, and it may represent a cost-effective intervention. Exercise may also be a promising treatment for depression. However, more methodologically sound research is needed from additional investigators to establish its efficacy in treating depression. Controlled studies are also needed to determine the efficacy of yoga and the potential mechanisms through which it may improve mood. BA and CBASP are relatively new treatments for depression that appear to be promising; however, more research is needed to determine their efficacy, as well.

TABLE 24.3. Evaluation of Psychological Interventions for Depression

Intervention	Treatment efficacy
CBT	Efficacious
IPT	Efficacious
Exercise	Possibly efficacious
Yoga	Further research needed to determine efficacy
CBASP	Possibly efficacious
BA	Possibly efficacious

Substance Abuse

The primary psychological treatments used to treat substance abuse are: CBT, motivational interviewing (MI), motivational enhancement therapy (MET), and self-help/12-step groups. CBT involves the use of coping skills training, which teaches patients to identify cues that trigger urges to use and to implement skills to resist these urges. CBT utilizes instruction, modeling, role plays, behavioral rehearsal techniques, and exposure to promote the use of coping skills in stressful situations (Morgenstern & Longabaugh, 2000; Rohsenow, Monti, Martin, Michalec, & Abrams, 2000). MI was originally developed by Miller and Rollnick (1991) as a treatment for substance abuse. MI utilizes a supportive, nonconfrontational approach that is intended to help clients resolve ambivalence to promote behavior change (Miller & Rollnick, 1991). MET is a brief therapy (four sessions over a 12-week period) that is based on the principles of MI. Twelve-step self-help groups are based on the model that alcoholism is a spiritual and medical disease that requires an individual's acceptance of the disease in order to overcome it. Transcendental meditation (TM), biofeedback, relaxation training, hypnosis, visualization, and forgiveness therapy have also been used as treatments for substance abuse, although there is less research evaluating their efficacy.

Cognitive-Behavioral Therapy

CBT has been shown to be one of the most efficacious treatments for substance abuse (Morgenstern & Longabaugh, 2000). In an RCT, Rohsenow et al. (2004) found that relapse rates for alcohol abuse were lower for those treated with coping skills training (a type of CBT) versus a drug education group, although the effect size was small. Monti, Rohsenow, Michalec, Martin, and Abrams (1997) conducted an RCT in which cocaine-addicted patients in a partial-hospital program were randomized to cocaine-specific coping skills training or to a control group using meditation/relaxation. Coping skills training significantly reduced cocaine use at 3-month follow-up. Among patients who had relapsed, those in the coping skills training group reported significantly fewer cocaine use days at 4- to 6-month follow-up. However, after 6 months, cocaine use increased in the coping skills training group, whereas the meditation/relaxation group remained the same, thereby eliminating these between-groups differences (Rohsenow et al., 2000). Therefore, treatments that can maintain long-term abstinence are needed.

Incorporating predictors of relapse into substance abuse treatment is an important tool for clinicians. Hall, Wasserman, and Havassy (1991) conducted a prospective study in which 104 cocaine-addicted patients were assessed at baseline, at 12 weeks, and at 6 months. The authors reported that a goal of complete abstinence and higher positive mood scores predicted lower risk of lapse at 12 weeks. These findings show the importance of accepting the goal of absolute abstinence. Additionally, treatments such as CBT, which aim to increase pleasant daily activities and challenge negative thoughts, may improve mood and thus lower the risk of relapse (Morgenstern & Longabaugh, 2000; Project MATCH Research Group, 1997). Despite the efficacy of CBT, there is often a disconnection between treatments that are empirically supported and those that are used clinically (Gordis, 1991). However, it has been shown that CBT can be disseminated to substance abuse counselors in the community (Morgenstern, Morgan, McCrady, Keller, & Carroll, 2001).

There is a well-established relationship between alcoholism and depression (Helzer & Pryzbeck, 1988; Ramsey, Brown, Stuart, Burgess, & Miller, 2002; Regier et al., 1990). Therefore, it is important for clinicians to understand how to effectively treat people diagnosed with both disorders. Ramsey et al. (2002) randomized patients with comorbid depression and alcoholism to CBT for depression (CBT-D) or to relaxation treatment, which consisted of daily tension monitoring, meditative and deep breathing techniques, PMR, and guided imagery. The CBT-D group displayed greater improvements on measures of alcohol-related expectancies than the relaxation group. Patients within the CBT-D group whose positive expectations of alcohol decreased drank significantly less at follow-up. Individuals in the CBT-D group may have been able to generalize the skills they learned and thus were more equipped to handle stress. The decrease in the level of depressive symptoms in the CBT-D group may have enabled these participants to benefit more from the alcohol treatment program (Ramsey et al., 2002). Therefore, changes in certain cognitive variables, such as expectations, may predict drinking outcomes.

Poor treatment adherence is a major barrier in the treatment of patients with substance abuse (Kirdorf, King, & Brooner, 1999; Brooner et al., 2004). One RCT evaluated the efficacy of motivated stepped care versus standard stepped care to increase adherence with a methadone treatment program among opioid-dependent outpatients (Brooner et al., 2004). The motivated stepped care condition utilized behavioral contingencies, such as less convenient methadone dosing times for those participants who missed counseling sessions, in order to motivate the participants to attend counseling. Behavioral contingencies were not used in the standard stepped care condition. Participants in the motivated stepped care group attended significantly more counseling sessions than those in standard care (94% vs. 70%). This finding suggests that behavioral contingencies may be an important tool for a clinician to utilize to increase adherence to substance abuse treatment programs.

Motivational Enhancement Therapy and Motivational Interviewing

MET has been shown to be efficacious in the treatment of addictive behaviors. Furthermore, MET appears to be most effective among patients with low levels of motivation to change their behavior. In one RCT (Rohsenow et al., 2004), cocaine-dependent patients in a partial-hospital setting were randomized either to two individual sessions of MET or to meditation/relaxation therapy. Individuals in the MET group with lower initial motivation levels had *lower* cocaine and alcohol relapse rates at 6-month and 1-year follow-up than patients who had higher initial levels of motivation. Patients in the meditation/relaxation group who had had lower initial motivation levels tended to have *higher* relapse rates at 3-month follow-up than patients who had higher initial motivation levels.

Sellman, Sullivan, Dore, Adamson, and MacEwan (2001) conducted an RCT with patients with mild to moderate alcohol dependence. All participants received a feedback/education session followed by a 6-week review session. Participants were then randomized into one of three conditions: MET, nondirective reflective listening, or no further counseling. Results showed that fewer patients treated with MET were classified as heavy drinkers at 6-month follow-up than in either the nondirective-reflective-listening or the no-further-counseling conditions. This study supports the efficacy and specificity of MET, although more research is needed to confirm the specificity.

Many clinical studies of MI have used adapted versions, which employ additional interviewing techniques or a feedback component, as well as the core components of MI (Burke, Arkowitz, & Menchola, 2003). The efficacy of adaptations of MI as a treatment for addictive behaviors has been supported in a meta-analytical review of 11 studies (Noonan & Moyers, 1997; Burke et al., 2003). Adaptations of MI treatment were superior to no-treatment or wait-list control groups for alcohol abuse, as measured by standard ethanol content (combined effect size: $d = 0.25$), blood alcohol concentration (combined effect size: $d = 0.53$) and drug addiction, as measured by the Addiction Severity Index, frequency of substance abuse, treatment days attended, opiate dependence, and drug-related problems (combined effect size: $d = 0.56$; Burke et al., 2003).

Twelve-Step Treatment and Self-Help Groups

Self-help groups may represent a cost-effective alternative to substance abuse treatment. Morgenstern et al. (2003) conducted an RCT to investigate whether 12-step treatment processes are active in improving outcome in substance abuse. Participation in 12-step treatment was associated with self-help affiliation, which, in turn, was associated with improvement in substance abuse outcomes, as measured by percentage of days abstinent. Additionally, a separate study showed that patients who were treated in a program that incorporated a self-help group were 40% less likely to relapse than those who received the usual aftercare (McAuliffe, 1990). These findings support 12-step programs as an efficacious treatment for substance abuse.

Project MATCH

Project MATCH is the largest multisite treatment outcome study of alcohol dependence to date (Project MATCH Research Group, 1997). It was hypothesized that matching individuals to treatment modalities based on many characteristics would produce greater treatment effects than simply having all alcohol-dependent patients receive the same treatment. Project MATCH consisted of two RCTs conducted in an outpatient and an aftercare setting following inpatient or partial-hospital treatment. Patients were randomly assigned to one of three 12-week, manual-guided treatment groups that were administered individually. The three treatment conditions were cognitive-behavioral coping skills therapy (CBT), MET, and Twelve-Step Facilitation Therapy (TSF). The CBT and TSF groups met weekly. The MET group consisted of four sessions, which took place in the 1st, 2nd, 6th, and 12th weeks of the study. Clients were assessed at posttreatment and at 3-, 6-, 9-, and 12-month follow-up. The primary outcome measures were self-reports and collateral reports of percent days abstinent (PDA) and drinks per drinking day (DDD).

Patients treated in both the outpatient and aftercare settings displayed significant within-group improvements in drinking outcomes, regardless of treatment modality (Project MATCH Research Group, 1997). These improvements were maintained at 1-year follow-up. Although the main hypothesis of treatment matching was not supported, there was some evidence that those with less psychiatric severity might benefit from TSF versus CBT (Project MATCH Research Group, 1997). This research shows that it is important to consider psychiatric severity level when matching alcohol-dependent patients to a type of treatment. Additionally, the efficacy of CBT, TSF, and MET as treatments for alcohol dependency was supported by this study, but treatment specificity was not.

Investigators identified between-group differences in alcohol consumption and alcohol-related negative consequences in the outpatient arm of the study (Project MATCH Research Group, 1998). Clients in both the CBT and TSF groups drank significantly less frequently than those in the MET group at postintervention. Thus it may be more efficient to place patients in a CBT or TSF group than an MET outpatient group when a quick treatment response is desired (Project MATCH Research Group, 1998). However, these between-group differences were not maintained at 1-year follow-up, essentially because the initial effects of CBT and TSF were weakened.

Other Stress Management Techniques

Comorbidity between anxiety and alcohol dependency is high (Kushner, Sher, & Beitman, 1990). Futterman and Shapiro (1986) propose that biofeedback and relaxation therapy may reduce anxiety symptoms and thus decrease the potential deleterious effects of anxiety on management of alcoholism. Additionally, biofeedback training may decrease the client's feelings of helplessness and increase his or her self-efficacy in controlling his or her drinking behavior (Denney & Baugh, 1992). Taub, Steiner, Weingarten, and Walton (1994) conducted a study on alcohol-dependent males, comparing the effects of TM (see Chapter 14, this volume); EMG biofeedback of the forehead; electronic neurotherapy, which is the application of low-intensity pulses of current to the head; and a control group of routine therapy. The control group received counseling and attended Alcoholics Anonymous (AA) meetings and optional occupational therapy. The TM and biofeedback groups had significantly more nondrinking days, as measured by self-report and blood alcohol level, than the routine therapy group at 6- and 12-month follow-up and in comparison with both the neurotherapy and routine therapy groups at 18-month follow-up. This study provides evidence to support biofeedback and TM as efficacious treatment methods; however, the study lacked a truly randomized design.

Multicomponent stress management techniques have also been used in the treatment of alcohol dependence. An uncontrolled study of alcohol-dependent males carried out a stress management program that included biofeedback (thermal and EMG feedback), autogenic training (see Chapter 8, this volume), PMR, meditation, breathing retraining, and systematic desensitization (Denney & Baugh, 1992). Reductions in stress-related symptoms were mildly correlated ($r = .22$) with sobriety, as measured by self-report and confirmed by a staff member or leader of AA (Denney & Baugh, 1992). This study was uncontrolled, and thus further research is needed to determine the efficacy of multicomponent stress management programs, as well as which specific components are most useful for the treatment of alcohol dependence.

Relaxation may be useful in the treatment of sleep disturbances, which are a side effect of alcoholism and alcohol withdrawal (Shinba, Murashima, & Yamamoto, 1994; Greeff & Conradie, 1998). Greeff and Conradie (1998) found that inpatient males in an alcohol rehabilitation center who received PMR reported significantly more improvements in their sleeping patterns than participants in a wait-list control group. Therefore, PMR may be a useful tool in reducing sleep disturbances and thus may aid in the management of alcoholism (Denney & Baugh, 1992; Futterman & Shapiro, 1986).

Anecdotal evidence has supported the use of hypnosis (see Karlin, Chapter 6, this volume, for a review of hypnotherapy) in the treatment of substance abuse. However, there is not yet sufficient empirical evidence to support its efficacy. A recent RCT assessed the efficacy of self-hypnosis on relapse rates following an intensive substance abuse program (Pekala et al., 2004). Hypnosis was not more efficacious than CBT based on stages of change (Prochaska, DiClemente, & Norcross, 1992) or than stress management group therapy consisting of relaxation training (conceptualized as an attention placebo) at 7-week follow-up. The study did have limitations, such as the loss of 46% of participants at follow-up and the use of self-report as the measure of sobriety. Therefore, further research is needed in order to label self-hypnosis as an efficacious treatment in relapse prevention.

Visualization is a cognitively focused technique that is derived from hypnosis, although it does not require an altered state. The theoretical rationale for visualization is based on the notion that it leads to behavior change by altering people's beliefs about themselves, the world, and the future (Kominars, 1997). A quasi-experimental study compared a psychoeducational addiction treatment group with a group-based intervention that combined visualization and progressive relaxation. Both groups displayed increases from pre- to posttreatment on emotional arousal, self-efficacy, and coping resources. However, there were no between-group differences, and this study was limited by lack of direct measurement of substance use. Thus this evidence does not support the efficacy of visualization as a treatment for substance abuse.

Forgiveness therapy (FT; Lin, Mack, Enright, Krahn, & Baskin, 2004) is a treatment that involves uncovering an individual's anger regarding a wrongdoing by someone else and making a decision about whether to forgive the person. The individual is taught, through the use of empathy and the forgiveness process, to view the perpetrator of the offense as a human being rather than just an injurer. Lin et al. (2004) used FT with individuals in a standard residential treatment program. The FT group improved significantly more than an adjunctive alcohol and drug counseling group on measures of trait anger, depression, anxiety, self-esteem, forgiveness, and vulnerability to drug use after 12 weeks of treatment and at 4-month follow-up on all measures except trait anger. This study suggests that FT is possibly efficacious in the treatment of substance abuse. However, conclusions are limited by small sample size and lack of direct measurement of substance use.

In summary, even the most efficacious of treatments for substance abuse, such as CBT, have only mild to moderate effect sizes (Morgenstern & Longabaugh, 2000). Table 24.4 lists the treatments that have already been established as efficacious for the treatment of substance abuse. TM, biofeedback, relaxation training, hypnosis, visualization, and FT are techniques with smaller bodies of research evaluating their efficacy that need further research in order to label them as efficacious.

Schizophrenia

Pharmacotherapy is regarded as the primary treatment for schizophrenia (Huxley, Rendall, & Sederer, 2000; Bellack & Muesser, 1993). However, the psychopharmacological agents have limited impact on the negative symptoms of schizophrenia, and they may not be sufficient to prepare patients for reentering the community (Huxley et al., 2000; Liberman,

TABLE 24.4. Efficacy of Stress Management Therapies for Substance Abuse

Intervention	Treatment efficacy
CBT	Efficacious
MI/MET	Efficacious
Self-help groups/twelve-step programs	Efficacious
Facial EMG biofeedback	Possibly efficacious
Transcendental meditation	Possibly efficacious
Hypnosis	Further research needed to establish efficacy
Visualization	Further research needed to establish efficacy
Forgiveness therapy	Possibly efficacious

1994). The diathesis–stress model posits that people develop schizophrenia because of the combined effects of genetic susceptibility and stress (McGuffin, Asherson, Owen, & Farmer, 1994). Therefore, these shortcomings of psychopharmacological treatments and the role of stress in relapse among patients with schizophrenia have led to increased interest in using psychosocial interventions as an adjunct to psychopharmacology (Falloon, Coverdale, & Booker, 1996; Huxley et al., 2000; Leff, Kuipers, Berkowitz, Vaughn, & Sturgeon, 1983; Liberman et al., 1998; Malla, Cortese, Shaw, & Ginsberg, 1990).

Evidence supports the diathesis–stress model for schizophrenia (Fowles, 1992; Nicholson & Neufeld, 1992; Nuechterlein & Dawson, 1984). Norman et al. (2002) assessed the effect of adding a multicomponent stress management program or a social activities group to a standard treatment program for patients with schizophrenia that included psychopharmacology. Patients in the stress management group received muscle relaxation, autogenic training, exercise training, nutritional education, and cognitive and behavioral skills. At 1-year follow-up, a significantly smaller percentage of patients (2 out of 32) with high attendance rates (i.e., $\geq 90\%$) in the stress management group were hospitalized compared with the percentage of patients with high attendance rates from the social activities group who were hospitalized (6 out of 27). This finding suggests that stress management is efficacious when added to standard treatment for schizophrenia, but only when patients have a high attendance rate for treatment.

Family therapy for schizophrenia was developed in response to evidence suggesting a strong correlation between negative family attitudes, stress, and increased relapse rates among patients with schizophrenia (Huxley et al., 2000; Berkowitz, Eberlein-Freis, Kuipers, & Leff, 1984; Brown, Birley, & Wing, 1972; Nugter, Dingemans, Van der Does, Linszen, & Gersons, 1997). Huxley et al. (2000) reviewed 18 studies on family therapy and concluded that it is efficacious in reducing relapse rates, improving symptomatology, improving social and vocational functioning, enhancing medication adherence, and limiting hospitalizations. The authors note, however, that empirical research comparing family therapy with group and individual therapy is needed in order to determine whether family therapy is the most efficacious psychosocial treatment. Hogarty and colleagues (1986; Hogarty et al., 1991) were the only researchers to combine multiple psychosocial treatment modalities. They found that the combination of social skills training and family therapy was superior to either of these therapies alone, as measured by relapse rates at 1-year follow-up, but not at 2-year follow-up.

In a meta-analysis that included 18 RCTs, Pilling et al. (2002b) assessed the effects of adding a family intervention to antipsychotic medication in the treatment of schizophrenia. The authors concluded that single-family therapy (as opposed to therapy with groups of families) had a preventative effect on relapse 1–2 years into treatment, as compared with all other treatments. Single-family interventions led to a reduction in hospital readmissions when assessed 1–2 years into treatment, as compared with standard care. However, the effect of family interventions on hospitalizations was not significant when group family interventions were included in the analysis. Additionally, the benefit of single-family therapy over standard care was not observed at 4- to 15-month follow-up after termination of treatment. Furthermore, there was no difference in suicide rates of patients treated with family therapy versus all other treatments. This is an important finding, because Pilling et al. (2002b) point out that there have been previous suggestions that family therapy leads to an increase in suicide among patients with schizophrenia.

Traditional social skills training utilizes behavioral techniques to teach interpersonal skills to patients with schizophrenia. Traditional social skills training has not been found to improve psychotic symptomatology or to decrease hospitalizations compared with standard care or group therapy (Benton & Schroeder, 1990; Huxley et al., 2000; Wallace et al., 1980). Furthermore, traditional social skills training has been shown to have a minimal effect on patients' social skills, and it has not led to improvements in relapse rates or quality of life. These findings raise questions regarding the clinical utility of traditional social skills training (Huxley et al., 2000; Marder et al., 1996; Liberman et al., 1998). However, poor methodology (e.g., small sample sizes and nonstandardized assessment tools) limits these conclusions concerning the efficacy of traditional social skills training.

The UCLA Social and Independent Living Skills (SILS) is a structured module that broadens the depth of traditional social skills training for patients with schizophrenia to include symptom management, basic conversational skills, and medication management (Wallace et al., 1992; Huxley et al., 2000; Liberman et al., 1998). Huxley et al. (2000) reviewed eight studies, four of which were controlled, that assessed the efficacy of the UCLA SILS program (Eckman & Liberman, 1990; Liberman et al., 1998; Marder et al., 1996; Wallace at al.,1992). The authors reported pre- to posttherapy improvements in social skills and medication and symptom management for the SILS program versus comparison treatments and standard care. However, no differences were found between the SILS group and control groups when relapse rates and quality of life were evaluated (Marder et al., 1996; Liberman et al., 1998).

Huxley et al. (2000) noted a recent increase in the use of individual psychoeducation and supportive psychotherapy and a decline in insight-oriented psychotherapy for patients with schizophrenia. Huxley et al. (2000) concluded that individual psychoeducation and supportive psychotherapy treatment is superior to standard care for improving medication knowledge and treatment adherence, but not symptomatology and hospitalization rates (Boczkowski, Zeichner, & DeSanto 1985; Kemp, Hayward, Applewhaite, Everitt, & David, 1996; MacPherson, Jerrom, & Hughes, 1996; Razali & Yahya, 1995; Robinson, Gilbertson, & Litwack, 1986).

The meta-analysis by Pilling et al. (2002a) also assessed the effects of CBT on schizophrenia. No evidence was found for the benefit of CBT during treatment, with the exception of one measure. Compared with all other treatments, CBT was associated with "important improvement" in mental state, as defined by a stabilization of positive symptoms, insight, and dysphoria, at a medium- to long-term point into treatment (Drury, Birchwood, Cochrane, & Macmillan, 1996). At 9- to 18-month follow-up this superior effect of CBT was noted only in comparison with standard care.

Gould, Mueser, Bolton, Mays, and Goff (2001) conducted a meta-analysis that reviewed controlled studies on the efficacy of CT (see Pretzer & Beck, Chapter 18, this volume) as an adjunctive treatment for the psychotic symptoms of schizophrenia. The authors reported a large effect size associated with the usefulness of CT in decreasing the severity of hallucinations and delusions. However, the authors noted that, although this meta-analysis supports CT as an efficacious treatment for positive psychotic symptoms of schizophrenia, the studies had limitations, including lack of blind evaluators and homogenous populations.

In their meta-analysis, Pilling et al. (2002a) also examined the effects of cognitive remediation on schizophrenia among RCTs. Cognitive remediation aims to improve cognitive skills and functioning through the use of behavioral and psychoeducational techniques (Medalia, Herlands, & Baginsky, 2003). The authors found no evidence of benefit of cognitive remediation on attention, verbal memory, visual memory, or mental state, as compared with controls. The authors concluded that cognitive remediation is not an efficacious treatment for schizophrenia.

In summary, it appears as though some forms of psychotherapy and stress management can be useful adjunctive treatments in the management of schizophrenia (see Table 24.5). Of all psychosocial treatments, individual family therapy has obtained the most empirical support for efficacy. Traditional social skills training and cognitive remediation have not been found to be efficacious in the management of schizophrenia. CBT has been found to be useful in improving mental state, and CT has been shown to be efficacious in managing positive psychotic symptoms.

TABLE 24.5. Summary of Treatment Efficacy for Schizophrenia

Treatment	Efficacy	Outcome measured
Multicomponent stress management therapy	Possibly efficacious	Relapse rate
Family therapy	Efficacious	Relapse rate; symptomatology; social and vocational functioning; medication adherence
Traditional social skills training	Further research needed to establish efficacy	Relapse rates, quality of life
UCLA SILS program	Efficacious	Social skills, medication and symptom management
	Further research needed to establish efficacy	Relapse rates, quality of life, hospitalization, positive symptoms
Individual psychoeducation and supportive therapy	Efficacious	Medical knowledge, treatment adherence
	Further research needed to establish efficacy	Symptomatology; hospitalization
CBT	Efficacious	Positive symptoms, insight, dysphoria
CT	Efficacious	Positive symptoms
Cognitive remediation	Further research needed to establish efficacy	Negative symptoms

STUDIES OF CHILDREN AND ADOLESCENTS

As noted in the previous edition of this volume (Lehrer et al., 1993), children and adolescents are able to learn and benefit from relaxation and biofeedback techniques, particularly when those techniques are presented in a developmentally appropriate manner (Culbert, Kajander, & Reaney, 1996; Koeppen, 1974; Lee & Olness, 1996; Powers & Spirito, 1998a, 1998b). This includes providing an understandable rationale for the treatment, avoiding threatening descriptor words (e.g., *electrodes*), and utilizing relaxation scripts that are attractive to children and adolescents. It also includes attending to the therapeutic relationship, as the quality of that relationship may affect treatment outcome.

Since the previous edition of this book, considerable attention has been given to evaluating the efficacy of these techniques in the treatment of emotional and behavioral problems among children and adolescents. In a large meta-analytic review of child and adolescent psychotherapy outcome research, Weisz, Weiss, Han, Granger, and Morton (1995) included 23 studies of relaxation training and three studies of biofeedback training. This review included studies of patients with a wide variety of psychological difficulties, and results for various forms of relaxation training or biofeedback were not reported separately. Effect sizes of 0.41 and 0.20 for the relaxation training and biofeedback, respectively, were reported, but the authors did not specify for which disorders relaxation and biofeedback were employed. Although such literature is not reviewed in this section, it should be noted that the efficacy of relaxation and biofeedback in the treatment of somatic complaints (e.g., headache; see Holden, Deichmann, & Levy, 1999, for a review) has also received substantial recent research.

There are at least three major differences between research conducted prior to the last edition of this volume and that conducted since. First, whereas studies reviewed previously more often implemented stress management interventions alone, current studies more often include relaxation or biofeedback procedures as one aspect of a more comprehensive treatment package, typically of a cognitive-behavioral nature. Second, and likely related to the first point, there is currently more research that focuses on treating childhood disorders rather than on subsyndromal symptoms. Third, there appears to have been a growing focus on the use of these strategies in the treatment of anxiety disorders and school refusal and less focus on externalizing disorders. Therefore, in the section that follows, the majority of the findings are related to the efficacy of CBT in the treatment of anxiety disorders and school refusal among children and adolescents. However, the section also addresses the substantially smaller amount of research related to stress management in the treatment of tic and habit disorders and attention-deficit/hyperactivity disorder (ADHD).

Anxiety Disorders

In 1998, Ollendick and King (1998) published a comprehensive review on the efficacy of behavioral and cognitive-behavioral treatments for phobia and anxiety disorders among children and adolescents. Specific treatments that included relaxation training (e.g., systematic desensitization and CBT) were reviewed and determined to be probably efficacious in the treatment of these disorders. With respect to the treatment of anxiety disorders, two RCTs conducted by Kendall and colleagues (Kendall, 1994; Kendall et al., 1997)—as well as others conducted since Ollendick and King's review that are discussed later—illustrate how relaxation training has been incorporated into CBT for children and adolescents with anxiety disorders. Briefly, relaxation training has been one component of a protocol (Kendall's is a 16-session protocol for children and young adolescents called "Coping Cat") during which patients are trained to recognize anxious feelings and somatic concomitants, to clarify cognitions that occur in anxiety-provoking situations, to develop a coping plan to manage anxiety responses in such situations, and to evaluate and reward performance. Practice of skills taught in-session occurs between sessions (see Hudson & Kendall, 2002, for a detailed discussion of the use of home practice in this treatment). Training in PMR (see Chapter 4, this volume), designed to help children recognize and respond to somatic effects of anxiety, is taught early in the treatment package, practiced, and then used during graduated exposure to anxiety-producing situations. Kendall (1994) and Kendall et al. (1997) studied children and young adolescents (ages 9–13) with a variety of DSM-III-R anxiety disorders (i.e., overanxious disorder, separation anxiety disorder, avoidant disorder), as determined by a structured clinical interview. Compared with wait-list controls, those who participated in the Coping Cat program showed decreases in self- and parent-reported measures of anxiety symptoms, as well as decreases in the percentages that continued to qualify for an anxiety disorder. These effects were maintained over follow-up periods of more than 3 years (Kendall & Southam-Gerow, 1996) and 7 years (Kendall, Safford, Flannery-Schroeder, & Webb, 2004). In one follow-up report (Kendall & Southam-Gerow, 1996), former patients were asked to recall and rate the importance of various aspects of the intervention. Interestingly, although only 14% of former patients spontaneously recalled the relaxation exercises, almost 70% recalled them when asked, and over 25% reported current use of them. In addition, remembering the relaxation exercises at follow-up was associated with positive changes on four of eight outcome variables of anxiety and depression, a greater number of relationships than for other components of the treatment.

Additionally, more recent research has expanded our knowledge of the efficacy of relaxation and biofeedback interventions for youths with anxiety disorders through inclusion of different intervention formats, treatment techniques, and patient populations. Studies of group interventions utilizing CBT (Ginsburg & Drake, 2002; Silverman et al., 1999), autogenic training (Goldbeck & Schmid, 2003), and biofeedback (Wenck, Leu, & D'Amato, 1996) within school (Ginsburg & Drake, 2002; Wenck et al., 1996) and outpatient settings (Goldbeck & Schmid, 2003; Silverman et al., 1999) have been conducted. All of these studies used random assignment, and one (Ginsburg & Drake, 2002) compared two active treatments. Silverman et al. (1999) reported that almost two-thirds of youths with DSM-III-R social phobia, overanxious disorder, or generalized anxiety disorder, diagnosed by a structured clinical interview, no longer met criteria for the disorder after completing group CBT (which also included a concurrent group for parents), whereas only 14% in the wait-list control group no longer met diagnostic criteria. The CBT group intervention utilized group processes (e.g., social comparison) and focused on parent facilitation of child exposure to anxiety-provoking situations, as well as on teaching children to observe their behavior, develop positive self-statements, and evaluate and reward themselves. These foci are comparable to those found in the Coping Cat intervention (Kendall, 1994). Ginsburg and Drake (2002) achieved similar results in a much smaller, school-based study of 11 African American adolescents with diagnosed anxiety disorders. Seventy-five percent (five out of six) of adolescents in the CBT group no longer met diagnostic criteria after treatment, whereas only 20% (one out of five) of adolescents in an attention-support control group no longer met diagnostic criteria. The group CBT in this study included relaxation training (PMR and diaphragmatic breathing), as well as CR, exposure to anxiety-provoking situations, and self-rewards. Although this is a very small study and certainly requires replication with a larger sample, it is the only study to demonstrate the superiority of CBT compared with another active intervention in the treatment of youths with anxiety disorders.

Two studies (Goldbeck & Schmid, 2003; Wenck et al., 1996) evaluated the effect of stress management techniques that were not embedded in a more comprehensive CBT protocol. Goldbeck and Schmid (2003) studied 50 children and adolescents with a variety of somatic, attentional, and anxiety complaints. These participants scored 1 SD above the normative mean on the Internalizing scale of the Child Behavior Checklist (CBCL; Achenbach, 1991) but in the average range on the Externalizing scale. Compared with those randomized to a wait-list control group, participants who received autogenic training (10 minutes a week for 8 weeks) showed a significant decrease in parent-reported internalizing and externalizing symptoms. Importantly, after treatment, scores on the Internalizing scale were within 1 *SD* of the normative mean, that is, in the average range. Effect sizes for differences between the groups were in the moderate range (e.g., 0.49). Children in both groups (treatment and wait-list control) reported decreased stress and somatic complaints. Wenck et al. (1996) reported that youths who received 12 sessions of biofeedback training (split evenly between thermal biofeedback and EMG biofeedback) had significantly lower self-reports of state and trait anxiety after treatment than did those in a wait-list control group.

Although all of the preceding studies focused on anxiety in youths, none included youths with PD or obsessive–compulsive disorder (OCD). Ollendick (1995) studied four adolescents with PD with agoraphobia using a multiple baseline design across participants. Treatment followed from behavioral programs developed for adults and included breathing retraining, applied relaxation, and other CBT components within an interoceptive conditioning exposure framework. Although treatment duration varied for participants, all exhibited an elimination of panic attacks and a lessening of agoraphobic avoidance, as well as of other anxiety and depressive symptoms.

As two independent research groups have shown CBT to be more efficacious than no treatment (i.e., wait-list control) in methodologically sound RCTs of children and adolescents with anxiety disorders (not including PD and OCD), CBT may be considered efficacious in the treatment of these disorders. However, CBT for these disorders cannot be considered efficacious and specific because it has not been shown to be more efficacious than other forms of treatment. Future studies should focus on comparing CBT with placebo and/or other active treatments. In addition, more research with samples of youths with PD and OCD is needed. Finally, more research is needed with respect to the specific effects of relaxation training and biofeedback for anxiety disorders. Although CBT protocols often include relaxation training, other than some evidence provided by Kendall and Southam-Gerow (1996), little is known about the specific effect of relaxation training among youths with anxiety disorders. In addition, although biofeedback has been utilized independently among youths with anxiety symptoms (Wenck et al., 1996), its effect in treating youths with anxiety disorders is unknown.

School Refusal

School refusal, defined as "difficulty attending school associated with emotional distress, especially anxiety and depression" (King & Bernstein, 2001, p. 197), is a problem for an estimated 5% of youths (King, Ollendick, & Tonge, 1995). Treatments for school refusal have been the focus of two recent reviews (King & Bernstein, 2001; King, Tonge, Heyne, & Ollendick, 2000). Based on the results of two randomized trials (King et al., 1998; Last, Hansen, & Franco, 1998), CBT for school refusal is efficacious, but not efficacious and specific, because it is not superior to an attention placebo (Last et al., 1998). In fact, when added to CBT, a pharmacological treatment (imipramine) has been shown to be more effective than CBT plus placebo (Bernstein et al., 2000).

School refusal is a heterogeneous behavior that may be associated with a variety of psychological symptoms. Although anxiety-related symptoms and disorders play a role in many cases, other psychiatric symptoms and disorders (e.g., oppositional defiant symptoms) may come into play when youths receive reinforcement for being out of school. Therefore, the majority of studies on the treatment of school refusal appear to contain samples of youths with more anxiety-based difficulties than other difficulties. As such, CBT for these youths closely resembles that developed for treatment of anxiety disorders discussed previously. For example, King and colleagues (1998) were influenced by Kendall's (1994) Coping Cat protocol in developing and implementing a six-session protocol that included relaxation training (specifically, cue-controlled relaxation and differential relaxation), coping skills training, and graduated exposure to school. Compared with those in a wait-list control condition, those who received the intervention showed less anxiety and improved school attendance, with almost 90% (vs. 30% in the control condition) attending school more than 90% of days. The CBT provided in the Last et al. (1998) trial does not appear to have included specific training in relaxation but instead focused on coping self-statements and graduated exposure. As alluded to earlier, this treatment was effective but not superior to an educational-support therapy control treatment.

One more recent study (Heyne et al., 2002) compared the efficacy of CBT, parent–teacher training, and CBT plus parent–teacher training. The CBT intervention included a relaxation training component specifically intended as a coping skill for children to use during exposure to school and for dealing with peer questions. The type of relaxation training was not specified. Although the combined treatment initially outperformed CBT, this was not the case at follow-up an average of 4.5 months later, at which time there was no difference in the efficacy of the treatments.

Thus, as with studies of the anxiety disorders previously discussed, CBT appears to be an efficacious treatment for school refusal. The specific role of stress management techniques (i.e., relaxation training) in the effectiveness of CBT for this population is unknown.

Tic and Habit Disorders

Habit reversal training (Azrin & Nunn, 1973) has been the primary nonpharmacological treatment for tic and habit disorders. Although relaxation is a component of the habit reversal protocol, the vast majority of treatment effort is aimed at increasing awareness of the behavior and learning an incompatible response to use to interrupt the behavior. Because relaxation is a less emphasized aspect of the treatment, we do not focus on studies of the effects of habit reversal training but on the few studies (Bergin, Waranch, Brown, Carson, & Singer, 1998; Cohen, Barzilai, & Lahat, 1999; Kohen, 1996) that have evaluated the efficacy of primarily using stress management techniques to treat these disorders.

Bergin et al. (1998) utilized a variety of general and specific relaxation techniques (e.g., diaphragmatic breathing, applied relaxation), as well as EMG biofeedback to facilitate awareness training and relaxation, in a study of the treatment of tics among 23 children and adolescents with Tourette disorder. Participants were randomized either to the treatment just described or to a "minimal therapy" group in which awareness training was taught and participants had "quiet time training" that consisted of sitting quietly while listening to music or environmental sounds. Although the study was relatively small, its two strengths were assessments of whether participants in the relaxation group learned relaxation and whether they practiced relaxation at home as directed (the latter was monitored electronically without the participants' awareness). Results indicated that although patients in the relaxation group practiced relaxation only 25% of the prescribed amount, a significantly greater percentage (73% vs. 45%) were found to be relaxed (using a validated behavioral relaxation scale; Norton, Holm, & McSherry, 1997; Poppen, 1988) at 6-week follow-up. Despite this finding, posttreatment differences between the groups in tic behavior (as measured by five separate severity rating instruments) were not significant. However, across both groups, the percentages of children showing improvement on each tic severity scale was over 40% and was 100% on one scale in the treatment group. It is possible that the failure to find a difference between the treatment groups resulted from the fact that the minimal treatment group received relaxation benefit from the "quiet time" portion of the treatment.

This study highlights an important and often neglected aspect of research in the area of stress management in the treatment of children and adolescents. Oftentimes, research has attempted to evaluate the efficacy of a treatment on an outcome behavior without determining whether changes in outcome (if they occur) are related to changes in mediating variables (e.g., cognitive changes, ability to achieve a relaxed state, ability to alter a parameter being measured by biofeedback) that are conceptualized as being changed by the treatment to influence outcome (Prins & Ollendick, 2003). The field could certainly be advanced by research that measures both mediating and outcome variables.

Two case study reports (Cohen et al., 1999; Kohen, 1996) have evaluated the efficacy of self-hypnosis (relaxation with guided imagery and suggestion directed at the habit behavior) among 8 children and young adolescents with trichotillomania, an impulse-control disorder characterized by habitual hair pulling that can lead to significant hair loss. Both studies showed that patients reported subjective improvement in symptoms (as rated on a 10-point scale). Although these studies represent a useful beginning, more controlled research is needed in which hypnotherapy is compared with other treatments and outcomes are measured with more diverse (and objective) methods.

Although biofeedback has not been widely studied in the treatment of tic and habit disorders, this is an area that could be pursued. Bergin et al. (1998) included EMG biofeedback in their protocol but did not report on patients' use of this part of the intervention. It would be interesting to know whether EMG biofeedback could be used to help children and adolescents increase awareness of the tic or habit behavior and help in the learning and training of an incompatible response.

ADHD and Learning Disorder

Lehrer et al. (1993), in the previous edition of this book, cited some research from the 1970s and 1980s (see Cobb & Evans, 1981 for a review) supporting the use of EMG biofeedback in the treatment of hyperactivity. However, two more recent comprehensive reviews of treatments for ADHD (Chan, 2002; Pelham, Wheeler, & Chronis, 1998) are not supportive of such treatment. Pelham et al. (1998) goes so far as to list biofeedback among treatments that have been shown *not* to be effective in treating ADHD. In her review of complementary and alternative medicine treatments for ADHD, Chan (2002) concludes that relaxation and biofeedback therapies may show some promise but are plagued by being understudied and by being evaluated in studies with small samples. It appears that since the 1980s relatively less research on the effects of relaxation and bio-

TABLE 24.6. Efficacy of Stress Management Therapies for Childhood Emotional and Behavioral Problems

Disorder/problem	Intervention	Treatment efficacy
Anxiety disorders		
GAD, SAD, social phobia	CBT[a]	Efficacious
Panic disorder	CBT[a]	More research needed
OCD	CBT[a]	More research needed
School refusal	CBT[a]	Efficacious
Tic and habit disorders	Relaxation training	More research needed
	EMG biofeedback	More research needed
ADHD	Relaxation training	More research needed
	EMG biofeedback	More research needed

[a] More research would be needed to determine the specific efficacy of relaxation training in the context of comprehensive CBT treatment.

feedback, as well as CBT, for ADHD has been conducted. (The same cannot be said for EEG biofeedback, which is beginning to be researched). Perhaps the reason is the demonstrated efficacy of pharmacological and behavioral (e.g., parent training) treatments and the difficulty in showing significant improvement over what those treatments can offer. Despite these challenges, there continues to be some interest in applying stress management techniques with children with ADHD (e.g., Gonzalez & Sellers, 2002), but more controlled research with larger samples is clearly needed before any positive conclusions about the efficacy of such intervention can be made (see Table 24.6).

CONCLUSIONS

The literature on stress management therapies for emotional and behavioral disorders has been dominated by studies of CBT. The field has advanced in the adult literature to examine the dismantling of CBT into its separate core components (e.g., cognitive restructuring, exposure, relaxation). Although the complete CBT package appears to be most effective for treatment of PD, individual components of CBT are efficacious for treatment of PTSD, GAD, and SAD. The combination of CBT and pharmacotherapy is not recommended at the present time for treatment of anxiety disorders due to higher relapse rates. CBT has been shown to be efficacious for treatment of anger; however, it is important to consider the dimension of anger that is being treated when selecting relaxation, CT, or the complete CBT package. CBT has also been established as an efficacious treatment for depression and substance abuse.

A number of alternatives to CBT have been developed and empirically tested. EMDR may be an efficacious treatment for PTSD, although the saccadic eye movements do not appear to be an active component of the treatment. Further research is needed to establish the efficacy of EMDR for treatment of other anxiety disorders. IPT has been established as an efficacious treatment for depression, and research is ongoing to determine whether IPT may be useful for anxiety disorders as well. Treatment for depression has also expanded to include exercise, CBASP, and BA, each of which has shown promising results in controlled studies. MI/MET and self-help/12-step groups are two types of treatments that have been established as efficacious for substance abuse. FT is a new treatment that has shown promising results in the treatment of substance abuse. Finally, there has been renewed interest in exploring adjunctive treatments to pharmacological management of patients with schizophrenia. Family therapy, CBT, and CT appear to be useful for improving outcome among various components of psychosis. Unfortunately, research on more traditional stress management approaches (e.g., yoga, meditation, biofeedback, hypnosis) continues to lag behind. Support for these therapies has primarily been derived from anecdotal evidence and uncontrolled studies.

Therapies for children and adolescents are relatively understudied compared with therapies for adults. Therefore, more research is needed to establish efficacy for most emotional and behavioral disorders among children. There is currently a concerted effort in the area of anxiety disorders to determine efficacy and specificity of CBT by comparing it with placebo and/or active treatment. With respect to determining the specific effects and efficacy of relaxation and/or biofeedback, this would require dismantling of treatment for patients whose symptoms reach the level of disorder. However, studying subsyndromal patients who do not require as comprehensive an approach may be more effective.

Finally, the notion of treatment matching has received increasing attention in recent years. The NIMH Treatment of Depression Collaborative Research Program showed that individuals might respond better to therapies that are more in line with their strengths than with their weaknesses (Sotsky et al., 1991). However, a multisite treatment outcome study of alcohol dependence was designed to examine treatment matching and failed to find support for its primary hypotheses (Project MATCH Research Group, 1997). Therefore, it is difficult to determine which subgroups of individuals will respond to specific treatment modalities. Since the previous edition of this volume (Lehrer et al., 1993), more nonpharmacological approaches have been established as efficacious treatments. Thus clinicians have more choices to consider in selecting efficacious treatments for emotional and behavioral disorders. A key area for future research will be to identify patient characteristics that predict differential responses to these treatments. Additionally, disseminating efficacious therapies to clinicians in the community also remains a top priority.

REFERENCES

Achenbach, T. M. (1991). *Integrative guide to the 1991 CBCL, YSR, and TRF profiles*. Burlington: University of Vermont, Department of Psychiatry.

Arntz, A. (2003). Cognitive therapy versus applied relaxation as treatment of generalized anxiety disorder. *Behaviour Research and Therapy, 41*, 633–646.

Arntz, A., & van Den Hout, M. (1996). Psychological treatments of panic disorder without agoraphobia: Cognitive therapy versus applied relaxation. *Behaviour Research and Therapy, 34*, 113–121.

Azrin, N. H., & Nunn, R. G. (1973). Habit reversal: A method of eliminating nervous habits and tics. *Behaviour Research and Therapy, 11*, 619–628.

Babyak, M., Blumenthal, J. A., Herman, S., Khatri, P., Doraiswamy, M., Moore, K., et al. (2000). Exercise treatment for major depression: Maintenance of therapeutic benefit at 10 months. *Psychosomatic Medicine, 62*, 633–638.

Barlow, D. H., Gorman, J. M., Shear, M. K., & Woods, S. W. (2000). Cognitive-behavioral therapy, imipramine, or their combination for panic disorder: A randomized controlled trail. *Journal of the American Medical Association, 283*, 2529–2536.

Beck, A. T., & Emery, G. (1985). *Anxiety disorders and phobias: A cognitive perspective*. New York: Guilford Press.

Beck, A. T., Rush, A. J., Shaw, B. F., & Emery, G. (1979). *Cognitive therapy of depression*. New York: Guilford Press.

Beck, A. T., Sokol, L., Clark, D. A., Berchick, R., & Wright, F. (1992). A crossover study of focused cognitive therapy for panic disorder. *American Journal of Psychiatry, 149*, 778–783.

Beck, J. G., Stanley, M. A., Baldwin, L. E., Deagle, E. A., & Averill, P. M. (1994). Comparison of cognitive therapy and relaxation training for panic disorder. *Journal of Consulting and Clinical Psychology, 62*, 818–826.

Beck, R., & Fernandez, E. (1998). Cognitive-behavioral therapy in the treatment of anger: A meta-analysis. *Cognitive Therapy and Research, 1*, 63–74.

Bellack, A. S., & Muesser, K. T. (1993). Psychosocial treatment of schizophrenia. *Schizophrenia Bulletin, 19*, 317–336.

Benton, M. K., & Schroeder, H. E. (1990). Social skills training with schizophrenics: A meta-analytic evaluation. *Journal of Consulting and Clinical Psychology, 58*, 741–747.

Bergin, A., Waranch, H. R., Brown, J., Carson, K., & Singer, H. S. (1998). Relaxation therapy in Tourette syndrome: A pilot study. *Pediatric Neurology, 18*, 136–142.

Berkowitz, R., Eberlein-Freis, R., Kuipers, L., & Leff, J. (1984). Educating relatives about schizophrenia. *Schizophrenia Bulletin, 10*, 418–429.

Bernstein, D. A., & Borkovec, T. D. (1973). *Progressive relaxation training.* Champaign, IL: Research Press.

Bernstein, G. A., Borchardt, C. M., Perwien, A. R., Crosby, R. K., Kushner, M. G., Thuras, P. D., et al. (2000). Imipramine plus cognitive-behavioral therapy in the treatment of school refusal. *Journal of the American Academy of Child and Adolescent Psychiatry, 39*, 276–283.

Blatt, S. J., Zuroff, D. C., Bondi, C. M., & Sanisolow, C. A., III. (2000). Short and long-term effects of medication and psychotherapy in the brief treatment of depression: Further analyses of data from NIMH TDCRP. *Journal of Psychotherapy Practice and Research, 10*, 215–234.

Blomhoff, S., Haug, T. T., Hellstrom, K., Holme, I., Humble, M., Madsbu, H. P., et al. (2001). Randomised controlled general practice trial of sertraline, exposure therapy and combined treatment in generalised social phobia. *British Journal of Psychiatry, 179*, 23–30.

Blumenthal, J. A., Babyak, M. A., Moore, K. A., Craighead, W. E., Herman, S., Khatri, P., et al. (1999). Effects of exercise training on older patients with major depression. *Archives of Internal Medicine, 159*, 2349–2356.

Boczkowski, J. A., Zeichner, A., & DeSanto, N. (1985). Neuroleptic compliance among chronic schizophrenic outpatients: An intervention outcome report. *Journal of Consulting and Clinical Psychology, 53*, 666–671.

Bolton, P., Bass, J., Neugebauer, R., Verdeli, H., Clougherty, K. F., Wickramaratne, P., et al. (2003). Group interpersonal psychotherapy for depression in rural Uganda: A randomized controlled trial. *Journal of the American Medical Association, 289*, 3117–3124.

Borkovec, T. D., & Costello, E. (1993). Efficacy of applied relaxation and cognitive-behavioral therapy in the treatment of generalized anxiety disorder. *Journal of Consulting and Clinical Psychology, 61*, 611–619.

Borkovec, T. D., Newman, M. G., & Castonguay, L. G. (2003). Cognitive-behavioral therapy for generalized anxiety disorder with integrations from interpersonal and experiential therapies. *CNS Spectrums, 8*, 382–389.

Borkovec, T. D., Newman, M. G., Pincus, A. L., & Lytle, R. (2002). A component analysis of cognitive-behavioral therapy for generalized anxiety disorder and the role of interpersonal problems. *Journal of Consulting and Clinical Psychology, 70*, 288–298.

Borkovec, T. D., & Ruscio, A. M. (2001). Psychotherapy for generalized anxiety disorder. *Journal of Clinical Psychiatry, 62*(Suppl. 11), 37–42.

Bouchard, S., Gauthier, J., Laberge, B., French, D., Pelletier, M. H., & Godbout, C. (1996). Exposure versus cognitive restructuring in the treatment of panic disorder with agoraphobia. *Behaviour Research and Therapy, 34*, 213–224.

Brooner, R. K., Kidorf, M. S., King, V. L., Stoller, K. B., Peirce, J. M., Bigelow, G. E., et al. (2004). Behavioral contingencies improve counseling attendance in an adaptive treatment model. *Journal of Substance Abuse Treatment, 27*, 223–232.

Brown, G. W., Birley, J. L. T., & Wing, J. K. (1972). Influences of family life on the course of schizophrenic disorders: A replication. *British Journal of Psychiatry, 121*, 241–258.

Buchman, B. P., Sallis, J. F., Criqui, M. H., Dimsdale, J. E., & Kaplan, R. M. (1991). Physical activity, physical fitness, and psychological characteristics of medical students. *Journal of Psychosomatic Research, 35*, 197–208.

Burke, B. L., Arkowitz, H., & Menchola, M. (2003). The efficacy of motivational interviewing: A meta-analysis of controlled clinical trials. *Journal of Consulting and Clinical Psychology*, *71*, 843–861.

Byrne, A., & Byrne, D. G. (1993). The effect of exercise on depression, anxiety and other mood states: A review. *Journal of Psychosomatic Research*, *37*, 565–574.

Camacho, T. C., Roberts, R. E., Lazarus, N. B., Kaplan, G. A., & Cohen, R. D. (1991). Physical activity and depression: Evidence from the Almeda County Study. *American Journal of Epidemiology*, *134*, 220–231.

Cameron, O. G., & Hudson, C. J. (1986). Influence of exercise on anxiety level in patients with anxiety disorders. *Psychosomatics*, *27*, 720–723.

Carlbring, P., Ekselius, L., & Andersson, G. (2003). Treatment of panic disorder via the Internet: A randomized trial of CBT vs. applied relaxation. *Journal of Behavior Therapy and Experimental Psychiatry*, *34*, 129–140.

Chambless, D. L., & Hollon, S. D. (1998). Defining empirically supported therapies. *Journal of Consulting and Clinical Psychology*, *66*, 7–18.

Chambless, D. L., & Hope, D. A. (1996). Cognitive approaches to the psychopathology and treatment of social phobia. In P. M. Salkovskis (Ed.), *Frontiers of cognitive therapy* (pp. 345–382). New York: Guilford Press.

Chambless, D. L., & Ollendick, T. H. (2001). Empirically supported psychological interventions: Controversies and evidence. *Annual Review of Psychology*, *52*, 685–716.

Chan, E. (2002). The role of complementary and alternative medicine in attention-deficit hyperactivity disorder. *Developmental and Behavioral Pediatrics*, *23*(1S), S37–S45.

Chang, P. P., Ford, D. E., Meoni, L. A., Wang, N. Y., & Klag, M. J. (2002). Anger in young men and subsequent premature cardiovascular disease: The precursors study. *Archives of Internal Medicine*, *22*, 901–906.

Clark, D. M. (1989). Anxiety states: Panic and generalized anxiety. In K. Hawton, P. Salkovskis, J. Kirk, & D. M. Clark (Eds.), *Cognitive behaviour therapy for psychiatric problems: A practical guide* (pp. 52–96). Oxford, UK: Oxford University Press.

Clark, D. M., Salkovskis, P. M., Hackmann, A., Middleton, H., Anastasiades, P., & Gelder, M. (1994). A comparison of cognitive therapy, applied relaxation and imipramine in the treatment of panic disorder. *British Journal of Psychiatry*, *164*, 759–769.

Clum, G. A., Clum, G. A., & Surls, R. (1993). A meta-analysis of treatments for panic disorder. *Journal of Consulting and Clinical Psychology*, *61*, 317–326.

Cobb, D. E., & Evans, J. R. (1981). The use of biofeedback techniques with school-age children exhibiting behavioral and/or learning problems. *Journal of Abnormal Child Psychology*, *9*, 251–281.

Cohen, H. A., Barzilai, A., & Lahat, E. (1999). Hypnotherapy: An effective treatment modality for trichotillomania. *Acta Paediatrica*, *88*, 407–410.

Coon, D. W., Thompson, L., Steffen, A., Sorocco, K., & Gallagher-Thompson, D. (2003). Anger and depression management: Psychoeducational skills training interventions for women caregivers of a relative with dementia. *Gerontologist*, *43*, 678–689.

Craske, M. G., Barlow, D. H., & Meadows, E. A. (2000). *Mastery of your anxiety and panic (MAP-3): Therapist guide for anxiety, panic, and agoraphobia*. San Antonio, TX: Psychological Corporation.

Craske, M. G., Brown, T. A., & Barlow, D. H. (1991). Behavioral treatment of panic: A two-year follow-up. *Behavior Therapy*, *22*, 289–304.

Craske, M. G., Maidenberg E., & Bystritsky, A. (1995). Brief cognitive-behavioral versus nondirective therapy for panic disorder. *Journal of Behavior Therapy and Experimental Psychiatry*, *26*, 113–120.

Culbert, T. P., Kajander, R. L., & Reaney, J. B. (1996). Biofeedback with children and adolescents: Clinical observations and patient perspectives. *Developmental and Behavioral Pediatrics*, *17*, 342–350.

Davidson, J. R., Foa, E. B., Huppert, J. D., Keefe, F. J., Franklin, M. E., Compton, J. S., et al. (2004). Fluoxetine, comprehensive cognitive-behavioral therapy, and placebo in generalized social phobia. *Archives of General Psychiatry*, *61*, 1005–1013.

Davidson, J. R. T., Miner, C. M., de Veaugh Geiss, J., Tupler, L. A., Colket, J. T., & Potts, N. L. S. (1997). The Brief Social Phobia Scale: A psychometric evaluation. *Psychological Medicine*, *27*, 161–166.

Deffenbacher, J. L., Dahlen, E. R., Lynch, R. S., Morris, C. D., & Gowensmith, W. N. (2000). An application of Beck's cognitive therapy to general anger reduction. *Cognitive Therapy and Research*, *24*, 689–697.

Deffenbacher, J. L., Filetti, L. B., Lynch, R. S., Dahlen, E. R., & Oetting, E. R. (2002). Cognitive-behavioral treatment of high anger drivers. *Behaviour Research and Therapy, 40*, 895–910.

Deffenbacher, J. L., Oetting, E. R., & Lynch, R. S. (1994). Development of a driving anger scale. *Psychological Reports, 74*, 83–91.

Del Vecchio, T., & O'Leary, K. D. (2004). Effectiveness of anger treatments for specific anger problems: A meta-analytic review. *Clinical Psychology Review, 24*, 15–34.

Denney, M. R., & Baugh, J. L. (1992). Symptom reduction and sobriety in the male alcoholic. *International Journal of the Addictions, 27*, 1293–1300.

Devilly, G. (2002). The psychological effects of a lifestyle management course on war veterans and their spouses. *Journal of Clinical Psychology, 58*, 1119–1134.

Devilly, G. J., & Spence, S. H. (1999). The relative efficacy and treatment distress of EMDR and a cognitive-behavior trauma treatment protocol in the amelioration of posttraumatic stress disorder. *Journal of Anxiety Disorders, 13*, 131–157.

Drury, V., Birchwood, M., Cochrane, R., & Macmillan, F. (1996). Cognitive therapy and recovery from acute psychosis: A controlled trial. I. Impact on psychotic symptoms. *British Journal of Psychiatry, 169*, 593–601.

Dua, J. K., & Swinden, M. L. (1992). Effectiveness of negative-thought reduction, meditation, and placebo training treatment in reducing anger. *Scandinavian Journal of Psychology, 33*, 135–146.

Eckman, T. A., & Liberman, R. P. (1990) A large-scale field test of a medication management skills training program for people with schizophrenia. *Psychosocial Rehabilitation Journal, 13*, 31–35.

Elkin, I., Shea, M. T., Watkins, J. T., Imber, S. D., Sotsky, S. M., Collins, J. F., et al. (1989). National Institute of Mental Health treatment of depression collaborative research program. *Archives of General Psychiatry, 46*, 971–982.

Eng, W., Coles, M. E., Heimberg, R. G., & Safren, S. A. (2001). Quality of life following cognitive-behavioral treatment for social anxiety disorder: Preliminary findings. *Depression and Anxiety, 13*, 192–193.

Eng, W., Coles, M. E., Heimberg, R. G., & Safren, S. A. (2005). Domains of life satisfaction in social anxiety disorder: Relation to symptoms and response to cognitive-behavioral therapy. *Journal of Anxiety Disorders, 19*, 143–156.

Falloon, I., Coverdale, J., & Booker, C. (1996). Psychosocial interventions in schizophrenia: A review. *International Journal of Mental Health, 25,*3–21.

Farmer, M. E., Locke, B. Z., Moscicki, E. K., Dannenberg, A. L., Larson, D. B., & Radloff, L. S. (1988). Physical activity and depressive symptoms: The NHANES I epidemiologic follow-up study. *American Journal of Epidemiology, 28*, 1320–1351.

Federoff, I. C., & Taylor, S. (2001). Psychological and pharmacological treatments of social phobia: A meta-analysis. *Journal of Clinical Psychopharmacology, 21*, 311–324.

Feiger, A. D., Bielski, R. J., Bremner, J., Heiser, J. F., Trivedi, M., Wilcox, C. S., et al. (1999). Double-blind, placebo-substitution study of nefazodone in the prevention of relapse during continuation treatment of outpatients with major depression. *International Clinical Psychopharmacology, 14*, 19–28.

Feske, U., & Chambless, D. L. (1995). Cognitive-behavioral versus exposure-only treatment for social phobia: A meta-analysis. *Behaviour Therapy, 26*, 695–720.

Feske, U., & Goldstein, A. J. (1997). Eye movement desensitization and reprocessing treatment for panic disorder: A controlled outcome and partial dismantling study. *Journal of Consulting and Clinical Psychology, 65*, 1026–1035.

Foa, E. B., Dancu, C. V., Hembree, E. A., Jaycox, L. H., Meadows, E. A., & Street, G. P. (1999). A comparison of exposure therapy, stress inoculation training, and their combination for reducing posttraumatic stress disorder in female assault victims. *Journal of Consulting and Clinical Psychology, 67*, 194–200.

Foa, E. B., Franklin, M. E., & Moser, J. (2002). Context in the clinic: How well do cognitive-behavioral therapies and medications work in combination? *Biological Psychiatry, 52*, 987–997.

Foa, E. B., Rothbaum, B. O., Riggs, D. S., & Murdock T. B. (1991). Treatment of posttraumatic stress disorder in rape victims: A comparison between cognitive-behavioral procedures and counseling. *Journal of Consulting and Clinical Psychology, 59*, 715–723.

Fowles, D. (1992). Schizophrenia: Diathesis–stress revisited. *Annual Review of Psychology, 43*, 303–336.

Futterman, A., & Shapiro, D. (1986). Review of biofeedback for mental disorders. *Hospital and Community Psychiatry, 34,* 27–33.

Galovski, T. E., Blanchard, E. B., Malta, L. S., & Freidenberg, B. M. (2003). The psychophysiology of aggressive drivers: Comparison to non-aggressive drivers and pre- to post-treatment change following a cognitive-behavioural treatment. *Behaviour Research and Therapy, 40,* 895–910.

Gillies, L. A. (2001). Interpersonal psychotherapy for depression and other disorders. In D. H. Barlow (Ed.), *Clinical handbook of psychological disorders* (pp. 309–331). New York: Guilford Press.

Ginsburg, G. S., & Drake, K. L. (2002). School-based treatment for anxious African-American adolescents: A controlled pilot study. *Journal of the American Academy of Child and Adolescent Psychiatry, 41,* 768–775.

Goldbeck, L., & Schmid, K. (2003). Effectiveness of autogenic relaxation training on children and adolescents with behavioral and emotional problems. *Journal of the American Academy of Child and Adolescent Psychiatry, 42,* 1046–1054.

Goldstein, A. J., de Beurs, E., Chambless, D. L., & Wilson, K. A. (2000). EMDR for panic disorder with agoraphobia: Comparison with waiting list and credible attention-placebo control conditions. *Journal of Consulting and Clinical Psychology, 68,* 947–956.

Gonzalez, L. O., & Sellers, E. W. (2002). The effects of a stress-management program on self-concept, locus of control, and the acquisition of coping skills in school-age children diagnosed with attention deficit hyperactivity disorder. *Journal of Child and Adolescent Psychiatric Nursing, 15,* 5–15.

Gordis, E. (1991). Linking research with practice: Common bonds, common progress. *Alcohol Health and Research World, 15,* 173–174.

Gould, R. A., Buckminster, S., Pollack, M. H., Otto, M. W., & Yap, L. (1997). Cognitive-behavioral and pharmacological treatment for social phobia: A meta-analysis. *Clinical Psychology: Science and Practice, 4,* 291–306.

Gould, R. A., Mueser, K. T., Bolton, E., Mays, V., & Goff, D. (2001). Cognitive therapy for psychosis in schizophrenia: An effect size analysis. *Schizophrenia Research, 48,* 335–342.

Gould, R. A., Otto, M. W., & Pollack, M. H. (1995). A meta-analysis of treatment outcome for panic disorder. *Clinical Psychology Review, 15,* 819–844.

Greeff, A. P., & Conradie, W. S. (1998). Use of progressive relaxation training for chronic alcoholics with insomnia. *Psychological Reports, 82,* 407–412.

Guy, W. (1976). *ECDEU assessment manual for psychopharmacology* (Revised ed., DHEW Publication No. ADM76-338). Washington, DC: U.S. Government Printing Office.

Hall, S. M., Wasserman, D. A., & Havassy, B. E. (1991). Effects of commitment to abstinence, positive moods, stress, and coping on relapse to cocaine use. *Journal of Consulting and Clinical Psychology, 59,* 526–532.

Hambrick, J. P., Weeks, J. W., Harb, G. C., & Heimberg, R. G. (2003). Cognitive-behavioral therapy for social anxiety disorder: Supporting evidence and future directions. *CNS Spectrums, 8,* 373–381.

Hamilton, M. (1959). The measurement of anxiety states by rating. *British Journal of Medical Psychology, 32,* 50–55.

Harburg, E., Julius, M., Kaciroti, N., Gleiberman, L., & Schork, M. A. (2003). Expressive/suppressive anger-coping responses, gender, and types of mortality: A 17-year follow-up (Tecumseh, Michigan, 1971–1988). *Psychosomatic Medicine, 65,* 588–597.

Hassmen, P., Koivula, N., & Uutela, A. (2000). Physical exercise and psychological well-being: A population study in Finland. *Preventive Medicine, 30,* 17–25.

Haug, T. T., Blomhoff, S., Hellstrom, K., Holme, I., Humble, M., Madsbu, H. P., et al. (2003). Exposure therapy and sertraline in social phobia: 1-year follow-up of a randomised controlled trial. *British Journal of Psychiatry, 182,* 312–318.

Hausenblas, H. A., Dannecker, E. A., & Focht, B. C. (2001). Psychological effects of exercise with general and diseased populations. *Journal of Psychotherapy in Independent Practice, 2,* 27–47.

Heimberg, R. G., Juster, H. R., Hope, D. A., & Mattia, J. I. (1995). Cognitive-behavioral group treatment: Description, case presentation, and empirical support. In M. B. Stein (Ed.), *Social phobia: Clinical and research perspectives* (pp. 293–321). Washington, DC: American Psychiatric Press.

Heimberg, R. G., Liebowitz, M. R., Hope, D. A., Schneier, F. R., Holt, C. S., Welkowitz, L. A., et al. (1998). Cognitive-behavioral group therapy vs. phenelzine therapy for social phobia: 12-week outcome. *Archives of General Psychiatry, 55,* 1133–1141.

Heimberg, R. G., Saltzman, D. G., Holt, C. S., & Blendell, K. A. (1993). Cognitive behavioral group treatment for social phobia: Effectiveness at five-year follow-up. *Cognitive Therapy and Research, 17*, 325–339.

Helzer, J. E., & Pryzbeck, T. R. (1988). The co-occurrence of alcoholism with other psychiatric disorders in the general population and its impact on treatment. *Journal of Studies on Alcohol, 49*, 219–224.

Heyne, D., King, N. J., Tonge, B. J., Rollings, S., Young, D., Pritchard, M., et al. (2002). Evaluation of child therapy and caregiver training in the treatment of school refusal. *Journal of the American Academy of Child and Adolescent Psychiatry, 41*, 687–695.

Hoehn-Saric, R., McLeod, D. R., Funderburk, F., & Kowalski, P. (2004). Somatic symptoms and physiologic responses in generalized anxiety disorder and panic disorder: An ambulatory monitor study. *Archives of General Psychiatry, 61*, 913–921.

Hofmann, S. G. (2004). Cognitive mediation of treatment change in social phobia. *Journal of Consulting and Clinical Psychology, 72*, 393–399.

Hogarty, G. E., Anderson, C. M., Reiss, D. J., Kornblith, S. J., Greenwald, P., Javna, C. D., et al. (1986). Family psychoeducation, social skills training, and maintenance chemotherapy in the aftercare treatment of schizophrenia: I. One-year effects of a controlled study on relapse and expressed emotion. *Archives of General Psychiatry, 43*, 633–642.

Hogarty, G. E., Anderson, C. M., Reiss, D. J., Kornblith, S. J., Greenwald, D. P., Ulrich, R. F., et al. (1991). Family psychoeducation, social skills training, and maintenance chemotherapy in the aftercare treatment of schizophrenia: II. Two-year effects of a controlled study on relapse and adjustment. *Archives of General Psychiatry, 48*, 340–347.

Holden, E. W., Deichmann, M. M., & Levy, J. (1999). Empirically supported treatments in pediatric psychology: Recurrent pediatric headache. *Journal of Pediatric Psychology, 24*, 91–99.

Hope, D. A., Heimberg, R. G., & Bruch, M. A. (1995). Dismantling cognitive-behavioral group therapy for social phobia. *Behaviour Research and Therapy, 33*, 637–650.

Hopko, D. R., Lejuez, C. W., Ruggiero, K. J., & Eifert, G. H. (2003). Contemporary behavioral activation treatments for depression: Procedures, principles, and progress. *Clinical Psychology Review, 23*, 699–717.

Hudson, J. L., & Kendall, P. C. (2002). Showing you can do it: Homework in therapy for children and adolescents with anxiety disorders. *Journal of Pediatric Psychology/In Session, 58*, 525–534.

Huxley, N. A., Rendall, M., & Sederer, L. (2000). Psychosocial treatments in schizophrenia: A review of the past 20 years. *Journal of Nervous and Mental Disease, 188*, 187–201.

Imber, S. D., Pilkonis, P. A., Sotsky, S. M., Elkin, I., Watkins, J. T., Collins, J. F., et al. (1990). Mode-specific effects among three treatments for depression. *Journal of Consulting and Clinical Psychology, 58*, 352–359.

Inouye, J., Flannelly, L., & Flannelly, K. J. (2001). The effectiveness of self-management training for individuals with HIV/AIDS. *Journal of the Association of Nurses in AIDS Care, 12*, 73–84.

Jacobson, N. S., Dobson, K. S., Truax, P. A., Addis, M. E., & Koerner, K. (1996). A component analysis of cognitive-behavioral treatment for depression. *Journal of Consulting and Clinical Psychology, 64*, 295–304.

Janakiramaiah, N., Gangadhar, B. N., Naga Venkatesha Murthy, P. J., Harish, M. G., Subbakrishna, D. K., & Vedamurthachar, A. (2000). Anti-depressant efficacy of sudarshan kriya yoga (SKY) in melancholia: A randomized comparison with electroconvulsive therapy (ECT) and imipramine. *Journal of Affective Disorders, 57*, 255–259.

Jerremalm, A., Jansson, L., & Öst, L. G. (1986). Cognitive and physiological reactivity and the effects of different behavioral methods in the treatment of social phobia. *Behaviour Research and Therapy, 24*, 171–180.

Kabat-Zinn, J., Massion, A. O., Kristeller, J., Peterson, L. G., Fletcher, K. E., Pbert, L., et al. (1992). Effectiveness of a meditation-based stress reduction program in the treatment of anxiety disorders. *American Journal of Psychiatry, 149*, 936–943.

Keller, M. B., McCullough, J. P., Klein, D. N., Arnow, B., Dunner, D. L., Gelenberg, A. J., et al. (2000). A comparison of nefazodone, the cognitive-behavioral-analysis system of psychotherapy, and their combination for the treatment of chronic depression. *New England Journal of Medicine, 342*, 1462–1470.

Kemp, R., Hayward, P., Applewhaite, G., Everitt, B., & David, A. (1996). Compliance therapy in psychotic patients: Randomised controlled therapy. *British Medical Journal, 312*, 345–349.

Kendall, P. C. (1994). Treating anxiety disorders in children: Results of a randomized clinical trial. *Journal of Consulting and Clinical Psychology, 62*, 100–110.

Kendall, P. C., Flannery-Schroeder, E., Panichelli-Mindel, S. M., Southam-Gerow, M., Henin, A., & Warman, M. (1997). Therapy for youths with anxiety disorders: A second randomized clinical trial. *Journal of Consulting and Clinical Psychology, 65*, 366–380.

Kendall, P. C., Safford, S., Flannery-Schroeder, E., & Webb, A. (2004). Child anxiety treatment: Outcomes in adolescence and impact on substance use and depression at 7.4 year follow-up. *Journal of Consulting and Clinical Psychology, 72*, 276–287.

Kendall, P. C., & Southam-Gerow, M. A. (1996). Long-term follow-up of a cognitive-behavioral therapy for anxiety-disordered youth. *Journal of Consulting and Clinical Psychology, 64*, 724–730.

Kennedy, J. E., Abbott, R. A., & Rosenberg, B. S. (2002). Changes in spirituality and well-being in a retreat program for cardiac patients. *Alternative Therapies in Health and Medicine, 8*, 64–73.

King, N., Tonge, B. J., Heyne, D., & Ollendick, T. H. (2000). Research on the cognitive-behavioral treatment of school refusal: A review and recommendations. *Clinical Psychology Review, 20*, 495–507.

King, N. J., & Bernstein, G. A. (2001). School refusal in children and adolescents: A review of the past 10 years. *Journal of the American Academy of Child and Adolescent Psychiatry, 40*, 197–205.

King, N. J., Ollendick, T. H., & Tonge, B. J. (1995). *School refusal: Assessment and treatment.* Boston: Allyn & Bacon.

King, N. J., Tonge, B. J., Heyne, D., Pritchard, M., Rollings, S., Young, D., et al. (1998). Cognitive-behavioral treatment of school-refusing children: A controlled evaluation. *Journal of the American Academy of Child and Adolescent Psychiatry, 37*, 395–403.

Kirdorf, M., King, V. L., & Brooner, R. K. (1999). Integrating psychosocial services with methadone treatment: Behaviorally contingent pharmacotherapy. In E. C. Strain & M. L. Stitzer (Eds.), *Treatment of opioid dependence: Methadone and alternative medications* (pp. 166–195). Baltimore: Hopkin Press.

Klein, M. H., Gresits, J. H., Gunman, A. S., Neimeyev, R. A., Lesser, D. P., Busuell, N. J., et al. (1985). A comparative outcome study of group psychotherapy vs. exercise treatments for depression. *International Journal of Emergency Mental Health, 13*, 148–177.

Klosko, J. S., Barlow, D. H., Tassinari, R., & Cemy, J. A. (1990). A comparison of alprazolam and behavior therapy in treatment of panic disorder. *Journal of Consulting and Clinical Psychology, 58*, 77–84.

Koeppen, A. S. (1974). Relaxation training for children. *Elementary School Guidance and Counseling, 9*, 41–55.

Koh, K. B., Kim, C. H., & Park, J. K. (2002). Predominance of anger in depressive disorders compared with anxiety disorders and somatoform disorders. *Journal of Clinical Psychiatry, 63*, 486–92

Kohen, D. P. (1996). Hypnotherapeutic management of pediatric and adolescent trichotillomania. *Developmental and Behavioral Pediatrics, 17*, 328–334.

Kominars, K. D. (1997). A study of visualization and addiction treatment. *Journal of Substance Abuse Treatment, 14*, 213–223.

Kushner, M. G., Sher, K. J., & Beitman, B. D. (1990). The relation between alcohol problems and the anxiety disorders. *American Journal of Psychiatry, 147*, 685–695.

Lamarre, B. W., & Nosanchuck, T. A. (1999). Judo–the gentle way: A replication of studies on martial arts and aggression. *Perceptual and Motor Skills, 88*, 992–996.

Last, C. G., Hansen, C., & Franco, N. (1998). Cognitive-behavioral treatment of school phobia. *Journal of the American Academy of Child and Adolescent Psychiatry, 37*, 404–411.

Lawlor, D. A., & Hopker, S. W. (2001). The effectiveness of exercise as an intervention in the management of depression: Systematic review and meta-regression analysis of randomized controlled trials. *British Medical Journal, 322*, 763–781.

Lee, C., Gavriel, H., Drummond, P., Richards, J., & Greenwald, R. (2002). Treatment of PTSD: Stress inoculation training with prolonged exposure compared to EMDR. *Journal of Clinical Psychology, 58*, 1071–1089.

Lee, L. H., & Olness, K. N. (1996). Effects of self-induced mental imagery on autonomic reactivity in children. *Developmental and Behavioral Pediatrics, 17*, 323–327.

Leff, J., Kuipers, L., Berkowitz, R., Vaughn, C., & Sturgeon, D. (1983). Life events, relative's expressed emotion and maintenance neuroleptics in schizophrenia relapse. *Psychosocial Medicine, 13*, 799–806.

Lehrer, P. M., Carr, R., Sargunaraj, D., & Woolfolk, R. L. (1993). Differential effects of stress management therapies on emotional and behavioral disorders. In P. M. Lehrer & R. L. Woolfolk (Eds.), *Principles and practice of stress management* (2nd ed., pp. 539–569). New York: Guilford Press.

Liberman, R. P. (1994). Psychosocial treatments for schizophrenia. *Psychiatry, 57,* 104–114.

Liberman, R. P., Wallace, C. J., Blackwell, G., Koplewicz, A., Vaccaro, J. V., & Mintz, J. (1998). Skills training versus psychosocial occupational therapy for persons with persistent schizophrenia. *American Journal of Psychiatry, 155,* 1087–1091.

Lin, W., Mack, D., Enright, R. D., Krahn, D., & Baskin, T. W. (2004). Effects of forgiveness therapy on anger, mood, and vulnerability to substance use among inpatient substance-dependent clients. *Journal of Consulting and Clinical Psychology, 72,* 1114–1121.

Linden, W., Lenz, J., & Con, A. (2001). Individualized stress management for primary hypertension. *Archives of Internal Medicine, 161,* 1071–1080.

Linkh, D. J., & Sonnek, S. M. (2003). An application of cognitive-behavioral anger management training in a military/occupational setting: Efficacy and demographic factors. *Military Medicine, 168,* 475–478.

Lipsitz, J. D., Markowitz, J. C., Cherry, S., & Fyer, A. J. (1999). Open trial of interpersonal psychotherapy for the treatment of social phobia. *American Journal of Psychiatry, 156,* 1814–1816.

Lipsitz, J. D., & Marshall, R. D. (2001). Alternative psychotherapy approaches for social anxiety disorder. *Psychiatric Clinics of North America, 24,* 817–829.

Lobstein, D. D., Mosbacher, B. J., & Ismail, A. H. (1983). Depression as a powerful discriminator between physically active and sedentary middle-aged men. *Journal of Psychosomatic Research, 27,* 69–76.

Macklin, M. L., Metzger, L. J., Lasko, N. B., Berry, N. J., Orr, S. P., & Pitman, R. K. (2000). Five-year follow-up study of eye movement desensitization and reprocessing therapy for combat-related posttraumatic stress disorder. *Comprehensive Psychiatry, 41,* 24–27.

MacPherson, R., Jerrom, B., & Hughes, A. (1996). A controlled study of education about drug treatment in schizophrenia. *British Journal of Psychiatry, 168,* 709–717.

Malla, A. K., Cortese, L., Shaw, T. S., & Ginsberg, B. (1990). Life events and relapse in schizophrenia: A one-year prospective study. *Social Psychiatry and Psychiatric Epidemiology, 25,* 221–224.

Manber, R., Allen, J. J. B., & Morris, M. M. (2002). Alternative treatments for depression: Empirical support and relevance to women. *Journal of Clinical Psychiatry, 63,* 628–640.

Marder, S. R., Wirshing, W. C., Mintz, J., McKenzie, J., Johnston, K., Eckman, T. A., et al. (1996). Two-year outcome of social skills training and group psychotherapy for outpatients with schizophrenia. *American Journal of Psychiatry, 153,* 1585–1592.

Marks, I., Lovell, K., Noshirvani, H., Livanou, M., & Thrasher, S. (1998). Treatment of posttraumatic stress disorder by exposure and/or cognitive restructuring. *Archives of General Psychiatry, 55,* 317–325.

McAuliffe, W. E. (1990). A randomized clinical trial of recovery training and self-help for opioid addicts in New England and Hong Kong. *Journal of Psychoactive Drugs, 22,* 197–209.

McCullough, J. P. (2003). Treatment for chronic depression: Cognitive behavioral analysis system of psychotherapy (CBASP). *Journal of Psychotherapy Integration, 13,* 241–263.

McDermut, W., Miller, I. W., & Brown, R. A. (2001). The efficacy of group psychotherapy for depression: A meta-analysis and review of the empirical research. *Clinical Psychology: Science and Practice, 8,* 98–116.

McGowan, R. W., Pierce, E. F., & Jordan, D. (1991). Mood alterations with a single bout of physical activity. *Perceptual and Motor Skills, 72,* 1203–1209.

McGuffin, P., Asherson, P., Owen, M., & Farmer, A. (1994). The strength of the genetic effect: Is there room for an environmental influence in the aetiology of schizophrenia? *British Journal of Psychiatry, 164,* 593–599.

McNair, D. M., Lorr, M., & Droppleman, L. F. (1992). *Manual for the Profile of Mood States.* San Diego, CA: Educational and Industrial Testing Service.

Medalia, A., Herlands, T., & Baginsky, C. (2003). Rehab rounds: Cognitive remediation in the supportive housing setting. *Psychiatric Services, 54,* 1219–1220.

Meichenbaum, D. (1975). Self-instructional methods. In F. H. Kanfer & A. P. Goldstein (Eds.), *Helping people change* (pp. 357–391). New York: Pergamon Press.

Meichenbaum, D. H. (1985). *Stress inoculation training.* New York: Pergamon Press.

Meuret, A. E., Wilhelm, F. H., & Roth, W. T. (2001). Respiratory biofeedback-assisted therapy in panic disorder. *Behavior Modification, 25,* 584–605.

Meuret, A. E., Wilhelm, F. H., & Roth, W. T. (2004). Respiratory feedback for treating panic disorder. *Journal of Clinical Psychology, 60,* 197–207.

Michelson, L., Mavissakalian, M., Marchione, K., Ulrich, R. F., Marchione, N., & Testa, S. (1990). Psychophysiological outcome of cognitive, behavioral and psychophysiologically-based treatments of agoraphobia. *Behaviour Research and Therapy, 28,* 127–139.

Miller, W. R., & Rollnick, S. (1991). *Motivational interviewing: Preparing people to change addictive behavior.* New York: Guilford Press.

Mizuno, E., Hosaka, T., Ogihara, R., Higano, H., & Mano, Y. (1999). Effectiveness of a stress management program for family caregivers of the elderly at home. *Journal of Medical and Dental Sciences, 46,* 145–153.

Monti, P. M., Rohsenow, D. J., Michalec, E., Martin, R. A., & Abrams, D. B. (1997). Brief coping skills treatment for cocaine abuse: Substance use outcomes at three months. *Addiction, 92,* 1717–1728.

Morgenstern, J., Bux, D. A., Labouvie, E., Morgan, T., Blanchard, K. A., & Muench, F. (2003). Examining mechanisms of action in 12-step outpatient treatment. *Drug and Alcohol Dependence, 72,* 237–247.

Morgenstern, J., & Longabaugh, R. (2000). Cognitive-behavioral treatment for alcohol dependence: A review of evidence for its hypothesized mechanisms of action. *Addiction, 95,* 1475–1490.

Morgenstern, J., Morgan, T. J., McCrady, B. S., Keller, D. S., & Carroll, K. M. (2001). Manual-guided cognitive-behavioral therapy training: A promising method for disseminating empirically supported substance abuse treatments to the practice community. *Psychology of Addictive Behaviors, 15,* 83–88.

Mowrer, O. H. (1939). A stimulus–response analysis of anxiety and its role as a reinforcement agent. *Psychological Review, 46,* 553–556.

Murphy, M. T., Michelson, L. K., Marchione, K., Marchione, N., & Testa, S. (1998). The role of self-directed *in vivo* exposure in combination with cognitive therapy, relaxation training, or therapist-assisted exposure in the treatment of panic disorder with agoraphobia. *Journal of Anxiety Disorders, 12,* 117–138.

Nicholson, I. R., & Neufeld, R. W. J. (1992). A dynamic vulnerability perspective on stress and schizophrenia. *American Journal of Orthopsychiatry, 62,* 117–130.

Noonan, W. C., & Moyers, T. B. (1997). Motivational interviewing: A review. *Journal of Substance Misuse, 2,* 8–16.

Norman, R. M., Malla, A. K., McLean, T. S., McIntosh, E. M., Neufeld, R. W., Voruganti, L. P., et al. (2002). An evaluation of stress management program for individuals with schizophrenia. *Schizophrenia Research, 58,* 293–303.

Norton, M., Holm, J., & McSherry, C. (1997). Behavioral assessment of relaxation: The validity of a behavior rating scale. *Journal of Behavior Therapy and Experimental Psychiatry, 28,* 129–137.

Novaco, R. W. (1975). *Anger control: The development and evaluation of an experimental treatment.* Lexington, MA: Heath.

Novaco, R. W. (1991). *The Novaco Anger Scale.* Irvine: University of California.

Nuechterlein, K. H., & Dawson, M. E. (1984). A heuristic vulnerability/stress model of schizophrenic episodes. *Schizophrenia Bulletin, 10,* 300–312.

Nugter, A., Dingemans, P., Van der Does, J. W., Linszen, D., & Gersons, B. (1997). Family treatment, expressed emotion and relapse in recent onset schizophrenia. *Psychiatry Research, 72,* 23–31.

Ollendick, T. H. (1995). Cognitive-behavioral treatment of panic disorder with agoraphobia in adolescents: A multiple baseline design analysis. *Behavior Therapy, 26,* 517–531.

Ollendick, T. H., & King, N. J. (1998). Empirically supported treatments for children with phobic and anxiety disorders: Current status. *Journal of Clinical Child Psychology, 27,* 156–167.

Öst, L.-G. (1987). Applied relaxation: Description of a coping technique and review of controlled studies. *Behaviour Research and Therapy, 25,* 397–409.

Öst, L.-G., & Breitholtz, E. (2000). Applied relaxation vs. cognitive therapy in the treatment of generalized anxiety disorder. *Behaviour Research and Therapy, 38,* 777–790.

Öst, L.-G., Jerremalm, A., & Johansson, J. (1981). Individual response patterns and the effects of different behavioral methods in the treatment of social phobia. *Behaviour Research and Therapy, 19,* 1–16.

Öst, L.-G., & Westling, B. E. (1995). Applied relaxation vs. cognitive behavior therapy in the treatment of panic disorder. *Behaviour Research and Therapy*, 33, 145–158.

Öst, L.-G., Westling, B. E., & Hellström, K. (1993). Applied relaxation, exposure *in vivo* and cognitive methods in the treatment of panic disorder with agoraphobia. *Behaviour Research and Therapy*, 31, 383–394.

Pasquini, M., Picardi, A., Biondi, M., Gaetano, P., & Morosini, P. (2004). Relevance of anger and irritability in outpatients with major depressive disorder. *Psychopathology*, 37, 155–160.

Pekala, R. J., Maurer, R., Kumar, V. K., Elliott, N. C., Masten, E., Moon, E., et al. (2004). Self-hypnosis relapse prevention training with chronic drug/alcohol users: Effects on self-esteem, affect, and relapse. *American Journal of Clinical Hypnosis*, 46, 281–297.

Pelham, W. E., Jr., Wheeler, T., & Chronis, A. (1998). Empirically supported psychosocial treatments for attention-deficit hyperactivity disorder. *Journal of Clinical Child Psychology*, 27, 190–205.

Pilling, S., Bebbington, P., Kuipers, E., Garety, P., Geddes, J., Martindale, B., et al. (2002a). Psychological treatments in schizophrenia: II. Meta-analyses of randomized controlled trials of social skills training and cognitive remediation. *Psychological Medicine*, 32, 783–791.

Pilling, S., Bebbington, P., Kuipers, E., Garety, P., Geddes, J., Orbach, G., et al. (2002b). Psychological treatments in schizophrenia: I. Meta-analysis of family intervention and cognitive-behaviour therapy. *Psychological Medicine*, 32, 763–782.

Pitman, R. K., Orr, S. P., Altman, B., Longpre, R. E., Poire, R. E., & Macklin, M. L. (1996). Emotional processing during eye movement desensitization and reprocessing therapy of Vietnam veterans with chronic posttraumatic stress disorder. *Comprehensive Psychiatry*, 37, 419–429.

Poppen, R. (1988). *Behavioral relaxation training and assessment*. New York: Pergamon Press.

Porter, J. F., Spates, R. C., & Smitham, S. (2004). Behavioral activation group therapy in public mental health settings: A pilot investigation. *Professional Psychology: Research and Practice*, 35, 297–301.

Power, K. G., Simpson, M. B., Swanson, V., & Wallace, L. A. (1990). A controlled comparison of cognitive-behaviour therapy, Diazepam, and placebo, alone and in combination, for the treatment of generalised anxiety disorder. *Journal of Anxiety Disorders*, 4, 267–292.

Powers, S., & Spirito, A. (1998a). Relaxation training. In J. D. Noshpitz (Ed.), *Handbook of child and adolescent psychiatry: Vol. 6. Basic psychiatric science and treatment* (pp. 411–417). New York: Wiley.

Powers, S., & Spirito, A. (1998b). Biofeedback. In J. D. Noshpitz (Ed.), *Handbook of child and adolescent psychiatry: Vol. 6. Basic psychiatric science and treatment* (pp. 417–422). New York: Wiley.

Prins, P. J. M., & Ollendick, T. H. (2003). Cognitive change and enhanced coping: Missing mediational links in cognitive behavior therapy with anxiety-disordered children. *Clinical Child and Family Psychology Review*, 6, 87–105.

Prochaska, J. O., DiClemente, C. C., & Norcross, J. C. (1992). In search of how people change: Applications to addictive behaviors. *American Psychologist*, 47, 1102–1114.

Project MATCH Research Group. (1997). Matching alcoholism treatments to client heterogeneity: Project MATCH posttreatment drinking outcomes. *Journal of Studies on Alcohol*, 58, 7–29.

Project MATCH Research Group. (1998). Matching alcoholism treatments to client heterogeneity: Treatment main effects and matching effects on drinking during treatment. *Journal of Studies on Alcohol*, 59, 631–639.

Ramsey, S. E., Brown, R. A., Stuart, G. L., Burgess, E. S., & Miller, I. W. (2002). Cognitive variables in alcohol-dependent patients with elevated depressive symptoms: Changes and predictive utility as a function of treatment modality. *Substance Abuse*, 23, 171–182.

Razali, M. S., & Yahya, H. (1995). Compliance with treatment in schizophrenia: A drug intervention program in a developing country. *Acta Psychiatrica Scandinavica*, 91, 331–335.

Regier, D. A., Farmer, M. E., Rae, D. S., Locke, B. Z., Keith, S. J., Judd, L. L., et al. (1990). Comorbidity of mental disorders with alcohol and other drug abuse. *Journal of the American Medical Association*, 264, 2511–2518.

Rice, K. M., Blanchard, E. B., & Purcell, M. (1993). Biofeedback treatments of generalized anxiety disorder: Preliminary results. *Biofeedback and Self-Regulation*, 18, 93–105.

Robinson, G. L., Gilbertson, A. D., & Litwack, L. (1986). The effects of a psychiatric patient education to medication program on post-discharge compliance. *Psychiatry Quarterly*, 58, 113–118.

Rohsenow, D. J., Monti, P. M., Martin, R. A., Colby, S. M., Myers, M. G., Gulliver, S. B., et al. (2004).

Motivational enhancement and coping skills training for cocaine abusers: Effects on substance use outcomes. *Addiction, 99,* 862–874.

Rohsenow, D. J., Monti, P. M., Martin, R. A., Michalec, E., & Abrams, D. B. (2000). Brief coping skills treatment for cocaine abuse: 12-month substance use outcomes. *Journal of Consulting and Clinical Psychology, 68*(3), 515–520.

Sellman, J. D., Sullivan, P. F., Dore, G. M., Adamson, S. J., & MacEwan, I. (2001). A randomized controlled trial of motivational enhancement therapy (MET) for mild to moderate alcohol dependence. *Journal of Studies on Alcohol, 62,* 389–396.

Shear, M. K., Brown, T. A., Barlow, D. H., Money, R., Sholomskas, D. E., Woods, S. W., et al. (1997). Multicenter collaborative Panic Disorder Severity Scale. *American Journal of Psychiatry, 154,* 1571–1575.

Shear, M. K., Pilkonis, P. A., Cloitre, M., & Leon, A. C. (1994). Cognitive-behavioral treatment compared with nonprescriptive treatment of panic disorder. *Archives of General Psychiatry, 51,* 395–401.

Shin, Y. (1999). The effects of a walking exercise program on physical function and emotional state of elderly Korean women. *Public Health Nursing, 16,* 146–154.

Shinba, T., Murashima, Y. L., & Yamamoto, K. I. (1994). Alcohol consumption and insomnia in a sample of Japanese alcoholics. *Addiction, 89,* 587–591.

Silverman, W. K., Kurtines, W. M., Ginsburg, G. S., Weems, C. F., Lumpkin, P. W., & Carmichael, D. H. (1999). Treating anxiety disorders in children with group cognitive-behavioral therapy: A randomized clinical trial. *Journal of Consulting and Clinical Psychology, 67,* 996–1003.

Sotsky, S. M., Glass, D. R., Shea, M. T., Pilkonis, P. A., Collins, J. F., Elkin, I., et al. (1991). Patient predictors of response to psychotherapy and pharmacotherapy: Findings in the NIMH Treatment of Depression Collaborative Research Program. *American Journal of Psychiatry, 148,* 997–1008.

Spielberger, C. D. (1988). *State–Trait Anger Expression Inventory.* Odessa, FL: Psychological Assessment Resources.

Spielberger, C. D. (1996). *State–Trait Anger Expression Inventory, research edition: Professional manual.* Odessa, FL: Psychological Assessment Resources.

Spielberger, C. D., Gorsuch, R. L., & Lushene, R. E. (1970). *Manual for the State–Trait Anxiety Inventory.* Palo Alto, CA: Consulting Psychologists Press.

Stephens, T. (1988). Physical activity and mental health in the United States and Canada: Evidence from four population surveys. *Preventive Medicine, 17,* 35–47.

Tafrate, R. C., Kassinove, H., & Dundin, L. (2002). Anger episodes in high- and low-trait-anger community adults. *Journal of Clinical Psychology, 58,* 1573–1590.

Taub, E., Steiner, S. S., Weingarten, E., & Walton, G. K. (1994). Effectiveness of broad spectrum approaches to relapse prevention in severe alcoholism: A long-term, randomized, controlled trial of transcendental meditation, EMG biofeedback, and electronic neurotherapy. *Alcoholism Treatment Quarterly, 11,* 187–220.

Taylor, S. (1996). Meta-analysis of cognitive-behavioral treatments for social phobia. *Journal of Behavior Therapy and Experimental Psychiatry, 27,* 1–9.

Taylor, S., Thordarson, D. S., Maxfield, L., Fedoroff, I. C., Lovell, K., & Ogrodniczuk, J. (2003). Comparative efficacy, speed, and adverse effects of three PTSD treatments: Exposure therapy, EMDR, and relaxation training. *Journal of Consulting and Clinical Psychology, 71,* 330–338.

Tivis, L. J., Parsons, O. A., & Nixon, S. J. (1998). Anger in an inpatient treatment sample of chronic alcoholics. *Alcoholism, Clinical and Experimental Research, 22,* 902–907.

Van Etten, M. L., & Taylor, S. (1998). Comparative efficacy of treatments for post-traumatic stress disorder: A meta-analysis. *Clinical Psychology and Psychotherapy, 5,* 126–144.

Wallace, C. J., Nelson, C. J., Liberman, R. P., Aitchison, R. A., Lukoff, D., Elder, J. P., et al. (1980). A review and critique of social skills training with schizophrenic patients. *Schizophrenia Bulletin, 6,* 42–63.

Wallace, C. J., Nelson, C. J., Liberman, R. P., MacKain, S. J., Blackwell, G., & Eckman, T. A. (1992). Effectiveness and replicability of modules for teaching social and instrumental skills to the severely mentally ill. *American Journal of Psychiatry, 149,* 654–658.

Weisz, J. R., Weiss, B., Han, S. S., Granger, D. A., & Morton, T. (1995). Effects of psychotherapy with children and adolescents revisited: A meta-analysis of treatment outcome studies. *Psychological Bulletin, 117,* 450–468.

Wenck, L. S., Leu, P. W., & D'Amato, R. C. (1996). Evaluating the efficacy of a biofeedback intervention to reduce children's anxiety. *Journal of Clinical Psychology, 52*, 469–473.

Williams, J. E., Nieto, F. J., Sanford, C. P., Couper, D. J., & Tyroler, H. A. (2002). The association between trait anger and incident stroke risk: The Atherosclerosis Risk in Communities (ARIC) study. *Stroke, 33*, 13–19.

Woolery, A., Myers, H., Sternlieb, B., & Zeltzer, L. (2004). A yoga intervention for young adults with elevated symptoms of depression. *Alternative Therapies, 10*, 60–63.

Young, J. E., Weinberger, A. D., & Beck, A. T. (2001). Cognitive therapy for depression. In D. H. Barlow (Ed.), *Clinical handbook of psychological disorders* (pp. 264–308). New York: Guilford Press.

Stress Management and Relaxation Therapies for Somatic Disorders

NICHOLAS D. GIARDINO
ANGELE McGRADY
FRANK ANDRASIK

The last 10 years have seen an enormous broadening of the application and acceptance of stress management intervention in medical settings. It is now difficult to find a somatic disorder for which stress management is not believed to be helpful. Empirical support for the effectiveness of these interventions varies greatly for specific interventions and for particular patient groups. In many cases, relaxation and stress management interventions have been shown to be useful adjunctive treatments for several somatic diseases. For some disorders (e.g., hypertension, primary insomnia, headache), behavioral stress management treatments may be as effective as or even more effective than pharmacological and other medical interventions. However, for others, evidence from well-designed clinical studies is scant or lacking altogether. In this chapter we review the application of behavioral stress management interventions in the treatment of several somatic disorders. A comprehensive review of research on all relaxation and stress management interventions used with every somatic disorder is now well beyond the scope of a single chapter. Therefore, we focus on only a subset of somatic illnesses for which stress management and relaxation interventions have demonstrated efficacy. As with other chapters in this volume, efficacy assessments follow the rating criteria developed and adopted by professional organizations in these fields (Chambless & Hollon, 1998; LaVaque et al., 2002).

RESPIRATORY DISORDERS

Asthma

Asthma is a chronic respiratory disease characterized by inflammation, irritability, and reversible obstruction of the airways (National Heart, Lung, and Blood Institute, 1997). Exacerbations of asthma may be affected by exposure to irritants, allergens, cold air, exercise, respiratory infections, and emotional stress (Lehrer, Isenberg, & Hochron, 1993).

Stress management and relaxation interventions have long been used in the treatment of asthma. But whereas a half-century ago asthma was considered a prototypical psychosomatic illness, more recently proposed mechanisms of therapeutic impact have included both direct physiological effects on airway function, as well as reduction in anxiety or panic that may be related to asthma attacks.

According to classical views of stress physiology and stress management mechanisms, the use of relaxation-based interventions for asthma would seem counterintuitive. For example, beta-sympathetic arousal and corticosteroid release, both components of the stress response, should be beneficial in asthma, producing bronchodilation and inflammatory suppression, respectively. Conversely, relaxation should then be counter-therapeutic. However, more recent conceptualizations of stress and health in terms of complex self-regulation, as well as a better understanding of the role of anxiety and stress in asthma-related behaviors, accommodate stress management and relaxation training as a logically consistent mode of intervention.

Several stress management and relaxation modalities, including progressive muscle relaxation (PMR), electromyogram (EMG) biofeedback, autogenic training, yoga, hypnotic suggestion, emotive writing, and functional, breathing-based, and music-based relaxation, have been studied in patients with asthma. Outcome measures have most commonly included lung function measurement (e.g., forced expiratory volume), prescription medication use, and health care visits. In all, most studies that were adequately designed (e.g., including randomization and appropriate control conditions) have shown no more than modest clinical effects for these interventions.

The effects of a very brief (1 day) functional relaxation intervention were tested in a within-subject control study design by Loew and colleagues (Loew, Siegfried, Martus, Tritt, & Hahn, 1996). Patients with asthma were taught functional relaxation techniques 1 day after they were given beta-agonist bronchodilator medication. The authors reported similar reductions in airway resistance in both conditions. But, because the conditions were not counterbalanced, carryover effects from the medication cannot be ruled out. A follow-up study (Loew et al., 2001) also yielded positive results for functional relaxation, but the crossover design was limited by the same drug carryover effects.

Autogenic training for asthma was tested in two controlled trials. Deter and Allert (Deter & Allert, 1983) compared autogenic training and functional relaxation, both in addition to group therapy, with a wait-list control group. Patients who completed the training program showed greater body awareness after 1 year but showed no significant changes on measures of lung function. However, use of beta-agonist medication decreased in the treatment groups. Some evidence of airway resistance increases during autogenic training session was also reported by the authors. Henry and colleagues (Henry, de Rivera, Gonzalez-Martin, & Abreu, 1993) compared autogenic training with a control group receiving supportive group therapy and asthma education. Significant improvements in lung function measurements from pre- to posttreatment were reported in the autogenic training but not in the control group.

Lehrer and colleagues (Lehrer, Hochron, McCann, Swartzman, & Reba, 1986) tested a multicomponent intervention on patients with "intrinsic" asthma (i.e., no obvious allergic component). Their treatment included PMR, EMG biofeedback, abdominal breathing, and systematic desensitization, which was compared with an elaborate control condition that included somatic awareness training, cognitive therapy techniques, subliminal message presentation (without any actual subliminal messages), and false EEG biofeedback. The relaxation treatment group showed a significant decrease in emotional asthma triggers, medication use, and response to methacholine challenge. Equivalent decreases in asthma symptoms were reported for both groups, and no changes in forced expiratory volume (FEV) were measured. In a second study, also with intrinsic asthma patients, Lehrer and colleagues (Lehrer et al., 1994) compared PMR and music relaxation with a wait-list control. Some lung function measurements (e.g., peak expiratory flow) showed improvements across sessions in the PMR group compared with music relaxation and wait-list control. But no treatment effects were found on measures of asthma symptoms, medication use, or medical care utilization.

The effect of yoga training on asthma has been examined in at least three controlled studies. Nagarathna and Nagendra (1985) randomly assigned participants with asthma to either a yoga intervention that emphasized slow breathing or a no-yoga control condition. Participants in the yoga group showed decreases in asthma symptoms, decreased use of asthma medication, and clinically significant increases in peak flow. Vijayalakshmi, Satyanarayana, Rao, and Prakesh (1988) also reported improvements in asthma compared with usual medical care using a combined yoga and psychotherapy treatment. However participants in this study were not randomly assigned to treatment group. Vedanthan and colleagues (Vedanthan et al., 1998) found no significant differences in lung function measurements, symptom ratings, or medication use between yoga and control groups after 4 and then 6 weeks of a 16-week training program (no posttreatment data were reported).

Smyth, Stone, Hurewitz, and Kaell (1999) reported statistical and clinical improvements in asthma after only three 20-minute sessions during which participants were asked to write about "the most stressful experience that they had ever undergone" (p. 1305). Participants in the control group wrote for the same amount of time about their plans for the day. At 4 months posttreatment, the active treatment group showed significant improvements in lung function compared with the control condition. The magnitude of improvement was quite impressive, especially given the nature of the intervention, with almost half of treatment participants showing a 15% or greater improvement in forced expiratory volume in 1 second (FEV_1). Disappointingly, a recent study that attempted to replicate and extend these findings failed to do so. Harris, Thoresen, Humphreys, and Faul (2005) found no differences between patients with asthma who were randomly assigned to one of three conditions in which they wrote for 20 minutes about either stressful, positive, or neutral experiences, respectively.

Although it is not explicitly a relaxation or stress management intervention, a novel biofeedback treatment for asthma has recently demonstrated efficacy in a well-designed, randomized controlled study. Lehrer and colleagues (2004) evaluated the effectiveness of heart rate variability (HRV) biofeedback as an adjunctive treatment for asthma. HRV is typically decreased in patients with asthma (Garrard, Seidler, McKibben, McAlpine, & Gordon, 1992; Kazuma, Otsuka, Matsuoka, & Murata, 1997) and may reflect reduced capacity for autonomic cardiopulmonary regulation. Previous uncontrolled and small pilot studies showed that HRV biofeedback improves pulmonary function (Lehrer, Smetankin, & Potapova, 2000) and decreases airway resistance (Lehrer et al., 1997) in children and adults, respectively, with asthma. In a larger, rigorously controlled trial of 94 patients with asthma, Lehrer et al. (2004) showed specific treatment effects on asthma severity, medication use, and pulmonary function with their biofeedback intervention. Although impressive, these results require replication in an independent research setting in order to meet the most stringent efficacy criteria.

Chronic Obstructive Pulmonary Disease

Chronic obstructive pulmonary disease (COPD) refers to a group of related disorders that are characterized by progressive, nonreversible airflow obstruction. Emphysema and chronic bronchitis are the two most common COPD diagnoses. Tobacco smoke accounts for 80–90% of the risk of developing COPD.

A number of breathing-based interventions have been used in COPD. However, they are designed to directly improve respiratory biomechanics in order to increase ventilatory capacity and flow rather than to manage stress. Therefore, although these interventions may also produce psychological benefits, they are not reviewed here.

Renfroe (1988) tested the effects of progressive muscle relaxation on anxiety, dyspnea, and respiratory function in 12 patients with COPD. Compared with the control group, treatment participants showed greater within-session reductions in dyspnea, anxiety, and respiration rate. However, at the end of the 4-week treatment, only changes in respiration rate differed between the two groups. Gift and colleagues (Gift, Moore, & Soeken, 1992) tested four weekly sessions of listening to a taped relaxation message on 26 patients with COPD randomly assigned to relaxation compared to a quietly sitting control group. Patients in the relaxation group showed decreases in dyspnea, anxiety, and airway obstruction. Control participants showed no improvements in outcome measures. Louie (2004) tested the effects of guided imagery relaxation in patients with COPD. In this randomized controlled study of 26 patients, guided imagery resulted in improved oxygen saturation in the treatment group but had no effect on other outcome variables, including dyspnea, EMG, skin conductance, and peripheral skin temperature.

CARDIOVASCULAR DISORDERS

Hypertension

Hypertension is defined as having systolic blood pressure (SBP) of 140 mm Hg or greater or having diastolic blood pressure (DBP) of 90 mm Hg or greater. However, the health significance of hypertension lies not so much in increased arterial pressure per se but rather in resultant structural cardiovascular changes that lead to additional morbidities, for example, in the heart, brain, and kidneys. Many studies have suggested that chronic stress may contribute to the development of hypertension, particularly in those with a genetic predisposition to the disease (e.g., Fredrikson & Matthews, 1990; Markovitz, Raczynski, Wallace, Chettur, & Chesney, 1998; Muldoon, Terrell, Bunker, & Manuck, 1993). The risk of cardiovascular disease doubles with each 20/10 mm Hg increase over 115/75 mm Hg. Therefore, the most recent guidelines target blood pressures well below the hypertension cutoff. According to the most recent guidelines of the Joint National Committee on Prevention, Detection, Evaluation and Treatment of High Blood Pressure (JNC7; Chobanian et al., 2003) individuals with an SBP of 120–139 mm Hg or a DBP of 80–89 mm Hg should be considered as prehypertensive and require health-promoting lifestyle modifications to prevent cardiovascular disease. These lifestyle modifications include physical activity, a healthy diet, weight loss (if necessary), and moderate alcohol consumption. Although not explicitly listed in the JNC7 guidelines, stress management is also a common target of biobehavioral interventions for hypertension. The absence of stress management from JNC7 is likely due to the relatively few large randomized controlled trials on the long-term effects of stress management therapies for hypertension.

Furthermore, no well-designed studies exist that demonstrate reductions in cardiovascular morbidity or mortality.

Nonetheless, there is good evidence that certain types of relaxation and stress-reduction programs are effective in significantly reducing blood pressure (BP) in individuals with hypertension. In a review of 12 randomized controlled studies of relaxation therapy, either alone or combined with biofeedback or other treatments, a meta-analysis by Kaufmann et al. (1988) found significant but modest DBP decreases in non-medicated, but not in medicated patients with hypertension. More recent randomized controlled trials have also shown positive effects of relaxation therapies. McGrady (1994) combined group relaxation with thermal biofeedback and reported that almost half showed a decrease in mean arterial pressure of at least 5 mm Hg at the posttreatment assessment. At 10-month follow-up, 37% of those continued to show similar improvements. Yung and Keltner (1996) compared muscle relaxation and cognitive relaxation therapies with placebo attention and measurement-only controls and found no significant differences between any of the groups at posttreatment or follow-up. Only 6 participants made up each group, however, so the study lacked the statistical power to detect all but very large effects.

In a comprehensive meta-analysis, Linden and Chambers (1994) compared 90 studies of stress-reduction hypertension therapy with 47 behavioral (e.g., diet modification, exercise) and 30 pharmacological interventions. Whereas single-component stress management therapies showed little or no effect on reducing BP, multicomponent stress reduction therapies significantly reduced BP (−9.7/−7.2 mm Hg) over short- and long-term assessments. Furthermore, the researchers found that individualized stress management therapies were equally as effective as pharmacological and exercise interventions at reducing SBP. In a more recent review of the evidence for the efficacy of behavioral treatments for hypertension, Linden and Moseley (2006) concluded that treatment effects from more than 100 randomized controlled study results have been highly variable and, overall, modest in size. More important, they point out several methodological issues that limit the strength of many of these studies, including failure to properly control for floor effects and other measurement confounds.

In more recent studies, Batey et al. (2000) found little or no benefit from their stress management intervention in a group of prehypertensive (DBP 80–89 mm Hg) men and women. Linden, Lenz, and Con (2001) reported that an individualized stress management intervention produced significant reductions in 24-hour ambulatory BP in a group of hypertensive men and women compared with controls. Interestingly, they found that office measurements of BP did not differ between groups. Habituation to measurement has been noted by several authors as a serious threat to the validity of office BP readings and may mask real treatment effects in some treatment studies.

McCraty, Atkinson, and Tomasino (2003) tested a workplace stress reduction program on employees with hypertension. The program involved 16 hours of instruction in "positive emotion refocusing and emotional restructuring techniques" (p. 355), with HRV feedback on 38 employees randomly assigned to the treatment or to a wait-list control group. Compared with control participants, employees in the treatment group showed a mean adjusted reduction of 10.6 mm Hg in SBP and of 6.3 mm Hg in DBP at 3 months postintervention. In addition to BP decreases, employees in the treatment group also showed significant reductions in stress symptoms, depression, and global psychological distress and significant increases in peacefulness, positive outlook, and workplace satisfaction.

CANCER

Most stress-reduction interventions for patients with cancer have targeted the reduction of symptoms common to cancer and the iatrogenic effects of cancer treatment, such as sleep disturbance, pain, nausea, and emotional distress. However, some studies have also examined effects on survival or medical recovery.

Spiegel and colleagues have published a number of studies on the effects of supportive group therapy that includes self-hypnosis for pain in women with breast cancer. In addition to effects on improving mood, coping, and anxiety, increased survival was evidenced over a 10-year follow-up period in the therapy group compared with the control participants who received usual care (Spiegel, Bloom, Kraemer, & Gottheil, 1989; Spiegel, Bloom, & Yalom, 1981). Stress management benefits on survival time have been reported in other studies. Fawzy and colleagues (Fawzy et al., 1993) found that participation in a 6-week early intervention to improve coping and reduce affective distress was associated with decreased mortality after 6 years among patients with malignant melanoma compared with control patients who received usual care. Spiegel and colleagues have also more recently shown that a 12-session supportive-expressive group therapy was effective in reducing mood and anxiety symptoms in female breast cancer patients who were within 1 year of their diagnoses (Spiegel et al., 1999).

Goodwin et al. (2001) studied the effect of a supportive–expressive group therapy that was added to routine care in women with metastatic breast cancer in a large randomized controlled trial. In this study, patients randomly assigned to group therapy showed no increase in survival time. However, group therapy patients with high levels of distress at baseline reported significant improvement in psychological symptoms and in pain. Women with low baseline distress showed no such benefit.

Recently the effects of mindfulness-based stress reduction (MBSR) on a number of different outcomes in heterogeneous groups of cancer patients have been studied. In a randomized controlled study (Speca, Carlson, Goodey, & Angen, 2000), a heterogeneous group of cancer patients receiving a 7-week mindfulness meditation-based stress reduction program showed decreased depression, anxiety, anger, and confusion symptoms and higher vigor than patients assigned to a wait-list control condition. In addition, the stress reduction group showed fewer stress and somatic symptoms posttreatment. In a follow-up study (Carlson, Ursuliak, Goodey, Angen, & Speca, 2001), improvements in mood and stress symptoms were largely maintained 6-months following treatment end. In another study (Carlson, Speca, Patel, & Goodey, 2003), patients with breast cancer or prostate cancer showed improvements in quality of life, stress symptoms, and sleep quality. No changes in cancer-relevant immune cell counts were observed following MBSR. However, changes in some cytokine profiles away from linked to depressive states were seen. In a third study from this group (Carlson & Garland, 2005), MBSR was shown to improve sleep disturbances and reduce self-reported stress, fatigue, and mood disturbance in a heterogeneous group of cancer patients. These latter studies used a more traditional MBSR program but did not, unfortunately, include a control group. In a subanalysis of data from a randomized controlled study of MBSR for women with breast cancer, Shapiro and colleagues (Shapiro, Bootzin, Figueredo, Lopez, & Schwartz, 2003) showed improvements in stress-related sleep problems, but only among participants who reported greater mindfulness practice.

SLEEP DISORDERS

According to DSM-IV-TR, the primary sleep disorders are divided into dyssomnias (disturbances in amount, timing, or quality of sleep) and parasomnias (abnormal behavioral or physiological events during sleep). Sleep disorders may also be due to another mental or medical condition or to intake of substances (American Psychiatric Association, 2000). Despite well-defined criteria for diagnosis, symptoms are variable. For example, patients report problems with: (1) sleep continuity, the balance between sleep and wakefulness during a night; (2) sleep latency, the number of minutes elapsed between bedtime and falling asleep; (3) intermittent wakefulness, the number of minutes spent awake after initial sleep onset; or (4) sleep efficiency, the percentage of time spent asleep compared with the time spent in bed (American Psychiatric Association, 2000). Sleep disruption also produces difficulties in daytime functioning, such as inability to finish tasks, loss of concentration resulting in accidents, and difficulties in interpersonal relationships (Doghramji, 2001).

The diagnosis of sleep disorders depends on self-report, history, physical examination, and polysomnography. Patients complete sleep diaries and provide detailed histories; sometimes a bed-partner interview is used for corroboration. Polysomnography is carried out in clinical settings in which multiple electrophysiological factors are assessed, resulting in a detailed analysis of sleep architecture, including the number of minutes spent and distribution of each sleep stage (Buscemi et al., 2005). The wrist actigraph monitors activity during the hours spent in bed and can also be part of the assessment of sleep disorders (Carney, Lajos, & Waters, 2004).

The overall prevalence rate of sleep disorders in adults is high, ranging from 30 to 40% during one year. Reports of insomnia are the most common, and primary insomnia represents 30% of the total. Psychiatric comorbidity, particularly mood and anxiety disorders, explain approximately 60% of insomnia symptoms (Roth & Drake, 2004). Chronic insomnia represents approximately 9–12% of sleeping problems reported; medical problems such as chronic pain are strong determinants of sleep disruption (Taylor, Lichstein, Durrence, Reidel, & Bush, 2005). Patients commonly present to their primary care providers and are treated in that setting; referrals to sleep medicine specialists are reserved for more complicated cases (Hauri, 1993). Multiple factors are associated with abnormal sleep pattern. For example, chronic insomnia is more likely in the elderly, in women, in those who consume excessive caffeine and alcohol, and in patients with medical and psychiatric illness (Buscemi et al., 2005). Treatment of sleep disorders in the elderly becomes complex; these patients may have other medical and psychiatric disorders that intensify the initial sleep disruption (Jagus & Benbow, 1999).

Multiple therapies have been used in the treatment of sleep disorders, as summarized by Stepanski (2003). Relaxation was first suggested as a means of decreasing insomnia due to excessive worry in the 1930s, and it was demonstrated to be effective in management of anxiety disorders in the 1950s. Biofeedback was tested in the 1980s and found to be helpful, but it is less used today. Interventions based on behavioral theory, such as stimulus control and sleep restriction, were advanced and refined in the 1980s and 1990s and remain mainstays in the treatment of insomnia. Stimulus control therapy consists of retraining patients to associate the bed and bedroom with sleep instead of with other activities or with anxiety-producing stimuli. Sleep restriction involves limiting the time in bed to approximate the actual hours spent asleep. The use of cognitive-behavioral therapy (CBT) was described in the previous edition of this volume (Lehrer, Carr, Sargunaraj, & Woolfolk, 1993), but controlled studies were few at that time. Since then, trials of CBT have proliferated and are currently viewed as equally effective as pharmacotherapy for insomnia (Stepanski, 2003).

Pharmacological therapy has been extensively studied in patients with primary insomnia, as well as insomnia due to psychiatric comorbidity. Two groups of prescription hypnotics, benzodiazepine receptor agonists and structurally nonbenzodiazepine hypnotics, are effective for short-term relief of insomnia (Buscemi et al., 2005). The long-term use of hypnotic drugs for insomnia is an area of controversy in behavioral medicine. But current consensus is that long-term management must include behavioral and cognitive changes, such as revision of patients' thoughts and beliefs, disassociation of anxiety from bedtime, treatment of clinical anxiety and depression if present, and changes in bedtime and daytime behaviors (Wilson & Nutt, 1999). Part of the effectiveness of CBT may be due to the increased sense of control that patients feel over the sleep problem (Verbeek, Schreuder, & Declerck, 1999). Continuous use of hypnotic medication causes problems that add to the initial sleep disorder, such as lower sleep efficiency, poorer daytime function, and drug dependence (Lichstein et al., 1999).

Medication was directly compared with five sessions of CBT in a randomized controlled trial in which 63 adults participated. CBT was most effective in improving sleep-onset latency and sleep efficiency. The drug produced moderate improvements during the active trial, but symptoms returned to baseline after the drug was discontinued (Jacobs, Pace-Schott, Stickgold, & Otto, 2004). CBT was as effective for insomnia as sedative hynotics in nine patients with acute psychophysiological insomnia. Self-reported improvements were backed up by sleep architecture; the durations of stage 2 sleep, REM sleep, and slow-wave sleep increased (Cervena et al., 2004). Another group of patients who were using hypnotics became drug-free at 1 year after CBT (Espie, Inglis, Tessier, & Harvey, 2001). According to the National Institutes of Health (2005) consensus statement, CBT was at least as effective as prescription drugs, with long-term benefit favoring CBT.

The behavioral and psychotherapeutic interventions, including sleep restriction, cognitive-behavioral therapy, relaxation, biofeedback, and stimulus control, have been studied singly or in multi-intervention behavioral packages. From a research perspective it is difficult to identify which of multiple treatment components are active, but clinically, several interventions are routinely provided, the choice depending on patient symptoms, preference accessibility, and the provider's familiarity with the therapies.

CBT was compared with PMR or placebo. CBT comprised education, stimulus control, and time-in-bed restrictions. Twenty-five patients were assigned to each group and were treated weekly for 6 weeks. Objective and subjective assessments were completed before and after treatment. CBT produced larger improvements in sleep fragmentation, increased sleep time by 30 minutes, and produced higher sleep efficiency than did PMR or placebo. CBT reduced awakenings by 54%. The results were stable at 6 months (Edinger, Wohlgemuth, Radtke, Marsh, & Quillian, 2001). Six sessions of CBT followed by booster sessions produced reductions in parameters related to insomnia, in addition to improved daytime functioning, compared with self-help information. Janson and Linton (2005) support early intervention for insomnia before the behaviors become firmly rooted in daily life. Short-term (6 weeks) CBT therapy combined with PMR, modified stimulus control, and bedtime restriction was tested for long-term results (3 years). Twenty patients with chronic primary insomnia improved their total sleep time and sleep efficiency and reduced sleep latency, in addition to achieving lower depression scores on standard questionnaires (Backhaus, Hohagen, Voderholzer, & Riemann, 2001).

Strategies are needed for detection and treatment of sleep disorders in primary care, as most patients will present to their family practice or internal medicine physician with complaints of poor sleep or daytime fatigue (National Institutes of Health [NIH], 2005). In one study, improvement in insomnia was tested at 12 months after CBT. Symptoms of anxiety, depression, and thinking errors positively predicted good outcome, but severity of symptoms or use of hypnotics did not (Espie et al., 2001). A structured 6-week primary care program, the Wilford Hall Program, for insomnia showed improvements in sleep-onset latency, wakefulness after sleep onset, and sleep efficiency (Hryshko-Mullen, Broeckl, Haddock, & Peterson, 2000). Hypnotic induction was added to CBT and was successful in improving sleep latency, sleep efficiency, and reduction in drug use. Older age was no barrier to success (Morgan, Dixon, Mathers, Thompson, & Tomeny, 2003).

Relaxation therapy, specifically PMR, has been studied alone and combined with other behavioral techniques. In comparison with untreated controls, PMR improved sleep in college students with insomnia but did not alter daytime functioning (Means, Lichstein, Epperson, & Johnson, 2000). Waters et al. (2003) found that certain interventions were effective for specific subtypes of insomnia. PMR and cognitive distraction had the greatest effect on sleep onset, whereas sleep restriction and stimulus control were better for sleep maintenance. Medication took effect quickly and improved sleep latency and quality and decreased restlessness. When PMR was tested against anxiety management training, both interventions were equally effective in reducing sleep onset, anxiety, and depression in a group of people with chronic insomnia (Viens, De Koninck, Mercier, St-Onge, & Lorrain, 2003). PMR was added to a drug withdrawal plan and compared with the withdrawal plan alone to assist patients who were long-term users of hypnotics. In the PMR group, sleep measures improved, and medication usage was decreased by 80%, but the sleep disruption during the withdrawal period was not shortened. Perhaps more important was the finding that when withdrawal was completed, sleep was either the same or improved. Usually, withdrawal of hypnotics leads to worsening of sleep disorder (Lichstein et al., 1999). Seventy-four adults over age 59 participated in 6 weeks of either passive relaxation, sleep compression, or placebo. At 1 year, sleep compression was the most successful in reducing symptoms. However, relaxation helped with daytime impairment, whereas sleep compression was most effective with sleep consolidation (Lichstein, Riedel, Wilson, Lester, & Aguillard, 2001).

CBT was provided in three formats to derive a model for clinically and cost effective therapy for insomnia. Group therapy was compared with individual sessions and phone consultations. All were effective at 6 months posttreatment (Bastien, Morin, Ouellet, Blais, & Bouchard, 2004). Patients who spontaneously sought help for insomnia benefited from a group multifactorial behavioral medicine program. Fifty-eight percent reported at least some improvement; 91% reduced or eliminated medication use. Long-term follow-up showed maintenance of the improvements with less medication (Jacobs, Benson, & Friedman, 1996). The effects of sequencing medical and behavioral interventions were tested in a small pilot study using sleep diaries and actigraph recordings (Vallieres, Morin, Guay, Bastien, & LeBlanc, 2004). The interventions combined medication and CBT in varying sequences for a total of 10 weeks. Regardless of whether CBT or medication was offered first, second, or at the same time, CBT was the essential component for positive outcome.

Sleep disruption can be a symptom of a psychiatric disorder, may exacerbate an existing psychiatric condition, or may be a harbinger of an impending illness (Jagus & Benbow, 1999). People with insomnia are more likely to have clinically significant anxiety and depression. In addition, insomnia and number of awakenings are related to depression, and anxious patients are more likely to have insomnia (Taylor et al., 2005). Frequently, insomnia is secondary to chronic pain. In a group of 50 persons with pain, 57% were statistically improved, but only 18% fully recovered from sleep problems associated with pain (Currie, Wilson, & Curran, 2002). In addition to pain, patients with other medical conditions such as heart disease, respiratory problems, and diabetes have sleep disruptions that affect daily functioning. Therefore Tsai (2004) tested several types of sleep-enhancing interventions with 41 patients with cardiac disease and compared the result to 59 control subjects. Audiovisual relaxation, deep breathing, exercise, and guided imagery were associated with better sleep quality while anxiety scores concomitantly decreased.

Morin et al. (1999) consulted 48 studies and 2 meta-analyses for data regarding behavioral interventions for chronic insomnia and were applied to the American Psychiatric Association (2000) criteria for empirically supported psychological treatments. Stimulus control and PMR were empirically validated and efficacious; sleep restriction, biofeedback, and CBT were found to be empirically validated and probably efficacious (Morin et al., 1999). In a more recent study, CBT was found to be superior to single-component therapy (Wang, Wang, & Tsai, 2005). A review of behavioral interventions in the management of chronic insomnia was conducted in order to develop practice guidelines for clinicians. Each therapy was rated according to the recommendations of the American Academy of Sleep Medicine (American Sleep Disorders Association Diagnostic Classification Steering Committee, 1990). The analysis showed that stimulus control was a standard therapy, that is, a strategy that "reflects a high degree of clinical certainty"; PMR and electromyographic feedback were both classified as guidelines, that is, strategies that reflect "a moderate degree of clinical certainty" (Chesson et al., 1999, p. 1130).

HEADACHE

Headache is a clinical syndrome that affects over 90% of the population at some time during their lives; thus it is considered a major public health issue (Mannix, 2001). The two most common forms of headache are migraine, experienced by about 18% of females and 7% of males, and tension-type headache, experienced by about 40% of the population at any point in time (Mannix, 2001).

Migraine incidence is higher among women than men at every age, except in the very young, and it peaks in the third and fourth decades of life (Bille, 1962; Lipton, Diamond, Reed, Diamond, & Stewart, 2001). Among all diseases worldwide that cause disability, migraine is ranked 19th by the World Health Organization. The impact of migraine is measurable, both at the individual and familial levels (Solomon & Dahlöf, 2000). For example, in a national sample of 4,000 U.S. households, approximately 60% of migraine sufferers noted that migraine had an impact on the family; 21% rated this impact as very or extremely serious (Smith, 1998). About one-third stated that migraines negatively affected relationships with their children, and over 70% reported missing activities with their children as a result of migraine. Finally, nearly 40% of those interviewed felt that migraine had a negative impact on their marriages. Michel (2000), on reviewing the socioeconomics of headache, concluded that the direct costs (those incurred by the health care system in diagnosing and treating headache), indirect costs (days of lost or diminished productivity), and intangible costs (pain, suffering) were all substantial. Migraine results in 112 million bedridden days each year (Hu, Markson, Lipton, Stewart, & Berger, 1999). The cost of migraine to the total American workforce is an estimated $13 billion a year in missed workdays and lost productivity. Direct medical costs (i.e., physician office visits, prescription medication claims, hospitalizations) for migraine care average $1 billion annually. Notably, patients with migraine generate twice the medical claims and 2½ times the pharmacy claims as other comparable patients without migraine in a health maintenance organization (Clouse & Osterhaus, 1994).

Tension-type headache (TTH) is far more common than migraine, with a lifetime prevalence of nearly 80% (Jensen, 1999). As with migraine, TTH peaks in the third and fourth decades, and females reveal higher rates of occurrence. The female preponderance is greater for chronic (a more difficult type to treat) than for episodic forms of TTH (Schwartz, Stewart, Simon, & Lipton, 1998). In comparison with migraine, much less is known about the impact of TTH. Schwartz et al. (1998) found that 8.3% of those with episodic forms of TTH lost days at work (average 9 per year), with 44% reporting reduced effectiveness at work, home, and school as a result of headache. For those with chronic forms of TTH, 11.8% lost days at work (average 20 per year), and 47% reported reduced productivity due to headache. Given the markedly increased prevalence of TTH, the total societal impact of lost workdays and decreased productivity may well rival that for migraine (Penzien, Rains, & Andrasik, 2002).

Migraine consists of two major subtypes—with and without aura (Olesen & Steiner, 2004). Migraine without aura is the most common, having a higher attack frequency and a greater level of disability. The prototypical migraine consists of a unilateral pain that is sudden in onset and pulsating in nature and that fairly quickly reaches a pain intensity that is judged to be moderate to severe. It is often accompanied by gastrointestinal distress and by photophobia (light sensitivity) and phonophobia (sound sensitivity). The attack may be brief (4 hours or so) or extended (72 hours if untreated or unsuccessfully treated). Some individuals experience a premonitory phase, which can occur hours or days before the headache attack, and a resolution phase. Symptoms experienced during the premonitory and resolution phases include hyper- or hypoactivity, depression, craving for particular foods, and repetitive yawning, among others. In younger children, the symptom presentation may depart from that described (headaches may be more frequent but briefer in duration, headache may be experienced bilaterally instead of unilaterally).

The auras that precede the other subtype of migraine typically develop gradually over 5–20 minutes and last for less than 60 minutes. The aura is a complex of fully reversible neurological symptoms, including visual (e.g., flickering lights, gaps in the visual field), sensory (i.e., numbness and feelings of pins and needles), and dysphasic speech disturbances. Additional premonitory symptoms may include fatigue, difficulty concentrating, neck stiffness, photo- and phonophobia, nausea, blurred vision, and pallor. The auras occur in about 10–15% of migraines.

TTH is the most common primary headache type, with a lifetime prevalence ranging from 30–78%. The prototypical TTH occurs frequently, in episodes lasting minutes to days. The pain is typically bilateral, pressing or tightening in nature, and of mild to moderate intensity. Nausea is absent, but photo- or phonophobia may be present. Current classification schemes distinguish between (1) *infrequent* (at least 10 episodes occurring on less than 1 day per month or 12 days per year on average), (2) *frequent* (at least 10 episodes occurring on 1 or more but less than 15 days per month for at least 3 months), and (3) *chronic* (occurring on 15 or more days per month on average for greater than 3 months) forms of TTH, and each of these is further subdivided according to the presence or absence of pericranial tenderness (identified by manual palpation). The frequency distinction is important because, all things remaining equal, the greater the frequency, the poorer the treatment response.

Although most headaches are relatively benign, for 1–3% of patients the etiology can be life-threatening (Evans, 2001). Consequently, nonphysician practitioners are urged to refer all patients with headache to a physician who is experienced with evaluating headache and who will maintain a close collaboration during treatment as necessary. Even after arranging a medical evaluation, the nonphysician therapist must be continually alert for evidence of a developing underlying physical problem.

Most individuals will experience a headache from time to time, yet few of these individuals seek regular treatment from a health care provider, even when headaches are severe and disabling (Mannix, 2001; Michel, 2000). More typically, headaches are tolerated, treated symptomatically with over-the-counter preparations, or managed by "borrowing" prescribed medications from friends and family members. When recurrent headache sufferers do visit a health care practitioner, their headaches are most commonly managed with a combination of medication and advice. For example, among primary care patients with headache, more than 80% reported the use of over-the-counter medications, and more than 75% reported the use of some form of prescription-only medications for management of their headaches (Von Korff, Galer, & Stang, 1995).

A number of effective pharmacological options are available to treat headaches, and they fall within three broad categories: symptomatic, abortive, and prophylactic.

Symptomatic medications are pharmacological agents with analgesic or pain-relieving effects. These include over-the-counter analgesics (i.e., aspirin, acetaminophen), nonsteroidal anti-inflammatory agents (i.e., ibuprofen), opioid analgesics, muscle relaxants, and sedative/hypnotic agents.

Abortive agents are consumed at the onset of a migraine headache in an effort to terminate or markedly lessen an attack. Ergotamine tartrate preparations were the mainstays of abortive care until the early 1990s, when triptans, designed to act on specific serotonin receptor subtypes, were introduced. Multiple triptan formulations are now available, differing with respect to potency, delivery mode (oral vs. other, for patients likely to vomit during attacks), time of peak onset, duration of sustained headache relief, rate of headache recurrence, improvement in associated symptoms, safety, and tolerability (Rapoport & Tepper, 2001; Tepper, 2001).

Prophylactic medications are consumed daily in an effort to prevent headaches or reduce the occurrence of attacks in the chronic sufferer. Beta blockers, calcium channel blockers, antidepressants (e.g., tricyclics, serotonin-specific reuptake inhibitors), and anticonvulsants are used most frequently (Chronicle & Mulleners, 2004; Tfelt-Hansen & Welch, 2000a, 2000b). Meta-analyses comparing various prophylactic agents, conducted with child as well as adult patients, have shown them to be superior to varied control conditions (waiting list, medication placebo, etc.; Hermann, Kim, & Blanchard, 1995; Holroyd & Penzien, 1990; Holroyd, Penzien, & Cordingley, 1991). These analyses showed that behavioral treatments achieved outcomes similar to those for varied prophylactic medications.

For TTH, the most commonly administered medications include tricyclic and newer generation antidepressants, muscle relaxants, nonsteroidal anti-inflammatory agents, and miscellaneous drugs (Mathew & Bendtsen, 2000). A recent, large-scale randomized controlled trial found stress management and drug prophylaxis to be equivalent in effectiveness (although time to response was quicker for medication). The combination of the two treatments was more effective than either treatment by itself (Holroyd et al., 2001).

Although a number of medications are effective in the treatment of recurring headache, concern exists regarding the risks of frequent, long-term use of certain medications. Major risks associated with pharmacological management include the potential for misuse and dependency (Mathew, 1987), development of drug-induced chronic headache, reduced efficacy of prophylactic headache medications, potential side effects, and acute symptoms associated with the cessation of headache medication (such as increased headache, nausea, cramping, gastrointestinal distress, sleep disturbance, and emotional distress). These potential risks, combined with the growing interest in self-management and alternative approaches, have helped to spur interest in the effectiveness of nonpharmacological treatment approaches.

The primary nonpharmacological approaches are designed (1) to promote general overall relaxation either by therapist instruction alone (e.g., PMR, autogenic training, meditation, etc.) or by therapist instruction augmented by feedback of various physiological parameters (e.g., temperature, electromyographic, or electrodermal response) indicative of autonomic arousal or muscle tension to help fine-tune relaxation, something Andrasik (2004) has termed "biofeedback-assisted relaxation"; (2) to control, in more direct fashion, those physiological parameters assumed to underlie headache (e.g., blood flow and electroencephalographic biofeedback, primarily); and (3) to enhance abilities to manage stressors and stress reactions to headache (e.g., cognitive and cognitive behavior therapy). With the exception of EEG biofeedback, nonpharmacological approaches have been the subject of extensive research. In assessing efficacy, the available literature has been examined from two perspectives: qualitative (evidence-based review panels evaluating level of design sophistication) and quantitative (via meta-analysis).

Evidence-based reviews have been conducted by multiple groups, including Division 12 of the American Psychological Association (Task Force on Promotion and Dissemination of Psychological Procedures, 1995), the U.S. Headache Consortium (composed of seven medical societies: the American Academy of Family Physicians, the American Academy of Neurology, the American Headache Society, the American College of Emergency Physicians, the American College of Physicians—American Society of Internal Medicine, the American Osteopathic Association, and the National Headache Foundation; Campbell, Penzien, & Wall, 2000), the Canadian Headache Society (Pryse-Phillips et al., 1998), the Task Force of the Society of Pediatric Psychology (Holden, Deichmann, & Levy, 1999), and the Association for Applied Psychophysiology and Biofeedback (Yucha & Gilbert, 2004).

The U.S. Headache Consortium's recommendations pertaining to behavioral interventions for migraine are as follows:

1. Relaxation training, thermal biofeedback combined with relaxation training, electromyographic biofeedback, and cognitive-behavioral therapy may be considered as treatment options for prevention of migraine (Grade A evidence).
2. Behavioral therapy may be combined with preventive drug therapy to achieve additional clinical improvement for migraine (Grade B evidence).
3. Evidence-based treatment recommendations are not yet possible regarding the use of hypnosis (Campbell et al., 2000).

The consortium concluded that behavioral treatments may be particularly well suited in one or more of the following cases: (1) the patient prefers such an approach; (2) pharmacological treatment cannot be tolerated or is medically contraindicated; (3) the response to pharmacological treatment is absent or minimal; (4) the patient is pregnant, has plans to become pregnant, or is nursing; (5) there is a long-standing history of frequent or excessive use of analgesics or acute medications that can exacerbate headache; and (6) the patient is faced with significant stressors or has deficient stress-coping skills.

The consortium also drew the following conclusions, which help to identify areas for further study.

1. Too few studies provide head-to-head comparisons of nondrug and drug treatments.
2. The integration of drug and nondrug treatments has not been adequately addressed.
3. Behavioral therapies are effective as sole or adjunctive therapy, but it is not yet established which specific patients are likely to be most responsive to specific behavioral modalities.
4. Component analysis is needed to determine the extent to which various elements of multimodal regimens contribute to efficacy.
5. Additional studies treating patients from primary care settings are needed.

Some of these issues are addressed in the concluding section.

The numerous meta-analyses that have been conducted for tension-type and migraine headache, some of which concern comparisons of pharmacological and non-pharmacological treatments, have been summarized by Andrasik and Walch (2003) and by Penzien et al. (2002), among other sources. The major conclusions that can be drawn are that (1) relaxation, biofeedback, and cognitive-behavior therapy produce significant improvements in headache activity, although a sizeable number of patients remain unhelped; (2) improvements are similar among these treatments, including those obtained for pharmacological treatment; (3) improvements exceed those obtained by various control conditions; and (4) effects appear to endure well over time. From a recent investigation, there is evidence to suggest that biofeedback can enhance medication treatment effects over time, particularly with difficult-to-treat patients (Grazzi et al., 2002).

The efficacy data reviewed here pertain primarily to typical or uncomplicated forms of migraine and TTH. As research evolves, we are finding that certain types of headache present particular challenges, calling at times for more extended treatment and incorporation of other allied modalities. These types include medication-overuse headaches; chronic, daily, high-intensity headaches; refractory headaches; cluster headaches; post-traumatic headaches; and headaches accompanied by comorbid conditions. For example, a number of medications routinely used for headaches (specifically, ergotamine, triptans, analgesics, and opioids) can induce or intensify existing headaches if taken improperly or to excess. Further, it is believed that medication overuse can result in a number of headaches evolving from episodic to chronic and becoming more resilient to treatment. As another example, patients whose headaches occur following trauma can experience a multitude of problems and significant disability that make treatment particularly challenging (Andrasik & Wincze, 1994; Marcus, 2003; Martelli, Grayson, & Zasler, 1999; Ramadan & Keidel, 2000). Furthermore, approximately one-third develop chronic forms of headaches, adding to the treatment challenge (Ramadan & Keidel, 2000). These headache types are discussed more fully by Andrasik (2003, 2004).

The meta-analyses reveal that a large percentage of patients with headache are helped in a meaningful way by various behavioral treatments. At the same time, a sizeable percentage of patients are left unhelped or are not helped sufficiently. This raises the question of what patient characteristics might bear on success. Thorn and Andrasik (2007) speculate that dysfunctional thinking might be a particularly relevant characteristic. This speculation is based on the finding that headache sufferers reveal higher levels of catastrophizing in comparison with headache-free controls and that pain-related catastrophizing significantly predicts treatment outcome (Hassinger, Semenchuk, & O'Brien, 1999; Ukestad & Wittrock, 1996). Perhaps treatments that specifically target catastrophizing (Thorn, 2004; Thorn, Boothby, & Sullivan, 2002), in addition to what has more typically been done in prior cognitive therapy treatments, may show heightened success.

Evidence- and meta-analytic-based reviews reveal similar levels of improvement for the various treatments attempted, leading some to suggest that patient and treatments may be interchangeable and that practitioners would be wise to use the simplest treatment for all patients. The designs used in most studies to date, unfortunately, have not produced the kind of data that can affirm or deny this interpretation. The most direct test of this assumption suggests that, at least for relaxation and biofeedback, patients may be responding in a different manner. Blanchard and colleagues (1982), using a sequential design, offered patients with migraine, TTH, and both headache types a comprehensive course of relaxation treatment. Those who did not achieve significant improvement were then offered a comprehensive trial of biofeedback (autogenic feedback for migraine and migraine combined with TTH, EMG biofeedback for TTH) to see whether some these relaxation failures could be helped to a meaningful degree by biofeedback. Such was the case, suggesting that patients and treatment are not interchangeable. Similar findings were obtained by Huber and Huber (1979).

The prevailing model accounting for all forms of chronic pain, including headache, is best termed the *biomedical model*, and it views pain as a direct transmission of impulses from the periphery to structures within the central nervous system (Turk & Flor, 1999). A model that is more fruitful and heuristic has been labeled the *biopsychosocial* or *biobehavioral* model. This model views pain (and any chronic illness, for that matter) as emanating from a complex interaction of biological, psychological, and social variables. From this perspective (Turk & Flor, 1999) the diversity in illness expression (including severity, duration, and consequences to the individual) can be accounted for by the complex interrelationships among predispositional, biological, and psychological characteristics (e.g., genetics, prior learning history), biological changes, psychological status, and the social and cultural contexts that shape the individual's perceptions and response to illness. This model stands in sharp contrast to the traditional biomedical perspective that conceptualizes illness in terms of more narrowly defined physiochemical dimensions. This alternative model differs in other key ways, as it is dynamic and recognizes reciprocal multifactorial influences over time. Andrasik, Flor, and Turk (2005) have applied this model to recurrent headache disorders, pointing out the role of behavioral, affective, and cognitive influences. Researchers in the field of headache have not fully exploited this model. Doing so may well enhance treatment outcome.

REFERENCES

American Psychiatric Association. (2000). *Diagnostic and statistical manual of mental disorders* (4th ed., text rev.). Washington, DC: Author.

American Sleep Disorders Association Diagnostic Classification Steering Committee. (1990). *The international classification of sleep disorders: Diagnostic and coding manual*. Rochester, MN: Author.

Andrasik, F. (2003). Behavioral treatment approaches to chronic headache. *Neurological Sciences*, 24(Suppl. 2), S80–85.

Andrasik, F. (2004). Behavioral treatment of migraine: current status and future directions. *Expert Review of Neurotherapeutics*, 4(3), 403–413.

Andrasik, F. (2004). The essence of biofeedback, relaxation, and hypnosis. In R. H. Dworkin & W. S.

Breitbart (Eds.), *Psychosocial aspects of pain: Handbook for healthcare providers. Progress in pain research and management* (Vol. 27, pp. 285–305). Seattle: International Association for the Study of Pain Press.

Andrasik, F., Flor, H., & Turk, D. C. (2005). An expanded view of psychological aspects in head pain: The biopsychosocial model. *Neurological Sciences*, 26(Suppl. 2), s87–91.

Andrasik, F., & Walch, S. E. (2003). Headaches. In A. M. Nezu, C. M. Nezu, & P. A. Geller (Eds.), *Handbook of psychology: Vol. 9. Health psychology* (pp. 245–266). New York: Wiley.

Andrasik, F., & Wincze, J. P. (1994). Emotional and psychosocial aspects of mild head injury. *Seminars in Neurology*, 14(1), 60–66.

Backhaus, J., Hohagen, F., Voderholzer, U., & Riemann, D. (2001). Long-term effectiveness of a short-term cognitive-behavioral group treatment for primary insomnia. *European Archives of Psychiatry and Clinical Neuroscience*, 251(1), 35–41.

Bastien, C. H., Morin, C. M., Ouellet, M.-C., Blais, F. C., & Bouchard, S. (2004). Cognitive-behavioral therapy for insomnia: Comparison of individual therapy, group therapy, and telephone consultations. *Journal of Consulting and Clinical Psychology*, 72(4), 653–659.

Batey, D. M., Kaufmann, P. G., Raczynski, J. M., Hollis, J. F., Murphy, J. K., Rosner, B., et al. (2000). Stress management intervention for primary prevention of hypertension: Detailed results from Phase I of Trials of Hypertension Prevention (TOHP-I). *Annals of Epidemiology*, 10(1), 45–58.

Bille, B. (1962). Migraine in school children. *Acta Paediatrica Scandinavica*, 51, 1–15.

Blanchard, E. B., Andrasik, F., Neff, D. F., Teders, S. J., Pallmeyer, T. P., Arena, J. G., et al. (1982). Sequential comparisons of relaxation training and biofeedback in the treatment of three kinds of chronic headache or, the machines may be necessary some of the time. *Behaviour Research and Therapy*, 20(5), 469–481.

Buscemi, N., Vandermeer, B., Friesen, C., Bialy, L., Tubman, M., Ospina, M., et al. (2005). Manifestations and management of chronic insomnia in adults. *Evidence Report/Technology Assessment (Summary)*, 125, 1–10.

Campbell, J. K., Penzien, D. B., & Wall, E. M. (2000). Evidence-based guidelines for migraine headaches: Behavioral and physical treatments. Available online at *aan.com/professionals/practice/pdfs/g10089.pdf*

Carlson, L. E., & Garland, S. N. (2005). Impact of mindfulness-based stress reduction (MBSR) on sleep, mood, stress and fatigue symptoms in cancer outpatients. *International Journal of Behavioral Medicine*, 12(4), 278–285.

Carlson, L. E., Speca, M., Patel, K. D., & Goodey, E. (2003). Mindfulness-based stress reduction in relation to quality of life, mood, symptoms of stress, and immune parameters in breast and prostate cancer outpatients. *Psychosomatic Medicine*, 65(4), 571–581.

Carlson, L. E., Ursuliak, Z., Goodey, E., Angen, M., & Speca, M. (2001). The effects of a mindfulness meditation-based stress reduction program on mood and symptoms of stress in cancer outpatients: 6-month follow-up. *Supportive Care in Cancer*, 9(2), 112–123.

Carney, C. E., Lajos, L. E., & Waters, W. F. (2004). Wrist actigraph versus self-report in normal sleepers: Sleep schedule adherence and self-report validity. *Behavioral Sleep Medicine*, 2(3), 134–143.

Cervena, K., Dauvilliers, Y., Espa, F., Touchon, J., Matousek, M., Billiard, M., et al. (2004). Effect of cognitive behavioural therapy for insomnia on sleep architecture and sleep EEG power spectra in psychophysiological insomnia. *Journal of Sleep Research*, 13(4), 385–393.

Chambless, D. L., & Hollon, S. D. (1998). Defining empirically supported therapies. *Journal of Consulting and Clinical Psychology*, 66(1), 7–18.

Chesson, A. L. J., Anderson, W. M., Littner, M., Davila, D., Hartse, K., Johnson, S., et al. (1999). Practice parameters for the nonpharmacologic treatment of chronic insomnia. *Sleep*, 22(8), 1128–1133.

Chobanian, A. V., Bakris, G. L., Black, H. R., Cushman, W. C., Green, L. A., Izzo, J. L., Jr., et al. (2003). The seventh report of the Joint National Committee on Prevention, Detection, Evaluation, and Treatment of High Blood Pressure: The JNC 7 report. *Journal of the American Medical Association*, 289(19), 2560–2572.

Chronicle, E., & Mulleners, W. (2004). Anticonvulsant drugs for migraine prophylaxis. *Cochrane Database of Systematic Reviews*, 3, CD003226.

Clouse, J. C., & Osterhaus, J. T. (1994). Healthcare resource use and costs associated with migraine in a managed healthcare setting. *Annals of Pharmacotherapy*, 28(5), 659–664.

Currie, S. R., Wilson, K. G., & Curran, D. (2002). Clinical significance and predictors of treatment response to cognitive-behavior therapy for insomnia secondary to chronic pain. *Journal of Behavioral Medicine, 25*(2), 135–153.

Deter, H. C., & Allert, G. (1983). Group therapy for asthma patients: A concept for the psychosomatic treatment of patients in a medical clinic—a controlled study. *Psychotherapy and Psychosomatics, 40*(1–4), 95–105.

Doghramji, P. P. (2001). Detection of insomnia in primary care. *Journal of Clinical Psychiatry, 62*(Suppl. 10), 18–26.

Edinger, J. D., Wohlgemuth, W. K., Radtke, R. A., Marsh, G. R., & Quillian, R. E. (2001). Cognitive behavioral therapy for treatment of chronic primary insomnia: A randomized controlled trial. *Journal of the American Medical Association, 285*(14), 1856–1864.

Espie, C. A., Inglis, S. J., Tessier, S., & Harvey, L. (2001). The clinical effectiveness of cognitive behaviour therapy for chronic insomnia: Implementation and evaluation of a sleep clinic in general medical practice. *Behaviour Research and Therapy, 39*(1), 45–60.

Evans, R. W. (2001). Diagnostic testing for headache. *Medical Clinics of North America, 85*(4), 865–885.

Fawzy, F. I., Fawzy, N. W., Hyun, C. S., Elashoff, R., Guthrie, D., Fahey, J. L., et al. (1993). Malignant melanoma: Effects of an early structured psychiatric intervention, coping, and affective state on recurrence and survival 6 years later. *Archives of General Psychiatry, 50*(9), 681–689.

Fredrikson, M., & Matthews, K. A. (1990). Cardiovascular responses to behavioral stress and hypertension: A meta-analytic review. *Annals of Behavioral Medicine, 12*, 30–39.

Garrard, C. S., Seidler, A., McKibben, A., McAlpine, L. E., & Gordon, D. (1992). Spectral analysis of heart rate variability in bronchial asthma. *Clinical Autonomic Research, 2*(2), 105–111.

Gift, A. G., Moore, T., & Soeken, K. (1992). Relaxation to reduce dyspnea and anxiety in COPD patients. *Nursing Research, 41*(4), 242–246.

Goodwin, P. J., Leszcz, M., Ennis, M., Koopmans, J., Vincent, L., Guther, H., et al. (2001). The effect of group psychosocial support on survival in metastatic breast cancer. *New England Journal of Medicine, 345*(24), 1719–1726.

Grazzi, L., Andrasik, F., D'Amico, D., Leone, M., Usai, S., Kass, S. J., et al. (2002). Behavioral and pharmacologic treatment of transformed migraine with analgesic overuse: Outcome at 3 years. *Headache, 42*(6), 483–490.

Harris, A. H., Thoresen, C. E., Humphreys, K., & Faul, J. (2005). Does writing affect asthma? A randomized trial. *Psychosomatic Medicine, 67*(1), 130–136.

Hassinger, H. J., Semenchuk, E. M., & O'Brien, W. H. (1999). Appraisal and coping responses to pain and stress in migraine headache sufferers. *Journal of Behavioral Medicine, 22*(4), 327–340.

Hauri, P. J. (1993). Consulting about insomnia: A method and some preliminary data. *Sleep, 16*(4), 344–350.

Henry, M., de Rivera, J. L., Gonzalez-Martin, I. J., & Abreu, J. (1993). Improvement of respiratory function in chronic asthmatic patients with autogenic therapy. *Journal of Psychosomatic Research, 37*(3), 265–270.

Hermann, C., Kim, M., & Blanchard, E. B. (1995). Behavioral and prophylactic pharmacological intervention studies of pediatric migraine: An exploratory meta-analysis. *Pain, 60*(3), 239–255.

Holden, E. W., Deichmann, M. M., & Levy, J. D. (1999). Empirically supported treatments in pediatric psychology: Recurrent pediatric headache. *Journal of Pediatric Psychology, 24*(2), 91–109.

Holroyd, K. A., O'Donnell, F. J., Stensland, M., Lipchik, G. L., Cordingley, G. E., & Carlson, B. W. (2001). Management of chronic tension-type headache with tricyclic antidepressant medication, stress management therapy, and their combination: A randomized controlled trial. *Journal of the American Medical Association, 285*(17), 2208–2215.

Holroyd, K. A., & Penzien, D. B. (1990). Pharmacological versus non-pharmacological prophylaxis of recurrent migraine headache: A meta-analytic review of clinical trials. *Pain, 42*(1), 1–13.

Holroyd, K. A., Penzien, D. B., & Cordingley, G. E. (1991). Propranolol in the management of recurrent migraine: A meta-analytic review. *Headache, 31*(5), 333–340.

Hryshko-Mullen, A. S., Broeckl, L. S., Haddock, C. K., & Peterson, A. L. (2000). Behavioral treatment of insomnia: The Wilford Hall Insomnia Program. *Military Medicine, 165*(3), 200–207.

Hu, X. H., Markson, L. E., Lipton, R. B., Stewart, W. F., & Berger, M. L. (1999). Burden of migraine in the United States: Disability and economic costs. *Archives of Internal Medicine, , 159*(8), 813–818.

Huber, H. P., & Huber, D. (1979). Autogenic training and rational-emotive therapy for long-term migraine patients: An explorative study of a therapy. *Behavioral Analysis and Modification*, *3*, 169–177.

Jacobs, G. D., Benson, H., & Friedman, R. (1996). Perceived benefits in a behavioral-medicine insomnia program: A clinical report. *American Journal of Medicine*, *100*(2), 212–216.

Jacobs, G. D., Pace-Schott, E. F., Stickgold, R., & Otto, M. W. (2004). Cognitive behavior therapy and pharmacotherapy for insomnia: A randomized controlled trial and direct comparison. *Archives of Internal Medicine*, *164*(17), 1888–1896.

Jagus, C. E., & Benbow, S. M. (1999). Sleep disorders in the elderly. *Advances in Psychiatric Treatment*, *5*, 30–38.

Jansson, M., & Linton, S. J. (2005). Cognitive-behavioral group therapy as an early intervention for insomnia: A randomized controlled trial. *Journal of Occupational Rehabilitation*, *15*(2), 177–190.

Jensen, R. (1999). Pathophysiological mechanisms of tension-type headache: A review of epidemiological and experimental studies. *Cephalalgia*, *19*(6), 602–621.

Kaufmann, P. G., Jacob, R. G., Ewart, C. K., Chesney, M. A., Muenz, L. R., Doub, N., et al. (1988). Hypertension Intervention Pooling Project. *Health Psychology* (7, Suppl.), 209–224.

Kazuma, N., Otsuka, K., Matsuoka, I., & Murata, M. (1997). Heart rate variability during 24 hours in asthmatic children. *Chronobiology International*, *14*(6), 597–606.

LaVaque, T., Hammond, D., Trudeau, D., Monastra, V., Perry, J., Lehrer, P., et al. (2002). Template for developing guidelines for the evaluation of the clinical efficacy of psychophysiological interventions. *Applied Psychophysiology and Biofeedback*, *27*(4), 273–281.

Lehrer, P., Carr, R. E., Smetankine, A., Vaschillo, E., Peper, E., Porges, S., et al. (1997). Respiratory sinus arrhythmia versus neck/trapezius EMG and incentive inspirometry biofeedback for asthma: A pilot study. *Applied Psychophysiology and Biofeedback*, *22*(2), 95–109.

Lehrer, P., Smetankin, A., & Potapova, T. (2000). Respiratory sinus arrhythmia biofeedback therapy for asthma: A report of 20 unmedicated pediatric cases using the Smetankin method. *Applied Psychophysiology and Biofeedback*, *25*(3), 193–200.

Lehrer, P. M., Carr, R., Sargunaraj, D., & Woolfolk, R. L. (1993). Differential effects of stress management therapies in behavioral medicine. In P. M. Lehrer & R. L. Woolfolk (Eds.), *Principles and practice of stress management* (2nd ed., pp. 571–605). New York: Guilford Press.

Lehrer, P. M., Hochron, S. M., Mayne, T., Isenberg, S., Carlson, V., Lasoski, A. M., et al. (1994). Relaxation and music therapies for asthma among patients prestabilized on asthma medication. *Journal of Behavioral Medicine*, *17*(1), 1–24.

Lehrer, P. M., Hochron, S. M., McCann, B., Swartzman, L., & Reba, P. (1986). Relaxation decreases large-airway but not small-airway asthma. *Journal of Psychosomatic Research*, *30*(1), 13–25.

Lehrer, P. M., Isenberg, S., & Hochron, S. M. (1993). Asthma and emotion: A review. *Journal of Asthma*, *30*(1), 5–21.

Lehrer, P. M., Vaschillo, E., Vaschillo, B., Lu, S. E., Scardella, A., Siddique, M., et al. (2004). Biofeedback treatment for asthma. *Chest*, *126*(2), 352–361.

Lichstein, K. L., Peterson, B. A., Riedel, B. W., Means, M. K., Epperson, M. T., & Aguillard, R. N. (1999). Relaxation to assist sleep medication withdrawal. *Behavior Modification*, *23*(3), 379–402.

Lichstein, K. L., Riedel, B. W., Wilson, N. M., Lester, K. W., & Aguillard, R. N. (2001). Relaxation and sleep compression for late-life insomnia: A placebo-controlled trial. *Journal of Consulting and Clinical Psychology*, *69*(2), 227–239.

Linden, W., & Chambers, L. (1994). Clinical effectiveness of non-drug treatment for hypertension: A meta-analysis. *Annals of Behavioural Medicine*, *16*, 35–45.

Linden, W., Lenz, J. W., & Con, A. H. (2001). Individualized stress management for primary hypertension: A randomized trial. *Archives of Internal Medicine*, *161*(8), 1071–1080.

Linden, W., & Moseley, J. V. (2006). The efficacy of behavioral treatments for hypertension. *Applied Psychophysiology and Biofeedback, 31*, 51–63.

Lipton, R. B., Diamond, S., Reed, M., Diamond, M. L., & Stewart, W. F. (2001). Migraine diagnosis and treatment: Results from the American Migraine Study II. *Headache*, *41*(7), 638–645.

Loew, T. H., Siegfried, W., Martus, P., Tritt, K., & Hahn, E. G. (1996). "Functional relaxation" reduces acute airway obstruction in asthmatics as effectively as inhaled terbutaline. *Psychotherapy and Psychosomatics*, *65*(3), 124–128.

Loew, T. H., Tritt, K., Siegfried, W., Bohmann, H., Martus, P., & Hahn, E. G. (2001). Efficacy of "functional relaxation" in comparison to terbutaline and a "placebo relaxation" method in patients with acute asthma: A randomized, prospective, placebo-controlled, crossover experimental investigation. *Psychotherapy and Psychosomatics*, 70(3), 151–157.

Louie, S. W. (2004). The effects of guided imagery relaxation in people with COPD. *Occupational Therapy International*, 11(3), 145–159.

Mannix, L. K. (2001). Epidemiology and impact of primary headache disorders. *Medical Clinics of North America*, 85(4), 887–895.

Marcus, D. A. (2003). Disability and chronic posttraumatic headache. *Headache*, 43(2), 117–121.

Markovitz, J. H., Raczynski, J. M., Wallace, D., Chettur, V., & Chesney, M. A. (1998). Cardiovascular reactivity to video game predicts subsequent blood pressure increases in young men: The CARDIA study. *Psychosomatic Medicine*, 60(2), 186–191.

Martelli, M. F., Grayson, R. L., & Zasler, N. D. (1999). Posttraumatic headache: Neuropsychological and psychological effects and treatment implications. *Journal of Head Trauma Rehabilitation*, 14(1), 49–69.

Mathew, N. (1987). Drugs and headache: Misuse and dependency. In C. S. Adler, S. M. Morrissey, & R. C. Packard (Eds.), *Psychiatric aspects of headache*. Baltimore: Williams & Wilkins.

Mathew, N. T., & Bendtsen, L. (2000). Prophylactic pharmacotherapy of tension-type headache. In J. Olesen, P. Tfelt-Hansen, & K. M. A. Welch (Eds.), *The headaches* (2nd ed., pp. 667–673). Philadelphia: Lippincott Williams & Wilkins.

McCraty, R., Atkinson, M., & Tomasino, D. (2003). Impact of a workplace stress reduction program on blood pressure and emotional health in hypertensive employees. *Joural of Alternative and Complementary Medicine*, 9(3), 355–369.

McGrady, A. (1994). Effects of group relaxation training and thermal biofeedback on blood pressure and related physiological and psychological variables in essential hypertension. *Biofeedback and Self-Regulation*, 19(1), 51–66.

Means, M. K., Lichstein, K. L., Epperson, M. T., & Johnson, C. T. (2000). Relaxation therapy for insomnia: Nighttime and day time effects. *Behaviour Research and Therapy*, 38(7), 665–678.

Michel, P. L. (2000). Socioeconomic costs of headache. In J. Olesen, P. Tfelt-Hansen, & K. M. A. Welch (Eds.), *The headaches* (2nd ed., pp. 33–40). Philadelphia: Lippincott Williams & Wilkins.

Morgan, K., Dixon, S., Mathers, N., Thompson, J., & Tomeny, M. (2003). Psychological treatment for insomnia in the management of long-term hypnotic drug use: A pragmatic randomised controlled trial. *British Journal of General Practice: The Journal of the Royal College of General Practitioners*, 53(497), 923–928.

Morin, C. M., Hauri, P. J., Espie, C. A., Spielman, A. J., Buysse, D. J., & Bootzin, R. R. (1999). Nonpharmacologic treatment of chronic insomnia: An American Academy of Sleep Medicine review. *Sleep*, 22(8), 1134–1156.

Muldoon, M. F., Terrell, D. F., Bunker, C. H., & Manuck, S. B. (1993). Family history studies in hypertension research: Review of the literature. *American Journal of Hypertension*, 6(1), 76–88.

Nagarathna, R., & Nagendra, H. R. (1985). Yoga for bronchial asthma: A controlled study. *British Medical Journal (Clinical Research Ed.)* , 291(6502), 1077–1079.

National Heart, Lung, and Blood Institute. (1997). *Expert panel report: 2. Guidelines for the diagnosis and management of asthma*. Washington, DC: U.S. Department of Health and Human Services.

National Institutes of Health. (2005, August). National Institutes of Health state-of-the-science conference statement on manifestations and management of chronic insomnia in adults. Retrieved November, 2005, from *consensus.nih.gov/2005/2005InsomniaSOS026html.htm*

Olesen, J., & Steiner, T. J. (2004). The international classification of headache disorders, 2nd ed. (ICDH-II). *Journal of Neurology, Neurosurgery, and Psychiatry*, 75(6), 808–811.

Penzien, D. B., Rains, J. C., & Andrasik, F. (2002). Behavioral management of recurrent headache: Three decades of experience and empiricism. *Applied Psychophysiology and Biofeedback*, 27(2), 163–181.

Pryse-Phillips, W. E., Dodick, D. W., Edmeads, J. G., Gawel, M. J., Nelson, R. F., Purdy, R. A., et al. (1998). Guidelines for the nonpharmacologic management of migraine in clinical practice. *Canadian Medical Association Journal*, 159(1), 47–54.

Ramadan, N. M., & Keidel, M. (2000). Chronic posttraumatic headache. In J. Olesen, P. Tfelt-Hansen, & K. M. A. Welch (Eds.), *The headaches* (2nd ed., pp. 771–780). Philadelphia: Lippincott Williams & Wilkins.

Rapoport, A. M., & Tepper, S. J. (2001). Triptans are all different. *Archives of Neurology, 58*(9), 1479–1480.

Renfroe, K. L. (1988). Effect of progressive relaxation on dyspnea and state anxiety in patients with chronic obstructive pulmonary disease. *Heart and Lung, 17*(4), 408–413.

Roth, T., & Drake, C. (2004). Evolution of insomnia: Current status and future direction. *Sleep Medicine, 5*(Suppl. 1), S23–30.

Schwartz, B. S., Stewart, W. F., Simon, D., & Lipton, R. B. (1998). Epidemiology of tension-type headache. *Journal of the American Medical Association, 279*(5), 381–383.

Shapiro, S. L., Bootzin, R. R., Figueredo, A. J., Lopez, A. M., & Schwartz, G. E. (2003). The efficacy of mindfulness-based stress reduction in the treatment of sleep disturbance in women with breast cancer: An exploratory study. *Journal of Psychosomatic Research, 54*(1), 85–91.

Smith, R. (1998). Impact of migraine on the family. *Headache, 38*(6), 423–426.

Smyth, J. M., Stone, A. A., Hurewitz, A., & Kaell, A. (1999). Effects of writing about stressful experiences on symptom reduction in patients with asthma or rheumatoid arthritis: A randomized trial. *Journal of the American Medical Association, 281*(14), 1304–1309.

Solomon, G. D., & Dahlöf, C. G. H. (2000). Impact of headache on the individual sufferer. In J. Olesen, P. Tfelt-Hansen, & K. M. A. Welch (Eds.), *The headaches* (2nd ed., pp. 25–31). Philadelphia: Lippincott Williams & Wilkins.

Speca, M., Carlson, L. E., Goodey, E., & Angen, M. (2000). A randomized, wait-list controlled clinical trial: The effect of a mindfulness meditation-based stress reduction program on mood and symptoms of stress in cancer outpatients. *Psychosomatic Medicine, 62*(5), 613–622.

Spiegel, D., Bloom, J. R., Kraemer, H. C., & Gottheil, E. (1989). Effect of psychosocial treatment on survival of patients with metastatic breast cancer. *Lancet, 2*(8668), 888–891.

Spiegel, D., Bloom, J. R., & Yalom, I. (1981). Group support for patients with metastatic cancer: A randomized outcome study. *Archives of General Psychiatry, 38*(5), 527–533.

Spiegel, D., Morrow, G. R., Classen, C., Raubertas, R., Stott, P. B., Mudaliar, N., et al. (1999). Group psychotherapy for recently diagnosed breast cancer patients: A multicenter feasibility study. *Psychooncology, 8*(6), 482–493.

Stepanski, E. J. (2003). Behavioral sleep medicine: A historical perspective. *Behavioral Sleep Medicine, 1*(1), 4–21.

Task Force on Promotion and Dissemination of Psychological Procedures. (1995). Training in and dissemination of empirically validated treatments: Report and recommendations. *Clinical Psychologist, 48*(1), 3–23.

Taylor, D. J., Lichstein, K. L., Durrence, H. H., Reidel, B. W., & Bush, A. J. (2005). Epidemiology of insomnia, depression, and anxiety. *Sleep, 28*(11), 1457–1464.

Tepper, S. J. (2001). Safety and rational use of the triptans. *Medical Clinics of North America, 85*(4), 959–970.

Tfelt-Hansen, P., & Welch, K. M. A. (2000a). General principles of pharmacological treatment of migraine. In J. Olesen, P. Tfelt-Hansen, & K. M. A. Welch (Eds.), *The headaches* (2nd ed., pp. 385–389). Philadelphia: Lippincott Williams & Wilkins.

Tfelt-Hansen, P., & Welch, K. M. A. (2000b). Prioritizing prophylactic treatment of migraine. In J. Olesen, P. Tfelt-Hansen, & K. M. A. Welch (Eds.), *The headaches* (2nd ed., pp. 499–500). Philadelphia: Lippincott Williams & Wilkins.

Thorn, B. E. (2004). *Cognitive therapy for chronic pain: A step-by-step guide.* New York: Guilford Press.

Thorn, B. E., & Adrasik, F. (2007). Psychological treatment of headache. In R. F. Schmidt & W. D. Willis (Eds.), *Encyclopedia of pain* (pp. 2034–2037). Heidelberg, Germany: Springer.

Thorn, B. E., Boothby, J. L., & Sullivan, M. J. (2002). Targeted treatment of catastrophizing for the management of chronic pain. *Cognitive and Behavioral Practice, 9*, 127–138.

Tsai, S.-L. (2004). Audio-visual relaxation training for anxiety, sleep, and relaxation among Chinese adults with cardiac disease. *Research in Nursing and Health, 27*(6), 458–468.

Turk, D. C., & Flor, H. (1999). Chronic pain: A biobehavioral perspective. In R. J. Gatchel & D. C. Turk (Eds.), *Psychosocial factors in pain.* New York: Guilford Press.

Ukestad, L. K., & Wittrock, D. A. (1996). Pain perception and coping in female tension headache sufferers and headache-free controls. *Health Psychology, 15*(1), 65–68.

Vallieres, A., Morin, C. M., Guay, B., Bastien, C. H., & LeBlanc, M. (2004). Sequential treatment for chronic insomnia: A pilot study. *Behavioral Sleep Medicine, 2*(2), 94–112.

Vedanthan, P. K., Kesavalu, L. N., Murthy, K. C., Duvall, K., Hall, M. J., Baker, S., et al. (1998). Clinical study of yoga techniques in university students with asthma: A controlled study. *Allergy and Asthma Proceedings*, 19(1), 3–9.

Verbeek, I., Schreuder, K., & Declerck, G. (1999). Evaluation of short-term nonpharmacological treatment of insomnia in a clinical setting. *Journal of Psychosomatic Research*, 47(4), 369–383.

Viens, M., De Koninck, J., Mercier, P., St-Onge, M., & Lorrain, D. (2003). Trait anxiety and sleep-onset insomnia: Evaluation of treatment using anxiety management training. *Journal of Psychosomatic Research*, 54(1), 31–37.

Vijayalakshmi, S., Satyanarayana, M., Krishna Rao, P. V., & Prakash, V. (1988). Combined effect of yoga and psychotherapy on management of asthma: Preliminary study. *Journal of Indian Psychology*, 7(2), 32–39.

Von Korff, M., Galer, B. S., & Stang, P. (1995). Chronic use of symptomatic headache medications. *Pain*, 62(2), 179–186.

Wang, M.-Y., Wang, S.-Y., & Tsai, P.-S. (2005). Cognitive behavioural therapy for primary insomnia: A systematic review. *Journal of Advanced Nursing*, 50(5), 553–564.

Waters, W. F., Hurry, M. J., Binks, P. G., Carney, C. E., Lajos, L. E., Fuller, K. H., et al. (2003). Behavioral and hypnotic treatments for insomnia subtypes. *Behavioral Sleep Medicine*, 1(2), 81–101.

Wilson, S., & Nutt, D. (1999). Treatment of sleep disorders in adults. *Advances in Psychiatric Treatment*, 5, 11–18.

Yucha, C., & Gilbert, C. (2004). *Evidence-based practice in biofeedback and neurofeedback*. Colorado Springs, CO: Association for Applied Psychophysiology and Biofeedback.

Yung, P. M., & Keltner, A. A. (1996). A controlled comparison on the effect of muscle and cognitive relaxation procedures on blood pressure: Implications for the behavioural treatment of borderline hypertensives. *Behavior Research and Therapy*, 34(10), 821–826.